Ethanol and the Liver

T0173994

Ethanol and the Liver

Mechanisms and management

Edited by

David I.N. Sherman

Department of Gastroenterology
Central Middlesex Hospital
London, UK

Victor R. Preedy

Department of Nutrition and Dietetics
King's College London
London, UK

and

Ronald Ross Watson

Division of Health Promotion Sciences
College of Public Health
University of Arizona, Tucson
Arizona, USA

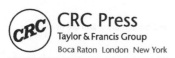
CRC Press
Taylor & Francis Group
Boca Raton   London   New York

CRC Press is an imprint of the
Taylor & Francis Group, an **informa** business

CRC Press
Taylor & Francis Group
6000 Broken Sound Parkway NW, Suite 300
Boca Raton, FL 33487-2742

First issued in paperback 2019

© 2010 by Taylor & Francis Group, LLC
CRC Press is an imprint of Taylor & Francis Group, an Informa business

No claim to original U.S. Government works

ISBN-13: 978-0-415-27582-8 (hbk)
ISBN-13: 978-0-367-39608-4 (pbk)

Library of Congress Card Number 2005053800

This book contains information obtained from authentic and highly regarded sources. Reasonable efforts have been made to publish reliable data and information, but the author and publisher cannot assume responsibility for the validity of all materials or the consequences of their use. The authors and publishers have attempted to trace the copyright holders of all material reproduced in this publication and apologize to copyright holders if permission to publish in this form has not been obtained. If any copyright material has not been acknowledged please write and let us know so we may rectify in any future reprint.

Except as permitted under U.S. Copyright Law, no part of this book may be reprinted, reproduced, transmitted, or utilized in any form by any electronic, mechanical, or other means, now known or hereafter invented, including photocopying, microfilming, and recording, or in any information storage or retrieval system, without written permission from the publishers.

For permission to photocopy or use material electronically from this work, please access www. copyright.com (http://www.copyright.com/) or contact the Copyright Clearance Center, Inc. (CCC), 222 Rosewood Drive, Danvers, MA 01923, 978-750-8400. CCC is a not-for-profit organization that provides licenses and registration for a variety of users. For organizations that have been granted a photocopy license by the CCC, a separate system of payment has been arranged.

Trademark Notice: Product or corporate names may be trademarks or registered trademarks, and are used only for identification and explanation without intent to infringe.

Visit the Taylor & Francis Web site at
http://www.taylorandfrancis.com

and the CRC Press Web site at
http://www.crcpress.com

Contents

Foreword

The liver is one of the most vital organs in the body. It plays a central role in the processing of fats, sugars and proteins, and in the body's defenses by marshalling an array of responses to trauma, stress, or inflammation.

Although the liver is capable of regeneration and repair, severe liver disease is life threatening. An association between heavy alcohol consumption and liver disease was recognized more than 200 years ago. However, it is only in the last three decades that our knowledge of how alcohol induces liver damage has been tremendously increased. Long-term heavy alcohol consumption is the leading cause of illness and death from liver disease in the Western World.

Alcoholic liver disease (ALD) is initially manifested as fatty liver, which is usually reversible with abstinence; alcoholic hepatitis, or liver inflammation; and cirrhosis, or scarring of the liver. Patients with both cirrhosis and alcoholic hepatitis have a death rate of more than 60 per cent over a 4-year period. New therapeutic tools for the treatment of ALD are sorely needed. To develop new therapies for ALD, a thorough understanding of the mechanisms for alcohol-induced liver injury is mandatory.

The *Ethanol and the Liver* monograph, edited by Drs Sherman, Preedy and Watson is not only timely, but also assembles under one roof a vast amount of knowledge in this area. The impressive talent end expertise recruited to contribute to this monograph is unparalleled. The book focuses on: (1) describing various pathological lesions following chronic alcohol consumption; (2) the role of alcohol metabolism in the genesis of ALD; (3) various mechanisms of ethanol-induced liver damage; (4) epidemiological data and diagnostic markers; (5) the interaction between ALD and extrahepatic consequences; and (6) management of ALD, including pharmacological treatment, and the role of other factors such as nutrition and viral hepatitis on the outcome.

Thus, this monograph is very valuable to students, researchers and health professionals in the fields of hepatology, alcohol metabolism, gastroenterology, and pathology, to name a few, and to clinicians. Each would find useful information that would no doubt propel the field forward. Since, the only treatment for liver cirrhosis is liver transplantation, advancing the field by developing early markers for liver damage, understanding the genetic factors involved in ALD, and developing appropriate medications are of paramount importance. This monograph is a significant step towards these goals.

Sam Zakhari, Ph.D.
Division of Basic Research, NIAAA
6000 Executive Blvd., Suite 402
Bethesda, MD 20852-7003

Preface

From the biological point of view, the human liver is one of the most well studied organs. Alcohol has been man's favored beverage for thousands of years, and liver damage due to alcohol has become one of the leading causes of morbidity and mortality in the Western World in the twentieth century. Ethanol remains the commonest cause of serious liver damage, although frequently in combination with other toxins such as drugs or hepatitis viruses. However, it is only comparatively recently that ethanol was shown to be a hepatotoxin and that liver damage was not merely a consequence of co-existent malnutrition. Although the mechanisms responsible for the spectrum of ethanol-induced liver disease have been the subject of numerous investigations, recent progress in the biomedical field indicate that the underlying mechanisms are complex and are still incompletely understood.

Thanks largely to a number of pioneers, the pace of progress in our understanding of clinical liver disease has increased markedly over the last thirty years, but rapid advances in various spheres of bio-molecular medicine have given rise to as many questions as answers. However, basic scientific advances have not, in general, been accompanied by great progress in treatment. Apart from improvements in the management of complications of chronic liver disease, the single most important therapeutic intervention remains abstinence from alcohol. In addition, the central role of the liver in many vital metabolic processes and the separate toxic effects of ethanol on other organ systems results in a number of diverse pathological processes in patients with alcoholic liver disease which may challenge physicians even further.

The aim of this book is to provide a comprehensive text embracing both pathogenic and clinical aspects of alcoholic liver disease (ALD), and to disseminate available knowledge on ethanol-induced liver damage, directly complementing the available bio-medical literature. Wherever possible, basic science has been related to pathogenesis as well as treatment modalities both in the present and with consideration of future developments. Attempts have been made to highlight areas where particular progress in understanding has occurred in the recent past, for example genetics, immunology and insulin-like growth factors. Areas often given low priority by clinicians such as the extrahepatic effects of alcoholic liver disease and the role of alcohol in potentiating liver damage due to other etiologies are covered in detail. Wherever possible, illustrations have been used to illuminate difficult concepts. As a result, we believe that *Ethanol and the Liver: Mechanisms and Management* provides a broader coverage of the subject than any available monograph. Inevitably, some duplication is inevitable, but this hopefully does not detract from the intention of a comprehensive approach to the subject.

The book starts with the major mechanisms thought to contribute to the pathogenesis of ALD before turning to clinical aspects and specific management . The first section defines the problem in terms of the specific histopathological lesions that characterise ALD, namely the classical segregation of fatty liver, alcoholic hepatitis and cirrhosis. An area of knowledge that has expanded rapidly is ethanol metabolism and its consequences. This is considered in depth in the next section along with the genetics of ALD, which encompasses the key area of varying individual susceptibility to liver damage. Detailed chapters follow in the third section on the major mechanisms involved in the pathogenesis of ALD, including free radicals; hyperdynamic circulation; inflammation including cytokines, endotoxin and adhesion molecules; growth factors, regeneration and carcinogenesis. In each case, the authors attempt to relate key advances in scientific knowledge to potential future treatments. As further work in these areas is undoubtedly still required, chapters on experimental models are included. The subsequent sections deal with the major clinical issues, namely epidemiology, diagnosis, extrahepatic features of ALD and treatment. In addition, the section on management discusses conventional therapeutic approaches to alcoholic hepatitis, cirrhosis and secondary complications, as well as possible future strategies and the thorny issue of transplantation. The interaction of alcohol with viral hepatitis is also considered in detail and the psychiatrist's viewpoint is also considered.

This book will be of interest to both basic scientists (from molecular biochemists to whole body physiologists) working in the field and allied areas, along with clinicians (hepatologists, gastroenterologists, general internists, psychiatrists and addiction specialists) and senior medical students. It would be a useful addition to the library of any unit where patients with alcohol-related problems are treated, and of any institution where biomedical research into the effects of alcohol is carried out.

David I.N. Sherman, Victor R. Preedy and Ronald Ross Watson

Abbreviations

%CDT	amount of CDT expressed as a percentage of total transferrin
‰	promille; per thousand; 1 ‰ = 1g/L
4-HNE	4-hydroxynonenal
5HIAA	5-hydroxyindole acetic acid
5HT	5-hydroxytryptamine (serotonin)
5-HTOL	5-Hydroxytryptophol
7-S	a domain of type IV collagen
AA	acetaldehyde
ACTH	adrenocorticotropic hormone
ADH	alcohol dehydrogenase
ADH⁻	alcohol dehydrogenase-deficient deer mice (*Peromyscus maniculatus*)
ADH	anti-diuretic hormone
aFGF	alpha fibroblastic growth factor
AIN	the American Institute of Nutrition
ALD	alcoholic liver disease
ALDH	aldehyde dehydrogenase
ALP	alkaline phosphatase
ALS	acid-labile subunit
ALT	alanine aminotransferase
AMA	antimitochondrial antibody
ANA	antinuclear autoantibody
Anti-HBs	antibody to hepatitis B surface antigen
AP-1	activating protein-1
APACHE	acute physiology and chronic health evaluation
Apo-B100	apolipoprotein-B100
APQ	alcohol problems questionnaire
AST	aspartate aminotransferase
ATP	adenosine triphosphate
AUDIT	Alcohol Use Disorders Identification Test
B	protein breakdown (Waterlow model)
BCAA	branched-chain amino acids
BLC	B lymphocyte chemokine
C	protein catabolism (Waterlow model)
CAGE	A four-question screening instrument for alcohol abuse
CBF	cerebral blood flow

CBT	cognitive behavioral therapy
CCl_4	carbon tetrachloride
CCLI	Combined Clinical and Laboratory Index
CD	cluster of differentiation
CDT	carbohydrate-deficient transferrin
CLD	chronic liver disease
CMR_A	cerebral metabolic rate for ammonia
$CMR_{glucose}$	cerebral metabolic rate for glucose
cNOS	constitutive nitric oxide synthetase
CNS	central nervous system
CoA	coenzyme A
Col1	a degradation product of PIIINP
COX	cyclooxygenase
CPM	central pontine myelinolysis
CRH	corticotropin releasing hormone
CSF	cerebrospinal fluid
CSHN	central sclerosing hyaline necrosis
CT	computed tomography
CTL	cytotoxic T-cell
CYP	cytochrome P450
CYP2E1	cytochrome P450 2E1
Cys	cysteine
d	day
D_2-receptors	dopamine$_2$ receptors
DARC	duffy associated red cell antigen
DAT	diacylglycerol transferase
DBI	diazepam binding inhibitor
DH	ductular hepatocytes
DNA	deoxyribonucleic acid
DSM-IV	diagnostic and statistical manual, 4th edition
DT	delirium tremens
EEG	electroencephalography
ELTR	European Liver Transplant Registry
ESPEN	European Society for Parenteral and Enteral Nutrition
ESR	electron spin resonance
ET-1	endothelin 1
EtOH	ethanol
Fab	antigen-binding fragment of an antibody
FABP	fatty acid binding protein
FAS	fetal alcohol syndrome
FRAMES	Feedback; Responsibility; Advice; Menu empathy; Self efficacy
FSR	fractional synthesis rate (fractional secretory rate for plasma proteins)
G	guanine
GABA	gaba-aminobutyric acid
$GdCl_3$	gadolinium chloride
GFAP	glial fibrillary acidic protein

GGT	gamma glutamyl transferase
GH	growth hormone
GHBP	growth hormone binding protein
GHR	growth hormone receptor
Gln	glutamine
GSH	reduced glutathione
GSSG	oxidized glutathione
HAV	hepatitis A virus
HBV	hepatitis B virus
HBV-DNA	hepatitis B virus deoxyribonucleic acid
HCC	hepatocellular carcinoma
HCV	hepatitis C virus
HCV-RNA	hepatitis C virus ribonucleic acid
HDL	high density lipoprotein
HGF	hepatocyte growth factor
HGV	hepatitis G virus
HGV-RNA	hepatitis G virus ribonucleic acid
HPLC	high performance liquid chromatography
HSC	hepatic stellate cell
HVPG	hepatic venous pressure gradient
I	intake (Waterlow model)
ICAM	intercellular adhesion molecule
ICD-10	international classification of diseases, 10th revision
ICTP	carboxyterminal telopeptide of type I collagen
ICU	intensive care unit
IFN	interferon
Ig	immunoglobulin
IGFBPs-1 to -6	insulin-like growth factor binding proteins -1 to -6
IGF-I	insulin-like growth factor-I
IgG	immunoglobulins G
IL	interleukin
IL-1	interleukin-1
iNOS	inducible nitric oxide synthetase
INSERM	Institut National de la Santé et de la Recherche Nationale
IRE	iron responsive element
IRP	iron regulatory protein
ISBRA	International Society for Biomedical Research on Alcoholism
ISMN	isosorbide-5-mononitrate
Italian MCP	Italian Multicentre Co-operative Project
KC	Kupffer cell
KIC	α-ketoisocaproic acid
K_m	substrate concentration producing enzyme half-maximal velocity (Michaelis constant)
LBP	lipopolysaccharide binding protein
LFA	lymphocyte function associated antigen
LH	luteinizing hormone
LPS	lipopolysaccharide

LV	left ventricle
MAA	malonyldialdehyde
MAA adduct	hybrid adduct with malonyldialdehyde and acetaldehyde
MAC	mid-arm circumference
MAdCAM	mucosal addressin cell adhesion protein
MAFA	mid-arm fat area
MAMA	mid-arm muscle area
MAMC	mid-arm muscle circumference
MAO-B	monoamine oxidase (B isoform)
MAPK	mitogen activated protein kinase
MAST	Michigan Alcoholism Screening Test
mAST	mitochondrial aminotransferase
MBs	mallory bodies
MCP	monocyte chemotactic protein
MCT	medium chain triglycerides
MCV	mean corpuscular volume of erythrocytes
MDA	malondialdehyde
MEOS	microsomal ethanol oxidizing system
MET	motivational enhancement therapy
MHC	major histocompatibility complex
MIP	macrophage inflammatory protein
MMP	matrix-metalloproteinase
MRI	magnetic resonance imaging
MRS	magnetic resonance spectroscopy
mtDNA	mitochondrial DNA
MTP	microsomal triglyceride protein
NAD	nicotinamide adenine dinucleotide
NAD+	nicotinamide adenine dinucleotide (oxidized)
NADH	nicotinamide adenine dinucleotide (reduced)
NADP+	nicotinamide adenine dinucleotide phosphate (oxidized)
NADPH	nicotinamide adenine dinucleotide phosphate (reduced)
NAPBQI	*N*-acetyl-*P*-benzoquinonimine
NASH	non-alcoholic steatohepatitis
NC1	a domain of type IV collagen
NCA	National Council of Alcoholism
NFκ-B	nuclear factor kappa-B
NIDDK	National Institute of Diabetes and Digestive and Kidney Diseases
NK	natural killer cell
NMDA	*N*-methyl-*D*-aspartate
NOLD	non-oxidative leucine disposal
NOS	nitric oxide synthase
NYHA	New York Heart Association
O_2^-	superoxide ion
PAF	platelet activating factor
PAH	phosphatidate phosphohydrolase
PB	peripheral blood
PBC	primary biliary cirrhosis

pC-collagen	collagen retaining its carboxyterminal end
PDGF	platelet-derived growth factor
PEG	percutaneous endoscopic gastrostomy
PET	positron emission tomography
PGD$_2$	prostaglandin D$_2$
PGE$_2$	prostaglandin E$_2$
PH	parial hepatectomy
pI	isoelectric point
PICP	carboxyterminal propeptide of type I collagen
PIIINP	aminoterminal propeptide of type III procollagen
PINP	aminoterminal propeptide of type I collagen
POBN	α-(4-pyridyl-1-oxide)N-t-butylnitrone
PS	permeability/surface area product
PSE	portal-systemic encephalopathy
PTBR	peripheral-type benzodiazepine receptor
PTU	propylthiouracil
Q	turnover rate or flux (Waterlow model)
Ra	rate of appearance
Rd	rate of disappearance
RDW	red cell distribution width
RES	reticuloendothelial system
RIA	radioimmunoassay
RNA	ribonucleic acid
ROS	reactive oxygen species
RP	relapse prevention
S	protein synthesis rate
SADQ	severity of alcohol dependence questionnaire
SAM	S-adenosylmethionine
SAPK	stress-activated protein kinase
SBP	spontaneous bacterial peritonitis
SCF	stem cell factor
SE	standard error of the mean
SEC	sinusoidal lining cell
sGOT	serum glutamic oxalacetic transaminase
sGPT	serum glutamic pyruvic transaminase
SHBG	sex-hormone-binding-globulin
SIAM	swift increase in alcohol metabolism
SMA	smooth muscle autoantibody
SMAST	Short Michigan Alcoholism Screening Text
SSRIs	Selective serotonin reuptake inhibitors
STAT-3	signal transducer and activator of transcription-3
T	thymidine
T$_3$	triiodothyronine
T$_4$	thyroxine
TBG	thyroxine-binding globulin
TCAs	tricyclic antidepressants
TGF	transforming growth factor

TGF-β1	transforming growth factor-β1
Th	T-helper
TIA	turbidimetric immunoassay
TIMP	preotease inhibitor
TIPS	transjugular intrahepatic porto-systemic shunt
TNF	tumor necrosis factor
TNFR	tumor necrosis factor-α receptor
TNF-α	tumor necrosis factor-alpha
TRH	thyroid releasing hormone
tRNA	transfer ribonucleic acid
TSF	triceps skinfold thickness
TSH	thyroid stimulating hormone
Tyr	tyrosine
UNOS	United Network for Organ Sharing
VAP	vascular adhesion protein
VCAM	vascular cell adhesion protein
VLA	very late after activation antigen
VLDL	very low density lipoproteins
WHO	World Health Organization

Contributors

Dr David H. Adams
Liver Research Laboratories
University of Birmingham
Queen Elizabeth Hospital
Birmingham B15 2TH

Prof Emanuele Albano
Department of Medical Sciences
University of Turin
Via Solaroli 17
28100 Novara
Italy

Dr Andrew J. Bathgate
Centre for Liver and
    Digestive Diseases
Royal Infirmary of Edinburgh
Lauriston Place
Edinburgh, EH3 9YW

Dr Roger F. Butterworth
Neuroscience Research Unit
CHUM Campus Saint-Luc
1058 St-Denis Street
Montreal, Quebec H2X 3J4
Canada

Dr David W. Crabb
Department of Medicine
Indiana University School
    of Medicine
975 West Walnut Street
Indianapolis IN 46202-5121
USA

Dr Christopher P. Day
Centre for Liver Research
Floor 4, William Leech Building
University of Newcastle Medical School
Framlington Place
Newcastle upon Tyne NE2 4HH

Dr H. Denk
Institute of Pathology
University of Graz School of Medicine
Auenbruggerplatz 25
A-8036 Graz
Austria

Dr Anthony J. Donaghy
The AW Morrow Gastroenterology
    and Liver Centre
Royal Prince Alfred Hospital and
    University of Sydney
Missenden Road
Camperdown 2050
Australia

Dr Samuel W. French
Department of Pathology
Harbor-UCLA Medical Center
1000 West Carson St
Torrance CA 90509, USA

Prof Christian Gluud
Copenhagen Trial Unit
Institute of Preventive Medicine
Kommunehospitalet
DK-1399 Copenhagen K
Denmark

Dr Robin Hughes
Institute of Liver Studies
Guy's, King's and St Thomas' School
  of Medicine
King's Denmark Hill Campus
Bessemer Road
London SE5 9PJ

Dr John Koskinas
Academic Department of Medicine
Hippokration Hospital
114 Vas. Sofias Street
Athens 11527, Greece

Prof F. Javier Laso
Servicio de Medicina Interna II
Hospital Universitario
Paseo de San Vicente 58-182
37007 Salamanca
Spain

Prof Kai O. Lindros
Alcohol Research Center
National Public Health Institute
PO Box 719
FIN-00101 Helsinki
Finland

Dr Angela Madden
School of Health and Sports Science
University of North London
Holloway Road
London N7 8DB

Dr E. Jane Marshall
National Alcohol Unit
Out Patient Department
Maudsley Hospital
Denmark Hill
London SE5 8AZ

Dr Philippe Mathurin
Service d'Hépatogastroentérologie
Hôpital Claude Huriez 2ème étage Est
Avenue Michel Polonovski
CHRU Lille
59037 Lille, France

Dr Robert S. McCuskey
Department of Cell Biology and
  Anatomy
University of Arizona College of
  Medicine
1501 N. Campbell Avenue
Tucson AZ 85724-5044, USA

Dr Onni Niemelä
EP Central Hospital Laboratory
FIN-60220 Seinäjoki
Finland

Dr John O'Grady
Institute of Liver Studies
King's College Hospital
Denmark Hill
London SE5 9RS

Dr Albert Parés
Liver Unit, Institut de Malaties
  Digestives
Hospital Clínic
Villarroel 170
08036 Barcelona
Spain

Dr Stephen P. Pereira
Gastroenterology Unit
4th Floor Thomas Guy House
Guy's Hospital
London Bridge
London SE1 9RT

Dr Martin Phillips
Institute of Liver Studies
King's College Hospital
Denmark Hill
London SE5 9PJ

Prof Thierry Poynard
Services d'HépatoGastroentérologie
Groupe Hospitalier
  Pitié-Salpêtrière
47-83 boulevard de l'Hôpital
75651 Paris cedex 13
France

Dr Victor R. Preedy
Department of Nutrition
   and Dietetics
King's College London
Franklin-Wilkins Building
150 Stamford Street
London SE1 9NN

Dr Stephen D. Ryder
Clinical Director,
   General Medicine
University Hospital
Queens Medical Centre
Nottingham NG7 2UH

Prof John B. Saunders
Centre for Drug and
   Alcohol Studies
Department of Psychiatry
Royal Brisbane Hospital
Herston QLD 4029
Australia

Dr David I.N. Sherman
Department of Gastroenterology
Central Middlesex Hospital
Acton Lane
Park Royal
London NW10 7NS

Dr Kenneth J. Simpson
Consultant Physician
Centre for Liver and Digestive
   Disorders

Royal Infirmary
Lauriston Place
Edinburgh EH3 9YW

Dr Ronald G. Thurman
Department of Pharmacology
University of North California
CB 7365 Mary Ellen Jones Bldg
Chapel Hill NC 27599-7365
USA

Dr Alvaro Urbano-Márquez
Department of Internal Medicine
Hospital Clínic
Villarroel 170
08036 Barcelona, Spain

Prof Elena Volpi
Division of Endocrinology
   and Diabetes
University of Southern California
1333 San Pablo Street, BMT-B11
Los Angeles CA 90033, USA

Prof Ronald Ross Watson
College of Public Health
University of Arizona
1501 N. Campbell
Tucson AZ 85749, USA

Prof Roger Williams
Institute of Hepatology
University College London
   Medical School
69-75 Chenies Mews
London WC1E 6HX

Color plates

monocyte, KC*: activated Kupffer cell, SC*: activated stellate cell. (*See page 141*)

Color plate 7   Marked steatosis and an inflammatory spot in a liver of a rat after consuming low-carbohydrate/high-fat ethanol liquid diet for 6 weeks. Note the high incidence of microvesicular steatosis. Details of the alcohol treatment are given in Lindros and Järveläinen (1998). (*See page 365*)

Color plate 8   Focal necrosis (arrow) and associated pericentral inflammation in a liver of a rat after six weeks of intragastric feeding. Note that the fatty changes are mainly macrovacuolar. HE staining. (Figures 15.2 and 15.3 are courtesy of Dr Samuel French, Harbor-UCLA Medical Center, Department of Pathology, Torrance, CA.) (*See page 367*)

Color plate 9   Central fibrotic changes (open arrows) and fat accumulation (F) in a liver of a rat after two months on intragastric ethanol liquid diet administration. The black arrow depicts a portal tract. The fibrotic changes are depicted by staining stellate cells for actin. (*See page 368*)

Color plate 10   Cirrhosis in a baboon fed alcohol for four years. Chromotrope-aniline blue staining. Reproduced with permission from Lieber and DeCarli (1974). (*See page 372*)

Biographies

Victor R. Preedy, Ph.D. DSc, FIBiol FRCPath. Reader in Clinical Biochemistry, King's College, University of London.

Dr Preedy is a Reader in Clinical Biochemistry and an international expert in the field of alcohol metabolism. He has published more than 450 articles and other scientific communications. He is on the Editorial Advisory Boards of five scientific Journals and a member of numerous Scientific Societies including both the International and the European Societies for Biomedical Research into Alcoholism. He lectures widely on the effects of alcohol at both International and National venues.

David Sherman MD FRCP, Consultant Physician and Gastroenterologist, Department of Gastroenterology & Nutrition, Central Middlesex Hospital, London, UK.

He trained in gastroenterology and general medicine at Charing Cross Hospital, London, and the Queen Elizabeth Hospital, Birmingham. He received training in liver disease at the Institute of Liver Studies, King's College Hospital, London, where he completed an MD thesis on susceptibility to alcoholic liver disease and other alcohol-related organ damage. Since 1996 he has been a Consultant Physician and Gastroenterologist at Central Middlesex Hospital, London, where his main interests have included liver disease.

Ronald Ross Watson, Ph.D., initiated and directed the National Institute of Alcohol Abuse and Alcoholism (NIAAA) Alcohol Research Center at the University of Arizona College of Medicine. The main goal of the Center was to understand the role of ethanol-induced immunosuppression on immune function and disease resistance in animals. Dr. Watson has edited 53 books, including 10 on alcohol abuse and 4 on other drugs of abuse. He has worked for several years on research for the U.S. Navy Alcohol and Substance Abuse Program.

Dr. Watson attended the University of Idaho but graduated from Brigham Young University in Provo, Utah, with a degre in Chemistry in 1966. He completed his Ph.D. degree in 1971 in Biochemistry from Michigan State University. His postdoctoral schooling was completed at the Harvard School of Public Health in Nutrition and Microbiology, including a two-year postdoctoral research experience in immunology. He was an Assistant Professor of Immunology and did research at the University of Mississippi Medical Center in Jackson from 1973 to 1974. He was an Assisstant Professor of Microbiology and Immunology at the Indiana University

Medical School from 1974 to 1978 and an Associate Professor at Purdue University in the Department of Food and Nutrition from 1978 to 1982. In 1982, he joined the faculty at the University of Arizona in the Department of Family and Community Medicine, and is also a Professor in the College of Public Health. He has published 450 research papers and review chapters.

Dr. Watson is a member of a several national and international nutrition, immunology, and cancer societies and research societies on alcoholism. He currently directs two National Institutes of Health (NIH) grants, one focusing on the Role of Alcohol in accentuating AIDS related heart and liver damage.

Part 1

Specific lesions

Chapter 1

Alcoholic fatty liver

Andrew J. Bathgate and Kenneth J. Simpson

Fatty Liver is the commonest pathological finding in patients who abuse alcohol. Patients are usually asymptomatic but may have evidence of hepatic decompensation and there is a risk of progression to cirrhosis in those continuing to drink alcohol.

The major accumulating lipid is triacylglycerol. The underlying mechanism of accumulation is not clearly understood. There is evidence suggesting that there is an increase in esterification of fatty acids and glycerol, an impairment of fatty acid oxidation and a reduction in hepatic secretion of triacylglycerol in very low density lipoprotein (VLDL).

The progression of fatty liver to cirrhosis may not require a stage of alcoholic hepatitis and the presence of lipid may lead to an increase in lipid peroxidation.

Fatty liver is reversible with abstinence although other therapies may be of benefit if drinking continues.

Microvesicular steatosis is less commonly seen and may be related to hepatocyte mitochondrial damage leading to a more pronounced impairment of fatty acid oxidation.

KEYWORDS: Fatty liver, triacylglycerol, esterification, beta oxidation, lipid peroxidation, microvesicular steatosis

INTRODUCTION

Fatty liver or hepatic steatosis is a common finding in liver biopsies from patients who abuse alcohol, occurring in up to 90% of patients presenting for treatment of chronic alcoholism (Edmondson *et al.*, 1967). Initially it was considered clinically benign but recent reports suggest that there is a risk of progression to cirrhosis in these patients (Sorenson *et al.*, 1984; Teli *et al.*, 1995).

Fatty liver is a common histological finding and is not exclusive to alcohol abusers, other common causes of acquired macrovesicular fatty liver are shown in Table 1.1. There are also a number of rarer inherited metabolic disorders which give rise to fatty liver e.g., abetalipoproteinemia, glycogen storage disease, galactosemia.

CLINICAL FEATURES

Patients found to have alcoholic fatty liver are mainly asymptomatic and present because of suspected heavy drinking or the incidental finding of abnormal liver

Table 1.1 Common causes of fatty liver

Alcohol
Non-insulin dependent diabetes mellitus
Obesity
Drugs e.g., methotrexate, zidovudine, perhexilene
Hyperlipidemia
Kwashiorkor
Rapid weight loss
Total parenteral nutrition
Intestinal bypass surgery

function tests (Brunt *et al.*, 1974; Levi and Chalmers, 1978; Morgan, 1985). In those who are symptomatic, the most common complaints are non-specific upper gastrointestinal symptoms (Leevy, 1962; Hislop *et al.*, 1983; Potter and James, 1987). However, 10–28% of patients with alcoholic fatty liver have at least one manifestation of hepatic decompensation (Brunt *et al.*, 1974; Hislop *et al.*, 1983) and occasionally hepatic failure may occur in the absence of any other pathology (Morgan *et al.*, 1978).

Mortality associated with alcoholic fatty liver is rare although some studies noted an increase in sudden death (Kuller *et al.*, 1974; Randall, 1980). There have also been some cases of fatal fat embolus in patients with steatosis reported (Lynch *et al.*, 1957). These cases are unusual and most patients have little systemic upset and if they abstain from alcohol the steatosis resolves.

Laboratory tests on the whole are not helpful in indicating the severity of steatosis in alcoholic fatty liver. There is often an increase in the serum gamma glutamyl transferase but the correlation with the degree of steatosis was demonstrated to be poor (Salaspuro, 1987).

Imaging of the liver with ultrasound or computerised tomography may indicate fatty liver. A recent study reported a good correlation of hepatic fat content determined by biopsy with ^{13}carbon nuclear magnetic resonance spectroscopy (Peterson *et al.*, 1996) as did a study involving calibrated CT (Ricci *et al.*, 1997) and these may prove to be useful in diagnosis and follow-up in the future but the definitive diagnosis of alcoholic fatty liver still requires liver biopsy.

PATHOLOGY

Fatty liver is a pathological diagnosis and has been defined as more than 5% of cells containing fat droplets (Underwood Ground, 1984) or total lipid exceeding 5% of liver weight (Hoyumpa *et al.*, 1975). The most common histopathological appearance in alcoholics is that of macrovacuolar steatosis where hepatocytes are distended with a single fat vacuole which displaces the nucleus. The microvesicular pattern of steatosis where microdroplets of fat surround the centrally placed nucleus is seen less commonly. The mixed pattern of steatosis along with the presence of giant mitochondria was shown to be more predictive of progression to cirrhosis (Teli *et al.*, 1995).

NATURE OF ACCUMULATING LIPID

In the normal human liver, lipid content ranges between 40–50 μmol/mg of DNA. The most abundant lipid is phospholipid, making up 53% of the total lipid content. Triacylglycerol makes up 19%, free fatty acids 20%, free cholesterol 7% and esterified cholesterol the remaining 1% of lipid (Cairns and Peters, 1983). In alcoholic fatty liver, the major accumulating lipid is triacylglycerol with the average increase being 10-fold (Cairns and Peters, 1983) although increases of 50-fold were observed in some patients. There are also increases in the esterified cholesterol content although to a lesser extent. Analysis of the individual fatty acids of the phospholpid fraction revealed reduced linoleic and arachidonic acid and increased palmitic acid. Increased free fatty acid content has been observed by some (Mavrelis *et al.*, 1983) but not others (Cairns and Peters, 1983).

HEPATOCYTE LIPID AND ETHANOL METABOLISM

Lipid metabolism

Triacylglycerols are the storage form of fatty acids, which are required for incorporation into phospholipids and glycolipids and also as a source of energy. The major body store of triacylglcerol is adipose tissue, but the synthesis of triacylglycerol occurs principally within hepatocytes. Triacylglycerol is then packaged and secreted within phospholipid membranes, as very low density lipoproteins (VLDL), and transported in the circulation to adipose tissue and muscle. The diagramatic structure of a triacylglycerol is shown in Figure 1.1. Triacylglycerols are synthesised from glycerol-3-phosphate and fatty acyl CoA (Figure 1.2). Phosphatidate phosphohydrolase, considered the rate limiting enzyme, catalyses the formation of diacylglycerol which is further acylated to triacylglycerol by diacylglycerol transferase. The triacylglycerol within the cytosol of hepatocytes is broken down by lipases into glycerol and fatty acid molecules. The fatty acid molecules then undergo beta oxidation within the mitochondria having been transferred across the outer mitochondrial membrane bound to carnitine. Beta oxidation producess acetyl CoA as a substrate for the tricarboxylic acid cycle as well as NADH,H^+ and $FADH_2$ (Figure 1.3) which transfer their electrons to O_2 by means of the respiratory chain.

Fatty acid synthesis is not the reverse of beta oxidation and occurs in the cytosol with the carboxylation of acetyl CoA to malonyl CoA by acetyl CoA carboxylase being

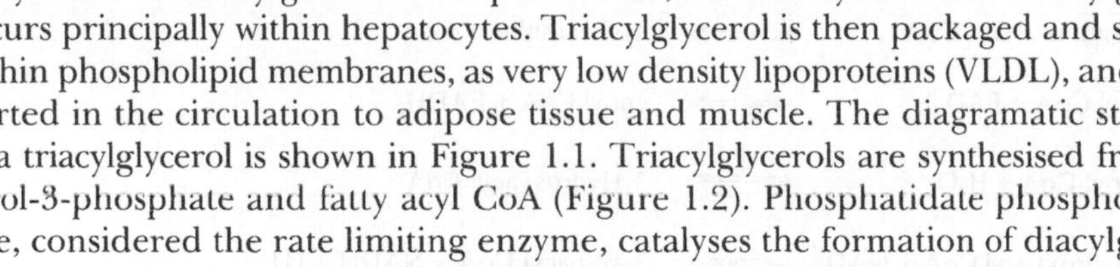

Figure 1.1 A triacylglycerol.

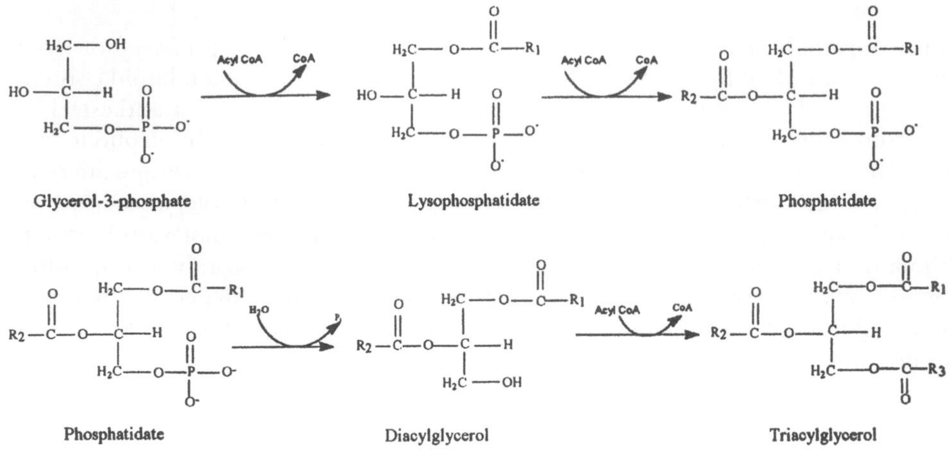

Figure 1.2 Triacylglycerol synthesis (R = acyl group).

1. Fatty acid + CoA + ATP $\rightleftharpoons$ acyl CoA + AMP + PP$_i$

2. Carnitine + acyl CoA $\rightleftharpoons$ acyl carnitine + CoA

3. Acyl CoA + FAD $\rightleftharpoons$ enoyl CoA + FADH$_2$

4. Enoyl CoA + H$_2$O $\rightleftharpoons$ 3-Hydroxyacyl CoA

5. 3-hydroxyacyl CoA + NAD* $\rightleftharpoons$ 3-ketoacyl CoA + NADH + H+

6. 3-ketoacyl CoA + CoA $\rightleftharpoons$ acetyl CoA + acyl CoA (shortened by C$_2$)

Figure 1.3 The principal reactions of fatty acid oxidation. Carnitine transferase (reaction 2) is responsible for transport across the outer mitochondrial membrane.

the committed step. This is followed by the sequential addition of two carbon units derived from acetyl CoA until the 16 carbon fatty acid palmitate is formed. This elongation process is carried out by the fatty acid synthetase complex. Further elongation and the insertion of double bonds to synthesize unsaturated fatty acids are carried out by other enzyme systems.

Ethanol metabolism

The subject of ethanol metabolism is covered in detail later on in this book, therefore only the two principal pathways of metabolism are briefly outlined in Figure 1.4.

Free radicals in the form of superoxide, hydroxyl radical, hydrogen peroxide and alcohol-derived radicals are generated within the cytosol, microsomes and

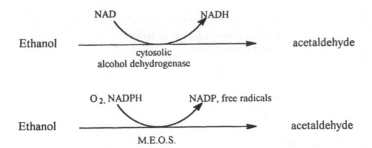

Figure 1.4 The principal metabolic pathways of ethanol (M.E.O.S. = microsomal enzyme oxidising system).

mitochondria as a result of ethanol metabolism. These free radicals can cause lipid peroxidation and may also initiate or amplify inflammation.

The redox hypothesis

As indicated above, the metabolism of ethanol alters the NADH/NAD$^+$ ratio within the cytosol. It has been suggested that this could lead to the accumulation of lipid in two ways. Firstly, the altered redox state within the mitochondria could impair β-oxidation of fatty acids and secondly, the increased NADH/NAD$^+$ ratio could lead to an increase in esterification by increasing the ratio of glycerol-3-phosphate/dihydroxyacetone phosphate (Lieber, 1974).

PATHOGENESIS

The pathogenesis of alcoholic fatty liver has been the subject of many studies both in humans and in experimental animals. The potential pathways leading to an increase in hepatic triacylglycerol are shown in Figure 1.5.

Enhanced substrate supply

As already discussed, triacylglycerol is synthesized from glycerol-3-phosphate and fatty acyl CoA esters. Ethanol may increase the supply of both of these precursors.

Glycerol-3-phosphate

Glycerol-3-phosphate is synthesized following the reduction of dihydroxyacetone phosphate by NADH-linked glycerol-3-phosphate reductase. This is the major pathway. Phosphorylation of glycerol by glycerol kinase is a minor pathway leading to glycerol-3-phosphate in human liver.

Ethanol oxidation by alcohol dehydrogenase forms NADH, therefore increasing the NADH/NAD ratio and forcing the reaction catalysed by glycerol-3-phosphate

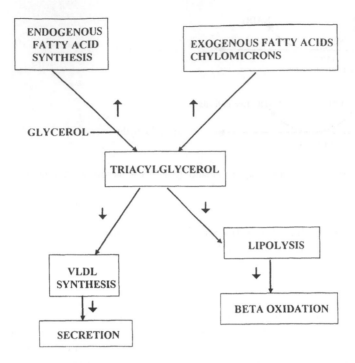

Figure 1.5 The possible pathways which could be disrupted in the pathogenesis of alcoholic fatty liver (↑ = increased, ↓ = impaired).

dehydrogenase in the direction of glycerol-3-phosphate synthesis. The increase in glycerol-3-phosphate concentration may then promote esterification of fatty acids rather than oxidation (Lieber, 1985).

Early studies in alcohol fed rats did show a correlation between esterification rate and the concentration of glycerol-3-phosphate (Ylikahri, 1970; Fellenius *et al.*, 1973). The reported effects of ethanol consumption on hepatic glycerol-3-phosphate however have been shown to be both increased (Nikkila and Otala, 1963) and reduced (Bustos *et al.*, 1970; Johnson *et al.*, 1971). Furthermore, the alteration of the hepatic redox state is not associated with increased triacylglycerol synthesis (Ryle *et al.*, 1985) and under most physiological conditions glycerol-3-phosphate concentrations do not limit fatty acid esterification (Zammit, 1984).

Fatty acids

In a study comparing free fatty acid content in liver biopsies from patients with alcoholic fatty liver and controls, there was a significant increase in fatty acid concentrations in patients with alcoholic fatty liver which were also higher than the levels found in morbidly obese patients (Mavrelis, 1983). The increase in free fatty acids could reflect an increase in supply, an increase in hepatic uptake, an increase in *de novo* synthesis or a reduction in β-oxidation.

In animal models of alcoholic fatty liver, acute ethanol administration led to an accumulation of liver triacylglycerol with fatty acids closely resembling those of adipose tissue (Lieber *et al.*, 1967). In chronic ethanol intake in man, the fat content of the diet affected the accumulating triacylglycerol (Lieber and Spritz, 1966). They reported that the fatty acids resembled those contained in a high fat diet. However, when a low fat diet was used the fatty acids were synthesized *de novo*.

The uptake of fatty acids by the liver may occur partly by carrier mediated processes (Stremmel *et al.*, 1992) as well as by diffusion. Recent evidence suggests that the most likely carrier protein is plasma membrane fatty acid binding protein (FABPpm) which is identical to mitochondrial aspartate aminotransferase (Isola *et al.*, 1995). This protein has been shown to be up-regulated in a human cell-line cultured with ethanol with a corresponding increase in fatty acid uptake (Zhou *et al.*, 1998).

The plasma level of fatty acids in acute ethanol administration to experimental animals has been reported as either reduced, unchanged or increased (Jauhonen *et al.*, 1975; Elko *et al.*, 1961; Savolainen *et al.*, 1977). In man, only very large doses of ethanol lead to an increase in plasma fatty acid levels (Lieber *et al.*, 1963; Bouchier and Dawson, 1964). Indeed, ethanol under certain circumstances may reduce the plasma fatty acid levels (Crouse *et al.*, 1968).

The role of hepatic blood flow may also influence fatty acid uptake in alcoholic fatty liver although reports are conflicting. In animal models, a reduction in hepatic blood flow was reported by Bravo *et al.* (1980) whereas Villeneuve *et al.* (1981) showed no change. A study in rats found the hepatic blood flow to vary with the infusion rate of ethanol (Jenkins *et al.*, 1986) but others found no difference in hepatic blood flow in chronic ethanol fed rats compared to pair-fed controls (Nott *et al.*, 1990). Studies in man reported a reduction in hepatic blood flow in patients with alcoholic fatty liver (Kasahara *et al.*, 1988).

Fatty acids are also transported in plasma within chylomicron remnants. Studies, again, have shown conflicting results with an increased uptake in chronic ethanol-fed rats found by some (Fraser *et al.*, 1980) while others found no difference in chylomicron remnant uptake between control and alcohol fed rats (Redgrave and Martin, 1977). A reduction in hepatic catabolism of chylomicron remnants has been reported (Lakshmanan and Ezekiel, 1986).

As previously mentioned chronic ethanol intake with a low fat diet led to the fatty acids contained within the triacylglycerol being synthesised *de novo*. This led to the hypothesis that ethanol directly stimulated hepatic fatty acid synthesis. Brunengraber *et al.* (1974) suggested that the catabolism of ethanol provided the two carbon units for fatty acid synthesis. However further studies reported that the majority of the acetate produced during ethanol oxidation is released from the liver for metabolism in the peripheral tissues, as acetate is a poor precursor for fatty acid synthesis due to the low activity of acetyl CoA carboxylase (Suokas *et al.*, 1984).

It has been suggested that the NADH produced during oxidation of ethanol may transfer the H^+ by transhydrogenation to NADPH which could then increase *de novo* fatty acid sythesis within the hepatocytes (Lieber, 1985). Initial studies carried out *in vitro* with rat liver slices did observe an increase in fatty acid synthesis following the addition of ethanol (Lieber and Schmid, 1961; Gordon, 1972).

This was supported initially in *in vivo* studies, in both acute and chronic ethanol administration (Scheig and Isselbacher, 1965; Cascles, 1983) but other studies have not confirmed these observations (Grunnet *et al.*, 1985; Venkatesan *et al.*, 1987; Simpson *et al.*, 1994). In 1986, Venkatesan *et al.* reported a reduced rate of fatty acid synthesis in liver biopsy tissue from patients with alcoholic fatty liver and the reduction correlated with the severity of lipid accumulation suggesting there may be feedback inhibition. The activity of acetyl CoA carboxylase, a major rate limiting enzyme, and other enzymes involved in fatty acid synthesis were found to be reduced in liver tissue from patients with alcoholic steatosis (Simpson *et al.*, 1987).

It appears that hepatic fatty acid synthesis is in fact not increased in alcoholic fatty liver but is reduced irrespective of the fat content of the diet and that the fatty acid supply to the liver is not significantly increased either by hepatic blood flow or an increase in lipolysis.

Impaired fatty acid oxidation

Fatty acid oxidation or β-oxidation takes place in the mitochondrial matrix and requires specific membrane transfer proteins for long chain fatty acids. The early evidence that these processes may be impaired by ethanol came from *in vitro* work with rat liver slices, perfused rat liver and isolated hepatocytes (Lieber and Schmid, 1961; Williamson *et al.*, 1969; Ontko, 1973). *In vivo* work in experimental animals (Reboucas and Isselbacher, 1961) and human work also supported this with decreased release of $^{14}CO_2$ release from $[^{14}C]$ triolein (Blomstrand and Kager, 1973) although others suggest this could reflect an increased esterification rather than diminished β-oxidation (Eaton *et al.*, 1996).

The mechanism by which β-oxidation may be impaired includes an effect on enzyme activity and in experimental animals chronic ethanol administration decreased carnitine palmitoyl transferase I activity and increased its sensitivity to malonyl-CoA inhibition (Guzman *et al.*, 1987; Guzman and Castro, 1990). Work done by Rabinowitz *et al.* (1991) also showed impairment of medium chain acyl CoA dehydrogenase in chronic ethanol feeding. Alternatively, the altered redox state of the hepatocyte as a consequence of ethanol metabolism may impair β-oxidation. The NAD^+-dependent enzyme 3-hydroxyacyl-CoA dehydrogenase is inhibited along with enzymes involved in the tricarboxylic acid cycle resulting in a marked decrease in the activity of the TCA cycle with a mild decrease in β-oxidation (Ontko, 1973; Grunnet and Kondrup, 1986).

The only study on homogenized human liver biopsies was carried out in 1986 by Leung and Peters and compared normal liver with alcoholic fatty liver in patients who had been abstinent. They observed no significant difference in β-oxidation of $[1-^{14}C]$ hexadecanoate to ketone bodies but did observe diminished $^{14}CO_2$ release possibly reflecting an attenuation in the Krebs cycle activity. They also found an increased esterification of $[1-^{14}C]$ hexadecanoate in patients with alcoholic fatty liver suggesting a mechanism distinct from substrate competition or short term redox changes.

A more recent study assessed the intermediates of β-oxidation from isolated mitochondria derived from needle biopsies of human liver (Eaton *et al.*, 1996). They reported no difference in β-oxidation flux but did find an increase in the proportion of 3-hydroxyacyl CoA and 2-enoyl-CoA esters in the alcoholic fatty liver mitochondria compared with normals. There was, however, no correlation between alterations in β-oxidation intermediates and the degree of steatosis. It was hypothesized that there could have been an effect on the respiratory chain resulting from a reduction of the antioxidant ubiquinone. This has been supported by the finding of reduced plasma levels of ubiquinone in human alcoholics (Bianchi *et al.*, 1994) and the reduction of ubiquinone in the mitochondrial membrane resulting from free radical damage (Forsmark Andree, 1995). Others, however have found the activity of mitochondrial enzymes to be normal or even increased in biopsy tissue from patients with alcoholic steatosis (Jenkins and Peters, 1978).

ESTERIFICATION

Fatty acids within the cytosol are usually bound to fatty acid binding protein (FABP) and the presence of these proteins is thought to increase esterification in rats (Burnett *et al.*, 1979). There is some evidence of a gender difference in the response of FABP to ethanol feeding in rats, with females having less of an increase than males suggesting a possible mechanism for the known gender difference in ethanol susceptibility (Shevchuk *et al.*, 1991).

The study by Leung and Peters (1986), already discussed above, indicated a chronic effect on the esterification pathway. The enzyme phosphatidate phosphohydrolase (PAH) is generally accepted as the rate limiting enzyme in the pathway of triacylglycerol synthesis. This enzyme is responsible for the formation of diacylglycerol and is present in two distinct forms in the hepatocyte – a metabolically active form present in the cytosol and microsomes and a cell-signaling form, predominantly found in the plasma membrane. The physiologically active metabolic form is associated with the membranous compartments and the translocation between microsomes and cytosol is increased by free fatty acids within the cytosol.

Animal studies revealed an increase in PAH activity following chronic ethanol feeding. Baboon studies demonstrated increased cytosolic and microsomal activity in the early stages of fatty liver (Savolainen *et al.*, 1984) and studies in the hamster reported similar findings (Lamb *et al.*, 1979). Acute ethanol administration has also been reported to increase enzyme activity in several animal studies (Brindley, 1988).

Two more recent studies involving liver tissue obtained from patients with alcoholic fatty liver have compared enzyme activity with controls. The study by Day *et al.* (1993) showed a correlation between degree of steatosis and metabolic PAH activity and the study of Simpson *et al.* (1995) showed an increased amount of PAH associated with membranous compartments in those patients with severe alcoholic steatosis. The mechanism by which alcohol may increase metabolic PAH activity is not clear. The corticosteroid/insulin ratio and glucagon have been shown to increase PAH activity at the level of enzyme synthesis. However, the acute effects of ethanol seen in hepatocyte cultures suggest that non-hormonal factors may also play a role and this is more fully reviewed by Day and Yeaman (1994).

The final step in the pathway of triacylglycerol synthesis is a transferase reaction catalyzed by diacylglycerol transferase (DAT). This is the only enzyme specific to triacylglycerol synthesis as diacylglycerol is also used in the synthesis of phospho-lipids. An increased activity of DAT was observed in chronically ethanol fed baboons but this was also accompanied by an increase in PAH (Savolainen *et al.*, 1984) and no study to date has found DAT activity increased without a concomitant increase in PAH activity.

HEPATOCYTE LIPID EXPORT

Lipid is exported from the hepatocyte in VLDL which are phospholipid and lipo-protein membranes containing triacylglycerol. Evidence suggests that cytosolic triacylglycerol must undergo lipolysis and subsequent re-esterification (Gibbons *et al.*, 1994; Yang *et al.*, 1995). If this process was impaired by ethanol then it may contribute to hepatic lipid accumulation. The experimental evidence from animals however suggests that acute ethanol ingestion has no uniform effect on hepatic lipase activities (Sturton *et al.*, 1978). In chronic ethanol feeding, both increased and unchanged activities have been reported (Mezey *et al.*, 1976, 1980). Human liver biopsies of alcoholic fatty liver revealed no change in the activities of lysosomal and endoplasmic reticulum lipases (Seymour and Peters, 1978).

Most alcoholic patients have normal levels of plasma triacylglycerols (Taskinen *et al.*, 1982). Therefore impaired export of VLDL triacylglycerol may contribute to lipid accumulation following ethanol consumption. *In vitro* work on cultured hepa-tocytes monolayers revealed a reduction in secretion of triacylglycerol and phos-pholipid when exposed to ethanol (Grunnet *et al.*, 1985). A reduction in VLDL triacylglycerol secretion has been reported in rats (Venkatesan *et al.*, 1988) although this may not be the case in baboons.

The proposed defect in VLDL secretion is in the Golgi apparatus, as human liver biopsy specimens revealed an accumulation of VLDL like particles in that site (Cairns and Peters, 1984). A reduction in the hepatic secretion of VLDL triacyl-glycerol in patients with alcoholic fatty liver has been observed (Simpson *et al.*, 1989). The proposed mechanism for the reduced VLDL secretion is inhibition of microtubular assembly by acetaldehyde produced during ethanol metabolism. This is supported by a study by Wood and Lamb (1979) in which inhibition of alcohol dehydrogenase prevented the alcohol induced reduction of triacylglycerol secretion.

Studies of patients with abetalipoproteinaemia have further elucidated the mechanisms involved in the assembly of packaging of VLDL triacylglycerol within the endoplasmic reticulum (Gregg and Wetterau, 1994). These patients have fatty liver and low plasma lipid concentrations. The apolipoprotein B and recently synthesized lipid form VLDL particles under the influence of micro-sosmal triglyceride protein (MTP) (Duerden *et al.*, 1990). It is mutations within the MTP genes which are responsible for the defective packaging and secretion of VLDL seen in the majority of patients with abetalipoproteinemia. The effect of ethanol on the assembly of VLDL within the endoplasmic reticulum has not been studied although animal studies failed to show altered MTP activity in con-ditions associated with decreased secretion of VLDL triacylglycerol (Brett *et al.*, 1995).

PROGRESSION OF FATTY LIVER

The early studies on progression of fatty liver to cirrhosis showed, firstly in baboons (van Waes and Lieber, 1977), that there was no necessity for alcoholic hepatitis for progression and that perivenular fibrosis started at the fatty liver stage. In a human study, patients with steatosis and perivenular fibrosis who continued to drink alcohol progressed over the course of 2 years, with 40% becoming precirrhotic or cirrhotic. In this study, only 1 out of 10 patients with pure steatosis progressed over 2 years (Nakano et al., 1982).

In the retrospective studies of progression in alcoholic liver disease, Sorenson et al. (1984) found over 20% of patients with moderate to severe steatosis without alcoholic hepatitis developed cirrhosis after 10–13 years. In the study of Teli et al. (1995), 9 out of 88 patients with pure fatty liver had progressed to cirrhosis and a further 7 to fibrosis. In this study, the patients who progressed drank significantly more than those who did not progress, and the presence of microvesicular steatosis as well as macrovesicular fat at initial biopsy predicted progression.

The absolute necessity of an intermediate alcoholic hepatitis for progression of steatosis to cirrhosis has been challenged further in the studies of Reeves et al. (1996). They showed, in human liver biopsies, that hepatic stellate cell activation correlated with the severity of steatosis in alcoholic patients and not with the number of Kupffer cells or degree of fibrosis. They conclude that non-inflammatory mediators such as the products of lipid peroxidation or acetaldehyde may be a common mechanism for the production of fatty liver and hepatic stellate cell activation.

Two studies by Lettèron et al. give further support for the role of lipid peroxidation as an underlying mechanism for fatty liver and its progression. The first (1993) showed a correlation between lipid peroxidation and histological score for steatosis in human alcohol abusers. The more recent study (1996) investigated chronic steatosis induced by alcohol and other drugs in experimental animals. This revealed evidence for chronic lipid peroxidation within the liver and the proposal that the mere presence of oxidizable fat within the liver triggers lipid peroxidation and may be a common mechanism for progression to other pathological entities such as steatohepatitis.

TREATMENT

In the early human work on alcoholic fatty liver, it became apparent that ethanol could produce a fatty liver in 8 days despite an adequate diet (Lieber et al., 1965). The same study showed a return to normal liver histology following 1 month abstinence. The best treatment therefore is abstinence from alcohol.

A recent report of restricted diet and exercise in fatty liver associated with obesity led to improvement in steatosis on biopsy (Ueno et al., 1997). There is also evidence that exercise in rats prevents ethanol-induced fatty liver as compared to sedentary ethanol fed rats (Trudell, 1995). The role of dietary fat in alcoholic fatty liver (Lieber and Spritz, 1966) suggests that there may be some benefit in a low fat diet although this has not been systematically assessed. Nanji et al. (1995) reported that the type of dietary fat consumed may be important suggesting that saturated fat reversed alcoholic fatty liver in rats while unsaturated fat made little difference to liver histology.

The addition of hepatocyte growth factor to an ethanol-containing diet in rats showed a marked reduction in hepatic lipid levels with a corresponding increase in serum levels of lipids and lipoproteins. This appears to be a result of increased synthesis of apolipoprotein B which then mobilizes lipids from hepatocytes (Tahara *et al.*, 1999). However no human work with hepatocyte growth factor has been undertaken as yet.

A recent randomized placebo controlled trial (Cabelleria *et al.*, 1998) reported an improvement in patients with alcoholic fatty liver, as measured by ultrasound, with a combination of pyridoxine and pyrrolidone carboxylate. This combination has been shown, in experimental animals, to restore the levels of reduced glutathione thus removing free radicals and also to accelerate the plasma clearance of ethanol and acetaldehyde. There was an improvement in steatosis and biochemical parameters in those patients who continued drinking.

MICROVESICULAR STEATOSIS

The coexistence of mixed macrovesicular and microvesicular steatosis in alcoholic fatty liver has already been mentioned. In Teli's study of the progression of pure alcoholic fatty liver, the presence of microvesicular steatosis indicated a poorer prognosis (1995). The basic pathogenic mechanisms of macrovesicular and microvesicular steatosis may be the same although the principal mechanism in each may differ (Fromenty and Pessayre, 1995).

Other causes of microvesicular steatosis such as acute fatty liver of pregnancy, Reyes syndrome and drugs such as sodium valproate, result from impaired β-oxidation of fatty acids within the mitochondria of hepatocytes. The evidence for impaired β-oxidation of fatty acids in experimental animals secondary to ethanol has already been discussed and at most appears moderate. There is, however, a condition termed alcoholic foamy degeneration (Uchida *et al.*, 1983) which is characterized by massive accumulation of microvesicular fat and can lead to coma and death (Rosmorduc *et al.*, 1992). It has been proposed that mutations within the maternally transmitted DNA (mtDNA) within mitochondria may lead to severe inhibition of β-oxidation by preventing reoxidation of NAD^+. Indirect evidence for this was reported by Fromenty *et al.* (1995). They found the common deletion of mtDNA in 6 out of 10 alcoholic patients with microvesicular steatosis, 2 out of 17 alcoholic patients with macrovesicular steatosis and no patients with alcoholic hepatitis, cirrhosis or nonalcoholic microvesicular steatosis.

Another hypothesis is that severe oxidative damage to mitochondria may cause both mutations in mtDNA and this may be representative of severe mitochondrial injury which may cause microvesicular steatosis. A recent study by Mansouri *et al.* (1997) reported other deletions in the mtDNA of alcoholic patients with 85% of those with microvesicular steatosis exhibiting deletions while only 7% of patients with other alcoholic lesions and only 3% of nonalcoholic controls, including 13 out of the 67 controls with microvesicular steatosis from other causes, exhibited deletions.

Further elucidation of the importance and mechanisms of alcoholic microvesicular steatosis is required.

CONCLUSION

Alcoholic fatty liver is a common finding and in most cases is asymptomatic. The pathogenetic mechanisms involved are not entirely clear. It is likely that there is some degree of inhibition of β-oxidation of fatty acids, an increase in esterification and reduced hepatic secretion of triacylglycerol. There is a risk of progression to cirrhosis in those patients who continue to abuse alcohol and patients should be advised to abstain.

REFERENCES

Bianchi, G.P., Fiorella, P.L., Bargossi, A.M., Grossi, G. and Marchesini, G. (1994) Reduced ubiquinone plasma levels in patients with liver cirrhosis and in chronic alcoholics. *Liver* **14**, 138–140.

Blomstrand, R. and Kager, L. (1973) The combustion of triolein-1-14C and its inhibition in man. *Life Sci* **13**, 113–123.

Bouchier, I.A.D. and Dawson, A.M. (1964) The effect of infusions of ethanol on the plasma free fatty acids in man. *Clin Sci* **26**, 47–54.

Bravo, I.R., Accudo, C.G. and Callards, V. (1980) Acute effects of ethanol on liver blood circulation in the anaesthetized dog. *Alc Clin Exp Res* **4**, 248–253.

Brett, D.J., Pease, R.J., Scott, J. and Gibbons, G.F. (1995) Microsomal triglyceride transfer protein activity remains unchanged in rat livers under conditions of altered very-low density lipoprotein secretion. *Biochem J* **310**, 11–14.

Brindley, D.N. (1988) What factors control hepatic triacylglycerol accumulation in alcohol abuse. *Biochem Soc Trans* **16**, 251–253.

Brunt, P.W., Kew, M.C., Scheuer, P.J. and Sherlock, S. (1974) Studies in alcoholic liver disease in Britain. 1. Clinical and pathological patterns related to natural history. *Gut* **15**, 52–58.

Brunengraber, H., Bountry, M., Lowenstein, L. and Lowenstein, J.M. (1974) *Alcohol and Acetaldehyde Metabolising Systems* pp. 329–337, New York: Academic Press.

Burnett, D.A., Lysenko, N., Manning, J.A. and Ockner, R.K. (1979) Utilization of long chain fatty acids by rat liver: studies of the role of fatty acid binding protein. *Gastroenterology* **77**, 241–249.

Bustos, G.O., Kalant, T., Khanna, J.M. and Loth, J. (1970) Pyrazole and induction of fatty liver by a single dose of ethanol. *Science* **168**, 1598–1599.

Caballeria, J., Pares, A., Bru, C., Mercader, J., Plaza, A.G., Caballeria, L., Clemente, G., Rodrigo, L. and Rodes, J. (1998) Metadoxine accelerates fatty liver recovery in alcoholic patients: results of a randomized double-blind, placebo-control trial. *J Hepatol* **28**, 54–60.

Cairns, S.R. and Peters, T.J. (1983) Biochemical accumulation of hepatic lipid in alcoholic, diabetic and control subjects. *Clin Sci* **65**, 645–652.

Cairns, S.R. and Peters, T.J. (1984) Isolation of micro and macrodroplet fractions from needle biopsy specimens of human liver and determination of the subcellular distribution of the accumulating liver lipids in alcoholic fatty liver. *Clin Sci* **67**, 337–345.

Cascles, C., Benito, M., Cascles, M., Caldes, J. and Santos-Ruiz, A. (1983) The effect of alcohol administraion on lipogenesis in the liver and adipose tissue in the rat. *Brit J Nutr* **50**, 549–553.

Crouse, J.R., Gerson, C.D., De Carli, L.M. and Lieber, C.S. (1968) Role of acetate on the reduction of plasma free fatty acids produced by ethanol in man. *J Lipid Res* **9**, 509–512.

Day, C.P., James, O.F.W., Brown, A.S., Bennett, M.K., Fleming, I.N. and Yeaman, S.J. (1993) The activity of the metabolic form of hepatic phosphatidate phosphohydrolase correlates with the severity of alcoholic fatty liver in human beings. *Hepatology* **18**, 832–838.

Day, C.P. and Yeaman, S.J. (1994) The biochemistry of alcohol-induced fatty liver. *Biochim Biophys Acta* **1215**, 33–48.

Duerden, J.M., Marsh, B., Burnham, F.J. and Gibbons, G.F. (1990) Regulation of hepatic synthesis and secretion of glycerolipids in animals maintained in different nutritional states. *Biochem J* **271**, 761–766.

Eaton, S., Zaitoun, A.M., Record, C.O. and Bartlett, K. (1996) β-oxidation in human alcoholic and non-alcoholic hepatic steatosis. *Clin Sci* **90**, 307–313.

Edmondson, H.A., Peters, R.L., Frankell, H.H. and Borowsky, S. (1967) The early stage of liver injury in the alcoholic. *Medicine* **46**, 119–129.

Elko, E.E., Wooles, W.R. and Di Luzio, N.R. (1961) Alterations and mobilisation of lipids in acute ethanol treated rats. *Am J Physiol* **201**, 923–926.

Fellenius, E., Bengtsson, G. and Kiessling, K.H. (1973) The influence of ethanol induced changes of the α-glycerophosphate level on hepatic triacylglycerol synthesis. *Acta Chem Scand* **27**, 2893–2901.

Forsmark Andree P., Lee C.P., Dallner G. and Ernster L. (1997) Lipid peroxidation and changes in ubiquinone content and the respiratory chain enzymes of submitochondrial particles. *Free Radic Biol Med* **22**, 391–400.

Fraser, R., Bowler, L.M. and Day, W.A. (1980) Damage of rat liver sinusoidal endothelium by ethanol. *Pathology* **12**, 371–376.

Fromenty, B., Grimbert, S., Mansouri, A., Beaugrand, M., Erlinger, S., Rotig, A. and Pessayre, D. (1995) Hepatic mitochondrial DNA deletion in alcoholics: association with microvesicular steatosis. *Gastroenterology* **108**, 193–200.

Gibbons, G.F., Khurana, R., Odwell, A. and Seelaender, M.C. (1994) Lipid balance in HepG2 cells: active synthesis and impaired mobilization. *J Lipid Res* **35**, 180–188.

Gordon, E.R. (1972) Effect of an intoxicating dose of ethanol on lipid metabolism in an isolated perfused rat liver. *Biochem Pharmacol* **21**, 2991–3004.

Gregg, R.E. and Wetterau, J.R. (1994) The molecular basis of abetalipoproteinemia. *Curr Opin Lipidol* **5**, 81–86.

Grunnet, N., Jensen, F., Kondrup, J. and Dich, F. (1985) Effect of ethanol on fatty acid metabolism in cultured hepatocytes. *Alcohol* **2**, 157–161.

Grunnet, N. and Kondrup, J. (1986) The effect of ethanol feeding on the β-oxidation of fatty acids. *Alc Clin Exp Res* **10**, 64S–68S.

Guzman, M. and Castro, J. (1990) Alterations in the regulatory properties of hepatic fatty acid oxidation and carnitine palmitoyltransferase I. *Alc Clin Exp Res* **14**, 472–477.

Guzman, M., Castro, J. and Maquedano, A. (1987) Ethanol feeding to rats reversibly decreases hepatic carnitine palmitoyltransferase activity and increases enzyme sensitivity to malonyl-CoA. *Biochem Biophys Res Comm* **149**, 443–448.

Hislop, W.S., Bouchier, I.A.D., Allan, J.G., Brunt, P.W., Eastwood, M., Finlayson, N.D.C., James, O.F.W., Russell, R.I. and Watkinson, G. (1983) Alcoholic liver disease in Scotland and northeastern England: presenting features in 510 patients. *QJM* **206**, 232–243.

Hoyumpa, A.M., Greene, H.L., Dunn, G.D. and Schenker, S. (1975) Fatty liver: biochemical and clinical considerations. *Am J Dig Dis* **20**, 1142–1170.

Isola, L.M., Zhou, S.L., Kiang, C.L., Stump, D.D., Bradbury, M.W., Berk, P.D. (1995) 3T3 fibroblasts transfected with cDNA for mitochondrial aspartate aminotransferase express plasma membrane fatty acid binding protein. *Proc Natl Acad Sci U.S.A.* **92**, 9866–9870.

Jauhonen, V.P., Savolainen, M.J. and Hassinen, I.E. (1975) Cyclic AMP linked mechanisms in ethanol induced derangements of lipid metabolism in rat liver and adipose tissue. *Biochem Pharmacol* **24**, 1879–1883.

Jenkins, S.A., Baxter, J.N., Devitt, P., Taylor, I. and Sheilds, R. (1986) Effects of alcohol on hepatic haemodynamics in the rat. *Digestion* **34**, 236–242.

Jenkins, W.J. and Peters, T.J. (1978) Mitochondrial enzyme activities in liver biopsies from patients with alcoholic liver disease. *Gut* **19**, 341–344.

Johnson, O., Hernell, O., Fex, G. and Olivecrona, T. (1971) Ethanol-induced fatty liver: the requirement of ethanol metabolism for the development of fatty liver. *Life Sci* **10**, 553–559.

Kasahara, A., Hayashi, N., Sasaki, Y., Katayama, K., Kono, M., Yashima, T., Fusamoto, H., Sato, N. and Kamada, T. (1988) Hepatic circulation and hepatic oxygen consumption in alcoholic and nonalcoholic fatty liver. *Am J Gastroenterol* **83**, 846–849.

Kuller, L.H., Perper, J.A., Cooper, M. and Fisher, R. (1974) An epidemic of deaths attributed to fatty liver in Baltimore. *Prev Med* **3**, 61–79.

Lakshmanan, M.R. and Ezekiel, M. (1986) Effect of chronic ethanol feeding on the catabolism of protein lipid moieties of chylomicrons and VLDL *in vivo* and in the perfused heart system. *Alc Clin Exp Res* **9**, 327–330.

Lamb, R.G., Wood, C.K. and Fallon, H.J. (1979) The effect of acute and chronic ethanol intake on hepatic glycerolipid biosynthesis in the hamster. *J Clin Invest* **63**, 14–20.

Leevy, C.M. (1962) Fatty liver: a study of 270 patients with biopsy proven fatty liver and a review of literature. *Medicine* **41**, 249–276.

Lettèron, P., Duchatelle, V., Berson, A., Fromenty, B., Fisch, C., Degott, C., Benhamou, J.P. and Pessayre, D. (1993) Increased ethane exhalation, an *in vivo* index of lipid peroxidation, in alcohol-abusers. *Gut* **34**, 409–414.

Lettèron, P., Fromenty, B., Terris, B., Degott, C. and Pessayre, D. (1996) Acute and chronic hepatic steatosis lead to *in vivo* lipid peroxidation in mice. *J Hepatol* **24**, 200–208.

Leung, N.N.Y. and Peters, T.J. (1986) Palmitic acid oxidation and incorporation into triglyceride by needle liver biopsy specimens from control subjects and patients with alcoholic fatty liver. *Clin Sci* **71**, 253–260.

Levi, A.J. and Chalmers, D.M. (1978) Recognition of alcoholic liver disease in a district general hospital. *Gut* **19**, 521–525.

Lieber, C.S. (1974) Effects of ethanol upon lipid metabolism. *Lipids* **9**, 103–116.

Lieber, C.S. (1985) Alcohol and the liver. *Acta Med Scand* **703**(Suppl. X), 11–55.

Lieber, C.S., Jones, D.P., Mendelson, J. and De Carli, L.M. (1963) Fatty liver, hyperlipemia and hyperuricemia produced by prolonged alcohol consumption, despite adequate dietary intake. *Trans Ass Am Physicians* **76**, 289–300.

Lieber, C.S., Lefevre, A., Spritz, N., Feinman, L. and De Carli, L.M. (1967) Difference in hepatic lipid metabolism of long and medium chain fatty acid. *J Clin Invest* **46**, 1451–1466.

Lieber, C.S., Jones, D.P. and De Carli, L.M. (1965) Effects of prolonged ethanol intake: production of fatty liver despite adequate diets. *J Clin Invest* **44**, 1009–1021.

Lieber, C.S. and Schmid, R. (1961) Effect of ethanol on fatty acid metabolism: stimulation of fatty acid synthesis *in vitro*. *J Clin Invest* **40**, 394–399.

Lieber, C.S. and Spritz, N. (1966) Effect of prolonged ethanol intake in man: role of dietary, adipose and endogenously synthesised fatty acids in the pathogenesis of the alcoholic fatty liver. *J Clin Invest* **45**, 1400–1411.

Lynch, Raphael, S.S.D. and Dixon, T.P. (1957) Fat embolism from fatty liver causing death. *Lancet* **ii**, 123–124.

Mansouri, A., Fromenty, B., Berson, A., Robin, M., Grimbert, S., Beaugrand, M., Erlinger, S. and Pessayre, D. (1997) Multiple hepatic mitochondrial DNA deletions suggest premature oxidative aging in alcoholic patients. *J Hepatol* **27**, 96–102.

Mavrelis, P.G., Ammon, H.L., Gleysteen, J.J., Komorowski, R.A. and Charaf, U.K. (1983) Hepatic free fatty acids in alcoholic liver disease and morbid obesity. *Hepatology* **3**, 226–231.

Mezey, E., Potter, J.J. and Ammon, R.A. (1976) Effect of choline deficient diet on the induction of drug and ethanol metabolizing enzymes and on the alteration of rates of ethanol degradation, by ethanol and phenobarbital. *Biochem Pharmacol* **25**, 1663–2667.

Mezey, E., Potter, J.J., Slusser, R.J., Brandes, D., Romero, J., Tamura, T. and Halsted, C.H. (1980) Effect of ethanol feeding on hepatic lysosomes in the monkey. *Lab Invest* **43**, 88–93.

Morgan, M.Y. (1985) Epidemiology of alcoholic liver disease: United Kingdom. In *Alcoholic liver disease: pathobiology, epidemiology and clinical aspects*, edited by P. Hall, pp. 193–229. London: Arnold.

Morgan, M.Y., Sherlock, S. and Scheuer, P.J. (1978) Acute cholestasis, hepatic failure and fatty liver in the alcoholic. *Scand J Gastroenterol* **13**, 299–303.

Nakano, M., Worner, T.M. and Lieber, C.S. (1982) Perivenular fibrosis in alcoholic liver injury: ultrastructure and histologic progression. *Gastroenterology* **83**, 777–785.

Nanji, A.A., Sadrzadeh, S.M.H., Yang, E.K., Fogt, F., Meydani, M. and Dannenberg, A.J. (1995) Dietary saturated fatty acids: a novel treatment for alcoholic liver disease. *Gastroenterology* **109**, 547–554.

Nikkila, E.A. and Otala, K. (1963) Role of hepatic L-α-glycerophosphate and triglyceride synthesis in production of fatty liver by ethanol. *Proc Soc Exp Biol Med* **113**, 814–817.

Nott, D.M., Yates, J., Preedy, V.R., Venkatesan, S., Peters, T.J. and Jenkins, S.A. (1990) Effects of chronic alcohol administration on hepatic haemodynamics and reticuloendothelial function in the rat. *Br J Surg* **77**, A703.

Ontko, J.A. (1973) Effects of ethanol on the metabolism of free fatty acids in isolated liver cells. *J Lipid Res* **14**, 78–86.

Petersen, K.F., West, A.B., Reuben, A., Rothman, D.L. and Shulman, G.I. (1996) Noninvasive assessment of hepatic triglyceride content in humans with ^{13}C Nuclear Magnetic Resonance Spectroscopy. *Hepatology* **24**, 114–117.

Potter, J.F. and James, O.F.W. (1987) Clinical features and progmosis of alcoholic liver disease in respect of advancing age. *Gerontology* **33**, 380–387.

Rabinowitz, J.L., Staeffen, J., Hall, C.L. and Brand, J.G. (1991) A probable defect in the β-oxidation of lipids in rats fed alcohol for 6 months. *Alcohol* **8**, 241–246.

Randall, B. (1980) Fatty liver and sudden death. A review. *Human Pathol* **11**, 147–153.

Reboucas, G. and Isselbacher, K.J. (1961) Studies on the pathogenesis of ethanol induced fatty liver. *J Clin Invest* **40**, 1355–1362.

Redgrave, T.G. and Martin, G. (1977) Effects of ethanol consumption on the catabolism of chylomicron triacylglycerol and cholesterol ester in the rat. *Atherosclerosis* **28**, 69–80.

Reeves, H., Burt, A.D., Wood, S. and Day, C.P. (1996) Hepatic stellate cell activation occurs in the absence of hepatitis in alcoholic liver disease and correlates with the severity of steatosis. *J Hepatol* **25**, 677–683.

Ricci, C., Longo, R., Gioulis, E., Bosco, M., Pollesello, P., Masutti, F., Croce, L.S., Paoletti, S., de Bernard, B., Tiribelli, C. and Dalla Palma, L. (1997) Noninvasive *in vivo* quantitative assessment of fat content in human liver. *J Hepatol* **27**, 108–113.

Rosmorduc, O., Richardet, J.P., Lageron, A., Munz, C., Callard, P. and Beaugrand, M. (1992) La stéatose hépatique massive: une cause de décès brutal chez la maladie alcoholique. *Gastronterol Clin Biol* **16**, 801–804.

Ryle, P.R., Chakraborty, J. and Thomson, A.D. (1985) Effect of methylene blue on the hepatocellular redox state and liver lipid content during chronic ethanol feeding in the rat. *Biochem J* **232**, 877–882.

Salaspuro, M. (1987) Use of enzymes for the diagnosis of alcohol-related organ damage. *Enzyme* **37**, 87–107.

Savolainen, M.J., Baraona, E., Pikkarainen, P. and Lieber, C.S. (1984) Hepatic triacylglycerol synthesising activity during progression of alcoholic liver injury in the baboon. *J Lipid Res* **25**, 813–820.

Savolainen, M.J., Jauhonen, V.P. and Hassinen, I.E. (1977) Effects of clofibrate on ethanol induced modification in liver and adipose tissue metabolism: role of hepatic redox state and hormonal mechanism. *Biochem Pharmacol* **26**, 425–431.

Scheig, R. and Isselbacher, K.J. (1965) Pathogenesis of ethanol-induced fatty liver III. *In vivo* and *in vitro* effects of ethanol on hepatic fatty acid metabolism in rat. *J Lipid Res* **6**, 269–277.

Seymour, C.A. and Peters, T.J. (1978) Changes in hepatic enzymes and organelles in alcoholic liver disease. *Clin Sci Mol Med* **55**, 383–389.

Shevchuk, O., Baraona, E., Ma, X., Pignon, J. and Lieber, C.S. (1991) Gender differences in the response of hepatic fatty acids and cytosolic fatty acid-binding capacity to alcohol consumption in rats. *Proc Soc Exp Biol Med* **198**, 584–590.

Simpson, K.J., Venkatesan, S., Martin, A., Brindley, D.N. and Peters, T.J. (1995) Phosphatidate phosphohydrolase activity in alcoholic liver disease. *Alcohol* **30**, 31–36.

Simpson, K.J., Venkatesan, S. and Peters, T.J. (1987) Fatty acid synthesis in alcoholic liver disease. *J Hepatol* **7**, 34P.

Simpson, K.J., Venkatesan, S. and Peters, T.J. (1994) Fatty acid synthesis by rat liver following chronic alcohol feeding with a low fat diet. *Clin Sci* **87**, 441–446.

Simpson, K.J., Venkatesan, S., Smith, G.D. and Peters, T.J. (1989) VLDL-triacylglycerol turnover in alcoholic subjects. *Biochem Soc Trans* **18**, 1189–1190.

Sorenson, T.I.A., Orholm, M., Bentsen, K.D., Hoybye, G., Echoje, K. and Christoffersen, P. (1984) Prospective evaluation of alcohol abuse and alcoholic liver injury in men as predictors of development of cirrhosis. *Lancet* **ii**, 241–244.

Stremmel, W., Kleinhert, H., Fischer, B.A., Gumaran, J., Klaaser-Schluter, C., Moller, K. and Wegener, M. (1992) Mechanism of cellular fatty acid uptake. *Biochem Soc Trans* **20**, 814–817.

Sturton, R.G., Pritchard, P.H., Han, L.Y. and Brindley, D.N. (1978) Involvement of phosphatidate phosphohydrolase and phospholipase A activities in the control of hepatic glycerolipid synthesis. *Biochem J* **174**, 667–670.

Suokas, A., Forsander, O. and Lindros, K. (1984) Distribution and utilisation of alcohol derived acetate in the rat. *J Stud Alc* **45**, 381–385.

Tahara, M., Matsumoto, K., Nukiwa, T. and Nakamura, T. (1999) Hepatocyte growth factor leads to recovery from alcohol-induced fatty liver in rats. *J Clin Invest* **103**, 313–320.

Taskinen, M.R., Valimaki, M., Nikkila, E.A., Kuusi, T., Ehnholm, C. and Ylikhari, R.H. (1982) High density lipoprotein subfraction and post heparin plasma lipases in alcoholic men before and after ethanol withdrawal. *Metabolism* **31**, 1168–1174.

Teli, M.R., Day, C.P., Burt, A.D., Bennett, M.K. and James, O.F.W. (1995) Determinants of progression to cirrhosis or fibrosis in pure alcoholic fatty liver. *Lancet* **346**, 987–990.

Trudell, J.R., Lin, W.Q., Chrystof, D.A., Kirsenbaum, G. and Ardies, C.M. (1995) Induction of HSP72 in rat liver by chronic ethanol consumption combined with exercise: association with the prevention of ethanol-induced fatty liver by exercise. *Alc Clin Exp Res* **19**, 753–758.

Uchida, T., Kao, H., Quispe-Sjogren, M. and Peters, R.L. (1983) Alcoholic foamy degeneration – a pattern of acute alcoholic injury of the liver. *Gastroenterology* **84**, 683–692.

Ueno, T., Sugarawa, H., Sujaku, K., Hashimoto, O., Tsuji, R., Tamaki, S., Torimura, T., Inuzaka, S., Sata, M. and Tanikawa, K. (1997) Therapeutic effects of restricted diet and exercise in obese patients with fatty liver. *J Hepatol* **27**, 103–107.

Underwood Ground, K.E. (1982) Prevalence of fatty liver in healthy male adults killed accidentally. *Aviat Space Environ Med* **53**, 14–18.

Van Waes, L. and Lieber, C.S. (1977) Early perivenular sclerosis in alcoholic fatty liver: an index of progressive liver injury. *Gastroenterology* **73**, 646–650.

Venkatesan, S., Leung, N.N.Y. and Peters, T.J. (1986) Fatty acid synthesis *in vitro* by liver tissue from control subjects and patients with alcoholic fatty liver. *Clin Sci* 723–728.

Venkatesan, S., Ward, R.J. and Peters, T.J. (1988) Effect on chronic ethanol feeding on the hepatic secretion of VLDL. *Biochim Biophys Acta* **960**, 61–66.

Venkatesan, S., Ward, R.J. and Peters, T.J. (1987) Fatty acid synthesis and triacylglycerol accumulation in rat liver after chronic ethanol feeding. *Clin Sci* **73**, 159–163.

Villeneuve, J.P., Pomier, G. and Huet, P.M. (1981) Effect of ethanol on hepatic blood flow in unanaesthetised dogs with chronic portal and hepatic vein catheterisation. *Can J Physiol Pharmacol* **59**, 598–603.

Williamson, J.R., Scholz, R., Browning, E.T., Thurman, R.G. and Fukami, M.H. (1969) Metabolic effects of ethanol in perfused rat liver. *J Bio Chem* **244**, 5044–5054.

Wood, C.K. and Lamb, R.G. (1979) The effect of ethanol on glycerolipid biosynthesis by primary monolayer cultures of adult rat hepatocytes. *Biochim Biophys Acta* **572**, 121–131.

Yang, L.Y., Kuksis, A., Myher, J.J. and Steiner, G. (1995) Origin of triacylglycerol moiety of plasma very low density lipoproteins in the rat: structural studies. *J Lipid Res* **36**, 125–136.

Ylikhari, R.H. (1970) Ethanol-induced changes in hepatic α-glycerophosphate and triglyceride concentration in normal and thyroxine-treated rats. *Metabolism* **19**, 1036–1045.

Zammit, V.A. (1984) Mechanisms of regulation of the partition of fatty acids between peroxidation and esterification in the liver. *Prog Lipid Res* **23**, 39–67.

Zhou, S.L., Gordon, R.E., Bradbury, M., Stump, D., Kiang, C.L. and Berk, P.D. (1998) Ethanol up-regulates fatty acid uptake and plasma memebrane expression and export of mitochondrial aspartate aminotransferase in HepG2 cells. *Hepatology* **27**, 1064–1074.

Chapter 2

Alcoholic hepatitis

H. Denk, K. Zatloukal and C. Stumptner

Alcoholic hepatitis is a severe form of chronic alcoholic liver disease and is associated with liver cell necrosis and inflammation. Its pathogenesis seems to be complex involving toxic effects of ethanol and its metabolites, oxidant stress, endotoxin action, cytokines as well as disturbance of the cytoskeleton. A complex network of interactions between hepatocytes, Kupffer cells, stellate cells, endothelial cells and inflammatory cells modulated by cytokines seems to be operative. Mallory bodies are characteristic, although not specific, morphologic features of alcoholic hepatitis and their appearance are associated with alterations of the intermediate filament cytoskeleton of hepatocytes. Analysis of Mallory bodies in human liver tissue as well as after experimental induction in mice disclosed a complex composition with abnormal cytokeratins and a diversity of non-cytokeratin components. Abnormal phosphorylation of cytokeratins seems to be one of the key events in Mallory body formation and associated cytoskeletal disturbance. Experiments with cytokeratin 8 and cytokeratin 18 knockout mice revealed that Mallory body formation in hepatocytes is an active process requiring protein synthesis and not a passive aggregation of preexisting hepatocytic cyto-skeletal cytokeratin intermediate filaments. These experiments not only disclosed the primary importance of cytokeratin 8 in contrast to cytokeratin 18 for Mallory body formation but also suggested that liver cytokeratins play a non-skeletal role in toxic liver injury in addition to the more static skeletal functions. Insight into the pathogenesis of Mallory body formation may provide clues concerning important pathogenetic aspects of liver cell damage associated with alcoholic and non-alcoholic steatohepatitis.

KEYWORDS: alcoholic hepatitis, Mallory bodies

INTRODUCTION

The spectrum of alcoholic liver disease comprises steatosis, alcoholic hepatitis, fibrosis and cirrhosis (Baptista *et al.*, 1981; Ishak *et al.*, 1991; Jensen and Gluud, 1994a,b; Hall, 1995; Burt *et al.*, 1998). Steatosis is a common and almost invariable consequence of heavy drinking and develops within a relatively short time. However, only in 20–40% of chronic drinkers more serious and life threatening chronic liver diseases, notably alcoholic hepatitis, fibrosis and cirrhosis, arise (Ishak *et al.*, 1991; Jensen and Gluud, 1994a,b; Lindros, 1995). These individual differences in susceptibility complicate studies on the pathogenesis of chronic alcoholic liver injury. Alcohol toxicity in humans does not seem to be strictly dose-dependent (Ishak *et al.*, 1991; Jensen and Gluud, 1994a,b; Weiner *et al.*, 1994). The extent of liver damage may, in addition to direct effects of ethanol and its metabolite, i.e., acetaldehyde, depend on a variety of factors and complex biochemical interactions. So far little is known about determinants of the individual sensitivity for chronic alcoholic liver disease (Bosron *et al.*, 1993). Besides the amount of ethanol ingested per day, genetic factors influencing ethanol metabolism, uptake and elimination, oxidant/antioxidant status, dietary habits, cell-to-cell interactions and cytokine networks, viral infections (e.g., hepatitis C virus), drugs and various additional toxins may be involved. It is well documented that females are more prone to develop alcoholic liver disease than males. In women, consumption of equal amounts of ethanol leads to higher ethanol blood levels as compared to men due to lower ethanol elimination rates. They often present with more severe liver damage and worse prognosis, even after shorter duration of alcohol abuse and lower daily intake.

Therefore, in addition to direct hepatotoxic effects, ethanol also seems to play a more indirect and permissive role allowing a variety of factors (genetic and environmental) to contribute to or aggravate liver damage. Insight into this complex situation is important for prevention and therapy.

MORPHOLOGY OF ALCOHOLIC HEPATITIS

Alcoholic hepatitis, alcoholic steatonecrosis and alcoholic steatohepatitis are synonyms indicating the presence of necrosis, steatosis and inflammation (Baptista *et al.*, 1981; Ishak *et al.*, 1991; French *et al.*, 1993; Hall, 1995; Burt *et al.*, 1998). Because of its rather variable clinical picture, alcoholic hepatitis can only be reliably diagnosed in the liver biopsy. Morphologic features are (macro- but also microvesicular) steatosis, liver cell degeneration, ballooning and necrosis, (predominantly neutrophil) leukocytic infiltration, fibrosis, and Mallory bodies (MBs), most pronounced, particularly in early stages, in perivenular zone 3 (Figure 2.1). However, MBs (Mallory, 1911) are considered to be diagnostically less important than parenchymal damage, inflammation and pericellular fibrosis (Ishak *et al.*, 1991). Polymorphonuclear leukocytes frequently surround and sometimes even penetrate hepatocytes containing MBs ("satellitosis"). Other morphologic features include apoptotic bodies, giant mitochondria in hepatocytes, cholestasis, siderosis, Kupffer cell enlargement and proliferation (activation), and infiltration to a variable degree by mononuclear cells (lymphocytes). Fibrosis may be minimal, perivenular and pericellular in zone 3 (central sclerosis), but also extensive with formation of fibrous septa, finally resulting in cirrhosis.

MBs are cytoplasmic inclusions in hepatocytes ranging in size from small granules to large irregular masses (Figure 2.1a–c; Mallory, 1911; Denk *et al.*, 1979; French *et al.*, 1993). At the electron microscopic level, they display a predominantly filamentous ultrastructure consisting of mostly haphazardly arranged, rarely parallel filaments, 10–20 nm thick, coated by fuzzy material (Figure 2.1d). Large and apparently older MBs usually contain a more electron dense granular core. Therefore, according to their ultrastructure, MBs can be classified as type I (bundles of filaments in parallel arrays), type II (clusters of randomly oriented filaments) and type III (granular and amorphous material; Yokoo *et al.*, 1972). Types II and III prevail, and are often seen as combination of type II at the periphery and type III in the center. MBs are usually present in enlarged,

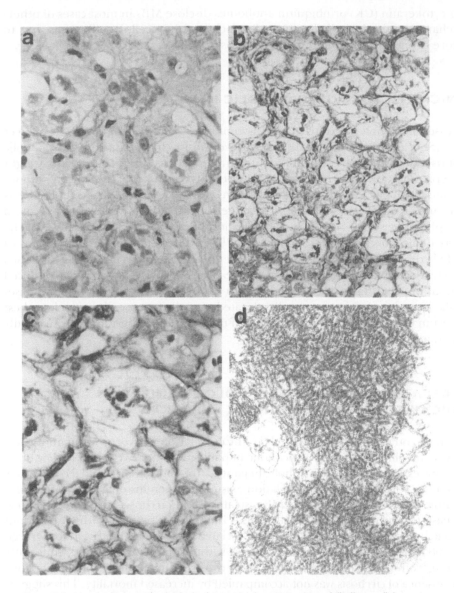

Figure 2.1 Human liver with alcoholic hepatitis showing enlarged (ballooned) hepatocytes containing Mallory bodies (MBs). Few polymorphonuclear leukocytes are present in the vicinity of MB-containing hepatocytes (**a**). MBs are eosinophilic in hematoxylin-eosin (**a**) and mostly blue in chromotrope aniline blue-stained sections (**b**, **c**). Note pericellular fibrosis (blue in **b** and **c**). At the ultrastructural level, MBs consist of mostly irregularly arranged filaments (**d**). a,c × 500; b × 200; d × 50,000. *(see Color Plate 1)*

ballooned hepatocytes, most of them with large nuclei and nucleoli. Most MB containing cells lack large fat vacuoles but may contain microvesicular fat. Although the presence of MBs in hematoxylin-eosin stained sections is not obligatory for the diagnosis of alcoholic hepatitis, more sensitive immunohistochemical stainings using cytokeratin (CK) or ubiquitin antibodies disclose MBs in most cases of otherwise characteristic alcoholic hepatitis. Parenchymal (pericellular) fibrosis seems to be more pronounced in the presence of MBs.

CLINICAL PICTURE OF ALCOHOLIC HEPATITIS

Mild cases of alcoholic hepatitis may be asymptomatic and the diagnosis rests on liver biopsy (Sherlock and Dooley, 1997). However, in its clinical appearance alcoholic hepatitis may also closely resemble acute viral hepatitis. Fatigue, anorexia, weight loss, hepatomegaly and pyrexia may follow periods of alcohol excess usually without adequate nutrition. The clinical manifestations closely resemble the metabolic effects of various cytokines (McClain et al., 1999). Peripheral leukocytosis as well as plasma neutrophil elastase levels, as signs of activation of granulocytes, correlate with the severity of alcoholic hepatitis (Stanley et al., 1996). There may also be symptoms of liver failure with ascites, bleeding and encephalopathy, diarrhea and steatorrhea caused by decreased bile salt excretion, pancreatic insufficiency and/or alcohol-induced intestinal mucosal damage. With respect to laboratory tests, serum transaminases and alkaline phosphatase are usually elevated, but disease severity correlates best with serum bilirubin levels and prothrombin time. Moreover, serum IgA is markedly elevated and serum albumin decreased.

CORRELATION BETWEEN MORPHOLOGY AND CLINICAL COURSE OF ALCOHOLIC HEPATITIS

As in many other liver diseases, a clear-cut correlation between histopathological findings and clinical severity of alcoholic hepatitis does not exist. In a review of 97 liver biopsies of patients with alcoholic hepatitis, 76% showed MBs and 97% steatosis (French et al., 1993), but little correlation existed between histopathologic findings, including presence or absence of MBs, steatosis and cirrhosis, and clinical course of disease (French et al., 1993; Hall, 1995). In cirrhotic patients with and without alcoholic hepatitis higher mortality was associated with the hepatitis group (Orrego et al., 1987), whereas mortality in cirrhotics without hepatitis was not significantly different from that of alcoholics without cirrhosis or hepatitis. Alcoholic hepatitis in the absence of cirrhosis was not accompanied by increased mortality. This suggests that capillarization of sinusoids and other vascular disturbances typical for cirrhosis sensitize the cirrhotic liver to further damage. For example, increased oxygen consumption induced by alcohol combined with impaired oxygen delivery could lead to liver cell necrosis (Ishak et al., 1991; Lieber and De Carli, 1991; Lieber, 1993, 1995). In contrast to earlier views, MBs do not seem to be signs of adverse prognosis and their presence does not influence mortality rates (Jensen and Gluud, 1994a,b). Therefore, on the basis of clinico-pathologic experience MBs seem to be indicators of a special type of liver cell injury rather than active players; but nevertheless, analysis of their composition and pathogenesis is essential for the understanding of pathogenetic principles involved in chronic alcoholic liver disease.

PATHOGENESIS OF ALCOHOLIC HEPATITIS: LESSONS FROM MORPHOLOGY

From the pathologist's point of view, morphology provides important clues to the pathogenesis of a disease. Thus, the morphologic features of alcoholic hepatitis, such as liver cell necrosis, apoptosis, degeneration and ballooning, steatosis, MB formation, inflammation, fibrosis as well as the behavior of non-parenchymal cells, are not only diagnostically relevant but also provide guidelines to the understanding of causes and evolution of the disease.

Liver cell necrosis and apoptosis

Several factors, alone and in combination, may be important for development of liver cell death (necrosis, apoptosis) in alcoholic hepatitis. Liver cell necrosis can largely be attributed to adverse effects of acetaldehyde, mitochondrial dysfunction and oxidative stress.

Oxidative stress seems to play a crucial role in alcoholic liver injury. It results from an imbalance between pro- and anti-oxidative processes. Free radicals and other highly reactive species (superoxide anion, hydrogen peroxide, hydroxyl radical, peroxy nitrite, ethanol-derived radicals) arise in hepatocytes from microsomal, mitochondrial, peroxisomal and cytosolic sources (Kurose *et al.*, 1997; Bautista, 1998; Rashid *et al.*, 1999; Clot *et al.*, 1994; Lauterburg and DeQuay, 1992; Nanji *et al.*, 1995; Bailey and Cunnigham, 1998; Rao *et al.*, 1996; Albano *et al.*, 1996; Dupont *et al.*, 1998; Thurman, 1998). They interact with all vital molecules of a cell (proteins, nucleic acids, lipids) leading to structural modification, metabolic disturbances and eventually cell death (Halliwell and Gutteridge, 1996, for review). Their effect is counteracted by enzymatic (superoxide dismutases, catalase, glutathione peroxidase) and non-enzymatic (glutathione, ascorbic acid, α-tocopherol, β-carotin) protective systems. Covalent binding of excess free radicals to proteins, including enzymes or receptors, leads to oxidative destruction of amino acids, unfolding of proteins, aggregation and cross-linking or depolymerization, and thus impairment of function. The interaction with nucleic acids initiates DNA damage and chromosomal breakage. Their reaction with lipids, particularly polyunsaturated fatty acids and cholesterol, initiates lipid peroxidation as a radical chain reaction, causing breakdown of cell membranes with membrane-bound enzymes, receptors and transporters. The microsomal ethanol oxidizing system (MEOS) with cytochrome P-450 2E1 (CYP 2E1) is a potential source of free radicals resulting from ethanol metabolism (Ingelman-Sundberg and Johansson, 1984; Ekström and Ingelman-Sundberg, 1989; Ishak *et al.*, 1991; Lieber and DeCarli, 1991; Castillo *et al.*, 1992; Lieber, 1993, 1995; Weiner *et al.*, 1994; Dilger *et al.*, 1997; Dupont *et al.*, 1998; Albano *et al.*, 1996; Rao *et al.*, 1996). CYP 2E1 is predominantly expressed in the perivenous (centrilobular) region where alcoholic liver cell damage usually starts in man as well as in experimental animals (Buhler *et al.*, 1992; Ingelman-Sundberg *et al.*, 1988; Tsutsumi *et al.*, 1989; Fang *et al.*, 1998; Nanji *et al.*, 1997). A diet high in polyunsaturated fat stimulates induction of CYP 2E1 and thus enhances radical formation and oxidant stress (Tsukamoto *et al.*, 1996). Ethanol-feeding to rats leads to depletion of mitochondrial glutathione levels, particularly in lobular zone 3 hepatocytes, preceding impairment of mitochondrial function and cell injury. Damage of mitochondrial DNA (Garcia-Ruiz *et al.*, 1994), proteins and lipids by reactive oxygen species causes impaired mitochondrial respiration (Kukielka *et al.*, 1994; Fromenti *et al.*, 1995; Wieland and Lauterburg, 1995). Reactive oxygen species may in addition to direct cytotoxic effects on hepatocytes activate transcription factors (e.g., NF-κB) and enhance cytokine and chemokine gene expression in Kupffer cells (Kamimura and Tsukamoto, 1995; Akira and Kishimoto, 1997; Tsukamoto, 1998). Experimental alcohol intoxication is also associated with decreased α-tocopherol levels as a sign of impaired antioxidant defense (Sadrzadeh *et al.*, 1994). Free radical formation can be enhanced by iron which explains the well-known synergistic hepatotoxic effects of ethanol and iron (Tsukamoto *et al.*, 1995). Moreover, the metabolism of ethanol increases the $NADH/NAD^+$ ratio leading to microsomal reduction of ferric to ferrous iron and initiation of lipid peroxidation (Lauterburg and DeQuay, 1992; Lieber, 1995). On the other hand, however, ethanol may also act as free radical scavenger and protector against lipid peroxidation or may directly inhibit radical formation by the MEOS. This could explain why sudden ethanol withdrawal could make hepatocytes even more vulnerable to further oxidant stress (Castillo *et al.*, 1992). This is consistent with clinical experience that patients may deteriorate after hospitalization and abstinence indicating that processes activated by ethanol, e.g., lipid peroxidation, can progress for some time in the absence of ethanol (Nanji *et al.*, 1997).

Ethanol itself affects Kupffer cell functions and particularly long term ethanol administration sensitizes Kupffer cells to secrete high levels of TNF-α after experimental lipopolysaccharide (LPS) injection (Hansen *et al.*, 1994; Thurman, 1998).

LPS (endotoxins) are components of the outer cell walls of most gram-negative bacteria and seem to play an important role in alcohol-induced liver injury. LPS circulates in a complex with the LPS binding protein (LBP) which has high affinity to the CD14 receptor on monocytes and macrophages, including Kupffer cells (Wright *et al.*, 1990; Järveläinen *et al.*, 1999). After binding of the LPS-LBP complex to the CD14 receptor release of cytokines is initiated. Long-term oral alcohol intake enhances CD14 expression and, in consequence, the endotoxin effect on cytokine production. Endotoxin may exert its toxic effects on hepatocytes directly by interference with transmembrane signaling and disturbance of mitochondrial function (Nolan, 1989), and/or indirectly through activation of Kupffer cells which then release potentially toxic products, such as reactive oxygen intermediates, nitric oxide, cytokines (TNF-α, IL-1, -6, -8), proinflammatory eicosanoids, and proteolytic enzymes, but also by its effects on microcirculation (Nolan, 1989; Kamimura *et al.*, 1992; McClain *et al.*, 1993; Hansen *et al.*, 1994; Adachi *et al.*, 1994; Simpson *et al.*, 1997; Nanji *et al.*, 1993). Plasma endotoxin levels are elevated in patients with chronic alcoholic liver disease as well as in rats fed alcohol by stomach tube, and correlate with the degree of liver injury. Several causes for endotoxinemia exist: increased intestinal mucosal permeability ("leaky gut syndrome"), elevated endotoxin production by intestinal bacteria, and reduced clearance by Kupffer cells (Bjarnson *et al.*, 1984; Bode *et al.*, 1987; Deaciuc, 1997; Iimuro *et al.*, 1997). Particularly TNF-α is a mediator of LPS-induced and other types of toxic cell injury, and plays a major role in the final common pathway involved in alcohol-related necroinflammation. Normal cells tolerate TNF-α, but are sensitized to TNF-α toxicity by agents interfering with RNA or protein synthesis. TNF-α exerts its biologic effects after binding to receptors and by subsequent activation of intracellular mechanisms, eventually leading to apoptosis or necrosis. Patients with severe alcoholic hepatitis have higher TNF-α levels than those with mild disease (Nolan, 1989; Akerman *et al.*, 1993; McClain *et al.*, 1993; Deaciuc, 1997; Grove *et al.*, 1997; Iimuro *et al.*, 1997).

As a consequence of pericellular fibrosis and fluctuating blood ethanol and oxygen levels ischemia/reoxigenation injury may also contribute to alcohol-induced liver cell damage (Tsukamoto *et al.*, 1985a, 1990; Jaeschke and Farhood, 1991; Arteel *et al.*, 1997; Horie *et al.*, 1997). Evidence exists that in the early phase of reperfusion injury, activated Kupffer cells and oxygen radicals are involved, whereas in the later phase cell damage seems to be executed by TNF-α and accumulated neutrophils. Thus TNF-α may also exert its detrimental effect indirectly by stimulating inflammation. The role of TNF-α in alcoholic liver disease is further supported by the observation that obesity, which is associated with high TNF-α levels, is a risk factor for the development of alcoholic hepatitis (Lelbach, 1976; Teli *et al.*, 1995; Rashid *et al.*, 1999; Yang *et al.*, 1997; Hoek, 1999).

The involvement of centrilobular hypoxia in alcoholic liver cell damage is substantiated by the observation that acute and chronic alcohol intoxication increase hepatic oxygen consumption together with depressed hepatic ATP level, and that centrilobular necrosis predominates in the livers of ethanol-fed rats (Videla *et al.*, 1973; Tsukamoto and Xi, 1989; Tsukamoto *et al.*, 1990; Lieber, 1995; Arteel *et al.*, 1997; Caraceni *et al.*, 1997; Thurman, 1998). Both alcohol dehydrogenase and the CYP 2E1-dependent MEOS require oxygen, but MEOS utilizes more oxygen to transform ethanol to acetate than alcohol dehydrogenase. Centrilobular hypoxia can, therefore, be related to MEOS concentrated in perivenular hepatocytes. Reduction of ATP synthesis, dysfunction of the mitochondrial respiratory chain and increased utilization of ATP are mechanisms leading to a low hepatic energy state during chronic ethanol intake, and this may further contribute to cell death by adverse effects on the cytoskeleton, on diverse ion pumps and on membrane permeability (Nicotera *et al.*, 1990, 1992).

Moreover, acetaldehyde adducts may adversely affect the function of diverse cellular components, including enzymes, but may also elicit immune responses leading to cell damage, inflammation and fibrosis (Paronetto, 1993; Yokoyama *et al.*, 1993, 1995; Klassen *et al.*, 1995; Tuma and Sorrell, 1995).

Apoptosis is also involved in alcoholic liver disease, as clearly revealed at the light microscopic level by the high number of apoptotic liver cells ("oxyphil bodies") and the demonstration of markers of apoptotic cells, e.g., by TUNEL assay, which seem to be most pronounced in hepatocytes containing MBs (Kawahara *et al.*, 1994; Zhao *et al.*, 1997; Nanji, 1998). Apoptosis of hepatocytes can be caused by TNF-α by activation of the type 1 TNF-α receptor initiation of signaling through the "death domain". Due to its high concentration of these receptors the hepatocyte is highly responsive to TNF-α. Moreover, chronic ethanol administration increases the receptor concentration on hepatocytes and thus the sensitivity to TNF-α. Similarly Fas ligand can engage its receptor on the cell membrane (CD95, Fas, APO-1) to activate downstream signaling, finally leading to apoptosis. Hepatocytes constitutively express Fas and are, therefore, sensitive to Fas ligand-induced apoptosis. Moreover, in alcoholic liver disease Fas ligand mRNA is upregulated in hepatocytes indicating that under these conditions the hepatocyte may represent target and effector as well. Thus, CD95 mediated apoptosis may be executed by direct interaction between neighboring cells via membrane bound ligand and receptor but also in an autocrine or paracrine fashion via a soluble form of the ligand (Galle and Krammer, 1998).

Steatosis

Negative effects of excess lipid in hepatocytes are only manifested if additional stress, e.g., due to inflammation, occurs (Caraceni *et al.*, 1997). Macrovesicular steatosis results from various combinations of enhanced mobilization of fat from adipose tissue, increased hepatic synthesis of fatty acids, increased esterification of fatty acids into triglycerides, impaired metabolization and decreased export of triglycerides from the liver (Weiner *et al.*, 1994; Lieber, 1995). In contrast to this mostly benign condition, microvesicular steatosis is regarded to be more serious and independent of its etiology. It results from mitochondrial damage with impairment of mitochondrial β-oxidation of fatty acids. Fatty acids are subsequently esterified into triglycerides, which accumulate. In addition, free fatty acids might impair assembly, cellular transport and secretion of very low density lipoproteins (Fromenty *et al.*, 1990; Fromenty and Passayre, 1995). Accumulation of oxidizable fat in the liver promotes lipid peroxidation independent of the causative mechanism (Letteròn *et al.*, 1996). Alcohol-induced fatty livers are particularly susceptible to endotoxin (Nanji *et al.*, 1993). Therefore, chronic lipid peroxidation might represent a link between chronic steatosis and steatohepatitis (Letteròn *et al.*, 1996). Chronic lipid peroxidation may lead to liver cell necrosis, stimulation of collagen production by stellate cells (via released malondialdehyde and 4-hydroxynonenal), chemotaxis (4-hydroxynonenal has strong chemotactic activity for neutrophils), but also crosslinking of proteins which may be exerted by malondialdehyde (Letteròn *et al.*, 1996). Reeves *et al.* (1996) found a correlation between alcohol-induced hepatic stellate cell activation and severity of steatosis, possibly attributable to a common pathogenetic mechanism in which acetaldehyde and free radicals with subsequent lipid peroxidation may be involved.

Inflammation

Infiltration by polymorphonuclear (neutrophil) leukocytes, particularly near ballooned MB containing hepatocytes, is a characteristic feature of alcoholic hepatitis (Denk *et al.*, 1979; Roll, 1991; Ishak *et al.*, 1991; Burt *et al.*, 1998). Neutrophils are rich sources of a variety of cytokines (Matsukawa and Yoshinaga, 1999; McClain *et al.*, 1999). Shiratori *et al.* (1989, 1993) observed the release of IL-8 from hepatocytes exposed to ethanol. IL-8 (or related protein) seems to be a major chemoattractant (chemokine) for neutrophil leukocytes and its release is regulated by IL-Iβ and TNF-α secreted by Kupffer cells (Mawet *et al.*, 1996). IL-8 is produced by hepatocytes as well as Kupffer cells in response to TNF-α stimulation (McClain *et al.*, 1999). Moreover, IL-8 plasma levels are increased in patients with alcoholic hepatitis and tissue levels correlate with neutrophil infiltration (Sheron *et al.*, 1993; McClain *et al.*, 1999). Neutrophils are recruited and activated by IL-8 to produce toxic substances, such as oxygen radicals and particularly proteases (Ganey *et al.*, 1994), causing hepatocyte necrosis (Mawet *et al.*, 1996; Sakamoto *et al.*, 1997). Consequently, neutrophil depletion has a protective effect (Hewett *et al.*, 1992). In rats, neutrophil infiltration is an early event after exposure to hepatotoxic doses of endotoxin and occurs before the onset of liver injury (Hewett *et al.*, 1992). In human alcoholic liver disease increased serum TNF-α as well as IL-6 levels have been detected which correlated with severity of disease (Khoruts *et al.*, 1991; Hill *et al.*, 1993; Schäfer *et al.*, 1995). In contrast, IL-10 acts as an anti-inflammatory cytokine. Exogenous IL-10 down-regulates release of proinflammatory IL-6 and TNF-α by Kupffer cells after LPS stimulation (Knolle *et al.*, 1995). Therefore, inflammation in alcoholic liver disease reflects an imbalance between pro- and anti-inflammatory cytokines. Increased expression of adhesion molecules on endothelial cells (e.g., E-selectins; ICAM-1, VCAM-1) promote binding and permeation of granulocytes but also lymphocytes into the liver (Fisher *et al.*, 1996). Öhlinger *et al.* (1993) found that ICAM-1 and neutrophils were preferentially associated with ballooned hepatocytes containing MBs suggesting that similar factors (e.g., oxidant stress) are responsible for hepatocyte damage, MB formation and inflammatory response. Neutrophil activation as measured by plasma neutrophil elastase levels seems to be a marker of disease severity in patients with chronic alcoholic liver disease (Stanley *et al.*, 1996). The pathogenetic role of inflammatory cytokines is the rationale for anticytokine therapy (McClain *et al.*, 1999).

In addition to neutrophils, mononuclear cells are also present in alcoholic hepatitis. In patients with alcoholic liver disease increased expression of the monocyte chemotactic protein 1 (MCP-1) and macrophage inflammatory proteins (MIP-1α and MIP-1β), which act on lymphocytes and monocytes, were detected. Composition and distribution of the inflammatory infiltrate, therefore, depends on the combination and relative proportions of chemokines present in the liver (Afford *et al.*, 1998; McClain *et al.*, 1999).

Enlargement and ballooning of hepatocytes

Enlargement of hepatocytes may result from disturbances of ion pumps with electrolyte and fluid retention, increased intracellular protein levels, but also from alterations of the cytoskeleton with adverse effects on cell stability and secretory processes. Microtubules play an important role in protein trafficking. Altered microtubular structure and function has been observed in livers of ethanol fed rats (Lieber and DeCarli, 1991). The α-tubulin subunit is prone to formation of stable adducts between its highly reactive lysine residues and acetaldehyde which block its polymerization to microtubules. This could be the basis of microtubular dysfunction in ethanol intoxicated livers leading to retention of secretory products and consecutive cell enlargement. Moreover, modifications of the microtubule associated tau protein could also interfere with microtubule assembly and stabilization (Kenner *et al.*, 1996). Since hepatocytes in alcoholic hepatitis and related non-alcoholic lesions show disturbance of the intermediate filament (IF) cytoskeleton impaired cellular stability can also be expected (Denk *et al.*, 1979; Denk and Lackinger, 1986; see also below). Perturbation of intracellular Ca^{++} homeostasis, which is a consequence of various stress situations including ethanol intoxication, may be an important initiating event of cytoskeletal damage (Nicotera *et al.*, 1990, 1992). Increased levels of intracellular proteins, at least partly resulting from a decline in protein degradation, may also contribute to cell enlargement (Pösö and Hirsimaki, 1991; Born *et al.*, 1996; Fataccioli *et al.*, 1999; Kharbanda *et al.*, 1995). Impairment of the proteasome pathway, in particular, could prevent the clearance of oxidized, cross-linked, or otherwise damaged proteins (Fataccioli *et al.*, 1999).

Fibrosis and cirrhosis

Although in most cases, fibrosis and cirrhosis can be regarded as part of a healing (scarring) process following acute or chronic necroinflammation, fibrosis and even cirrhosis can also arise in the absence of necroinflammation (Reeves *et al.*, 1996). It is now widely accepted that activated stellate cells are the major source of extracellular matrix, which accumulates in response to chronic liver injury (Schmitt-Gräff *et al.*, 1991; Maher and Friedman, 1995; Friedman, 1996; Hautekeete and Geerts, 1997). Under these conditions, stellate cells acquire a myofibroblastic phenotype and this is associated with fibrosis in alcoholic patients as well as in related animal models. Activation of stellate cells involves retinoid loss, proliferation, migration into regions of injury, contraction, fibrogenesis and cytokine release. Kupffer cells are also major effector cells in alcoholic liver fibrogenesis (Tsukamoto *et al.*, 1990a,b) by releasing cytokines (TNF-α, IL-6, TGF-β1) capable of inducing proliferation of and matrix gene expression by hepatic stellate cells. In this context, TGF-β is a major fibrogenic cytokine released by Kupffer cells (Matsuoka and Tsukamoto, 1990; Matsuoka *et al.*, 1990; Kamimura and Tsukamoto, 1995; Tsukamoto *et al.*, 1996). Moreover, the extent of experimental alcoholic liver fibrosis correlates with hepatic levels of lipid peroxidation products, such as malondialdehyde and 4-hydroxynonenal, suggesting stimulation of collagen production by stellate cells by these aldehydes (Tsukamoto *et al.*, 1995). Oxidant stress may also enhance hepatic fibrogenesis by induction of transcription factors in stellate cells, alteration of cytosolic calcium homeostasis and effects on intracellular signaling (Tsukamoto *et al.*, 1995). However, in addition to causing fibrosis stellate cells are also involved in matrix degradation and remodeling, particularly during tissue repair after injury by expressing matrix degrading metalloproteinases as well as potent inhibitors (e.g., TIMP-1) (Hautekeete and Geerts, 1997).

Taken together, a complex network of interactions between activated Kupffer cells, stellate cells, hepatocytes, endothelial cells and inflammatory cells modulated by cytokines is responsible for the alterations observed in alcoholic liver disease.

Mallory bodies (MBs) and alterations of the IF cytoskeleton of hepatocytes

MBs have originally been regarded as specific and essential for the diagnosis of alcoholic hepatitis since the first description of their association with alcoholic liver cirrhosis by Mallory (1911). However, alcoholic hepatitis may also be diagnosed in alcoholic patients with steatosis, hepatocyte necrosis, ballooning, and neutrophil granulocytic inflammation in the absence of MBs, and, on the other hand, if present, they are not specific for alcoholic liver injury since they are also associated with a diversity of non-alcoholic conditions (Zimmerman and Ishak, 1995). However, they are certainly not a non-specific and stereotypical response, but index structures of a peculiar type of liver cell injury. Analysis of MB composition and pathogenesis may contribute to our understanding of pathogenetic principles characteristically, although not exclusively, involved in alcoholic hepatitis. MBs are closely related to the IF CK filament cytoskeleton of the hepatocyte. The problem of MB composition and formation and associated IF cytoskeleton alterations will, therefore, be discussed in greater detail below.

ROLE OF CYTOSKELETON ALTERATIONS IN ALCOHOLIC HEPATITIS AND RELATED ANIMAL MODELS

Cytoskeleton of the hepatocyte

The cytoskeleton of the hepatocyte comprises three major components, IFs of the CK type, microfilaments and microtubules. The hepatocytic IFs are arranged in bundles in the cytoplasm, and are composed of equimolar amounts of type I (CK18) and type II (CK8) CK polypeptides (Franke *et al.*, 1979a, 1981; Moll *et al.*, 1982). A 1:1 ratio of type I and type II CKs is essential for correct IF assembly. Because of its simple CK composition, the hepatocyte is regarded as "simple" epithelial cell whereas most other, particularly stratified, epithelia have a more complex CK pattern and express more than two different CK polypeptides (Moll *et al.*, 1982; Fuchs and Weber, 1994). In addition to the cytoplasmic CKs, IF proteins are also found in the nucleus of hepatocytes, namely the nuclear lamins, which form the nuclear lamina (Krohne and Benavente, 1986). The microfilaments are concentrated beneath the cell membrane, particularly surrounding the bile canaliculus, which reflects their role in canalicular motility and as modulators of canalicular bile flow (Phillips *et al.*, 1994). One of the major functions of microtubules in the liver cell is to guide vesicular transport thus being essential for endocytosis and secretion as well as for maintenance of organelle position (Satir, 1994).

Mallory body

The first evidence that MBs are related to the IF-CK cytoskeleton was based on the observation that MBs react with antibodies directed to CKs (Denk *et al.*, 1979a,b, 1981, 1982; Franke *et al.*, 1979b) (Figure 2.2a–c). In their ultrastructure, MBs resemble aggregates of rod-shaped fimbriated filaments with diameters of 10–20 nm, which was originally interpreted as evidence that MBs result from the collapse of IFs (Figure 2.3). Studies performed with monoclonal antibodies which recognize conformation-dependent epitopes on CKs revealed, however, that the CK polypeptides in MBs are not organized as in true IFs (Denk *et al.*, 1979b; Franke *et al.*, 1979b; Kimoff and Huang, 1981; Okanoue *et al.*, 1985; Hazan *et al.*, 1986). This is in line with data obtained by biochemical analysis of isolated MBs which showed that in MBs, the equimolar ratio of type I and type II CKs (i.e., CK8

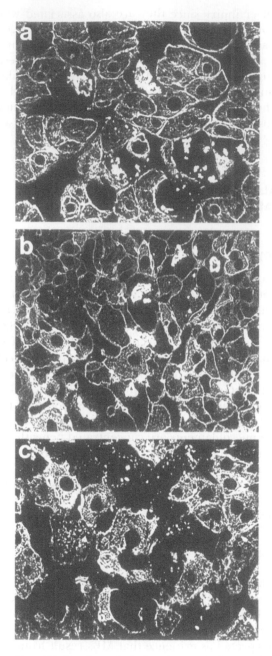

Figure 2.2 Sections of a human liver with alcoholic hepatitis (**a**) and of mouse livers intoxicated with DDC for 2.5 months (**b**) and GF for 4 months (**c**) immunostained (indirect immunofluorescence microscopy) with polyclonal antibodies to mouse liver CKs 8 and 18. Note specific staining of MBs in different stages of development (small granular to large irregular cytoplasmic inclusions). Most MB-containing hepatocytes show irregular, diminished or even missing cytoskeletal network, which, on the other hand, is clearly demonstrable in surrounding hepatocytes lacking MBs. (×450)

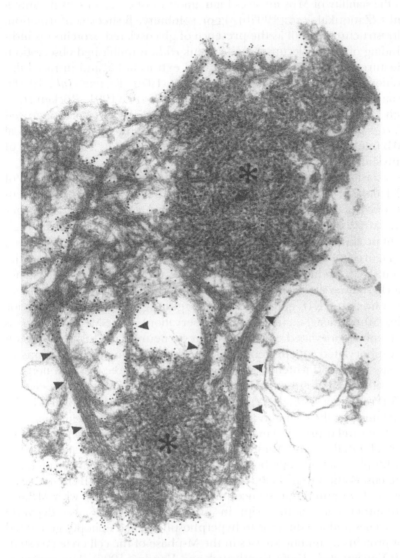

Figure 2.3 Small MBs (asterisks) lying within a network of bundles of intermediate filaments of the CK type (arrowheads). The CK content of MBs and intermediate filaments is indicated by deposition of gold particles after immunostaining with polyclonal antibodies to mouse liver CKs 8 and 18 (immunoelectron microscopy). (×36,000)

and CK18) is not maintained and that CK8 prevails over CK18 (Denk *et al.*, 1982; Hazan *et al.*, 1986; Zatloukal *et al.*, 1991). Analysis of MBs by infrared spectroscopy further demonstrated an increase in β-sheet conformation as compared to normal IFs, which are predominantly α-helical (Cadrin *et al.*, 1991). The transition in secondary structure to β-sheet could also, at least in part, be responsible for the poor solubility of MB proteins even under highly aggressive solubilizing conditions (French *et al.*, 1972; Kimoff and Huang, 1981; Zatloukal *et al.*, 1991). Another factor contributing to the stability of MBs involves high amounts of covalent ϵ-(γ-glutamyl)-lysine cross-links (Zatloukal *et al.*, 1992b). Poor solubility, β-sheet conformation, filamentous ultrastructure as well as the presence of glycosylated proteins (as indicated by the binding of certain lectins to MBs; Denk *et al.*, unpublished observation) are common features of a diversity of filamentous extracellular and intracellular amyloid depositions (French *et al.*, 1972; Denk *et al.*, 1979; Franke *et al.*, 1979b; Kimoff and Huang, 1981; Breathnach, 1985; Zatloukal *et al.*, 1991; Röcken *et al.*, 1996). Although MBs do not show the apple green birefringence after Congo red staining (Denk *et al.*, unpublished observation), which is characteristic for classical amyloid, the MB fulfills enough of the criteria to be considered as a special type of intracellular amyloid.

Besides CKs, a variety of non-CK components were identified as constituents of MBs (Figures 2.4 and 2.5; Table 2.1). They include the M_M120-1 and SMI 31 antigens and ubiquitin (Lowe *et al.*, 1988; Otha *et al.*, 1988; Zatloukal *et al.*, 1990a,b; Preisegger *et al.*, 1992). The M_M120-1 antigen is associated with a not yet characterized high molecular weight protein that *in vivo* is an exclusive MB component (Zatloukal *et al.*, 1990b, 1991) (Figure 2.2). *In vitro* studies have shown that accumulation of the M_M120-1 antigen can be induced by a variety of stress treatments (e.g., Ca^{++}-ionophore, heat shock, sodium arsenite) but also by transfection of various types of cultured cells with a human CK18 gene construct suggesting similarities in behavior to stress proteins (Stumptner *et al.*, unpublished observation). The SMI 31 antibody is directed against a phosphorylated epitope present on neurofilaments as well as on abnormally phosphorylated tau protein of neurofibrillary tangles in neurons of Alzheimer's disease patients (Lichtenberg-Kraag *et al.*, 1992). It recognizes a non-CK MB component with an apparent molecular mass of 62 to 65 kDa and an isoelectric pH around 4.5 (Preisegger *et al.*, 1992). Although the nature of the SMI 31 MB component is still unclear, the common phospho-epitope in MBs and neurofibrillary tangles indicate that similar protein kinases (i.e., proline-directed kinases) are active in both diseases (Mandelkow and Mandelkow, 1993). A further indication for the similarities in phosphorylation state between MBs and neurofibrillary proteins is provided by the observation that the 62–65 kDa MB protein and MBs *in situ* react in immunoblots and immunofluorescence microscopy, respectively, with MPM-2 antibodies (Stumptner *et al.*, manuscript in preparation), which also decorate neurofibrillary tangles and are directed to hyperphosphorylated epitopes generated on a number of proteins by mitotic kinases in the M-phase of the cell cycle (Westendorf *et al.*, 1994; Vincent *et al.*, 1996; Kondratick and Vandré, 1996). This supports the assumption that M-phase specific kinases are involved in creating this epitope. This SMI 31- and MPM-2-reactive MB component is identical in its electrophoretic coordinates with p62 which has recently been identified as a major protein constituent of intracellular hyaline bodies present in hepatocellular carcinoma cells (Stumptner *et al.*, 1999). p62 is induced under a variety of stress conditions, it interacts with protein kinases and is a cytoplasmic ubiquitin chain-binding protein (Vadlamudi *et al.*, 1996; Joung *et al.*, 1996; Vadlamudi and Shin, 1998; Shin, 1998).

Low and high molecular weight heat shock proteins (HSP) are also components of MBs (Stumptner *et al.*, manuscript in preparation). HSP70 belongs to a family of ubiquitous chaperone proteins that assist in correct protein folding in order to prevent aggregation or promote refolding of conformationally altered proteins

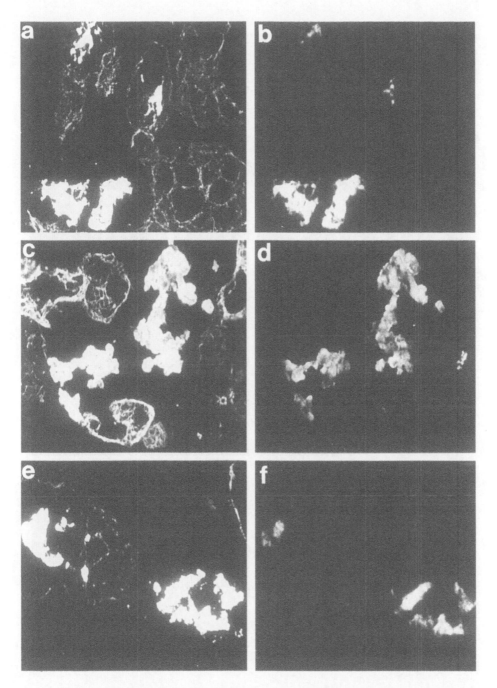

Figure 2.4 Immunohistochemical analysis of MBs in human alcoholic hepatitis (double immunofluorescence microscopy) with polyclonal antibodies to mouse liver CKs 8 and 18 (**a, c, e**) and monoclonal antibodies to M_M120-1 antigen (**b**), ubiquitin (**d**) and the SMI 31 epitope (**f**). Note specific reactivity of MBs for M_M120-1, ubiquitin and SMI 31. (×1300)

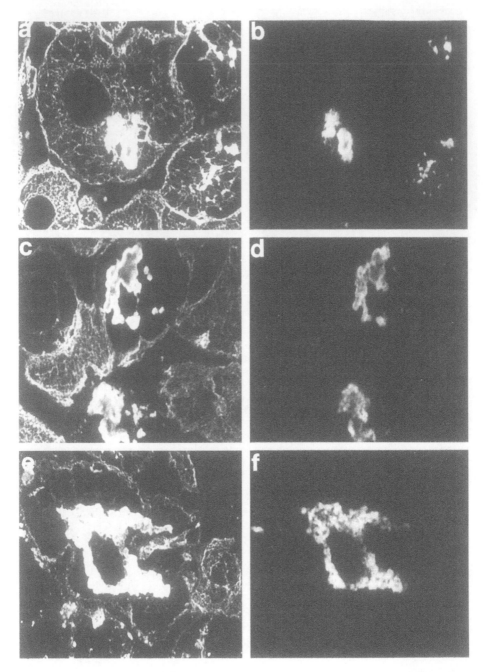

Figure 2.5 Immunohistochemical analysis of MBs in chronically (2.5 months) DDC-treated mouse liver (double immunofluorescence microscopy) with polyclonal antibodies to mouse liver CKs 8 and 18 (**a, c, e**) and monoclonal antibodies to $M_M120\text{-}1$ antigen (**b**), ubiquitin (**d**) and the SMI 31 epitope (**f**). Note specific reactivity of MBs for $M_M120\text{-}1$, ubiquitin and SMI 31. (×1300)

Table 2.1 Antigenic composition of Mallory bodies

Antibodies/antigens	Alcoholic hepatitis	DDC/GF mice
cytokeratin 8	+++	+++
cytokeratin 18	+++	+++
ubiquitin	+++	++
mAb M$_M$ 120-1	+++	+++
mAb SMI 31	++[*]	+++[*]
mAb RT 97	++[*]	+++[*]
mAb MPM-2	++[*]	+++[*]
phosphoserine	+++	−
phosphothreonine	−	+++
αB-crystallin	+	−

[*] only large MBs are reactive.
mAb = monoclonal antibody.

(Hartl, 1996; Rassow *et al.*, 1997). These chaperones bind to exposed hydrophobic surfaces of proteins, that in the native state are buried by forming noncovalent interactions, and thus prevent irreversible multimeric aggregation. The expression of stress proteins is triggered by the intracellular accumulation of altered proteins resulting from a variety of stresses, including oxygen radicals, heat shock, toxins and heavy metals, i.e., conditions which are, or may be, associated with alcohol intoxication. The capacity of the cell to degrade damaged proteins or prevent their appearance is a major opponent to the expression of stress proteins. Therefore, if protein degradation is blocked, e.g., by inhibition of proteasome action, heat shock and damaged proteins accumulate. Thus the presence of HSP70 (and ubiquitin) in association with MBs implies impairment of proteasome function. Indeed, chronic ethanol administration to rats as well as oxidative stress inhibit proteasome activity in hepatocytes (Fataccioli *et al.*, 1999).

Similar to chronic human alcoholic liver disease, experimental induction of MBs requires long-term intoxication with griseofulvin (GF) or 3,5-diethoxycarbonyl-1,4-dihydrocollidine (DDC) indicating that the metabolic conditions leading to MBs are related to chronic liver damage (Denk *et al.*, 1975; Tsunoo *et al.*, 1987). Analyses of mice allowed to recover from intoxication showed that most MBs disappeared within 4 weeks and only remnants of MBs were seen at the cell periphery, preferentially associated with desmosomes (Denk *et al.*, 1979b, 1981, 1985; Zatloukal *et al.*, 1990a). Complete disappearance of MBs, however, required up to 8 months of drug withdrawal. Surprisingly, if mice were re-exposed to the toxin after a 4 week recovery period, newly formed MBs rapidly (within 2 days) appeared in many hepatocytes (Figure 2.6; Denk *et al.*, 1976). Reinduction of MBs is not only achieved by readministration of the original inducers, e.g., GF or DDC, but also by colchicine, which is inactive in the "naive" mouse, suggesting an antimicrotubular effect to be involved in MB reinduction (Denk *et al.*, 1976; Denk and Eckerstorfer, 1977). In agreement with this assumption is the observation that lumicolchicine, which lacks antimicrotubular properties, lacks MB reinducing capacity in DDC- as well as GF-primed livers (Stumptner *et al.*, manuscript in preparation). This rapid reappearance of MBs, which is also observed in humans

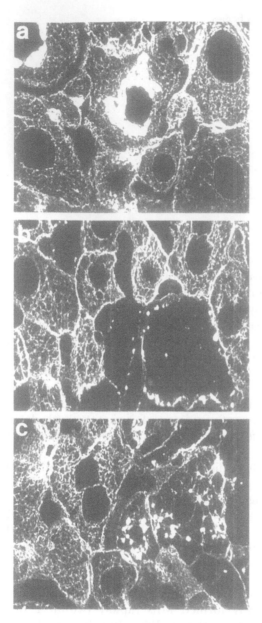

Figure 2.6 Immunohistochemical demonstration (indirect immunofluorescence microscopy) of MBs and the CK cytoskeletal network of hepatocytes with polyclonal antibodies to mouse liver CKs 8 and 18 in mouse liver after 2.5 months intoxication with DDC (**a**), after 4 weeks recovery following 2.5 months DDC intoxication (**b**) and after 72 hours of DDC reintoxication following 2.5 months DDC feeding and 4 weeks recovery (**c**). Note that after 4 weeks recovery, large MB have disappeared and only small MB granules are present at the periphery of still enlarged and "empty" hepatocytes (**b**). After 72 hours of DDC reintoxication, small MB granules reappear, particularly at intersections of the CK cytoskeletal network (**c**). (×1100)

upon re-exposure to ethanol, is reminiscent of an immunological memory response (Klassen *et al.*, 1995). This means that chronic intoxication "primes" the livers to respond differently than "naive" livers to toxin re-exposure. The "primed" state persists in the mouse for at least two months after recovery (Stumptner *et al.*, manuscript in preparation). Since, at least in the mouse model, no evidence exists that immune mechanisms are responsible for this phenomenon, we coined the term "toxic memory" response (Zatloukal *et al.*, 1996).

Because reinduction of MBs in "primed" livers is a rapid process in contrast to MB formation in the "naive" mouse, the different phases of MB development could be investigated in more detail. We found that CKs and the $M_M 120$-1 antigen were the earliest detectable MB components, whereas the SMI 31/MPM-2 epitopes and ubiquitin appeared later during MB formation (Stumptner *et al.*, manuscript in preparation; Zatloukal *et al.*, manuscript in preparation). This suggests that in the process of MB formation an "initiation" (accumulation of CKs and $M_M 120$-1 antigen) and a "maturation" phase (appearance of the SMI 31 and MPM-2 epitopes and ubiquitination) exist. The central role of CKs in MB formation was further underlined by the observation that MB appearance was accompanied by an up to 5-fold increase in the mRNA concentrations for CK8 and CK18 (Stumptner *et al.*, manuscript in preparation). A causal relationship between CK mRNA over-expression and MB formation was further suggested by the correlation of increased CK mRNA and presence of MBs at the single cell level, as revealed by *in situ* hybridization. However, overproduction of CK proteins alone is not sufficient for MB formation as shown with short-time intoxicated naive and primed mice. Despite rapid increase of CK mRNA and protein levels as well as hyperphosphorylation, MBs developed only in primed mice. The $M_M 120$-1 antigen appeared only in the latter situation, suggesting that the final trigger of MB formation is more closely related to occurrence of the $M_M 120$-1 antigen than to increased CK levels and hyperphosphorylation (Stumptner *et al.*, manuscript in preparation).

The phenomenon of "priming" and "triggering" has recently been studied in detail by French and coworkers (Yuan *et al.*, 1995, 1996, 1998a,b). These authors showed that a variety of treatments such as ethanol feeding, treatment by protein phosphatase inhibitors, and heat shock treatment were able to reinduce MB formation in primed recovered mice. The mechanisms involved are still unclear. French and coworkers emphasized that necrosis and consecutive regeneration play an essential role in MB reinduction, although no direct correlation at the cellular level between regeneration (as assessed by PCNA immunostaining of nuclei) and MB formation could be found (Yuan *et al.*, 1995, 1996; Zhang-Gouillon *et al.*, 1998). Oxidative stress also seems to be a good candidate as trigger of MBs. Oxidative stress is a major responsible factor for abnormal protein folding (Johnson *et al.*, 1999; Ando *et al.*, 1998). Several inducers of MBs, such as GF, DDC, ethanol and okadaic acid are inducers of free radicals and thus initiate oxidative stress (Ortiz de Montellano *et al.*, 1981; Knasmüller *et al.*, 1997; Yuan *et al.*, 1998a; Ingelman-Sundberg *et al.*, 1984; Kukielka *et al.*, 1994; Lauterburg and DeQuay, 1992; Rouach *et al.*, 1997; Wieland and Lauterburg, 1995; Bailey and Cunnigham, 1998; Castillo *et al.*, 1992; Weltman *et al.*, 1998). In addition, free radicals are generated by activated Kupffer cells (Adachi *et al.*, 1994; Jaeschke and Farhood, 1991).

Alteration of CK IF cytoskeleton

In alcoholic hepatitis as well as in the animal models of chronic intoxication with GF or DDC, the hepatocytic CK IF network is disrupted concomitant with the occurrence of MBs. The disturbance of the CK architecture is preferentially seen in ballooned hepatocytes, and occasionally hepatocytes without any detectable cytoplasmic CK filaments ("empty hepatocytes") are observed (Denk *et al.*, 1979a,b, 1981; Denk and Franke, 1981; Morton *et al.*, 1981; Barbatis *et al.*, 1986; Zatloukal *et al.*, 1990a). It was a matter of debate for several years whether the phenomenon of empty hepatocytes reflects a real loss of CK IF or is a consequence of lack of immunolabeling because of epitope masking. There are several lines of evidence in favor of a real loss: (i) empty hepatocytes were demonstrated with a variety of mono- and polyclonal antibodies, so that in the case of epitope masking all epitopes would have to be lost simultaneously (Preisegger *et al.*, 1991); (ii) electron microscopy revealed desmosomes without attached CK IF, thus demonstrating the absence of IF at locations where CK IF are present under normal conditions (Denk and Franke, 1981; Zatloukal *et al.*, 1990a); (iii) *in situ* hybridization showed increased CK mRNA concentrations in MB-containing cells with normal or reduced CK content ("active hepatocytes") but no signal for CK mRNA was obtained in ballooned hepatocytes without MBs and without an immunohistochemically detectable CK network (Stumptner *et al.*, manuscript in preparation); and (iv) in CK8 gene knockout mice (see below) the loss of the CK network does not affect the integrity and distribution of desmosomes (like in the GF-intoxicated mice) and is compatible with survival of hepatocytes.

Besides the cytoplasmic CK cytoskeleton, the nuclear lamins, which also belong to the IF family, are altered in intoxicated mice. The loss of lamins B1 and B2 from the nuclear lamina was demonstrable by immunohistochemistry and confirmed by protein analysis (Zatloukal *et al.*, 1992a). Two-dimensional gel electrophoresis not only revealed markedly reduced amounts of lamins B1 and B2 in relation to lamins A and C (which were not affected), but also showed an increase in the more acidic isoelectric variants of CKs and lamins, characteristic of increased phosphorylation. In human, alcoholic hepatitis phosphorylation of CKs at multiple sites and accumulation of phosphorylated CKs in MBs was detected by antibodies that selectively recognize phosphorylated epitopes of CKs 8 or 18 (Stumptner *et al.*, 2000). Two-dimensional gel electrophoresis of CK preparations derived from GF-treated animals showed an increase of the more acidic isoelectric CK variants reminiscent of phosphorylation (Zatloukal *et al.*, 1992; Salmhofer *et al.*, 1994). Increased phosphorylation of CKs in response to GF intoxication was furthermore confirmed *in vivo* by ^{32}P-incorporation (Salmhofer *et al.*, 1994). In DDC-intoxicated mice, hyperphosphorylation occurred rapidly already after 1 day of DDC intoxication and preceded architectural changes of the cytoskeleton. In chronically DDC-treated mice with MB-containing livers, phosphorylated CKs were preferentially associated with MBs but not with the residual CK network adjacent to MBs suggesting that hyperphosphorylation of CKs contributes to aggregation and MB formation (Stumptner *et al.*, 2000). Phosphorylation (in addition to proteolysis) is one of the most important regulators of protein function, particularly in response to external stimuli. Hyperphosphorylation of CKs is involved in the cellular stress response and seems to play a role in protection from hepatotoxic injury (Ku *et al.*, 1996a; Omary and Ku, 1997).

In addition to the formation of MBs and the disturbance of the CK network, another phenomenon, namely the aberrant expression of bile duct type CKs (i.e., CK7 and CK19) has been observed in hepatocytes of livers with alcoholic hepatitis (Van Eyken *et al.*, 1988; Dinges *et al.*, 1992). This phenomenon is not specific for alcoholic hepatitis, and can also be seen in cholestatic liver disease (Van Eyken *et al.*, 1989). Because of the occurrence of CK19-positive hepatocytes in close association with adjacent bile ducts and since some of these hepatocytes phenotypically resembled bile duct epithelia, this phenomenon was regarded as a sign of bile duct (ductular) metaplasia of hepatocytes (Van Eyken *et al.*, 1988). Moreover, it has been postulated, that the expression of bile duct type CKs may compensate for the loss of CK8 and CK18 in hepatocytes (French *et al.*, 1993). Investigation of snap frozen human liver biopsies as well as the analysis of CK8 and CK18 gene knockout mice revealed, however, that the aberrant expression of CK7 was independent of the morphologic feature of ductular metaplasia (Dinges *et al.*, 1992) and CK7 or CK19 did not compensate for the absence of CK8 and CK18, respectively (see below).

Clues from CK gene knockout mice

Analyses of human livers with alcoholic hepatitis and livers of chronically GF- or DDC-intoxicated mice revealed profound alterations of the hepatocytic cytoskeleton as well as accumulation of a variety of altered cellular proteins in MBs. The relevance of these changes with respect to the pathogenesis of alcoholic hepatitis and hepatocyte damage was unclear until recently. New insights into the role of CKs in MB formation and the consequences of the loss of the CK network on hepatocyte function were obtained with the help of mice in which the gene for CK8 had been disrupted (Baribault *et al.*, 1993, 1994). Since CK8 and CK18 are the only CKs expressed in hepatocytes, no CK-IF can be formed in the absence of CK8. The remaining partner of CK8, i.e., CK18, is rapidly degraded and does not accumulate in hepatocytes. Although the hepatocytes lack a CK cytoskeleton, homozygous CK8 gene knockout FVB/N mice (–/–) develop normally and have no evidence of liver defects (Baribault *et al.*, 1994). However, CK8 –/– mice were much more sensitive to DDC intoxication than wild-type (+/+) mice. Mortality was significantly increased (Figure 2.7; Zatloukal *et al.*, manuscript submitted). Serologic as well as histologic analyses revealed that porphyria in intoxicated CK8 –/– mice lacking a hepatocellular CK cytoskeleton was more severe than in wild-type mice. The altered response of CK8 –/– mice to DDC suggests that CK exerts in simple epithelia additional (i.e., non-skeletal) functions than just providing structural stability as shown in the epidermis (Fuchs and Weber, 1994; Fuchs, 1996; McLean and Lane, 1995). Analysis of livers of CK8 –/– mice fed DDC by double immunofluorescence microscopy showed that in the absence of CK8 no MBs were formed (Figure 2.8a,b). Moreover, none of the non-CK MB components accumulated in these livers, indicating that CK8 is indeed the core protein of MBs and that all other MB components either bind to or coassemble with CK. These *in vivo* data are in line with observations made *in vitro* where overexpression of CK by transient transfection of

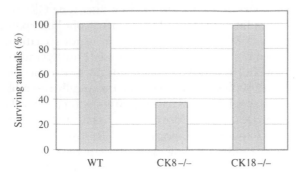

Mortality in DDC-intoxicated mice

(within 3 months of DDC intoxication)

Figure 2.7 CK8 knockout (CK8 –/–) mice show significantly increased mortality in contrast to wild type (WT) and CK18 knockout (CK18 –/–) mice.

cells leads to induction of the $M_M 120$-1 protein and to its association with CK aggregates, mimicking the initial phase of MB formation (Stumptner *et al.*, unpublished observations). Surprisingly, DDC intoxication of mice with only one inactivated CK8 +/– allele, which are able to form a regular CK network, did not result in the appearance of MBs although all other signs of DDC intoxication, such as the loss of the B-type lamins from the nuclear lamina, development of porphyria and bile ductular reaction were present. This different behavior of wild-type and CK8 +/– mice has, therefore, to be attributed to the loss of one CK8 allele. In the absence of the second CK8 allele the DDC-induced overexpression of CK8 mRNA was only approximately 2.5-fold, whereas in wild-type mice a 5-fold overexpression was found. This suggests that the excess of CK18 prevented CK8 from interacting with other MB components to initiate MB formation. Moreover, these results indicate that the effect of DDC intoxication on CK mRNA expression is independent of the status of the CK cytoskeleton since, like in CK8 +/+ mice, an upregulation of CK18 mRNA was seen in CK8 –/– mice, which were devoid of a CK cytoskeleton, thus excluding feedback regulation.

Further important clues on the role of CKs in MB formation came from experiments with CK18 knockout –/– mice (Magin *et al.*, 1998). Hepatocytes of CK18 –/– mice also lacked a CK-IF cytoskeleton. However, CK18 –/– mice responded differently to DDC intoxication than CK8 –/– mice since they showed no increased sensitivity to DDC (Figure 2.7; Stumptner *et al.*, unpublished observations). Therefore, the mortality seen in DDC-treated CK8 –/– mice cannot be attributed to impaired mechanical stability due to the loss of the CK cytoskeleton but has to be related to the non-assembled CK polypeptides or oligomeres. This suggests a novel mechanism of involvement of CKs in cellular metabolic processes, and that CK8 and CK18 fulfil different functions in this respect. Another difference between CK8- and CK18-deficient mice was that DDC intoxication of CK18 –/– mice led to the formation of classical MBs consisting of CK8 and non-CK components (Figure 2.8c). These findings show that CK8 can be stabilized in cells under certain conditions even without the corresponding type I partner. Moreover, the observation that mice able to form

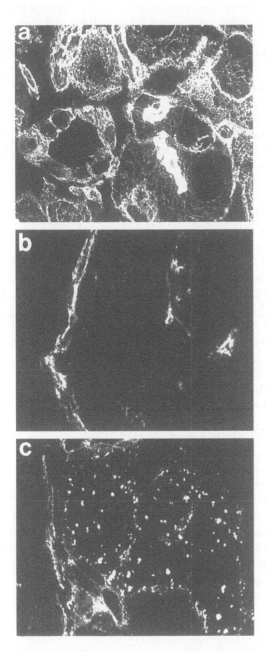

Figure 2.8 Immunofluorescence microscopy (indirect immunofluorescence) using polyclonal antibodies to mouse liver CKs 8 and 18. Feeding of CK8 knockout (CK8 −/−) mice with DDC for 2.5 months did not result in MB formation (**b**) in contrast to the situation with wild type mice (**a**). Note that in CK8 −/− mice, only bile duct epithelia show a lumen-oriented staining, reflecting residual CK18. In contrast, in CK18 knock out (CK18 −/−) mice MBs (demonstrated as small granules) are readily induced by prolonged DDC intoxication (**c**). (×1100)

MBs had less signs of toxicity than those unable to do so, implies that the MB itself does not damage the hepatocyte but is rather the result of a cellular defense response. In this context, it is interesting that overexpression of CKs by transfection of cells *in vitro* resulted in up to 450-fold higher resistance against a variety of toxins, such as colcemid (Baumann *et al.*, 1994).

CK8 −/− and CK18 −/− mice also provided new insights into the regulation of CK expression in the liver cell. mRNA concentrations of CK partners are controlled independently without any evidence of feedback regulation. In CK8 −/− as well as in CK18 −/− mice, the mRNA concentration of the non-inactivated partner CK was not significantly different from wild-type mice. Moreover, no compensatory expression of CK7 or CK19 was found in hepatocytes. Even in bile duct epithelia, which normally express CK7 and CK19 in addition to CKs 8/18, no compensation was seen although it has been shown *in vitro* that CK7 can interact with CK18 (Hatzfeld and Franke, 1985). CKs 8/18 were found in the whole cytoplasm whereas CKs 7/19 were restricted to the apical cell compartment. In the absence of CK8, CK7 did not substitute for CK8, and CK7 was still exclusively detectable in the apical region of bile duct epithelia. This observation further indicates that the yet unknown mechanisms which direct the subcellular distribution of CK pairs are highly specific (and probably related to function) and do not allow a compensatory redistribution to maintain the CK network.

Further clues on potential roles of CKs in liver disease came from transgenic mice expressing a mutated CK18 (R89C) (Ku *et al.*, 1996b). Because of the mutation in CK18, which corresponded to the mutation found in epidermal CKs causing epidermolysis bullosa simplex in humans (Fuchs, 1996), no CK-IF are formed and mutated CK polypeptides accumulate in the hepatocytes. In contrast to CK knockout mice, where the consequences of the absence of individual CK proteins can be investigated, the R89C-CK18 transgenic mice expressing the mutated CK allow to study the effects of the deposition of abnormal CK material in cells. These abnormal CK aggregates were associated with hepatocyte necrosis and inflammation, indicating that accumulation of abnormal CK material and/or the disturbance of CK function can damage hepatocytes. These effects were interpreted, at least in part, as a consequence of increased hepatocyte fragility due to the loss of the CK-IF cytoskeleton which, however, is in contrast to the findings in CK8 or CK18 knockout mice. In addition to these spontaneous lesions observed in the R89C-CK18 transgenic mice, a markedly increased sensitivity to liver toxins was found (Ku *et al.*, 1996b).

The general importance of CKs in hepatocytes and the role of CK alterations in human liver disease has recently been supported by the detection of a mutation in the CK18 gene (H127L) in one patient with cryptogenic liver cirrhosis (Ku *et al.*, 1997; Omary and Ku, 1997).

NON-ALCOHOLIC STEATOHEPATITIS (NASH) AND OTHER LIVER LESIONS ASSOCIATED WITH MB FORMATION

Alcoholic hepatitis shares many morphologic features, including development of MBs, with a variety of non-alcoholic disorders, collectively termed non-alcoholic steatohepatitis (NASH) (Zimmerman and Ishak, 1995; James and Day, 1998; Diehl, 1999), although not all disorders included under this term express all features of classical alcoholic hepatitis. The term "NASH" was introduced by Ludwig *et al.* (1980), but in the German literature "Fettleberhepatitis" has been used earlier to indicate that identical or similar morphologic features may have alcoholic as well as non-alcoholic causes (Thaler, 1982). Zimmerman and Ishak (1995) proposed the classification of NASH in three categories: (i) lesions associated with morbid obesity and surgical treatment of it and/or diabetes mellitus; (ii) lesions associated with toxic agents, including copper toxicity (e.g., Wilson's disease), and drugs; and (iii) miscellaneous group comprising hepatic neoplasms, chronic cholestasis and metabolic disorders.

Principal histologic features of NASH include macrovesicular (rarely microvesicular) steatosis, focal liver cell necrosis, ballooning of hepatocytes, MBs and apoptosis, most pronounced in acinar zone 3. Acinar inflammation is predominantly mononuclear (but may also be granulocytic). MBs may be less distinct than in alcoholic hepatitis but most often are indistinguishable from their alcoholic counterparts by light and electron microscopy. Similar to alcoholic liver disease fibrosis is almost invariably present, predominantly in zone 3 in pericellular ("chicken wire") fashion. In different types of NASH, the different morphologic features may be present in different proportions.

Liver lesions associated with morbid obesity after treatment by intestinal bypass operation and type II diabetes mellitus closely resemble alcoholic liver disease, including an alcoholic hepatitis-like picture and progression to cirrhosis, whereas in untreated morbidly obese patients steatosis and inflammation prevail. Drugs (amiodarone, perhexiline maleate, 4,4-diethylaminoethoxyhexestrol) as well as experimental agents, like GF or DDC, and diseases of still unknown etiology (presumably copper toxicity), like Indian childhood cirrhosis, closely resemble alcoholic hepatitis with respect to the presence of MBs and inflammation but usually show less pronounced fibrosis. MBs associated with chronic cholestatic conditions, e.g., primary biliary cirrhosis, may also be related to chronic copper toxicity since they are associated with zone 1 hepatocytes in which also copper overload can be demonstrated histochemically.

Little is known about the pathogenetic mechanisms involved in the development of NASH, and how apparently diverse etiologies can be responsible for identical or almost identical morphologic features (James and Day, 1998; Diehl, 1999; Burt *et al.*, 1998). However, several findings in humans as well as animal models suggest a pathogenesis similar to that of alcoholic liver disease (James and Day, 1998).

Similar pathogenetic principles may be involved in MB formation in Wilson's disease and Indian childhood cirrhosis where chronic copper overload and toxicity may play a major role. It remains to be established whether copper acts by initiating free radical damage or indirectly, e.g., by antimicrotubular action. It is noteworthy in this context, that all these toxic agents, copper included, are inactive with respect to MB formation in acute intoxication but exert their effect after chronic administration. This is comparable to alcohol which in its effects also differs significantly after acute and chronic exposure. This clearly indicates that a morphologic picture resembling alcoholic or non-alcoholic (pseudoalcoholic) steatohepatitis results from profound and possibly accumulating metabolic alterations.

NASH observed in association with amiodarone, 4,4-diethylaminoethoxyhexestrol and perhexiline maleate administration is often accompanied by phospholipidosis. This does not seem to be a causal relationship since either one lesion may be present separately (Guigui *et al.*, 1988; for review see Zimmerman and Ishak, 1995). Moreover, phospholipidosis may be induced by agents without accompanying pseudoalcoholic liver disease (Zimmerman and Ishak, 1995), whereas, for example, diethylstilbestrol leads to pseudoalcoholic liver disease without phospholipidosis. The pathogenesis of these drug effects is still unclear. Perhexiline inhibits mitochondrial oxidative phosphorylation as well as mitochondrial β-oxidation of fatty acids similar to ethanol (Deschamps *et al.*, 1994). It also inhibits the export of triglycerides from the hepatocyte. Similar effects have been reported for amiodarone and diethylaminoethoxyhexestrol. Perhexiline is eliminated from the body mainly after hydroxylation of its cyclohexane rings, a process in which cytochrome P-450 2D6 is involved. Genetic defects of this isoenzyme leads to longer half life and increased risks of hepato- and neuropathy (Deschamps *et al.*, 1994). From clinical observations it can be concluded that phospholipidosis is a predictable drug effect whereas NASH results from a less predictable individual reaction of the patient (Zimmerman and Ishak, 1995). Abnormal metabolism of the drug in individual patients may be the reason for the differences in individual susceptibility. It is interesting that CYP 2E1 is induced in NASH liver as in alcoholic liver disease (Weltmann *et al.*, 1998). Like in MEOS-catalyzed ethanol oxidation, the formation of reactive oxygen metabolites (predominantly in acinar zone 3) may result in oxidative stress and peroxidative destruction of cell membranes and other cellular components (Weltmann *et al.*, 1998). Induction of CYP 2E1 seems to be specific and not part of a generalized increase in hepatic cytochrome P-450 proteins in NASH patients, since it is accompanied by decreased cytochrome P-450 3A and antipyrine metabolism.

ANIMAL MODELS

Animal models are indispensable tools to study pathogenetic mechanisms despite the inherent disadvantage that usually not all features associated with human disease can be reproduced. Numerous animal models for human alcoholic liver disease have been designed. The problem can be approached from different angles, one emphasizing etiology and the effects of chronically administered high amounts of ethanol, eventually supported by dietary modifications, and the other starting from morphologic features irrespective of the etiology. Both approaches and particularly their combination are valuable to uncover mechanisms involved in alcoholic hepatitis, NASH and its sequelae. The diversity of models clearly provide clues for better understanding of alcoholic and pseudoalcoholic liver lesions.

Alcohol (ethanol) models

After several attempts in the past to reproduce pathologic alterations resembling those in human chronic drinkers by administration of excessive amounts of ethanol, often without consideration of adequate dietary conditions, to dogs and rodents, models for alcohol-associated liver disease now exist which take into account adequate nutritional status of the animals. This review will briefly comment on animal models which are presently used and will neglect historical ones (French et al., 1995). Major obstacles encountered with animal models, particularly the rat, are the natural aversion of animals to ethanol, the relatively high metabolic rate of ethanol, and the greater tolerance to toxic ethanol effects.

Liquid diet – alcohol model (Lieber et al., 1989)

In this model, ethanol incorporated into a liquid diet is administered. The rat is the usual experimental animal. By this regimen relatively high blood alcohol levels are achieved and local and systemic alterations such as fatty liver, hyperlipidemia and various metabolic and endocrine disturbances can be produced. In baboons, fatty liver, necrosis, inflammation, fibrosis and cirrhosis were produced by feeding this diet but in contrast to initial reports classical alcoholic hepatitis, particularly associated with MBs, did not appear and the results in different laboratories were variable. The major advantage of this model is that it is practical and easily adaptable to different experimental situations. Pair-feeding an isocaloric diet with carbohydrates instead of ethanol to control animals corrects for the lower total calories intake of the ethanol-treated group. However, as a disadvantage, this model reproduces predominantly the acute alcohol effects, such as fatty liver, and only inconstantly pathologic alterations typical for severe chronic human alcoholic liver injury.

Intragastric tube feeding model

This model developed by Tsukamoto and French (Tsukamoto et al., 1990; French et al., 1995) is based on the continuous administration through gastric tube of an ethanol containing liquid diet to rats. By this procedure, high blood ethanol levels in the range of 0.4–0.5 g% and a certain degree of cycling between higher and lower blood levels (maximum levels of 10 mmol/L every 6th to 7th day) are achieved which correlate with CYP 2E1 induction (Tsukamoto et al., 1985b). When ethanol was administered together with low fat diet fatty liver, necrosis and inflammation were found in correlation with blood alcohol levels. Amount and type of fat in the diet had a significant influence on liver pathology. Particularly long-term administration of polyunsaturated fat (olive oil, sunflower oil, corn or fish oil) together with alcohol markedly exaggerated fatty liver, centrilobular necrosis, inflammation (mostly mononuclear cells) and perivenular and bridging fibrosis. Thus, a diet rich in polyunsaturated fat seems to be the key for induction of experimental alcohol-induced liver fibrosis and is accompanied by activation of stellate cells (Tsukamoto et al., 1996). This diet may not only enhance oxidant stress by induction of CYP 2E1 but also sensitize stellate cells and stimulate Kupffer cells. On the other hand, saturated dietary fat (e.g., beef fat with low levels of linoleic acid) in association with ethanol supressed lipid peroxidation, CYP 2E1, synthesis of vasoactive and proinflammatory eicosanoids by cyclooxygenase, fibrosis and liver cell necrosis. This suggests that induction of the MEOS and resulting lipid peroxidation driven by MEOS-derived free radicals, centrilobular hypoxia due to induction of MEOS, activation of macrophages and sensitization of stellate cells play a role either alone or in combination (Nanji *et al.*, 1997). Moreover, pathologic changes (including fibrosis) were even more pronounced with nutritionally (with respect to protein, vitamins, choline) borderline diets. The correlation of severity of lesions with fluctuation of blood alcohol levels may, at least partly, reflect hypoxia-reoxygenation injury.

Recently, Enomoto *et al.* (1999) proposed a simple new rat model of early alcohol-induced liver injury based on the sensitization of Kupffer cells to endotoxin by alcohol pretreatment. In this model steatosis, inflammation and necrosis were achieved by administration of ethanol once every 24 hours intragastrally for several weeks.

Griseofulvin intoxication and related models

The alcohol models briefly discussed above produce lesions closely resembling acute alcohol effects in humans, particularly steatosis, but also necrosis, inflammation, fibrosis and cirrhosis. However, MBs, still the most characteristic features of human alcoholic hepatitis, and associated liver cell alterations, such as ballooning and pronounced accumulation of polymorphonuclear leukocytes ("satellitosis") are not induced by these treatment regimens. In contrast, chronic GF- and DDC-feeding to mice leads to accumulation of MBs in enlarged and hydropic (ballooned) hepatocytes, liver fibrosis, steatosis and ductular reaction, as well as liver cell necrosis in addition to protoporphyrin accumulation, whereas neutrophil infiltration is less pronounced than in human alcoholic hepatitis or even absent (Denk *et al.*, 1975, 1976, 1979; Tsunoo *et al.*, 1987). Thus, although these models are not alcohol models in the strict sense, they reproduce important features of alcoholic hepatitis and NASH and thus allow studies on their pathogenesis. The common pathways between alcoholic and non-alcoholic steatohepatitis remain to be uncovered. It is, however, noteworthy in this context that oxidant stress also seems to be involved in GF- and DDC-related liver toxicity (Ortiz de Montellano *et al.*, 1981; Knasmüller *et al.*, 1997).

The ideal model?

To date, no ideal animal model exists which exactly reproduces the human situation, namely alcohol as inducer of the classical morphologic picture of alcoholic hepatitis, fibrosis and cirrhosis. The experimental reproduction of human alcoholic hepatitis is the more difficult since chronic ethanol intoxication in man does not simply reflect repetition of episodes of acute intoxication (Akerman *et al.*, 1993; Deaciuc, 1997). Consequently, like in many other animal models of human disease, only certain aspects can be studied with the help of model systems and the results finally "compiled" to a more complete picture of human disease. This approach is justified because of the multifaceted pathogenesis of chronic human alcoholic liver disease, depending in addition to ethanol and metabolites, on a diversity of genetic, environmental and dietary factors. That alcoholic hepatitis may indeed reflect the complex interaction of different pathogenetic principles is suggested not only by the variability of its morphologic picture but also its clinical manifestation. Moreover, the information derived from different models (not only from those where alcohol is used as toxin) may also help to understand pathogenetic principles of NASH as well as of diverse other liver lesions associated with MBs, like chronic cholestasis, metabolic disorders and copper intoxication.

REFERENCES

Adachi, Y., Bradford, B.U., Gao, W., Bojes, H.K. and Thurman, R.G. (1994) Inactivation of Kupffer cells prevents early alcohol-induced liver injury. *Hepatology* **20**, 453–460.

Afford, S.C., Fisher, N.C., Neil, D.A.H., Fear, J., Brun, P., Hubscher, S.G. and Adams, D.H. (1998) Distinct patterns of chemokine expression are associated with leukocyte recruitment in alcoholic hepatitis and alcoholic cirrhosis. *J Pathol* **186**, 82–89.

Akerman, P.A., Cote, P.M., Yang, S.Q., McClain, C., Nelson, S., Bagby, G. and Diehl, A.M. (1993) Long-term ethanol consumption alters the hepatic response to the regenerative effects of tumor necrosis factor-α. *Hepatology* **17**, 1066–1073.

Akira, S. and Kishimoto, T. (1997) NF-IL6 and NF-kB in cytokine gene regulation. *Advances Immunol* **65**, 1–46.

Albano, E., Clot, P., Morimoto, M., Tomasi, Ingelman-Sundberg, M. and French, S. (1996) Role of cytochrome P4502E1-dependent formation of hydroxyethyl free radicals in the development of liver damage in rats intragastrically fed with ethanol. *Hepatology* **23**, 155–163.

Ando, Y., Suhr, O. and El-Salhy, M. (1998) Oxidative stress and amyloidosis. *Histol Histopathol* **13**, 845–850.

Arteel, G.E., Iimuro, Y., Yin, M., Raleigh, J.A. and Thurman, R.G. (1997) Chronic enteral ethanol treatment causes hypoxia in rat liver tissue *in vivo*. *Hepatology* **25**, 920–926.

Bailey, S.M. and Cunningham, C.C. (1998) Acute and chronic ethanol increase reactive oxygen species generation and decrease viability in fresh isolated rat hepatocytes. *Hepatology* **28**, 1318–1326.

Baptista, A., Bianchi, L., deGroote, J., Desmet, V.J., Gedigk, P., Korb, G., Mac Sween, R.N.M., Popper, H., Poulsen, H., Scheuer, P.J., Schmid, M., Thaler, H. and Wepler, W. (1981) Alcoholic liver disease: morphological manifestations. Review by an international group. *Lancet* **i**, 707–711.

Barbatis, C., Morton, J., Woods, J.C., Burns, J., Bradley, J. and McGee, J.O'D. (1986) Disorganisation of intermediate filament structure in alcoholic and other liver diseases. *Gut* **27**, 765–770.

Baribault, H., Penner, J., Iozzo, R.V. and Wilson-Heiner, M. (1994) Colorectal hyperplasia and inflammation in keratin 8-deficient FVB/N mice. *Genes Dev* **8**, 2964–2974.

Baribault, H., Price, H., Miyai, K. and Oshima, R.G. (1993) Mid-gestational lethality in mice lacking keratin 8. *Genes Dev* **7**, 1191–1202.

Baumann, P.A., Dalton, W.S., Anderson, J.M. and Cress, A.E. (1994) Expression of cytokeratin confers multiple drug resistance. *Proc Natl Acad Sci USA* **91**, 5311–5314.

Bautista, A.P. (1998) The role of Kupffer cells and reactive oxygen species in hepatic injury during acute and chronic alcohol intoxication. *Alcohol Clin Exp Res* **22**, 255S–259S.

Bjarnson, I., Ward, K. and Peters, T.J. (1984) The leaky gut of alcoholism: possible route of entry for toxic compounds. *Lancet* **i**, 179–182.

Bode, C., Kugler, V. and Bode, J.C. (1987) Endotoxemia in patients with alcoholic and non-alcoholic cirrhosis and in subjects with no evidence of chronic liver disease following acute ethanol excess. *J Hepatol* **4**, 8–14.

Born, L.J., Kharbanda, K.K., McVicker, D.L., Zetterman, R.K. and Donohue Jr., T.M. (1996) Effects of ethanol administration on components of the ubiquitin proteolytic pathway in rat liver. *Hepatology* **23**, 1556–1563.

Bosron, W.F., Ehrig, T. and Li, T.K. (1993) Genetic factors in alcohol metabolism and alcoholism. *Sem Liver Dis* **13**, 126–135.

Breathnach, S.M. (1985) The cutaneous amyloidoses. Pathogenesis and therapy. *Arch Dermatol* **121**, 470–475.

Buhler, R., Lindros, K.O., Nordling, A., Johansson, I. and Ingelman-Sundberg, M. (1992) Zonation of cytochrome P450 isozyme expression and induction in rat liver. *Eur J Biochem* **204**, 407–412.

Burt, A.D., Mutton, A. and Day C.P. (1998) Diagnosis and interpretation of steatosis and steatohepatitis. *Seminars in Diagnostic Pathology* **15**, 246–258.

Cadrin, M., French, S.W. and Wong, T.T. (1991) Alteration in molecular structure of cytoskeleton proteins in griseofulvin-treated mouse liver: a pressure tuning infrared spectroscopy study. *Exp Mol Pathol* **55**, 170–179.

Caraceni, P., Ryu, H.S., Subbotin, V., De Maria, N., Colantoni, A., Roberts, L., Trevisani, F., Bernardi, M. and Van Thiel, D.H. (1997) Rat hepatocytes isolated from alcohol-induced fatty liver have an increased sensitivity to anoxic injury. *Hepatology* **25**, 934–949.

Castillo, T., Koop, D.R., Kamimura, S., Triadafilopoulos, G. and Tsukamoto, H. (1992) Role of cytochrome P-450 2E1 in ethanol-, carbon tetrachloride- and iron-dependent microsomal lipid peroxidation. *Hepatology* **16**, 992–996.

Clot, P., Tabone, M., Aricò, S. and Albano, E. (1994) Monitoring oxidative damage in patients with liver cirrhosis and different daily alcohol intake. *Gut* **35**, 1637–1643.

Deaciuc, I.V. (1997) Alcohol and cytokine networks. *Alcohol* **14**, 421–430.

Denk, H. and Eckerstorfer, R. (1977) Colchicine-induced Mallory body formation in the mouse. *Lab Invest* **36**, 563–565.

Denk, H., Eckerstorfer, R., Gschnait, F., Konrad, K. and Wolff, K. (1976) Experimental induction of hepatocellular hyalin (Mallory bodies) in mice by griseofulvin treatment. I. Light microscopic observations. *Lab Invest* **35**, 377–382.

Denk, H. and Franke, W.W. (1981) Rearrangement of the hepatocyte cytoskeleton after toxic damage: Involution, dispersal and peripheral accumulation of Mallory body material after drug withdrawal. *Eur J Cell Biol* **23**, 241–249.

Denk, H., Franke, W.W., Eckerstorfer, R., Schmid, E. and Kerjaschki, D. (1979a) Formation and involution of Mallory bodies (alcoholic hyalin) in murine and human liver revealed by immunofluorescence microscopy with antibodies to prekeratin. *Proc Natl Acad Sci USA* **76**, 4112–4116.

Denk, H., Franke, W.W., Dragosics, B. and Zeiler, I. (1981) Pathology of cytoskeleton of liver cells: Demonstration of Mallory bodies (alcoholic hyalin) in murine and human hepatocytes by immunofluorescence microscopy using antibodies to cytokeratin polypeptides from hepatocytes. *Hepatology* **1**, 9–20.

Denk, H., Franke, W.W., Kerjaschki, D. and Eckersdorfer, R. (1979b) Mallory bodies in experimental animals and man. *Int Rev Exp Pathol* **20**, 77–121.

Denk, H., Gschnait, F. and Wolff, K. (1975) Hepatocellular hyalin (Mallory bodies) in long term griseofulvin-treated mice: a new experimental model for the study of hyalin formation. *Lab Invest* **32**, 773–776.

Denk, H., Krepler, R., Lackinger, E., Artlieb, U. and Franke, W.W. (1982) Immunological and biochemical characterization of the keratin-related component of Mallory bodies: A pathological pattern of hepatocytic cytokeratins. *Liver* **2**, 165–175.

Denk, H. and Lackinger, E. (1986) Cytoskeleton in liver diseases. *Sem Liver Dis* **6**, 199–211.

Denk, H., Lackinger, E., Cowin, P. and Franke, W.W. (1985) Maintenance of desmosomes in mouse hepatocytes after drug-induced rearrangement of cytokeratin filament material. *Exp Cell Res* **161**, 161–171.

Deschamps, D., DeBeco, V., Fisch, C., Fromenty, B., Guillouzo, A. and Pessayre, D. (1994) Inhibition by perhexiline of oxidative phosphorylation and the β-oxidation of fatty acids: possible role in pseudoalcoholic liver lesions. *Hepatology* **19**, 948–961.

Diehl, A.M. (1999) Nonalcoholic steatohepatitis. *Sem Liver Dis* **19**, 221–229.

Dilger, K., Metzler, J., Bode, J.C. and Klotz, V. (1997) CYP 2E1 activity in patients with alcoholic liver disease. *J Hepatol* **27**, 1009–1014.

Dinges, H.P., Zatloukal, K., Denk, H., Smolle, J. and Mair, S. (1992) Alcoholic liver disease. Parenchyma to stroma relationship in fibrosis and cirrhosis as revealed by three-dimensional reconstruction and immunohistochemistry. *Am J Pathol* **141**, 69–83.

Dupont, I., Lucas, D., Clot, P., Ménez, C. and Albano, E. (1998) Cytochrome P450 2E1 inducibility and hydroxyethyl radical formation among alcoholics. *J Hepatol* **28**, 564–571.

Ekström, G. and Ingelman-Sundberg, M. (1989) Rat liver microsomal NADPH-supported oxidase activity and lipid peroxidation dependent on ethanol-inducible cytochrome P-450 (P-450 IIE1). *Biochem Pharmacol* **38**, 1313–1319.

Enomoto, N., Yamashina, S., Kono, H., Schemmer, P., Rivera, C.A., Enomoto, A., Nishiura, T., Nishimura, T., Brenner, D.A. and Thurman, R.G. (1999) Development of a new, simple rat model of early alcohol-induced liver injury based on sensitization of Kupffer cells. *Hepatology* **29**, 1680–1689.

Fang, C., Lindros, K.O., Badger, T.M., Ronis, M.J.J. and Ingelman-Sundberg, M. (1998) Zonated expression of cytokines in rat liver: effect of chronic ethanol and the cytochrome P450 2E1 inhibitor, chlormethiazole. *Hepatology* **27**, 1304–1310.

Fataccioli, V., Andrand, E., Gentil, M., French, S.W. and Rouach, H. (1999) Effects of chronic ethanol administration on rat liver proteasome activities: relationship with oxidative stress. *Hepatology* **29**, 14–20.

Fisher, N., Afford, S. and Adams, D.H. (1996) Adhesion molecules and alcoholic liver disease. *Hepato-Gastroenterol* **43**, 1113–1116.

Franke, W.W., Denk, H., Kalt, R. and Schmid, E. (1981) Biochemical and immunological identification of cytokeratin proteins present in hepatocytes of mammalian liver tissue. *Exp Cell Res* **131**, 299–318.

Franke, W.W., Schmid, E., Kartenbeck, J., Mayer, D., Hacker, H.J., Bannasch, P., Osborn, M., Weber, K., Denk, H., Wanson, J.-C. and Drochmans, P. (1979a) Characterization of the intermediate-sized filaments in liver cells by immunofluorescence and electron microscopy. *Biol Cell* **34**, 99–110.

Franke, W.W., Denk, H., Schmid, E., Osborn, M. and Weber, K. (1979b) Ultrastructural, biochemical and immunologic characterization of Mallory bodies in livers of griseofulvin-treated mice. Fimbriated rods of filaments containing prekeratin-like polypeptides. *Lab Invest* **40**, 207–220.

French, S.W., Ihrig, T.J. and Norum, M.L. (1972) A method of isolation of Mallory bodies in a purified fraction. *Lab Invest* **26**, 240–244.

French, S.W., Morimoto, M. and Tsukamoto, H. (1995) Animal models of alcohol-associated liver injury. In *Alcoholic Liver Disease: Pathology and Pathogenesis*, 2nd edn, edited by P. Hall, pp. 279–296, London: Edward Arnold.

French, S.W., Nash, J., Shitabata, P., Kachi, K., Hara, C., Chedid, A., Mendenhall, C.L. and the VA Cooperative Study Group 119 (1993) Pathology of alcoholic liver disease. *Sem Liver Dis* **13**, 154–169.

Friedman, S.L. (1996) Hepatic stellate cells. *Progr Liver Dis* **14**, 101–130.

Fromenty, B., Fisch, C., Labbe, G., Degott, C., Deschamps, D., Letteròn, P. and Pessayre, D. (1990) Amiodarone inhibits the mitochondrial β-oxidation of fatty acids and produces microvesicular steatosis of the liver in mice. *J Pharmacol Exp Ther* **255**, 1371–1376.

Fromenty, B., Grimbert, S., Mansouri, A., Beaugrand, M., Erlinger, S., Röting, A. and Passayre, D. (1995) Hepatic mitochondrial DNA deletion in alcoholics: association with microvesicular steatosis. *Gastroenterology* **108**, 193–200.

Fromenty, B. and Passayre, D. (1995) Inhibition of mitochondrial β-oxidation as a mechanism of hepatotoxicity. *Pharmacol Ther* **67**, 101–154.

Fuchs, E. (1996) The cytoskeleton and disease: genetic disorders of intermediate filaments. *Annu Rev Genet* **30**, 197–231.

Fuchs, E. and Weber, K. (1994) Intermediate filaments: structure, dynamics, function and disease. *Annu Rev Biochem* **63**, 345–382.

Galle, P.R. and Krammer P.H. (1998) CD95-induced apoptosis in human liver disease. *Sem Liver Dis* **18**, 141–151.

Ganey, P.E., Bailie, M.B., VanCise, S., Colligan, M.E., Madhukar, B.V., Robinson, J.P. and Roth, R.A. (1994) Activated neutrophils from rat injured isolated hepatocytes. *Lab Invest* **70**, 53–60.

Garcia-Ruiz, C., Morales, A., Ballesta, A., Rodes, J., Kaplowitz, N. and Fernandez-Checa, J.C. (1994) Effect of chronic ethanol feeding on glutathione and functional integrity of mitochondria in periportal and perivenous hepatocytes. *J Clin Invest* **94**, 193–201.

Grove, J., Daly, A.K., Bassendine, M.F. and Day, C.P. (1997) Association of a tumor necrosis factor promoter polymorphism with susceptibility to alcoholic steatohepatitis. *Hepatology* **26**, 143–146.

Guigui, B., Perrot, S., Berry, J.P., Fleury-Feith, J., Martin, N., Métreau, J.M., Dhumeaux, D. and Zafrani, E.S. (1988) Amiodarone-induced hepatic phospholipidosis: a morphological alteration independent of pseudoalcoholic liver disease. *Hepatology* **8**, 1063–1068.

Hall, P. (1995) Pathological spectrum of alcoholic liver disease. In *Alcoholic Liver Disease: Pathology and Pathogenesis*, 2nd edn, edited by P. Hall, pp. 41–68, London: Edward Arnold.

Halliwell, B. and Gutteridge, J.M.C. (1996) *Free Radicals in Biology and Medicine*, 2nd edn, Oxford: Clarendon Press.

Hansen, J., Cherwitz, D.L. and Allen, J.I. (1994) The role of tumor necrosis factor-α in acute endotoxin-induced hepatotoxicity in ethanol-fed rat. *Hepatology* **20**, 461–474.

Hartl, F.U. (1996) Molecular chaperones in cellular protein folding. *Nature* **381**, 571–580.

Hatzfeld, M. and Franke, W.W. (1985) Pair formation and promiscuity of cytokeratins: formation *in vitro* of heterotypic complexes and intermediate-sized filaments by homologous and heterologous recombinations of purified polypeptides. *J Cell Biol* **101**, 1826–1841.

Hautekeete, M.L. and Geerts, A. (1997) The hepatic stellate (Ito) cell: its role in human liver disease. *Virchows Arch* **430**, 195–207.

Hazan, R., Denk, H., Franke, W.W., Lackinger, E. and Schiller, D.L. (1986) Change of cytokeratin organization during development of Mallory bodies as revealed by a monoclonal antibody. *Lab Invest* **54**, 543–553.

Hewett, J.A., Schultze, E., VanCise, S. and Roth, R.A. (1992) Neutrophil depletion protects against liver injury from bacterial endotoxin. *Lab Invest* **3**, 347–361.

Hill, D.B., Marsano, L.S. and McClain, C.J. (1993) Increased plasma interleukin-8 concentration in alcoholic hepatitis. *Hepatology* **18**, 576–580.

Hoek, J.B. (1999) Endotoxin and alcoholic liver disease: tolerance and susceptibility (Editorial). *Hepatology* **29**, 1602–1604.

Horie, Y., Wolf, R., Russell, J., Shanley, T.P. and Granger, D.N. (1997) Role of Kupffer cells in gut ischemia/reperfusion-induced hepatic microvascular dysfunction in mice. *Hepatology* **26**, 1499–1505.

Hutter, H., Zatloukal, K., Winter, G., Stumptner, C. and Denk, H. (1993) Disturbance of keratin homeostasis in griseofulvin-intoxicated mouse liver. *Lab Invest* **69**, 576–582.

Iimuro, Y., Gallucci, R.M., Luster, M.I., Kono, H. and Thurman, R.G. (1997) Antibodies to tumor necrosis factor alfa attenuate hepatic necrosis and inflammation caused by chronic exposure to ethanol in the rat. *Hepatology* **26**, 1530–1537.

Ingelman-Sundberg, M. and Johansson, I. (1984) Mechanisms of hydroxyl radical formation and ethanol oxidation by ethanol-inducible and other forms of rabbit liver microsomal cytochrome P-450. *J Biol Chem* **259**, 6447–6458.

Ingelman-Sundberg, M., Johansson, I., Penttila, K.E., Glaumann, H. and Lindros, K.O. (1988) Centrilobular expression of ethanol-inducible cytochrome P-450(IIE1) in rat liver. *Biochem Biophys Res Commun* **157**, 55–60.

Ishak, K.G., Zimmerman, H.J. and Ray, M.B. (1991) Alcoholic liver disease: pathologic, pathogenetic and clinical aspects. *Alcoholism: Clin Exp Res* **15**, 45–66.

Jaeschke, H. and Farhood, A. (1991) Neutrophil and Kupffer cell-induced oxidant stress and ischemia-reperfusion injury in rat liver. *Am J Physiol* **260**, G355–G362.

James, O.F.W. and Day, C.P. (1998) Non-alcoholic steatohepatitis (NASH): a disease of emerging identity and importance. *J Hepatol* **29**, 495–501.

Järveläinen, H.A., Fang, C., Ingelman-Sundberg, M. and Lindros, K.O. (1999) Effect of chronic coadministration of endotoxin and ethanol on rat liver pathology and proinflammatory and anti-inflammatory cytokines. *Hepatology* **29**, 1503–1510.

Jensen, K. and Gluud, C. (1994a) The Mallory body: morphological, clinical and experimental studies (part 1 of a literature survey). *Hepatology* **20**, 1061–1077.

Jensen, K. and Gluud, C. (1994b) The Mallory body: theories on development and pathological significance (part 2 of a literature survey). *Hepatology* **20**, 1330–1342.

Johnson, F.B., Sinclair, D.A. and Guarente, L. (1999) Molecular biology of aging. *Cell* **96**, 291–302.

Joung, I., Strominger, J.L. and Shin, J. (1996) Molecular cloning of a phosphotyrosine-independent ligand of the p56[lck] SH2 domain. *Proc Natl Acad Sci USA* **93**, 5991–5995.

Kamimura, S., Gaal, K., Britton, R.S., Bacon, B.R., Triadafilopoulos, G. and Tsukamoto, H. (1992) Increased 4-hydroxynonenal levels in experimental alcoholic liver disease: association of lipid peroxidation with liver fibrogenesis. *Hepatology* **16**, 448–453.

Kamimura, S. and Tsukamoto, H. (1995) Cytokine gene expression by Kupffer cells in experimental alcoholic liver disease. *Hepatology* **21**, 1304–1309.

Kawahara, H., Matsuda, Y. and Takase, S. (1994) Is apoptosis involved in alcoholic hepatitis? *Alcohol* **29**, 113–118.

Kenner, L., Zatloukal, K., Stumptner, C., Eferl, R. and Denk, H. (1999) Altered microtubule associated tau messenger RNA isoform expression in livers of griseofulvin- and 3,5-diethoxycarbonyl-1,4-dihydrocollidine-treated mice. *Hepatology* **29**, 793–800.

Kharbanda, K.K., McVicker, D.L., Zetterman, R.K. and Donohue, T.M. (1995) Ethanol consumption reduces the proteolytic capacity and protease activities of hepatic lysosomes. *Biochim Biophys Acta* **1245**, 421–429.

Khoruts, A., Stahnke, L., McClain, C.J., Logan, G. and Allen, J.I. (1991) Circulating tumor necrosis factor, interleukin-1 and interleukin-6 concentrations in cirrhotic alcoholic patients. *Hepatology* **13**, 267–276.

Kimoff, R.J. and Huang, S.N. (1981) Immunocytochemical and immunoelectron microscopic studies on Mallory bodies. *Lab Invest* **45**, 491–503.

Klassen, L.W., Tuma, D. and Sorrell, M.F. (1995) Immune mechanisms in alcohol-induced liver disease. *Hepatology* **22**, 355–357.

Knasmüller, S., Parzefall, W., Helma, C., Kassie, F., Ecker, S. and Schulte-Hermann, R. (1997) Toxic effects of griseofulvin: disease models, mechanisms, and risk assessment. *Crit Reviews Toxicol* **27**, 495–537.

Knolle, P., Schlaak, J., Uhrig, A., Kempf, P., Meyer zum Büschenfelde, K.H. and Gerken, G. (1995) Human Kupffer cells secrete IL-10 in response to lipopolysaccharide (LPS) challenge. *J Hepatol* **22**, 226–229.

Kondratick, C.M. and Vandre, D.D. (1996) Alzheimer's disease neurofibrillary tangles contain mitosis-specific phosphoepitopes. *J Neurochem* **67**, 2405–2416.

Krohne, G. and Benavente, R. (1986) The nuclear lamins: amultigene family of proteins in evolution and differentiation. *Exp Cell Res* **162**, 1–10.

Ku, N.-O., Liao, J., Chon, C.F. and Omary, M.B. (1996a) Implications of intermediate filament protein phosphorylation. *Cancer Metastasis Rev* **15**, 429–444.

Ku, N.-O., Michie, S.A., Soetikno, R.M., Resurreccion, E.Z., Broome, R.L., Oshima, R.G. and Omary, M.B. (1996b) Susceptibility to hepatotoxicity in transgenic mice that express a dominant-negative human keratin 18 mutant. *J Clin Invest* **98**, 1034–1046.

Ku, N.-O., Wright, T.L., Terrault, N.A., Gish, R. and Omary, M.B. (1997) Mutation of human keratin 18 in association with cryptogenic cirrhosis. *J Clin Invest* **99**, 19–23.

Kukielka, E., Dicker, E. and Cederbaum, A.I. (1994) Increased production of reactive oxygen species by rat liver mitochondria after chronic ethanol treatment. *Arch Biochem Biophys* **309**, 377–386.

Kurose, I., Higuchi, H., Miura, S., Saito, H., Watanabe, N., Hokari, R., Hirokawa, M., Takaishi, M., Zeki, S., Nakamura, T., Ebinuma, H., Kato, S. and Ishii, H. (1997) Oxidative stress-mediated apoptosis of hepatocytes exposed to acute ethanol intoxication. *Hepatology* **25**, 368–378.

Lauterburg, B.H. and DeQuay, B. (1992) Radicals and oxidants in ethanol induced liver injury. In *Free Radical Mechanisms of Tissue Injury*, edited by M.T. Moslen and C.V. Smith, pp. 33–43, London: CRC Press.

Lelbach, W.K. (1976) Epidemiology of alcoholic liver disease. *Prog Liv Dis* **5**, 494–513.

Letteròn, P., Fromenty, B., Terris, B., Degott, C. and Pessayre, D. (1996) Acute and chronic hepatic steatosis lead to *in vivo* lipid peroxidation in mice. *J Hepatol* **24**, 200–208.

Lichtenberg-Kraag, B., Mandelkow, E.M., Biernat, J., Steiner, B., Schröter, C. and Gustke, N. (1992). Phosphorylation – dependent epitopes of neurofilament antibodies on tau protein and relationship with Alzheimer tau. *Proc Natl Acad Sci USA* **89**, 5384–5388.

Lieber, C.S. (1993) Biochemical factors in alcoholic liver disease. *Sem Liver Dis* **13**, 136–153.

Lieber, C.S. (1995) Metabolism of alcohol: an update. In *Alcoholic Liver Disease: Pathology and Pathogenesis*, 2nd edn, edited by P. Hall, pp. 17–40, London: Edward Arnold.

Lieber, C.S. and DeCarli, L.M. (1991) Hepatotoxicity of ethanol. *J Hepatol* **12**, 394–401.

Lieber, C.S., DeCarli, L.M. and Sorrell, M.F. (1989) Experimental methods of ethanol administration. *Hepatology* **10**, 501–510.

Lindros, K.O. (1995) Alcoholic liver disease: pathobiological aspects. *J Hepatol* **23**(Suppl), 7–15.

Lowe, J., Blanchard, A., Morell, K., Lennox, G., Reynolds, L., Billet, M., Landon, M. and Mayer, R.J. (1988) Ubiquitin is a common factor in intermediate filament inclusion bodies of diverse type in man, including those of Parkinson's disease, Pick's disease, and Alzheimer's disease, as well as Rosenthal fibers in cerebellar astrocytomas, cytoplasmic bodies in muscle and Mallory bodies in alcoholic liver disease. *J Pathol* **155**, 9–15.

Ludwig, J., Viggiano, T.R., McGill, D.B. and Ott, B.J. (1980) Non alcoholic steatohepatitis: Mayo Clinic experiences with a hitherto unnamed disease. *Mayo Clin Proc* **55**, 434–438.

Magin, T.M., Schröder, R., Leitgeb, S., Wanninger, F., Zatloukal, K., Grund, C. and Melton, D.W. (1998) Lessons from keratin 18 knockout mice: formation of novel keratin filaments, secondary loss of keratin 7 and accumulation of liver-specific keratin 8-positive aggregates. *J Cell Biol* **140**, 1441–1451.

Maher, J.J. and Friedman, S.L. (1995) Pathogenesis of hepatic fibrosis. In *Alcoholic Liver Disease: Pathology and pathogenesis*, 2nd edn, edited by P. Hall, pp. 71–88, London: Edward Arnold.

Mallory, F.B. (1911) Cirrhosis of the liver: five different lesions from which it may arise. *Bull Johns Hopkins Hosp* **22**, 69–75.

Mandelkow, E.-M. and Mandelkow, E. (1993) Tau as a marker for Alzheimer's disease. *TIBS* **18**, 480–483.

Matsukawa, A. and Yoshinaga, M. (1999) Neutrophils as a source of cytokines in inflammation. *Histol Histopathol* **14**, 511–516.

Matsuoka, M. and Tsukamoto, H. (1990) Stimulation of hepatocyte collagen production by Kupffer cell-derived transforming growth factor α: implication for a pathogenetic role in alcoholic liver fibrosis. *Hepatology* **11**, 599–605.

Matsuoka, M., Zhang, M.Y. and Tsukamoto, H. (1990) Sensitization of hepatic lipocytes by high-fat diet to stimulatory effects of Kupffer cell derived factors: implication in alcoholic liver fibrogenesis. *Hepatology* **11**, 173–182.

Mawet, E., Shiratori, Y., Hikiba, Y., Takada, H., Yoshida, H., Okano, K., Komatsu, Y., Matsumura, M., Niwa, Y. and Omata, M. (1996) Cytokine-induced neutrophil chemoattractant release from hepatocytes is modulated by Kupffer cells. *Hepatology* **23**, 353–358.

McClain, C.J., Barve, S., Barve, S., Deaciuc, I. and Hill D.B. (1998) Tumor necrosis factor and alcoholic liver disease. *Alcohol Clin Exp Res* **22**, 248S–252S.

McClain, C.J., Barve, S., Deaciuc, I., Kugelmas, M. and Hill, D. (1999) Cytokines in alcoholic liver disease. *Sem Liver Dis* **19**, 205–219.

McClain, C., Hill, D., Schmidt, J. and Diehl, A.M. (1993) Cytokines and alcoholic liver disease. *Sem Liver Dis* **13**, 170–182.

McLean, W.H.I. and Lane, E.B. (1995) Intermediate filaments in disease. *Current Opinion Cell Biol* **7**, 118–125.

Moll, R., Franke, W.W., Schiller, D., Geiger, B. and Krepler, R. (1982) The catalog of human cytokeratins: patterns of expression in normal epithelia, tumors and cultured cells. *Cell* **31**, 11–24.

Morton, J.A., Bastin, J., Fleming, K.A., McMichael, A., Burns, J. and McGee, J.O'D. (1981) Mallory bodies in alcoholic liver disease: identification of cytoplasmic filament/cell membrane and unique antigenic determinants by monoclonal antibodies. *Gut* **22**, 1–7.

Nanji, A.A. (1998) Apoptosis and alcoholic liver disease. *Sem Liver Dis* **18**, 187–190.

Nanji, A.A., Griniuviene, B., Sadrzadeh, S.M.H., Levitsky, S. and McCeelly, J.D. (1995) Effect of type of dietary fat and ethanol on antioxidant enzyme mRNA induction in rat liver. *J Lipid Res* **36**, 736–744.

Nanji, A.A., Khettry, U., Sadrzadeh, S.M.H. and Yamanaka, T. (1993) Severity of liver injury in experimental alcoholic liver disease. Correlation with plasma endotoxin, prostaglandin E2, leukotriene B4, and thromboxane B2. *Am J Pathol* **142**, 167–373.

Nanji, A.A., Zakim, D., Rahemtulla, A., Daly, T., Miao, L., Zhao, S., Khwaja, S., Tahan, S.R. and Dannenberg, A.J. (1997) Dietary saturated fatty acids down-regulate cyclooxygenase-2 and tumor necrosis factor alfa and reverse fibrosis in alcohol-induced liver disease in the rat. *Hepatology* **26**, 1538–1545.

Nicotera, P., Bellano, G. and Orrenius, S. (1990) The role of Ca^{2+} in cell killing. *Chem Res Toxicol* **3**, 484–494.

Nicotera, P., Bellano, G. and Orrenius, S. (1992) Calcium-mediated mechanisms in chemically induced cell death. *Annu Rev Pharmacol Toxicol* **32**, 449–470.

Nolan, J.P. (1989) Intestinal endotoxins as mediators of hepatic injury – an idea whose time has come again. *Hepatology* **10**, 887–891.

Öhlinger, W., Dinges, H.P., Zatloukal, K., Meir, S., Gollowitsch, F. and Denk, H. (1993) Immunohistochemical detection of tumor necrosis factor-alpha, other cytokines and adhesion molecules in human livers with alcoholic hepatitis. *Virchows Arch A Pathol Anat* **423**, 169–176.

Ohta, M., Marceau, N., Perry, G., Manetto, V., Gambetti, P., Autilio-Gambetti, L., Metuzals, J., Kawahara, H., Cadrin, M. and French, S.W. (1988) Ubiquitin is present on the cytokeratin filaments and Mallory bodies of hepatocytes. *Lab Invest* **59**, 848–856.

Okanoue, T., Ohta, M., Ou, O., Kachi, K., Kagawa, K., Yuki, T., Okuno, T., Takino, T. and French, S.W. (1985) Relationship of Mallory bodies to intermediate filaments in hepatocytes. A scanning electron microscopy study. *Lab Invest* **53**, 534–540.

Omary, M.B. and Ku, N.-O. (1997) Intermediate filament proteins of the liver: emerging disease association and function. *Hepatology* **25**, 1043–1048.

Orrego, H., Blake, J.E., Blendis, L.M. and Medline, A. (1987) Prognosis of alcoholic cirrhosis in the presence and absence of alcoholic hepatitis. *Gastroenterology* **92**, 208–214.

Ortiz de Montellano, P.R., Beilan, H.S. and Kunze, K.L. (1981) *N*-alkylprotoporphyrin IX formation in 3,5-dicarbethoxy-1,4-dihydrocollidine-treated rats. Transfer of the alkyl group from the substrate to the porphyrin. *J Biol Chem* **256**, 6708–6713.

Paronetto, F. (1993) Immunologic reactions in alcoholic liver disease. *Sem Liver Dis* **13**, 183–195.

Phillips, M.J. (1994) Biology and pathobiology of actin in the liver. In *The Liver Biology and Pathobiology*, 3rd edn, edited by I. Arias, J.L. Boyer, N. Fausto, W.B. Jakoby, D. Schachter and D.A. Shafritz, pp. 19–32. New York: Raven Press.

Pösö, A.R. and Hirsimäki, P. (1991) Inhibition of proteolysis in the liver by chronic ethanol feeding. *Biochem* **273**, 149–152.

Preisegger, K.-H., Zatloukal, K., Spurej, G. and Denk, H. (1991) Changes in cytokeratin filament organization in human and murine Mallory body – containing livers as revealed by a panel of monoclonal antibodies. *Liver* **11**, 300–309.

Preisegger, K.-H., Zatloukal, K., Spurej, G., Riegelnegg, D. and Denk, H. (1992) Common epitopes of human and murine Mallory bodies and Lewy bodies as revealed by a neuro-filament antibody. *Lab Invest* **66**, 193–199.

Rashid, A., Wu, T.C., Huang, C.-C., Chen, C.-H., Lin, H.Z., Yang, S.Q., Lee, F.Y.J. and Diehl, A.M. (1999) Mitochondrial proteins that regulate apoptosis and necrosis are induced in mouse fatty liver. *Hepatology* **29**, 1131–1138.

Rassow, J., Ahsen, O., Boiner, U. and Pfanner, N. (1997) Molecular chaperones: towards a characterization of the heat-shock protein 70 family. *Trend Cell Biol* **7**, 129–133.

Reeves, H.L., Burt, A.D., Wood, S. and Day, C.P. (1996) Hepatic stellate cell activation occurs in the absence of hepatitis in alcoholic liver disease and correlates with the severity of steatosis. *J Hepatol* **25**, 677–683.

Roll, F.J. (1991) The pathogenesis of inflammation in alcoholic liver disease. In *Drug and Alcohol Abuse Reviews, Vol 2, Liver Pathology and Alcohol*, edited by R.R. Watson, pp. 61–89, The Humana Press Inc.

Rouach, H., Fataccioli, V., Gentil, M., French, S.W., Morimoto, M. and Nordmann, R. (1997) Effect of chronic ethanol feeding on lipid peroxidation and protein oxidation in relation to liver pathology. *Hepatology* **25**, 351–355.

Röcken, C., Schwotzer, E.B., Linke, R.P. and Saeger, W. (1996) The classification of amyloid deposits in clinicopathological practice. *Histopathol* **29**, 325–335.

Sadrzadeh, S.M.H., Nanji, A.A. and Meydani, M. (1994) Effect of chronic ethanol intake on plasma and liver alpha and gamma tocopherol levels in normal and vitamin E deficient rats: relationship to lipid peroxidation. *Biochem Pharmacol* **47**, 2005–2010.

Sakamoto, S., Okanoue, T., Itoh, Y., Sakamoto, K., Nishioji, K., Nakagawa, Y., Yoshida, N., Yoshikawa, T. and Kashima, K. (1997) Intercellular adhesion molecule-1 and CD18 are involved in neutrophil adhesion and its cytotoxicity to cultured sinusoidal endothelial cells in rats. *Hepatology* **26**, 658–663.

Salmhofer, H., Rainer, I., Zatloukal, K. and Denk, H. (1994) Posttranslational events involved in griseofulvin-induced keratin cytoskeleton alterations. *Hepatology* **20**, 731–740.

Satir, P. (1994) Motor molecules of the cytoskeleton. Possible functions in the hepatocyte. In *The Liver Biology and Pathobiology*, 3rd edn, edited by I. Arias, J.L. Boyer, N. Fausto, W.B. Jakoby, D. Schachter and D.A. Shafritz, pp. 45–52, New York: Raven Press.

Schäfer, C., Schips, I., Landig, J., Bode, J.C. and Bode, C. (1995) Tumor-necrosis-factor and interleukin-6 response of peripheral blood monocytes to low concentrations of lipopolysaccharide in patients with alcoholic liver disease. *Z Gastroenterol* **33**, 503–508.

Schmitt-Gräff, A., Krüger, S., Borchard, F., Gabbiani, G. and Denk, H. (1991) Modulation of alpha smooth muscle actin and desmin expression in perisinusoidal cells of normal and diseased human livers. *Am J Pathol* **138**, 1233–1242.

Sherlock, S. and Dooley, J. (1997) *Diseases of the liver and biliary system*, 10th edn, pp. 385–403. Oxford: Blackwell Science Ltd.

Sheron, N., Bird, G., Koskinas, J., Portmann, B., Ceska, M., Lindley, I. and Williams, R. (1993) Circulating and tissue levels of the neutrophil chemotaxin interleukin-8 are elevated in severe acute alcoholic hepatitis and tissue levels correlate with neutrophil infiltration. *Hepatology* **18**, 41–46.

Shin, J. (1998) P62 and the sequestosome, a novel mechanism for protein metabolism. *Arch Pharm* **21**, 629–633.

Shiratori, Y., Takada, H., Hikiba, Y., Nakata, R., Okano, K., Komatsu, Y., Niwa, Y., Matsumura, M., Shiina, S., Omata, M. and Kamii, K. (1993) Production of chemotactic factor interleukin 8 from hepatocytes exposed to ethanol. *Hepatology* **18**, 1477–1482.

Simpson, K.J., Lukaes, N.W., Colletti, L., Strieter, R.M. and Kunkel, S.L. (1997) Cytokines and the liver. *J Hepatol* **27**, 1120–1132.

Stanley, A.J., McGregor, I.R., Dillon, J.F., Bouchier, I.A.D. and Hayes, P.C. (1996) Neutrophil activation in chronic liver disease. *Europ J Gastroenterol Hepatol* **8**, 135–138.

Stumptner, C., Heid, H., Fuchsbichler, A., Hauser, H., Mischinger, H.J., Zatloukal, K. and Denk, H. (1999) Analysis of intracytoplasmic hyaline bodies in a hepatocellular carcinoma. Demonstration of p62 as major constituent. *Am J Pathol* **154**, 1701–1710.

Stumptner, C., Omary, M.B., Fickert, P., Denk, H. and Zatloukal, K. (2000) Hepatocyte cytokeratins are hyperphosphorylated at multiple sites in human alcoholic hepatitis and in a Mallory body mouse model. *Am J Pathol* **156**, 77–90.

Teli, M., James, O.F., Burt, A.D., Bennet, M.K. and Day, C.P. (1995) A natural history of nonalcoholic fatty liver: a follow-up study. *Hepatology* **22**, 1714–1717.

Thaler, H. (1982) *Leberkrankheiten, Histologie, Pathophysiologie, Klinik*. Berlin: Springer-Verlag.

Thurman, R.G. (1998) Mechanisms of hepatic toxicity. II. alcoholic liver injury involves activation of Kupffer cells by endotoxin. *Am J Physiol* **275**, (*Gastrointest Liver Physiol* 38), G605–G611.

Tsukamoto, H. (1998) Molecular mechanism of induced hepatic macrophage cytokine gene expression in experimental alcoholic liver injury. *Alcohol Clin Exp Res* **22**, 253S–254S.

Tsukamoto, H., Cheng, S. and Blaner, W.S. (1996) Effects of dietary polyunsaturated fat on ethanol-induced Ito cell activation. *Am J Physiol* **270**, (*Gastrointest Liver Physiol* 33), G581–G586.

Tsukamoto, H., French, S.W., Benson, N., Delgado, G., Rao, G.A., Larkin, E.C. and Largman, C. (1985a) Severe and progressive steatosis and focal necrosis in rat liver induced by continuous intragastric infusion of ethanol and low fat diet. *Hepatology* **5**, 224–232.

Tsukamoto, H., French, S.W., Reidelberger, R.D. and Largman, C. (1985b) Cyclical pattern of blood alcohol levels during continuous intragastric ethanol infusion in rats. *Alcoholism. Clin Exp Res* **9**, 31–37.

Tsukamoto, H., Gad, K. and French, S.W. (1990a) Insights into the pathogenesis of alcoholic liver necrosis and fibrosis: status report. *Hepatology* **12**, 599–608.

Tsukamoto, H., Matsuoka, M. and French, S.W. (1990b) Experimental models of hepatic fibrosis: a review. *Sem Liver Dis* **10**, 56–65.

Tsukamoto, H., Horne, W., Kamimura, S., Niemelä, O., Parkkila, S., Yiä-Herttuala, S. and Brittenham, G.M. (1995) Experimental liver cirrhosis induced by alcohol and iron. *J Clin Invest* **96**, 620–630.

Tsukamoto, H. and Xi, X.P. (1989) Incomplete compensation of enhanced hepatic oxygen consumption in rats with alcoholic centrilobular liver necrosis. *Hepatology* **9**, 302–306.

Tsunoo, C., Harwood, T.R., Arak, S. and Yokoo, H. (1987) Cytoskeletal alterations leading to Mallory body formation in livers of mice fed 3,5-diethoxycarbonyl-1,4-dihydrocollidine. *J Hepatol* **5**, 85–97.

Tsutsumi, M., Lasker, J.M., Shimizu, M., Rosman, A.S. and Lieber, C.S. (1989) The intralobular distribution of ethanol-inducible P450 IIE1 in rat and human liver. *Hepatology* **10**, 437–446.

Tuma, D.J. and Sorrell, M.F. (1995) The role of acetaldehyde adducts in liver injury. In *Alcoholic Liver Disease: Pathology and Pathogenesis*, 2nd edn, edited by P. Hall, pp. 89–90, London: Edward Arnold.

Vadlamudi, R.K., Joung, I., Strominger, J.L. and Shin, J. (1996) p62, a phosphotyrosine-independent ligand of the SH2 domain of p56[lck] belongs to a new class of ubiquitin-binding proteins. *J Biol Chem* **271**, 20235–20237.

Vadlamudi, R.K. and Shin, J. (1998) Genomic structure and promoter analysis of the p62 gene encoding a non-proteasomal multi-ubiquitin chain binding protein. *FEBS Lett* **435**, 138–142.

Van Eyken, P., Sciot, R. and Desmet, V.J. (1988) A cytokeratin immunohistochemical study of alcoholic liver disease: evidence that hepatocytes can express "bile duct-type" cytokeratins. *Histopathology* **13**, 605–617.

Van Eyken, P., Sciot, R. and Desmet, V.J. (1989) A cytokeratin immunohistochemical study of cholestatic liver disease: evidence that hepatocytes can express "bile duct-type" cytokeratins. *Histopathology* **15**, 125–135.

Videla, L., Bernstein, J. and Israel, Y. (1973) Metabolic alteration produced in the liver by chronic ethanol administration. Increased oxidative capacity. *Biochem J* **134**, 507–514.

Vincent, I., Rosado, M. and Davies, P. (1996) Mitotic mechanisms in Alzheimer's disease. *J Cell Biol* **132**, 413–425.

Weiner, F.R., Degli Esposti, S. and Zern, M.A. (1994) Ethanol and the liver. In *The Liver: Biology and Pathobiology*, 3rd edn, edited by I.M. Arias, J.L. Boyer, N. Fausto, W.B. Jakoby, D.A. Schachter and D.A.Shafritz, pp. 1383–1411, New York: Raven Press.

Weltman, M.D., Farrell, G.C., Hall, P., Ingelman-Sundberg, M. and Liddle. C. (1998) Hepatic cytochrome P450 2E1 is increased in patients with non alcoholic steatohepatitis. *Hepatology* **27**, 128–133.

Westendorf, J.M., Rao, P.N. and Gerace, L. (1994) Cloning of cDNAs for M-phase phosphoproteins recognized by the MPM2 monoclonal antibody and determination of the phosphorylated epitope. *Proc Natl Acad Sci USA* **91**, 714–718.

Wieland, P. and Lauterburg, B.A. (1995) Oxidation of mitochondrial proteins and DNA following administration of ethanol. *Biochem Biophys Res Comm* **213**, 815–819.

Wright, S.D., Ramos, R.A., Tobias, P.S., Ulevitch, R.J. and Mathison, J.C. (1990) CD14, a receptor of lipopolysaccharide-binding protein. *Science* **249**, 1429–1433.

Yang, S.Q., Lin, H.Z., Lane, M.D., Clemens, M. and Diehl, A.M. (1997) Obesity increases sensitivity to endotoxin liver injury: implications for pathogenesis of steatohepatitis. *Proc Natl Acad Sci USA* **94**, 2557–2562.

Yokoo, H., Minick, O.T., Batti, F. and Kent, G. (1972) Morphologic variants of alcoholic hyalin. *Am J Pathol* **69**, 25–40.

Yokoyama, H., Ishii, H., Nagata, S., Kato, S., Kamegaya, K. and Tsuchiya, M. (1993) Experimental hepatitis induced by ethanol after immunization with acetaldehyde adducts. *Hepatology* **17**, 14–19.

Yokoyama, H., Nagata, S., Moriya, S., Kato, S., Ito, T., Kamegaya, K. and Ishii, H. (1995) Hepatic fibrosis produced in guinea pigs by chronic ethanol administration and immunization with acetaldehyde adducts. *Hepatology* **21**, 1438–1442.

Yuan, Q., French, B.A. and French, S.W. (1998b) Tautomycin induces extensive Mallory body formation in drug primed mouse livers. *Hepatology* **28**, 256A.

Yuan, Q.X., Marceau, N., French, B.A., Fu, P. and French, S.W. (1995) Heat shock *in vivo* induces Mallory body formation in drug primed mouse liver. *Exp and Mol Pathol* **63**, 63–76.

Yuan, Q.X., Marceau, N., French, B.A., Fu, P. and French, S.W. (1996) Mallory body induction in drug-primed mouse liver. *Hepatology* **24**, 603–612.

Yuan, Q.X., Nagao, Y., Gaal, K., Hu, B. and French, S.W. (1998a) Mechanism of Mallory body formation induced by okadaic acid in drug-primed mice. *Exp Mol Pathol* **65**, 87–103.

Zatloukal, K., Boeck, G., Rainer, I., Denk, H. and Weber, K. (1991) High molecular weight components are main constituents of Mallory bodies isolated with a fluorescence activated cell sorter. *Lab Invest* **64**, 200–206.

Zatloukal, K., Denk, H., Spurej, G. and Hutter, H. (1992a) Modulation of protein composition of nuclear lamina. *Lab Invest* **66**, 589–597.

Zatloukal, K., Denk, H., Spurej, G., Lackinger, E., Preisegger, K.-H. and Franke, W.W. (1990b) High molecular weight component of Mallory bodies detected by a monoclonal antibody. *Lab Invest* **62**, 427–434.

Zatloukal, K., Fesus, L., Denk, H., Tarcsa, E., Spurej, G. and Böck, G. (1992b) High amount of ε-(γ-glutamyl) lysine cross-links in Mallory bodies. *Lab Invest* **66**, 774–777.

Zatloukal, K., Spurej, G., Rainer, I., Lackinger, E. and Denk, H. (1990a) Fate of Mallory body-containing hepatocytes: disappearance of Mallory bodies and restoration of the hepatocytic intermediate filament cytoskeleton after drug withdrawal in the griseofulvin-treated mouse. *Hepatology* **11**, 652–661.

Zatloukal, K., Stumptner, C., Fuchsbichler, A., Lehner, M. and Denk, H. (1996) Induction of Mallory bodies reflects a toxic memory response and is linked to overexpression of cytokeratin mRNA in hepatocytes. *Hepatology* **24**, 601A.

Zhang-Gouillon, Z.Q., Yuan, Q.X., Hu, B., Marceau, N., French, B.A., Gaal, K., Nagao, Y., Wan, Y.J.Y. and French, S.W. (1998) Mallory body formation by ethanol feeding in drug-primed mice. *Hepatology* **27**, 116–122.

Zhao, M., Laissue, J. and Zimmermann, A. (1997) TUNEL-positive hepatocytes in alcoholic liver disease: a retrospective biopsy study using DNA nick end-labelling. *Virchows Arch* **431**, 337–344.

Zimmerman, H.J. and Ishak, K.G. (1995) Non-alcoholic steatohepatitis and other forms of pseudo-alcoholic liver disease. In *Alcoholic Liver Disease: Pathology and Pathogenesis*, 2nd edn, edited by P. Hall, pp. 175–198, London: Edward Arnold.

Chapter 3

Fibrosis in alcoholic cirrhosis

Samuel W. French

CLINICAL ALCOHOLIC LIVER DISEASE: PATTERNS OF LIVER FIBROSIS

Alcoholic liver disease (ALD) is characterized by liver fibrosis, starting in the fatty liver stage and progressing to cirrhosis as the result of activation of the stellate cells to proliferate, contract, migrate and synthesize and secrete extracellular matrix including collagen, proteases and protease inhibitors. Fibrosis that leads to scar formation, architectural distortion and liver cell replacement to form cirrhosis occurs when the balance between the formation and removal of extracellular matrix is tipped to favor formation over removal of collagen by the stellate cells. Research utilizing the experimental animal models of liver fibrosis and cirrhosis as well as tissue culture models of stellate cell activation has shown that the dynamics of collagen synthesis is highly regulated and fine tuned by numerous cytokines and receptor–ligand interactions, particularly the integrins. The role of the stellate cell in fibrosis is analogous to the pericyte in wound healing and fibrosis that occurs anywhere in the body. Numerous reviews have shown how advanced this sophicated system of fibrosis induction is at the experimental level (Kovacs and Difietro, 1994; Raghow, 1994; Gressner and Bachem, 1990; Ramadori, 1991; Friedman, 1993; Bissell *et al.*, 1990; Hogemann and Domschke, 1993; Reid *et al.*, 1997; Biagni and Ballardini, 1989; Rockey, 1997; Maher and Friedman, 1995). However, there is a big gap between what is known experimentally in animals and *in vitro* compared with the complex *in vivo* mechanisms involved in human alcoholic liver disease. In this chapter, an attempt will be made to bridge this gap so as to apply the experimental breakthroughs to the human condition. In this attempt, it is well to remember that the end stage of alcoholic liver disease is cirrhosis (Figure 3.1) as defined by diffuse fibrosis where all fibrous bands connect with each other to dissect the liver cell parenchyma into small isolated nodular compartments. Such a pattern of scarring and nodularity of the parenchyma has not been replicated in any animal model of alcoholic liver disease.

Central and focal lobular fibrosis

There are three main types of scarring which predominate in human ALD: (1) centrilobular scarring; (2) sinusoidal "capillarization" (pericellular fibrosis); and (3) periportal fibrosis. In the case of centrilobular fibrosis, the first feature is an

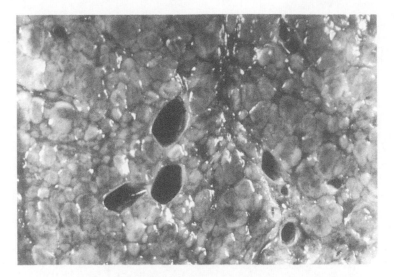

Figure 3.1 Gross photo of alcoholic cirrhosis. The nodules of liver are small but irregular in shape and size. They protrude above the contracted scars that distort the liver architecture.

increase in the central vein collagen with extension of collagen out into the parenchyma in a radial and perisinusoidal location which culminates in central vein-central vein bridging fibrosis. This begins in the fatty liver stage and worsens in the alcoholic hepatitis stage when Mallory bodies (MBs) appear in the centrilobular location, the so called central sclerosing hyaline necrosis (CSHN) stage (Edmondson *et al.*, 1963). CSHN is encountered in 4% of liver biopsies in the fatty liver stage and 68% in the alcoholic hepatitis stage of ALD (Chedid *et al.*, 1991).

Centrilobular fibrosis is commonly found in the fatty liver stage of ALD. It is important to make a distinction between centrilobular fibrosis and perivenular fibrosis since the latter has been identified as a better predictor of eventual cirrhosis development (Worner and Lieber, 1985). Electron microscopic examination of this lesion reveals activated stellate cells (Okanoue *et al.*, 1983) associated with MB formation by hepatocytes (Figure 3.2). In the wall of the central vein, myofibroblasts that resemble stellate cells are found. However, stellate cells should not be confused with the normal resident smooth muscle present in the wall of the central vein. Similar fibrotic foci are seen within the lobule apart from the central vein, usually associated with mononuclear infiltrate and hepatocellular balloon degeneration (Figure 3.3). This lesion shows increased collagen scarring surrounding hepatocytes as seen by the sirus red stain. When these foci are stained for α smooth muscle actin, they stain strongly positive (Figure 3.4), indicating that the stellate cells are activated (Friedman, 1993). The surrounding stellate cells, apart from the scars, do not stain for α actin indicating the activation of the stellate cells is limited to the scars (Figure 3.4). It has been reported that the activation of stellate cells is diffuse based on morphologic measurement of the percentage cell volume of fat in the stellate cells (Mak and Lieber, 1988). When the stellate cells contained a cell volume of fat droplets which was under 20% of the total cell volume, the cells were

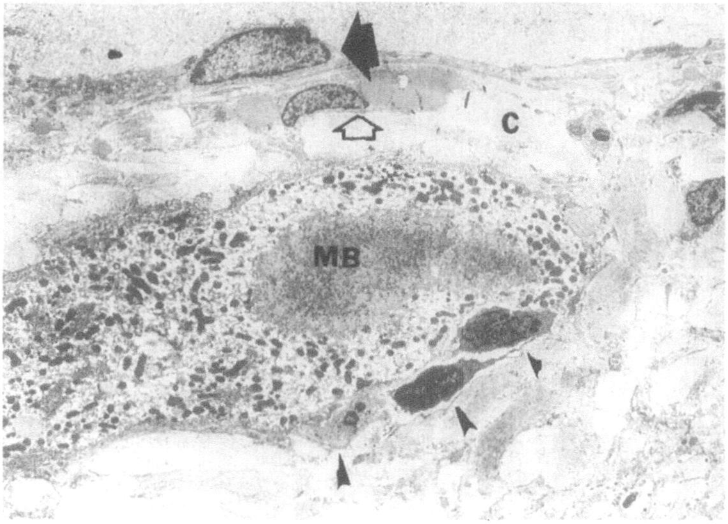

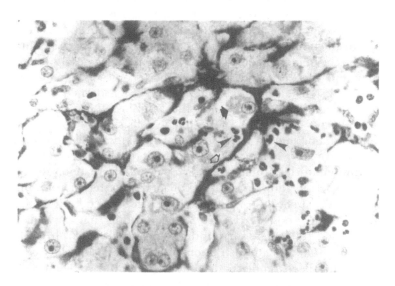

Figure 3.2 Electron microscopic view of central sclerosing hyaline necrosis (CSHN), a typical feature of ALD. Note the Mallory body (MB), the stellate cell (open arrow), the endothelium (closed arrow), collagen (C) and the inflammatory cells at the cell border of the hepatocyte (H) which contains the MB. The inflammatory cells abut against the part of the hepatocyte that is near the MB (peripolesis) (arrow heads). Permission to publish was granted by Dr. Okanoue and the Archives of Pathology and Laboratory Medicine (Oranoue *et al.*, 1983).

Figure 3.3 Liver biopsy section stained for α smooth muscle actin indicating stellate cell activation (open arrow). The hepatocytes contain MBs (closed arrow) and emperipolesis (arrow heads). (× 624)

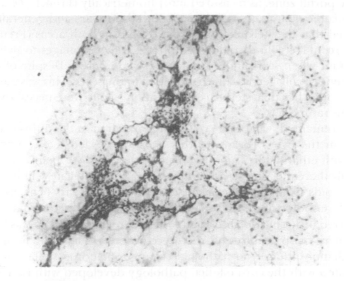

Figure 3.4 Liver biopsy section stained for a smooth muscle actin. There is an extensive focal activation of the stellate cells around the central vein. (×312)

designated transitional cells. The transitional cells were associated with a significantly increased collagen score in the space of Disse. The number of transitional cells was not increased in the fatty liver and perivenular fibrosis stages but they were significantly increased in the cirrhotic stage.

To further investigate the question of whether stellate cell activation, as measured by electron microscopic morphologic criteria, was localized only in scars or was also present throughout the sinusoids, we quantified the activation of stellate cells by morphometric measurements in liver biopsies from 43 patients with ALD (French *et al.*, 1988a). The percentage volume of fat per stellate cell was significantly greater in the random sinusoidal location than in the scars ($p = <0.001$). This was true regardless of which stage of ALD was present, i.e., fatty liver, alcoholic hepatitis or cirrhosis. The same was true when stellate cell rough endoplasmic reticulum was measured instead of fat percentage volume. There was no correlation between percentage volume of collagen in the sinusoidal wall with the volume of fat in the associated stellate cells. Likewise, when the criteria for "transitional" stellate cells was filled and this was correlated with the volume of associated collagen in the perisinusoidal space, no positive correlation was found. It was concluded that "activation" of stellate cells was limited to scarred areas and was not present diffusely throughout the sinusoids in the lobule (French *et al.*, 1988a). Thus, stellate cell activation must occur due to local factors such as cytokines involved in the scarring process rather than systemic mediators such as ethanol or acetaldehyde. These cytokines probably are secreted by "activated" macrophages involved as scavengers in the localized inflammatory or necrotizing process (Kovacs and Difietro, 1994).

Using an experimental rat model where rats were fed ethanol and a borderline deficient diet for 4–5 months, where liver biopsies were done before and during ethanol feeding, we observed an increase in collagen, both in the centrilobular zone and in the portal zone, as measured morphometrically (French *et al.*, 1988b). Electron microscopic quantitation of the stellate cells in scars and generally in the sinusoids showed that the stellate cells were activated in both areas (French *et al.*, 1988b). The percentage volume ratio of Kupffer cell-macrophages to stellate cells remained constant when scars and sinusoids were compared. Despite of this, the percentage volume of collagen was much increased in the scars. This was interpreted to mean that factors other than stellate cell "activation" alone were necessary for scar formation in this rat model.

The question remained, what is the role of malnutrition in the diffuse activation of stellate cells in the liver. To answer this question we fed rats a nutritionally adequate diet with ethanol for 5 months. We biopsied the liver before feeding the diet and monthly thereafter and measured the activation of stellate cells in scars and in random sinusoids using electron microscopy morphometrics (Takahashi *et al.*, 1991). Two different diets were fed, one with tallow as the source of fat where no pathology occurred including no fibrosis, and the other where corn oil was fed as the source of fat where many features of ALD were observed including focal fibrosis. With tallow, ethanol induced no pathologic change including stellate activation. On the other hand with the corn oil diet, pathology developed with focal scarring and evidence of stellate cell activation in scars early and in random sinusoids later (Takahashi *et al.*, 1991). These results indicate that stellate cells are not activated directly by ethanol or acetaldehyde since no activation occurred over 5 months of feeding with tallow and ethanol. More important, diffuse stellate cell activation by ethanol and corn oil did not occur until long after scarring was observed indicating that centrilobular scarring is a result of localized injury to hepatocytes, not due to activation of stellate cells generally. Thus short term (i.e., 2–4 months) ethanol feeding experiments using rodents may not provide relevant data on stellate cell activation *in vitro* in ALD because stellate cells are not diffusely activated *in vivo* in this model.

There are many circumstances where stellate cell activation occurs in the human liver *in vivo* where no scarring is associated. These include the embryonic, fetal, infant and adolescent as well as adult liver (Schmitt-Graff *et al.*, 1991). In disease states such as circulatory shock, septic shock and chronic congestion of the liver, stellate cells are diffusely activated as indicated by the expression of α smooth muscle (SM) actin and desmin. Likewise, they are activated in various liver diseases such as fatty liver, alcoholic hepatitis, chronic active hepatitis, extrahepatic bile duct obstruction, primary biliary cirrhosis, stage 1 and 2, and acute liver rejection. Thus, stellate cell activation in adult liver may be a systemic response to injury as well as a localized response to liver damage.

Studies have been done on stellate cells *in situ* and stellate cells and fibroblasts isolated from human liver biopsies or soft tissue to determine the type of collagen synthesized and the modulating factors which regulate the production of the extracellular matrix by stellate cells. In alcoholic livers with fibrosis or cirrhosis, stellate cells in the scars showed increased type I, III, and IV collagen as well as fibronectin *in situ* (Clement *et al.*, 1986). Immunohistochemical studies showed that transforming growth factor (TGF) was also localized to the site of fibrosis (Nagy *et al.*, 1991). Stellate cells isolated and cultured from normal human livers responded to TGF-β in a dose dependent way to produce procollagen I and III and fibronectin (Casini *et al.*, 1993). The mitogenic response to TGF-β_1 by human stellate cells is mediated by endogenous platelet-derived growth factor (PDGF) (Win *et al.*, 1993) due to induction of autocrine PDGF secretion by stellate cells. These results differ from stellate cells isolated from rat liver where TGF-β was shown to inhibit the proliferation of stellate cells in culture (Matsuoka *et al.*, 1989; David, 1988). This mitogenic effect of PDGF applies only to the PDGF-receptor-β (PDGF-R) subunit which is induced by TGF-β as are PDGF-BB binding sites in cultured human stellate cells (Pinzani *et al.*, 1985). In human cirrhotic liver, PDGF and PDGF-R subunit mRNA expression is markedly increased in PDGF-AA and -BB in foci of inflammation and within fibrous septae. PDGF-Rα and β subunit mRNAs were also over expressed in α-SM actin positive stellate cell (Pinzani *et al.*, 1996). Cultured Kupffer cells derived from rats fed ethanol to produce fibrosis generate factors in the culture medium which stimulate stellate cell formation of collagen. This effect is blocked by an antibody to TGF-β (Matsuoka and Tsukamoto, 1990). Thus stellate cell activation by Kupffer cells in man and rats fed ethanol may be a mechanism to stimulate the scarring process *in vivo* and this process appears to require PDGF in man. These observations are important because they focus on which factors can be inhibited through therapeutic intervention to prevent liver scarring in ALD. For instance IFN-α and γ inhibit human stellate cell proliferation and collagen synthesis *in vitro* stimulated by PDGF-BB and AA as well as TGF-$β_1$ (Mallat *et al.*, 1995). Another potential candidate for therapy is osteonectin (SPARC) which is expressed in stellate cells (myofibroblasts) in human liver scars (Blazejewskin *et al.*, 1997). This mediator is mitogenic to activated stellate cells.

Central sclerosing hyaline necrosis (CSHN)

CSHN is a more severe variant of central fibrosis where hepatocellular degenerative changes, MB formation and acute and chronic inflammation dominate and central fibrosis ranges from mild to severe (French *et al.*, 1993). Characteristically, there is a gradient in the cytokeratin (CK8 and 18) positive staining of hepatocytes by the monoclonal antibody CAM5.2. The periportal hepatocytes stain the most positive whereas most of the centrilobular hepatocytes either do not stain positive (Figure 3.5) or a mosaic of darkly stained and unstained hepatocytes are seen to form a mosaic pattern centrally (Figure 3.6). MBs are prominent in both stained and unstained hepatocytes (Figure 3.6). The phenomenon where the liver cells fail to stain positive for cytokeratin, first described by Denk's group (Denk and Krepler, 1982), is termed "empty cells" because the affected cells appear as ghost cells where only the nucleus and MBs are seen within what otherwise appears as an empty space when the stain for cytokeratins is used (Denk and Krepler, 1982; Kimoff and Huang, 1981; Ray *et al.*, 1988; French, 1994). The cytokeratins expressed are usually CK8 and 18 but sometimes bile duct cytokeratins are also found (Van Eyken *et al.*, 1988; Katsuma *et al.*, 1987). The MB forming cells are round instead of polyhedral in shape, which is why these cells have been referred to as showing balloon degeneration (French *et al.*, 1993a).

CSHN provokes a mixed inflammatory response, predominantly lymphocytes and macrophages (Figure 3.3) but sometimes predominantly neutrophils (Figure 3.4) (Okanoue *et al.*, 1983; French *et al.*, 1977, 1979; Yuan *et al.*, 1995, 1996). The

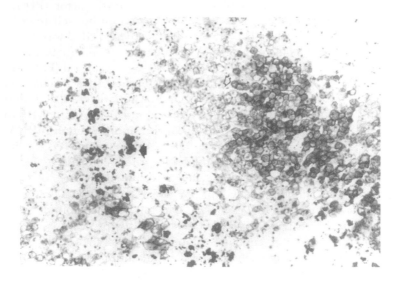

Figure 3.5 Liver biopsy section from a case of CSHN stained for liver cell cytokeratins (CK8 and 18). The hepatocytes in the periportal area (open arrow) stain positive but fail to stain centrally. Note the MBs stain positive (closed arrow). (× 156)

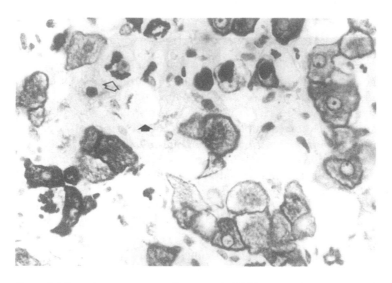

Figure 3.6 Liver biopsy section of a case of CSHN stained for CK8 and 18. Note variability in staining of the hepatocytes and MBs (open arrow). Swollen "empty" hepatocytes show balloon degeneration (closed arrow). (× 156)

inflammatory response may induce stellate cell activation (Figure 3.7) through a variety of mechanisms involving oxidative stress signals (Casini *et al.*, 1997), cytokines such as TNF-α, TGF-β, PDGF, prostanoids, leukocyte mediators, acute phase components, mitogens, vasoactive compounds and growth factors (Friedman, 1997).

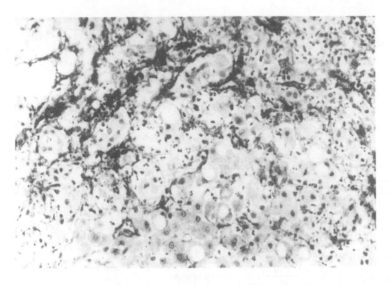

Figure 3.7 Liver biopsy section from a case of CSHN stained for α smooth muscle actin. There is extensive inflammatory infiltrate of mixed cell type associated with focal stellate cell activation. (×312).

Activated stellate cells produce chemokines which are chemotaxic for neutrophils (Sprenger *et al.*, 1997) which could explain why the neutrophilic infiltrate is sometimes prominent if MBs are present (Figure 3.2). MB formation incites satellitosis of inflammatory cells which leads to peripolesis (Figure 3.2) and emperipolesis and death of the hepatocytes presumably through immune mechanisms, either through sensitized CD8 cytotoxic lymphocytes or antibody dependent cytotoxicity (Figure 3.8). In one series of patients with alcoholic hepatitis, expression of class I and II MHC correlated with liver pathology severity (Chedid *et al.*, 1993a) which included MB formation and necrosis suggesting that T cell mediated injury by T lymphocytes may perpetuate ALD through autoimmune mechanisms initiated by MBs (Hasumura *et al.*, 1988) or products of lipid peroxidation such as malondialdyde (MDA) and hydroxynonenal (HNE) adduct or formation of adducts with acetaldehyde or hydroxyethyl radical (Albano *et al.*, 1996; Israel, 1997; Clot *et al.*, 1997; Vitala *et al.*, 1997). Antibodies to cytoskeletal antigens which are common in ALD (Kurki *et al.*, 1983) may injure liver cells through antibody dependent cytotoxicity (Figure 3.8). In ALD, hepatocytes show enhanced expression of the β1 chain of the integrins (CD29) and the isoform of leukocytic common antigen (CD45RA) (Chedid *et al.*, 1993b). The lymphocytes in the liver of ALD express CD45R0 indicating they are of the "memory" type which supports the concept that cell–cell contact proceeds to a cell mediated cytotoxic mechanism in the hepatocellular injury observed in CSHN.

   The scarring in CSHN progresses in severity, widening and extending to connect with neighboring central veins to form central–central bridging fibrosis. The sirus red stain for scar collagen highlights this type of scarring as distinct from the periportal scarring which may develop later (Figure 3.9). The central vein appears narrowed

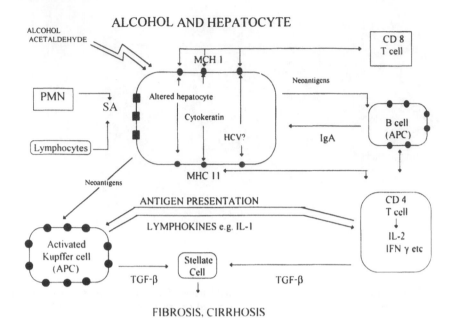

Figure 3.8 To illustrate the complex nature of the immune system and the role that it plays in alcoholic liver disease, this figure shows the cast of characters that are involved. This includes two types of T lymphocytes (CD4 and 8) and their interaction with class I and II MHC molecules (HLA equivalent), as mediators of antigen dependent cellular injury. Neoantigens such as hydroxyethyl protein adducts of liver cell cytokeratins or HCV processed by Kupffer cells or B lymphocyte antigen presenting cells (APC) stimulate the formation of humoral antibodies (IgA) by B lymphocytes or sensitize T lymphocytes (CD4). Activated Kupffer cells and sensitized lymphocytes generate lymphokines (IL-1, IL-2, IFNγ) and cytokines (TGF-β) which activate stellate cells to form fibrous scars. Lymphocytes and PMNs bind to the liver surface antigens (SA) to injure the hepatocytes in antibody dependent or cell mediated reactions. This scheme is a modification of one by Ian McKay, Melbourne, Australia.

or obliterated. Often it is not possible to locate the central vein. The scarring is pericellular at first but as liver cells are lost the collagen fibers collapse together to form a matt which is directionally oriented, that is, the fibers run parallel to each other at a 90° angle to the direction of the portal tract (Figure 3.9 and 3.10). This feature is helpful in identifying CSHN late in the course of ALD when incomplete cirrhosis develops. The stellate cells in CSHN remain active even when the hepatocellular degenerative changes have subsided (Figure 3.10). Activity is indicated when the bundles of stellate cells stain strongly positive for α smooth muscle actin (Figure 3.10). Patients with CSHN often have clinical evidence of portal hypertension (Edmondson *et al.*, 1963) in the absence of cirrhosis because the venous drainage of the sinusoids is ostensibly blocked by the interposition of the mass of stellate cells at the central vein location.

The CSHN lesion with increased concentrations of stellate cells may be the result of the proliferation and migration of these stellate cells in response to growth

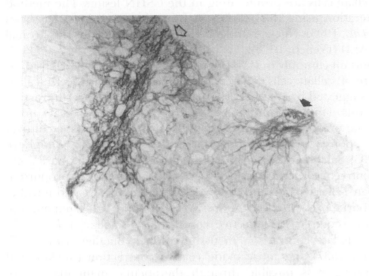

Figure 3.9 Liver biopsy section from a case of CSHN stained for collagen with sirus red. Note there is scarring around the central vein (open arrow) and the portal tract (closed arrow). (× 10)

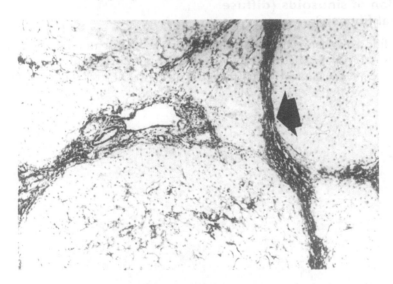

Figure 3.10 Liver biopsy section from a case of central and periportal fibrosis stained for α smooth muscle actin. Note the stellate cells run parallel to each other in the central area (solid arrow). (× 156)

factors such as PDGF (Pinzani *et al.*, 1985, 1996; Win *et al.*, 1993) in a way that is analogous to the formation of a smooth muscle arteriosclerotic plaque in the aorta. Stains for proliferating cell nuclear antigen (PCNA/cyclin), an auxillary protein of DNA polymerase (Bravo and MacDonald-Bravo, 1985) synthesized during late G1 and S phase, show that both hepatocytes and nonparenchymal cells such as endothelium and stellate cells are proliferating in the CSHN lesion. The method of measuring proliferation using this marker in formalin fixed tissue has been validated (Tamaka *et al.*, 1993). Nuclear antigen Ki-67 (MIB) confirms the stromal cell proliferation in ALD (French, 1996).

What may be important clinically in CSHD to explain the portal hypertension is the contractile nature of stellate cells. The contractile nature of these cells (called myofibroblasts) was suggested by Bhathal (1972) as a mechanisms for contraction of scar tissue in cirrhosis. This was found to be the case in pharmacological studies of contractility of tissue preparations (Irle *et al.*, 1980) and later in tissue cultures of stellate cells in response to endothelin-1, substance P and Ca^{++} ionophore (Kawahara *et al.*, 1993; Sakamoto *et al.*, 1993; Bauer *et al.*, 1995; Kawahara *et al.*, 1995). Stellate cell contractility increases with progressive liver injury in proportion to the degree of stellate cell activation and this may contribute to increased intrahepatic resistance and portal pressure (Rockey and Wesiger, 1996). Collagen binding integrins ($\alpha 1$ $\beta 1$) are required for effective contraction (Bataller *et al.*, 1997). Vasopressin induces stellate contraction in tissue culture (Bataller *et al.*, 1997; Racine-Sampson *et al.*, 1997) and nitric oxide relaxes contraction (Rockey and Chung, 1995) indicating it is possible through therapeutic manipulations of stellate contraction to relieve portal hypertension.

Capillarization of sinusoids (diffuse perisinusoidal fibrosis)

Uncommonly, diffuse thickening of collagen in the space of Disse develops in ALD ("florid cirrhosis"). It usually occurs in the presence of periportal and central fibrosis and provides one mechanism of central-portal bridging fibrosis (Figure 3.11).

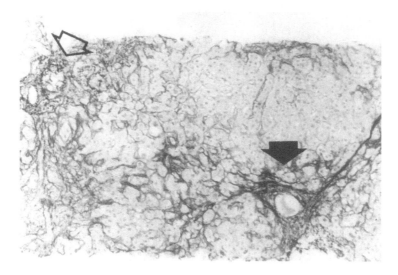

Figure 3.11 Liver biopsy section from a case of pericellular fibrosis and capillarization due to diffuse activation of stellate cells stained with sirus red. There is central (solid arrow) portal (open arrow) bridging fibrosis. (×156)

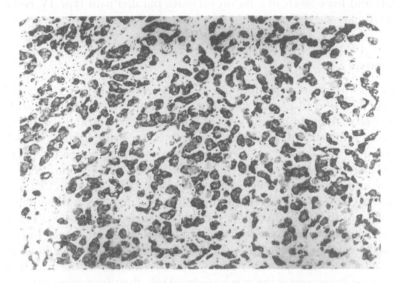

Figure 3.12 Liver biopsy section from a case of diffuse perisinusoidal fibrosis stained for hepatocyte CK8 and 18. Note the pericellular fibrosis has interrupted the liver cell cords. (×312)

When diffused, it breaks up the liver plates causing the hepatocytes to be dissociated from each other (Figure 3.12) (Biagni and Ballardini, 1989). A diffusion barrier is postulated so that exchange of plasma nutrients and secretory products of hepatocytes is theoretically impaired as is sinusoidal blood flow. The phenomenon is referred to as a capillarization of the sinusoids (Schaffner and Popper, 1963). In this condition there is an increase in the deposition of type III and IV collagen, and fibronectin and hyaluronic acid in the space of Disse (Hahn *et al.*, 1980; Gressner and Schafer, 1989; Horn *et al.*, 1985; Ericksson *et al.*, 1983). The increase in type IV collagen precedes the increase in total collagen content in ALD, differing in this way from liver fibrosis caused by other liver conditions (Tsutsumi *et al.*, 1993a). When the liver is stained immunohistochemically for the type IV collagen early in ALD there is an increase in diffuse staining that outlines the sinusoids and this persists as fibrosis progresses (Tsutsumi *et al.*, 1993b). It is associated with the development of basal lamina between the endothelial cell and the stellate cell in the space of Disse (Hahn *et al.*, 1980; Horn *et al.*, 1985). Stellate cells synthesize the extracellular matrix of the space of Disse including type III and IV collagen, fibronectin, laminin (Friedman, 1997) and hyaluronic acid (Gressner and Shafer, 1989). Hyaluronic acid is secreted by the stellate cells and cleared by the endothelial cells (Ericksson *et al.*, 1983). Thus serum levels of hyaluronate has proven to be a good measure of liver sinusoidal capillarization (Veno *et al.*, 1993; Urashima *et al.*, 1993; Pares *et al.*, 1996). In ALD, hyaluronate levels correlate with type III procollagen levels in the blood and are a marker of the severity of liver inflammation, fibrosis and fibrogenesis (Pares *et al.*, 1996). Serum levels of type IV collagen are a sensitive marker of early perisinusoidal fibrosis which plateau as fibrosis progresses in ALD (Tsutsumi *et al.*, 1993). Stellate cells secrete laminin M subunit (Maher and

Tzagarakis, 1994) and liver levels of laminin increase parallel with type IV collagen in ALD (Tsutsumi *et al.*, 1993).

Periportal fibrosis

Periportal fibrosis is the product of limiting plate erosion, ductular piecemeal
type, similar to the reaction to extrahepatic bile duct obstruction (Baptista *et al.*,
1988). The earliest change noted may be seen in the fatty liver stage and consists of
mixed inflammatory infiltrate and the beginning of ductular proliferation (French
et al., 1993a) (Figure 3.13). Limiting plate erosion of some degree is seen in 79% of
liver biopsies showing alcoholic hepatitis (Chedid *et al.*, 1991). The lesion is easier
to detect using the immunostain for bile duct cytokeratins which stain CK19 and 7
(AE_{1-3} keratin cocktail, DAKO). This stain identifies the bile ductules at the limiting
plate which extends into the parenchyma for variable distances (Figure 3.13). These
ductules were first regarded as ductules derived from hepatocytes and termed ductular metaplasia (Desmet, 1986), analogous to the ductal plate that forms bile ducts in
the embryo and fetal liver (Cocjin *et al.*, 1996). Transformation of the liver cell
plates into biliary type structures is the mechanism of bile duct formation prior to
birth (Desmet, 1985). This change in ALD has been analyzed and illustrated by
Ray *et al.* (1993). Recently, the concept of intralobular ductule change at the interface
between the portal tracts and limiting plate has been changed to indicate that the
"metaplastic" change represents a bipotential progenitor epithelium with phenotypic markers of hepatocytes, bile duct cells, oval cells and stem cells accounts for

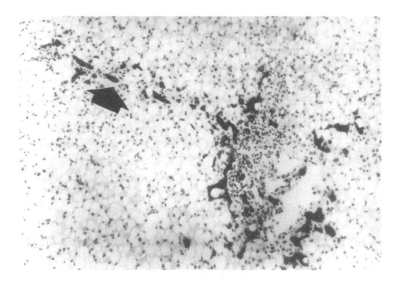

Figure 3.13 Liver biopsy section of early fibrosis in the steatohepatitis stage of ALD stained for
bile duct keratins CK7 and 19. Note the ductal hepatocytes are formed at the limiting plate of the portal tract (small arrow) and extend out into the parenchyma
(large arrow) in the direction of a neighboring portal tract. (× 156)

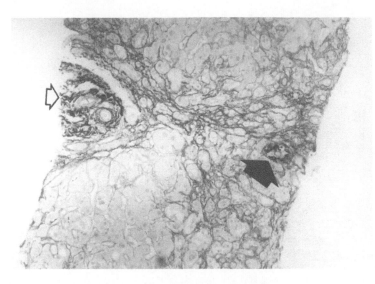

Figure 3.14 Liver biopsy section of central-portal bridging fibrosis stained with sirus red. The portal tract (open arrow) and central vein (closed arrow) are embedded in scar. (× 312)

this interface ductal change in chronic liver disease (Cocjin *et al.*, 1996; Desmet, 1985; Ray *et al.*, 1993; DeVos and Desmet, 1992; Demetris *et al.*, 1996; Thorgiersson, 1996; Hsia *et al.*, 1992; Factor *et al.*, 1994; Sarraf *et al.*, 1994; Lenzi *et al.*, 1992; Thorgiersson *et al.*, 1993). This change is present in submassive necrosis in humans who had a hepatectomy in order to perform a liver transplant 2–14 days after the onset of liver injury (Demetris *et al.*, 1996). As early as 2 days after liver damage was initiated, ductular hepatocytes (DHs) appeared at the limiting plate–portal tract interface. DHs were tubular or bilayered structures that resembled bile duct cells. The number of DHs increased with the extent of necrosis and the time after insult. They were intermixed with hepatocytes that were smaller than normal and had more basophilic cytoplasm. Special marker stains identified CK19 positive ductular hepatocytes (DHs). Using a marker for Ki-67 (MIB) to identify proliferating cells, the DHs had the highest proliferative rate. These cells were surrounded by a laminin rich matrix (basal lamina similar to that found with bile ducts), focally expressed vimentin and Lewis[x] and showed up-regulation of bcl-2 and type IV collagenase mRNA. They were CD34 and α-1-antitrypsin positive indicating, they had some phenotypic features of both duct and liver cell epithelium. Thus, this ductular change may represent a transient amplification of a population of progenitor cells located in or near the canals of Herring (cholangioles). The rate of apoptosis was less in the DH cells compared with bile duct and liver cells. With increased proliferation and decrease in cell death by apoptosis, these cells had a growth advantage in response to injury. In ALD, these cells stain for CK19 and 7 (AE_{1-3}), extend into the lobular parenchyma radially around the portal tract and induce stellate cells to proliferate and form collagen (Figure 3.14) (see Figure 3.13 in French *et al.*, 1993a to visualize stellate cell proliferation around portal tracts where DH-like ductules are formed). The cells connect with liver cells and canaliculi and when they form

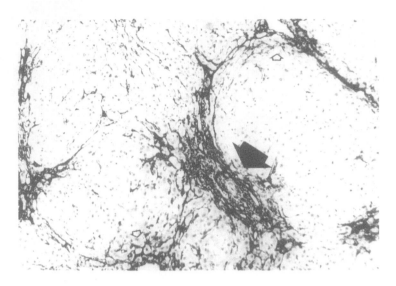

Figure 3.15 Liver biopsy section from a case of ALD showing central (open arrow) – portal (closed arrow) bridging fibrosis stained for a smooth muscle actin. The stellate cells remain active in the scars. (× 156)

lumens, they are a functional conduit for bile flow. The DH cells at the rim of the portal tract extend into the parenchyma (Figure 3.13). Since these extensions are associated with stellate cells and collagen, these extensions form radiating spurs which project into the parenchyma from the portal tract (ductule piecemeal necrosis). These extensions appear to be directional in that they extend along the periphery of zone 1 in the direction of adjacent portal tracts or central veins (Figures 3.12–3.14). When they meet extensions from adjacent portal tracts, they form a bridge, known as bridging fibrosis (see Figure 3.14 in French *et al.*, 1993a). The DH cell extensions bridge portal tracts to portal tracts or portal tracts to central veins. Stellate cells form these bridges (Figure 3.15) and lay down collagen to form fibrous bridges. The DHs may persist (Figure 3.16) or may disappear through apoptosis leaving only a fibrous bridge containing stellate cells. The periportal scar may become devoid of DH cells to form fibrous collars around portal tracts (periportal fibrosis). When all of the bridges hook up to form septa separating hepatocellular nodules, cirrhosis has developed. The formation of DH cells may persist however in the cirrhotic stage of ALD, either because alcoholic hepatitis continues (in a series of 281 biopsies of patients with alcoholic hepatitis 149 had cirrhosis and of these, 111 had alcoholic hepatitis as well (Chedid *et al.*, 1997)) or ischemic necrosis occurs in liver regenerative nodules due to acute blood loss from bleeding varices. Figure 3.16 shows extensive DH proliferation with scarring seen in cirrhosis. Due to the attrition of hepatocytes to form DH cells, few hepatocytes remain. Such is the vicious cycle of liver injury-DH formation-scar formation that results in cirrhosis.

To stop this cycle, we need to understand the mechanism of the general response to liver injury where induction of DH cells formation develops. What is known about

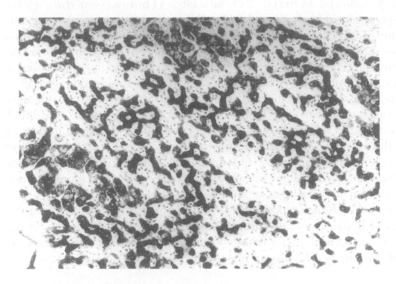

Figure 3.16 Liver biopsy section from a case of ALD in the cirrhosis stage stained for liver cell cytokeratin CK8 and 18. Note two islands of hepatocytes remain but the rest have been converted into ductal hepatocytes. (× 156)

the DH cell response begins with the understanding that it is initiated by nonspecific liver injury and the degree of the response is proportional to the severity of the liver injury. If the liver injury is mild, the DH response may not occur or it may be too subtle to be detected by staining the liver with special markers. It does not appear to be initiated by partial hepatectomy where hepatocytes regenerate without forming DH cells. Acute ethanol ingestion does not induce the DH cell response. Acute severe necrosis induced by any toxin will induce the DH cell response, especially if liver cell regeneration is inhibited (Thorgiersson, 1996) or if the injury is chronic or recurrent such as in chronic hepatitis due to a viral infection (Hsia *et al.*, 1992). Experimental induction of DH cells (oval cells, stem cells) is achieved by chemical carcinogenic compounds followed by partial hepatectomy (PH), i.e., dipin (Factor *et al.*, 1994), acetylaminofluorene (AAF) (Sarraf *et al.*, 1994). Choline-deficient ethionine-containing diet (Lenzi *et al.*, 1992) achieves the same response. The use of these models to study the factors which induce the proliferation of DH cells (oval cells-stem cells) has revealed first the transient activation of the stem cell factor (SCF)/c-kit system (Fuji *et al.*, 1994), i.e., 12–11 hours after AAF/PH (Thorgiersson *et al.*, 1993). The expression of both SCF and c-kit genes is increased in both oval cells and stellate cells whereas expression of c-kit transcripts was only found in oval cells (Fuji *et al.*, 1994). Hepatocyte growth factor (HGF) transcripts increase from 4–96 hours after PH. Ascitic fibroblastic growth factor (αFGF) transcripts increase from 24–96 hours, PH/TGF-α increases from 4–96 hours and TGF-β1 increases from 4–96 hours after AAF/PH (Thorgiersson *et al.*, 1993). The first cells entering DNA synthesis after AAF/PH are the oval cells and stellate cells in the periportal area (Thorgiersson, 1996). Coincidental with the appearance and expansion of these cell populations is an increase in the transcripts for TGF-α,

HGF and TGF-β, followed by αFGF 24 hours later (Thorgiersson *et al.*, 1993). TGF-α transcripts are found in both oval and stellate cells. HGF transcripts are only found in stellate cells (Thorgiersson *et al.*, 1993). TGF-β₁ transcripts are found mainly in stellate cells. The transcripts for the receptors for all these growth factors are located in the oval cells (Thorgiersson *et al.*, 1993). Teleologically, these observations suggest a communication system between growth and migration stimuli of the DH cells and stellate cells. The growth response to injury exists through autocrine and paracrine mechanisms (see Figures 3.17 and 3.18 in French *et al.*, 1988b). *In vitro* HGF, IL-6 and EGF stimulate growth of biliary duct epithelium indicating that these growth factors may participate in growth regulation of human biliary duct epithelium through paracrine and autocrine stimulation (Matsumoto *et al.*, 1994). The triggering mechanism which initiates the activation of the DH-oval cell proliferation and stellate cell periportal scarring system is the key.

Liver parenchymal cells at the limiting plate are converted to DH cells. In this way the number of hepatocytes are diminished during periportal fibrosis. As this process continues during and after cirrhosis formation, the number of hepatocytes are progressively diminished relative to the scar formed.

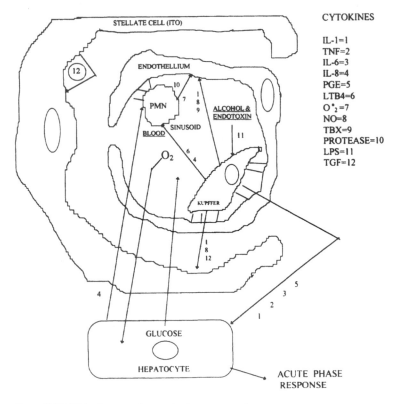

Figure 3.17 This diagram shows the liver sinusoid and perisinusoidal cells including a stellate cell. Cytokines and other reactive factors provide communication between cell types. (see *Color Plate 2*)

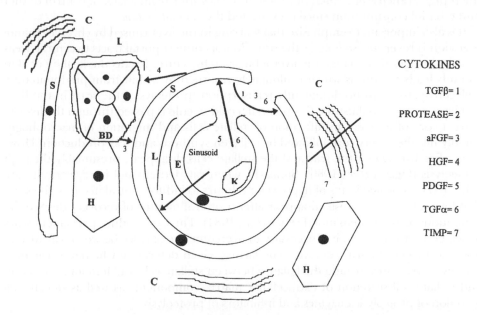

CYTOKINES

TGFβ= 1

PROTEASE= 2

aFGF= 3

HGF= 4

PDGF= 5

TGFα= 6

TIMP= 7

Figure 3.18 Perisinusoidal and periportal scar formation in alcoholic liver disease. The stellate cells (S) secrete collagen and collagenase (C). The collagenase (protease) digests the collagen to maintain a balance in the normal liver but it is inhibited by tissue inhibitor metalloprotease (TIMP) during scarring so that collagen accumulates. Laminin (L) accumulates under the endothelium (E) around the hepatic ductules (BD). Kupffer cells (K) secrete transforming growth factor β (TGF-β) which stimulates stellate cells to make collagen. Stellate cells also make TGF-β, acid fibroblastic growth factor (αFGF) and transforming growth factor alpha (TGF-α) and hepatocyte growth factor (HGF). The latter stimulates stellate cells to proliferate by secreting αFGF. (see *Color Plate 3*)

EXPERIMENTAL LIVER FIBROSIS IN ALD

It is important to review the experimental evidence derived from tissue culture and test these findings using *in vivo* models in order to determine their relevance to the pathology observed *in vivo*. The concepts described in *in vitro* systems can only be tested using *in vivo* models where pathology is observed, i.e., fibrosis. The intragastric tube feeding model is such a model since focal fibrosis is observed as early as 1 month into ethanol feeding and increases in severity over a 6 month period of feeding ethanol (French *et al.*, 1986, 1988a; Tsukamoto *et al.*, 1986, 1990a,b; Takahashi *et al.*, 1990, 1991), especially when fed a borderline deficient diet (French *et al.*, 1988a) or a diet rich in polyunsaturated fatty acids (Morimoto *et al.*, 1994; French *et al.*, 1988c), or when iron is added to the diet (Tsukamoto *et al.*, 1995), when isoniazide (INH) is fed with ethanol (French *et al.*, 1993b) or CCl$_4$ is given with ethanol (Hall *et al.*, 1991). Other models exist, i.e., dog, baboon and micropig (French *et al.*, 1995) but these models suffer from a lack of control of diet and ethanol consumption since they are fed the diet *ad libitum*.

It is also important to emphasize that scarring in the liver caused by chronic ethanol ingestion is reversible so long as the scars do not connect portal tracts to central areas to form bridges that change the liver lobular architecture. Just as the healing of skin wounds leads to fibrosis which is ultimately resorbed by a shift from predominantly collagen synthesis to predominantly reabsorption (proteolysis), the scars in the liver can be resorbed. To illustrate this point, if a cold needle is passed through the liver to leave a core of necrosis, proliferation of stellate cells and migration of macrophages rapidly fills the empty core followed by collagen synthesis and scar production. However, after two weeks, the scar and the stellate cells disappear, presumably through proteolysis (Ogawa *et al.*, 1986). Similarly, when rats fed ethanol intragastrically are subjected to repeated bouts of hypoxia for 5 hours to induce central necrosis, the scars that form after the necrosis disappear after a several months of recovery despite the continuous feeding of ethanol (French *et al.*, 1984). Thus, to produce permanent scars which go on to cirrhosis, it is necessary to overcome the balance between scar formation and proteolytic scar removal. The factors which determine whether a scar progresses or regresses include the balance between stellate cell proliferation, migration and stellate cell secretion of extracellular matrix components as well as stellate cell secretion of proteolytic enzymes and inhibitors of proteolysis.

Stellate cell migration, proliferation and secretion of extracellular matrix

The factors which activate stellate cells to migrate, proliferate and secrete collagen and other extracellular matrix components are outlined in Figures 3.17 and 3.18. These include cytokines and growth factors derived from Kupffer cells, neutrophils, and hepatocytes. The sequence of events after hepatic necrosis, where these cells play a role in the scarring process (wound healing), is as follows: (1) necrotic areas become permeated with plasma within 24 hours; (2) The areas become strongly positive for fibronectin and become infiltrated with inflammatory cells positive for lysozyme; (3) By 3 days stellate cells proliferate in the peripheral zone between the viable hepatocytes and the necrotic areas. The stellate cells stain positive for actin and desmin and negative for lysozyme; (4) Collagen fibers and matrix stained positive for collagen types I and IV, laminin and fibronectin beginning 3 days after necrosis; (5) They were located at the interface between stellate cells and bordering viable hepatocytes; (6) Basal lamina associated with capillaries and bile ducts increased after a 1 day delay; (7) The necrotic areas were replaced by granulation tissue by day 5; (8) Rapid diminution of the granulation tissue followed and normal hepatic tissue was restored in 7–10 days after injury (Ogawa *et al.*, 1986). This sequence of events after injury sets the stage for the stellate cell's role in scarring, healing and restitution in this reaction to injury in the liver and illustrates the dynamics of the process. It is important to realize that it is impossible to create this process *in vitro* in tissue culture experiments even if two cell types such as Kupffer cells and stellate cells are cocultured. Despite these limitations, it is possible to gain insight into the process by examining individual components by perturbing isolated stellate cells in tissue culture under controlled experimental conditions.

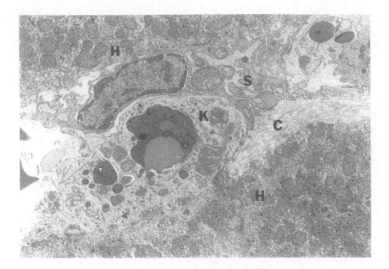

Figure 3.19 Liver from a rat fed ethanol chronically showing the apposition of a Kupffer cell (K) against an activated stellate cell (S) in pericellular fibrosis (collagen C). Hepatocytes (H) appear normal. (Electron micrograph × 60,000)

Activation of stellate cells is the result of a cascade of events which occur in two phases, initiation and perpetuation (Friedman, 1993). In the inhibition stage, the stellate cells are stimulated by substances released by neighboring endothelium, Kupffer cells, and hepatocytes in a paracrine manner (Friedman, 1993) (see Figures 3.17 and 3.18). The close apposition of these cells to stellate cells is seen by electron microscopy of the hepatic sinusoids (Figure 3.19). Initiation may result from the release of lipid peroxides from injured hepatocytes undergoing oxidative stress (Bedossa *et al.*, 1994). However, since lipid peroxidation regularly occurs in hepatocytes, some modulating factors must prevent resting stellate activation by this mechanism. Vitamin E and superoxide dismutase are modulating factors since antioxidants block the activation of stellate cells by lipid peroxidases (Casini *et al.*, 1997). Other sources of free radicals in the sinusoids which may initiate stellate cell activation are Kupffer cells and neutrophils (Casini *et al.*, 1997) (Figure 3.17).

Acetaldehyde has been postulated to activate stellate cells to form collagen *in vitro* (Shiratori *et al.*, 1986; Moshage *et al.*, 1990; Casini *et al.*, 1991; Anania *et al.*, 1995). This phenomenon observed *in vitro* may not be applicable *in vivo*, however (Maher *et al.*, 1994). This is especially apparent where ethanol is fed to maintain high blood alcohol levels for 5 months with a diet where tallow is the source of fat calories. In this model, ethanol is metabolized to acetaldehyde *in vivo* but stellate cells are not activated (Takahashi *et al.*, 1991). Clearly, if acetaldehyde stimulates stellate cells to form collagen *in vivo* the conditions for activation require more than a simple increase in acetaldehyde formation by hepatocytes.

Early activation of stellate cells appears to result from rapid deposition of cellular fibronectin and release of soluble components from Kupffer cells (Friedman and Arthur, 1989). These changes sensitize the stellate cells which become responsive to

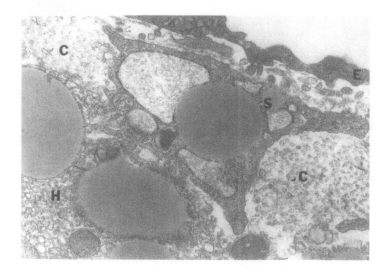

Figure 3.20 Electron micrograph of an activated stellate cell (S) between an endothelial cell (E) and hepatocyte (H). This is an example of perisinusoidal fibrosis and capillarization in the liver of a rat fed ethanol. The stellate cell is activated since the rough endoplasmic reticulum is dilated and filled with flocculent product. Collagen (C) is increased. Basal lamina has formed under the endothelium (arrow). (Electron micrograph ×100,000)

cytokines and growth factors such as PDGF. TGF-β, probably released from Kupffer cells, induces PDGF-BB receptor mRNA (Pinzani *et al.*, 1985). In cirrhosis both α and β subunits are overexpressed in stellate cells (Pinzani *et al.*, 1996). Cellular fibronectin increases in the liver prior to the increase in αSM actin in experimental ethanol fed rats (Gillis and Nagy, 1997). However, in the rat model, cellular location of these two changes was not determined.

Activated stellate cells are identified by numerous changes in cellular morphology, cellular metabolism and gene expression (Hellerbrand *et al.*, 1996). These changes include the development of myofibroblast-like cells inducing the formation of microfilaments along the cell borders (α smooth muscle actin), a loss of vitamin A and triglyceride stores in fat globules and an increase in rough endoplasmic reticulum (Figure 3.20).

Kupffer cells and macrophages are the primary cells involved in the early activation of stellate cells (Johnson *et al.*, 1992). Activation of Kupffer cells in experimental ALD in rats fed ethanol is a key element in the development of liver pathology which precedes fibrosis (Thurman *et al.*, 1997). Conditioned medium from cultures of Kupffer cells speeds up the process of activation which normally occurs in the tissue culture of stellate cells (Matsuoka and Tsukamoto, 1990; Matsuoka *et al.*, 1989) including proliferation and collagen synthesis. Importantly, this stimulation is greater in injured liver compared to normal liver, derived Kupffer cells (Friedman and Arthur, 1989; Shiratori *et al.*, 1986). This was dramatically shown in ethanol-fed rats where collagen synthesis was enhanced by a high fat diet and further enhanced by ethanol feeding, indicating that the stellate cells from ethanol-fed rats were sensitize to an element in the conditioned medium (Matsuoka and Tsukamoto, 1990). This element was most liklely TGF-β secreted by the Kupffer cells since the response was blocked by anti TGF-β antibody added to the medium (Matsuoka and Tsukamoto, 1990). TGF-β is a cytokine derived from macrophages which has been shown to enhance stellate cell production of extra-cellular matrix *in vitro* (Matsuoka *et al.*, 1989; Weiner *et al.*, 1990; Meyer *et al.*, 1990). TGF-β derived from both paracrine and autocrine sources, increases collagen gene expression at the transcriptional level which probably requires binding of the tran-scriptional factor AP-1. Thus, Kupffer cell activation with secretion of TGF-β fol-lowing endothelial secretion of fibronectin is an important initiator of the early activation of stellate cells in ALD (Figure 3.20). The activation of Kupffer cells to initiate fibrosis focally is most likely hepatocellular necrosis (Friedman, 1997) and diffuse activation may be initiated by endotoxemia (Thurman *et al.*, 1997). As explained earlier, the hepatocellular injury must be chronic because fibrosis due to liver damage is soon resolved leaving no residual scar.

During initiation, stellate cells undergo a number of phenotypic changes which prepare them for proliferation, extracellular matrix secretion, migration and contraction. The endoplasmic reticulum dilates and proliferates and its lumen fills up with newly formed protein (Figure 3.20). The lipid droplets in the cytoplasm diminish in volume in concert with a decrease in vitamin A stores. Microfilaments composed of α smooth muscle actin accumulate along the cell borders, i.e., myofibroblast transformation as seen in wound healing. Receptors for PDGF and TGF receptors are expressed making the stellate cell more sensitive in response to extracellular matrix components like fibronectin (Bissell, 1997). Transcription factors including CREB, c-myb and NFKB are activated by oxidative stress mechanisms (Lee *et al.*, 1995; Friedman, 1996). Initially, activated stellate cells also respond to fibroblastic growth factor, transforming growth factor-α, epidermal growth factor (Pinzani *et al.*, 1989), interleukin-1 and tumor necrosis factor-α (Matsuoka *et al.*, 1989).

Stellate cell activation perpetuation

After initial activation, the stellate cell phenotype responds to various stimuli in an autocrine and paracrine way to proliferate, migrate and contract, secreting extra-cellular matrix components, cytokines, proteases and growth factors, as well as expressing signaling molecules and transcription factors, at least as assessed in tissue culture (Friedman, 1997). Of these functions of the activated stellate cells, secretion of extracellular matrix components is the most important, especially secre-tion of collagen type I (Rojkind *et al.*, 1979; Seyer *et al.*, 1979). Sulfated proteogly-cans (Arenson *et al.*, 1988) and glycoproteins such as laminin (Mayer *et al.*, 1988), cellular fibronectin (Martinez-Hernandez, 1985) and tenascin (Ramadori *et al.*, 1991) are also secreted. Laminin together with collagen IV make up the basal lamina which when formed accounts for the capillarization seen in ALD and men-tioned earlier. These components are normal constituents of the space of Disse but form basal lamina which constitutes an abnormal diffuse barrier to the diffusion of nutrients from the sinusoidal lumens when capillarization occurs in ALD. Additional collagens produced by stellate cells in the space of Disse include collagen type III, V, VI and XIV. Proteoglycans produced by stellate cells include heparan, dermatan and chondroitin sulfates, perlecan, syndecan-1, biglycan and decorin (Meyer *et al.*, 1992; Krull *et al.*, 1993). Glycoproteins besides cellular fibronectin, laminin and tenascin include merosin, nidogen/entactin, undulin (Knittel *et al.*, 1992) and hyaluronic acid (Friedman, 1997). The latter is normally taken up by endothelial cells but in hepatic fibrosis, in ALD, the endothelial cells fail to clear it and it increases in the blood, making it a serum marker for active fibrosis in ALD as mentioned earlier. This is also true in the early stages of ALD in the rat model (Nanji *et al.*, 1996). The CD44 receptor isoform (CD9, 44, V6+) for hyaluronate in the extracellular matrix is expressed by stellate cells as well as Kupffer cells and endothelial cells (Bissell *et al.*, 1997) in liver injury and this may be a factor in migration of stellate cells to the site of injury in localized fibrosis in ALD. The binding of CD44 to hyaluronic acid in the matrix provides the mechanism for migration of stellate cells in tissue cultures (Bissell *et al.*, 1997). Cellular fibronectin in the matrix induces special isoforms of integrins to be expressed at the cell membrane of stellate cells (Bissell, 1997) and this interaction could play a role in down regulating stellate cell secretion of collagens and thus reverse the scarring process.

Since liver cell fibrosis is reversible in the absence of cirrhosis, the role of proteases secreted by stellate cells to bring a balance to counter act and reverse the scarring process is vital. Such proteases include type IV collagenase (gelatinase A) and matrix-metalloproteinase 2 (Arthur *et al.*, 1992), stromelysin-1 (transin), interstitial collagenase (MMP-1) and membrane type-matrix metaloproteinases secreted by stellate cells (Friedman, 1997; Takahara *et al.*, 1995, 1997; Theret *et al.*, 1997). The latter are triggered by hepatocytes (Theret *et al.*, 1997). The activities of these proteases are tempered by the secretion of protease inhibitors such as TIMP-1, TIMP-2, PAI-I by stellate cells (Herbst *et al.*, 1997; Iredale *et al.*, 1996) which further adds to the remodeling of the extracellular matrix. The inhibitors increase in the blood during active scarring in ALD and therefore they have been used as markers of fibrosis (Friedman, 1997; Tsutsumi *et al.*, 1996; Li *et al.*, 1994).

Stellate cells proliferate (French, 1992) and migrate to increase their numbers in scars stimulated by PDGF partly because activated stellate cells express PDGF receptors as noted earlier (Wong *et al.*, 1994). Epidermal growth factor (Mullhaupt *et al.*, 1994), fibroblast growth factor (Pinzani *et al.*, 1989), endothelin 1 (Hausset *et al.*, 1993), insulin-like growth factor (Pinzani *et al.*, 1990) and transforming growth factor alpha (Pinzani *et al.*, 1989) can all stimulate stellate cell proliferation which amplifies and perpetuates the stellate cell scarring process. Some of these growth factors originate in activated stellate cells. One of these is hepatocyte growth factor (Thorgiersson, 1996), which is important as the instigator of bile ductular proliferation. Also stem cell factor (SCF) and its receptor c-kit are expressed differentially. SCF is expressed by stellate cells and c-kit is expressed by ductular hepatocytes (putative stem cells) (Fuji *et al.*, 1994). Thus growth factors from stellate cells stimulate the proliferation of ductules during regeneration of the liver following injury. Since bile ductular proliferation induces stellate cell proliferation and activation, this represents a self perpetuating scarring process in the periportal area.

Finally, activated stellate cells may contribute to the focal inflammatory response to liver injury by secreting cytokines which are chemotactic to granulocytes. These cytokines and chemokines include colony-stimulating factor (Pinzani *et al.*, 1989) and monocyte chemotactic peptide 1 (Marra *et al.*, 1993), PGF2α, PGD2, PG12, PGE2, LTC4, LTB4, PAF, α2-macroglobulin, IL-6, and nitric oxide (Friedman, 1997). Thus, stellate cells may induce leukocyte accumulations and leukocytes may in turn produce factors which activate stellate cells to perpetuate the scarring process.

CONCLUSION

Fibrosis in human ALD and in the experimental rat model develops late in the course of chronic ethanol ingestion. In both human and rat, the fibrosis is at first focal and reversible until bridging fibrosis develops. This means that a balance of factors are at work, where stimulation of stellate cells to secrete extracellular matrix, structural proteins, degradation enzymes and protease inhibitors, can lead to resolution or progression of the scarring process. Liver fibrosis results from a relative imbalance between synthesis and degradation of matrix proteins. Modulating factors including focal inflammatory and hepatocellular degenerative changes as well as ductular proliferation lead to persistent activation, proliferation and migration of stellate cells. Stellate cell secretion of growth factors stimulates the proliferation of ductular cells. All these factors contribute to the progression of the scarring process. Contractions of the stellate cells within the scars further distort the liver architecture to force surviving hepatocytes to ball up into nodules at which point irreversible cirrhosis is formed.

REFERENCES

Albano, E., Clot, P., Morimoto, M., Tomashi, A., Ingelman-Sundberg, M. and French, S.W. (1996) Role of cytochrome P450 2E1-dependent formation of hydroxyethyl free radicals in the development of liver damage in rats intragastrically fed with ethanol. *Hepatology* **23**, 155–163.

Anania, F.A., Potter, J.J., Rennie-Tankarsley, L. and Mezey, E. (1995) Effects of acetaldehyde on nuclear protein binding to the nuclear factor I consensus sequence in the αz (I) collagen promoter. *Hepatology* **21**, 1640–1648.

Arenson, D.M., Friedman, S.L. and Bissell, D.M. (1988) Formation of extracellular matrix in normal liver: lipocytes as major source of proteoglycans. *Gastroenterology* **95**, 441–447.

Arthur, M.J., Stanley, A., Iredale, J.P., Rafferty, J.A., Hembry, R.M. and Friedman, S.L. (1992) Secretion of 72KD a type IV collagenase/gelatinase by cultured human lipocytes analysis of gene expression, protein synthesis and proteinase activity. *Biochem J* **287**, 701–707.

Baptista, A., Bianchi, L., DeGroote, J., Desmet, V.J., Ishak, K.G., Korb, G. *et al.* (1988) The diagnostic significance of periportal hepatic necrosis and inflammation. *Histopathology* **12**, 569–579.

Bataller, R., Nicolas, J.M., Gines, P., Esteve, A., Gorbig, M.N., Garcia-Ramallo *et al.* (1997) Arginine vassopressin induces contraction and stimulates growth of cultured human stellate cells. *Gastroenterology* **113**, 615–624.

Bauer, M., Paquette, N.C., Zhang, J.X., Bauer, I., Pannen, B.H.J., Kleeberger, S.R. *et al.* (1995) Chronic ethanol consumption increases hepatic sinusoidal contractile response to endothilin-1 in the rat. *Hepatology* **22**, 1565–1576.

Bhathal, P.S. (1972) Presence of modified fibroblasts in cirrhotic livers in man. *Pathology* **4**, 139–144.

Bedossa, P., Houglum, K., Holstege, A. and Chojkier, M. (1994) Stimulation of collagen α, (I) gene expression is associated with lipid peroxidation in hepatocellular injury: a link to tissue fibrosis. *Hepatology* **19**, 1262–1271.

Biagni, G. and Ballardini, G. (1989) Liver fibrosis and extracellular matrix. *J Hepatol* **8**, 115–124.

Bissell, D.M. (1997) Regulation of fibronectin (FN) expression in sinusoidal endothelial cells and hepatocytes distinct patterns of binding to the proximal promoter region. *Hepatology* **26**, 336A.

Bissell, D.M., Friedman, S.L., Maher, J.J. and Roll, F.J. (1990) Connective tissue biology and hepatic fibrosis: report of a conference. *Hepatology* **11**, 488–498.

Bissell, D.M., Wang, F.S. and Timmons, C. (1997) Expression of the hyaluronate receptor CD44 by liver stellate cells: splice isoforms in wound repair and role in cell migration. *Molec Biol Cell* **8**, 396A.

Blazejewskin, S., LeBoil, B., Boussarie, L., Blanc, J.-F., Malaval, L., Okubo, K. *et al.* (1997) Osteonectin (SPARC) expression in human liver and in cultured human liver myofibroblasts. *Am J Pathol* **151**, 651–657.

Bravo, R. and MacDonald-Bravo, H. (1985) Changes in the nuclear distribution of cyclin (PCNA) but not its synthesis depend on DNA replication. *EMBO J* **4**, 655–661.

Casini, A., Cunningham, M., Rojkind, M. and Lieber, C.S. (1991) Acetaldehyde increases procollagen type I and fibronectin gene transcription in cultured rat fat-storing cells through a protein synthesis-dependent mechanism. *Hepatology* **13**, 758–765.

Casini, A., Pinzani, M., Milani, S., Gappone, C., Galli, G., Jezequel, A.M. *et al.* (1993) Regulation of excellular matrix synthesis by transforming growth factor β_1 in human fat-storing cells. *Gastroenterology* **105**, 245–253.

Casini, A., Cani, E., Salzano, R., Biondi, P., Paola, M., Galli, A. *et al.* (1997) Neutrophil-derived superoxide anion induces lipid peroxidation and stimulates collagen synthesis in human hepatic stellate cells: role of nitric oxide. *Hepatology* **25**, 361–367.

Chedid, A., Mendenhall, C.L., Gartside, P., French, S.W., Chen, T., Robin, L. and the VA Cooperative Study Group (1991) Prognostic factors in alcoholic liver disease. *Am J Gastroenterol* **86**, 210–216.

Chedid, A., Mendenhall, C.L., Moritz, T.E., French, S.W., Morgan, T.R., Rosell, G.A. *et al.* and Veterans Affairs Cooperative Study Group 275 (1993a) Cell-mediated hepatic injury in alcoholic liver disease. *Gastroenterology* **105**, 254–266.

Chedid, A., Mendenhall, C.L., Moritz, T.E., French, S.W., Chen, T.S., Morgan, T.R. *et al.* and the VA Cooperative Study Group No. 275 (1993b) Expression CD29 (β1) integrin in receptor and CD45 in alcoholic liver disease. *Am J Gastroenterol* **88**, 1920–1927.

Clement, B., Grimand, J.-A., Campion, J.-P., Dengnier, Y. and Gouillouzo, A. (1986) Cell types involved in collagen and fibronectin production in normal and fibrotic human liver. *Hepatology* **6**, 225–234.

Clot, P., Parola, M., Bellomo, G., Dianzani, U., Carini, R., Tabone, M. *et al.* (1997) Plasma membrane hydroxyethyl radical adducts cause antibody-dependent cytotoxicity in rat hepatocytes exposed to alcohol. *Gastroenterology* **113**, 265–276.

Cocjin, J., Rosenthal, P., Buslon, V., Luk Jr., L., Barajas, L., Geller, S.A. *et al.* (1996) Bile ductule formation in fetal, neonatal, and infant livers compared with extrahepatic biliary atresia. *Hepatology* **24**, 568–574.

David, B.H. (1988) Transforming growth factor β responsiveness is modulated by the extracellular collagen matrix during hepatic Ito cell culture. *J Cell Physiol* **136**, 547–553.

Demetris, A.J., Seaberg, E.C., Wennerberg, A., Lonellie, J. and Michalopoulos, G. (1996) Ductular reaction after submassive necrosis in humans: special emphasis on analysis of ductular hepatocytes. *Am J Pathol* **149**, 439–448.

Denk, H. and Krepler, R. (1982) The cytoskeleton in pathological conditions. *Pathol Res Proct* **175**, 180–195.

Desmet, V.J. (1985) Intrahepatic bile ducts under the lens. *J Hepatol* **1**, 545–559.

Desmet, V.J. (1986) Current problems in diagnosis of biliary disease and cholestasis. *Semin Liver Dis* **6**, 233–245.

DeVos, R. and Desmet, V. (1992) Ultrastructural characteristics of novel epithelial cell types identified in human pathologic liver specimens with chronic ductular reaction. *Am J Pathol* **140**, 1441–1450.

Edmondson, H.A., Peter, R.L., Reynolds, T.B. and Kuzma, O.T. (1963) Sclerosing hyaline necrosis of the liver in the chronic alcoholic: a recognizable clinical syndrome. *Ann Intern Med* **59**, 646–672.

Ericksson, S., Fraser, J.R.E., Laurent, T.C., Pertoft, H. and Smedsrod, B. (1983) Endothelial cells are a site of uptake and degradation of hyaluronic acid: a whole body autoradiographic study. *Cell Tissue Res* **222**, 285–293.

Factor, V.M., Radaeva, S.A. and Thorgiersson, S.S. (1994) Origin and fate of oval cells in dipin-induced hepatocarcinogenesis in the mouse. *Am J Pathol* **145**, 409–422.

French, S.W., Sim, J.S., Franks, K.E., Burbige, E.J., Denton, T. and Caldwell, M.G. (1977) Alcoholic hepatitis. In *Alcohol and the Liver*, edited by M.M. Fisher and J.G. Rankin, pp. 261–286. New York: Plenum Publ Corp.

French, S.W., Burbige, E.J., Tarder, G., Bourke, E., Harkin, C.G. and Denton, T. (1979) Lymphocyte sequestration by the liver in alcoholic hepatitis. *Arch Pathol Lab Med* **103**, 146–152.

French, S.W., Benson, N.C. and Sun, P.S. (1984) Centrilobular liver necrosis induced by hypoxia in chronic ethanol-fed rats. *Hepatology* **4**, 912–917.

French, S.W., Miyamoto, K. and Tsukamoto, H. (1986) Ethanol-induced hepatic fibrosis in the rat: role of the amount of dietary fat. *Alcoholism: Clin Exp Res* **10**, 13S–19S.

French, S.W., Wong, K., Nanji, A., Arseneau, R. and Mendenhall, C. (1988a) The role of the Ito cell in fibrogenesis in alcoholic liver disease. In *Biomedical and Social Aspects of Alcohol and Alcoholism*, edited by K. Kuriyama, A. Takada and H. Ishii, pp. 767–773. Elsevier Sci Publ.: Biomedical Division.

French, S.W., Miyamoto, K., Wong, K., Jui, L. and Briere, L. (1988b) Role of the Ito cell in liver parenchymal fibrosis in rats fed alcohol and a high fat low protein diet. *Am J Pathol* **132**, 73–85.

French, S.W., Nanji, A., Shannon, J. and Mendenhall, C.L. (1988c) Effect of the type of dietary fat on experimentally induced alcoholic liver injury in the rat. *Biomedical and Social Aspects of Alcohol and Alcoholism* edited by K. Kuriyama, A. Takada and H. Ishii, pp. 643–649. Elsevier Sci Publ BV (Biomedical Division).

French, S.W. (1992) Nutritional factors in the pathogenesis of alcoholic liver disease. In *Nutrition and Alcohol*, edited by B. Watzl and R. Watson, pp. 337–362. Boca Raton: CRC Press Inc.

French, S.W., Nash, J., Shitabata, P., Kachi, K., Hara, C., Chedid, A. *et al.* and the VA Cooperative Study Group 119 (1993a) Pathology of alcoholic liver disease. *Semin Liver Dis* **13**, 154–169.

French, S.W., Kim, W., Jui, L., Albano, E., Hagbjork, A.-L. and Ingelman-Sundberg, M. (1993b) Effect of ethanol on cytochrome P450 2E1 (CYP2E1), lipid peroxidation and serium protein adduct formation in relation to liver pathology pathogenesis. *Exp Molec Pathol* **58**, 61–75.

French, S.W. (1994) Cytoskeleton: intermediate filaments. In *The Liver: Biology and Pathobiology*, 3rd edn, edited by I.M. Arias, J.L. Boyer, N. Fausto, W.B. Jakoby, D.A. Schachter and D.A. Shafritz, pp. 33–44, New York: Raven Press, Ltd.

French, S.W., Morimoto, M. and Tsukamoto, H. (1995) Animal models of alcohol-associated liver injury. In *Alcoholic Liver Disease*, 2nd edn, edited by P. Hall, pp. 279–296. London: Edward Arnold.

French, S.W. (1996) Ethanol and hepatocellular injury. *Clin Lab Med* **16**, 289–306.

Friedman, S.L. and Arthur M.J.P. (1989) Activation of cultured rat hepatic lipocytes by Kupffer cell conditioned medium: direct enhancement of matrix synthesis and stimulation of cell proliferation via induction of platelet derived growth factor receptors. *J Clin Invest* **84**, 1780–1785.

Friedman, S.L. (1993) The cellular basis of hepatic fibrosis: mechanisms and treatment strategies. *NEJ Med* **328**, 1828–1835.

Friedman, S.L. (1996) Hepatic stellate cells. *Progress Liver Dis* **14**, 101–130.

Friedman, S.L. (1997) Molecular mechanisms of hepatic fibrosis and principals of therapy. *J Gastroenterol* **32**, 420–424.

Fuji, K., Evarts, R.P., Hu, Z., Marsden, E.R. and Thorgeirsson, S.C. (1994) Expression of stem cell factor and its receptor c-kit during liver regeneration from putative stem cells in adult rat. *Lab Invest* **70**, 511–516.

Gillis, S.E. and Nagy, L.E. (1997) Deposition of cellular fibronectin increases before stellate cell activation in rat liver during ethanol feeding. *Alcoholism: Clin Exp Res* **21**, 857–861.

Gressner, A.M. and Bachem, M.G. (1990) Cellular sources of noncollagenous matrix proteins: role of fat-storing cells in fibrogenesis. *Seminar Liver Dis* **10**, 30–40.

Hall, P., de la, M., Plummer, J.L., Ilsley, A.H. and Cousins, M.J. (1991) Hepatic fibrosis and cirrhosis after chronic administration of alcohol and "low-dose" carbon tetrachloride vapor in the rat. *Hepatology* **13**, 815–819.

Hasumura, Y., Izumi, N., Sakai, Y. and Takeuchi, J. (1988) Lymphocyte infiltration in the liver in patients with alcoholic hepatitis. In *Biomedical and Social Aspects of Alcohol and Alcoholism*, edited by K. Kuriyama, A. Takada and H. Ishii, pp. 779–782, Elsevier Sci Publ BV: Biomedical Division.

Hausset, C., Rockey, D.C. and Bissell, D.M. (1993) Endothelin receptors in rat liver: lipocytes as a contractile target for endothelin 1. *Proc Nat Acad Sci USA* **90**, 9266–9270.

Hellerbrand, C., Wang, S.C., Tsukamoto, H., Brenner, D.A. and Rippe, R.A. (1996) Expression of intercellular adhesion molecule 1 by activated hepatic stellate cells. *Hepatology* **24**, 670–676.

Herbst, H., Wege, T., Milani, S., Pellegrini, G., Orzechowski, H.-D., Bechstein, W.O. *et al.* (1997) Tissue inhibitor of metalloproteinase-1 and 2 RNA expression in rat and human liver fibrosis. *Am J Pathol* **150**, 1647–1659.

Hogemann, B. and Domschke, W. (1993) Hepatic fibrosis-current concepts of pathogenesis and therapy. *Gastroenterol Jap* **28**, 570–579.

Horn, T., Junge, J. and Christoffersen, P. (1985) Early alcoholic liver injury: changes of the Disse space in acinar zone 3. *Liver* **5**, 301–310.

Iredale, J.P., Benyon, R.C., Arthur, M.J.P., Ferris, W.F., Alcolado, R., Winwood, P.J. *et al.* (1996) Tissue inhibitor of metalloproteinase-1 messenger RNA expression is enhanced relative to interstitial collagenase messenger RNA in experimental liver injury and fibrosis. *Hepatology* **24**, 176–184.

Irle, C., Kocher, O. and Gabbiani, G. (1980) Contractility of myofibroblasts during experimental liver cirrhosis. *J Submicrosc Cytol* **12**, 209–217.

Israel, Y. (1997) Antibodies against ethanol-derived protein adducts: pathogenic implications. *Gastroenterology* **113**, 353–355.

Johnson, S.J., Hines, J.E. and Burt, A.D. (1992) Macrophage and perisinusoidal cell kinetics in acute liver injury. *J Pathol* **166**, 351–358.

Katsuma, Y., Swierenga, S.H.H., Khettey, U., Marceau, N. and French, S.W. (1987) Changes in the cytokeratin intermediate filament cytoskeleton associated with Mallory body formation in mouse and human liver. *Hepatology* **7**, 1215–1223.

Kawada, N., Kuroki, T., Kobayashi, K., Inoue, M., Kanida, K. and Decker, K. (1995) Action of endothelins on hepatic stellate cells. *J Gastroenterol* **30**, 731–738.

Kawahara, H., Matsuda, Y., Takase, S. and Takada, A. (1993) Migration and contraction of cultured Ito cells. *Intern Hepatol Commun* **1**, 307.

Kimoff, R.J. and Huang, S. (1981) Immunocytochemical and immunoelectron microscopic studies on Mallory bodies. *Lab Invest* **45**, 491–453.

Knittel, T., Armbrust, T., Schwogler, S., Schuppan, D. and Ramadori, G. (1992) Distribution and cellular origin of induction in rat liver. *Lab Invest* **67**, 779–787.

Kovacs, E.J. and Difietro, L.A. (1994) Fibrogenic cytokines and connective tissue production. *FASEB J* **8**, 854–861.

Krull, N.B., Zimmermann, T. and Gressner, A.M. (1993) Special and temporal patterns of gene expression for hte proteoglycans biglycan and deiorin and for transforming growth factor B_1 revealed by *in situ* hybridization during experimentally induced liver fibrosis in the rat. *Hepatology* **18**, 581–589.

Kurki, P., Miettinen, A., Salaspuro, I., Virtanen, I. and Stenman, S. (1983) Cytoskeleton antibodies in chronic active hepatitis, primary biliary cirrhosis and alcoholic liver disease. *Hepatology* **3**, 297–302.

Lee, K.S., Buck, M., Houglum, K. and Chojkier, M. (1995) Activation of hepatic stellate cells by TGF alpha and collagen type I is mediated by oxidative stress through c-myb expression. *J Clin Invest* **96**, 2461–2168.

Lenzi, R., Liu, M.H., Tarsetti, F., Slott, P.A., Alpini, G., Zhai, W.-R. *et al.* (1992) Histogenesis of bile duct-like cells proliferating during ethionine hepatocarcinogenesis: evidence for a biliary eptihelial nature of oval cells. *Lab Invest* **66**, 390–402.

Li, J., Rosman, A.S., Leo, M.A., Nagai, Y. and Lieber, C.S. (1994) Tissue inhibitor of mella-proteinase is increased in the serum of precirrhotic alcoholic patients and can serve as a marker of fibrosis. *Hepatology* **19**, 1418–1423.

Maher, J.J. and Friedman, S.L. (1995) Pathogenesis of hepatic fibrosis. In *Alcoholic Liver Disease: Pathology and Pathogenesis,* 2nd edn, edited by P. Hall, pp. 71–88. London: Edward Arnold.

Maher, J.J., Shaheen, Z. and Tzogarakis, C. (1994) Acetaldehyde-induced stimulation of collagen synthesis and gene expression is dependent on conditions of cell culture: Studies with rat lipocytes and fibroblasts. *Alcoholism: Clin Exp Res* **18**, 403–409.

Maher, J.J. and Tzagarakis, C. (1994) Partial cloning of the M subunit of laminin from adult rat lipocytes: Expression of the M subunit by cells isolated from normal and injured liver. *Hepatology* **19**, 764–770.

Mak, K.M. and Lieber, C.S. (1988) Lipocytes and transitional cells in alcoholic liver disease: a morphometric study. *Hepatology* **8**, 1027–1033.

Mallat, A., Preaux, A.-M., Blazejewski, S., Rosenbaum, J., Dhumeaux, D. and Mavier, P. (1995) Interferon alfa and gamma inhibit proliferation and collagen synthesis of human Ito cells in culture. *Hepatology* **21**, 1003–1010.

Marra, F., Valente, A.J., Pinzani, M. and Abboud, H.E. (1993) Cultured human liver fat-storing cells by proinflammatory cytokines. *J Clin Invest* **92**, 1674–1680.

Martinez-Hernandez, A. (1985) The hepatic extracellular matrix. II Electron immuno-histochemical studies in rats with CCl_4-induced cirrhosis. *Lab Invest* **53**, 166–186.

Matsumoto, K., Fujii, H., Michalopoulos, G., Feng, J.J. and Demtris, A.J. (1994) Human biliary epithelial cells secrete and respond to cytokines and hepatocyte growth factors *in vitro*: interleukin-6, hepatocyte growth factor and epidermal growth factor promote DNA synthesis *in vitro*. *Hepatology* **20**, 376–382.

Matsuoka, M., Pham, N.-T. and Tsukamoto, H. (1989) Differential effects of interleukin-1 alpha, tumor necrosis factor alpha and transforming growth factor beta 1 on cell prolifera-tion and collagen formation by cultured fat-storing cells. *Liver* **9**, 71–78.

Matsuoka, M. and Tsukamoto, H. (1990) Stimulation of hepatic lipocyte collagen production by Kupffer cell-derived transforming growth factor β: implication for a pathogenetic role in alcoholic liver fibrogenesis. *Hepatology* **11**, 599–605.

Mayer, J.J., Friedman, S.L., Roll, F.J. and Bissell, D.M. (1988) Immunolocalization of laminin in normal rat liver and biosynthesis of laminin by hepatic lipocytes in primary culture. *Gastroenterology* **94**, 1053–1062.

Meyer, D.H., Bachem, M.G. and Gressner, A.M. (1990) Modulation of hepatic lipocyte proteoglycan synthesis and proliferation by Kupffer cell-derived transforming growth factors type β1 and α1. *Biochem Biophys Res Commun* **171**, 1122–1129.

Meyer, D.H., Krull, N., Dreher, K.L. and Gressner, A.M. (1992) Biglycan and decorin gene expression in normal and fibrotic rat liver: cellular localization and regulatory factors. *Hepatology* **16**, 204–216.

Morimoto, M., Zern, M.A., Hagbjork, A.-L., Ingelman-Sundberg, M. and French, S.W. (1994) Fish oil alcohol and liver pathology: role of cytochrome P450 2E1. *Proc Soc Exp Biol Med* **207**, 197–205.

Moshage, H., Casini, A. and Lieber, C.S. (1990) Acetaldehyde selectively stimulates collagen production in cultured rat liver fat-storing cells but not in hepatocytes. **12**, 511–518.

Mullhaupt, B., Feren, A., Fodor, E. and Jones, A. (1994) Liver expression of epidermal growth factor RNA: rapid increases in immediate-early phase of liver regeneration. *J Biol Chem* **269**, 19667–19670.

Nagay, P., Schaft, Z. and Lapis, K. (1991) Immunohistochemical detection of transforming growth factor-β1 in fibrotic liver diseases. *Hepatology* **14**, 269–273.

Nakano, M., Worner, T.M. and Lieber, C.S. (1982) Perivenular fibrosis in alcoholic liver injury: ultrastructure and histologic progression. *Gastroenterology* **83**, 777–785.

Nanji, A.A., Tahan, S.R., Khwaja, S., Yacoub, L.K. and Sadrzadeh, S.M.H. (1996) Elevated plasma levels of hyaluronic acid indicate endothelial dysfunction in the initial stages of alcoholic liver disease in the rat. *J Hepatol* **24**, 368–374.

Ogawa, K., Suzuki, J.-I., Mukai, H. and Mori, M. (1986) Sequential changes of extracellular matrix and proliferation of Ito cells with enhanced expression of desmin and actin in focal hepatic injury. *Am J Pathol* **125**, 611–619.

Okanoue, T., Burbige, E.J. and French, S.W. (1983) The role of the Ito cell in perivenular and intralobular fibrosis in alcoholic hepatitis. *Arch Pathol Lab Med* **107**, 459–463.

Pares, A., Deulofeu, R., Gimenez, A., Caballeria, L., Bruguera, M., Caballeria, J. *et al.* (1996) Serum hyaluronate reflects hepatic fibrogenesis in alcoholic liver disease and is useful as a marker of fibrosis. *Hepatology* **24**, 1399–1403.

Pinzani, M., Gentilini, A., Cliquiri, A., DeFranco, R., Pellegrini, G., Milani, S. *et al.* (1985) Transforming growth factor β1 regulates platelet-derived growth factor receptor β subunit in human liver fat-storing cells. *Hepatology* **21**, 232–239.

Pinzani, M., Gesualdo, L., Sabbah, G.M. and Abboud, H.E. (1989) Effects of platelet-derived growth factor and other polypetide mitogens on DNA synthesis and growth of cultured rat liver fat-storing cells. *J Clin Invest* **84**, 1786–1793.

Pinzani, M., Abboud, H.E. and Aron, D.C. (1990) Secretion of insulin-like growth factor-1 and binding proteins by rat liver fat-storing cells: regulatory role of platelet-derived growth factor. *Endocrinology* **127**, 2343–2349.

Pinzani, M., Milani, S., Herbst, H., DeFranco, R., Grappone, C., Gentilini, A. *et al.* (1996) Expression of platelet-derived growth factor and its receptors in normal human liver and during active hepatic fibrogenesis. *Am J Pathol* **148**, 785–800.

Racine-Sampson, R., Rockey, D.C. and Bissell, D.M. (1997) Expression of the collagen-binding integrins α1, β1 and α2 β1 during activation of rat hepatic stellate cells *in vivo*. *J Biol Chem*.

Raghow, R. (1994) The role of extracellular matrix in post inflammatory wound healing and fibrosis. *FASEB J* **8**, 823–831.

Ramadori, G. (1991) The stellate cell (Ito-cell, fat-storing cell, lipocyte, perisinusoidal cell) of the liver: new insights into pathophysiology of an intriguing cell. *Virochows Archiv B Cell Pathol* **61**, 147–158.

Ramadori, G., Schwogler, S., Veit, T., Rieder, H., Chiquet-Ehrismann, R., Mackie, E.J. *et al.* (1991) Tensascin gene expression in rat liver and rat liver cells. *Virch Arch B Cell Pathol* **60**, 145–153.

Ray, M.B., Mendenhall, C.L., French, S.W., Gartside, P.S. and Veterans Administration Cooperative Study Group (1988) Serum vitamin A deficiency and increased intrahepatic expression of cytokeratin antigen in alcoholic liver disease. *Hepatology* **8**, 1019–1026.

Ray, M.B., Mendenhall, C.L., French, S.W., Gartside, P.S. and the Veterans Administration Cooperative Study Group (1993) Bile duct changes in alcoholic liver disease. *Liver* **13**, 36–45.

Reid, L.M., Fiorino, A.S., Sigal, S.H., Brill, S. and Holst, P.A. (1997) Extracellular matrix gradients in the space of Disse: relevance to liver biology. *Hepatology* **15**, 1198–1203.

Rockey, D. (1997) The cellular pathogenesis of portal hypertension: stellate cell contractility, endothelin, and nitric oxide. *Hepatology* **25**, 2–5.

Rockey, D.C. and Chung, J.J. (1995) Inducible nitric oxide synthase in rat hepatic lipocytes and the effect of nitric oxide on lipocyte contractility. *J Clin Invest* **95**, 1199–1206.

Rockey, D.C. and Wesiger, R.A. (1996) Endothelin induced contractility of stellate cells from normal and cirrhotic rat liver: implications for regulation of portal pressure and resistance. *Hepatology* **24**, 233–240.

Rojkind, M., Giambrone, M.A. and Biempica, L. (1979) Collagen types in normal and cirrhotic human liver. *Gastroenterology* **76**, 710–719.

Sakamoto, M., Veno, T., Kin, M., Ohira, H., Torimura, T., Inuzuka, S. *et al.* (1993) Ito cell contraction in response to endothelin-1 and substance P. *Hepatology* **18**, 978–983.

Sarraf, C.E., Lalani, E.-N., Golding, M. *et al.* (1994) Cell behavior in acetalminofluorene-treated regenerating rat liver: light and electron microscopic observations. *Am J Pathol* **145**, 1114–1126.

Schaffner, F. and Popper, H. (1963) Capillarization of hepatic sinusoids in man. *Gastroenterology* **44**, 239–242.

Schmitt-Gräff, A., Grüger, S., Bochard, F., Gabbiani, G. and Denk, H. (1991) Modulation of alpha smooth muscle actin and desmin expression in perisinusoidal cells of normal and diseased human livers. *Am J Pathol* **138**, 1233–1242.

Seyer, J.M., Huheson, E.T. and Kang, A.H. (1979) Collagen polymorphism in normal and cirrhotic human liver. *J Clin Invest* **59**, 241–248.

Shiratori, Y., Ichida, T., Kawase, T. and Wisse, E. (1986) Effect of acetaldehyde on collagen synthesis by fat-storing cells isolated from rats treated with carbon tetrachloride. *Liver* **6**, 246–251.

Sprenger, H., Kaufmann, A., Garn, H., Lahine, B., Gemsa, D. and Gressner, A.M. (1997) Induction of neutrophil-attracting chemokines in transforming rat hepatic stellate cells. *Gastroenterology* **113**, 277–285.

Takahara, T., Furui, K., Funaki, J., Nakayama, Y., Itoh, H., Miyabayashi, C. *et al.* (1995) Increased expression of matrix metalloproteinase-II in experimental liver fibrosis in rats. *Hepatology* **21**, 787–795.

Takahara, T., Furui, K., Yata, Y., Jin, B., Zhang, L.P., Nambu, S. *et al.* (1997) Dual expression of matrix metalloproteinase-Z and membrane-type matrix metalloproteinase in fibrotic human livers. *Hepatology* **26**, 1521–1529.

Takahashi, H., Geoffrion, Y., Butler, K.W. and French, S.W. (1990) *In vivo* hepatic energy metabolism during the progression of alcoholic liver disease: a noninvasive ^{31}P nuclear magnetic resonance study in rats. *Hepatology* **11**, 65–73.

Takahashi, H., Wong, K., Jui, L., Nanji, A.A., Mendenhall, C.S. and French, S.W. (1991) Effect of dietary fat on Ito cells activation by chronic ethanol intake: a long-term serial morphometric study on alcohol-fed and control rats. *Alcoholism: Clin Exp Res* **15**, 1060–1066.

Tamaka, K., Yamashita, A. and Okita, K. (1993) Immunohistological detection of PCNA/ cyclic in paraffin-embedded liver tissue. *Intern Hepatol Commun* **1**, 97–103.

Theret, N., Musso, O., L'Helgoulch, A. and Clement, B. (1997) Activation of matrix metalloproteinase-Z from hepatic stellate cells requires interactions with hepatocytes. *Am J Pathol* **150**, 51–58.

Thorgeirsson, S.S., Evarts, R.P., Bisgaard, H.C., Fujio, K. and Hu, Z. (1993) Hepatic stem cell compartment: activation and lineage commitment. *Proc Soc Exp Biol Med* **204**, 253–260.

Thorgiersson, S.S. (1996) Hepatic stem cells in liver regeneration. *FASEB J* **10**, 1249–1256.

Thurman, R., Bradford, B.U., Iimuro, Y., Knecht, K.T., Connor, H.D., Adachi, Y. *et al.* (1997) Role of Kupffer cells, endotoxin and free radicals in hepatotoxicity due to prolonged alcohol consumption: studies in female and male rats. *J Nutr* **127**, 903S–906S.

Tsukamoto, H., Towner, S.J., Ciofalo, L.M. and French, S.W. (1986) Ethanol-induced liver fibrosis in rats fed high fat diet. *Hepatology* **6**, 814–822.

Tsukamoto, H., Gaal, K. and French, S.W. (1990) Insights into the pathogenesis of alcoholic liver necrosis and fibrosis: status report. *Hepatology* **12**, 599–608.

Tsukamoto, H., Matsuoka, M. and French, S.W. (1990) Experimental models of hepatic fibrosis: a review. *Semin Liver Dis* **10**, 56–65.

Tsukamoto, H., Horne, W., Kamimura, S., Niemela, O., Parkkila, S., Yla-Herttuala, S. *et al.* (1995) Experimental liver cirrhosis induced by alcohol and iron. *J Clin Invest* **96**, 620–630.

Tsutsumi, M., Urashima, S., Matsuda, Y., Takase, S. and Takada, A. (1993a) Changes in type IV collagen content in livers of patients with alcoholic liver disease. *Hepatology* **17**, 820–827.

Tsutsumi, M., Urashima, S., Nakase, K., Takase, S. and Takada, A. (1993b) Type IV collagen and laminin contents of livers from patients with alcoholic liver disease. *Alcohol Alcoholism* **28**, 45–52.

Tsutsumi, M., Takase, S., Urashima, Y., Ueshima, Y., Kawahara, H. and Takada, A. (1996) Serum markers for hepatic fibrosis in alcoholic liver disease: which is the best marker, type III procollagen, type IV collagen, laminin, tissue inhibitor of metalloproteinase, or prolyl hydroxylase? *Alcoholism: Clin Exp Res* **20**, 1512–1517.

Urashima, S., Tsutsumi, M., Nakase, K., Wang, J.-S. and Takada, A. (1993) Studies on capillarization of the hepatic sinusoids in alcoholic liver disease. *Alcohol Alcoholism* **28**, 77–84.

Van Eyken, P., Sciot, R. and Desmet, V.J. (1998) A cytokeratin immunohistochemical study of alcohol liver disease: evidence that hepatocytes can express 'bile duct-type' cytokeratins. *Histopathology* **13**, 605–617.

Veno, T., Inuzuka, S., Torimura, T., Tamaki, S., Koh, H., Kin, M. *et al.* (1993) Serum hyaluronate reflects hepatic sinusoidal capillarization. *Gastroenterology* **105**, 475–481.

Vitala, K., Israel, Y., Blake, J.E. and Niemela, O. (1997) Serum IgA, IgG and IgM antibodies directed against acetaldehyde-derived epitopes: relationship to liver disease severity and alcohol consumption. *Hepatology* **25**, 1418–1424.

Weiner, F.R., Giambone, M.A., Czaja, M.J., Shah, A., Annoni, G., Takahashi, S. *et al.* (1990) Ito-cell gene expression and collagen regulation. *Hepatology* **11**, 111–117.

Win, K.M., Charlotte, F., Mallat, A., Cherqui, D., Martin, N., Mavier, P. *et al.* (1993) Mitogenic effect of transforming growth factor-β_1 on human Ito cells in culture: evidence for mediation by endogenous plated-derived growth factor. *Hepatology* **18**, 137–145.

Wong, L., Yamasaki, G., Johnson, R.J. and Friedman, S.L. (1994) Induction of betal-platelet-derived growth factor receptor in rat hepatic lipocytes during cellular activation *in vivo* and in culture. *J Clin Invest* **94**, 1563–1569.

Worner, T.M. and Lieber, C.S. (1985) Perivenular fibrosis as precursor lesion of cirrhosis. *JAMA* **253**, 627, 630.

Yuan, Q.X., Marceau, N., French, B.A., Fu, P. and French, S.W. (1995) Heat shock *in vivo* induces Mallory body formation in drug primed mouse liver. *Exp Molec Pathol* **63**, 63–76.

Yuan, Q.X., Marceau, N., French, B.A., Fu, P. and French, S.W. (1996) Mallory body induction in drug-primed mouse liver. *Hepatology* **24**, 603–612.

Direct and indirect consequences of alcohol metabolism

Part IV

Direct and indirect
consequences of
alcohol metabolism

Chapter 4

Genetics of ethanol metabolism and alcoholic liver disease

Paul Y. Kwo and David W. Crabb

The metabolism of ethanol in part determines its pharmacological properties and toxicity. Ethanol metabolizing systems, including alcohol and aldehyde dehydrogenases and cytochrome P450 2E1, are genetically polymorphic. Inheritance of high activity ADH2*2 has been associated with decreased drinking and risk of alcoholism, and is probably associated with increased risk of liver damage with heavy drinking. Inheritance of the dominant negative ALDH2*2 allele markedly reduces alcohol consumption and risk of alcoholism, but also may predispose to increased hepatic toxicity of alcohol. ALDH2*2 is also associated with increased risk of esophageal and upper airway cancer. Thus, inheritance of enzyme variants which would be expected to lead to increased intrahepatic production of acetaldehyde (high activity ADH) or reduced disposal of acetaldehyde (inactive ALDH2) appear to correlate with aversion to drinking. Individuals who persist in heavy drinking despite the aversive reactions may be at increased risk of liver injury. Promoter variants of cytochrome P450 2E1 have been studied in many populations for association with alcoholic liver disease or alcoholism, but the results have been controversial. A number of other genetic variations have been reported in association with alcoholic liver disease, and these findings need to be confirmed.

KEYWORDS: ethanol, pharmacokinetics, genetics, stomach, liver, alcohol dehydrogenase, aldehyde dehydrogenase, cytochrome P450, pharmacogenetics, liver disease, alcoholism, enzyme

ETHANOL METABOLISM

The genetic factors modulating ethanol metabolism are important for several reasons. To date, these factors are the best understood genes that influence susceptibility to alcoholism; second, they are the only factors so far identified that appear to alter the risk of alcoholic liver disease. The metabolism of ethanol and its long-term effects on the liver and other organs can be considered from at least two standpoints. First, ethanol is a drug and its absorption, pharmacokinetics, pharmacodynamics and toxicity can and have been studied like those of other drugs. Inherited differences in the metabolism of ethanol might predispose certain individuals to toxic effects of ethanol. Inherited risk of ethanol toxicity could therefore be considered as a pharmacogenetic problem. However, unlike any other drug, ethanol is also a nutrient. It is ingested in far larger quantities than any other drug, and it shares the metabolic pathways used for catabolism of macronutrients such as carbohydrate and lipids. Thus, the effects of ethanol include both primary effects on the central nervous system as well as secondary effects on a variety of other pathways. These secondary effects, being influenced by the rate of alcohol metabolism, may also be subject to inter-individual variation. This chapter will review the disposition of ethanol, emphasizing particularly the hepatic and gastric enzymes involved in its metabolism. The regulation of this short metabolic pathway will be discussed as well as the genetic variants of the enzymes that can contribute to differences among individuals in ethanol metabolism. It will also examine the notion that alcoholic liver disease represents a pharmacogenetic disorder for which certain individuals are predisposed because of their inherited complement of ethanol metabolizing enzymes.

Gastrointestinal absorption and first pass metabolism

First pass metabolism is the difference between the amount of a drug administered orally and the amount reaching the systemic circulation. Conceptually, it refers to metabolism of the drug by the gut during absorption or liver during the "first pass" of the drug through that organ. The gastrointestinal tract, just like the liver, expresses drug metabolizing enzymes such as cytochrome P450s and alcohol dehydrogenases. First pass metabolism is important because it reduces the amount of drug reaching the target organs. Ingested ethanol is absorbed slowly from the stomach and very rapidly from the upper small intestine. The fraction absorbed transgastrically may be subject to metabolism. Ethanol leaving the gut is then carried to the liver, where a fraction is metabolized before leaving that organ.

Lieber's group pioneered studies on first pass metabolism of ethanol in animals and humans. They established that first pass metabolism was the easiest to detect with low doses of ethanol (0.3 g/kg, equivalent to approximately 20 grams of ethanol or two social drinks for a 70 kg individual) when gastric emptying is not rapid, for example, when the ethanol is taken with a meal. Experimentally, the concentration of ethanol in the blood (BAC, blood alcohol concentration) at various times after ethanol administration is measured and the areas under the blood alcohol concentration curves (AUC) are calculated for ethanol administered orally or intravenously (Julkunen et al., 1985; Caballeria et al., 1987). The area under the BAC curve was greater for the intravenous dose than for the oral dose, indicating the existence of first pass metabolism. Larger doses of ethanol make the difference between the AUCs, too small to measure accurately.

The phenomenon of first pass metabolism is well established, but the organ in which it occurs is not (Figure 4.1). Many findings favor the stomach as a major site (Lim et al., 1993). Gastric mucosa contains several ADHs (γ-ADH, χ-ADH and σ-ADH, discussed in more detail, see below) that could be involved in metabolism of ethanol. Under circumstances in which gastric ADH activity was reported to be decreased (e.g., in women (Frezza et al., 1990; Seitz et al., 1993), individuals with atrophic gastritis, alcoholics (DiPadova et al., 1987) and individuals taking certain medications (Cabelleria et al., 1991; Roine et al., 1990)), first pass metabolism was reduced. σ-ADH, a major gastric ADH isozyme, has been reported to be absent in the stomach of about 30% of Asian subjects, and as a group, those lacking this enzyme had lower first pass metabolism of ethanol (Dohmen et al., 1996), suggesting that σ-ADH is important in gastric oxidation of ethanol. First pass metabolism is strongly affected by the rate of gastric emptying, since slow gastric emptying, especially after eating, permits prolonged contact of the alcohol solution with the stom-

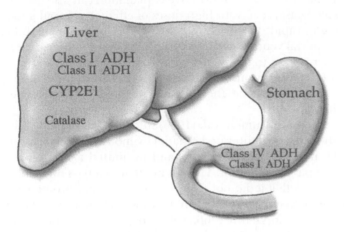

Figure 4.1 Metabolism of ethanol in stomach and liver. The various enzymes capable of oxidizing ethanol in the stomach and liver are indicated, as are the classes of ADH expressed in each organ. (see *Color Plate 4*)

ach and absorption of a greater fraction of the alcohol transgastrically. This would favor oxidation of ethanol in the stomach mucosal cells in transit. Rapid gastric emptying reduces first pass metabolism of alcohol, especially in the fasting state. Oral administration of alcohol resulted in a significantly higher blood alcohol level and AUC in the fasted as compared with the fed state (DiPadova *et al.*, 1987). All of these facts are consistent with an important role for the stomach mucosa in first pass metabolism of ethanol.

However, whether or not the stomach is the major site of first pass metabolism remains controversial. The assertion that gastric ADH (Yin *et al.*, 1997) or first pass metabolism (Ammon *et al.*, 1996) is reduced in women is contested, and other studies have found no correlation between gastric ADH activity and first pass metabolism (Brown *et al.*, 1995). In addition, calculation of the total ADH activity in the stomach, even when large surgical specimens are utilized for the assays, does not seem to account for the amount of ethanol that needs to be metabolized in order to observe the noted differences between oral and intravenous AUCs (Yin *et al.*, 1997). Another problem is the fact that the human and the rat σ-ADHs have markedly different kinetic properties. The K_m for ethanol for the human enzyme is 40 mmol/L, whereas for the rat enzyme is 80 times greater. Yet, first pass metabolism in the two species is similar. This has led to the suggestion that first pass metabolism of ethanol also occurs in the liver. Hepatic first pass metabolism is postulated to be dependent on the rate at which ethanol is absorbed; at lower rates (lower portal venous ethanol concentrations) ethanol is efficiently extracted whereas at higher rates (higher portal ethanol concentrations) the relatively low K_m hepatic ADH isozymes are saturated and ethanol reaches the systemic circulation sooner (Levitt, 1994). The area under the BAC curve is very sensitive to the rate of portal venous administration of ethanol. Slower rates of alcohol adminstration resulted in smaller areas under the curve in systemic venous blood samples, and very slow rates of administration resulted in virtually no ethanol reaching the bloodstream

(Levitt *et al.*, 1994; Smith *et al.*, 1992). This alternative explanation can also account for the lack of first pass metabolism seen with high doses of ethanol or rapid gastric emptying, thereby leading to rapid delivery of ethanol to the liver. On the other hand, it was reported that portal venous administration of ethanol to rats at a rate previously measured to correspond to the rate of gastric disappearance of ethanol resulted in higher blood ethanol concentrations than occurred after oral dosing (Lim *et al.*, 1993). This would argue that the stomach was able to metabolize a substantial amount of ethanol.

In an attempt to clarify this issue, Ammon *et al.* (1996) studied ethanol metabolism by giving ethanol intravenously and deuterated ethanol by mouth or into the duodenum. This reduced the intra-subject variability, and permitted an estimate of both gastric and hepatic first pass metabolism. They found that first pass metabolism was about 8–9% of the oral dose, that it did not differ between men and women, and that the gastric contribution to first pass metabolism was about 6% of the oral dose. Even this elegant study can be criticized (Crabb, 1997). It seems safe to conclude that first pass metabolism of oral ethanol is usually a small fraction (perhaps 10%) of total body ethanol elimination and when gastric emptying is rapid or the ethanol dose consumed is high, it is quantitatively even less important. Gender differences in first pass metabolism are probably not major (Ammon *et al.*, 1996; Schenker, 1997). It is not clear how all the data can be reconciled. The overall importance of first pass metabolism might lie in the potential for gastric first pass metabolism to protect the liver from low doses of ethanol, and for certain drugs to block first pass metabolism (Roine *et al.*, 1990; Caballeria *et al.*, 1991), resulting in intoxication from smaller than expected doses of ethanol.

Hepatic ethanol metabolism

Systemic ethanol metabolism is almost entirely hepatic, and until recently was exclusively quantified by following BAC after oral or IV bolus dosing. After blood alcohol concentration peaks, there is a pseudo-linear decline in blood alcohol concentration. This pseudo-linear phase results from the major alcohol oxidizing enzymes having relatively low K_m for ethanol; thus, they are saturated with respect to this substrate until its concentration falls below 40–50 mg%. At this point, the rate of alcohol disappearance begins to slow in a manner consistent with Michaelis-Menton enzyme kinetics. Alcohol elimination rates are typically expressed as the amount of alcohol cleared from the blood per unit time ($\beta 60$, mg/dl/hour) or as alcohol elimination rate (AER, mg/kg body weight/hour). Two aspects of alcohol elimination have attrracted substantial interest, gender differences and differences between individuals.

Many studies have compared alcohol elimination rates between genders because of the increased vulnerability of women to alcoholic liver disease (Schenker, 1997). However, these studies are difficult to compare because of lack of standardization of pharmacokinetic measurements, different concentrations of administered alcohol and different times of administration. Clearly, there are differences in body composition (Sutker *et al.*, 1983; Marshall *et al.*, 1983; Thomasson, 1995). Men have greater body water and less body fat than women of similar weight. As alcohol distributes in body water, there is a larger compartment in men than women for alcohol distribution. As a result, there is a tendency for oral dosing to result in higher BAC in women then men, which may increase alcohol clearance rates. As reviewed by Thomasson (1995), several of the gender studies concluded that women have faster alcohol metabolic rates than men as determined by β60 and by calculated elimination rates (Cole-Harding and Wilson, 1987; Thomasson *et al.*, 1995). Other studies have concluded that no gender differences occur (Sutker *et al.*, 1983; Marshall *et al.*, 1983; Goist and Sutker, 1985; Jones and Jones, 1996), including a large twin study (Martin *et al.*, 1985). The obvious hormonal differences between women and men have been invoked to explain the difference in alcohol metabolic rates in humans based on gender differences in rodents. Female rats have higher liver ADH activity than males. The differences are sex steroid-dependent (Rachamin *et al.*, 1980; Lumeng and Crabb, 1984), but probably mediated by differences in growth hormone secretion. This difference in enzyme activity has not been documented in humans.

There are two studies examining gender differences using intravenous administration of alcohol, thereby bypassing some of the gastric metabolism issues. In one study, ethanol was administered intravenously to nine brother-sister sibling pairs. This design reduced the amount of genetic variation between the subjects. There was a significantly higher rate of ethanol elimination in the nine women than in the men (Mishra *et al.*, 1989). However, the dose of alcohol was not adjusted for differences in lean body mass. Another study observed higher mean blood alcohol concentrations in females and noted a significantly lower apparent volume of distribution in females (Arthur *et al.*, 1984). No differences in ethanol elimination rates were found by this group.

More recently, two techniques have been combined to address this problem. First was a new method to simplify the measurement of ethanol oxidation rate. If alcohol is infused at a steady-state infusion rate that maintains a constant blood alcohol concentration (BAC), a so-called "alcohol clamp", that infusion rate is equal to the rate at which ethanol is removed from the vascular space. This measurement is independent of total body water. This technique is made possible by the ability to estimate arterial ethanol concentrations accurately and rapidly from the breath alcohol concentration (BrAC). Alcohol clamping can be achieved after an oral or IV loading dose and can achieve a clamping window of ±5 milligram per cent (mg%). The rate of alcohol administration in the equilibrated steady state yields a direct measure of the AER, and changes in the AER are reflected in different rates of administration (O'Connor *et al.*, 1998). The second method was the determination of liver volume using computed tomography. The correlation between CT scan measurement and measurement of cadaveric liver volume was strong, and the intra-observer and inter-observer correlation was extremely high. While men demonstrated a larger mean body weight and lean body mass than females, there was no significant difference in liver volume between genders, indicating that women have a larger liver volume per unit of lean body mass than men. Determination of AER by the alcohol clamp and expressed on the basis of liver size showed no significant difference between men and women in AER per unit liver volume, but a 33% greater AER per kilogram lean body mass in the women (Kwo *et al.*, 1997). This is consistent with reports of increased AER in women. However, it does not explain their susceptibility to alcoholic liver injury, since it suggests that the rate of ethanol oxidation per cell is similar.

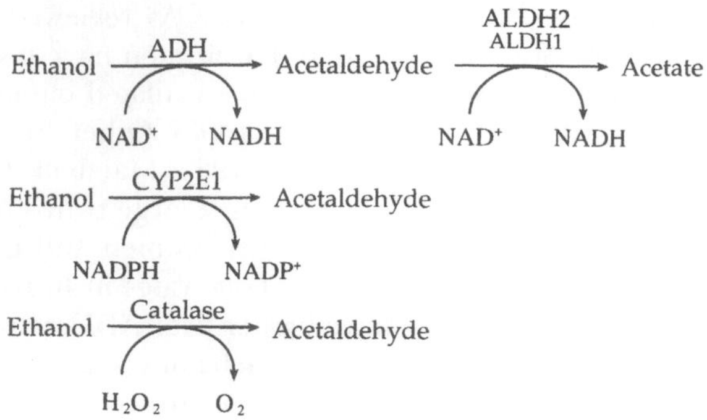

Figure 4.2 Pathways for the oxidation of ethanol and acetaldehyde in the liver. Note that the three ethanol oxidizing enzymes use different cofactors, while the aldehyde dehydrogenases all utilize NAD^+.

The second important aspect of alcohol elimination is the variability observed between individuals. The rate of ethanol clearance from the blood in the pseudo-linear segment of the elimination curve varies by 2- to 3-fold between individuals (Martin *et al.*, 1985; Kopun and Propping, 1997). The test-retest reliability in the oral ethanol challenge method of determining AER is open to criticism, but significant variation between individuals was recently confirmed using the alcohol clamp technique (O'Conner *et al.*, 1998). The reasons for this variation are incompletely understood. The likeliest explanation for the difference is variation in the activity of enzymes catalyzing alcohol oxidation. Ethanol metabolism in the liver proceeds along two or three parallel pathways. The best established pathways are those catalyzed by ADHs and cytochrome P450 IIE1. These enzymes oxidize ethanol to acetaldehyde in the cytosol and endoplasmic reticulum, respectively. Catalase, localized mainly in the peroxisomes, may contribute to ethanol oxidation, although its contribution may be limited by the availability of its other substrate hydrogen peroxide (Figure 4.2). Acetaldehyde derived from ethanol can then be oxidized by several different pathways. Cytosolic aldehyde dehydrogenase (ALDH1) and mitochondrial aldehyde dehydrogenase (ALDH2) are the best characterized aldehyde oxidizing enzymes. These broad specificity enzymes utilize NAD^+ and acetaldehyde in micromolar concentrations, generating acetate in a physiologically irreversible reaction. Most of this acetate leaves the liver for oxidation in extra-hepatic tissues (Lumeng and Davis, 1970). Examination of these isozymes and their genes has revealed a substantial number of functional polymorphisms which contribute to responses to ethanol. These will be considered in turn.

Alcohol dehydrogenases

The enzymes responsible for the bulk of alcohol oxidation are the alcohol dehydrogenase (ADHs). This ancient family of enzymes is expressed in all vertebrates, insects, many plants and microbes. The isozymes are given in Greek letter designations. α, β, and γ were the first of these to be purified and studied. Pi ADH was named for its *p*yrazole-*i*nsensitivity (pi or π). Chi ADH was originally named

ADH X, which was changed to Greek χ. Sigma ADH was named for its expression in stomach (it is referred to as μ (mucosal) ADH by another laboratory, since it is also expressed in mucosae other than that in stomach). All are dimeric enzymes with subunit molecular weight of about 40 kDa. The oldest form, in evolutionary terms appears to be χ ADH, from which π, σ, and finally α, β, and γ ADHs evolved (Danielsson and Jornvall, 1992; Kaiser *et al.*, 1993, Jornvall, 1994). These enzymes have been grouped into classes based upon enzymatic properties and the degree of sequence similarities. Classes I, II, and possibly IV are likely to participate in ethanol oxidation *in vivo*. The general properties of the enzymes in each of these classes are summarized in Table 4.1 (Bosron and Li, 1986, 1987). Class I contains α, β, and γ isozymes. These enzymes have a low K_m for ethanol and are highly sensitive to inhibition by pyrazole derivatives. Class I enzymes are very abundant in liver, and are therefore believed to play a major role in hepatic alcohol metabolism. Class II ADH (π ADH) was first found in human liver, has a higher K_m for ethanol and as mentioned, is less sensitive to pyrazole inhibition than class I enzymes (Ehrig *et al.*, 1990). Because of its high K_m, it may contribute to increased rates of alcohol elimination (that is, a steeper blood ethanol disappearance curve) sometimes observed at high blood ethanol concentrations. Class III ADH (χ ADH) is relatively abundant in all tissues studied, is virtually inactive with ethanol, but is capable of metabolizing longer chain alcohols and ω-hydroxy-fatty acids (Pares and Vallee, 1981). This enzyme also exhibits glutathione-dependent formaldehyde dehydrogenase activity (Koivusalo *et al.*, 1989).

Recent additions to this family of enzymes are class IV and (tentatively) classes V and VI. The class IV enzyme has been purified from stomach and esophagus.

Table 4.1 Properties of alcohol dehydrogenases in humans

Gene locus	Subunit type	K_m (ethanol)	V_{max}	Tissue distribution
Class I				
ADH1	α	4	54	Liver
ADH2	β	0.05–34**	–	Liver, lung
ADH3	γ	0.6–1**	–	Liver, stomach
Class II				
ADH4	π	34	40	Liver, cornea
Class III				
ADH5	χ	1000	–	Most tissues
Class IV*				
ADH7	σ, μ	20	1510	Stomach, esophagus, other mucosae
Class V*				
ADH6	–	30	?	Liver, stomach
Class VI*				
ADH8	–	–	?	Not detected in humans, found in deermouse and rat liver

*Tentative assignments based upon sequence homologies. Details about the class IV, V, and VI enzymes are given in the text. K_m values are given in mM and V_{max} values are given in terms of turnover number (min⁻¹).

** Kinetic constants vary with isozyme, see Table 4.2.

Designated either μ ADH (Yin *et al.*, 1990) or σ-ADH (Moreno and Pares, 1991), it is structurally distinct from classes I, II, and III (Stone *et al.*, 1993; Pares *et al.*, 1994; Farres *et al.*, 1994a; Satre *et al.*, 1994). Its high K_m for ethanol may be speculated to be appropriate for high concentrations of ethanol, to which the gastric mucosa is exposed after ethanol consumption; however, the actual concentration of ethanol present in the gastric epithelial cells after drinking is difficult to ascertain. The fact that this enzyme has such a high K_m for ethanol suggests that other alcohols may be its physiological substrates. σ-ADH has the highest V_{max} of any of the known alcohol dehydrogenases and is very active with retinol as substrate (Stone *et al.*, 1993). Its expression in a variety of epithelial (esophagus, stomach, vagina, nasopharynx, and cornea) and the importance of retinol in the integrity of these tissues suggest that σ-ADH has a role in retinol conversion to retinal. The gene and its promoter were recently cloned, but control of expression of this gene is not well understood (Satre *et al.*, 1994). It appears to be the first ADH expressed in the embryonic mouse and its sites of expression correlate with the first appearance of retinoic acid (Ang *et al.*, 1996a,b). Class V ADH, encoded by the ADH6 gene, remains poorly characterized. It was cloned by screening genomic and cDNA libraries with oligonucleotides corresponding to conserved regions of ADH enzymes. The protein sequence deduced from the cDNA indicates about 60% homology to class I, II, III, and IV enzymes (Yasunami *et al.*, 1991). The mRNA for this enzyme was found in liver and in stomach, but the enzyme itself has not been purified. *In vitro* expressed enzyme had a pI of about 8.6, a high K_m for ethanol (about 30 mM), and moderate sensitivity to pyrazole inhibition (Cheng and Yoshida, 1991). An additional class of ADH (tentatively designated class VI) was reported in liver of deermice (Zheng *et al.*, 1993) and rats (Hoog and Brandt, 1995); and class VII ADH was cloned from chicken (Kedishvili *et al.*, 1997); to date the human homologs have not been found.

These enzymes and their mRNAs are quite abundant in liver, indicating that the genes are transcriptionally very active. The structure of the ADH genes and the tissue-specificity of the promoters have been studied extensively. They are typically 15 kb in size and are organized into 9 exons (Duester *et al.*, 1986; Crabb *et al.*, 1989). The ADH promoters contain binding sites for both ubiquitous transcription factors (e.g., TATAA binding factors, upstream stimulatory factor (USF) (Potter *et al.*, 1991), CTF/NF-I, which appears to function as a negative factor (Edenberg *et al.*, 1993), and Sp1-like factors (Brown *et al.*, 1992)) as well as tissue-specific factors (hepatocyte nuclear factor 1 (HNF-1), D-box binding protein (DBP), and CCAAT-enhancer binding proteins (C/EBPα and β)) (Stewart *et al.*, 1990, 1991; Potter *et al.*, 1991). C/EBP may be the most important in establishing high level liver expression of class I, II, and IV ADHs. Exceptions are the ADH5 and ADH7 promoters, which lack TATAA boxes. The ADH5 promoter is G+C rich, a characteristic of "housekeeping" genes. The affinities of the various binding sites for their respective transcription factors differ between the isozyme types and appear to explain the developmentally-regulated activation of ADH1, 2 and 3 during fetal hepatogenesis (van Ooij *et al.*, 1992). ADH1 is the first ADH gene to be activated in the liver during fetal development, probably due to the early expression of HNF-1 in the fetal liver cells. The subsequent activation of ADH2 follows the onset of expression of C/EBPα; ADH3 is activated by DBP, a homolog of C/EBP, which also increases the expression of ADH1 and ADH2 in the growing animal.

Binding sites for thyroid hormone, retinoic acid (Duester *et al.*, 1991; Harding and Duester, 1992) and glucocorticoid receptors (Winter *et al.*, 1990) have been identified in the upstream regions of ADH genes. These hormones affect promoter activity *in vitro*, with retinoic acid and glucocorticoids activating transcription and thyroid hormone antagonizing the effect of retinoic acid (Harding and Duester, 1992). However, much less pronounced effects of these hormones are seen *in vivo*, apparently because of multiple effects of the hormones on protein synthesis and turnover as well as on transcription (Qulali and Crabb, 1992; Dipple *et al.*, 1993). Other hormones have been studied but fewer details of the molecular mechanisms of action on ADH expression are understood. Growth hormone increased ADH activity in intact animals and cultured hepatocytes (Mezey and Potter, 1979; Mezey *et al.*, 1986b; Mezey and Yang, 1989; Potter *et al.*, 1993), while androgens (Mezey *et al.*, 1986a) and thyroid hormones (Mezey and Potter, 1981; Dipple *et al.*, 1993) decreased it. Ethanol itself clearly does not induce ADH; however, by reducing blood levels of testosterone, ethanol increases ADH activity in male rats (Rachamin *et al.*, 1980). Although there are controversial data about women having higher alcohol elimination rates, orchiectomy increased alcohol elimination rates in humans (Mezey *et al.*, 1988).

ADHs are also expressed in a variety of other tissues, albeit at lower levels than in the liver. Relatively high levels of class I ADH mRNA were found in kidney, stomach, duodenum, colon, and uterus of rats (Estonius *et al.*, 1993). Lower levels were found in many organs including the lung and small intestine, as well as in hepatic Ito cells (Yamauchi *et al.*, 1998b). Very low levels were found in brain, thymus, muscle or heart (Estonius *et al.*, 1993). Class I ADH has also been found in blood vessels (Allali-Hassani *et al.*, 1997), a finding of potential relvance to the alcohol-induced flush reaction (below). Class II ADH was detected in liver and duodenum (Estonius *et al.*, 1993). The acinar distribution of ADHs has also been reported with disparate results. Perivenous (Gumucio *et al.*, 1978; Yamauchi *et al.*, 1988a; Kato *et al.*, 1990), periportal (Bengtsson *et al.*, 1981) and continuous distributions (Vaananen *et al.*, 1984; Chen *et al.*, 1992) have been reported. Some of the discrepancy may have resulted from lack of specificity of the antisera utilized in some of the studies. In rats, there was no difference in ADH mRNA or protein levels in extracts from isolated perivenous and periportal liver cells (Chen *et al.*, 1992). Additional study in humans is warranted because of the numerous ADH isozymes. There may be different acinar distributions for the different isozymes that would be obscured when total ADH activity or immunoreactive protein levels are studied. The high degree of specificity needed for these studies will probably be achieved using oligonucleotide probes specific for each mRNA.

Cytochrome P450 IIE1

Another well-established ethanol oxidizing pathway is catalyzed by cytochrome P450 IIE1 (CYP 2E1). This cytochrome was initially designated the microsomal ethanol oxidizing system (MEOS; Lieber, 1994). It consists of cytochrome P450 reductase and the CYP2E1 enzyme embedded in the endoplasmic reticulum membrane. This enzyme system was originally identified as a cytochrome inducible by chronic ethanol administration. It has a molecular weight of about 54,000, a moderately high K_m for ethanol (10 mM or higher) and utilizes NADPH and oxygen as cofactors (Morgan *et al.*, 1982). In effect, ethanol serves as an electron donor for the reduction of O_2 to water, resulting in the oxidation of ethanol to acetaldehyde. The gene is 11 kb in length and divided into 9 exons (Uemeno *et al.*, 1988). Strong promoter activity was detected in the proximal 5′ flanking region up to about −130 bp in *in vitro* transcription assays (Uemeno *et al.*, 1988). This region contains a TATAA box and sites for binding HNF-1 (Ueno and Gonzales, 1990; Liu and Gonzales, 1995); an NFY/CP1 site was also detected but is of unknown physiological importance (Ueno and Gonzales, 1990). As mentioned, HNF-1 is expressed early in fetal development, and the CYP 2E1 gene is apparently active in the human fetus at 16–24 weeks (Carpenter *et al.*, 1996). The gene is expressed in a highly tissue-specific manner, with highest levels in liver, and lower levels in lung, gut and esophagus (Farinati *et al.*, 1985; Shimizu *et al.*, 1990; Lieber, 1994).

This enzyme, in contrast to ADH isozymes, is expressed in a zonal distribution. It is more abundant in the centrilobular zone of the liver acinus (Tsutsumi *et al.*, 1989). Induction of CYP 2E1 is most pronounced in the central zone, and can be dramatic, with increases up to 10-fold in enzyme mass. It occurs both by way of stabilization of the enzyme by ethanol, as well as other physiological subtrates such as ketone bodies (Johansson *et al.*, 1988; Song *et al.*, 1990). Increased levels of CYP 2E1 mRNA were reported in starved or diabetic animals (Song *et al.*, 1987; Yun *et al.*, 1992), possibly due to stabilization of the transcript rather than to increased rate of transcription. Very high concentrations of ethanol appear to increase levels of CYP 2E1 mRNA (Takahaski *et al.*, 1993), possibly due to increased transcription of the gene (Badger *et al.*, 1993). In alcohol-naive individuals, CYP 2E1 may mediate a small fraction of total alcohol metabolism. A greater contribution at high blood alcohol concentrations is possible due to the high K_m of this system. In heavy drinkers, in whom CYP 2E1 is induced, it probably accounts for a greater proportion of alcohol elimination.

Levels of CYP 2E1 are reported to vary up to 50-fold in different human liver samples, in part due to the environmental variables mentioned above (Wrighton *et al.*, 1986). CYP 2E1 metabolizes a variety of compounds in addition to alcohol, including acetaldehyde (Terelius *et al.*, 1991), acetaminophen (Sato *et al.*, 1981), isoniazide, nitrosamines, benzene, butadiene and urethane (Lieber, 1990; Stephen *et al.*, 1994). It is postulated that metabolism of carcinogens by CYP 2E1 (e.g., *N*-nitrosodimethylamine) is enhanced in alcoholics, resulting in increased risk of cancers of the oropharynx and esophagus in alcoholics. CYP 2E1 could also contribute to the increased risk for hepatocellular carcinoma in alcoholic cirrhosis. It certainly contributes to the increased susceptibility of heavy drinkers to the hepatotoxicity of acetaminophen (Sato *et al.*, 1981; Seeff *et al.*, 1986). It is now clear that heavy drinkers are susceptible to acetaminophen hepatotoxicity from doses that are quite safe in the non-drinker (as low as 3 to 5 g per 24 hours (Seeff, 1986)). CYP 2E1 oxidizes acetaminophen to *N*-acetyl-*p*-benzoquinonimine, the major toxic metabolite in acetaminophen poisoning. CYP 2E1 is also important for many drug-alcohol interactions. Generally, alcoholics, when sober, have increased rates of metabolism of certain drugs (e.g., propranolol, benzodiazepines, phenobarbital, phenytoin, theophylline), but when they are intoxicated, the alcohol competes with the drug for metabolism and slows their elimination, often with adverse or even fatal consequences.

Catalase

Catalase is a tetrameric, glycosylated protein with 60 kDa subunits and a single heme moiety per tetramer. It is expressed in all tissues, with highest levels in liver, kidney, heart and red blood cells; in liver, it is present predominantly in the peroxisomes, with lesser amounts in mitochondria. The gene for catalase is about 34 kb in length and consists of 13 exons. The promoter lacks a TATAA box; instead, it is GC rich and contains several GT and CCAAT boxes (Quan *et al.*, 1986; VanRemmen *et al.*, 1998). There are known, but quite rare, examples of hypocatalasemia in Swiss, Hungarian and Japanese populations. These appear to be due to point mutations in the gene. There are no reports of effects of this deficiency on alcohol metabolic rate. The enzyme is capable of oxidizing ethanol to acetaldehyde in the presence of hydrogen peroxide, but the availability of hydrogen peroxide probably limits this reaction. The contribution of catalase to systemic ethanol elimination remains controversial, with some recent data indicating that catalase may oxidize a substantial fraction of ethanol under physiological conditions. For instance, deermice lacking class I ADH were shown to oxidize ethanol and methanol, the latter being a good substrate for catalase but not for most ADHs or CYP2E1 (Bradford *et al.*, 1993b). However, these animals are now known to express class VI ADH which could conceivably oxidize these alcohols (Zheng *et al.*, 1993). In the past, 4-methylpyrazole, an inhibitor of ADH, was shown to markedly reduce ethanol oxidation in liver. This supported the importance of ADH in ethanol oxidation. However, 4-methylpyrazole also inhibits fatty acyl-CoA synthetase, an enzyme needed for activation of fatty acids prior to oxidation. Since peroxisomal fatty acid oxidation is a major source of hydrogen peroxide, 4-methylpyrazole may simultaneously inhibit ADH- and catalase-mediated ethanol oxidation. This could result in underestimating the contribution of catalase to alcohol oxidation (Bradford *et al.*, 1993a). In support of this notion, induction of peroxisomal β oxidation and catalase, but not ADH, with bezafibrate was shown to be accompanied by an increase in ethanol elimination rates in rats (Tsukamoto *et al.*, 1996). Thus, a role for catalase in ethanol oxidation cannot be disregarded.

Aldehyde dehydrogenases

Acetaldehyde is generated in cytosol, endoplasmic reticulum or peroxisomes by the enzymes described above. This reactive and highly toxic compound is further metabolized predominantly by NAD^+-dependent aldehyde dehydrogenases (ALDHs) (Table 4.2). These enzymes have broad substrate specificity for aliphatic and aromatic aldehydes, which are oxidized via a thiohemiacetal intermediate to their corresponding carboxylic acids (Lindahl, 1992). The reaction is irreversible under physiological conditions. The ALDHs are expressed in a wider range of tissues than are the ADH isozymes or cytochrome P450s. Moreover, many enzymes with

Table 4.2 Properties of human aldehyde dehydrogenases

Gene locus	Structure	K_m (Ach)*	Tissue distribution
Class 1			
ALDH1	α4	30 μM	Many tissues, liver > kidney
Class 2			
ALDH2	α4	1 μM	Low levels in most tissues
			Liver > kidney > muscle > heart
ALDH5**	?	?	Low levels in most tissues
			Liver > kidney > muscle
Class 3			
ALDH3	α2	11 mM	Stomach, liver, cornea
Other enzymes			
ALDH9	α4	30 μM	Liver
ALDH6–8	?	?	?

The various classes of aldehyde dehydrogenases characterized in humans are shown. ALDH5–8 have been cloned, but the kinetic properties of the enzymes have not been studied. ALDH9 is the gene locus encoding ALDHE3.
* Ach indicates acetaldehyde.
** ALDH5 is tentatively assigned to class 2 because of sequence similarities to ALDH2 and the presence of a potential mitochondrial leader sequence. The structure of the enzymes is indicated by α2 for dimers and α4 for tetramers. It is not known if ALDH6–9 play any role in metabolism of acetaldehyde.

a specific aldehyde substrate, e.g., glyceraldehyde 3-phosphate dehydrogenase, can oxidize acetaldehyde when it is present at high concentrations. These enzymes do not participate in acetaldehyde metabolism. The nomenclature for ALDHs is confusing. The original designations assigned numbers based on electrophoretic mobility, although different laboratories used different systems. To reduce confusion and to group them according to function, they have been tentatively classified as class 1 (low K_m, cytosolic), class 2 (low K_m, mitochondrial) and class 3 (high K_m ALDHs such as those expressed in tumors, stomach and cornea) based upon kinetic properties and sequence similarities.

The most important enzymes for acetaldehyde oxidation are cytosolic ALDH1 and mitochondrial ALDH2 (Greenfield and Pietruszko, 1977). Both are tetrameric enzymes composed of 54 kDa subunits. ALDH1 has a very low K_m for NAD^+, a low K_m for acetaldehyde (about 30 μM) and is exquisitely sensitive to disulfiram (Antabuse) *in vitro* (Greenfield and Pietruszko, 1977; Dickinson *et al.*, 1981). ALDH2 has a submicromolar K_m for acetaldehyde, and is less sensitive to disulfiram *in vitro*. The inhibition of this enzyme *in vivo* is thought to depend on the metabolism of disulfiram to other compounds such as diethyldithiocarbamic acid ethanethiol and other mixed disulfides (MacKerell *et al.*, 1985; Kitson, 1989), which then covalently modify the active site cysteine. These enzymes have high inhibition constants for NADH, unlike many hepatic dehydrogenases that are inhibited during the oxidation of ethanol. Thus, these enzymes ALDHs remain active despite the high $NADH/NAD^+$ ratio that is established in cytosol and mitochondria during alcohol metabolism. The enzymes are distributed evenly across the liver acinus as demonstrated by immunohistochemistry (Maeda *et al.*, 1988), while determination of enzyme activity and Western blots of isolated periportal and perivenous hepato-cytes suggested a slight periportal predominance. Unfortunately, this distribution fails to match the increased acetaldehyde generation via CYP 2E1 in the pericen-tral zone (Tsutsumi *et al.*, 1989). ALDH1 and ALDH2 mRNAs are expressed in a variety of human tissues besides liver (Stewart *et al.*, 1996b); ALDH2 mRNA was particularly abundant in kidney, muscle and heart. Low levels of ALDH1 and ALDH2 mRNAs were found in placenta brain and pancreas; these are obviously target organs for alcoholic pathology, consistent with the hypothesis that the presence of ALDHs is protective against acetaldehyde toxicity.

The control of expression of these enzymes has been studied. The ALDH1 gene was cloned (Hsu *et al.*, 1989) and the promoter was studied in transfection and DNA binding assays. 2.6 kb of 5′ flanking DNA permitted expression of reporter constructs in hepatoma cells; a minimal promoter was shown to bind NF-Y/CP1 and octamer factors (Yanagawa *et al.*, 1995). The ALDH2 gene has been more intensively studied in our laboratories. It has no TATAA box (Hsu *et al.*, 1988); similar to ALDH1, it has a binding site for the ubiquitous CCAAT-box binding protein NF-Y/CP1 near the transcription start site (Stewart *et al.*, 1996a). Addi-tional factors binding upstream promoter sites are found at high level in the liver and kidney. These have been identified as members of the nuclear receptor superfamily, and include retinoid X receptor, ARP-1, COUP-TF1, hepatocyte nuclear factor 4 (HNF-4), and peroxisome proliferator-activated receptors (PPARs). HNF-4 probably determines the high level of expression in liver and kidney, while the other receptors may modulate extrahepatic expression of the gene. Additional ALDH enzymes have been reported in recent years. Pietruszko's laboratory has purified and cloned an enzyme designated ALDHE3. This enzyme has properties similar to ALDH1: it is expressed in the cytosol and has a K_m for aliphatic aldehydes of about 30–50 µM (Kurys *et al.*, 1989), but is only 40% similar to ALDH1 or ALDH2 at the amino acid level (Kurys *et al.*, 1993). This enzyme has a uniquely low K_m for aminoaldehydes such as 4-aminobutyraldehyde and hence may play a role in the metabolism of compounds derived from polyamines such as spermine. It also oxidizes betaine aldehyde efficiently (Chern and Pietruszko, 1995). Its gene (designated ALDH9) was recently cloned (Lin *et al.*, 1996). ALDH5 (originally called ALDH$_x$) was cloned by screening a genomic library with an oligonucleotide corresponding to a conserved region of ALDHs (Hsu and Chang, 1991). This gene is unique among the ALDH genes in that it lacks introns. The deduced amino acid sequence indicates that it is closely related to ALDH2 (with about 70% sequence similarity). The N-terminus of the protein may form an amphipathic helix, and hence may be a mitochondrial leader sequence. If so, ALDH5 may be classified as the second class 2 ALDH. The ALDH5 gene is also polymorphic at two different residues: valine or alanine at position 69 and leucine or arginine at position 120 (Hsu and Chang, 1991; Sherman *et al.*, 1993). It is not known at present if these substitutions alter the enzymatic properties of ALDH5. ALDH5 mRNA is expressed in liver, kidney and skeletal muscle at high-est levels (Stewart *et al.*, 1996b). Nothing is really known about the regulation of these genes.

ALDH3 and ALDH4 are also present in liver extracts. These isozymes have considerably higher K_m for aliphatic aldehydes than the class 1 and 2 enzymes and have higher affinity for aromatic aldehyde substrates. The class 3 ALDH3 family includes the cytosolic, TCDD (dioxin)-inducible ALDH, the hepatoma-associated ALDH, and the corneal and stomach ALDH3 (Lin *et al.*, 1984; Lindahl, 1986; Jones *et al.*, 1988; Algar *et al.*, 1993). The stomach form might participate in the oxidation of acetaldehyde generated during gastric metabolism of ethanol. The ALDH3 promoter has been studied in some detail because of its interesting induction by dioxin (Lindahl, 1986, 1992), but since this enzyme is not involved in ethanol metabolism, it will not be discussed further. ALDH4 appears to be glutamic γ-semialdehyde dehydrogenase. ALDH6, ALDH7 and ALDH8 have been cloned (Hsu *et al.*, 1995), but enzymological characteristics for these enzymes are not yet known.

REGULATION OF ETHANOL METABOLISM

The rate of ethanol metabolism may be critical in determining its toxicity because the intermediates of this pathway are themselves potentially toxic. The ADH pathway is the quantitatively major pathway. The maximal activities of alcohol and aldehyde dehydrogenases are similar, so that each enzyme contributes to the overall control of the rate of alcohol oxidation. Modeling of alcohol oxidation in rat liver indicated that ADH activity was controlled in part by the total activity of the enzyme as well as product inhibition by NADH and acetaldehyde (Crabb *et al.*, 1983). Liver NADH levels are higher during alcohol oxidation because the first enzyme in the malate-aspartate shuttle, malate dehydrogenase, has a high K_m for NADH, not because the shuttle or mitochondrial reoxidation of NADH is limiting (Crow *et al.*, 1982, 1983). Thus, in a steady state, ADH is operating below its V_{max}. Flux though the pathway is also sensitive to the total activity of ADH. Reduction in total ADH activity (as occurs in fasting) reduced the ability of the liver to oxidize ethanol in rats, but increases in activity did not increase the metabolic rate proportionally (Crabb *et al.*, 1987). This is presumed to be due to the inability to increase acetaldehyde oxidation, and therefore an increase in steady state acetaldehyde concentration limits the activity of ADH. CYP 2E1 or catalase act in parallel with ADH; under conditions in which they become more active, they may produce excess acetaldehyde. As a result, oxidation of ethanol by these enzymes may result in lower flux through ADH, with no net increase in alcohol elimination rate. This raises the possibility that under certain conditions, pathways of alcohol metabolism and the concentrations of metabolic intermediates change, but the alcohol elimination rate does not. This may be the case with several naturally occurring ADH, CYP 2E1 and ALDH2 variants; their effects on alcohol metabolism will be considered in turn.

Alcohol dehydrogenase

The ADH enzymes function as dimers. Enzyme subunits belonging to the same class can heterodimerize, but dimers do not form between subunits of different classes. The heterodimers have kinetic properties described by the active sites

Table 4.3 Properties of polymorphic forms of human alcohol dehydrogenase

Gene locus	Subunit type	K_m (ethanol)	V_{max}	Population
ADH2*1	β1	0.05	9	Caucasians, African-Americans
ADH2*2	β2	0.9	400	Asians
ADH2*3	β3	34	300	African-Americans
ADH3*1	γ1	1.0	87	All groups
ADH3*2	γ2	0.63	35	Caucasians

The kinetic constants are noted for the homodimers of the subunits listed (Bosron and Li, 1986b; Bosron and Li, 1987a; Ehrig *et al.*, 1990). Heterodimers behave as if the active sites were independent. The K_m values are in mM and the V_{max} values are given in terms of turnover numbers (min^{-1}), as in Table 4.1. The column labeled population indicates which populations have high allele frequencies for these variants. The alleles are not limited to those populations.

acting independently. The isozymes in class I are polymorphic; two alleles exist for ADH3 and three for ADH2 (Burnell and Bosron, 1989). The kinetic properties and population distribution of these allelic enzymes are shown in Table 4.3. The isozymes encoded by the three ADH2 alleles, each differing from the others at a single amino acid residue, vary markedly in K_m for ethanol and V_{max}. β1 is the most common in Caucasians, has a relatively low V_{max} and a very low K_m for ethanol. β2 is found commonly in Asians and was originally designated "atypical" ADH (von Wartburg *et al.*, 1964). It has a substantially higher V_{max} and somewhat higher K_m compared with β1. The β3 isozyme was first detected in liver extracts from African-Americans (Bosron *et al.*, 1980) because of its lower pH optimum than the other ADH isozymes. It has a high K_m for ethanol, and high V_{max}. Smaller differences in enzymatic properties are observed between the products of the ADH3 alleles. The γ1 isozyme has about twice the V_{max} of the γ2 isozyme, while the K_ms for ethanol are similar. γ1 ADH is found at high frequency in Asians and African-Americans; Caucasians have about equal frequency of γ1 and γ2 ADH alleles (Burnell and Bosron, 1989). The other ADH loci have not been found to be polymorphic to date.

The widely varying V_{max} and Michaelis constants of the ADH2 and ADH3 isozymes suggests the possibility that individuals with different combinations of isozymes would have different alcohol elimination rates. The presence of more active ADH isozymes was predicted to increase ethanol metabolic rates. This has been difficult to demonstrate, in part because a given isozyme will constitute only a fraction of the total alcohol oxidizing capacity of the liver and because alcohol elimination rates are rather variable even among individuals of the same ADH genotypes, or even twins (Kopun and Propping, 1977; Martin *et al.*, 1985). To date, different ADH2*2 genotypes have been related at most to only a small portion of the differences between-individual in alcohol elimination rates (Thomasson *et al.*, 1990; Mizoi *et al.*, 1994). The ADH2*3 polymorphism has been shown to be associated with a 10% increase in the rate of ethanol metabolism (Thomasson *et al.*, 1995). ADH3 polymorphism did not affect alcohol elimination (Couzigou *et al.*, 1991).

Cytochrome P450 2E1

Although the contribution of CYP 2E1 to ethanol metabolism is likely to be greatest after the induction of the enzyme by chronic ethanol use, there are also polymorphisms in the gene. The best studied is an *Rsa* I polymorphism at −1019 bp upstream has been correlated with different levels of expression of the gene in transient transfection assays (Hayashi *et al.*, 1991). The allele referred to as c2 is associated with higher promoter activity *in vitro*. Transfection studies suggested that promoters with the c2 sequence fail to suppress expression compared with the c1 sequence (Watanabe *et al.*, 1994). The mutation occurs in a consensus sequence for HNF-1α (Uemeno *et al.*, 1988; Liu and Gonzalez, 1995). The c2 allele is rather common among Asians, but uncommon in Caucasian and African-American populations (Stephen *et al.*, 1994). Studies aimed at determining the effect of this polymorphism have followed the rate of acetaminophen or chlorzoxazone elimination, since these compounds are oxidized by the CYP 2E1 enzyme. A recent paper indicated that acetaminophen metabolism was faster in the c2 homozygotes and slower in the c1 homozygotes (Ueshima *et al.*, 1996), consistent with the notion that the c2 allele is transcriptionally more active; however, several other groups found no correlation of CYP 2E1 genotype with CYP 2E1 protein levels in liver or chlorzoxazone metabolic rate (Kim and O'Shea, 1995; Carriere *et al.*, 1996; Kim *et al.*, 1996). Recently, two coding sequence variants (CYP 2E1*2 due to a R76H mutation and CYP 2E1*3 due to a V289I mutation) were discovered. The CYP 2E1*3 variant appeared to have the same enzymatic properties as the wild-type enzyme, while CYP 2E1*2 protein seemed to be less stable, predicting lower activity in individuals with this allele (Hu *et al.*, 1997). These variants are rare, and there is no information to suggest that they affect alcohol metabolic rates. It is interesting that there is wide (4–5-fold) variation in chlorzoxazone metabolic rate (Kim and O'Shea, 1995; Kim *et al.*, 1996), suggesting variation in CYP 2E1 expression that could be due to other genetic or environmental factors.

Aldehyde dehydrogenase

The importance of ALDH2 in ethanol oxidation is demonstrated by an inborn error of metabolism. It had long been known that alcohol consumption resulted in facial flushing in certain individuals. A large proportion of Japanese, Chinese and Koreans had visible facial flushing accompanied by increased skin blood flow after consuming a small amount of alcohol, while similar reactions were rare among Caucasians (Wolff, 1972, 1973). Since the reaction was also observed in Asian infants given alcohol, it was apparently genetically determined. A family study carried out in Hawaii suggested that the flush reaction was inherited as a dominant trait (Schwitters *et al.*, 1982). The flushing was correlated with the accumulation of acetaldehyde to high levels (Zeiner *et al.*, 1979; Goedde *et al.*, 1983; Enomoto *et al.*, 1991b). In non-flushers, drinking elicited a small increase in acetaldehyde levels (to 5–10 μM); in flushers the levels are variable, but may exceed 100 μM (Enomoto *et al.*, 1991b). Since this is similar to the disulfiram-flush reaction (Asmussen *et al.*, 1948), the activity of ALDH was examined in flushing individuals using electrophoretic assays. A large proportion (about 40%) of Japanese were found to lack

ALDH2 activity (Harada *et al.*, 1981, 1982) and most of these individuals flushed when they drank. This implies that ALDH2 plays a crucial role in maintaining low levels of acetaldehyde during alcohol oxidation.

The mutation responsible for the deficiency is a G to A substitution that results in replacement of glutamate with lysine at position 487 of the ALDH2 polypeptide (Yoshida *et al.*, 1984; Hempel *et al.*, 1984). The normal allele is called ALDH2*1 and the mutant allele is designated ALDH2*2. It is interesting that ALDH2 deficiency is a dominant trait. The ALDH2*2 heterozygotes as well as homozygotes are ALDH2 deficient in all populations studied. The dominance of is only partial, as the homozygotes have far higher acetaldehyde levels after they drink than the heterozygotes, and heterozygotes have residual low K_m ALDH activity on liver biopsies (Enomoto *et al.*, 1991b). Measurement of ALDH activity in livers of controls and individuals with ALDH2 deficiency suggested that about 40% of total liver ALDH activity is ALDH2 and 60% is contributed by other forms (ALDH1, ALDHE3 and possibly ALDH5) (Yin, S.J., personal communication). Both alleles of ALDH2 have been expressed in bacteria and their kinetic behavior was studied. The ALDH2*2 allele encodes an enzyme with a much increased K_m for NAD^+ and a reduced V_{max} when compared with the wild-type enzyme (Farres *et al.*, 1994). Thus, although it is active *in vitro*, it is predicted to be virtually inactive under conditions occurring in liver mitochondria. Our laboratory has expressed the two ALDH2 alleles in tissue culture cells (Xiao *et al.*, 1995). Transduction of ALDH2*1 resulted in expression of a low K_m ALDH with the expected isoelectric point. The ALDH2*2 allele directed expression of an inactive, immunoreactive protein. Transduction of ALDH2*2 into ALDH2*1 expressing cells reduced the low K_m activity substantially. The degree of reduction in activity suggested that only tetramers containing either three or four wild-type subunits are active. Moreover, the ALDH2*2 polypeptides were less stable in the transduced cell lines, further reducing the level and thus activity of heterotetramers (Xiao *et al.*, 1996) and contributing to the dominance of the ALDH2*2 allele. The X-ray crystal structure of ALDH2 was reported recently. The mutation at position 487 occurs in a region of the protein that is involved in subunit-subunit interactions (Steinmetz *et al.*, 1997). Introduction of a positive charge at 487 disrupts ionic bonds with arginines normally neutralized by the glutamate; this may suffice to inactivate the adjacent subunits and explain the dominance of the mutation.

Studies on the effect of ALDH2 deficiency on alcohol metabolic rates are limited by the adverse effects of alcohol for these subjects. Small early studies failed to show a difference in alcohol elimination rates between flushers and non-flushers (Mizoi *et al.*, 1979; Inoue *et al.*, 1984), but a more recent study detected reduced rates of alcohol elimination in individuals with ALDH2 deficiency when the groups were controlled for ADH genotype (Mizoi *et al.*, 1994). This would be consistent with product inhibition of ADH by elevated intrahepatic acetaldehyde levels.

Other ALDH variants

There have been isolated reports of abnormal ALDH1 isozymes in Asians and Caucasians. One laboratory observed a single Japanese liver that was deficient in ALDH1 activity despite the presence of immunologically cross-reacting material

(Yoshida *et al.*, 1983). Another laboratory reported additional variants of ALDH1 (Eckey *et al.*, 1986). Flushing after drinking is reported rather uncommonly among Caucasians (6–10%) (Wolff, 1972), and a small number of Caucasians who flush and have an ALDH1 with altered mobility on gel electrophoresis have been reported (Yoshida *et al.*, 1989). The basis for the altered mobility is unknown and the presence of flushing was not unequivocally established. One additional rare mutation of ALDH2 is known that substitutes lysine for glutamate at position 479 (Novoradovsky *et al.*, 1995); the effect on enzyme activity is unknown since the subject in which it was identified was also heterozygous for ALDH2*2. ALDHE3 has the same electrophoretic mobility as ALDH1 (Kurys *et al.*, 1989), which may explain why ALDH1 deficiency, if it exists, has not been conclusively detected by electrophoretic methods.

GENETIC INFLUENCES ON ALCOHOLISM AND ALCOHOLIC LIVER DISEASE

Twin studies have provided evidence that there is a genetic component both to alcohol elimination rates (Kopun and Propping, 1977; Martin *et al.*, 1985) and susceptibility to alcoholic liver disease (Hrubec and Omenn, 1981). However, follow-up analysis of the VA twin panel indicated that much of the previously observed genetic risk of cirrhosis (largely due to alcohol) could be accounted for by the genetic risk of alcoholism per se (Reed *et al.*, 1996). Since ethanol metabolism is thought to contribute to the pathogenesis of alcoholic liver disease, the polymorphic genes discussed above have been examined as candidate genes accounting for these genetic differences. The main hypothesis has been that the presence of high activity ADH isozymes or high activity of CYP 2E1, or lower activity of ALDHs, results in increased rates of production or decreased rates of oxidation of acetaldehyde, respectively (Figure 4.3). Either process would result in increased steady-state acetaldehyde concentrations, which might be aversive to heavy drinking and alcoholism, but

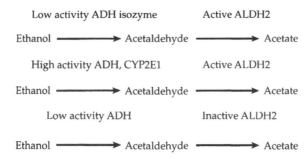

Figure 4.3 Potential mechanisms for liver injury related to genetically altered rates of ethanol and acetaldehyde metabolism. It is hypothesized that increase of acetaldehyde production by high activity ADH or CYP 2E1, or decreased acetaldehyde removal by ALDH2 would lead to accumulation of acetaldehyde, a highly reactive intermediate capable of forming numerous adducts with hepatic proteins.

also might increase the risk of developing alcoholic liver disease (Lumeng and Crabb, 1994). A small number of other genes have been implicated in risk of alcohol induced liver injury but these have yet to be confirmed.

Alcohol dehydrogenase

Effects on risk of alcoholism

Despite the small effect that ADH genotype has on alcohol elimination rate, the ADH genotypes have been related to differences in alcohol drinking behavior. This is best documented for the ADH2*2 allele found in Asians. Chinese living in Taiwan were genotyped at the ADH loci to see if there was an association between ADH2 genotype and drinking behavior. The ADH2*2 allele was significantly more common in the non-alcoholic group than in the alcoholics (Thomasson et al., 1991). The ADH2*2 allele encodes the highly active β2 ADH isozyme that may permit faster conversion of alcohol to acetaldehyde; hence, this has been postulated as a mechanism by which this gene could be "protective" against heavy drinking and alcoholism. However, alcohol elimination rates and peak blood acetaldehyde levels were not influenced by ADH2*2 genotype in a study of Japanese individuals (Mizoi et al., 1994). The finding that individuals without alcohol drinking problems have a higher frequency of the ADH2*2 allele compared with alcoholics has been confirmed in the Atayal natives of Taiwan (Thomasson et al., 1994), the Maori of New Zealand (Marshall and Chambers, 1994), and in Spanish patients (Pares et al., 1992). There was no apparent effect of ADH2 alleles on quantity and frequency of drinking in Japanese men (Takeshita et al., 1994), although the number of individuals with the genotypes expected to predispose to highest drinking (individuals homozygous for both ALDH2*1 and ADH2*1) is small due to the allele frequencies in this population. A more recent study indicated that ADH2*1 was more common in heavy drinkers than in moderate drinkers (Tanaka et al., 1997). Moreover, the ADH3*1 allele was also more prevalent among non-alcoholics than alcoholics (Shen et al., 1997) in Asians, but there is no apparent effect of the ADII3 locus on alcohol consumption or alcoholism rates in Caucasians (Gilder et al., 1993).

Effect on risk of liver disease

The effect of ADH variants on the risk of alcoholic liver disease is potentially complex (Lumeng and Crabb, 1994). High activity variants such as ADH2*2 appear to decrease alcoholism risk, but if the individual persisted in drinking, it might potentiate the hepatic insult by generating high intrahepatic concentrations of acetaldehyde. To date, there has been a single study from Japan, demonstrating increased risk of alcoholic liver diseases among ADH2*2 hetero- or homozygotes (Yamauchi et al., 1995). Moreover, if two other studies are pooled with it (Chao et al., 1994; Tanaka et al., 1996), there was a significantly increased risk of cirrhosis in the subjects with ADH2*2. The ADH3 locus is the only ADH gene subject to variation in Caucasian populations and hence it has been evaluated for a possible role in modifying the risk of alcoholic liver disease. Two studies of the prevalence of ADH3*1 and

ADH3*2 in alcoholics with and without liver disease have suggested that ADH3*1, encoding the more active enzyme, may be more common in those with alcoholic liver diseases. This was observed in patients from the United Kingdom (Day *et al.*, 1991) and from France (Poupon *et al.*, 1992). When the data from the two studies were pooled, the prevalence of ADH3*1 was 0.65 in alcoholics with cirrhosis and 0.55 in controls (Day *et al.*, 1993) and the difference approached significance. This suggested that higher rates of acetaldehyde production by the γ1 ADH enzyme encoded by ADH3*1 may contribute to an increased risk of organ damage in heavy drinkers. However, a reduction in ADH3*1 allele frequency was reported in cirrhotics by another laboratory (Sherman *et al.*, 1994). Summarizing the three studies showed an allele frequency for ADH3*1 of 0.58 in cirrhotics and 0.56 in controls among a total of 137 controls and 108 patients with cirrhosis. Thus, this polymorphism may not play a role in determining risk for liver disease.

An additional ADH genetic variant is a *Pvu* II RFLP in the ADH2 gene. The nucleotide variation occurs within an intron of the gene, and so it is not likely to alter expression of the gene itself, but may be linked to another polymorphism that does. The B allele was found at considerably higher frequency in alcoholics and seemed to be more common in patients with cirrhosis rather than alcoholic hepatitis (Sherman *et al.*, 1993). Since most of the patients studied had liver disease, and the total number was small, this study will need to be replicated in other populations to see if the variant is more closely associated with alcoholism or with alcoholic liver disease. If confirmed, this test could be useful to predict risk for alcoholic liver disease.

Effects on other health risks

There are data available on relatively small numbers of patients indicating that ADH2*2 may be more prevalent in individuals with alcoholic pancreatitis than in control alcoholics (Matsumoto *et al.*, 1996). There may also be an association of the homozygous ADH3*1 genotype with risk of oral cancer (Harty *et al.*, 1997; Coutelle *et al.*, 1997). Both of these findings await confirmation.

Cytochrome P450 IIE1

Effects on risk of alcoholism

There is no evidence that individuals with different promoter variants of CYP 2E1 have different drinking patterns (Tanaka *et al.*, 1997) or risks of alcoholism (Ball *et al.*, 1995; Carr *et al.*, 1995, 1996; Savolainen *et al.*, 1997). This might be expected based on the high K_m of this enzyme and its small contribution to alcohol metabolism in light or moderate drinkers.

Effect on risk of liver disease

The polymorphism in the promoter of CYP 2E1 suggested the possibility that individuals with the high activity allele might be at higher risk for alcoholic liver injury, since this would generate both higher acetaldehyde and possibly free radical levels in the centrilobular zone of the liver acinus. The results of studies of allele frequencies in Japanese subjects have been contradictory, with two groups reporting higher prevalence of the c2 allele in patients with alcoholic liver disease (Maezawa *et al.*, 1994; Tsutsumi *et al.*, 1994) and another group reporting the opposite finding (Chao *et al.*, 1995). In Caucasians, the c2 allele is rare, and no significant differences in c2 allele frequency could be seen between alcoholics with and without cirrhosis in several cohorts (Maezawa *et al.*, 1994; Ball *et al.*, 1995; Carr *et al.*, 1995, 1996; Agundez *et al.*, 1996; Savolainen *et al.*, 1997); however, a single study suggested an increased risk of alcoholic liver disease in c2 heterozygotes (Pirmohamed *et al.*, 1995). These findings must be interpreted in light of reports that the polymorphism does not correlate well with enzyme activity or chlorzoxazone metabolism rate.

Effects on other health risks

The CYP 2E1 polymorphism has been examined for association with Korsakoff syndrome (Ball *et al.*, 1995), alcoholic pancreatitis (Chao *et al.*, 1995), gastric cancer (Kato *et al.*, 1995), or hepatocellular carcinoma (Kato *et al.*, 1995). No correlation has been observed with any of these conditions.

Aldehyde dehydrogenase 2

Effects on risk of alcoholism

Elegant studies from Japan have demonstrated that among men, ALDH2 deficiency reduced quantity and frequency of alcohol consumption and the risk of alcoholism (Higuchi *et al.*, 1992). This was reflected further in several Asian populations in which it was observed that individuals who were alcoholic (Goedde *et al.*, 1983; Harada *et al.*, 1983, 1985; Lumeng and Crabb, 1994) or who had alcoholic liver disease (Shibuya and Yoshida, 1989) rarely had ALDH2 deficiency (determined by electrophoresis of hair root extracts) or an ALDH2*2 allele (determined by genotyping). Among Japanese subjects, about 41% of controls were ALDH2 deficient, while only 2–5% of alcoholics were deficient (Harada *et al.*, 1983). In a study performed on Taiwanese males, the frequency of the ALDH2*2 allele was 30% in a non-alcoholic control group, and 6% in a group of alcoholic individuals (Thomasson *et al.*, 1991). Similar results were seen by other groups. Although the differences in allele frequencies have been repeatedly demonstrated, the actual reasons for reduced drinking in individuals with ALDH2*2 alleles may not be as simple as initially thought (reviewed in Chao, 1995a). It is also interesting to note that among Japanese, the protective effect of being heterozygous for ALDH2*2 appears to be decreasing over time (Higuchi *et al.*, 1994), i.e., the frequency of finding ALDH2*2 heterozygotes among alcoholics is increasing, presumably because of environmental and cultural changes. However, homozygotes for ALDH2*2 appear to be absolutely protected against alcoholism, presumably because of the severity of their flushing (Chao, 1995a; Higuchi *et al.*, 1994). This phenomenon does not seem to be limited to Japan, as it has been observed in other countries (China and Pacific islands (Agarwal *et al.*, 1981; Goedde *et al.*, 1983,

1989; Goedde and Agarwal, 1987) with somewhat different prevalence of the ALDH2*2 allele, as well as in Asians living in Canada, suggesting that it is a bio-chemical and not purely a cultural phenomenon (Tu and Israal, 1995).

Effect on risk of liver disease

ALDH2 deficiency may be a double-edged sword for the reasons mentioned above for ADH2*2, namely the individuals with mild flushing may tolerate heavy drinking and suffer from the hepatic effects of elevated acetaldehyde concentrations. For example, alcoholic Caucasians exhibited elevated acetaldehyde levels after drinking (up to as high as 60 μM) and may flush (Korsten *et al.*, 1975; Lindros *et al.*, 1980), but apparently do not experience this as an aversive reaction. The elevation in acetaldehyde level probably results from higher rates of acetaldehyde formation by CYP 2E1, which is induced by heavy drinking, and reduced ability of the mito-chondria to oxidize the acetaldehyde due to toxic effects of ethanol or acetaldehyde itself. This increase in acetaldehyde level may perpetuate the alcoholic liver injury. There has been one small study suggesting that ALDH2*2 heterozygotes who drink heavily may develop alcoholic liver injury, especially alcoholic hepatitis, at lower cumulative alcohol consumption (Enomoto *et al.*, 1991a). When the results of several studies are combined, the prevalence of ALDH2*2 was significantly higher in the alcoholic patients with cirrhosis than those without (Chao *et al.*, 1994; Yamauchi *et al.*, 1995; Tanaka *et al.*, 1996). With the apparent increase in the number of alcoholics heterozygous for ALDH2*2 in Japan, this may become an important risk factor in that population.

Effects on other health risks

ALDH2 deficiency is associated with alcohol-induced asthma, thought to result from the effect of increased circulating acetaldehyde on the airways (Takada *et al.*, 1994). Several papers have recently been published that associate ALDH2 defi-ciency with increased risk of esophageal and oro-pharyngeal cancer (Yokoyama *et al.*, 1996a,b,c). This is difficult to explain since esophageal and upper airway tissues normally have low levels of ALDH2 (Yin *et al.*, 1997). An additional associ-ation with ALDH2 deficiency is a mitochondrial DNA mutation that has been found to be associated with diabetes in Japanese subjects. It was hypothesized that ALDH2 deficiency predisposed the patients to mutagenic effects of acetaldehyde on mitochondrial DNA (Suzuki *et al.*, 1996). No effect on the risk of stomach cancer has been reported.

Other genetic variants

A few other genetic variants have been investigated for their association with alco-holic liver disease. The glutathione S transferase M1 null genotype was more com-mon in alcoholics with liver injury and fibrosis than in alcoholics without liver disease (Savolainen *et al.*, 1996). A variant in the TNF-α promoter that is thought to confer increased expression of that gene was found more often in patients with alcoholic steatohepatitis (Grove *et al.*, 1997a). The frequencies of apolipoprotein E alleles differs between cirrhotics and control Caucasians (Iron *et al.*, 1994). Lastly, the newly identified hemochromatosis alleles have been investigated for interactions with alcohol toxicity, but hemochromatosis heterozygotes were not at higher risk of liver injury than other alcoholics (Grove *et al.*, 1997b). The positive findings await confirmation in other populations.

SUMMARY

The elucidation of nucleotide and amino acid sequences of the genes and enzymes involved in the metabolism of ethanol has led to the ability to genotype individuals simply and rapidly. Although the different isozymes were once thought to be a likely explanation for differences between individuals in alcohol elimination rates, this has not been found to be the case. Other explanations that remain to be investigated include potential regulatory variants in the genes that alter the level of expression of the enzymes, and genetic influences on activity of the malate-aspartate shuttle and rates of mitochondrial NADH reoxidation.

However, the isozymes encoded by ADH2*2, ADH3*1 and ALDH2*2 have been found to influence alcohol drinking behavior and alcoholism substantially. This supports the original premise that the metabolic disposition of ethanol affects individuals' responses to it. The results suggest that any additional variants, such as those recently found in the CYP2E1 gene, might also contribute to the spectrum of individual drinking preferences. On the other hand, the influence of the different isozymes on risk of alcoholic liver disease, while real, is small in magnitude, suggesting that many other factors, such as those controlling responses to oxidative stress, cytokine expression, and fibrogenic reactions, perhaps interacting with the enzyme polymorphisms, are involved in determining susceptibility.

REFERENCES

Agarwal, D.P., Harada, S. and Goedde, H.W. (1981) Racial differences in biological sensitivity to ethanol: the role of alcohol dehydrogenase and aldehyde dehydrogenase isozymes. *Alcohol Clin Exp Res* **5**, 12–16.

Agundez, J., Ladero, J., Diaz-Rubio, M. and Benitez, J. (1996) Rsa I polymorphism at the cytochrome P450 2E1 locus is not related to the risk of alcohol-related severe liver disease. *Liver* **16**, 380–383.

Algar, E.M., Cheung, B., Hayes, J., Holmes, R.S. and Beacham, I.R. (1993) Bovine corneal aldehyde dehydrogenases: evidence for multiple gene products (ALDH3 and ALDHx). *Adv Exp Med Biol* **328**, 153–157.

Allali-Hassani, A., Martinez, S.E., Peralba, J.J., Vaglenova, J., Vidal, F., Richart, C. *et al.* (1997) Alcohol dehydrogenase of human and rat blood vessels: role in ethanol metabolism. *FEBS Lett* **405**, 26–30.

Ammon, E., Schafer, C., Hoffman, U. and Klotz, U. (1996) Disposition and first pass metabolism of ethanol in humans: is it gastric or hepatic and does it depend on gender? *Clin Pharmacol Toxicol* **59**, 503–513.

Ang, H.L., Deltour, L., Hayamizu, T.F., Zgombic-Knight, M. and Duester, G. (1996a) Retinoic acid synthesis in mouse embryos during gastrulation and craniofacial development linked to class IV alcohol dehydrogenase gene expression. *J Biol Chem* **271**, 9526–9534.

Ang, H.L., Deltour, L., Zgombic-Knight, M., Wagner, M.A. and Duester, G. (1996b) Expression patterns of class I and class IV alcohol dehydrogenase genes in developing epithelia suggest a role for ADH in local retinoic acid synthesis. *Alcohol Clin Exp Res* **20**, 1050–1064.

Arthur, M.J., Lee, A. and Wright, R. (1984) Sex differences in the metabolism of ethanol and acetaldehyde in normal subjects. *Clin Sci* **67**, 397–401.

Asmussen, E., Hald, J. and Larsen, V. (1948) The pharmacological action of acetaldehyde on the human organism. *Acta Pharmacol Toxicol* **4**, 311–320.

Badger, T.M., Huang, J., Rans, M. and Lumpkin, C.K. (1993) Induction of cytochrome P450 2E1 during chronic ethanol exposure occurs via transcription of the CYP 2E1 gene when blood alcohol concentrations are high. *Biochem Biophys Res Comm* **190**, 780–785.

Ball, D.M., Sherman, D., Gibb, R., Powell, J.F., Hillman, A., Peters, T. *et al.* (1995) No association between the c2 allele at the cytochrome P450 2E1 gene and alcohol-induced liver disease, alcohol Korsakoff's syndrome, or alcohol dependence syndrome. *Drug Alcohol Depend* **39**, 181–184.

Bengtsson, B.G., Kiessling, K.H., Smith-Kielland, A. and Morland, J. (1981) Partial separation and biochemical characteristics of periportal and perivenous hepatocytes from rat liver. *Eur J Biochem* **118**, 591–597.

Bosron, W.F., Li, T.-K. and Vallee, B.L. (1980) New molecular forms of human liver alcohol dehydrogenase: isolation and characterization of ADH Indianapolis. *Proc Nat Acad Sci USA* **77**, 5784–5788.

Bosron, W.F. and Li, T.-K. (1986) Genetic polymorphism of human liver alcohol and aldehyde dehydrogenases, and their relationship to alcohol metabolism and alcoholism. *Hepatol* **6**, 502–510.

Bosron, W.F. and Li, T.-K. (1987) Catalytic properties of human liver alcohol dehydrogenase isoenzymes. *Enzyme* **37**, 19–28.

Bradford, B.U., Forman, D.T. and Thurman, R.G. (1993a) 4-Methyl pyrazole inhibits fatty acyl coenzyme A synthetase and diminishes catalase-dependent alcohol metabolism: has the contribution of alcohol dehydrogenase to alcohol metabolism been previously over-estimated? *Mol Pharmacol* **43**, 115–119.

Bradford, B.U., Seed, C.B., Handler, J.A., Forman, D.T. and Thurman, R.G. (1993b) Evidence that catalase is a major pathway for ethanol oxidation *in vivo*: dose-response studies in deer mice using methanol as a selective substrate. *Arch Biochem Biophys* **303**, 172–176.

Brown, A.St.J.M., Flatatrone, J.R., Wood, P., Nennett, M.K., Kelly, P.J., Rawlins, M.D. *et al.* (1995) The effect of gastritis on human gastric alcohol dehydrogenase activity and ethanol metabolism. *Aliment Pharmacol Ther* **9**, 57–61.

Brown, C.J., Baltz, K.A. and Edenberg, H.J. (1992) Expression of the human ADH2 gene: an unusual Sp1-binding site in the promoter of a gene expressed at high levels in the liver. *Gene* **121**, 313–320.

Burnell, J.C. and Bosron, W.F. (1989) Genetic polymorphism of human liver alcohol dehydrogenase and kinetic properties of the isoenzymes. In *Human metabolism of alcohol*. 11th edn, edited by K.E. Crow and R.D. Batt, pp. 65–75. Boca Raton, FL: CRC Press.

Cabelleria, J., Baraona, E., Deulafeu, R., Hernandez-Munoz, R., Rodes, J. and Lieber, C.S. (1991) Effects of H2-receptor antagonists on gastric alcohol dehydrogenase activity. *Dig Dis Sci* **36**, 1673–1679.

Caballeria, J., Baraona, E. and Lieber, C.S. (1987) The contribution of the stomach to ethanol oxidation in the rat. *Life Sci* **41**, 1021–1027.

Carpenter, S.P., Lasker, J.M. and Raucy, J.L. (1996) Expression, induction, and catalytic activity of the ethanol inducible cytochrome P450 (CYP 2E1) in human fetal liver and hepatocytes. *Mol Pharmacol* **49**, 260–268.

Carr, L.G., Hartleroad, J.R., Liang, Y., Mendenhall, C., Moritz, T. and Thomasson, H.R. (1995) Polymorphism at the P450 IIE1 locus is not associated with alcoholic liver disease in Caucasian men. *Alc Clin Exp Res* **19**, 182–184.

Carr, L.G., Yi, I.S., Li, T.-K. and Yin, S.J. (1996) Cytochrome P450 2E1 genotypes, alcoholism, and alcoholic cirrhosis in Han Chinese and Atayal natives of Taiwan. *Alcohol Clin Exp Res* **20**, 43–46.

Carriere, V., Verthou, F., Baird, S., Belloc, C., Beaune, P. and De Waziers, I. (1996) Human cytochrome P450 2E1 (CYP 2E1): from genotype to phenotype. *Pharmacogenetics* **6**, 203–211.

Chao, H.M. (1995) Alcohol and the mystique of flushing. *Alcohol Clin Exp Res* **19**, 104–109.

Chao, Y.-C., Liou, S.-R., Chung, Y.-Y., Tang, H.-S., Hsu, C.-T., Li, T.-K. *et al.* (1994) Polymorphism of alcohol and aldehyde dehydrogenase genes and alcoholic cirrhosis in Chinese patients. *Hepatology* **19**, 360–366.

Chao, Y.C., Young, T.H., Chang, W.K., Tang, T.S. and Hsu, C.T. (1995) An investigation of whether polymorphisms of cytochrome P4502E1 are genetic markers of susceptibility to alcoholic end-stage organ damage in a Chinese population. *Hepatology* **22**, 1409–1414.

Chen, L., Sidner, R.A. and Lumeng, L. (1992) Distribution of alcohol dehydrogenase and the low K_m form of aldehyde dehydrogenase in isolated perivenous and periportal hepatocytes in rats. *Alcohol Clin Exp Res* **16**, 23–29.

Cheng, C.-S. and Yoshida, A. (1991) Enzymatic properties of the protein encoded by newly-cloned human alcohol dehydrogenase ADH6 gene. *Biochem Biophys Res Comm* **181**, 743–747.

Chern, M.K. and Pietruszko, R. (1995) Human aldehyde dehydrogenase E3 isozyme is a betaine aldehyde dehydrogenase. *Biochem Biophys Res Commun* **213**, 561–568.

Cole-Harding, S. and Wilson, J.R. (1987) Ethanol metabolism in men and women. *J Stud Alcohol* **48**, 380–387.

Coutelle, C., Ward, P.J., Fleury, B., Quattrorocchi, P., Chambrin, G., Iron, A. Couzigou, P. *et al.* (1997) Laryngeal and oropharyngeal cancer and alcohol dehydrogenase 3 and glutathione S-transferase M1 polymorphisms. *Hum Genet* **99**, 319–325.

Couzigou, P., Fleury, B., Groppi, A., Iron, A., Coutelle, C., Cassaigne, A. *et al.* (1991) Role of alcohol dehydrogenase polymorphism in ethanol metabolism and alcohol-related diseases. *Adv Exp Med Biol* **284**, 263–270.

Crabb, D.W. (1997) First pass metabolism of ethanol: gastric or hepatic, mountain or molehill. *Hepatology* **25**, 1292–1294.

Crabb, D.W., Bosron, W.F. and Li, T.-K. (1983) Steady-state kinetic properties of purified rat liver alcohol dehydrogenase: application to predicting alcohol elimination rates *in vivo*. *Arch Biochem Biophys* **224**, 299–309.

Crabb, D.W., Bosron, W.F. and Li, T.-K. (1987) Ethanol metabolism. *Pharmacol Ther* **34**, 59–73.

Crabb, D.W., Stein, P.M., Dipple, K.M., Hittle, J.B., Sidhu, R., Qulali, M. *et al.* (1989) Structure and expression of the rat class I alcohol dehydrogenase gene. *Genomics* **5**, 906–914.

Crow, K.E., Braggins, T.J., Batt, R.D. and Hardman, M.J. (1982) Rat liver cytosolic malate dehydrogenase: purification, kinetic properties, and role in control of free cytosolic NADH concentration. *J Biol Chem* **257**, 14217–14225.

Crow, K.E., Braggins, T.J. and Hardman, M.J. (1983) Human liver cytosolic malate dehydrogenase: purification, kinetic properties, and role in ethanol metabolism. *Arch Biochem Biophys* **225**, 621–629.

Danielsson, O. and Jornvall, H. (1992) Enzymogenesis: classical liver alcohol dehydrogenase origin from the glutathione-dependent formaldehyde dehydrogenase line. *Proc Natl Acad Sci USA* **89**, 9247–9251.

Day, C.P., Bashir, R., James, O.F.W., Bassendine, M.F., Crabb, D.W., Thomasson, H.R. *et al.* (1991) Investigation of the role of polymorphisms at the alcohol and aldehyde dehydrogenase loci in genetic predisposition to alcohol-related end-organ damage. *Hepatology* **798**, 801.

Day, C.P., James, O.F., Bassendine, M.F., Crabb, D.W. and Li, T.-K. (1993) Alcohol dehydrogenase polymorphism and predisposition to alcoholic cirrhosis (Letter). *Hepatology* **18**, 230–232.

Dickinson, F.M., Hart, G.J. and Kitson, T.M. (1981) The use of pH-gradient ion-exchange chromatography to separate sheep liver cytoplasmic aldehyde dehydrogenase from mitochondrial enzyme contamination, and observations on the interaction between the pure cytoplasmic enzyme and disulfiram. *Biochem J* **199**, 573–600.

DiPadova, D., Worner, T.M., Julkunen, R.J.K. and Lieber, C.S. (1987) Effects of fasting and chronic alcohol consumption on the first-pass metabolism of ethanol. *Gastroenterology* **92**, 1169–1173.

Dipple, K.M., Qulali, M., Ross, R.A. and Crabb, D.W. (1993) Effects of thyroxine on the expression of alcohol dehydrogenase in rat liver and kidney. *Hepatology* **17**, 701–706.

Dohmen, K., Baraona, E., Ishibashi, H., Pozzato, G., Moretti, M., Matsunaga, C. *et al.* (1996) Ethnic differences in gastric sigma alcohol dehydrogenase and ethanol first pass metabolism. *Alcohol Clin Exp Res* **20**, 1569–1576.

Duester, G., Shean, M.L., McBride, M.S. and Stewart, M.J. (1991) Retinoic acid response element in the human alcohol dehydrogenase gene ADH3: implications for regulation of retinoic acid synthesis. *Mol Cell Biol* **11**, 1638–1646.

Duester, G., Smith, M., Bilanchone, V. and Hatfield, G.W. (1986) Molecular analysis of the human class I alcohol dehydrogenase gene family and nucleotide sequence of the gene encoding the β subunit. *J Biol Chem* **261**, 2027–2033.

Eckey, R., Agarwal, D.P., Saha, N. and Goedde, H.W. (1986) Detection and partial characterization of a variant form of cytosolic aldehyde dehydrogenase isozyme. *Hum Genet* **72**, 95–97.

Edenberg, H.J., Brown, C.J. and Zhang, L. (1993) Regulation of the human alcohol dehydrogenase genes ADH1, ADH2, and ADH3: differences in cis-acting sequences at CTF/NF-I sites. *Adv Exp Med Biol* **328**, 561–570.

Ehrig, T., Bosron, W.F. and Li, T.-K. (1990) Alcohol and aldehyde dehydrogenase. *Alcohol Alcohol* **25**, 105–116.

Enomoto, N., Takase, S., Takada, N. and Takada, A. (1991a) Alcoholic liver disease in heterozygotes of mutant and normal dehydrogenase-2 genes. *Hepatology* **13**, 1071–1075.

Enomoto, N., Takase, S., Yasuhara, M. and Takada, A. (1991b) Acetaldehyde metabolism in different aldehyde dehydrogenase 2 genotypes. *Alcohol Clin Exp Res* **15**, 141–144.

Estonius, M., Danielsson, O., Karlsson, C., Person, H., Jornvall, H. and Hoog, J.-O. (1993) Distribution of alcohol and sorbitol dehydrogenases assessment of mRNA species in mammalian tissues. *Eur J Biochem* **215**, 497–503.

Farinati, F., Zhou, Z., Bellah, J., Lieber, C.S. and Garro, A.J. (1985) Effect of chronic ethanol consumption on activation of nitrosopyrrolidine to a mutagen in the rat upper alimentary tract, lung, and hepatic tissue. *Drug Metab Disp* **13**, 210–214.

Farres, J., Moreno, A., Crosas, B., Peralbe, J.M., Allali-Hassani, A., Hjelmqvist, L. *et al.* (1994a) Alcohol dehydrogenase of class IV (sigma ADH) from human stomach: cDNA sequence and structure/function relationships. *Eur J Biochem* **224**, 549–557.

Farres, J., Wang, X., Takahashi, K., Cunningham, S.J., Wang, T.T. and Weiner, H. (1994b) Effects of changing glutamate 487 to lysine in rat and human liver mitochondrial aldehyde dehydrogenase. *J Biol Chem* **269**, 13854–13860.

Frezza, M., DiPadova, C., Pozzato, G., Terpin, K.M., Baraona, E. and Lieber, C.S. (1990) High blood alcohol levels in women: the role of decreased gastric alcohol dehydrogenase activity and first-pass metabolism. *N Eng J Med* **322**, 95–99.

Gilder, F.J., Hodgkinson, S. and Murray, R.M. (1993) ADH and ALDH genotype profiles in Caucasians with alcohol-related problems and controls. *Addiction* **88**, 383–388.

Goedde, H.W. and Agarwal, D.P. (1987) Polymorphism of aldehyde dehydrogenase and alcohol sensitivity. *Enzyme* **37**, 29–44.

Goedde, H.W., Agarwal, D.P., Harada, S., Meier-Tackmann, D., Ruofo, D., Bienzle, U. *et al.* (1983) Population genetic studies of aldehyde dehydrogenase isozyme deficiency and alcohol sensitivity. *Am J Hum Genet* **35**, 769–772.

Goedde, H.W., Singh, S., Agarwal, D.P., Fritze, G., Stapel, K. and Paik, Y.K. (1989) Genotyping of mitochondrial aldehyde dehydrogenase in blood samples using allele-specific oligonucleotides: comparison with phenotyping in hair roots. *Hum Genet* **81**, 305–307.

Goist Jr., K.C. and Sutker, P.B. (1985) Acute alcohol intoxication and body composition in women and men. *Pharmacol Biochem Behav* **22**, 811–814.

Greenfield, N.J. and Pietruszko, R. (1977) Two aldehyde dehydrogenases from human liver: isolation via affinity chromatography and characterization of the isozymes. *Biochim Biophys Acta* **483**, 35–45.

Grove, J., Daly, A.K., Bassendine, M.F. and Day, C.P. (1997a) Association of a tumor necrosis factor promoter polymorphism with susceptibility to alcoholic steatohepatitis. *Hepatology* **26**, 143–146.

Grove, J., Daly, A.K., Burt, A.D., Guzail, M., Bassendine, M.F. and Day, C.P. (1997b) HLA-H mutations, hepatic iron content, and risk of advanced liver in alcoholics. *Hepatology* **26**, 275A.

Gumucio, J.J., DeMason, L.J., Miller, D.L., Krezoski, S.O. and Keener, M. (1978) Induction of cytochrome P-450 in a selective subpopulation of hepatocytes. *Am J Physiol* **234**, C102–C109.

Harada, S., Agarwal, D.P. and Goedde, H.W. (1981) Aldehyde dehydrogenase deficiency as cause of facial flushing reaction to alcohol in Japanese. *Lancet* **2**, 982.

Harada, S., Agarwal, D.P. and Goedde, H.W. (1985) Aldehyde dehydrogenase and alcohol metabolism in alcoholics. *Alcohol* **2**, 391–392.

Harada, S., Agarwal, D.P., Goedde, H.W. and Ishikawa, B. (1983) Aldehyde dehydrogenase isozyme variation and alcoholism in Japan. *Pharmacol Biochem Behav* **18**, 151–153.

Harada, S., Agarwal, D.P., Goedde, H.W., Tagaki, S. and Ishikawa, B. (1982) Possible protective role against alcoholism for aldehyde dehydrogenase isozyme deficiency in Japan. *Lancet* **2**, 827.

Harding, P.P. and Duester, G. (1992) Retinoic acid activation and thyroid hormone repression of the human alcohol dehydrogenase gene ADH3. *J Biol Chem* **267**, 14145–14150.

Harty, L.C., Caporaso, N.E., Hayes, R.B., Winn, D.M., Bravo-Otero, E., Blot, W.J. *et al.* (1997) Alcohol dehydrogenase 3 genotype and risk of oral cavity and pharyngeal cancers. *J Natl Canc Inst* **89**, 1698–1705.

Hayashi, S.I., Watanabe, J. and Kawajiri, K. (1991) Genetic polymorphism in the 5′ flanking region changes transcriptional regulation of the human cytochrome P450 IIE1 gene. *J Biochem* **110**, 559–565.

Hempel, J., Kaiser, R. and Jornvall, H. (1984) Human liver mitochondrial aldehyde dehydrogenase: a C-terminal segment positions and defines the structure corresponding to the one reported to differ in the Oriental enzyme variant. *FEBS Lett* **173**, 367–373.

Higuchi, S., Matsushita, S., Imazeki, H., Kinoshita, T., Takagki, S. and Kono, H. (1994) Aldehyde dehydrogenase genotypes in Japanese alcoholics. *Lancet* **343**, 741–742.

Higuchi, S., Muramatsu, T., Shigemori, K., Saito, M., Kono, H., Dufour, M.C. *et al.* (1992) The relationship between low K_m aldehyde dehydrogenase phenotype and drinking behavior in Japanese. *J Stud Alcohol* **53**, 170–175.

Hoog, J.O. and Brandt, M. (1995) Mammalian class VI alcohol dehydrogenase: novel types of the rodent enzymes. *Adv Exp Med Biol* **373**, 355–364.

Hrubec, Z. and Omenn, G.S. (1981) Evidence of genetic predisposition to alcoholic cirrhosis and psychosis: twin concordances for alcoholism and its biological endpoints by zygosity among male veterans. *Alcohol Clin Exp Res* **5**, 207–215.

Hsu, L.C., Bendel, R.E. and Yoshida, A. (1988) Genomic structure of the human mitochondrial aldehyde dehydrogenase gene. *Genomics* **2**, 57–65.

Hsu, L.C. and Chang, W.C. (1991) Cloning and characterization of a new functional human aldehyde dehydrogenase gene. *J Biol Chem* **266**, 12257–12265.

Hsu, L.C., Chang, W., Lin, S.W. and Yoshida, A. (1995) Cloning and characterization of genes encoding four additional human aldehyde dehydrogenase isozymes. *Adv Exp Med Biol* **372**, 159–168.

Hsu, L., Chang, W.-C. and Yoshida, A. (1989) Genomic structure of the human cytosolic aldehyde dehydrogenase gene. *Genomics* **5**, 857–865.

Hu, Y., Oscarson, M., Johansson, I., Yue, Q.Y., Dahl, M.L., Tabone, M. *et al.* (1997) Genetic polymorphism of human CYP 2E1: characterization of two variant alleles. *Mol Pharmacol* **51**, 370–376.

Inoue, K., Fukunaga, M., Kiriyama, T. and Komura, S. (1984) Accumulation of acetaldehyde in alcohol-sensitive Japanese: relationship to ethanol and acetaldehyde oxidizing capacity. *Alcohol Clin Exp Res* **8**, 319–322.

Iron, A., Richard, P., Pascual De Zulueta, M., Dumas, F., Cassaigne, A. *et al.* (1994) Genetic polymorphism of apolipoprotein E in Caucasian alcoholic cirrhosis. *Alcohol* **29**, 715–718.

Johansson, I., Ekstrom, G., Scholte, B., Puzyck, D., Jornvall, H. and Ingelman-Sundberg, M. (1988) Ethanol-, fasting- and acetone-inducible cytochromes P-450 in rat liver: regulation and characteristics of enzymes belonging to the IIB and IIE gene subfamilies. *Biochemistry* **27**, 1925–1934.

Jones, B.M. and Jones, M.K. (1976) Alcohol effects in women during the menstrual cycle. *Ann N Y Acad Sci* **273**, 576–587.

Jones, D.E., Brennan, M.D., Hempel, J. and Lindahl, R. (1988) Cloning and complete nucleotide sequence of a full-length cDNA encoding a catalytically functional tumor-associated aldehyde dehydrogenase. *Proc Nat Acad Sci USA* **85**, 1782–1786.

Jornvall, H. (1994) The alcohol dehydrogenase system. *EXS* **71**, 221–229.

Julkunen, R.J.K., DiPadova, C. and Lieber, C.S. (1985) First pass metabolism of ethanol – a gastrointestinal barrier against the systemic toxicity of ethanol. *Life Sci* **37**, 567–573.

Kaiser, R., Fernandez, M.R., Pares, X. and Jornvall, H. (1993) Origin of the human alcohol dehydrogenase system: implications from the structure and properties of the octopus protein. *Proc Nat Acad Sci USA* **90**, 11222–11226.

Kato, S., Ishii, H., Aiso, S., Yamashita, S., Ito, D. and Tsuchiya, M. (1990) Histochemical and immunohistochemical evidence for hepatic zone 3 distribution of alcohol dehydrogenase in rats. *Hepatology* **12**, 66–69.

Kato, S., Onda, M., Matsukura, N., Tokunaga, A., Tajiri, T., Kim, D.Y. *et al.* (1995) Cytochrome P4502E1 (CYP2E1) genetic polymorphism in a case-control study of gastric cancer and liver disease. *Pharmacogenetics* **5**, S141–S144.

Kedishvili, N.Y., Gough, W.H., Chernoff, E.A.G., Hurley, T.D., Stone, C.L., Bowman, K.D. *et al.* (1997) cDNA sequence and catalytic properties of a chick embryo alcohol dehydrogenase that oxidizes retinol and 3β,5α-hydroxysteroids. *J Biol Chem* **272**, 7494–7500.

Kim, R.B. and O'Shea, D. (1995) Inter-individual variability of chlorzoxazone 6-hydroxylation in men and women and its relationship to CYP 2E1 genetic polymorphisms. *Clin Pharmacol Ther* **57**, 645–655.

Kim, R.B., Yamazaki, H., Chiba, K., O'Shea, D., Mimura, M., Guengerich, F.P. *et al.* (1996) *In vivo* and *in vitro* characterization of CYP 2E1 activity in Japanese and Caucasians. *J Pharmacol Exp Ther* **279**, 4–11.

Kitson, T.M. (1989) Reactions of aldehyde dehydrogenase with disulfiram and related compounds. In *Human Metabolism of Alcohol*, edited by K.E. Crow and R.D. Badd, pp. 117–132. Boca Raton, Florida: CRC Press.

Koivusalo, M., Baumann, M. and Uotila, L. (1989) Evidence for the identity of glutathione-dependent formaldehyde dehydrogenase and class III alcohol dehydrogenase. *FEBS Lett* **257**, 105–109.

Kopun, M. and Propping, P. (1977) The kinetics of ethanol absorption and elimination in twins and supplementary repetitive experiments in singleton subjects. *Eur J Clin Pharmacol* **11**, 337–344.

Korsten, M.A., Matsuzaki, S., Feinman, L. and Lieber, C.S. (1975) High blood acetaldehyde levels after ethanol administration: differences between alcoholic and non-alcoholic subjects. *N Eng J Med* **292**, 386–389.

Kurys, G., Ambrosiak, W. and Pietruszko, R. (1989) Human aldehyde dehydrogenase. Purification and characterization of a third isozyme with low Km for gamma-aminobutyraldehyde. *J Biol Chem* **264**, 4715–4721.

Kurys, G., Shah, P.C., Kikonyogo, A., Reed, D., Ambrosiak, W. and Pietruszko, R. (1993) Human aldehyde dehydrogenase: cDNA cloning and primary structure of the enzyme that catalyzes dehydrogenation of 4-aminobutyraldehyde. *Eur J Biochem* **218**, 311–320.

Kwo, P.Y., Ramchandani, V.A., Amann, D., Carr, L.G., Sandrasegaran, K., Kopecky, K. *et al.* (1997) Gender differences in alcohol metabolism are explained in part by computed liver volume and lean body mass. *Alcohol Clin Exp Res* **21**, 51A.

Levitt, M.D. (1994) Antagonist: the case against first pass metabolism in the stomach. *J Lab Clin Med* **123**, 28–31.

Levitt, M.D. and Levitt, D.G. (1994) The critical role of the rate of ethanol absorption in the interpretation of studies purporting to demonstrate gastric metabolism of ethanol. *J Pharmacol Exp Ther* **269**, 297–304.

Lieber, C.S. (1990) Interaction of ethanol with drugs, hepatotoxic agents, carcinogens and vitamins. *Alcohol Alcohol* **25**, 157–176.

Lieber, C.S. (1994) Alcohol and the liver: 1994 Update. *Gastroenterology* **106**, 1085–1105.

Lim, R.T., Gentry, R.T., Ito, D., Yokoyama, H., Baraona, E. and Lieber, C.S. (1993) First-pass metabolism of ethanol is predominantly gastric. *Alcohol Clin Exp Res* **17**, 1337–1344.

Lin, K.-H., Winters, A.L. and Lindahl, R. (1984) Regulation of aldehyde dehydrogenase activity in 5 rat hepatoma cell lines. *Cancer Res* **44**, 5219–5226.

Lin, S.W., Chen, J.C., Hsu, L.C., Hsieh, C.L. and Yoshida, A. (1996) Human γ-aminobutyraldehyde dehydrogenase (ALDH9): cDNA sequence, genomic organization, chromosomal localization, and tissue expression. *Genomics* **34**, 376–380.

Lindahl, R. (1986) Identification of hepatocarcinogenesis-associated aldehyde dehydrogenase in normal rat urinary bladder. *Cancer Res* **46**, 2502–2506.

Lindahl, R. (1992) Aldehyde dehydrogenases and their role in carcinogenesis. *Crit Rev Biochem Mol Biol* **27**, 283–335.

Lindros, K.O., Stowell, A., Pikkarainen, P. and Salaspuro, M. (1980) Elevated blood acetaldehyde in alcoholics with accelerated ethanol elimination. *Pharmacol Biochem Behav* **13**, 119–125.

Liu, S.Y. and Gonzalez, F.J. (1995) Role of liver-enriched transcription factor HNF-1α in expresion of the CYP 2E1 gene. *DNA Cell Biol* **14**, 285–293.

Lumeng, L. and Crabb, D.W. (1984) Rate determining factors for ethanol metabolism in fasted and castrated male rats. *Biochem Phamacol* **22**, 811–814.

Lumeng, L. and Crabb, D.W. (1994) Genetic aspects and risk factors in alcoholism and alcoholic liver disease. *Gastroenterology* **107**, 572–578.

Lumeng, L. and Davis, E.J. (1970) Oxidation of acetate by liver mitochondria. *FEBS Lett* **29**, 124–134.

MacKerell, A.D., Vallari, R.C. and Pietruszko, R. (1985) Human mitochondrial aldehyde dehydrogenase inhibition by diethyldithiocarbamic acid ethanethiol mixed disulfide: a derivative of disulfiram. *FEBS Lett* **179**, 77–81.

Maeda, M., Husumura, Y. and Takeuchi, J. (1988) Localization of cytoplasmic and mito-chondrial aldehyde dehydrogenase isozymes in human liver. *Lab Invest* **59**, 75–81.

Maezawa, Y., Yamauchi, M. and Toda, G. (1994) Association between restriction fragment length polymorphism of the human cytochrome P450 IIE1 gene and susceptibility to alcoholic liver cirrhosis. *Am J Gastroenterol* **89**, 561–565.

Marshall, A.W., Kingstone, D., Boss, M. and Morgan, M.Y. (1983) Ethanol elimination in males and females: relationship to menstrual cycle and body composition. *Hepatology* **3**, 701–706.

Marshall, S.J. and Chambers, G.K. (1994) Alcohol dehydrogenase and aldehyde dehydrogen-ase gene variants in New Zealand alcoholic patients. *Alcohol Clin Exp Res* **18**, 58A (Abstract).

Martin, N.G., Perl, J., Oakeshott, J.G., Gibson, J.B., Starmer, G.A. and Wilks, A.V. (1985) A twin study of ethanol metabolism. *Behav Genet* **15**, 93–109.

Matsumoto, M., Takahashi, H., Maruyama, K., Higuchi, S., Matsushita, S., Muramatsu, T. *et al.* (1996) Genotypes of alcohol-metabolizing enzymes and the risk for alcoholic pan-creatitis in Japanese alcoholics. *Alcohol Clin Exp Res* **20**, 289A–292A.

Mezey, E., Oesterling, J.E. and Potter, J.J. (1988) Influence of male hormones on rates of ethanol elimination in man. *Hepatology* **8**, 742–744.

Mezey, E. and Potter, J.J. (1979) Rat liver alcohol dehydrogenase activity: effects of growth hormone and hypophysectomy. *Endocrinology* **104**, 1667–1673.

Mezey, E. and Potter, J.J. (1981) Effects of thyroidectomy and triiodothyronine administra-tion on rat liver alcohol dehydrogenase. *Gastroenterology* **80**, 566–574.

Mezey, E., Potter, J.J. and Diehl, A.M. (1986a) Depression of alcohol dehydrogenase activity in rat hepatocyte culture by dihydrotestosterone. *Biochem Pharmacol* **35**, 335–339.

Mezey, E., Potter, J.J. and Rhodes, D.L. (1986b) Effect of growth hormone on alcohol dehydrogenase activity in hepatocyte culture. *Gastroenterology* **91**, 1271–1278.

Mishra, L., Sharma, S., Potter, J.J. and Mezey, E. (1989) More rapid elimination of alcohol in women as compared with their male siblings. *Alcohol Clin Exp Res* **13**, 552–554.

Mizoi, Y., Ijiri, I., Tatsuno, Y., Kijima, T., Fujiwara, S. and Adachi, J. (1979) Relationship between facial flushing and blood acetaldehyde levels after alcohol intake. *Pharmacol Biochem Behav* **10**, 303–311.

Mizoi, Y., Yamamoto, K., Ueno, Y., Fukunaga, T. and Harada, S. (1994) Involvement of genetic polymorphism of alcohol and aldehyde dehydrogenases in individual variation of alcohol metabolism. *Alcohol* **29**, 707–710.

Moreno, A. and Pares, X. (1991) Purification and characterization of a new alcohol dehydro-genase from human stomach. *J Biol Chem* **266**, 1128–1133.

Morgan, E.T., Koop, D.R. and Coon, M.J. (1982) Catalytic activity of cytochrome P450 isoenzyme 3a isolated from liver microsomes of ethanol-treated rabbits. *J Biol Chem* **257**, 13951–13957.

Novoradovsky, A., Tsai, S.J., Goldfarb, L., Peterson, R., Long, J.C. and Goldman, D. (1995) Mitochondrial aldehyde dehydrogenase polymorphism in Asian and American Indian populations: detection of new ALDH2 alleles. *Alcohol Clin Exp Res* **19**, 1105–1110.

O'Connor, S., Morzorati, S., Christian, J. and Li, T.K. (1998) Clamping BrAC reduces experimental variance: application to the study of acute tolerance to alcohol and alcohol elimination rate. *Alcohol Clin Exp Res* **22**, 202–210.

Pares, X., Cederlund, E., Moreno, A., Hjelmqvist, L. and Jornvall, H. (1994) Mammalian class IV alcohol dehydrogenase (stomach alcohol dehydrogenase): structure, origin, and correlation with enzymology. *Proc Nat Acad Sci USA* **91**, 1893–1897.

Pares, X., Moreno, A., Farres, J., Soler, X., Panes, J., Pares, A. *et al.* (1992) Liver and stomach alcohol dehydrogenase in normal and alcoholic individuals from Barcelona. *Proceedings of the ISBRA Satellite Symposium: Genetics and Alcohol Related Diseases*, June 18–19, 1992 Bordeaux, France (Abstract).

Pares, X. and Vallee, B.L. (1981) New human liver alcohol dehydrogenase forms with unique kinetic characteristics. *Biochem Biophys Res Comm* **98**, 122–130.

Pirmohamed, M., Kitteringham, N.R., Quest, L.J., Allott, R.L., Green, V.J., Gilmore, I.T. *et al.* (1995) Genetic polymorphism of cytochrome P450 2E1 and risk of alcoholic liver disease in Caucasians. *Pharmacogenetics* **5**, 351–357.

Potter, J.J., Cheneval, D., Dang, C.V., Resar, L.M., Mezey, E. and Yang, V.W. (1991a) The upstream stimulatory factor binds to and activates the promoter of the rat class I alcohol dehydrogenase gene. *J Biol Chem* **266**, 15457–15463.

Potter, J.J., Mezey, E., Christy, R.J., Crabb, D.W., Stein, P.M. and Yang, V.W. (1991b) CCAAT/enhancer binding protein binds and activates the promoter of the rat class I alcohol dehydrogenase gene. *Arch Biochem Biophys* **285**, 246–251.

Potter, J.J., Mezey, E. and Yang, V.W. (1989) Influence of growth hormone on the synthesis of rat liver alcohol dehydrogenase in primary hepatocyte culture. *Arch Biochem Biophys* **274**, 548–556.

Potter, J.J., Yang, V.W. and Mezey, E. (1993) Regulation of the rat class I alcohol dehydrogenase gene by growth hormone. *Biochem Biophys Res Comm* **191**, 1040–1045.

Poupon, R.E., Nalpas, B., Coutelle, C., Fleury, B., Couzigou, P. and Higueret, D. (1992) Polymorphism of alcohol dehydrogenase, alcohol and aldehyde dehydrogenase activities: implication in alcoholic cirrhosis in white patients. *Hepatology* **15**, 1017–1022.

Quan, F., Korneluk, R.G., Tropak, M.B. and Bravel, R.A. (1986) Isolation and characterization of the human catalase gene. *Nucl Acids Res* **14**, 5321–5332.

Qulali, M. and Crabb, D.W. (1992) Corticosterone induces rat liver alcohol dehydrogenase mRNA but not enzyme protein or activity. *Alcohol Clin Exp Res* **16**, 427–431.

Rachamin, G., MacDonald, J.A., Wahid, S., Clapp, J.J., Khanna, J.M. and Israel, Y. (1980) Modulation of alcohol dehydrogenase and ethanol metabolism by sex hormones in the spontaneously hypertensive rat effect of chronic ethanol administration. *Biochem J* **186**, 489–490, 70.

Reed, R., Page, W.F., Viken, R.J. and Christian, J.C. (1996) Genetic predisposition to organ-specific endpoints of alcoholism. *Alcohol Clin Exp Res* **20**, 1528–1533.

Roine, R., Gentry, R.T., Hernandez-Munoz R., Baraona, E. and Lieber, C.S. (1990) Aspirin increases blood alcohol concentration in humans after ingestion of ethanol. *JAMA* **264**, 2406–2408.

Sato, C., Matsuda, Y. and Lieber, C.S. (1981) Increased hepatotoxicity of acetaminophen after chronic ethanol consumption in the rat. *Gastroenterology* **80**, 140–148.

Satre, M.A., Zgombic-Knight, M. and Duester, G. (1994) The complete structure of human class IV alcohol dehydrogenase (retinol dehydrogenase) determined from the ADH7 gene. *J Biol Chem* **269**, 15606–15612.

Savolainen, V.T., Pjarinen, J., Perola, M., Penttila, A. and Karhunen, P.J. (1996) Glutathione-S-transferase GST M1 "null" genotype and the risk of alcoholic liver disease. *Alcohol Clin Exp Res* **20**, 1340–1345.

Savolainen, V.T., Pajarinen, J., Perola, M., Tenttila, A. and Karhunen, P.J. (1997) Polymorphism of the cytochrome P450 2E1 gene and the risk of alcoholic liver disease. *J Hepatol* **216**, 55–61.

Schenker, S. (1997) Medical consequences of alcoholism: is gender a factor? *Alcohol Clin Exp Res* **21**, 179–181.

Schwitters, S.Y., Johnson, R.C., Johnson, S.B. and Ahern, F.M. (1982) Familial resemblances in flushing following alcohol use. *Behavior Genet* **12**, 349–352.

Seeff, L.B., Cuccherini, B.A., Zimmerman, H.J., Adler, E. and Benjamin, S.B. (1986) Acetaminophen toxicity in alcoholics. *Ann Intern Med* **104**, 399–404.

Seitz, H.K., Egerer, G., Simanowski, U.A., Waldherr, R., Eckey, R., Agarwal, D.P. *et al.* (1993) Human gastric alcohol dehydrogenase activity: effect of age, sex, and alcoholism. *Gut* **34**, 1433–1437.

Shen, Y.-C., Fan, J.-H., Edenberg, H.J., Li, T.-K., Cui, Y.-H., Wang, Y.-F. *et al.* (1997) Polymorphism of ADH and ALDH genes among four ethnic groups in China and effects upon the risk for alcoholism. *Alcohol Clin Exp Res* **21**, 1272–1277.

Sherman, D., Dave, V., Hsu, L.C., Peters, T.J. and Yoshida, A. (1993a) Diverse polymorphism within a short coding region of the human aldehyde dehydrogenase-5 (ALDH5) gene. *Hum Genet* **92**, 477–480.

Sherman, D.I.N., Ward, R.J., Warren-Perry, M., Williams, R. and Peters, T.J. (1993b) Association of restriction fragment length polymorphism in alcohol dehydrogenase 2 gene with alcohol-induced liver damage. *Br Med J* **307**, 1388–1390.

Sherman, D.I., Ward, R.J., Yoshida, A. and Peters, T.J. (1994) Alcohol and acetaldehyde dehydrogenase gene polymorphism and alcoholism. *EXS* **71**, 291–300.

Shibuya, A. and Yoshida, A. (1989) Genotypes of alcohol metabolizing enzymes in Japanese with alcoholic liver diseases: a strong correlation of the usual Caucasian type aldehyde dehydrogenase gene (ALDH2-1) with the disease. *Am J Hum Genet* **43**, 744–748.

Shimizu, M., Lasker, J.M., Tsutsumi, M. and Lieber, C.S. (1990) Immunohistochemical localization of ethanol-inducible P450 IIE1 in the rat alimentary tract. *Gastroenterology* **99**, 1044–1053.

Smith, T., DeMaster, E.G., Furne, J.K., Springfield, J. and Levitt, M.D. (1992) First-pass gastric mucosal metabolism of ethanol is negligible in the rat. *J Clin Invest* **89**, 1801–1806.

Song, B.J., Matsunaga, T., Hardwick, J.P., Park, S.S., Veech, R.L., Yang, C.-S. *et al.* (1987) Stabilization of cytochrome P450j messenger ribonucleic acid in the diabetic rat. *Mol Endocrinol* **1**, 542–547.

Song, B.J., Veech, R.L., Park, S.S., Gelboin, H.V. and Gonzales, F.J. (1990) Induction of rat hepatic N-nitrosodimethylamine demethylase by acetone is due to protein stabilization. *J Biol Chem* **264**, 3568–3572.

Steinmetz, C.G., Xie, P., Weiner, H. and Hurley, T.D. (1997) Structure of mitochondrial aldehyde dehydrogenase: the genetic component of ethanol aversion. *Structure* **5**, 701–711.

Stephen, E.A., Taylor, J.A., Kaplan, N., Yang, C.-H., Hsieh, L.L., Lucier, G.W. *et al.* (1994) Ethnic variation in the CYP 2E1 gene: polymorphism analysis of 695 African-Americans, European-Americans, and Taiwanese. *Pharmacogenetics* **4**, 185–192.

Stewart, M.J., Dipple, K.M., Stewart, T.R. and Crabb, D.W. (1996a) The role of nuclear factor NF-Y/CP1 in the transcriptional regulation of the human aldehyde dehydrogenase 2-encoding gene. *Gene* **173**, 155–161.

Stewart, M.J., Malek, K. and Crabb, D.W. (1996b) Distribution of messenger RNAs for aldehyde dehydrogenase 1, aldehyde dehydrogenase 2, and aldehyde dehydrogenase 5 in human tissues. *J Investig Med* **44**, 42–46.

Stewart, M.J., McBride, J.S., Winter, L.A. and Duester, G. (1990) Promoters for the human alcohol dehydrogenase genes ADH1, ADH2, and ADH3: interactions of CCAAT/enhancer binding protein with elements flanking the TATA box. *Gene* **90**, 271–279.

Stewart, M.J., Shean, M.L., Paeper, B.W. and Duester, G. (1991) The role of C/EBP in the differential transcriptional regulation of a family of human liver alcohol dehydrogenase genes. *J Biol Chem* **266**, 11594–11603.

Stone, C.L., Thomasson, H.R., Bosron, W.F. and Li, T.-K. (1993) Purification and partial amino acid sequence of a high activity human alcohol dehydrogenase. *Alcohol Clin Exp Res* **17**, 911–917.

Sutker, P.B., Tabakoff, B., Goist Jr., K.C. and Randall, C.L. (1983) Acute alcohol intoxication, mood states and alcohol metabolism in women and men. *Pharmacol Biochem Behav* **18** (Suppl 1), 349–354.

Suzuki, Y., Muramatsu, Y., Taniyama, M., Atsumi, Y., Suematswu, M., Kawaguchi, R. *et al.* (1996) Mitochondrial aldehyde dehydrogenase in diabetes associated with mitochondrial tRNA [Leu(UUR)] mutation at position 3243. *Diabetes Care* **12**, 1432–1425.

Takada, A., Tsutsumi, M. and Kobayashi, Y. (1994) Genotypes of ALDH2 related to liver and pulmonary diseases and other genetic factors related to alcoholic liver disease. *Alcohol* **29**, 719–727.

Takahashi, T., Lasker, J.M., Rosman, A.S. and Lieber, C.S. (1993) Induction of cytochrome P450 2E1 in the human liver by ethanol is caused by a corresponding increase in encoding mRNA. *Hepatology* **17**, 236–245.

Takeshita, T., Morimoto, K., Mao, X.Q., Hashimoto, T. and Furuyama, J.I. (1994) Characterization of the three genotypes of low Km aldehyde dehydrogenase in a Japanese population. *Hum Genet* **94**, 217–223.

Tanaka, F., Shiratori, Y., Yokosuka, O., Imazeki, F., Tsukada, Y. and Omata, M. (1996) High incidence of ADH2*1/ALDH2*1 genes among Japanese alcohol dependents and patients with alcoholic liver disease. *Hepatology* **23**, 234–239.

Tanaka, F., Shiratori, Y., Yokosuka, O., Imadzeki, F., Tsukada, Y. and Omata, M. (1997) Polymorphism of alcohol-metabolizing genes affects drinking behavior and alcoholic liver disease in Japanese men. *Alcohol Clin Exp Res* **21**, 596–601.

Terelius, Y., Norstenhoog, C., Cronholm, T. and Ingelman-Sundberg, M. (1991) Acetaldehyde as an efficient substrate for ethanol-inducible cytochrome P450 (CYP 2E1). *Biochem Biophys Res Comm* **179**, 689–694.

Thomasson, H.R. (1995) Gender differences in alcohol metabolism: physiological responses to ethanol. *Recent Dev Alcohol* **12**, 163–179.

Thomasson, H.R., Beard, J. and Li, T.-K. (1995) ADH gene polymorphisms are determinants of alcohol pharmacokinetics. *Alcohol Clin Exp Res* **19**, 1494–1499.

Thomasson, H.R., Crabb, D.W., Edenberg, H.J., Li, T.-K., Hwu, H.-G., Chen, C.-C. *et al.* (1994) Low frequency of the ADH2*2 allele among Atayal natives of Taiwan with alcohol use disorders. *Alcohol Clin Exp Res* **18**, 640–643.

Thomasson, H.R., Edenberg, H.J., Crabb, D.W., Mai, X.-L., Jerome, R.E., Li, T.-K. *et al.* (1991) Alcohol and aldehyde dehydrogenase genotypes and alcoholism in Chinese men. *Am J Hum Genet* **48**, 677–681.

Thomasson, H.R., Li, T.-K. and Crabb, D.W. (1990) Correlations between alcohol-induced flushing, genotypes for alcohol and aldehyde dehydrogenases, and alcohol elimination rates. *Hepatology* **12**, 903A.

Tsukamoto, A., Kanegae, T., Isobe, E., Hireose, M., Shimamua, M. and Nagoya, T. (1996) Effects of bezafibrate on ethanol oxidation in rats. *Alcohol Clin Exp Res* **20**, 1599–1603.

Tsutsumi, M., Lasker, J.M., Shimizu, M., Rosman, A.S. and Lieber, C.S. (1989) The intralobular distribution of ethanol-inducible P450IIE1 in rat and human liver. *Hepatology* **10**, 437–446.

Tsutsumi, M., Takada, A. and Wang, J.-S. (1994) Genetic polymorphisms of cytochrome P450 2E1 related to the development of alcoholic liver disease. *Gastroenterology* **107**, 1430–1435.

Tu, G.C. and Israel Y. (1995) Alcohol consumption by Orientals in North American is predicted largely by a single gene. *Behav Genet* **25**, 59–65.

Uemeno, M., McBride, O.W., Yang, C.S., Gelboin H.V. and Gonzales, F.J. (1988) Human ethanol-inducible P450IIE1: complete gene sequence, promoter characterization, chromosome mapping and cDNA-directed expression. *Biochemistry* **27**, 9006–9013.

Ueno, T. and Gonzales, F.J. (1990) Transcriptional control of the rat hepatic CYP 2E1 gene. *Mol Cell Biol* **10**, 4495–4505.

Ueshima, Y., Tsutsumi, M., Takase, S., Matsuda, Y. and Kawahara, H. (1996) Acetaminophen metabolism in patients with different cytochrome P-450 2E1 genotypes. *Alcohol Clin Exp Res* **20**, 25A–28A.

Vaananen, H., Salaspuro, M. and Lindros, K. (1984) The effect of chronic ethanol ingestion on ethanol metabolizing enzymes in isolated periportal and perivenous rat hepatocytes. *Hepatology* **4**, 862–866.

van Ooij, C., Snyder, R.C., Paeper, B.W. and Duester, G. (1992) Temporal expression of the human alcohol dehydrogenase gene family during liver development correlates with differential promoter activation by hepatocyte nuclear factor 1, CCAAT/enhancer-binding protein α, liver activator protein, and D-element-binding protein. *Mol Cell Biol* **12**, 3023–3031.

VanRemmen, H., Williams, M.D., Yang, H., Walter, C.A. and Richardson A. (1998) Analysis of the transcriptional activity of the 5' flanking region of the rat catalase gene in transiently transfected cells and in transgenic mice. *J Cell Physiol* **174**, 18–26.

von Wartburg, J.P., Papenberg, J. and Aebi, H. (1964) An atypical alcohol dehydrogenase. *Can J Biochem* **43**, 889–898.

Watanabe, J., Hayashi, S. and Kawajiri, K. (1994) Different regulation and expression of the human CYP 2E1 gene due to the Rsa I polymorphism in the 5'-flanking region. *J Biochem* **16**, 321–326.

Winter, L.A., Stewart, M.J., Shean, M.L., Dong, Y., Poellinger, L., Okret, S. *et al.* (1990) A hormone response element upstream from the human alcohol dehydrogenase gene ADH2 consists of three tandem glucocorticoid receptor binding sites. *Gene* **91**, 233–240.

Wolff, P.H. (1972) Ethnic differences in alcohol sensitivity. *Science* **449**, 451.

Wolff, P.H. (1973) Vasomotor sensitivity to alcohol in diverse mongoloid populations. *Am J Hum Genet* **25**, 193–199.

Wrighton, S.A., Thomas, P.E., Molowa, D.T., Haniu, M., Shively, J.E., Maines, S.L. *et al.* (1986) Characterization of ethanol-inducible human liver *N*-nitrosodimethylamine demethylase. *Biochemistry* **25**, 6731–6735.

Xiao, Q., Weiner, H. and Crabb, D.W. (1996) The mutation in the mitochondrial aldehyde dehydrogenase (ALDH2) gene responsible for alcohol-induced flushing increases turnover of the enzyme tetramers in a dominant fashion. *J Clin Invest* **98**, 2027–2032.

Xiao, Q., Weiner, H., Johnson, T. and Crabb, D.W. (1995) The aldehyde dehydrogenase ALDH2*2 allele exhibits dominance over ALDH2*1 in HeLa cells. *J Clin Invest* **96**, 2180–2186.

Yamauchi, M., Maezawa, Y., Toda, G., Suzuki, H. and Sakurai, S. (1995) Association of a restriction fragment length polymorphism in the alcohol dehydrogenase-2 gene with Japanese alcoholic liver cirrhosis. *J Hepatol* **23**, 519–523.

Yamauchi, M., Potter, J.J. and Mezey, E. (1988a) Lobular distribution of alcohol dehydrogenase in the rat liver. *Hepatology* **2**, 243–247.

Yamauchi, M., Potter, J.J. and Mezey, E. (1988b) Characteristics of alcohol dehydrogenase in fat-storing (Ito) cells of rat liver. *Gastroenterology* **94**, 163–169.

Yanagawa, Y., Chen, J.C., Hsu, L.C. and Yoshida, A. (1995) The transcriptional regulation of human aldehyde dehydrogenase I gene. The structure and functional analysis of the promoter. *J Biol Chem* **270**, 17521–17527.

Yasunami, M., Chen, C.-S. and Yoshida, A. (1991) A human alcohol dehydrogenase gene (ADH6) encoding an additional class of isozyme. *Proc Nat Acad Sci USA* **88**, 7610–7614.

Yin, S.-J., Liao, C.-S., Wu, C.-W., Li, T.-T., Chen, L.-L., Lai, C.-L. and Tsao, T.-Y. (1997) Human stomach alcohol and aldehyde dehydrogenases: comparison of expression pattern and activities in alimentary tract. *Gastroenterology* **112**, 766–775.

Yin, S.-J., Wang, M.-F., Liao, C.-S., Chen, C.-M. and Wu, C.-W. (1990) Identification of a human stomach alcohol dehydrogenase with distinctive kinetic properties. *Biochem Int* **22**, 829–835.

Yokoyama, A., Muramatsu, T., Ohmori, T., Higuchi, S., Hayashida, M. and Ishii, H. (1996a) Esophageal cancer and aldehyde dehydrogenase-2 genotypes in Japanese males. *Cancer Epidemiol Biomarkers Prev* **5**, 99–102.

Yokoyama, A., Muramatsu, T., Ohmori, T., Makuuchi, H., Higuchi, S., Matsushita, S. *et al.* (1996b) Multiple primary esophageal and concurrent upper aerodigestive tract cancer and the aldehyde dehydrogenase-2 genotype of Japanese alcoholics. *Cancer* **77**, 1986–1990.

Yokoyama, A., Ohmori, T., Muramatsu, T., Higuchi, S., Yokoyama, T., Matsushita, S. *et al.* (1996c) Cancer screening of upper aerodigestive tract in Japanese alcoholics with reference to drinking and smoking habits and aldehyde dehydrogeanse 2 genotype. *Int J Cancer* **68**, 313–316.

Yoshida, A., Dave, V., Ward, R.J. and Peters, T.J. (1989) Cytosolic aldehyde dehydrogenase (ALDH1) variants found in alcohol flushers. *Ann Hum Genet Lond* **53**, 1–7.

Yoshida, A., Huang, I.-Y. and Ikawa, M. (1984) Molecular abnormality of an inactive aldehyde dehydrogenase variant commonly found in Orientals. *Proc Nat Acad Sci USA* **81**, 258–261.

Yoshida, A., Wang, G. and Dave, V. (1983) Determination of genotypes of human liver aldehyde dehydrogenase ALDH2 locus. *Am J Hum Genet* **35**, 1107–1116.

Yun, Y.P., Casazza, J.P., Sohn, D.H., Veech, R.L. and Song, B.J. (1992) Pretranslational activation of cytochrome P450 IIE during ketosis induced by a high fat diet. *Mol Pharmacol* **41**, 474–479.

Zeiner, A.R., Paredes, A. and Christiansen, D.H. (1979) The role of acetaldehyde in mediating reactivity to an acute dose of ethanol among different racial groups. *Alcohol Clin Exp Res* **3**, 11–18.

Zheng, Y.W., Bey, M., Liu, H. and Felder, M.R. (1993) Molecular basis of the alcohol dehydrogenase-negative deermouse: evidence for deletion of the gene for class I enzyme and identification of a possible new enzyme class. *J Biol Chem* **268**, 24933–24939.

Chapter 5

Acetaldehyde adducts: role in ethanol-induced liver disease

John Koskinas

Acetaldehyde, the main product of ethanol metabolism in the liver, is a highly reactive compound which is able to react with proteins to form both stable and unstable adducts. The chemistry of acetaldehyde–protein interaction mainly involves unstable Schiff base adducts formed by binding of acetaldehyde to lysine residues of a protein which are further stabilized by reduction. Acetaldehyde adducts could be involved in alcohol induced liver injury either by modifying the biological function of the protein or by changing its antigenicity. Proteins with reactive lysine residues involved in their biological activity are subjected to acetaldehyde induced impaired function. Stable acetaldehyde adducts have been found to act as antigens eliciting immune responses. Circulating antibodies, mainly IgA isotype, to synthetic adducts have been detected predominantly in alcoholics with liver disease and to a lesser extent in patients with non-alcoholic liver disease and in heavy drinkers without liver injury. Additionally, a few target antigenic proteins in animals fed alcohol and in alcoholics have been identified using either antibodies to synthetic adducts or circulating antibodies. Patients with non-alcohol liver damage and alcoholics without liver disease exhibited these antigens in their livers much less frequently. Immunohistochemical studies have also established the presence of acetaldehyde adducts in the liver in a high proportion of alcoholics with liver disease. In conclusion, acetaldehyde adducts generated *in vivo* are immunogenic and could induce both inflammation and fibrosis.

KEYWORDS: acetaldehyde adducts, pathogenesis, liver disease

INTRODUCTION

The conversion of ethanol to acetaldehyde involves two metabolic pathways; the alcohol dehydrogenase and the P450 2E1 which becomes more important in chronic alcohol consumption (Lieber and DeCarli, 1968). In alcoholic subjects, it is known that tissue and blood levels of acetaldehyde are high (Lindros, 1982), as a result of an enhanced rate of metabolism of ethanol to acetaldehyde (Lieber and DeCarli, 1970) by the MEOS, and a reduction in activity of hepatic acetaldehyde dehydrogenase (Takase *et al.*, 1989). Among alcoholics, only about 20% develop serious liver disease; furthermore, ethanol hepatotoxicity does not show a direct correlation with dose, suggesting that other host specific factors may be crucial in the development of liver injury (Mezey, 1982). In patients with acute alcoholic hepatitis, there is clinical and laboratory evidence of liver damage progressing for a period of 2–4 weeks after cessation of alcohol ingestion (Marshall *et al.*, 1983; Reynolds *et al.*, 1989). Based on these data, it has been suggested that immune mechanisms might be involved and that formation of acetaldehyde adducts can both incite an inflammatory response and also generate specific antigen antibody reaction. The formation of acetaldehyde adducts in the liver during the metabolism of ethanol is a very crucial element in the evaluation of their role in alcoholic liver damage. Early studies have shown that alcohol in cell free liver homogenates (Donohue *et al.*, 1983a) and in liver slices (Medina *et al.*, 1985) is metabolized to acetaldehyde which subsequently binds to proteins forming both unstable and stable adducts.

CHEMISTRY OF ACETALDEHYDE–PROTEIN INTERACTIONS

Acetaldehyde is a highly reactive compound which is able to react with a variety of nucleophilic groups because of the electrophilic nature of the carbonyl carbon (O'Donnell, 1982). The ϵ-amino group of internal lysine residues and the α-amino group of N-terminal amino acids of proteins are the major nucleophilic groups that participate in acetaldehyde binding. Covalent binding of acetaldehyde to proteins yields both unstable and stable adducts (Gaines *et al.*, 1977; Nomura and Lieber, 1981; Stevens *et al.*, 1981; Kenny, 1982; Donohue *et al.*, 1983b; Tuma and Sorrell, 1985, Tuma *et al.*, 1987a,b). Unstable adducts can easily dissociate when exposed to conditions such as dialysis, gel filtration or treatment with weak acids or bases, whereas stable ones are irreversible products characterized by their resistance to various conditions (Donohue *et al.*, 1983b; Tuma and Sorrell, 1985; Tuma *et al.*, 1987b). Unstable Schiff base adducts are subject to stabilization through various metabolic pathways. Adducts generated by binding of acetaldehyde to the α-amino group of an N-terminal amino acid of a protein are stabilized by a cyclization reaction forming a 2-methyl-imidazolidin-4 product (San George and Hoberman, 1986). Unstable Schiff base adducts formed by binding of acetaldehyde to the ϵ-amino group of the internal lysine residues of a protein, which seems to be the most important mechanism of acetaldehyde adduct formation, can be stabilized either by reduction or by addition of a thiol group (Sorrell and Tuma, 1985; Tuma and Sorrell, 1985) (Figure 5.1). Reduction and subsequent formation of *N*-ethyllysine residues take place in the presence of reducing agents such as sodium cyanoborohydride or ascorbate (Donohue *et al.*, 1983b; Tuma *et al.*, 1984, 1987b). Additionally, ethanol oxidation in liver also generates reducing equivalents (increased NADH/NAD ratio) which can enhance the reduction of Schiff bases to form stable secondary amines (Sorrell and Tuma, 1985; Tuma and Sorrell, 1985). However, further studies showed that stable adducts formed in the absence of strong reducing agents were different from the *N*-ethylated amino groups generated under reductive conditions (Tuma *et al.*, 1987b) and also that reduction by ascorbic acid did not involve the classical reduction pathway (Tuma *et al.*, 1987b). Therefore, the addition of thiol groups was proposed as another possible mechanism of stabilization (Sorrell and Tuma, 1985; Tuma and Sorrell, 1985). This was based on the observation that cysteine, which contains an amino group and a thiol group, can easily form stable adducts when reacted with acetaldehyde (Cederbaum and Rubin, 1976). However, additional studies revealed that proteins lacking free thiol groups are

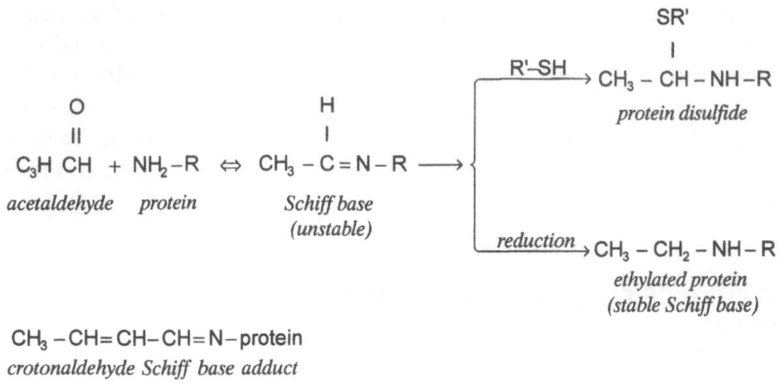

Figure 5.1 Formation of acetaldehyde–protein adduct and stabilization of Schiff bases by reduction or thiol addition. Crotonaldehyde Schiff base adduct with proteins.

able to form stable adducts with acetaldehyde (Tuma *et al.*, 1987b, 1991; Jennett *et al.*, 1990). One such mechanism that has been proposed involves an amine-catalyzed aldol condensation reaction with another molecule of acetaldehyde resulting in the formation of a crotonaldehyde Schiff base derivative (Kikugawa *et al.*, 1985, 1988, 1989; Hoffmann *et al.*, 1993) (Figure 5.1). The presence of the conjugated double bond system in this product is expected to react with other reactive compounds generating a wide variety of conjugated products with proteins.

Regulation of acetaldehyde adduct formation is also dependent on the levels of thiol compounds, glutathione and cysteine, which decrease the binding of acetaldehyde to proteins (Donohue *et al.*, 1983a; Medina *et al.*, 1985). Therefore, conditions such as fasting (Pessayre *et al.*, 1979), intake of drugs (Gillette, 1981) and chronic alcohol consumption (MacDonald *et al.*, 1977; Vina *et al.*, 1980; Fernandez and Videla, 1981), all of which lower hepatic thiol compounds, could promote the formation of acetaldehyde protein adducts in the liver. Furthermore, recent studies have shown that the acetaldehyde adducts are taken up and degraded by the scavenger receptor of liver endothelial cells and that long-term ethanol consumption severely impairs this degradation (Thiele *et al.*, 1996).

In conclusion, binding of acetaldehyde to proteins generates unstable adducts that are further stabilized by various mechanisms. These adducts have been considered to play a major role in alcohol induced liver damage either by modifying the biological function of the proteins involved or by generating an immune response to the modified proteins (neoantigens).

FUNCTIONAL ALTERATIONS OF PROTEINS FORMING ACETALDEHYDE ADDUCTS

The identification of target proteins and the precise alterations in their function due to formation of acetaldehyde conjugates are key factors in understanding the role of adducts in alcohol liver injury. Proteins vary in their ability to generate acetaldehyde adducts and the impaired function of a specific protein depends on the particular alterations which the acetaldehyde induces. These alterations could involve the displacement of pyridoxal phosphate from its binding site on proteins (Lumeng, 1978) and interference with the activity of certain enzymes, particularly those forming Schiff base–enzyme complexes as intermediates in their catalytic activity (Grazi *et al.*, 1963). However, since acetaldehyde–protein Schiff bases are readily reversible and high concentrations of acetaldehyde are needed to produce extensive Schiff base formation, the possibility of significant long lasting dysfunction of proteins is questionable. In favor of their role in alcoholic liver injury, the fact that unstable adducts can be reduced to stable ones and longer the protein is exposed to acetaldehyde lower the concentration needed to form adducts – a more realistic condition in chronic alcohol consumption. The stable adducts are not easily reversible and they persist in the liver cells even when all of acetaldehyde has been metabolized. In this context, acetaldehyde–albumin adducts may explain altered drug binding in alcoholics (Karp *et al.*, 1985) and acetaldehyde–hemoglobin formation changes in erythrocyte-oxygen affinity (Tsuboi *et al.*, 1981).

Enzymes harboring essential lysine residues, i.e., glucose-6-phosphate dehydrogenase and ribonuclease A, are especially susceptible to inhibition of their catalytic activity as a result of acetaldehyde adduct formation (Mauch *et al.*, 1985, 1986). Ribonuclease A has ten lysyl residues including one at its active site (Jentoft *et al.*, 1981). Other examples of biological alterations include the accelerated low density lipoprotein catabolism (Kesaniemi *et al.*, 1987), the inhibition of O6-methylquanine transferase (Espina *et al.*, 1988), the decreased prostaglandin binding to hepatic plasma membrane (Buko and Zavodnik, 1990), the altered DNA methylation (Garro *et al.*, 1991), the impaired histone binding to DNA (Niemela *et al.*, 1990b), the altered function of calmodulin (Jennett *et al.*, 1989a) and the impaired cilia motion (Sisson *et al.*, 1991). Tubulin is a preferred target protein for acetaldehyde binding because it contains a highly reactive lysine residue (Jennett *et al.*, 1987, 1989b). The α-chain generates 2–3 times more stable adducts than the β-chain at low concentration of acetaldehyde despite the fact that both chains have equal amounts of lysine residues. This observation suggests that other factors may be important for the increased reactivity of certain lysine sites such as the neighboring amino acids and the three dimensional structure (Acharya *et al.*, 1983; Watkins *et al.*, 1985). Free tubulin dimers also form 100–200% more acetaldehyde adducts than the polymerized tubulin in the microtubules (Smith *et al.*, 1992). Formation of acetaldehyde–tubulin adduct significantly decreases the ability of tubulin to assemble into microtubules, an integral component of cellular cytoskeleton, by direct interference with tubulin dimer-dimer interactions. These alterations of tubulin polymerization significantly impair intracellular protein trafficking and secretion leading to ballooning of hepatocytes and other structural changes (Tuma and Sorrell, 1984; Volentine *et al.*, 1984; Lieber, 1990, 1991). In addition to tubulin, another component of the cytoskeleton, actin, is a target of acetaldehyde binding (Xu *et al.*, 1989). Therefore, acetaldehyde induced cytoskeleton dysfunction is a major contributing factor in the pathogenesis of alcohol liver injury (Tuma and Sorrell, 1984; Lieber, 1991).

In summary, acetaldehyde selectively or preferentially binds to certain proteins and particularly those with key lysine residues in their polypeptide chain. This binding even at a relatively low level can ultimately impair protein function, particularly if the reactive lysine residues are directly involved in the biological activity of a protein, which contributes to liver injury.

EFFECT OF ACETALDEHYDE ADDUCTS ON THE ANTIGENICITY OF PROTEINS

Protein targets of acetaldehyde binding

Early studies suggested that autoimmune mechanisms are implicated in the induction or perpetuation of alcoholic liver damage (Zinnemann, 1975; Zetterman and Sorrell, 1981; Zetterman, 1990). A role of ethanol or its metabolite acetaldehyde in the induction of a new or an altered antigen on the membrane of the hepatocyte has been suggested (MacSween *et al.*, 1981; Burt *et al.*, 1982; Anthony *et al.*, 1983; Izumi *et al.*, 1985; Crossley *et al.*, 1986). Therefore, if such immunological reactions are involved, it would be important to demonstrate the presence of modified proteins acting as neoantigens in the hepatocytes. Early studies have shown that antibodies recognizing the acetaldehyde hapten are expressed in animals and humans which have been exposed chronically to ethanol *in vivo* (Israel *et al.*, 1986; Hoerner *et al.*, 1986, 1988; Niemela *et al.*, 1987; Worrall *et al.*, 1989, 1990, 1991). These investigations were undertaken using a variety of stable acetaldehyde–protein adducts as test antigens. The adducts were produced *in vitro* by reaction of acetaldehyde with a protein carrier (either keyhole limpet hemocyanin, albumin, prothrombin or hemoglobin) in the presence of reducing agent (sodium cyanoborohydride or borohydride). These studies, however, provide no information as to the nature of the protein adducts eliciting and/or being recognized by the humoral immune response.

Various research groups have investigated the liver target proteins to which acetaldehyde binds using either antibodies raised against synthetic acetaldehyde protein conjugates or sera from alcoholic patients (Table 5.1). Lin *et al.* (1988, 1989) reported that a stable acetaldehyde–protein adduct of molecular mass 37 kDa was expressed in cytosolic fractions prepared from livers of rats fed ethanol chronically,

Table 5.1 Acetaldehyde adducts in liver acting as neoantigens

Investigators	Method	Adduct (kDa)	Antigen	Antibodies
Lin *et al.* (1988, 1990, 1993a)	Rats fed EtOH and hepatocytes + EtOH	37	aldehyde reductase?	rabbit IgG anti-hemocyanin-AA
Behrens *et al.* (1988)	Rats fed EtOH	52	P450 2EI?	rabbit IgG anti-hemocyanin-AA
Koskinas *et al.* (1992)	Rat and human cytosol incubated with AcH + CN	200	?	sera from patients with ALD
Ramsay *et al.* (1995)	Liver tissue from patients with ALD	200	?	sera from patients with ALD
Svegliati-Baroni *et al.* (1994)	Liver tissue from patients with ALD	200	collagen I?	rabbit IgG anti-rat P450 2EI-AA

EtOH: ethanol, AcH: acetaldehyde, CN: cyanoborohydride, ALD: alcoholic liver disease.

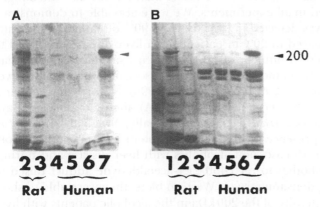

Figure 5.2 Production of the acetaldehyde modified 200 kDa protein in human and rat liver cytosol *in vitro*. Human and rat liver cytosol were incubated for 2 hours at 21°C, with or without 2.5 mM acetaldehyde and/or 100 mM cyanoborohydride and then analysed by immunoblotting for reactivity with IgA antibodies from serum of two patients with alcoholic hepatitis (**A, B**). Sample loading was 42.5 μg per track. The position of the 200 kDa rat liver antigen which co-migrated with a 200 kDa human liver, is indicated. Lanes: (1) −acetaldehyde, −cyanoborohydride, no incubation; (2) +acetaldehyde, +cyanoborohydride; (3) +acetaldehyde, −cyanoborohydride; (4) −acetaldehyde, −cyanoborohydride, no incubation; (5) +acetaldehyde, −cyanoborohydride; (6) −acetal-dehyde, +cyanoborohydride; (7) +acetaldehyde, +cyanoborohydride.

and also in isolated rat hepatocytes which had been cultured with ethanol for several days (Lin *et al.*, 1990). However, the same workers reported that many different acetaldehyde–protein adducts, exhibiting a wide range of molecular masses which included the 37 kDa region, were produced *in vitro* when rat liver cytosol was incubated with acetaldehyde in the presence of sodium cyanoborohydride (Lin *et al.*, 1988). The latter adducts were unstable, and could not be detected unless cyanoborohydride was present (Lin *et al.*, 1988). The same group has provided evidence that the cytosolic 37 kDa protein is the Δ4-3-ketosteroid 5β-reductase (Lin *et al.*, 1993a; Zhu *et al.*, 1996). In contrast, Behrens *et al.* (1988) failed to detect the 37 kDa adduct in livers from rats treated chronically with ethanol, but instead reported a single major adduct of 52 kDa, which by immunoadsorption was found to be the microsomal cytochrome P-450 isozyme responsible for microsomal ethanol metabolism (2E1). Both workers have used antibodies raised against synthetic acetaldehyde protein conjugates. Our group have reported a novel 200 kDa protein antigen expressed when cytosolic fractions from both rat and human liver had been incubated with acetaldehyde and cyanoborohydride (Koskinas *et al.*, 1992) (Figure 5.2). This 200 kDa antigen was recognized by IgA antibodies in sera from a high proportion of patients with alcoholic hepatitis (70%), compared to patients with alcoholic cirrhosis without hepatitis (30%), heavy drinkers without overt liver disease (20%), non-alcoholic liver disease (35%) or normal controls consuming moderate quantities of alcohol (25%) (Koskinas *et al.*, 1992). Expression of several acetaldehyde-induced protein antigens which exhibited molecular masses of markedly less than 200 kDa was noted in a number of experiments but they were recognized much more weakly by patients' antibodies than was the 200 kDa antigen and they were not detected in all experiments. We were also able to demonstrate that the 200 kDa protein was detected in liver tissue in 90% of patients with acute alcoholic hepatitis as compared to 20% in patients with liver disease unrelated to alcohol (Ramsay *etal.*, 1995). A number of other antigens, smaller or larger than the 200 kDa protein, were also found to be exclusively associated with alcoholic liver disease but were not common (<20%) (Ramsay *etal.*, 1995). Nevertheless, patients positive for both antigen (200 kDa) and antibody (IgA) almost exclusively have alcoholic liver disease (Ramsay *etal.*, 1995). Additionally, Svegliati-Baroni *etal.* (1994) have reported the presence of the 200 kDa protein in liver biopsies from patients with alcoholic liver disease, non-alcoholics with liver disease and normal controls by using IgG antibodies to rat P450 2E1-acetaldehyde adduct raised in rabbits. By using scanning densitometry on Western blots, they were able to show that the immunostaining intensity of the 200 kDa in the alcoholic patients with liver disease was greater than in non-alcoholic patients with liver disease and very weak in normal livers. They have also presented data suggesting that this 200 kDa protein could be a form of collagen type I. The last two studies strongly suggest that the 200 kDa antigen is generated *in vivo* in patients with acute alcoholic hepatitis and can elicit a humoral immune response.

In addition to acetaldehyde adducts acting as antigens, Clot *etal.* (1995, 1996) reported a major 52 kDa antigenic protein, by incubating human liver microsomes with NADPH and ethanol, which is recognized by circulating class IgA and IgG antibodies that differ from those antibodies recognizing acetaldehyde adducts. They have also demonstrated by immunoblotting and immunoprecipitation that the 52 kDa protein is the microsomal P450 2E1 that becomes antigenic after binding with hydroxyethyl free radicals generated by this enzyme during ethanol metabolism.

In summary, it is well established that acetaldehyde adducts, generating *in vivo* during ethanol metabolism, are antigenic and capable of eliciting strong humoral immune reactions. As to the nature of these neo-antigens, there are conflicting data as to which is/are the most likely candidate protein/s for such immune responses. This could be attributed to different ways that the investigators have approached the target, the variable assays utilized for acetaldehyde adduct production and the source and specificity of antibodies used. The development of more sophisticated techniques, the identification of the precise antigenic proteins and the production of more specific antibodies to specifically defined acetaldehyde generated epitopes will clarify the role of acetaldehyde adducts in the pathogenesis of ethanol induced liver disease.

Cellular and tissue expression of acetaldehyde adducts

To further elucidate the extent and the zonal distribution of acetaldehyde adducts within the liver, immunohistochemical studies using antibodies to synthetic acetaldehyde-adducts were performed. Niemela *etal.* (1990a) were able to demonstrate for the first time that acetaldehyde adducts are present in the liver of individuals with a history of excessive alcohol consumption. They have used in their immunohistochemical studies anti-acetaldehyde-albumin antibodies raised in rabbits. The acetaldehyde adducts were predominantly in zone III – the perivenular zone – which is involved early in alcohol induced liver damage. No extracellular staining was observed. Subsequently, Lin *et al.* (1993c) detected acetaldehyde adducts in the liver of rats fed alcohol by using anti-hemocyanin–acetaldehyde antibodies. They have also demonstrated that distribution of immunostaining was mainly in the perivenous region in rats fed alcohol for 2 weeks and more diffuse in the livers of rats fed alcohol for longer periods (e.g., 11 weeks). An additional observation was that rats fed alcohol-containing diet supplemented with cyanamide had more liver cells producing protein acetaldehyde adducts. In a more extensive study, Holstege *et al.* (1994) investigated the presence and localization of acetaldehyde adducts in the livers of alcoholics by using polyclonal antibodies produced against low-density lipoprotein-acetaldehyde conjugate and they have correlated the presence of adducts with the progression or subsequent occurrence of liver fibrosis in those patients who had a second liver biopsy. They have been able to detect acetaldehyde adducts in biopsy specimens by immunohistochemistry in 85% of patients with a history of alcohol abuse, in none of the non-alcoholic individuals with normal liver histology and in a high proportion (65%) of patients with non-alcoholic liver disease. The immunostaining was predominantly in zone III but no correlation was found between the intensity and the histologically assessed severity of liver damage. Extracellular detection of acetaldehyde adducts was also seen, particularly in patients with alcoholic hepatitis (85%), and was significantly correlated to progression of liver fibrosis. Our group was also able to detect acetaldehyde adducts in liver specimens of alcoholics with liver disease by using antibodies against albumin-acetaldehyde adduct raised in rabbits (Koskinas *et al.*, unpublished data). The distribution of immunostaining was perivenous in patients with mild features of liver disease and more diffuse in patients with advanced or acute liver disease (Figure 5.3). Furthermore, when liver tissue specimens taken from patients who expressed acetaldehyde adducts in their livers were analyzed by Western transfer and blotting, using either antibodies

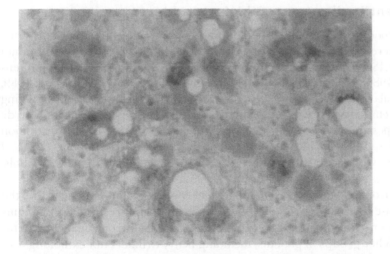

Figure 5.3 Immunostaining for acetaldehyde adducts in alcoholic hepatitis, showing pleomorphic hepatocytes with strong cytoplasmic immunoreactivity. The anti-acetaldehyde antibodies to synthetic acetaldehyde–albumin adduct were raised in rabbits. (*see Color Plate 5*)

to synthetic acetaldehyde adducts or circulating antibodies from their own serum, they were found to express predominantly the 200 kDa protein (Ramsay *et al.*, 1995).

In another study, the cellular and subcellular localization of acetaldehyde adducts were examined by ultrastructural immunohistochemical study in liver specimens from patients with liver disease (Paradis *et al.*, 1996). The investigators have shown that adducts were detected in the rough endoplasmic reticulum, in some peroxisomes and in the cytosol of hepatocytes. Interestingly, in patients with fibrosis acetaldehyde adducts were also detected in Ito cells and in the cytoplasmic processes of myofibroblasts in areas of fibrogenesis. Additionally, adducts were detected in isolated rat Ito cells incubated with acetaldehyde (Paradis *et al.*, 1996). These data point to the possible role of acetaldehyde adducts in liver fibrogenesis and, they also support previous studies showing that adducts increase collagen gene transcription in fibroblasts (Brenner and Chojkier, 1987) and in activated Ito cells (Casini *et al.*, 1991). In summary, all these experiments clearly show that acetaldehyde adducts are present in liver biopsies of patients with alcoholic liver disease and are recognized by anti-acetaldehyde antibodies. The perivenous distribution is characteristic in the early stages and is clearly associated with the lobular distribution of the inducible cytochrome P450 2E1 which catalyzes the oxidation of ethanol to acetaldehyde. And also, it is zone III which is impaired early by alcohol, suggesting that these acetaldehyde adducts could be involved in the pathogenesis of liver damage. The finding that some patients with non-alcoholic liver disease express acetaldehyde adducts in their livers could be explained by the increased production or impaired elimination of endogenous acetaldehyde. The differences with regard to the extracellular distribution of the acetaldehyde modified proteins could be attributed to different synthetic acetaldehyde adducts used to develop antibodies that may cross react with different proteins.

Circulating antibodies to acetaldehyde adducts

Circulating antibodies to acetaldehyde modified epitopes (presumably the *N*-ethyl lysine group) were detected in mice or rats fed ethanol chronically and in human alcoholics by ELISA using various synthetic acetaldehyde adducts as test antigens (Hoerner *et al.*, 1986, 1988; Israel *et al.*, 1986; Niemela *et al.*, 1987; Worrall *et al.*, 1989, 1990, 1991; Viitala *et al.*, 1997). These studies have also demonstrated that circulating antibodies to acetaldehyde modified proteins were able to recognize acetaldehyde generated epitopes independent of the carrier protein (Israel *et al.*, 1986). In addition to ELISA studies, Western blot analysis demonstrated high frequency (70%) of antibodies to the cytosolic 200 kDa antigen in sera from patients with acute alcoholic hepatitis (Koskinas *et al.*, 1992; Ramsay *et al.*, 1995).

The findings from all these experiments reveal two important issues. Firstly, the antibody response to acetaldehyde modified epitopes was not restricted to patients with alcoholic liver disease, although of higher titer and frequency in such patients than in various other groups of patients, including heavy drinkers not exhibiting liver disease (Niemela *et al.*, 1987; Hoerner *et al.*, 1988; Koskinas *et al.*, 1992; Viitala *et al.*, 1997). Secondly, analysis with isotype-specific second antibodies demonstrated that patients with alcoholic liver disease, drinkers with no liver disease and patients with non-alcoholic liver disease, all exhibited an IgA response to acetaldehyde modified epitopes. However, these antibodies were of markedly higher titer in alcoholic liver disease than in the other patient groups (Worrall *et al.*, 1991; Koskinas *et al.*, 1992; Viitala, 1997). An attempt was also made to correlate the expression of the different isotypic variants of the antibodies against acetaldehyde derived adducts with the amount of alcohol consumed or with the presence of liver disease. Worral *et al.* (1991) have reported that the antibody responses to adducts is exclusively of IgA and titers were found to correlate with the amount of alcohol consumed but not with the degree of liver disease as assessed by biochemical parameters; none of the groups of patients exhibited a significant IgG response to acetaldehyde induced epitopes, whereas both alcoholics and social drinkers exhibited a high-titer acetaldehyde specific IgM response. In the study of Viitala and his colleagues (1997), increased titers of IgA were found in 70% of patients with alcoholic liver disease and these titers were significantly higher than those from patients with non-alcoholic liver disease, nondrinking controls and heavy drinkers without evidence of liver disease. In contrast, IgG and IgM titers to acetaldehyde adducts were elevated both in patients with alcoholic liver disease and in heavy drinkers without liver disease suggesting that IgA responses to acetaldehyde adducts are more likely to be related with liver disease than ethanol consumption. Furthermore, titers of IgA were found to be correlated with the severity of liver disease as assessed by the combined clinical and laboratory index and titers of anti-adduct IgG were found to correlate with the presence of inflammation and necrosis (Viitala *et al.*, 1997). The high frequency (70%) of class IgA antibodies to the cytosolic 200 kDa antigen in sera from patients with alcoholic hepatitis as compared with the significantly lower frequency found in other patient groups, with no evidence of an IgG response to the antigen or to other acetaldehyde modified liver antigens, are in agreement with the ELISA findings (Koskinas *et al.*, 1992). As mentioned before, patients with non-alcoholic liver disease and social drinkers exhibit antibodies reacting with acetaldehyde–protein conjugates, albeit less frequently and in low titer (Niemela *et al.*, 1987; Hoerner *et al.*, 1988; Koskinas *et al.*, 1992; Viitala *et al.*, 1997). In these individuals, the antibody response may be elicited as a consequence of occasional ethanol ingestion, perhaps in combination with endogenous ethanol production by microorganisms present in the gastrointestinal tract (Krebs and Perkins, 1970; Baraona *et al.*, 1986) and/or the decreased hepatic acetaldehyde dehydrogenase activity in chronic non-alcoholic liver disease (Mathewson *et al.*, 1986).

In conclusion, all these data, in addition to the observation that there is no relation between total IgA and anti-adduct IgAs in various groups with elevated levels of total IgA concentration (Worrall *et al.*, 1991; Viitala *et al.*, 1997), support the hypothesis that increased levels of IgA in alcoholic patients may be, at least in part, antigen driven rather than a non-specific increased synthesis and/or decreased catabolism. Candidates for neo-antigens within the liver are the acetaldehyde adducts but also other liver proteins, such as the 65 kDa heat shock protein (HSP) to which circulating IgA antibodies have been found in 65% of patients with alcoholic hepatitis (Koskinas *et al.*, 1993). As to the reported differences regarding the isotype specific antibodies to acetaldehyde modified proteins, particularly class IgM and IgG, these could be related to variations in the assays for immune responses, the different antigenic characteristics of the proteins used and the concentration of acetaldehyde used for the preparation of adducts. Relevant to the last option is the finding that high concentration of acetaldehyde readily crosslinks proteins and generate antigenic epitopes that are different from those prepared at lower concentration (Lin *et al.*, 1993b). Consistent with these observations are the characteristic findings of IgA abnormalities found in patients with alcoholic liver disease. Firstly, increased serum IgA levels are seen particularly in patients with alcoholic hepatitis (Delacroix *et al.*, 1983; Van de Wiel *et al.*, 1987, 1988) and secondly, a characteristic pattern of IgA deposition in the liver has been described (Kater *et al.*, 1979; Swerdlow *et al.*, 1982; Amano *et al.*, 1988). There are also reports of circulating immune complexes containing IgA and undefined ethanol modifed proteins (Bjorneboe *et al.*, 1972; Coppo *et al.*, 1985).

Acetaldehyde adducts in other tissues

Acetaldehyde adducts seem to play a role in the dysfunction of other organs seen in alcoholics. Studies in animals have shown that homogenates from immature rat brains can generate acetaldehyde via a catalase mediated reaction and that acetaldehyde adducts are expressed in neonatal brains exposed to ethanol as shown by immunohistochemical staining (Hamby-Mason *et al.*, 1997). These adducts could play an important role in the neurotoxic effects of *in utero* ethanol exposure. Acetaldehyde–DNA neuroadducts have been detected in the brain of an intoxicated alcoholic driver, who sustained fatal motor vehicle injuries by 32P prelabeled DNA and two dimensional thin layer chromatography (Steinberg *et al.*, 1997). The observation that the brain regions in which acetaldehyde adducts have been identified had normal histology suggests that the mechanism of neurotoxicity could be related to biochemical nonenzymatic changes of DNA at the nucleic acid level which can alter gene function and stability. DNA-acetaldehyde adducts have also been detected in granulocyte and lymphocyte DNA isolated from alcoholic patients (Fang *et al.*, 1991). In our laboratory, circulating antibodies to acetaldehyde modified cardiac cytosolic proteins that have been detected in 33% of patients with alcoholic heart muscle disease (Harcombe *et al.*, 1995). The molecular sizes of the protein antigens observed ranged from 58 to 120 kDa and the antibodies were either IgA or IgG isotype. In contrast, circulating IgG antibodies to the same proteins have been observed in a very small number of control subjects with and without heart disease who were not drinking and in subjects with only alcoholic liver disease.

ACETALDEHYDE ADDUCTS AND PATHOGENESIS OF LIVER INJURY

Experiments in animals have shown that acetaldehyde adducts are related to liver injury and can also elicit T cell responses. Murine splenic cells whose surface is modified by acetaldehyde can generate MHC class I dependent CTL responses when injected in a synergetic host (Terabayashi and Kolber, 1990). The importance of acetaldehyde adducts in producing liver injury has been highlighted by a Japanese study showing the development of hepatic necrosis and infiltration of mononuclear cells into the lobules in guinea pigs immunized with hemoglobin–acetaldehyde adducts and simultaneously given ethanol for 40 days (Yokoyama *et al.*, 1993). Titers of antibody against acetaldehyde adducts were elevated and blast formation of lymphocytes was shown by stimulation with adducts. By contrast, the combination of ethanol and immunization with unmodified hemoglobin produced only fatty changes and animals immunized with the adducts alone had minimal inflammatory changes. Although the histological features are not typical of alcohol induced liver damage in humans, these experiments suggest that acetaldehyde adducts can induce liver damage under certain conditions.

Circulating and sinusoidal IgA – as a response to acetaldehyde adducts can be involved in macrophage/monocyte activation, leading to the secretion of various cytokines such as IL-6, TNF, TGFb and IL-1 (Deviere *et al.*, 1991, 1992) (Figure 5.4). Increased TNF levels were found in the plasma of patients with severe acute alcoholic hepatitis and titers were correlated with disease activity and short-term survival (Bird *et al.*, 1990; Felver *et al.*, 1990). Deviere and colleagues (1989) reported an increase in IL-6 activity in patients with alcoholic cirrhosis and a positive correlation between IL-6 levels and serum IgA. Similarly, increased levels of IL-6 were found in patients with acute alcoholic hepatitis and a strong correlation was found between circulating levels of IL-6 and indicators of disease severity (Sheron *et al.*, 1991). Secretion of IL-8 by activated macrophage/monocyte is also an important factor for the chemotaxis and activation of neutrophils; high circulating levels correlate with blood neutrophilia and increased synthesis in the liver, leading to high tissue concentration, mediate neutrophil invasion which is a characteristic feature of alcoholic hepatitis (Sheron *et al.*, 1993) (Figure 5.4). Superoxide secretion and other cytotoxic factors such as TGF1 from activated Kupffer cells could potentiate fibrogenesis. Anti-acetaldehyde adduct antibodies could also initiate antibody mediated hepatotoxicity (Neuberger *et al.*, 1984) (Figure 5.4). Although intracellular proteins that form adducts are unlikely to act as antigens unless they

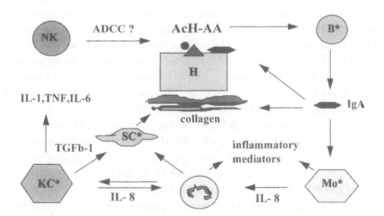

Figure 5.4 Pathogenesis of alcohol induced liver disease. Possible pathogenetic mechanisms involved in alcohol induced liver injury based on the immune response to acetaldehyde adducts [AcH-AA] generated from ethanol metabolism. NK: natural killer, ADCC: antibody dependent cytotoxicity, B*: activated B lymphocyte, Mo*: activated monocyte, KC*: activated Kupffer cell, SC*: activated stellate cell. (*see Color Plate 6*)

are expressed on the surface of the hepatocyte, it is possible that under alcohol toxicity either these modified intracellular proteins are expressed on the membrane or antibodies reacting to certain intracellular proteins could cross react with other acetaldehyde adducts expressed on the membrane of hepatocytes. It has also been demonstrated that physical presentation of the hapten can affect antibody recognition. (Truddel *et al.*, 1990).

CONCLUSION

Acetaldehyde, the main product of ethanol metabolism, has the ability to form unstable and stable adducts with various proteins. The predominant acetaldehyde protein formation involves the generation of Schiff bases that under certain metabolic pathways become more stable adducts. Certain proteins selectively form acetaldehyde adducts due to specific amino acid sequences and conformational factors at their binding site. However, further studies are needed to evaluate the precise mechanisms of stable acetaldehyde adduct formation *in vivo* and to define the factors which are contributing to enhanced production or decreased catabolism of adducts. Binding of acetaldehyde to proteins could induce liver injury by either modifying the biological function of the protein or by changing its antigenicity. The biological function of certain proteins has been found to be severely impaired, particularly in proteins in which the site of enzymatic activity contains lysine residues. Although the altered biological function of some proteins has been extensively investigated, further experimental proof is still required in order to implicate them in the pathogenesis of liver injury. Identification of other target proteins critically involved in cell metabolism and integrity remain a challenging goal for the future.

Stable acetaldehyde adducts also represent the best candidates to act as antigens to elicit immune responses. In this area of research, the approach followed two paths. The first one was the demonstration of circulating antibodies to synthetic acetaldehyde adducts in alcohol fed animals and in alcoholics. These antibodies although they were found in alcoholics without liver injury and in patients with non-alcoholic liver disease, their frequency and titers were significantly lower as compared with those seen in alcoholics with liver disease. The second approach was to identify the liver target proteins to which acetaldehyde binds by using antibodies raised against synthetic acetaldehyde adducts or serum from patients. Although a few candidate proteins have been identified, more studies are necessary to clarify the identity and the specificity of these proteins. Immunohistochemical studies have also established the presence of acetaldehyde adducts in the liver in a higher proportion of patients with alcohol induced liver disease than in patients with non-alcoholic liver disease. It is therefore well documented that acetaldehyde adducts generated *in vivo* are able to elicit an immune response that mainly involves IgA antibody production. This antigen antibody reaction could trigger the production of various cytokines inducing inflammation or fibrosis. However, future studies are required to establish the causal effect of acetaldehyde adducts in liver damage.

REFERENCES

Acharya, A.S., Sussman, L.G. and Manning, J.M. (1983) Schiff base adducts of glyceralde-hyde with hemoglobin. *Journal of Biological Chemistry* **258**, 2296–2302.

Amano, K., Tsukada, K., Takeuchi, T., Fukuda, Y. and Nagura, H. (1988) IgA deposition in alcoholic liver disease. *American Journal of Clinical Pathology* **89**, 728–734.

Anthony, R.S., Farquharson, M. and MacSween, R.N.M. (1983) Liver membrane antibodies in alcoholic liver disease II. Antibodies to ethanol altered hepatocytes. *Journal of Clinical Pathology* **36**, 1302–1308.

Baraona, E., Julkunen, R., Tannenbaum, L. and Lieber, C.S. (1986) Role of intestinal bacterial overgrowth in ethanol production and metabolism in rats. *Gastroenterology* **90**, 103–110.

Behrens, U.J., Hoerner, M., Lasker, J.M. and Lieber, C.S. (1988) Formation of acetaldehyde adducts with ethanol inducible P450 IIE1 *in vivo*. *Biochemical and Biophysical Research Communications* **154**, 584–590.

Bird, G.L.A., Sheron, N., Goka, A.K.J., Alexander, G.J.M. and Williams, R. (1990) Increased plasma tumor necrosis factor in severe alcoholic hepatitis. *Annals of Internal Medicine* **112**, 917–920.

Bjorneboe, M., Prytz, H. and Orskov, F. (1972) Antibodies to intestinal microbes in serum of patients with cirrhosis of the liver. *Lancet* **1**, 58–60.

Brenner, D.A. and Chojkier, M. (1987) Acetaldehyde increases collagen gene transcription in cultured human fibroblasts. *Journal of Biological Chemistry* **262**, 17690–17695.

Buko, V.U. and Zavodnik, I.B. (1990) Effect of acetaldehyde on binding of prostaglandins by receptors of liver plasma membranes. *Alcohol and Alcoholism* **25**, 483–487.

Burt, A.D., Anthony, R.S., Hislop, W.S., Bouchier, I.A.D. and MacSween, R.N.M. (1982) Liver membrane antibodies in alcoholic liver disease. I. Prevalence and immunoglobulin class. *Gut* **23**, 221–225.

Casini, A., Cunningham, M., Rojkind, M. and Lieber, C.S. (1991) Acetaldehyde increases procollagen type I and fibronectin gene transcription in cultured rat fat storing cells through aprotein synthesis dependent mechanism. *Hepatology* **13**, 758–765.

Cederbaum, A.I. and Rubin, E. (1976) Protective effect of cysteine on the inhibition of mitochondrial functions by acetaldehyde. *Biochemical Pharmacology* **25**, 963–973.

Clot, P., Bellomo, G., Tabone, M., Arico, S. and Albano, E. (1995) Detection of antibodies against proteins modified by hydroxyethyl free radicals in patients with alcoholic cirrhosis. *Gastroenterology* **108**, 201–207.

Clot, P., Albano, E., Eliasson, E., Tabone, M., Arico, S., Israel, Y. and Moncada, C. (1996) Cytochrome P450 IIE1 hydroxyethyl radical adducts as the major antigen in autoantibody formation among alcoholics. *Gastroenterology* **111**, 206–216.

Coppo, R., Arico, S., Piccoli, G., Basolo, B., Roccattelo, D., Amore, A., Tabone, M., De la Pierre, M., Sessa, A., Delacroix, D.L. and Vaerman, J.P. (1985) Presence and origin of IgA1- and IgA2-containing circulating immune complexes in chronic alcoholic liver diseases with and without glomerulonephritis. *Clinical Immunology and Immunopathology* **35**, 1–8.

Crossley, I.R., Neuberger, J., Davis, M., Williams, R. and Eddleston, A.L.W.F. (1986) Ethanol metabolism in the generation of new antigenic determinants on liver cells. *Gut* **27**, 186–189.

Delacroix, D.L., Elkon, K.B., Geubel, A.P., Hodgson, H.F., Dive, C. and Vaerman, J.P. (1983) Changes in size, subclass and metabolic properties of serum immunoglobulin A in liver diseases and in other diseases with high serum immunoglobulin A. *American Journal of Clinical Investigation* **71**, 358–367.

Deviere, J., Content, J., Denys, C., Vandenbussche, P., Schandene, L. and Wybran, J. (1989) High interleukin-6 serum levels and increased production by leukocytes in alcoholic liver disease: correlation with IgA serum levels and lymphokines production. *Clinical and Experimental Immunology* **77**, 221–225.

Deviere, J., Vaerman, J.P., Content, J., Denys, C., Schandene, L., Vandenbussche, P., Sibille, Y. and Dupont, E. (1991) IgA triggers TNFa secretion by monocytes: a study in normal subjects and patients with alcoholic liver cirrhosis. *Hepatology* **13**, 670–675.

Deviere, J., Content, J., Denys, C., Vandenbussche, P., Le Moine, O., Schandene, L., Vaerman, J.P. and Dupont, E. (1992) Immunoglobulin A and interleukin 6 form a positive secretory feedback loop: a study of normal subjects and alcoholic cirrhotics. *Gastroenterology* **103**, 1296–1301.

Donohue, T.M., Tuma, D.J. and Sorrell, M.F. (1983a) Binding of metabolically derived acetaldehyde to hepatic proteins *in vitro*. *Laboratory Investigation* **49**, 226–229.

Donohue, T.M., Tuma, D.J. and Sorrell, M.F. (1983b) Acetaldehyde adducts with proteins: binding of (14C) acetaldehyde to serum albumin. *Archives of Biochemistry and Biophysics* **220**, 239–246.

Espina, N., Lima, V., Lieber, C.S. and Garro, A.J. (1988) *In vitro* and *in vivo* inhibitory effect of ethanol and acetaldehyde on O^6-methylguanine transferase. *Carcinogenesis* **9**, 761–766.

Fang, J.L. and Vaca, C.E. (1991) Detection of DNA adducts of acetaldehyde in peripheral white blood cells of alcohol abusers. *Alcohol and Alcoholism* **1**(Suppl), 305–310.

Felver, M.E., Mezey, E., McGuire, M., Mitchell, M.C., Herlong, H.F., Veech, G.A. and Veech, R.L. (1990) Plasma tumour necrosis factor predicts decreased long term survival in severe alcoholic hepatitis. *Alcoholism: Clinical and Experimental Research* **14**, 255–259.

Fernandez, V. and Videla, L.A. (1981) Effect of acute and chronic ethanol ingestion on the content of reduced glutathione of various tissues of the rat. *Experientia* **37**, 392–393.

Gaines, K.C., Salhany, D.J., Tuma, D.J. and Sorrell, M.F. (1977) Reactions of acetaldehyde with human erythrocytes membrane proteins. *FEBS Letters* **75**, 115–119.

Garro, A.J., McBeth, D.L., Lima, V. and Lieber, C.S. (1991) Ethanol consumption inhibits fetal DNA methylation in mice: implications for the fetal alcohol syndrome. *Alcoholism: Clinical and Experimental Research* **15**, 395–398.

Gillette, J.R. (1981) An integrated approach to the study of chemically reactive metabolites of acetaminophen. *Archives of Internal Medicine* **141**, 375–379.

Grazi, E., Melochi, H., Martinez, G., Wood, W.A. and Horecker, B.L. (1963) Evidence for Schiff base formation in enzymatic aldol condensations. *Biochemical and Biophysical Research Communication* **10**, 4–10.

Hamby-Mason, R., Chen, J.J., Schenker, S., Perez, A. and Henderson, G.I. (1997) Catalase mediates acetaldehyde formation from ethanol in fetal and neonatal rat brain. *Alcoholism: Clinical and Experimental Research* **21**, 1063–1072.

Harcombe, A.A., Ramsay, L., Kenna, J.G., Koskinas, J., Why, H.J., Richardson, P.J., Weissberg, P.L. and Alexander, G.J. (1995) Circulating antibodies to cardiac protein acetaldehyde adducts in alcoholic heart muscle disease. *Clinical Science* **88**, 263–268.

Hoerner, M.U., Behrens, U.J., Worner, T. and Lieber, C.S. (1986) Humoral immune response to acetaldehyde adducts in alcoholic patients. *Research Communications in Chemical Pathology and Pharmacology* **54**, 3–12.

Hoerner, M.U., Behrens, U.J., Worner, T., Blacksberg, I., Braly, L.F., Schaffner, F. and Lieber, C.S. (1988) The role of alcoholism and liver disease in the appearance of serum antibodies against acetaldehyde adducts. *Hepatology* **8**, 569–574.

Hoffmann, T., Meyer, R.J., Sorrell, M.F. and Tuma, D.J. (1993) Reaction of acetaldehyde with proteins: formation of stable fluorescent adducts. *Alcoholism: Clinical and Experimental Research* **17**, 69–74.

Holstege, A., Bedossa, P., Poynard, T., Kollinger, M., Chaput, J.C., Houglum, K. and Chojkier, M. (1994) Acetaldehyde modified epitopes in liver biopsy specimens of alcoholic and non-alcoholic patients: localization and association with progression of liver fibrosis. *Hepatology* **19**, 367–374.

Israel, Y., Hurwitz, E., Niemela, O. and Arnon, R. (1986) Monoclonal and polyclonal antibodies against acetaldehyde containing epitopes in acetaldehyde proteins adducts. *Proceedings of National Academy of Science* **83**, 7923–7927.

Izumi, N., Sato, C., Hasumura, Y. and Takeuchi, J. (1985) Serum antibodies against alcohol treated rabbit hepatocytes in patients with alcoholic liver disease. *Clinical and Experimental Immunology* **61**, 585–592.

Jennett, R.B., Sorrell, M.F., Johnson E.L. and Tuma, D.J. (1987) Covalent binding of acetaldehyde to tubulin: evidence for preferential binding to the α-chain. *Archives of Biochemistry and Biophysics* **256**, 10–18.

Jennett, R.B., Saffari-Fard, A., Sorrell, M.F., Smith S.L. and Tuma, D.J. (1989a) Increased covalent binding of acetaldehyde to calmodulin in the presence of calcium. *Life Sciences* **45**, 1461–1466.

Jennett, R.B., Sorrell, M.F., Saffari-Fard, A., Ockner, J.L. and Tuma, D.J. (1989b) Preferential covalent binding of acetaldehyde to the α-chain of purified rat liver tubulin. *Hepatology* **9**, 57–62.

Jennett, R.B., Tuma, D.J. and Sorrell, M.F. (1990) Effects of acetaldehyde on hepatic proteins. In *Progress in Liver Diseases*, edited by H. Popper and F. Schaffner, Vol IX, pp. 325–333. W.B. Saunders, Philadelphia, PA.

Jentoft, J.E., Gerken, T.A., Jentoft, N. and Dearborn, D.G. (1981) (^{13}C) methylated ribonuclease A. ^{13}C NMR studies of the interaction of lysine 41 with active site ligands. *Journal of Biological Chemistry* **256**, 231–236.

Karp, W.B., Kinsley, M., Subramanyam, S.B. and Robertson, A.F. (1985) Binding properties of glycosylated albumin and acetaldehyde albumin. *Alcoholism: Clinical and Experimental Research* **9**, 429–432.

Kater, L., Jobsis, A.C., Baart de La Faille-Kuyper, E.H., Vogten, A.J.M. and Grijm, R. (1979) Alcoholic hepatic disease: specificity of IgA deposits in the liver. *American Journal of Pathology* **71**, 51–75.

Kenny, W.C. (1982) Acetaldehyde adducts of phospholipids. *Alcoholism: Clinical and Experimental Research* **6**, 412–416.

Kesaniemi, Y.A., Kervinen, K. and Miettinen, T.A. (1987) Acetaldehyde modification of low density lipoprotein accelerates its catabolism in man. *European Journal of Clinical Investigation* **17**, 29–36.

Kikugawa, K., Takayanagi, K. and Watanabe, S. (1985) Polylysines modified with malonaldehyde, hydroperoxylinoleic acid and monofunctional aldehydes. *Chemical and Pharmaceutical Bulletin* **33**, 5437–5444.

Kikugawa, K., Iwata, A. and Beppu, M. (1988) Formation of cross-links and fluorescence in polylysine, soluble proteins and membrane proteins by reaction with 1-butanal. *Chemical and Pharmaceutical Bulletin* **36**, 685–692.

Kikugawa, K., Kato, T. and Iwata, A. (1989) A tetrameric dialdehyde formed in the reaction of butyraldehyde and benzylamine: a possible intermediate component for protein cross-linking induced by lipid oxidation. *Lipids* **24**, 962–969.

Kolber, M.A. and Terabayashi, H. (1991) Cytotoxic T lymphocytes can be generated aginst acetaldehyde modified syngeneic cells. *Alcohol and Alcoholism* **1**(Suppl), 277–280.

Koskinas, J., Kenna, J.G., Bird, G.L., Alexander, G.J.M. and Williams, R. (1992) Immunoglobulin A antibody to a 200 kilodalton cytosolic acetaldehyde adduct in alcoholic hepatitis. *Gastroenterology* **103**, 1060–1067.

Koskinas, J., Winrow, V., Bird, G., Alexander, G.J.M. and Williams, R. (1993) Hepatic 65 kDa heat shock protein in alcoholic hepatitis. *Hepatology* **17**, 1047–1053.

Krebs, H.A. and Perkins, J.R. (1970) The physiologic role of liver alcohol dehydrogenase. *Biochemical Journal* **118**, 635–644.

Lieber, C.S. and DeCarli, L.M. (1968) Ethanol oxidation by hepatic microsomes: adaptive increase after ethanol feeding. *Science* **162**, 917–918.

Lieber, C.S. and DeCarli, L.M. (1970) Hepatic microsomal ethanol oxidizing system: *in vitro* characteristics and adaptive properties *in vivo*. *Journal of Biological Chemistry* **245**, 2505–2512.

Lieber, C.S. (1990) Mechanism of ethanol induced hepatic injury. *Pharmacological Therapy* **46**, 1–413.

Lieber, C.S. (1991) Hepatic, metabolic and toxic effects of ethanol: 1991 update. *Alcoholism: Clinical and Experimental Research* **15**, 573–592.

Lin, R.C., Smith, R.S. and Lumeng, L. (1988) Detection of a protein acetaldehyde adduct in the liver of rats fed alcohol chronically. *Journal of Clinical Investigation* **81**, 615–619.

Lin, R.C. and Lumeng, L. (1989) Further studies on the 37 kD liver protein acetaldehyde adduct that forms *in vivo* during chronic alcohol ingestion. *Hepatology* **10**, 807–814.

Lin, R.C., Fillenwarth, J., Minter, R. and Lumeng, L. (1990) Formation of the 37 kD protein acetaldehyde adduct in primary cultured rat hepatocytes exposed to alcohol. *Hepatology* **11**, 401–407.

Lin, R.C., Fillenworth, M.J. and Lumeng, L. (1993a) Identification of the 37 kDa liver protein that forms acetaldehyde adduct in alcohol-fed rats. *Alcoholism: Clinical and Experimental Research* **17**, 477.

Lin, R.C., Shahidi, S. and Lumeng, L. (1993b) Production of antibodies that recognise the heterogeneity of immunoreactive sites in human hemoglobin chemically modified by acetaldehyde. *Alcoholism: Clinical and Experimental Research* **17**, 822–886.

Lin, R.C., Zhou, F.C., Fillenworth, M.J. and Lumeng, L. (1993c) Zonal distribution of protein acetaldehyde adducts in the liver of rats fed alcohol for long periods. *Hepatology* **18**, 864–869.

Lindros, K.O. (1982) Human blood acetaldehyde levels: with improved methods a clearer picture emerges. *Alcoholism: Clinical and Experimental Research* **4**, 70–75.

Lumeng, L. (1978) The role of acetaldehyde in mediating the deleterious effect of ethanol on pyridoxan 5 phosphate metabolism. *Journal of Clinical Investigation* **62**, 286–293.

MacDonald, C.M., Dow, J. and Moore, M.R. (1977) A possible protective role for sulphydryl compounds in acute alcoholic liver injury. *Biochemical Pharmacology* **26**, 1529–1531.

MacSween, R.N.M., Anthony, R.S. and Farquharson, M. (1981) Antibodies to alcohol altered hepatocytes in patients with alcoholic liver disease. *Lancet* **2**, 803–804.

Marshall, J.B., Burnett, D.A., Zetterman, R.K. and Sorrell, M.F. (1983) Clinical and biochemical course of alcoholic liver disease following sudden discontinuation of alcoholic consumption. *Alcoholism: Clinical and Experimental Research* **7**, 312–315.

Mathewson, K., Mardini, H.A.L., Bartlett, K. and Record, C.O. (1986) Impaired acetaldehyde metabolism in patients with non-alcoholic liver disorders. *Gut* **27**, 756–764.

Mauch, T.J., Donohue, T.M., Zetterman, R.K., Sorrell, M.F. and Tuma, D.J. (1985) Covalent binding of acetaldehyde to lysine-dependent enzymes can inhibit catalytic activity. *Hepatology* **5**, 1056.

Mauch, T.J., Donohue, T.M., Zetterman, R.K., Sorrell, M.F. and Tuma, D.J. (1986) Covalent binding of acetaldehyde selectively inhibits the catalytic activity of lysine-dependent enzymes. *Hepatology* **6**, 263–269.

Medina, V.A., Donohue, T.M., Sorrell, M.F. and Tuma, D.J. (1985) Covalent binding of acetaldehyde to hepatic proteins during ethanol oxidation. *Journal of Laboratory and Clinical Medicine* **105**, 5–10.

Mezey, E. (1982) Alcoholic liver disease. *Progress in Liver Diseases* **7**, 555–572.

Neuberger, J., Crossley, I.R., Saunders, J.B., Davis, M., Portmann, B., Eddleston, A.L.W.F. and Williams, R. (1984) Antibodies to alcohol-altered liver cell determinants in patients with alcoholic liver disease. *Gut* **25**, 300–304.

Niemela, O., Klajner, F., Orrego, H., Vidins, E., Blendis, L. and Israel, Y. (1987) Antibodies against acetaldehyde modified protein epitopes in human alcoholics. *Hepatology* **7**, 1210–1214.

Niemela, O., Juvonen, T. and Parkkita, S. (1990a) Immunohistochemical demonstration of acetaldehyde-modified epitopes in human liver after alcohol consumption. *Journal of Clinical Investigation* **87**, 1367–1374.

Niemela, O., Mannermaa, R.-M. and Oikarinen, J. (1990b) Impairment of histone H' DNA binding by adduct formation with acetaldehyde. *Life Sciences* **47**, 2241–2249.

Nomura, F. and Lieber, C.S. (1981) Binding of acetaldehyde to rat liver microsomes: enhancement after chronic alcohol consumption. *Biochemical and Biophysical Research Communications* **100**, 131–137.

O'Donnell, J.P. (1982) The reaction of amines with carbonyls: its significance in the non-enzymatic metabolism of xenobiotics. *Drug Metabolism Reviews* **13**, 123–159.

Paradis, V., Scoazec, J.Y., Kollinger, M., Holstege, A., Moreau, A., Feldmann, G. and Bedossa, P. (1996) Cellular and subcellular localization of acetaldehyde protein adducts in liver biopsies from alcoholic patients *Journal of Histochemistry and Cytochemistry* **44**, 1051–1057.

Pessayre, D., Dolder, A., Artigou, J.Y., Andscheer, J.C., Descatoire, V., Degott, C. and Benhamou, J.P. (1979) Effect of fasting on metabolite-mediated hepatotoxicity in the rat. *Gastroenterology* **77**, 264–271.

Ramsay, L., Kenna, J.G., Koskinas, J., Allison, M., Carter, M., Wight, D. and Alexander, G. (1995) Acetaldehyde modified hepatic antigens in alcoholic liver disease. *Journal of Hepatology* **23** (Abstract), 67.

Reynolds, T.B., Benhamou, J.P., Blake, J., Naccarato, R. and Orrego, H. (1989) Treatment of acute alcoholic hepatitis. *Gastroenterology International* **2**, 208–216.

San George, R.C. and Hoberman, H.D. (1986) Reaction of acetaldehyde with hemoglobin. *Journal of Biological Chemistry* **261**, 6811–6821.

Sheron, N., Bird, G.L.A., Goka, A.K.J., Alexander, G.J.M. and Williams, R. (1991) Elevated plasma interleukin 6 and increased severity and mortality in alcoholic hepatitis. *Clinical and Experimental Immunology* **84**, 449–453.

Sheron, N., Bird, G.L.A., Koskinas, J., Ceska, M., Lindley, I., Portmann, B. and Williams, R. (1993) Circulating and tissue levels of the neutrophil chemotaxin interleukin-8 are elevated in severe acute alcoholic hepatitis and tissue levels correlate with neutrophil infiltration. *Hepatology* **18**, 41–46.

Sisson, J.H., Tuma, D.J. and Rennard, S.I. (1991) Acetaldehyde-mediated cilia dysfunction in bovine bronchial epithelial cells. *American Journal of Physiology* **260**, 20–36.

Smith, S.L., Jennett, R.B., Sorrell, M.F. and Tuma, D.J. (1992) Substoichiometric inhibition of microtubule formation by acetaldehyde-tubulin adducts. *Biochemical Pharmacology* **44**, 65–72.

Sorrell, M.F. and Tuma, D.J. (1985) Hypothesis: alcoholic liver injury and the covalent binding of acetaldehyde. *Alcoholism: Clinical and Experimental Research* **9**, 306–309.

Steinberg, J.J., Oliver, G.W.J. and Cajigas, A. (1977) The formation and measurement of DNA neuroadduction ion alcoholism: case report. *American Journal of Forensic Medical Pathology* **18**, 84–91.

Stevens, V.J.W., Fantl, W.J., Newman, C.B., Sims, R.V., Cerami, A. and Peterson, C.M. (1981) Acetaldehyde adducts with hemoglobin. *Journal of Clinical Investigation* **67**, 361–369.

Svegliati-Baroni, G., Baraona, E., Rosman, A.S. and Lieber, C.S. (1994) Collagen acetaldehyde adducts in alcoholic and nonalcoholic liver diseases. *Hepatology* **20**, 111–118.

Swerdlow, M.A., Chowdhury, L.N. and Horn, T. (1982) Pattern of IgA deposition in liver tissues in alcoholic liver disease. *American Journal of Clinical Pathology* **77**, 259–266.

Swerdlow, M.A. and Chowdhury, L.N. (1983) IgA subclasses in liver tissues inalcoholic liver disease. *American Journal of Clinical Pathology* **80**, 283–289.

Takase, S., Takada, A., Yasuhara, M. and Tsutsumi M. (1989) Hepatic aldehyde dehydrogenase activity in liver diseases, with particular emphasis on alcoholic liver disease.
Hepatology **9**, 704–709.

Terabayashi, H. and Kolber, M.A. (1990) The generation of cytotoxic T lymphocytes against
acetaldehyde-modified syngeneic cells. *Alcoholism: Clinical and Experimental Research* **14**,
893–899.

Thiele, G.M., Miller, J.A., Klassen, L.W. and Tuma, D.J. (1996) Long term ethanol administration alters the degradation of acetaldehyde adducts by liver endothelial cells. *Hepatology*
24, 643–648.

Truddel, J.R., Ardies, C.M. and Anderson, W.R. (1990) Cross reactivity of antibodies raised
against acetaldehyde adducts of protein with acetaldehyde adducts of phosphatidyl-
ethanolamine: possible role in alcoholic cirrhosis. *Molecular Pharmacology* **38**, 587–593.

Tsuboi, K.K., Thompson, D.J., Rush, E.M. and Schwartz, H.C. (1981) Acetaldehyde-dependent
changes in hemoglobin and oxygen affinity of human erythrocytes. *Hemoglobin* **5**, 241–250.

Tuma, D.J. and Sorrell, M.F. (1984) Effect of ethanol on hepatic secretory proteins. In *Recent
Developments in Alcoholism*, edited by M. Galanter, Vol. 2, 159–180, New York, NY: Plenum
Press.

Tuma, D.J., Donohue, T.M., Medina, V.A. and Sorrell, M.F. (1984) Enhancement of acetaldehyde protein adduct formation by L-ascorbate. *Archives of Biochemistry and Biophysics* **234**,
377–381.

Tuma, D.J. and Sorrell, M.F. (1985) Covalent binding of acetaldehyde to hepatic proteins:
role in alcoholic liver injury. In *Aldehyde Adducts in Alcoholism*, edited by M.A. Collins, *Prog
Clin Biol Res*, Vol. 183, 3–17. Alan R. Liss, Inc. New York, NY.

Tuma, D.J., Jennett, R.B., Sorrell, M.F. (1987a) The interaction of acetaldehyde with
tubulin. *Annals of the New York Academy of Sciences* **492**, 277–286.

Tuma, D.J., Newman, M.R., Donohue, T.M. and Sorrell, M.F. (1987b) Covalent binding of
acetaldehyde to proteins: participation of lysine residues. *Alcoholism: Clinical and Experimental
Research* **11**, 579–584.

Tuma, D.J., Hoffmann, T. and Sorrell, M.F. (1991) The chemistry of acetaldehyde protein
adducts. *Alcohol and Alcoholism* **1**, 271–276.

Van de Wiel, A., Seifert, W.J., Van der Linden, J.A., Gmelig Meyling, F.H.J., Kater, L. and
Schuurman, H.J. (1987) Spontaneous IgA synthesis by blood mononuclear cells in alcoholic
liver disease. *Scandinavian Journal of Immunology* **25**, 181–187.

Van de Wiel, A., Van Hattum, J., Schurman, H.J. and Kater, L. (1988) Immunoglobulin A
in the diagnosis of alcoholic liver disease. *Gastroenterology* **94**, 457–462.

Viitala, K., Israel, Y., Blake, J.E. and Niemela, O. (1997) Serum IgA, IgG and IgM antibodies
directed against acetaldehyde-derived epitopes: relationship to liver disease severity and
alcohol consumption. *Hepatology* **25**, 1418–1424.

Vina, J., Estrela, J.M., Guerri, C. and Romero, F.J. (1980) Effect of ethanol on glutathione
concentration in isolated hepatocytes. *Biochemical Journal* **188**, 549–552.

Volentine, G.D., Tuma, D.J. and Sorrell, M.F. (1984) Acute effects of ethanol on hepatic
glycoprotein secretion in the rat *in vivo*. *Gastroenterology* **86**, 225–229.

Watkins, N.G., Thorpe, S.R. and Baynes, J.W. (1985) Glycation of amino groups in protein.
Journal of Biochemical Chemistry **260**, 10629–10636.

Worrall, S., De Jersey, J., Shanley, B.C. and Wilce, P.A. (1989) Ethanol induces the production
of antibodies to acetaldehyde modified epitopes in rats. *Alcohol and Alcoholism* **24**, 217–223.

Worrall, S., De Jersey, J., Shanley, B.C. and Wilce, P.A. (1990) Antibodies against acetaldehyde modified epitopes: presence in alcoholics, non alcoholic liver disease and control
subjects. *Alcohol and Alcoholism* **25**, 509–517.

Worrall, S., De Jersey, J., Shanley, B.C. and Wilce, P.A. (1991) Antibodies against acetaldehyde modified epitopes: an elevated IgA response in alcoholics. *European Journal of Clinical Investigation* **21**, 90–95.

Xu, D.S., Jennett, R.B., Smith, S.L., Sorrell, M.F. and Tuma, D.J. (1989) Covalent interactions of acetaldehyde with the actin/microfilament system. *Alcohol and Alcohoslim* **24**, 281–289.

Yokoyama, H., Ishii, H., Nagata, S., Kato, S., Kamegaya, K. and Tsuchiya, M. (1993) Experimental hepatitis induced by ethanol after immunization with acetaldehyde adducts. *Hepatology* **17**, 14–19.

Zetterman, R.K. and Sorrell, M.F. (1981) Immunologic aspects of alcoholic liver disease. *Gastroenterology* **81**, 616–624.

Zetterman, R. (1990) Autoimmunity and alcoholic liver disease. *American Journal of Medicine* **89**, 127–128.

Zhu, Y., Fillenwarth, M.J., Crabb, D., Lumeng, L. and Lin, R.C. (1996) Identification of the 37 kDa rat liver protein that forms an acetaldehyde adduct *in vivo* as 4-3-ketosteroid 5-reductase. *Hepatology* **23**, 115–122.

Zinnemann, H.H. (1975) Autoimmune phenomena in alcoholic cirrhosis. *American Journal of Digestive Diseases* **20**, 337–345.

Part III

Mechanisms of damage

Chapter 6

Free radicals and alcohol-induced liver injury

Emanuele Albano

The possible involvement of free radicals in causing some of the toxic effects of alcohol has been suggested by the detection of biochemical signs of oxidative damage in the liver and in the serum of alcoholic patients and experimental animals exposed to ethanol. Such an hypothesis has recently been supported by experiments using rats fed ethanol by intragastric nutrition that have demonstrated a relationship between alcohol-induced oxidative stress and the development of either hepatocyte damage or liver fibrosis. Oxidative stress associated with ethanol intoxication can be the consequence of the depletion of antioxidants as well as an increased production of reactive oxygen species (superoxide anion and hydrogen peroxide) by mitochondrial electron transport chain, alcohol-inducible cytochrome P450 2E1 (CYP 2E1), xanthine oxidase, aldehyde oxidase and activated phagocytes. Furthermore, during ethanol metabolism by CYP 2E1, hydroxyethyl free radicals are also generated. The mechanisms by which oxidative damage contribute to alcohol toxicity are still poorly understood. The data so far obtained suggest three main possible pathogenetic roles for alcohol-mediated oxidative injury: (i) promotion of hepatocellular damage; (ii) induction of immunological reactions; (iii) stimulation of collagen deposition. Hepatocellular damage by oxidative events appears to primarily involve mitochondria promoting the development of micro-vesicular steatosis and leading to hepatocyte necrosis and/or apoptosis. The involvement of free radical processes in stimulating immune reaction is demonstrated by the capacity of adducts between hydroxyethyl radical and liver proteins to induce the production of specific antibodies. Anti-hydroxyethyl radical antibodies present in the serum of patients with alcoholic liver disease recognize these epitopes in the plasma membranes of hepatocytes exposed to ethanol and are able to cause cell-mediated antibody-dependent cytotoxicity. Oxidative stress can also promote liver fibrosis by triggering the release of pro-fibrotic cytokines as well as by directly activating collagen gene expression in hepatic stellate cells. Although further studies are required to better characterize the role of free radical mechanisms in alcohol liver damage, the possible application of antioxidants in therapy for alcoholic liver disease can be proposed.

KEYWORDS: free radicals, oxidative injury, ethanol, hydroxyethyl radicals, lipid peroxidation, alcoholic liver disease

EVIDENCE FOR THE INVOLVEMENT OF FREE RADICALS IN ALCOHOLIC LIVER DISEASES

The possibility that free radical-mediated oxidative injury might contribute to ethanol hepatotoxicity was first proposed by Di Luzio in the early 1960s following the observation that pre-treatment of rats with antioxidants alleviated ethanol-induced fat accumulation in the liver (Di Luzio, 1963). In the subsequent years, a number of experimental studies supporting the association between oxidative damage and alcohol toxicity have been obtained in rats (Dianzani, 1985; Albano *et al.*, 1991a; Nordmann *et al.*, 1992). These findings are not limited to rodents, since signs of oxidative injury have also been detected in mini-pigs, baboons and rhesus monkeys chronically fed with alcohol (Niemelä *et al.*, 1995; Lieber *et al.*, 1997; Pawlosky *et al.*, 1997). Nonetheless, the most relevant contribution in establishing a connection between free radical-mediated oxidative damage and alcohol-induced liver injury has been recently obtained by the use of a new experimental model developed by Tsukamoto and French (Tsukamoto *et al.*, 1985). This model is based on the continuous intragastric administration of alcohol along with a liquid diet rich in fat and poor in carbohydrates (Tsukamoto *et al.*, 1986). Using intragastric ethanol feeding, it is possible to reproduce in rats several pathological features of human alcoholic liver disease (ALD), including steatosis, inflammatory infiltrates and focal necrosis (Tsukamoto *et al.*, 1985). Extending alcohol treatment up to 16 weeks, it is also possible to obtain the onset of liver fibrosis (Tsukamoto *et al.*, 1986). The studies performed using this experimental model have provided important information concerning the possible mechanisms involved in the pathogenesis of ALD. In particular, Nanji and French (Nanji and French, 1989; Nanji *et al.*, 1998) have shown that while rats on ethanol-beef fat diet had no liver injury, the combination of ethanol and corn oil, which is rich in linoleic acid, promoted the development of ALD. This effect was associated with a stimulation of oxidative damage, as monitored by an increase in lipid peroxidation and protein carbonyls (Kamimura *et al.*, 1992; Nanji *et al.*, 1994a; Rouach *et al.*, 1997; Polavarapu *et al.*, 1998), suggesting that the high dietary content of polyunsaturated fatty acids favors ethanol-induced generation of harmful aldehydic endproducts of peroxidative lipid breakdown. Indeed, increased hepatic levels of 4-hydroxynonenal (4-HNE), an highly reactive aldehydic lipid peroxidation product have been observed in the livers of rats receiving the alcohol-containing diet (Kamimura *et al.*, 1992; Li *et al.*, 1997; Niemelä *et al.*, 1998). The association between the stimulation of lipid peroxidation and alcohol toxicity is further strengthened by the observation that the replacement of corn oil with rich omega-3 unsaturated fatty acid fish oil, further stimulates lipid peroxidation and worsens liver pathology (Nanji *et al.*, 1994b). Interestingly, when ethanol administration to rats is discontinued after 6 weeks of combined feeding of alcohol and fish oil, replacing fish oil with saturated fatty acids rich palm oil, or with medium chain tryglycerides lowers lipid peroxidation by greatly improves the recovery from liver damage (Nanji *et al.*, 1995a, 1996).

The possible implication of oxidative damage in human alcoholic liver disease (ALD) is suggested by several clinical studies showing that lipid peroxidation products (conjugated dienes, malonildialdehyde, 4-hydroxynonenal, F_2-isoprostanes) and protein carbonyls, are higher in liver biopsies or in the sera obtained from patients with ALD as compared to specimens from non-drinker subjects or patients with non-alcoholic liver diseases (Suematzu *et al.*, 1981; Shaw *et al.*, 1983; Situnayake *et al.*, 1990; Baldi *et al.*, 1993; Lecompte *et al.*, 1994; Grattagliano *et al.*, 1996; Aleynik *et al.*, 1998; Hill and Awad, 1999). Patients with alcoholic cirrhosis also exhale more pentane, a volatile end product of lipid peroxidation (Letteron *et al.*, 1993). Furthermore, lipid hydroperoxides and malonildialdehyde (MDA), were about 3-fold higher in ALD subjects drinking more than 100 g ethanol/day than in those drinking below 100 g ethanol/day, irrespective of the extent of liver injury (Clot *et al.*, 1994).

The causal relationship between oxidative events and the development of alcoholic liver injury is further supported by morphological studies performed in the liver of ethanol-fed rats and mini-pigs as well as in liver biopsies obtained from patients with ALD. Immunohistochemical staining has revealed, in fact, the presence of aldehydes derived from lipid peroxidation in the areas of fatty infiltration, focal necrosis and fibrosis (Niemelä *et al.*, 1994, 1995, 1999; Tsukamoto *et al.*, 1995; Ohhira *et al.*, 1998).

MECHANISMS REPONSIBLE FOR CAUSING OXIDATIVE LIVER INJURY BY ALCOHOL

One feature characterizing the involvement of free radicals in alcoholic liver disease concerns the possible contribution of different free radical intermediates (oxygen-derived radicals, hydroxyethyl radicals, nitric oxide, lipid derived radicals) in causing tissue damage (Table 6.1). These radical species are produced not only by hepatocytes, but also by Kupffer cells, endothelial cells and by infiltrating inflammatory leucocytes. Besides stimulating free radical production, ethanol is also responsible for the impairment of liver antioxidant defences. The combination of increased free radical production and decreased cellular antioxidants is probably responsible for the development of oxidative injury associated with ALD.

Formation of reactive oxygen species

The formation of reactive oxygen species such as superoxide anion (O_2^-) and hydrogen peroxide (H_2O_2) represents an important cause of oxidative injury in many diseases associated to free radical formation. In the presence of trace

Table 6.1 Free radical species possibly involved in alcoholic liver disease

Species	Chemical structure	Possible sources
Superoxide anion	O_2^-	Cytochrome P450 2E1 Mitochondrial respiratory chain Xanthine oxidase Aldehyde oxidase Oxidative burst of phagocytes
Hydroxyl radical	$OH^\bullet$	Iron-mediated degradation of H_2O_2
Nitric oxide	NO	Nitroxide synthetases of hepato-cytes, Kupffer and endothelial cells
Peroxinitrite	$ONOO^\bullet$	Reaction of NO with O_2^-
α-Hydroxyethyl radical	$CH_3C^\bullet HOH$	Ethanol oxidation by CYP 2E1 Reaction with O_2^- or $OH^\bullet$ Kupffer cells?
Methylcarbonyl radical	$CH_3C^\bullet O$	Acetaldehyde oxidation by xanthine oxidase or aldehyde oxidase

amounts of transition metals, most frequently iron, O_2^- and H_2O_2 generate highly reactive hydroxyl radicals (OH$^\bullet$), which are responsible for the oxidation of biological constituents (Aust et al., 1985).

Several enzymatic systems have been proposed as sources of O_2^- and H_2O_2 in parenchymal cells during ethanol intoxication and include the microsomal mono-oxygenase system, the mitochondrial respiratory chain and the cytosolic enzymes xanthine oxidase and aldehyde oxidase (Table 6.1). The mechanisms responsible for the formation of reactive oxygen species by alcohol are discussed below. However, it should be considered that most of the evidence so far available has been obtained in vitro, while comparatively little is known about the capacity of ethanol to induce oxygen free radical production in vivo. For instance, only recently, Thome and coworkers (1997) reported preliminary data indicating that OH$^\bullet$-mediated conversion of acetylsalicilic acid to 2,3-dihydrobenzoic acid is significantly increased in alcoholic patients as compared to healthy controls.

Role of cytochrome P450 system

The induction of CYP 2E1-dependent monoxygenase activity by chronic alcohol exposure can represent an important source of oxygen radicals, since CYP 2E1 has an especially high rate of NADPH oxidase activity and produces large quantities of O_2^- and H_2O_2 (Ronis et al., 1996). Microsomes obtained from rats chronically exposed to alcohol are more active than microsomes from untreated animals in producing O_2^-, H_2O_2 and OH$^\bullet$ (Cederbaum, 1989; Persson et al., 1990). Antibodies directed against CYP 2E1 selectively inhibit such an excess formation of oxygen radicals (Ekström and Ingelman-Sundberg, 1989). Interestingly, NADH can replace NADPH as a cofactor for the microsomal production of reactive oxygen species (Dicker and Cederbaum, 1992). Such a peculiarity can be important during ethanol intoxication because alcohol metabolism leads to an excess generation of NADH (Lieber, 1994). Although human liver microsomes produce O_2^- and H_2O_2 at rates that are 20–30% lower than those observed in rat liver microsomes (Rabshabe-Step and Cederbaum, 1994), NADPH-oxidase activity in human microsomes is positively correlated with CYP 2E1 content (Ekström et al., 1989). Moreover, in human liver microsomes, NADH is equally effective as NADPH in promoting oxidative reactions (Rabshabe-Step and Cederbaum, 1994). Thus, the high efficiency of CYP 2E1 in reducing oxygen to superoxide anion and hydrogen peroxide could be regarded as one of the key factors contributing to the stimulation of lipid peroxidation during chronic exposure to alcohol (Ingelman-Sundberg et al., 1993). Consistently, experiments performed using rats chronically fed with alcohol by the Tsukamoto-French model have demonstrated that the induction of CYP 2E1 by ethanol is associated with the stimulation of lipid peroxidation, while compounds that interfere with CYP 2E1 induction significantly reduced peroxidative damage (French et al., 1993; Morimoto et al., 1995; Albano et al., 1996).

Role of mitochrondria

It is well known that the respiratory chain of mitochondria represents one of the main sources of superoxide anions in the cells (Forman and Boveris, 1988). Acute alcohol exposure increases O_2^- production by liver sub-mitochrondrial particles (Sinaceur *et al.*, 1985), while chronic intoxication appears to depress superoxide generation (Ribiére *et al.*, 1994). Kukielka and coworkers (1994) reported that chronic alcohol intake stimulates the production of reactive oxygen species by intact liver mitochondria through a pathway independent from the respiratory chain which involves the activity of a rotenone-insensitive NADH-cytochrome c reductase. The importance of this enzyme in causing ethanol-induced oxidative injury to the mitochondria could be even greater than that of the respiratory chain, since the enzyme involved is located in the outer mitochondrial membrane and does not require the transfer of NADH through the mitochondrial membranes. An additional mechanism contributing to the mithochondrial formation of reactive oxygen species during ALD might be represented by the effect of tumor necrosis factor α (TNF-α). During ALD, the stimulation of Kupffer cells and infiltrating inflammatory cells results in an increased secretion of this cytokine (Lands, 1995). Recent evidence indicates that TNF-α induces the release of *N*-acetylsphingosine (C_2-ceramide) from sphingomyelin (Fernandez-Checa *et al.*, 1997). The interaction of C_2-ceramide with hepatocyte mitochondrial respiratory chain at a site between complex II and complex III is then responsible for stimulating the leakage of O_2^- and H_2O_2 (Fernandez-Checa *et al.*, 1997). Accumulation of lipid peroxidation products and oxidative modifications of mitochondrial proteins and DNA (mtDNA) (Kamimura *et al.*, 1992; Weiland and Lautemburg, 1995; Cahill *et al.*, 1997) can be observed following both acute and chronic exposure of rats to ethanol confirming that ethanol-mediated oxidative injury of mitochondria can take place *in vivo*.

Role of cytosolic enzymes

The generation of O_2^- by xanthine oxidase is one of the mechanisms believed to be responsible for increased oxygen radical production during post-ischemic tissue damage (McCord, 1985). Following both acute and chronic ethanol intoxication, an increase in purine degradation leading to excess formation of xanthine and hypoxanthine can be observed (Kato *et al.*, 1990) along with the conversion of xanthine dehydrogenase to the O_2^--producing oxidase form (Sultatos, 1988; Abbondanza *et al.*, 1989). Consistently, xanthine oxidase inhibition by allopurinol prevents ethanol-induced lipid peroxidation (Kato *et al.*, 1990). However, the contribution of this metabolic pathway in causing alcohol-mediated oxidative damage requires further confirmation, since the protection given by allopurinol might be due to the scavenging of hydroxyl radicals (Moorhouse *et al.*, 1978).

Acetaldehyde oxidation by xanthine oxidase has also been suggested as an alternative pathway in the generation of oxygen radicals during ethanol metabolism (Shaw and Jayatilleke, 1990a; Grattegliano *et al.*, 1996). However, the possibility that acetaldehyde might be an effective substrate for xanthine oxidase is still under debate because of the high K_m of the enzyme for acetaldehyde (about 30 mM) (Fridovich, 1989). Nonetheless, Puntarulo and Cederbaum (1989) have reported that xanthine oxidase is capable of inducing the formation of reactive oxygen species at concentrations of acetaldehyde close to those present in the liver following alcohol intake (about 0.1 mM) (Stowel *et al.*, 1980). The molybdenum-containing enzyme aldehyde oxidase has a much lower K_m for acetaldehyde (1 mM), thus might represent a potential source of reactive oxygen species (Shaw and Jayatilleke, 1990a). Recently, Mira and coworkers (1995) have reported that NADH is a better substrate (K_m 28 μM) than acetaldehyde for O_2^- generation by aldehyde oxidase. The possible contribution of aldehyde oxidase in promoting oxidative injury by alcohol comes from the observation that the enzyme stimulates lipid peroxidation when added to rat liver microsomes incubated with ethanol in the presence of NAD^+ and alcohol dehydrogenase (Mira *et al.*, 1995). Conversely, menadione, an inhibitor of aldehyde oxidase, significantly decreased lipid peroxidation in isolated rat hepatocytes incubated with ethanol or acetaldehyde (Shaw and Jayatilleke, 1990b).

Phagocytic cells as source of reactive oxygen species

The formation of superoxide anion by activated phagocytes represents an important source of oxidizing species in inflammated tissues (Smith, 1994). Bautista and Spitzer (1992) have observed that both acute and chronic ethanol administration stimulates O_2^- production by *in situ* perfused rat liver and have suggested that Kupffer cells are likely to be responsible for this effect. Short-term *in vitro* exposure of macrophages to low doses of ethanol is capable of directly stimulating O_2^- production (Dorio *et al.*, 1988). However, the release of prostanoids can also be involved, since cyclooxygenase inhibition by ibuprofen abolishes the production of superoxide anion by Kupffer cells in perfused livers exposed to ethanol (Bautista and Spitzer, 1992). Interestingly, an increased production of O_2^- by rat livers has been demonstrated during the recovery period after 12 hours of continuous ethanol infusion (Bautista and Spitzer, 1996). Such a post-binge stimulation in O_2^- generation involves Kupffer and endothelial cells and can be significantly attenuated following liver depletion of Kupffer cells with gadolinium chloride (Bautista and Spitzer, 1996).

Liver infiltration by granulocytes and monocytes is a common feature of alcoholic hepatitis and these cells might substantially contribute to oxygen radical production during ALD. Roll and collaborators have suggested that lipid peroxidation is responsible for the generation of a chemotactic factor for neutrophils by rat hepatocytes exposed to alcohol (Hultcrantz *et al.*, 1991). Other studies have shown that powerful chemotactic agents, such as interleukin-8 (IL-8) (Shiratori *et al.*, 1993) and leucotriene B_4 (Shirley *et al.*, 1992) are also produced by hepatocytes exposed to ethanol. In this respect, peroxidized fatty acids have been reported to stimulate IL-8 secretion (Jayatilleke and Shaw, 1998). Increased circulating levels of IL-8, tumor necrosis factor-α (TNF-α), and interleukin-1 (IL-1) are a common feature in ALD patients (McClain *et al.*, 1993; Sheron *et al.*, 1993). These pro-inflammatory cytokines can promote liver leucocyte infiltration in ALD patients by inducing the expression of leucocyte adhesion molecules in liver endothelial cells (Adams, 1994). In addition, chronic ethanol administration in rats is associated with an increased production of macrophage inflammatory protein-2 (MIP_2) as well as with the up-regulation in CD18 adhesion molecule expression in neutrophils and of its counter receptor ICAM-1 in endothelial and hepatic cells (Bausista, 1997). These events account for the increased hepatic sequestration of neutrophils observed in ethanol-treated animals and for the priming of neutrophils to O_2^- production (Bausista *et al.*, 1992).

During ALD, Kupffer cell activation can be also favored by the presence of endotoxemia. Low levels of circulating endotoxins can, in fact, be observed in humans (Bode *et al.*, 1987; Fukii *et al.*, 1991) and in ethanol-fed rats (Nanji *et al.*, 1993; Adachi *et al.*, 1995). In the plasma endotoxins bind to a 60 kD protein, known as lipopolysaccaride-binding protein (LBP), that interacts with a receptor (CD14) on the plasma membrane of Kupffer cells triggering the synthesis and the release of cytokines (IL-1, IL-6, IL-8, IL-10, TNF-α, TGF-β1) platelet activating factor (PAF), eicosanoids, reactive oxygen species and nitrogen oxide (NO) (Lands, 1995). Recent studies by Thurman's group have pointed out the importance of endotoxin-mediated activation of Kupffer cells in the development of liver damage in the intragastric ethanol feeding model (Thurman, 1998). Nonetheless, more studies are required to evaluate the actual importance of activated Kupffer cells in ALD, since chronic co-administration of ethanol and endotoxins to rats does not promote alcohol toxicity (Järveläinen *et al.*, 1999). Moreover, the inactivation of Kupffer cells by gadolinium chloride does not affect O_2^- generation following ethanol infusion in *in situ* perfused rat livers (Nakano *et al.*, 1995).

Role of iron in ethanol-induced oxidative stress

It is well known that the presence of trace amounts of iron represents a critical factor in the generation of hydroxyl radicals as well as in the catalysis of lipid peroxidation (Aust *et al.*, 1985). Alcohol abuse in humans is often associated with an impaired utilization and with an increased deposition of iron in the liver (Chapman *et al.*, 1983; Irving *et al.*, 1988). Experiments performed in rats have shown that dietary supplementation with iron increases alcohol toxicity (Tsukamoto *et al.*, 1995; Stål *et al.*, 1996) and promotes ethanol-induced lipid peroxidation (Tsukamoto *et al.*, 1995). Conversely, the administration of the oral iron chelator 1,2-dimethyl-3-hydroxypyrid-4-one, but not of long acting parenteral iron chelator hydroxy-ethyl-starch-desferrioxamine, has been reported to reduce non-hem iron levels, lipid peroxidation and fat accumulation following intragastric ethanol feeding of rats (Sadrzadeh *et al.*, 1994a, 1997).

Free radical reactions appear to be promoted by a small pool of low molecular weight non-protein iron complexes (Minotti *et al.*, 1991). Acute ethanol intake can increase liver low molecular weight iron content by increasing the uptake of transferrin (Rouach *et al.*, 1994). Moreover, experiments *in vitro* have shown that the rise in the cytosolic levels of NADH (Tophan *et al.*, 1989) or the generation of O_2^- promote the release catalytically active iron from ferritin (Shaw and Jayatilleke, 1990a). The addition of ferritin to liver microsomes from ethanol-fed rats greatly stimulates both NADPH and NADH dependent lipid peroxidation. This effect is prevented by the addition of superoxide dismutase, iron chelators and anti-CYP 2E1 antibodies (Kulielka and Cederbaum, 1996), indicating that CYP 2E1-generated O_2^- might also contribute to the mobilization redox reactive iron from ferritin. However, the contribution of iron released from ferritin in causing ethanol-induced oxidative stress in the whole liver has not been proven unequivocally. The cytosolic levels of low molecular weight iron increases following acute alcohol administration (Rouach *et al.*, 1990), but they are decreased (Rouach *et al.*, 1997) or unchanged (Kamimura *et al.*, 1992) in rats chronically treated with ethanol by intragastric

feeding. These findings might be explained by the fact that hepatocyte iron homeostasis is finely tuned by cytosolic iron regulatory protein (IRP). By interacting with
the metal, IRP changes its affinity for the iron responsive elements (IRE) in mRNAs
coding for ferritin and transferrin receptor. Thus, in the presence of low molecular
weight iron, IRP does not bind to IRE and this stimulates ferritin synthesis and iron
sequestration, while iron uptake by the transferrin receptor is depressed (Mascotti
et al., 1995). During long-term alcohol exposure, an increase in ferritin synthesis
might also be stimulated by cytokines such as IL-1 and TNF-α (Mascotti *et al.*, 1995).
Furthermore, Cairo and coworkers (1996) have recently reported that O_2^- and H_2O_2
are able to reversibly inhibit IRP binding to IRE, suggesting that an increased
formation of reactive oxygen species can stimulate iron chelation by ferritin in order
to prevent the spreading of iron dependent oxidative events.

Free radical species derived from ethanol or acetaldehyde

Hydroxyethyl free radicals

In 1987, two independent studies using Electron Spin Resonance (ESR) spectroscopy
in combination with spin trapping technique, have reported the formation of
1-hydroxyethyl free radicals ($CH_3C^{\bullet}HOH$) by rat liver microsomes incubated in the
presence of ethanol and NADPH (Albano *et al.*, 1987; Reinke *et al.*, 1987). These
observations have been confirmed by several other reports (Albano *et al.*, 1988;
Reinke *et al.*, 1990; Rao *et al.*, 1996) and by the demonstration that hydroxyethyl
radicals can be generated *in vivo* in the liver of ADH deficient deer-mice (Knecht
et al., 1990) as well as of alcohol-fed rats (Moore *et al.*, 1995; Knecht *et al.*, 1995;
Reinke *et al.*, 1997a) receiving an acute dose of ethanol. Free radical intermediates
are similarly produced during microsomal oxidation of propanol, butanol and penta-
nol, indicating a common metabolic pathway producing free radicals intermediates from aliphatic alcohols (Albano *et al.*, 1994a). The formation of hydroxyethyl
radicals in liver microsomes and in reconstituted monoxygenase systems strictly
requires NADPH (Albano *et al.*, 1991), but in human liver microsomes NADH can
also support hydroxyethyl radicals production (Rao *et al.*, 1996). The involvement
of CYP 2E1 in the generation of free radical metabolites from ethanol and other
aliphatic alcohols is suggested by the following observations: (i) a strong correlation
between the capacity of liver microsomes from ethanol-fed rats to form hydroxyethyl radicals and their individual content of CYP 2E1 (Albano *et al.*, 1996); (ii) the
high efficiency of reconstituted monoxygenase systems containing purified CYP 2E1
in generating alcohol-derived radicals (Albano *et al.*, 1991); (iii) the inhibition
exerted by anti-CYP 2E1 antibodies or CYP 2E1 inhibitors in the generation of
hydroxyethyl free radicals by liver microsomes from alcohol-fed rats (Albano *et al.*,
1991, 1994a).

So far the mechanisms responsible for hydroxyethyl radical production by CYP 2E1
have not yet been completely elucidated. The results of *in vitro* experiments indicate
that superoxide dismutase, catalase, hydroxyl radical scavengers and desferroxamine
lower hydroxyethyl radical generation by rodent and human liver microsomes
(Albano *et al.*, 1988, 1991; Reinke *et al.*, 1990; Knecht *et al.*, 1993; Rao *et al.*, 1996).

Similar effects are also exerted by tryptamine, isoniazid and octylamine (Albano *et al.*, 1991), compounds that interfere with the NADPH oxidase activity of CYP 2E1 (Persson *et al.*, 1990). Conversely, the addition of iron or the inhibition of endogenous catalase by azide stimulate the ethanol-radical production (Albano *et al.*, 1988). Thus, the interaction of iron with reactive oxygen species (O_2^-, H_2O_2) originating as a result of CYP 2E1-mediated NADPH-oxidase activity might be responsible for hydroxyethyl radical formation (Figure 6.1). Alternatively, the direct one-electron oxidation of ethanol by superoxide anion has also been proposed to account for hydroxyethyl free radical formation (Knecht *et al.*, 1993; Rao *et al.*, 1996; Reinke *et al.*, 1997b). Recently Stoyanovsky and Cederbaum (1998) have determined that the rate of hydroxyethyl radical formation by pyrazole-treated rat liver microsomes is about 1–1.5 nmol/minute/mg of protein, 10 times lower compared to the rate of acetaldehyde formation by two-electron ethanol oxidation.

It has been reported that the stimulation of Kupffer cells by rat pre-treatment with endotoxins caused a three-fold increase in the secretion of hydroxyethyl spin

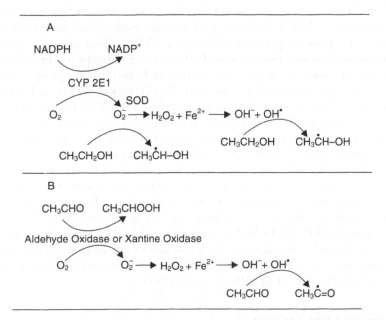

Figure 6.1 Reactions possibly involved in the formation of ethanol-derived hydroxyethyl free radicals (panel A) and acetaldehyde-derived methyl-carbonyl free radicals (panel B) in hepatocytes exposed to ethanol. The interaction of iron with reactive oxygen species (O_2^-, H_2O_2) originating by NADPH-oxidase activity of CYP 2E1 has been proposed to generate hydroxyethyl radical in rat and human liver microsomes. Alternatively, a direct one-electron oxidation of ethanol by superoxide anion might also account for hydroxyethyl free radical formation. Experiments using purified enzymes have shown that O_2^- and H_2O_2 are produced during the oxidation of acetaldehyde by xanthine oxidase. In the presence of iron, O_2^- and H_2O_2 can lead to the formation of $OH^•$ radicals that are then responsible for attacking an other molecule of acetaldehyde giving rise to methyl carbonyl radical. Thus, acetaldehyde might act at the same time as source of reactive oxygen species, being substrate for xanthine oxidase, as well as target for $OH^•$ radicals.

adducts into the bile (Chamulitrat *etal.*, 1998). Endotoxin-induced stimulation in ethanol radical formation was reduced by 50% by the animal treatment with dexferrioxamine or following Kupffer cells destruction by gadolinium chloride (Chamulitrat *etal.*, 1998). Similarly, gadolinium chloride decreases the trapping of hydroxyethyl radicals in intragastric ethanol-fed rats (Knecht *etal.*, 1995). Although chronic ethanol treatment can induce CYP 2E1 expression in Kupffer cells (Koivisto *etal.*, 1996), reactive oxygen species produced during phagocyte activation are more likely to be responsible for the formation of hydroxyethyl radicals. Nonetheless, the actual role of non-parenchymal cells in generating ethanol-derived radicals requires further investigations.

Hydroxyethyl free radicals are quite reactive species and can interact with a number of organic compounds including ascorbic acid, glutathione, α-tocopherol, proteins and DNA (Schuessler, 1981; Schuessler *etal.*, 1992; Stoyanovsky *etal.*, 1998). 8-hydroxyethyl-guanine has been characterized as the product of hydroxyethyl radical interaction with DNA (Nakao and Augusto, 1998), while tyrosine and tripto-phan residues appear to be the preferential targets of hydroxyethyl radicals in proteins (Anni and Israel, 1999). Upon incubation of rat liver microsomes with NADPH and radioactive ethanol, hydroxyethyl radical residues can be recovered covalently bound to microsomal proteins (Albano *etal.*, 1993; Moncada *etal.*, 1994). Immunoblots using antibodies raised against hydroxyethyl radical-protein adducts have demonstrated the association of hydroxyethyl radical-derived epitopes with at least four microsomal proteins of, respectively, 78 kD, 60 kD, 52 kD and 40 kD (Clot *etal.*, 1996). The 52 kD protein has been identified as CYP 2E1 by combined immunoblotting and immunoprecipitation techniques (Clot *etal.*, 1996), while the identity of the other proteins is presently unknown. It is likely that these proteins are intimately associated with CYP 2E1, although the 78 kD protein is not NADPH-cytochrome P450 reductase. The formation of hydroxyethyl-CYP 2E1 adducts has been shown to occur also *in vivo* and can be detected in immunoblots of micro-somal proteins obtained from rats acutely treated with a large dose of ethanol, as well as in microsomes from rats receiving ethanol by intragastric feeding (Clot *etal.*, 1996). The alkylation of CYP 2E1 by hydroxyethyl free radicals suggests the possib-ility that these radicals could originate at the active site of the enzyme, possibly as a result of the interaction between ethanol and O_2^- or the ferric cytochrome P450-oxygen complex (CYP 2E1-Fe^3+O_2) (Albano *etal.*, 1991).

Acetaldehyde-derived free radicals

As mentioned above, xanthine oxidase and aldehyde oxidase metabolize acetalde-hyde with the formation of reactive oxygen species. During the oxidation of acetalde-hyde by xanthine oxidase a carbon centered free radical, identified as methyl carbonyl species ($CH_3C^•O$) is produced (Albano *etal.*, 1994b). Superoxide dismut-ase, catalase and hydroxyl radical scavengers are able to inhibit the formation of methyl carbonyl radicals, indicating that $OH^•$ radicals are likely to be responsible for the free radical activation of acetaldehyde (Albano *etal.*, 1994b) (Figure 6.1). Interestingly, the formation of methyl carbonyl radicals by xanthine oxidase is evident at concentrations of acetaldehyde as low as 0.1 mM and when acetalde-hyde is generated from ethanol by alcohol dehydrogenase (Albano *etal.*, 1994b).

Thus, the formation of methyl carbonyl radicals might contribute to the covalent binding of acetaldehyde to proteins (Nicholls *et al.*, 1992) that has been implicated in causing cell toxicity and immunological reactions associated with alcohol abuse (Lieber, 1994; Paronetto, 1993).

Nitrogen oxide and alcohol-induced oxidative injury

Nitric oxide (NO) is a nitrogen centered free radical produced from *L*-arginine by constitutive (cNOS) and inducible (iNOS) NO synthetase enzymes (Moncada *et al.*, 1991). In hepatocytes, endothelial and Kupffer cells' membrane-bound cNOS produces pulses of NO for short periods in response to specific stimuli and NO formed in this way, is believed to mediate intra- and inter-cellular communication and signaling (Li and Billiar, 1999). Once stimulated by cytokines, prostaglandins or endotoxins the same cells respond with the activation of cytosolic iNOS that leads to the continuous formation of large amounts of NO (Li and Billiar, 1999). Wang and coworkers (1995) have reported that increased levels of NO metabolites in the plasma and in the liver perfusate following chronic ethanol administration in combination or not with acute endotoxin treatment. They also demonstrated that Kupffer cells were responsible for the NO increase in the animals receiving alcohol alone, while the combination of ethanol and endotoxins also stimulated hepatocyte NO synthesis (Wang *et al.*, 1995). However, the actual capacity of alcohol intake to stimulated NO production, has been questioned by more recent studies demonstrating that ethanol can interfere at the transcriptional and post-transcriptional level with iNOS induction (Zhao *et al.*, 1997).

It is known that the reaction of NO with O_2^- leads to the formation of highly reactive peroxynitrite radicals (ONOO•), which can inactivate several enzymes, impair mitochondrial functions and exert cytotoxic actions (Beckman and Koppenol, 1996; Grisham *et al.*, 1999). The generation of ONOO• by activated Kupffer cells has been proposed to be responsible for hepatocyte damage during endotoxemia (Li and Billiar, 1999). However, the actual role of NO and ONOO• in the development of liver injury by ethanol is still controversial. In a recent study by Chamulitrat and Spitzer (1996), rats chronically exposed to ethanol and receiving 12 hours endotoxin infusion showed a 3-fold increase in NO generation as compared to rats receiving endotoxins alone. This effect was associated with a 2–3-fold stimulation in transaminase release, that was attenuated by the inhibition of iNOS with aminoguanidine (Chamulitrat and Spitzer, 1996). On the other hand, other evidence indicates that NO may have remarkable antioxidant capabilities (Grisham *et al.*, 1999). The *in vivo* inhibition of liver NO formation enhances O_2^- release by Kupffer cells (Bautista and Spitzer, 1994), while NO formation by hepatocytes is associated with an increased resistance to oxygen radical-mediated injury (Kuo and Slivka, 1994; Li and Billiar, 1999). Recently, Sergent and coworkers (1997) have proposed that the capacity of NO to decrease cytosolic low molecular weight iron complexes can be responsible for the resistance to ethanol-induced oxidative stress observed in isolated hepatocyte following the stimulation of NO production by endotoxins. The inhibition of CYP 2E1 activity by NO (Gergel *et al.*, 1997) might be important in this respect, considering the ability of CYP 2E1 to generate reactive oxygen species. It is noteworthy that the development of liver injury during intragastric alcohol feeding is associated with the lowering of iNOS in non-parenchymal cells while the treatment with NO-inhibitor, N-nitro-L-arginine methyl ester (L-NAME) worsens liver damage (Nanji et al., 1995c). It is possible that these contrasting results might depend upon different effects exerted by NO in relation to the timing, location and rate of production of NO itself and reactive NO-derived species (Grisham et al., 1999). Thus, further studies are needed before any conclusion is drawn on the actual role of NO in the pathogenesis of ALD.

Lowering of antioxidant defenses in ethanol-induced oxidative injury

The lowering of liver antioxidant defences, along with the formation of free radical intermediates, might significantly contribute to the development of ethanol-induced oxidative damage. A decrease in hepatic glutathione (GSH) levels (about 30–50% of the control values) is one of the most constant features of acute alcohol intoxication in experimental animals (Guerri and Grisolia, 1980; Videla and Valenzuela, 1982; Israel et al., 1992). These changes are not associated with a significant elevation in the hepatic levels of oxidized glutathione (GSSG) (Lauterburg et al., 1984) and are independent from ethanol metabolism. Thus, the lowering of GSH is not a direct effect of free radical formation (Speisky et al., 1988), but is more likely due to the combination of an increased GSH efflux from hepatocytes and an interference with GSH re-synthesis (Lauterburg et al., 1984; Speisky et al., 1985). Rats fed alcohol chronically also exhibit an increased rate of GSH efflux that is associated with a marked enhancement in the ecto-activity of gamma-glutamyl transferase (GGT) (Israel et al., 1992). Speisky and coworkers (1990) have demonstrated that GGT induction occurs mostly in the sinusoidal surface of hepatocytes where GGT is responsible for the degradation of circulating GSH into precursors for the re-synthesis of the tripeptide. They have proposed that GGT induction, along with a stimulation of cysteine synthesis from methionine via S-adenosyl-methionine synthetase and cystathionine synthetase, might provide a compensatory response to the increase in GSH demand due to ethanol-induced oxidative stress (Israel et al., 1992). In this respect, GSH turnover increases by 30–40% in the liver of rats fed alcohol by the Lieber-De Carli diet, while GSH content is normal or slightly modified (Israel et al., 1992).

Although total hepatocyte GSH content is not appreciably affected by chronic alcohol intake, a progressive lowering of mitochondrial GSH up to 50–85% of the control values is instead evident in the livers of rats receiving alcohol either by traditional pair feeding (Fernandez-Checa et al., 1987) or by intragastric nutrition (Tacheshi et al., 1992). The selective depletion of the mitochondrial GSH pool is likely to depend upon a defect in the transport of the tripeptide from cytosol to the mitochondrial matrix (Fernandez-Checa et al., 1991) due to the decreased efficiency of a specific ATP-dependent GSH transporter in the inner mitochondrial membrane (Colell et al., 1997). This effect is more evident in centrilobular hepatocytes (Garcia-Ruitz et al., 1994) and precedes the development of lipid peroxidation and of alterations in ATP production (Tacheshi et al., 1992). Thus, the effect of ethanol on mitochondrial glutathione (GSH) homeostasis might significantly contribute to the development of oxidative damage to these organelles (Fernandez-Checa et al., 1997).

The compensatory mechanisms able to maintain hepatic GSH in rodents are not as efficient in primates, since a decrease on liver GSH independently from the nutritional status or the degree of liver disease is a common feature in ethanol-fed baboons (Shaw *et al.*, 1981) as well as in alcoholic patients (Shaw *et al.*, 1983; Jewell *et al.*, 1986; Situnayake *et al.*, 1990). The importance of GSH homeostasis in preventing alcohol-mediated oxidative injury is supported by the observation that the depletion of liver GSH enhances lipid peroxidation and acute alcohol toxicity (Kera *et al.*, 1989; Strubelt *et al.*, 1987), while stimulation of GSH re-synthesis by treatment with *S*-adenosyl-*L*-methionine (SAM) reduces alcohol toxicity (Vendemiale *et al.*, 1989; Lieber *et al.*, 1990).

Chronic alcohol administration to rats either by the Lieber-De Carli diet or the intragastric infusion model is associated with a decrease in the liver and plasma levels of the lipid soluble antioxidant vitamin E (Bjørneboe *et al.*, 1987; Kawase *et al.*, 1989; Sadrzadeh *et al.*, 1994b; Rouach *et al.*, 1997). Such an effect involves both the α-tocopherol (20–50% decrease) and γ-tocopherol isoforms (65–75% decrease) of the vitamin (Sadrzadeh *et al.*, 1994b). The plasmatic and hepatic levels of α-tocopherol are also often reduced in patients with alcohol abuse with or without overt signs of liver disease (Tanner *et al.*, 1986; Bell *et al.*, 1992; Lecompte *et al.*, 1994; Clot *et al.*, 1994). The mechanisms responsible for the lowering in vitamin E associated with alcohol intake have not yet been completely elucidated, but an interference with the uptake of the vitamin in the gut or by the hepatocytes does not appear to play a major role (Bjørneboe *et al.*, 1987). Conversely, microsomes from ethanol-fed rats have shown a decrease in the ratio between α-tocopherol and its oxidation product, α-tocopherol quinone (Kawase *et al.*, 1989), suggesting an increased oxidation of α-tocopherol. This interpretation is consistent with the inverse correlation between the α-tocopherol and γ-tocopherol levels and the content of lipid peroxidation products observed in the liver of intragastric ethanol-fed rats (Sadrzadeh *et al.*, 1994b; Rouach *et al.*, 1997), as well as in the plasma of patients with alcoholic cirrhosis (Clot *et al.*, 1994). Although vitamin E deficient rats are more susceptible to alcohol toxicity (Sadrzadeh *et al.*, 1994b), the actual contribution of vitamin E loss to the development of alcohol liver damage is still uncertain. Rats receiving intragastric ethanol feeding supplemented with high doses of α-tocopherol acetate are not protected against liver injury (Sadrzadeh *et al.*, 1995). However, upon discontinuation of alcohol feeding, the administration of vitamin E contributes to reducing the severity of hepatic lesions (Nanji *et al.*, 1996).

A number of studies have also investigated the effect of ethanol on the enzymes involved in the detoxification of reactive oxygen species or lipid peroxidation products. The results of these studies are rather inconclusive since, while acute alcohol intoxication lowers liver catalase, superoxide dismutase and glutathione *S*-transferase activities, these effects were not constantly observed following chronic treatments (Nordmann *et al.*, 1991; Nordmann, 1994). More recent investigations using the intragastric alcohol nutrition model have shown a significant decline in either the enzymatic activity and the immunoreactive protein concentrations of liver (Cu-Zn)-superoxide dismutase, catalase and glutathione peroxidase (Rouach *et al.*, 1997; Polavarapu *et al.*, 1998). These effects were found to be inversely correlated with the extent of, respectively, lipid peroxidation or hepatic injury (Polavarapu *et al.*, 1998). Nonetheless, an induction in liver glutathione peroxidase and catalase mRNA expression has been previously observed in the same experimental model (Nanji *etal.*, 1995b). This suggests the possibility that ethanol might interfere at the post-transcriptional level with the synthesis of antioxidant enzymes or might stimulate their intracellular degradation. Ethanol-fed animals developing liver injury also showed increased protein levels of the mitochondrial manganese-containing form of superoxide dismutase, without modifications of the overall enzymatic activity (Polavarapu *etal.*, 1998). It is noteworthy, that these changes in liver antioxidant enzymes can be seen also in a pig model of ALD (Zindenberg-Cherr *etal.*, 1991). This suggests the possible relevance of impaired antioxidant enzyme activities in the development of oxidative injury during alcohol-induced liver damage.

ROLE OF OXIDATIVE INJURY IN THE PATHOGENESIS OF ALCOHOLIC LIVER DISEASE

In recent years, several studies using intragastric ethanol-fed rats have clearly demonstrated that markers of oxidative stress are positively correlated with the extent of histological liver lesions (Kamimura *etal.*, 1992; Nanji *etal.*, 1994a; Albano *etal.*, 1996; Rouach *etal.*, 1997; Polavarapu *etal.*, 1998). However, the mechanisms by which free radical reactions contribute to the pathogenesis of alcoholic liver disease are still largely unknown.

Oxidative mechanisms in ethanol-induced hepatocyte injury

Morphological and functional abnormalities of mitochondria represent one of the earliest manifestations of hepatocyte injury following chronic ethanol intoxication (Ishak *etal.*, 1991). As discussed above, in the presence of ethanol, mitochondria can represent an important source of reactive oxygen species. Moreover, they undergo a selective decrease of GSH content that makes them more susceptible to oxidative damage (Fernandez-Checa *etal.*, 1997). Indeed, GSH decrease and lipid hydroperoxide accumulation are associated with the decline of membrane potential in mitochondria of rats acutely treated with ethanol (Masini *etal.*, 1994). Mitochondrial GSH loss also precedes the development of functional alterations on these organelles during chronic ethanol feeding which can be partially prevented by restoring mitochondrial GSH by rat supplementation with SAM (Fernandez-Checa *etal.*, 1997). Mitochondria obtained from either acute or chronic alcohol-treated rats show oxidative modifications to protein and mitochondrial DNA (mtDNA) (Weiland and Lautemburg, 1995; Cahill *etal.*, 1997). Single or multiple deletions of mtDNA are also 8-fold more frequent in the liver of alcoholics as compared to age-matched controls (Mansouri *etal.*, 1997). These alterations might be responsible for the impairment of several mitochondrial enzymes as well as for the lowering of mitochondrially-encoded sub-units of the electron transport chain observed in animals exposed to ethanol (Coleman *etal.*, 1994). Recently, the formation of adducts between cytochrone c oxidase and 4-hydroxynonenal has also been reported to be responsible for the inhibition of enzyme activity in the liver of alcohol-treated animals (Chen *etal.*, 1999). Moreover, ethanol-stimulated lipid peroxidation is also linked to the impairment of mitochondrial phosphorylating capacity and with the appearance of megamitochondria (Matsuhashi *et al.*, 1998). Indeed, the daily administration of the free radical scavenger 4-hydroxy-2,2,6,6-tetramethyl-piperidine-1-oxyl (4-OH-TEMPO) improves mitochondrial function and completely prevents the formation of megamitochondria (Matsuhashi *et al.*, 1998).

Hepatic steatosis is one of the most constant consequences of alcohol intoxication (Ishak *et al.*, 1991) and the impairment of mitochondrial oxidation of fatty acids is regarded as one of the key factors in causing hepatocyte fat accumulation (Dianzani, 1991; Fromenty and Pessayre, 1995). Early work by Di Luzio has shown that rat pre-treatment with antioxidants partially prevents fatty liver caused by acute alcohol poisoning (Di Luzio, 1964). This effect might be related to the prevention of oxidative mitochondrial damage, since oxidative stress might contribute to lowering the activity of the enzymes involved in mitochondrial fatty acid β-oxidation (Fromenty and Pessayre, 1995). Moreover, by causing mutations in mtDNA, reactive oxygen species might affect the efficiency of NADH oxidation by the respiratory chain enzymes (Figure 6.2), thus contributing to metabolic imbalances responsible for hepatocyte steatosis (Fromenty and Pessayre, 1995). Supporting this view, mtDNA deletions show a very high prevalence (about 85% of the cases) in alcoholics with hepatic microvesicular steatosis (Fromenty *et al.*, 1995; Mansouri *et al.*, 1997), a lesion that is ascribed to impaired mitochondrial β-oxidation of fatty acids (Fromenty and Pessayre, 1995). However, it must be noted that oxidative damage can contribute to causing alcoholic steatosis by affecting lipoprotein secretion (Dianzani, 1991). Ethanol, in fact, interferes with lipoprotein glycosylation in the Golgi apparatus (Nanni *et al.*, 1978; Cottalasso *et al.*, 1996) possibly through the direct impairment of glycosyl-transferase activities by aldehydic products of lipid peroxidation (Marinari *et al.*, 1987) or by inducing the oxidative degradation of dolichols that act as glycosyl sugar carriers in the Golgi membrane (Cottalasso *et al.*, 1998).

The induction of oxidative stress within the liver is often associated with the permeability transition of mitochondria, the inhibition of protein synthesis, the derangement of the cytoskeleton and with alterations in hepatocyte ion homeostasis (Rosser and Gores, 1995). The role of oxidative stress in causing ethanol-induced hepatic cell death is suggested by a recent study using a human hepatoblastoma cell line (HepG2) transfected with the human CYP 2E1 gene. Ethanol cytotoxicity, in fact, can be observed only in the cells expressing CYP 2E1 gene, but not in those infected with the retrovirus lacking CYP 2E1 cDNA. CYP 2E1 inhibitors, antioxidants (Vitamin E, Trolox C, diphenylphenilen-diamine and *N*-acetylcysteine), oxygen radical scavengers (thiourea, uric acid) and superoxide dismutase or catalase reduce the killing of CYP 2E1-transfected HepG2 cells receiving ethanol (Wu and Cederbaum, 1996). Kurose and coworkers (1997a) have observed that following ethanol treatment, a 50% decrease in the mitochondrial membrane potential does not result in an appreciable cytotoxicity in cultured rat hepatocytes or isolated perfused livers. However, hepatocyte death is instead appreciable when extensive mitochondrial damage is promoted by the combined treatment with ethanol and the GSH-depleting agent diethylmaleate (Kurose *et al.*, 1997a). Thus, oxidative mitochondrial damage may well play a role in the development of ethanol-mediated hepatotoxicity (Rosser and Gores, 1995) (Figure 6.2). Nonetheless, even when ethanol-induced mitochondrial damage is not so extensive to be the primary

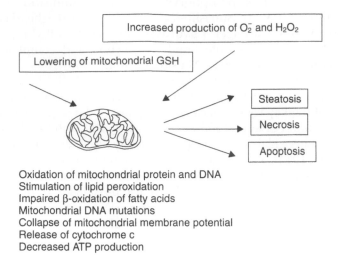

Oxidation of mitochondrial protein and DNA
Stimulation of lipid peroxidation
Impaired β-oxidation of fatty acids
Mitochondrial DNA mutations
Collapse of mitochondrial membrane potential
Release of cytochrome c
Decreased ATP production

Figure 6.2 Possible involvement of oxidative injury of mitochondria in the development of hepatocyte injury during ALD. The impairment of mitochondrial fatty acids oxidation is regarded as one of the key factors in causing hepatocyte fat accumulation. Oxidative mitochondrial damage might affect the activity of the enzymes involved in mitochondrial fatty acid β-oxidation. Moreover, by causing mutations in mtDNA, reactive oxygen species might reduce the efficiency NADH oxidation by the respiratory chain enzymes, thus contributing to the metabolic unbalances responsible for hepatocyte steatosis. Oxidative mitochondrial damage is associated with the decline of mitochondrial membrane potential, the lowering in ATP production, and the permeability transition of inner mitochondrial membranes. All these alterations can be regarded as possible cause for hepatocyte killing during ALD. It has also been shown that oxidative mitochondrial damage, by releasing cytochrome c and other intramitochondrial proteins, can trigger liver cell apoptosis. On the other hand, oxidative modifications of mitochondrial proteins and mutations of mtDNA resulting from oxidative attack are likely responsible for the decrease in the activity of several mitochondrial enzymes and for the depression in the levels of mitochondrially-encoded sub-units of the electron transport chain observed in animals exposed to ethanol. These events can affect ATP production and lead to a premature ageing of mitochondria that respond less efficiently to ethanol-induced centrilobular hypoxia.

cause of cell death, the impairment of ATP production, might enhance the liver cells susceptibility to alcohol-induced centrilobular hypoxia (Ji *et al.*, 1982) (Figure 6.2).

In recent years, increasing interest has been devoted to the occurrence of cell death by apoptosis in several hepatobiliary diseases (Patel and Gores, 1995; Galle, 1997). The use of immunofluorescence techniques has revealed that chronic alcohol feeding of rats, mice and pigs is associated with the detection of an increased number of apoptotic bodies within the liver (Goldin *et al.*, 1993; Svegliati-Baroni *et al.*, 1994; Halsted *et al.*, 1996). Moreover, evidence for the expression of apoptosis-related Lewis antigen in association with the presence of Mallory bodies has been reported in hepatic biopsies from patients with alcoholic hepatitis (Kawahara *et al.*, 1994). Several mechanisms might account for the stimulation of apoptotic hepatocyte death during alcoholic liver disease and include the action of TGF-β, TNF-α and

TNF-related proteins, the activation of CD95 (APO-1/Fas) receptor and the induction of cell-mediated immunotoxic reactions (Patel and Gores, 1995; Galle, 1997). However, it is now apparent that, under certain conditions, cell exposure to low level of oxidants might also induce apoptosis (Buttke and Sanderstrom, 1994; Slater *et al.*, 1995). Following intragastric ethanol feeding, a significant increase in apoptotic hepatocytes has been detected in association with lipid peroxidation in the liver of rats receiving corn oil or fish oil, but not in those receiving ethanol and saturated fat (Yacoub *et al.*, 1995). Moreover, Kurose and colleagues (1997b) have reported that cultured hepatocytes exposed *in vitro* to ethanol undergo apoptotic changes in association with the formation of reactive oxygen species. Cell killing by apoptosis has also been observed in CYP 2E1-transfected HepG2 cell incubated with ethanol in association with an increased activity of caspase 1 and 3 (Wu and Cederbaum, 1999). The ethanol effect in these cells can be prevented by antioxidants and by the over-expression of anti-apoptotic protein Bcl-2 (Wu and Cederbaum, 1999). Although these observations indicate that ethanol-induced oxidative stress might cause liver cell apoptosis, the mechanisms involved have not yet been elucidated. Increasing evidence obtained with different experimental systems suggests that stimulation of oxygen radical formation within the mitochondria triggers the release of cytochrome c and of apoptosis inducing factor (AIF), probably by inducing mitochondria permeability transition (Green and Kroemer, 1998). The release in the cytosol of cytochrome c and AIF can then activate caspases 9 and 3 that are responsible for the progression of the apoptotic programme (Green and Kroemer, 1998). The release of cytochrome c from the mitochondrial matrix is prevented by the over-expression of anti-apoptotic protein Bcl-2 (Kroemer, 1997). An increase in Bcl-2 has been reported in the liver of intragastric ethanol-fed rats with a good correlation with lipid peroxidation, but it was mainly localized in bile duct epithelial cells and in infiltrating inflammatory cells (Yacoub *et al.*, 1995).

Recent studies have implicated increased secretion of cytotoxic cytokines (TNF-α, IL-1) by Kupffer cells as mediators of hepatocyte injury by alcohol (Thurman, 1998). Indeed, rats receiving intragastric alcohol feeding are protected against liver damage by antibodies to TNF-α (Iimuro *et al.*, 1997). Many cell types, including hepatocytes, are, however, resistant to TNF-α pro-apoptotic action in relation to the activation of a specific signaling pathway that involves both nuclear factor kB (NFkB) dependent and independent gene transcription (Van Antwerp *et al.*, 1998; Natoli *et al.*, 1998). Colell and coworkers (1998) have reported that hepatocytes obtained from chronically ethanol-fed rats which develop a selective deficiency of mitochondrial GSH, undergo cell death by necrosis following TNF-α addition, despite NFkB activation. The susceptibility to TNF-α can be reproduced in control hepatocytes by selectively depleting mitochondrial GSH pool with 3-hydroxyl-4-pentanoate, while restoration of mitochondrial GSH with SAM or glutathione-ethyl ester prevents TNF-α killing of hepatocytes from ethanol-treated rats (Colell *et al.*, 1998). Cytosolic GSH depletion has also been shown to increase TNF-α-induced apoptosis in rat and mouse hepatocytes primed to respond to the cytokine by protein synthesis inhibition with actinomycin D or galactosamine (Xu *et al.*, 1998b). These observations suggest the possibility that modulation of hepatocyte resistance to TNF-α might represent an additional mechanism by which oxidative stress induced by ethanol can contribute to alcohol liver damage.

Oxidative mechanisms in the onset of alcohol-induced liver fibrosis

Liver fibrosis and cirrhosis represent the terminal stage of ALD and one of the main causes of death among patients with alcohol abuse. Research performed in recent years has given new insight into the mechanisms responsible for liver fibrosis, showing that hepatic stellate cells (perisinusoidal fat-storing cells or Ito cells) are the main connective tissue producing cells in the liver. Under the influence of inflammatory stimuli stellate cells become activated and transform to myofibroblast-like cells producing collagen and extracellular matrix components (Gressner, 1991; Lissoos *et al.*, 1992). The activation and the transformation of hepatic stellate cells are mediated by paracrine and autocrine stimuli that mainly involve transforming growth factor β1 (TGF-β1) and platelet-derived growth factor (PDGF) (Gressner, 1991; Lissoos *et al.*, 1992).

As recently pointed out by Poli and Parola (1996), events associated with oxidative stress are involved in the evolution of fibrotic processes consequent to chronic inflammatory lung diseases and atherosclerosis as well as in the stimulation of experimental liver fibrosis induced by iron or copper overload, by chronic cholestasis and by long-term CCl_4 administration to animals. In all these conditions, intracellular redox changes in tissue macrophages have been shown to activate nuclear factor kB (NFkB) and activator protein-1 (AP-1), triggering the transcriptional up-regulation of the genes' encoding for pro-inflammatory or fibrogenetic cytokines, such as granulocyte-macrophage colony stimulation factor (GM-CSF), tumor necrosis factor-β (TNF-β), interleukin-6 (IL-6) and TGF-β1. The increased secretion of these cytokines is then responsible for the stimulation of matrix producing cells (Poli and Parola, 1996) (Figure 6.3). Apart from these mechanisms, recent studies in cultured human and rat hepatic stellate cells have shown that MDA and 4-HNE derived from lipid peroxidation are able to stimulate collagen type 1 production by activating gene transcription (Poli and Parola, 1996). The mechanisms responsible for 4-HNE stimulation of procollagen gene expression involve the binding of 4-HNE to the 46 kD and 54 kD isoforms of c-Jun terminal kinase and the subsequent activation and translocation of these proteins into the nucleus where they induce AP-1 activation (Parola *et al.*, 1998).

Despite the difficulties in reproducing alcoholic fibrosis in experimental models, several studies have shown that the biochemical and immunohistochemical detection of MDA and 4-HNE in the liver of intragastric alcohol-fed rats or alcohol-fed mini-pigs precedes the appearance of the initial signs of hepatic fibrosis (Kamimura *et al.*, 1992; Kaminura and Tsukamoto, 1995; Niemelä *et al.*, 1995). Using intragastric alcohol-fed rats, Kaminura and Tsukamoto (1995) have also observed that stimulation of lipid peroxidation is associated with a marked induction of TNF-α, IL-6 and TGF-β1 production by Kupffer cells. Moreover, the same group has reported that the dietary supplementation with carbonyl iron greatly stimulates alcoholic fibrosis and that this effect is closely associated with the promotion of MDA and 4-HNE formation and with an increase in the levels of TGF-β1 and procollagen-α-1 mRNA in the whole liver and in freshly isolated hepatic stellate cells (Tsukamoto *et al.*, 1995). On the other hand, inhibition of CYP 2E1 induction by rat treatment with chlormethiazole is able to reduce ethanol-stimulated liver TNF-α, IL-1β and

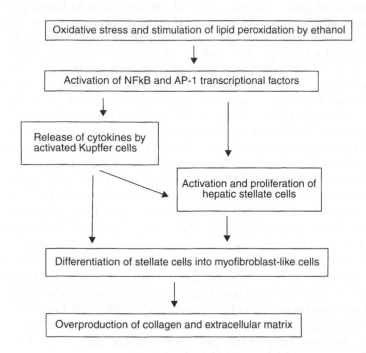

Figure 6.3 Proposed mechanisms involved in the stimulation of fibrogenesis by ethanol-induced oxidative injury. Changes in the intracellular redox equilibrium in Kupffer cells or in macrophages infiltrating the liver can induce the activation of nuclear factor kB (NFkB) and activator protein-1 (AP-1) leading to the transcriptional up-regulation of gene encoding for pro-inflammatory or fibrogenetic cytokines such as granulocyte-macrophage colony stimulation factor (GM-CSF), tumor necrosis factor-β (TNF-β), interleukin-6 (IL-6) and TGF-β1, that on their term, cause the stimulation of matrix producing hepatic stellate cells. Furthermore, MDA and 4-HNE derived from lipid peroxidation, by directly inducing AP-1 activation in hepatic stellate cells, are able to directly stimulate the gene transcription and the protein synthesis of procollagene type 1.

TGF-β1 expression (Fang *et al.*, 1998). Alcohol-induced liver fibrosis, TNF-α and cyclooxygenase-2 mRNA expression can also be reversed after ethanol discontinuation by feeding rats with medium-chain triglycerides that also lower lipid peroxidation (Nanji *et al.*, 1997a). These data are far from conclusive, but the hypothesis that ethanol-induced oxidative stress might contribute to the stimulation of liver fibrogenesis is very attractive.

Free radical mechanisms in immune reactions associated with alcoholic liver disease

Alcoholic liver disease is often associated with immune reactions involving lymphocyte-mediated reactions to alcoholic hyalin or to autologous human hepatocytes as well as with the presence of circulating antibodies directed against hepatocytes from ethanol-treated animals (Paronetto, 1993). These immunological reactions have been ascribed to the formation of new antigens as a result of acetaldehyde binding to proteins (Nicholls *et al.*, 1992). Either experimental animals exposed to alcohol (Israel *et al.*, 1986) or alcoholic patients display, in fact, high titers of immunoglobulins reacting with acetaldehyde–protein adducts (Koskinas *et al.*, 1992; Teare *et al.*, 1993; Viitala *et al.*, 1997). However, the antibody response towards acetaldehyde adducts can not completely explain the immuno-allergic reactions associated with alcoholic liver disease, since anti-acetaldehyde antibodies can also be found in patients with liver diseases unrelated to alcohol (Worrall *et al.*, 1990).

Moncada and coworkers (1994) have demonstrated that proteins alkylated by hydroxyethyl radicals became immunogenic and lead to the formation of antibodies that specifically recognize hydroxyethyl radical epitopes. Similar antibodies have been detected in rats chronically fed with ethanol (Albano *et al.*, 1996). The sera of patients with ALD, but not those from patients with non-alcoholic liver diseases, also contain both IgG and IgA specifically recognizing proteins modified by hydroxyethyl radicals (Clot *et al.*, 1995). In alcohol-fed rats, the presence of anti-hydroxyethyl radical antibodies shows a strict correlation with hydroxyethyl free radical production and CYP 2E1 activity (Albano *et al.*, 1996). A similar relationship has also been detected in alcoholic patients since heavy drinkers who did not display CYP 2E1 induction by the chlorzoxasone oxidation test (Lucas *et al.*, 1996) have levels of anti-hydroxyethyl radical IgG similar to those of abstainers and significantly lower than those of drinkers with normally induced CYP 2E1 activity (Dupont *et al.*, 1998).

Experiments using immunofluorescence and laser confocal microscopy have demonstrated that human anti-hydroxyethyl radical IgG reacts with epitopes present in the outer edge of the plasma membrane of intact hepatocytes incubated *in vitro* with ethanol (Clot *et al.*, 1997). Three main protein bands, one of which corresponds to CYP 2E1 can be shown by Western blot analysis in the plasma membranes from ethanol-treated hepatocytes (Clot *et al.*, 1997). The presence of CYP 2E1-hydroxyethyl radical adducts on hepatocyte plasma membranes has also been confirmed by the co-localization of the immunofluorescence staining due to anti-hydroxyethyl radical antibodies and anti-CYP 2E1 IgG (Clot *et al.*, 1997). Circulating antibodies recognizing, respectively, trifluoroacetyl-CYP 2E1 and tienilic acid-CYP 2C11 adducts on hepatocyte surface have been detected in the sera of patients suffering from halothane- or tienilic acid-induced hepatitis (Elliasson and Kenna, 1996; Robin *et al.*, 1996) and are thought to be critical for the development of immuno-mediated hepatotoxicity (van Pelt *et al.*, 1995; Manns and Obermayer-Straub, 1997). We have similarly observed that isolated rat hepatocytes exposed *in vitro* to ethanol are killed by antibody-dependent cell-mediated cytotoxicity (ADCC) upon the addition of the sera from ALD patients and normal human blood mononuclear cells (Clot *et al.*, 1997). Thus, during alcohol abuse, the development of immuno-toxic reaction towards hydroxyethyl radical-derived antigens might contribute to liver damage (Figure 6.4). Indeed, a clinical survey among alcoholic patients has associated the presence of antibodies toward alcohol-modified hepatocytes with an increased risk of developing liver cirrhosis (Takase *et al.*, 1993).

Oxidative protein modification due to direct free radical attack or reaction with lipid peroxidation products has been detected in the liver of intragastric alcohol-fed rats and is associated with a reduced cytosolic proteolysis by proteasome activity (Rouach *et al.*, 1997; Fataccioli *et al.*, 1999). The possibility that these oxidatively

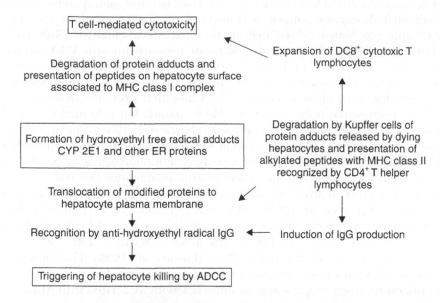

Figure 6.4 Possible role of hydroxyethyl free radicals in causing immunotoxic reactions during ALD. Hydroxyethyl free radicals formed during CYP 2EI-mediated ethanol oxidation covalent bind to CYP 2EI and other proteins of the hepatocyte endoplasmic reticulum. Following hepatocyte death, the degradation of alkylated proteins by endothelial and Kupffer cells or by other phagocytes can lead to the presentation of modified peptides in association with the major histocompatibility complex (MHC) class II molecules to CD4[+] helper T lymphocytes. The activation of CD4[+] lymphocyte may provide help for further events involving either cytotoxic CD8[+] T lymphocytes or immature B lymphocytes clones. The presence of hydroxyethyl radical-modified proteins on the plasma membranes of hepatocytes can, in fact, stimulate B cells recognizing this epitope to differentiate to plasmocytes secreting anti-hydroxyethyl radical antibodies. The reaction of anti-hydroxyethyl radical IgG with CYP 2EI and other modified proteins on the hepatocyte surface then results in antibody-mediated cell-depended cytotoxic reactions involving hepatocyte killing by macrophages and NK cells. Alternatively, intracellular degradation of hydroxyethyl radical modified proteins may lead to the presentation of alkylated peptides on the hepatocyte surface in association with MHC class I proteins. The recognition as non-self of these peptides by cytotoxic CD8[+] T lymphocytes in association with the help of stimulated CD4[+] cells leads to the clonal expansion of T lymphocytes that will be then became capable to kill all hepatocytes expressing hydroxyethyl modified peptides.

modified proteins might became immunogenic has been recently confirmed by the observation that either chronic alcohol-fed rats and alcoholic patients develop antibodies recognizing protein-MDA adducts (Albano *et al.*, 1996; Dupont *et al.*, 1998). Tuma and Thiele have also demonstrated that MDA and acetaldehyde react together with ε-amino group of lysine residues in proteins to form a group of compounds named malonildialdehyde-acetaldehyde (MAA) adducts (Tuma *et al.*, 1996; Xu *et al.*, 1997). MAA adducts have been detected in livers of ethanol-fed rats (Tuma *et al.*, 1996) and their presence is associated with the development of circulating anti-MAA antibodies in alcohol-treated rats (Xu *et al.*, 1998a). IgG recognizing MAA-modified proteins are also significantly increased in ALD patients (Rolla *et al.*,

2000). The human anti-MAA antibodies are unrelated to those against acetaldehyde-
or malondialdehyde-derived antigens and mainly recognized a specific, cyclic MAA
epitope identified as 4-methyl-1,4-dihydropyridine-2,5-dicarbaldehyde (Rolla *et al.*,
1999). The interest in the detection of an immune response towards MAA adducts
in ALD patients is not limited to the possibility that these antibodies might promote
hepatotoxic reactions by targeting specific epitopes on liver cells. Recent evidence
demonstrates that mice immunized with MAA-modified proteins produce antibodies that recognize not only the specific MAA epitope, but also immunological
determinants on the unmodified carrier proteins (Thiele *et al.*, 1998). Similar findings
have also been obtained in ethanol-fed rats in which the development of antibodies
vs. MAA antigens is associated with an increased immunoreactivity towards self
epitopes in hepatic cytosol, microsomes and plasma membranes (Xu *et al.*, 1998a).
Autoimmune reactions to liver cell antigens have been repeatedly reported in
patients with ALD (Paronetto, 1993) and shown to involve an as yet unidentified
plasma membrane lipoprotein, (Perperas *et al.*, 1981) as well as 65 kD heath shock
protein (Winrow *et al.*, 1994), alcohol dehydrogenase (Ma *et al.*, 1997) and cytochrome P450 isoenzymes CYP2E1 and CYP3A4 (Litton *et al.*, 1999). Thus, it is possible that also in humans MAA antigens might act as a stimulus for the breaking of
immuno-tolerance, triggering the autoimmune reactions associated with ALD.

POSSIBLE USE OF ANTIOXIDANTS IN THE PHARMACOLOGICAL APPROACH TO ALCOHOLIC LIVER DISEASE

The use of antioxidants has been proposed in the therapy of a number of diseases
involving free radical mechanisms (Maxwell, 1995). In spite of the increasing evidence about the implication of free radicals in the development of liver injury by
alcohol, relatively few studies have investigated a possible therapeutical use of
antioxidants in ALD.

On the basis of the data concerning the effects of ethanol on hepatocellular
antioxidant defences, the most likely candidates for testing a possible use of antioxidants in ALD therapy would be α-tocopherol and GSH-precursors. Supplementation
with α-tocopherol is able to reduce liver fibrosis induced by CCl_4 or iron overload
(Parola *et al.*, 1992; Pietrangelo *et al.*, 1995a) and to inhibit collagen α1 (I) gene
expression in control animals (Chojkier *et al.*, 1998). The treatment with α-tocopherol
has also been successfully tested in the prevention of hepatic stellate cell activation
in chronic hepatitis C (Houglum *et al.*, 1997). However, dietary supplementation
with high doses of α-tocopherol acetate does not ameliorate liver damage in intragastric alcohol-fed rats (Sadrazadeh *et al.*, 1995). This observation is not surprising
since *in vitro* the addition of α-tocopherol acetate also fails to prevent oxidative injury
in isolated hepatocytes (Farris, 1990), suggesting that, in this form, α-tocopherol is
probably not active as an antioxidant in rodents. Thus, further experiments using
different formulations of α-tocopherol are required before drawing definitive conclusions on the possible use of vitamin E supplements in the prevention of ALD.

Better results have been obtained by modulating GSH homeostasis with SAM. The
increase in hepatic GSH and the normalization of serum transaminases can be

observed following the administration of SAM to either ALD patients (Vendemiale *et al.*, 1989) or alcohol-fed babbons (Lieber *et al.*, 1990). The recovery of hepatic GSH levels following SAM administration may occur because SAM is both a precursor of homocysteine and an activator cystathionine synthetase, a key enzyme in cysteine synthesis (Israel *et al.*, 1991). The importance of SAM in maintaining liver GSH homeostasis during chronic alcohol exposure is also suggested by the observation that hepatic *S*-adenosyl-methionine synthetase activity is severely depressed in alcoholic cirrhotics (Duce *et al.*, 1988). Furthermore, SAM, but not *N*-acetylcysteine, appears especially effective in preserving the mitochondrial GSH pool. SAM-supplemented ethanol-fed rats display 40–50% more mitochondrial GSH than non-supplemented animals and this effect is accompanied by the preservation of mitochondrial function (Fernandez-Checa *et al.*, 1997). The action of SAM on mitochrondrial GSH is related to the maintenance of mitochondrial membrane fluidity that critically influences the activity of the GSH transporter in the inner mitochondrial membrane (Colell *et al.*, 1997). It is possible that the capacity of SAM to act as a donor of methyl groups in the synthesis of phosphatidylcholine from phoshatidylethanolamine might influence liver membrane fluidity (Hirata *et al.*, 1978). In this later respect, it is interesting to note that dietary phosphatidylcholine supplementation is able to lower lipid peroxidation and to prevent the development of liver fibrosis and cirrhosis in alcohol-fed baboons (Lieber *et al.*, 1994, 1997). The beneficial effect of SAM in the treatment of ALD has recently been investigated by a 2 year randomized placebo-controlled double-blind clinical study carried out on 123 patients, that has demonstrated an improved survival or delayed liver trans-plantation in patients with alcoholic liver cirrhosis receiving SAM, especially in those with less advanced liver disease (Mato *et al.*, 1999).

A successful use of antioxidants in the prevention of alcoholic liver damage has been recently reported by Sadrzadeh and Nanji (1998) by using 21-aminosteroid-16-desmethyl-tirilazad mesylate (U74389), a member of the 21-aminosteroid (lazaroids) compound family. Lazaroids are a group of non-glucocorticoid amino-steroids that are effective in the therapy of acute injury of the central nervous system (Hall *et al.*, 1994). The beneficial effects of lazaroids have been ascribed to their antioxidant and free radical scavenging capability (Hall *et al.*, 1994). In intragastric alcohol-fed rats, daily administration of tirilazad mesylate greatly reduced MDA and 8-isoprostane formation and completely prevented the development of necro-inflammatory changes, without affecting liver steatosis (Sadrzadeh and Nanji, 1998). Considering the still limited number of effective antioxidant drugs available for human therapy, these results open a potential new area for clinical testing in ALD.

Among other antioxidants that have been proposed for use in ALD, flavonoids derived from silymarin might deserve some attention. Silymarin is a standardized extract of the milk thistle, *Silybum Marianum*, that has been shown to prevent etha-nol-induced lipid peroxidation (Valenzuela *et al.*, 1985) and to retard collagen accumulation in an experimental model of biliary fibrosis (Boigk *et al.*, 1997). In an early double blind randomized clinical trial, silymarim significantly reduced the mortality by alcoholic cirrhosis (Ferenci *et al.*, 1989). However, these results have not been confirmed by more recent investigations (Parés *et al.*, 1998). Silybin is the main constituent (about 60%) of silymarin and also exhibits hepatoprotective activity connected with the antioxidant proprieties (Valenzuela and Guerra, 1985;

Pietrangelo *et al.*, 1995b). The poor enteral absorption of silybin has recently been overcome by complexation with phosphatidylcholine (Morazzoni *et al.*, 1993) and the silybin-phosphatidylcholine complex (Silipide) displays antioxidant activity and prevents cytotoxicity induced by oxidative stress when administered orally to rats (Carini *et al.*, 1992). Interestingly, *in vivo* rat pre-treatment with Silipide decreases the spin trapping of hydroxyethyl radicals in either microsomal preparations *in vitro* or the whole liver *in vivo* (Comoglio *et al.*, 1995). Other constituents of silymarin have been investigated recently and among them silibinin has been shown to inhibit leukotriene formation by Kupffer cells (Dehmlow *et al.*, 1996). Thus, silymarin-derived flavonoids are compounds of potential interest for further trials in ALD treatment.

The antithyroid drug propylthiouracyl (PTU) has been proposed for the treatment of ALD on the basis of the hepatoprotective properties observed in animal experimental systems (Israel *et al.*, 1975) and the results of clinical studies demonstrating a 50–60% reduction in the mortality rates from ALD (Orrego *et al.*, 1987, 1994). The beneficial effects of PTU have been ascribed to the suppression of the increase in hepatic oxygen consumption induced by ethanol and in the amelioration of liver blood flow (Carmichael *et al.*, 1993; Rojter *et al.*, 1995). However, the lack of a better understanding in the biochemical mechanisms of PTU action has so far limited its clinical use. In chemical systems PTU displays strong hydroxyl radical scavenging and antioxidant actions (Hicks *et al.*, 1992). Another effect of PTU that has been recently unravelled concerns the selective inhibition of hypochlorous acid (HOCl) generation by granulocyte myeloperoxidase (Ross *et al.*, 1998). Hypochlorous acid is an highly oxidizing species produced during the oxidative burst of phagocytes that contributes along with reactive oxygen species and NO to tissue damage during inflammation (Smith *et al.*, 1994). Since Kupffer cell activation and neutrophil infiltration are common in ALD, and particularly in alcoholic hepatitis, it is possible that the inhibition of HOCl generation and the antioxidant action of PTU might have a relevant role in the therapeutic action of this drug.

A further reason for interest in the use of antioxidants in the therapy of ALD comes from recent observations about the role of cellular redox equilibrium in the signal transduction and in the modulation of gene expression in many cell types (Sen and Packer, 1997; Dalton *et al.*, 1999). Modifications of intracellular thiol redox state and oxidative stress activate gene expression by influencing NFκB and AP-1 functions (Sen and Packer, 1997; Dalton *et al.*, 1999). Conversely, liposoluble antioxidants such as vitamin E, α-lipoate and butylhydroxyanisole down-regulate NFkB activation induced by a wide range of stimuli (Sen and Packer, 1997). On this basis, it is possible that antioxidants might favourably modulate cytokine and growth factor gene expression in liver non-parenchymal cells and reduce inflammatory cell activation. Indeed, it has been reported that rat supplementation with vitamin E down-regulates liver TGF-β1 gene expression (Parola *et al.*, 1992), while the *in vitro* addition of *N*-acetylcysteine and α-tocopherol to Kupffer cells reverses endotoxin-induced stimulation of cytokine production (Fox *et al.*, 1997). Moreover, stimulation of lipid peroxidation during experimental alcoholic liver injury is associated with an up-regulation of TNF-α and cyclooxygenase-2 (COX-2) gene expression (Nanji *et al.*, 1997b) that can be reversed by treatments affecting ethanol-induced peroxidative damage (Nanji *et al.*, 1997a; Sadrzadeh and Nanji, 1998).

CONCLUSION

The presence of free radical-mediated oxidative damage following the exposure to alcohol has been demonstrated by a large number of experimental and clinical studies. The depletion of antioxidants and the production of reactive oxygen species by several enzymatic sources and by activated phagocytes might account for the oxidative stress associated to ethanol intoxication. Oxidative modification of cellular components and stimulation of lipid peroxidation are likely to represent the mechanisms by which free radical-mediated reactions can cause hepatocyte death. Immunological reactions against hepatic proteins modified by the reaction with hydroxyethyl radical or lipid oxidation products can be regarded as a possible additional mechanism in the pathogenesis of alcoholic liver injury. Moreover, by modulating gene expression, oxidative events might contribute to the development of hepatic fibrosis. On this basis, the possible application of antioxidant drugs in the therapeutical approach to ALD can be proposed.

REFERENCES

Abbondanza, A., Battelli, M.G., Soffritti, M. and Cessi, C. (1989) Xanthine oxidase status in ethanol-intoxicated rat liver. *Alcohol Clin Exp Res* **13**, 841–844.

Adachi, Y., Moore, L., Bradford, B.U., Gao, W. and Thurman, R.G. (1995) Antibiotics prevent liver injury in rats following long-term exposure to ethanol. *Gastroenterol* **108**, 218–224.

Adams, D.H. (1994) Leucocyte adhesion molecules and alcoholic liver disease. *Alcohol Alcoholism* **29**, 249–260.

Albano, E., Tomasi, A., Goria-Gatti, L., Poli, G., Vannini, V. and Dianzani, M.U. (1987) Free radical metabolism of alcohols in rat liver microsomes. *Free Rad Res Communs* **3**, 243–249.

Albano, E., Tomasi, A., Goria-Gatti, L. and Dianzani, M.U. (1988) Spin trapping of free radical species produced during the microsomal metabolism of ethanol. *Chem Biol Inter* **65**, 223–234.

Albano, E., Ingelman-Sundberg, M., Tomasi, A. and Poli, G. (1991a) Free radical mediated reactions and ethanol toxicity: some considerations on the methodological approaches. In *Alcoholism: A Molecular Perspective*, edited by T.N. Palmer, pp. 45–55. New York: Plenum Press.

Albano, E., Tomasi, A., Goria-Gatti, L., Persson, J.O., Terelius, Y., Ingelman-Sundberg, M. and Dianzani, M.U. (1991b) Role of ethanol-inducible cytochrome P-450 (P450IIE1) in catalysing the free radical activation of aliphatic alcohols. *Biochem Pharmacol* **41**, 1895–1902.

Albano, E., Parola, M., Comoglio, A. and Dianzani, M.U. (1993) Evidence for the covalent binding of hydroxyethyl radicals to rat liver microsomal proteins. *Alcohol Alcohol* **28**, 453–459.

Albano, E., Tomasi, A. and Ingelman-Sundberg, M. (1994a) Spin trapping of alcohol-derived radicals in microsomes and recostituted systems by electron spin resonance. *Meth Enzymol* **233**, 117–127.

Albano, E., Clot, P., Comoglio, A., Dianzani, M.U. and Tomasi, A. (1994b) Free radical activation of acetaldehyde and its role in protein alkylation. *FEBS Lett* **384**, 65–70.

Albano, E., Clot, P., Morimoto, M., Tomasi, A., Ingelman-Sundberg, M. and French, S.W. (1996) Role of cytochrome P4502E1-dependent formation of hydroxyethyl free radicals in the development of liver damage in rats intragastrically fed with ethanol. *Hepatol* **23**, 155–163.

Aleynik, S.I., Leo, M.A., Aleynik, M.K. and Lieber, C.S. (1998) Increased circulating products of lipid peroxidation in patients with alcoholic liver disease. *Alcohol Clin Exp Res* **22**, 192–196.

Anni, H. and Israel, Y. (1999) Characterisation of adducts of ethanol metabolites with cytochrome c. *Alcohol Clin Exp Res* **23**, 26–37.

Aust, S.D., Morehouse, L.A. and Thomas, C.E. (1985) Role of metals in oxygen radical reactions. *J Free Rad Biol Med* **1**, 3–25.

Baldi, E., Burra, P., Plebani, M. and Salvagnini, M. (1993) Serum malondialdehyde and mitochondrial aspartate amino transferase activity as markers of chronic alcohol intake and alcoholic liver disease. *J Gastroenterol* **25**, 429–432.

Bautista, A. (1997) Chronic alcohol intoxication induces hepatic injury through enhanced macrophage inflammatory protein-2 production and intracellular adesion molecule-1 expression in the liver. *Hepatol* **25**, 335–342.

Bautista, A.P., D'Souza, N.B., Lang, C.H. and Spitzer, J.J. (1992) Modulation of f-met-leu-phe-induced chemotactic activity and superoxide production by neutrophils during chronic ethanol intoxication. *Alcoholism Clin Exp Res* **16**, 788–794.

Bautista, A.P. and Spitzer, J.J. (1992) Ethanol intoxication stimulates superoxide anion production by *in situ* perfused rat liver. *Hepatol* **15**, 892–898.

Bautista, A.P. and Spitzer, J.J. (1994) Inhibition of nitric oxide formation *in vivo* enhances superoxide release by the perfused liver. *Am J Physiol* **266**, G783–G788.

Bautista, A.P. and Spitzer, J.J. (1996) Postbinge effects of acute alcohol intoxication on hepatic free radical formation. *Alcoholism Clin Exp Res* **20**, 502–509.

Beckman, J.S. and Koppenol, W.H. (1996) Nitric oxide, superoxide and peroxynitrite: the good, the bad and the ugly. *Am J Physiol* **271**, C1424–C1437.

Bell, H., Bjørneboe, A., Eidsvoll, B., Norum, K.R., Raknerud, N., Try, K., Thomassen, Y. and Drevon, A.C. (1992) Reduced concentration of hepatic α-tocopherol in patients with alcoholic liver cirrhosis. *Alcohol Alcohol* **27**, 39–46.

Bjørneboe, G.-E.Aa., Bjørneboe, A., Hagen B.F., Mørland, J. and Drevon C.A. (1987) Reduced hepatic α-tocopherol content after long-term administration of ethanol to rats. *Biochem Biophys Res Communs* **918**, 236–241.

Bode, C., Kugler, V. and Bode, J.C. (1987) Endotoxemia in patients with alcoholic and non-alcoholic cirrhosis and in subjects with no evidence of chronic liver disease following acute alcohol excess. *J Hepatol* **4**, 8–14.

Boigk, G., Stroedter, L., Herbst, H., Waldschmidt, J., Rienken, E.O. and Schuppan, D. (1997) Silymarin retards collagen accumulation in early and advanced biliary fibrosis secondary to complete bile duct obliteration in rats. *Hepatol* **26**, 643–649.

Buttke, T.M. and Sandstrom, P.A. (1994) Oxidative stress as a mediator of apoptosis. *Immunol Today* **15**, 7–10.

Cahill, A., Wang, X. and Hoek, J.B. (1997) Increased oxidative damage to mitochondrial DNA following chronic ethanol consumption. *Biochim Biophys Res Commun* **235**, 286–290.

Cairo, G., Castrusini, E., Minotti, G. and Bernelli-Zazzera A. (1996) Superoxide and hydrogen peroxide-dependent inhibition of iron regulatory protein activity: a protective stratagem against oxidative injury. *FASEB J* **10**, 1326–1335.

Carini, R., Comoglio, A., Albano, E. and Poli, G. (1992) Lipid peroxidation and irreversible damage in the rat hepatocyte model: protection by the silybin-phospholipid complex IdB 1016. *Biochem Pharmacol* **43**, 2111–2115.

Carmichael, F.J., Orrego, H., Saldivia, V. and Israel, Y. (1993) Effect of propylthiouracil on the ethanol-induced increase in liver oxygen consumption in awake rats. *Hepatol* **18**, 415–421.

Cederbaum, A.I. (1989) Oxygen radical generation by microsomes: Role of iron and implications for alcohol metabolism and toxicity. *Free Rad Biol Med* **7**, 559–562.

Chamulitrat, W. and Spitzer, J.J. (1996) Nitric oxide and liver injury in alcohol-fed rats after lipopolysaccaride administration. *Alcohol Clin Exp Res* **20**, 1065–1070.

Chamulitrat, W., Carnal, J., Reed, N.M. and Spitzer, J.J. (1998) *In vivo* endotoxin enhances biliary ethanol-dependent free radical generation. *Am J Physiol* **274**, G653–G661.

Chapman, R.W., Morgan, M.J., Bell, R. and Sherlock, S. (1983) Hepatic iron uptake in alcoholic liver disease. *Gastroenterol* **84**, 143–148.

Chen, J., Robinson, N.C., Schenker, S., Frosto, T.A. and Henderson G.I. (1999) Formation of 4-hydroxynonenal adducts with cytochrome c oxidase in rats following short-term ethanol intake. *Hepatol* **29**, 1792–1798.

Chojkier, M., Houglum, K., Lee, K.S. and Buck, M. (1998) Long- and short-term D-α-tocopherol supplementation inhibits liver collagen α1(I) gene expression. *Am J Physiol* **275**, G1480–G1485.

Clot, P., Tabone, M., Aricò, S. and Albano, E. (1994) Monitoring oxidative damage in patients with liver cirrhosis and different daily alcohol intake. *Gut* **35**, 1637–1643.

Clot, P., Bellomo, G., Tabone, M., Aricò S. and Albano E. (1995) Detection of antibodies against proteins modified by hydroxyethyl free radicals in patients with alcoholic cirrhosis. *Gastroentrol* **108**, 201–207.

Clot, P., Albano, E., Elliasson, E., Tabone, M., Aricò, S., Israel, Y., Moncada, Y. and Ingelman-Sundberg, M. (1996) Cytochrome P4502E1 hydroxyethyl radical adducts as the major antigenic determinant for autoantibody formation among alcoholics. *Gastroenterol* **111**, 206–216.

Clot, P., Parola, M., Bellomo, G., Dianzani, U., Carini, R., Tabone, M., Aricò, S., Ingelman-Sundberg, M. and Albano, E. (1997) Plasma membrane hydroxyethyl radical adducts cause antibody-dependent cytotoxicity in rat hepatocytes exposed to alcohol. *Gastroenterol* **113**, 265–276.

Colell, A., Garcia-Ruiz, C., Morales, A., Ballesta, A., Ookhtens, M., Rodes, J., Kaplowitz, N. and Fernandez-Checa, J.C. (1997) Transport of reduced glutathione in hepatic mitochondria and mitoplasts from ethanol-treated rats: effect of membrane physical properties and S-adenosyl-L-methionine. *Hepatol* **26**, 699–708.

Colell, A., Garcia-Ruiz, C., Miranda, M, Ardite, E., Marì, M., Morales, A., Corrales, F., Kaplowitz, N. and Fernandez-Checa, J.C. (1998) Selective glutathione depletion of mitochondria by ethanol sensitizes hepatocytes to tumor necrosis factor. *Gastroenterol* **115**, 1541–1551.

Coleman, W.B., Cahill, A., Ivester, P. and Cunningham (1994) Differential effects of ethanol consumption on synthesis of cytoplasmic and mitochondrial encoded subunits of the ATP synthase. *Alcohol Clin Exp Res* **18**, 947–950.

Comoglio, A., Tomasi, A., Malandrino, S., Poli, G. and Albano, E. (1995) Scavenging effect of silipide, a new silybin-phospholipid complex, on ethanol-derived free radicals. *Biochem Pharmacol* **50**, 1313–1316.

Cottalasso, D., Gazzo, P., Dapino, D., Domenicotti, C., Pronzato, M.A., Traverso, N., Bellocchio, A., Nanni, G. and Marinari, U.M. (1996) Effect of chronic ethanol consumption on glycosylation processes in rat liver microsomes. *Alcohol Alcohol* **31**, 51–59.

Cottalasso, D., Bellocchio, A., Pronzato, M.A., Domenicotti, C., Traverso, N., Gianelli, M.V., Marinari, U.M. and Nanni, G. (1998) Effect of ethanol administration on the levels of dolichol in rat liver microsomes and Golgi apparatus. *Alcohol Clin Exp Res* **22**, 730–737.

Dalton, T.P., Shertzer, H.G. and Puga, A. (1999) Regulation of gene expression by reactive oxygen. *Annu Rev Pharmacol Toxicol* **39**, 67–101.

Dehmlow, C., Erhard, J. and de Groot, H. (1996) Inhibition of Kupffer cell functions as an explanation for the hepatoprotective properties of silibinin. *Hepatol* **23**, 749–754.

Di Luzio, N.R. (1963) Prevention of acute ethanol-induced fatty liver by antioxidants. *Physiologist* **6**, 169–173.

Dianzani, M.U. (1985) Lipid peroxidation in ethanol poisoning: a critical reconsideration. *Alcohol Alcohol* **20**, 161–173.

Dianzani, M.U. (1991) Biochemical aspects of fatty liver. In *Hepatotoxicology*, edited by E.G. Meeks, S.D. Harrison and R.J. Bull, pp. 327–400. Boca Raton: CRC Press.

Dicker, E. and Cederbaum, A.I. (1992) Increases NADH-dependent production of reactive oxygen intermediates by microsomes after chronic ethanol consumption: comparisons with NADPH. *Arch Biochem Biophys* **293**, 274–280.

Dorio, R.J., Hoek, J.B., Rubin, E. and Forman, H.J. (1988) Ethanol modulation of rat alveolar macrophage superoxide production. *Biochem Pharmacol* **37**, 3528–3533.

Duce, A.M., Ortiz, P., Cabrero, C. and Mato, J. (1988) S-adenosyl-L-methionine synthetase and phosholipid methyltransferase are inhibited in human cirrhosis. *Hepatol* **8**, 65–68.

Dupont, I., Lucas, D., Clot, P., Ménez, C. and Albano, E. (1998) Cytochrome P4502E1 inducibility and hydroxyethyl radical formation among alcoholics. *J Hepatol* (in press).

Ekström, G. and Ingelman-Sundberg, M. (1989) Rat liver microsomal NADPH-supported oxidase activity and lipid peroxidation dependent on ethanol-inducible cytochrome P450. *Biochem Pharmacol* **38**, 1313–1319.

Ekström, G., Von Bahr, C. and Ingelman-Sundberg M. (1989) Human liver microsomal cytochrome P450IIE1: immunological evaluation of its contribution to microsomal ethanol oxidation, carbon tetrachloride reduction and NADPH oxidase activity. *Biochem Pharmacol* **38**, 689–693.

Eliasson, E. and Kenna, J.G. (1996) Cytochrome P450 2E1 is a cell surface autoantigen in halothane hepatitis. *Mol Pharmacol* **50**, 573–582.

Fang, C., Lindros, K.O., Badger, T.M., Ronis, J.J. and Ingelman-Sundberg, M. (1998) Zonated expression of cytokines in rat liver: effect of chronic ethanol and cytochrome P4502E1 inhibitor, chlormethiazole. *Hepatol* **27**, 1304–1310.

Fariss, M.W. (1990) Oxygen toxicity: unique cytoprotective properties of vitamin E succinate in hepatocytes. *Free Rad Biol Med* **9**, 333–343.

Fataccioli, V., Andraud, E., Gentil, M., French, S.W. and Rouach, H. (1999) Effects of chronic ethanol administration on rat liver proteasome activities: relationship with oxidative stress. *Hepatol* **29**, 14–20.

Ferenci, P., Dragosics, B., Dittrich, H., Frank, H., Benda, L., Locks, H., Meryn, S., Base, W. and Schneider, B. (1989) Randomised controlled trial of silymarin treatment in patients with cirrhosis of liver. *J Hepatol* **9**, 105–113.

Fernandez-Checa, J.C., Ookhtens, M. and Kaplowitz, N. (1987) Effect of chronic ethanol feeding on rat hepatocytic glutathione compartimentation, efflux and response to incubation with ethanol. *J Clin Invest* **80**, 57–62.

Fernandez-Checa, J.C., Garcia-Ruiz, C., Ookhtens, M. and Kaplowitz, N. (1991) Impaired uptake of glutathione by hepatic mitochondria from ethanol fed rats. *J Clin Invest* **87**, 397–405.

Fernandez-Checa, J.C., Kaplowitz, N., Garcia-Ruiz, C., Collel, A., Miranda, M., Marì, M., Ardite, E. and Morales, A. (1997) GSH transport in the mitochondria: defence against TNF-induced oxidative stress and alcohol-induced defect. *Am J Physiol* **273**, G7–G17.

Forman, H.J. and Boveris, A. (1988) Superoxide radical and hydrogen peroxide in mitochondria. In *Free Radicals in Biology*, edited by W.A. Pryor, Vol. V, pp. 65–82. New York: Academic Press.

Fox, E.S., Brower, J.S. and Leingang, K.A. (1997) N-acethylcysteine and alpha-tocopherol reverse the inflammatory response in activated rat Kupffer cells. *J Immunol* **158**, 5418–5423.

French, S.W., Wong, K., Jui, L., Albano, E., Hagbjörk, A.-L. and Ingelman-Sundberg, M. (1993) Effect of ethanol on cytochrome P450 (CYP2E1), lipid peroxidation and serum protein adduct formation in relation to liver pathology pathogenesis. *Exp Mol Pathol* **58**, 61–75.

Fridovich, I. (1989) Oxygen radicals from acetaldehyde. *Free Rad Biol Med* **7**, 557–559.

Fromenty, B. and Pessayre, D. (1995) Inhibition of mitochondrial beta-oxidation as a mechanism of hepatotoxicity. *Pharmacol Ther* **67**, 101–154.

Fromenty, B., Grimbert, S., Mansouri, A., Beaugrand, M., Erlinger, S., Röting, A. and Pessayre, D. (1995) Hepatic mitochondrial DNA deletion in alcoholics: association with microvesicular steatosis. *Gastroenterol* **108**, 193–200.

Fukui, H., Brauner, B., Bode, J.C. and Bode, C. (1991) Plasma endotoxin concentrations in patients with alcoholic and non-alcoholic liver disease: re-evaluation with an improved chromogenic assay. *J Hepatol* **12**, 162–169.

Galle, P.R. (1997) Apoptosis in liver disease. *Gut* **27**, 405–412.

Garcia-Ruiz, C., Morales, A., Ballesta, A., Rhodes, J., Kaplowitz, N. and Fernandez-Checa, J.C. (1994) Effect of chronic ethanol feeding on glutathione and functional integrity of mitochondria in periportal and perivenous rat hepatocytes. *J Clin Invest* **94**, 193–201.

Gergel, D., Nisik, V., Riesz, P. and Cederbaum, A.I. (1997) Inhibition of rat and human cytochrome P4502E1 catalytic actitity and reactive oxygen radical formation by nitric oxide. *Arch Biochem Biophys* **337**, 239–250.

Goldin, R.D., Hunt, N.C., Clark, J. and Wickramaisinghe, S.N. (1993) Apoptotic bodies in a murine model of alcoholic liver disease: reversibility of ethanol-induced changes. *J Pathol* **171**, 73–76.

Grattagliano, I., Vendemiale, G., Sabbà, G., Buonamico, P. and Altomare E. (1996) Oxidation of circulating proteins in alcoholics: role of acetaldehyde and xanthine oxidase. *J Hepatol* **25**, 28–36.

Green, D. and Kroemer G. (1998) The central executioners of apoptosis: caspases or mitochondria? *Trends Cell Biol* **8**, 267–271.

Gressner, A.M. (1991) Liver fibrosis: perspectives in pathobiochemical research and clinical outlook. *Eur J Clin Chem Clin Biochem* **29**, 293–311.

Guerri, C. and Grisolia, S. (1980) Changes in glutathione in acute and chronic alcohol intoxication. *Pharmacol Biochem Behav* **13**, 53–61.

Hall, E.D., McCall, J.M. and Means, E.D. (1994) Therapeutical potential of the lazaroids (21-aminosteroids) in acute central nervous system trauma, ischemia and subarachnoid hemorrhage. *Adv Pharmacol* **28**, 221–268.

Halsted, C.H., Villanuova, J., Chandler, C.J., Stabler, S.P., Allen, R.H., Muskhelishvili, L., James, S.J. and Poinrier, L. (1996) Ethanol feeding of micropigs alters methionine metabolism and increase hepatocellular apoptosis and proliferation. *Hepatol* **23**, 497–505.

Hicks, M., Wong, L.S. and Day, R.O. (1992) Antioxidant activity of propylthiouracil. *Biochem Pharmacol* **43**, 439–444.

Hill, D.B. and Awad, J.A. (1999) Increased urinary F_2-isoprostane excretion in alcoholic liver disease. *Free Rad Biol Med* **26**, 656–660.

Hirata, F., Viveros, O.H., Diliberto, E.J. and Axelrod, J. (1978) Identification and properties of two methyltransferases in conversion of phosphatidylethanolamine to phosphatidylcholine. *Proc Natl Acad Sci USA* **75**, 1718–1721.

Houglum, K., Venkataramani, A., Lyche, K. and Chojkier, M. (1997) A pilot study of the effects of d-α-tocopherol on hepatic stellate cell activation in chronic hepatitis C. *Gastroenterol* **113**, 1069–1073.

Hultcrantz, R., Bissell, D.M. and Roll, F.J. (1991) Iron mediates production of a neutrophil chemoattractant by rat hepatocytes metabolizing ethanol. *J Clin Invest* **87**, 45–49.

Iimuro, Y., von Frankenberg, M., Arteel, G.E., Bradford, B.U. and Thurman, R.G. (1997) Antibodies to tumor necrosis factor-α attenuate hepatic necrosis and inflammation due to chronic exposure to ethanol in the rat. *Am J Physiol* **272**, G1186–G1194.

Ingelman-Sundberg, M., Johansson, I., Yin, H., Terelius, Y., Eliasson, E., Clot, P. and Albano, E. (1993) Ethanol-inducible cytochrome P4502E1: genetic polymorphism, regulation and possible role in the etiology of alcohol-induced liver disease. *Alcohol* **10**, 447–452.

Irving, M.G., Halliday, J.W. and Powell L.W. (1988) Association between alcoholism and increased hepatic iron store. *Alcohol Clin Exp Res* **12**, 7–12.

Ishak, K.G., Zimmerman, H.J. and Ray, M.B. (1991) Alcoholic liver disease: pathology, pathogenetic and clinical aspects. *Alcohol Clin Exp Res* **15**, 45–66.

Israel, Y., Kalant, H., Khanna, J.M., Orrego, H. and Phillips, M.J. (1975) Experimental alcohol-induced hepatic necrosis: suppression by propylthiouracil. *Proc Natl Acad Sci USA* **72**, 1137–1141.

Israel, Y., Speisky, H., Lança, A.J., Iwamura, S., Hirai, M. and Vargese, G. (1992) Metabolism of hepatic glutathione and its relevance in alcohol induced liver damage. In *Cellular and Molecular Aspects of Cirrhosis*, Colloque INSERM/J, Vol. 216, edited by B. Clément and A. Guillouzo, pp. 25–37. London: John Libbey Eurotest Ldt.

Järveläinen, H.A., Fang, C., Ingelman-Sundberg, M. and Lindros, K.O. (1999) Effect of chronic coadministration of endotoxin and ethanol on rat liver pathology and proinflammatory and anti-inflammatory cytokines. *Hepatol* **29**, 1503–1520.

Jewell, S.A., Di Monte, D., Gentile, A., Guglielmini, A., Altomare, E. and Albano, O. (1986) Decreased hepatic glutathione levels in chronic alcoholic patients. *J Hepatol* **3**, 1–6.

Ji, S., Lemasters, J.J., Christerson, V.R. and Thurman R.G. (1982). Periportal and pericentral pyridine nucleotide fluorescence from the surface of perfused liver: evaluation of the hypothesis that chronic treatment with ethanol produces pericentral hypoxia. *Proc Natl Acad Sci USA* **79**, 5415–5419.

Kamimura, S., Gall, K., Britton, S.R., Bacon, B.R., Triadafilopulos, G. and Tsukamoto, H. (1992) Increased 4-hydroxynonenal levels in experimental alcoholic liver disease: Association of lipid peroxidation with liver fibrogenesis. *Hepatol* **16**, 448–453.

Kato, S., Kavase, T., Alderman, J., Inatomi, N. and Lieber, C.S. (1990) Role of xanthine oxidase in ethanol-induced lipid peroxidation. *Gastroenterol* **98**, 203–210.

Kawahara, H., Matsuda, Y. and Takase, S. (1994) Is apoptosis involved in alcoholic hepatitis? *Alcohol Alcohol* **29** (suppl. 1), 113–118.

Kawase, T., Kato, S. and Lieber, C.S. (1989) Lipid peroxidation and antioxidant defense systems in rat liver after chronic ethanol feeding. *Hepatol* **10**, 815–821.

Kera, Y., Ohbora, Y. and Komura, S. (1982) Buthionine sulfoximine inhibition of glutathione biosynthesis enhances hepatic lipid peroxidation in rats during acute ethanol intoxication. *Alcohol Alcohol* **24**, 519–524.

Knecht, K.T., Bradfort, B.U., Mason, R.P. and Thurman, R.G. (1990) *In vivo* formation of free radical metabolite of ethanol. *Mol Pharmacol* **38**, 26–30.

Knecht, K.T., Thurman, R.G. and Mason, R.P. (1993) Role of superoxide and trace transition metals in the production of α-hydroxyethyl radical from ethanol by microsomes from alcohol dehydrogenase-deficient deermice. *Arch Biochem Biophys* **303**, 339–348.

Knecht, K.T., Adachi, Y., Bradfort, B.U., Iimuro, Y., Kadiiska, M., Qun-Hui, X. and Thurman, R.G. (1995) Free radical adducts in the bile of rats treated chronically with intragastric alcohol: inhibition by destruction of Kupffer cells. *Mol Pharmacol* **47**, 1028–1034.

Koivisto, T., Mishin, V.M., Mak, K.M., Cohen, A.P. and Lieber, C.S. (1996) Induction of cytochrome P-4502E1 by ethanol in rat kupffer cells. *Alcohol Clin Exp Res* **20**, 207–212.

Koskinas, J., Kenna, J.G., Bird, G.L., Alexander, G.J.M. and Williams, R. (1992) Immunoglobulin A antibody to a 200-kilodalton cytosolic acetaldehyde adduct in alcoholic hepatitis. *Gastroenterol* **103**, 1860–1867.

Kroemer, G. (1997) The proto-oncogene Blc-2 and its role in regulating apoptosis. *Nature Genetic* **3**, 614–620.

Kukielka, E., Dicker, E. and Cederbaum, A.I. (1994) Increased production of reactive oxygen species by rat liver mitochondria after chronic ethanol treatment. *Arch Biochem Biophys* **309**, 377–386.

Kukielka, E. and Cederbaum, A.I. (1996) Ferritin stimulation of lipid peroxidation by microsomes after chronic ethanol treatment. Role of cytochrome P4502E1. *Arch Biochem Biophys* **332**, 121–127.

Kuo, P.C. and Slivka, A. (1994) Nitric oxide decreases oxidant-mediated hepatocyte injury. *J Surg Res* **56**, 549–600.

Kurose, I., Higuchi, H., Kato, S., Miura, S., Watanabe, N., Kamegaya, Y., Tomita, K., Takaishi, M., Horie, Y., Fukuda, M., Mizukami, K. and Ishii, H. (1997a) Oxidative stress on mitochondria and cell membrane of cultured rat hepatocytes and perfused liver exposed to ethanol. *Gastroenterol* **112**, 1331–1343.

Kurose, I., Higuchi, H., Miura, S., Saito, H., Watanabe, N., Hokari, R., Hirokawa, M., Takaishi, M., Zeki, S., Nakamura, T., Ebinuma, H., Kato, S. and Ishii, H. (1997b) Oxidative stress-mediated apoptosis of hepatocytes exposed to acute ethanol intoxication. *Hepatol* **25**, 368–378.

Lands, W. (1995) Cellular signals in alcohol-induced liver injury: a review. *Alcohol Clin Exp Res* **19**, 928–938.

Lauterburg, B.H., Davies, S. and Mitchell, J.R. (1984) Ethanol suppresses hepatic glutathione synthesis in rats *in vivo*. *J Pharmacol Exp Ther* **230**, 7–11.

Lecompte, E., Herberth, B., Pirrolet, P., Chancerelle, Y., Arnaud, J., Musse, N., Paille, F., Siest, G. and Artur, Y. (1994) Effect of alcohol consumption on blood antioxidant nutrients and oxidative stress indicators. *Am J Clin Nutr* **60**, 255–261.

Letteron, P., Duchettelle, V., Berson, A., Fromenty, B., Fish, C., Degott, C., Benhamou, P.J. and Pessayre, D. (1993) Increased ethane exhalation, an *in vivo* index of lipid peroxidation, in alcohol abusers. *Gut* **34**, 409–414.

Lieber, C.S., Casini, A., De Carli, L.M., Kim, C.-I., Lowe, N., Sasaki, R. and Leo, M.A. (1990) S-adenosyl-L-methionine attenuates alcohol-induced liver injury in baboon. *Hepatol* **11**, 165–172.

Lieber, C.S. (1994) Alcohol and the liver: 1994 update. *Gastroenterol* **106**, 1085–1105.

Lieber, C.S., Leo, M.A., Aleynik, S.I., Aleynik, M.K. and De Carli, L. (1997) Polyenylphosphatidylcholine decreases alcohol-induced oxidative stress in baboon. *Alcohol Clin Exp Res* **21**, 375–379.

Li, C.J., Nanji, A.A., Siakotos, A.N. and Lin, R.C. (1997) Acataldehyde-modified and 4-hydroxynonenal-modified proteins in the liver of rats with alcoholic liver disease. *Hepatol* **26**, 650–657.

Lissoos, T.W., Beno, D.W.A. and Davis, B.H. (1992) Hepatic fibrogenesis and its modulation by growth factors. *J Pediat Gastroenterol Nutr* **15**, 225–231.

Lucas, D., Ménez, J.F. and Berthou, F. (1996) Chlorozazone: an *in vivo* and *in vitro* substrate probe for liver CYP2E1. *Meth Enzymol* **272**, 115–123.

Lytton, S.D., Hellander, A., Zhang-Gouillon, Z.Q., Stokkeland, K., Bordone, R., Aricò, S. Albano, E., French, S.W. and Ingelman-Sundberg, M. (1999) Autoantibodies against cytochromes P-4502E1 and P4503A in alcoholics. *Mol Pharmacol* **55**, 223–233.

Ma, Y., Garken, J., McFarlane, B.M., Foss, Y., Farzaneh, F., McFarlane, I.G., Mieli-Vergani, G. and Vergani, D. (1997) Alcohol dehydrogenase: A target of humoral autoimmune response in liver disease. *Gastroenterol* **112**, 483–492.

Mansouri, A., Fromenty, B., Berson, A., Robin, M.A., Grimbert, S., Beaugrand, M., Erlinger, S. and Pessayre, D. (1997) Multiple hepatic mitochondrial DNA deletions suggest premature oxidative aging in alcoholics. *J Hepatol* **27**, 96–102.

Marinari, U.M., Pronzato, M.A., Cottalasso, D., Rolla, C., Biasi, F., Nanni, G. and Dianzani, M.U. (1987) Inhibition of liver Golgi glycosylation activities by carbonyl products of lipid peroxidation. *Free Rad Res Commun* **3**, 319–324.

Mascotti, D.P., Rup, D. and Thach, R.E. (1995) Regulation of iron metabolism. Effect mediated by iron, heme and cytokines. *Annu Rev Nutr* **15**, 239–261.

Masini, A., Ceccarelli, D., Gallesi, D., Giovannini, F. and Trenti, T. (1994) Lipid hydroperoxide induced mitochondrial dysfunction following acute ethanol intoxication in rats. *Biochem Pharmacol* **47**, 217–224.

Mato, J.M., Cámara, J., Fernández de Paz, J., Caballeria, L., Coll, S., Caballero, A., Garcia-Buey, L., Beltrán, J., Benita, V., Caballeria, J., Solà, R., Moreno-Otero, R., Barrao, F., Martin-Duce, A., Correa, J.A., Parés, A., Barrao, E., Garcia-Margaz, I., Puerta, J.L., Moreno, J., Boissard, G., Ortiz, P. and Rodés, J. (1999) S-adenosylmethionine in alcoholic liver cirrhosis: a randomized, placebo-controlled, double-blind, multicenter clinical trial. *J Hepatol* **30**, 1081–1089.

Matsuhashi, T., Karbowski, M., Liu, X., Usukura, J., Wozniak, M. and Wakabayashi, T. (1998) Complete suppression of ethanol-induced formation of megamitochondria by 4-hydroxy-2,2,6,6,-tetramethyl-piperidine-1-oxyl (4-OH-TEMPO). *Free Rad Biol Med* **24**, 139–147.

Maxwell, S.R. (1997) Prospects for the use of antioxidant therapies. *Drug* **49**, 345–361.

McCord, J. (1985) Oxygen derived free radicals in postischemic tissue damage. *N Engl J Med* **321**, 159–165.

McClain, C.J, Hill, D., Schmidt, J. and Diehl, A.M. (1993) Cytokines and alcoholic liver disease. *Sem Liver Dis* **13**, 170–181.

Minotti, G., Di Gennaro, M., D'Ugo, D. and Granone, P. (1991) Possible source of iron for lipid peroxidation. *Free Rad Res Comms* **12**, 99–110.

Moncada, C., Torres, V., Vargese, E., Albano, E. and Israel, Y. (1994) Ethanol-derived immunoreactive species formed by free radical mechanisms. *Mol Pharmacol* **46**, 786–791.

Moncada, S., Palmet, R.M.J. and Higgs, E.A. (1991) Nitric oxide: physiology, pathophysiology and pharmacology. *Pharmacol Rev* **43**, 109–142.

Moore, D.R., Reinke, L.A. and McCay, P.B. (1995). Metabolism of ethanol to 1-hydroxyethyl radicals *in vivo*: detection with intravenous administration of α-(4-pyridyl-1-oxide)N-t-butylnitrone. *Mol Pharmacol* **47**, 1224–1230,

Moorhouse, P.C., Grootveld, M., Halliwell, B., Quinlan, J.G. and Gutteridge, J.M. (1978) Allopurinol and oxypurinol are hydroxyl radical scavengers. *FEBS Lett* **213**, 23–28.

Morazzoni, P., Montalbetti, A., Malandrino, S. and Pifferi, G. (1993) Comparative pharmaco-kinetics of silipide and silymarin in rats. *Eur J Drug Metab Pharmacokin* **18**, 289–297.

Morimoto, M., Hagbjvrk, A.-L., Wan, Y.J.Y., Fu, P.C., Ingelman-Sundberg, M., Albano, E., Clot, P. and French, S.W. (1995) Modulation of alcoholic liver disease by cytochrome P4502E1 inhibitors. *Hepatol* **21**, 1610–1617.

Nakano, M., Kikuyama, M., Hasegawa, T., Ito, T., Sakurai, K., Hiraishi, K., Hashimura, E. and Adachi, M. (1995) The first observation of O_2^- generation at real time *in vivo* from non-kupffer sinusoidal cells in perfused rat liver during acute ethanol intoxication. *FEBS Lett* **372**, 140–143.

Nakao, L.S. and Augusto, O. (1998) Nucleic acid alkylation by free radical metabolites of ethanol. Formation of 8-(1-hydroxyethyl)guanine and 8-(2-hydroxyethyl)guanine adducts. *Chem Res Toxicol* **11**, 888–894.

Nanji, A.A. and French, S.W. (1989) Dietary linoleic acid is requires for development of experimentally induced alcoholic liver disease. *Life Sci* **44**, 223–227.

Nanji, A.A., Mendenhall, C.L. and French, S.W. (1989) Beef fat prevents alcoholic liver disease in the rat. *Alcohol Clin Exp Res* **13**, 15–19.

Nanji, A.A., Khettry, U., Sadrzadeh, S.M.H and Yamanaka, T. (1993) Severity of liver injury in experimental alcoholic liver disease. Correlation with plasma endotoxin, prostaglandin E2, leukotriene B_4 and thromboxane B_2. *Am J Pathol* **142**, 367–373.

Nanji, A.A., Khwaja, S., Tahan, S.R. and Sadrzadeh, H.S.M. (1994a) Plasma levels of a novel noncyclooxygenase-derived prostanoid (8-isoprostane) correlate with severity of liver injury in experimental alcoholic liver disease. *J Pharmacol Exp Ther* **269**, 1280–1285.

Nanji, A.A., Zhao, S., Sadrzadeh, S.M.H., Dannenberg, A.J., Tahan, S.R. and Waxman, D.J. (1994b) Markedly enhanced cytochrome P4502E1 induction and lipid peroxidation is associated with severe liver injury in fish oil-treated ethanol-fed rats. *Alcohol Clin Exp Res* **18**, 1280–1285.

Nanji, A.A., Sadrzadeh, S.M.H., Yang, E.K., Fogt, F., Maydani, M. and Dannenberg, A.J. (1995a) Dietary saturated fatty acids: A novel treatment for alcoholic liver disease. *Gastroenterol* **109**, 547–620.

Nanji, A.A., Griniuviene, B., Sadrzadeh, S.M.H., Levitsky, S. and McCully, J.D. (1995b) Effect of dietary fat and ethanol on antioxidant enzyme mRNA induction in rat liver. *J Lipid Res* **36**, 736–744.

Nanji, A.A., Greenberg, S.S., Tahan, S.R., Fogt, F., Loscalzo, J., Sadrzadeh, S.M.H., Xie, J. and Stamler, J.S. (1995c) Nitric oxide production in experimental alcoholic liver disease in the rat: role in protection from injury. *Gastroenterol* **109**, 899–907.

Nanji, A.A., Yang, E.K., Fogt, F., Sadrzadeh, S.M.H. and Dannenberg, A.J. (1996) Medium chain triglycerides and vitamin E reduce the severity of established experimental alcoholic liver disease. *J Pharmacol Exp Ther* **277**, 1694–1700.

Nanji, A.A., Zakim, D., Rahemtulla, A., Daly, T., Miao, L., Zhao, S., Khwaja, S., Tahan, S.R. and Dannenberg, A.J. (1997a) Dietary saturated fatty acids down-regulate cycloxygenase-2 and tumor necrosis factor alpha and reverse fibrosis in alcohol-induced liver disease in rats. *Hepatol* **26**, 1538–1545.

Nanji, A.A., Miao, L., Thomas, P., Rahemtulla, T., Khwaja, S., Zhao, S., Peters, D., Tahan, S.R. and Dannenberg, A.J. (1997b) Enhanced cycloxygenase-2 gene expression in alcoholic liver disease in rats. *Gastroenterol* **109**, 547–554.

Nanni, G., Pronzato, M.A., Avarame, M.M., Gambella, G.R., Cottalasso, D. and Marinari, U.M. (1978) Influence of acute ethanol intoxication on rat Golgi apparatus glycosylation activities. *FEBS Lett* **93**, 242–246.

Natoli, G., Costanzo, A., Guido, F., Moretti, F. and Levrero, M. (1998) Apoptotic, non-apoptotic and anti-apoptotic pathways of tumor necrosis factor signaling. *Biochem Pharmacol* **56**, 915–920.

Nicholls, R., De Jersey, J., Worrall, S. and Wilce, P. (1992) Modification of proteins and other biological molecules by acetaldehyde: adduct structure and functional significance. *Int J Biochem* **24**, 1899–1906.

Niemelä, O., Parkkila, S., Ylä-Herttuala, S., Halsted, C., Witztum, J.L., Lanca, A. and Israel, Y. (1994) Covalent protein adducts in the liver as a result of ethanol metabolism and lipid peroxidation. *Lab Invest* **70**, 537–546.

Niemelä, O., Parkkila, S., Ylä-Herttuala, S., Villanueva, J., Ruebner, B. and Halsted, C.H. (1995) Sequential acetaldehyde production, lipid peroxidation and fibrogenesis in micropigs model of alcohol-induced liver disease. *Hepatol* **22**, 1208–1214.

Niemelä, O., Parkkila, S., Britton, R.S., Brunt, E., Janney, C. and Bacon, B. (1999) Hepatic lipid peroxidation in hereditary hemochromatosis and alcoholic liver injury. *J Lab Clin Med* **133**, 451–460.

Niemelä, O., Parkkila, S., Pasanen, M., Imuro, Y., Bradford, B. and Thurman, R.G. Early alcoholic liver injury: formation of adducts with acetaldehyde and lipid peroxidation products and expression of CYP2E1 and CYP3A. *Alcohol Clin Exp Res* **22**, 2118–2124.

Nordmann, R., Ribière, C. and Rouach, H. (1992) Implication of free radical mechanisms in ethanol induced cellular injury. *Free Rad Biol Med* **12**, 219–240.

Nordmann, R. (1994) Alcohol and antioxidant systems. *Alcohol Alcohol* **29**, 513–522.

Ohhira, M., Ohtake, T., Matsumoto, A., Saito, H., Ikuta, K., Fujimoto, Y., Ono, M., Toyokuni, S. and Kohgo, Y. (1998) Immunohistochemical detection of 4-hydroxy-2-nonenal-modified protein adducts in human alcoholic liver disease. *Alcohol Clin Exp Res* **22**, 145S–149S.

Orrego, H., Blake, J.E., Blendis, L.M., Compton, K.V. and Israel, Y. (1987) Long-term treatment of alcoholic liver disease with propylthiouracil. *N Engl J Med* **317**, 1421–1427.

Orrego, H., Blake, J.E., Blendis, L.M., Compton, K.V., Volpe, R. and Israel, Y. (1994) Long-term treatment of alcoholic liver disease with propylthiouracil. Part 2: Influence of the drop-out rates of continued alcohol consumption on a clinical trial. *J Hepatol* **20**, 343–349.

Parés, A., Planas, R., Tores, M., Caballeira, J., Vivier, J.M., Acaro, D., Panés, J., Rigau, J., Santos, J. and Rodés, J. (1998) Effect of silymarin in alcoholic patients with cirrhosis of the liver: results of a controlled, double-blind, randomized and multicenter trial. *J Hepatol* **28**, 615–621.

Park, K.M., Rouach, H., Orfanelli, M.T., Janvier, B. and Nordmann, R. (1988) Influence of allopurinol and desferrioxamine on the ethanol-induced oxidative stress in rat liver and cerebellum. In *Alcohol Toxicity and Free Radical Mechanisms*, edited by R. Nordmann, C. Ribière and H. Rouach, pp. 135–139. Oxford: Pergamon Press.

Parola, M., Leonarduzzi, G., Biasi, F., Albano, E., Biocca, M.E., Poli, G. and Dianzani, M.U. (1992) Vitamin E dietary supplementation protects against carbon tetrachloride-induced chronic liver damage and cirrhosis. *Hepatol* **16**, 1014–1021.

Parola, M., Muraca, R., Dianzani, I., Barrera, G., Leonarduzzi, G., Bendinelli, P., Piccoletti, R. and Poli, G. (1992) Vitamin E dietary supplementation inhibits trasforming growth factor β1 gene expression. *FEBS Lett* **308**, 267–270.

Parola, M., Robino, G., Marra, F., Pinzani, M., Bellomo, G., Leonarduzzi, G., Chiarugi, P., Camandola, S., Poli, G., Waeg, G., Gentilini, P. and Dianzani, M.U. (1998) HNE interacts directly with JNK isoforms in human hepatic stellate cells. *J Clin Invest* **102**, 1942–1950.

Paronetto, F. (1993) Immunologic reactions in alcoholic liver disease. *Sem Liver Dis* **13**, 183–195.

Patel, T. and Gores, G.J. (1995) Apoptosis and hepatobiliary disease. *Hepatol* **21**, 1725–1744.

Pawlosky, R.J., Flynn, B.M. and Salem, N. (1997) The effects of low dietery levels of poly-unsaturateds on alcohol-induced liver disease in rhesus monkeys. *Hepatol* **26**, 1386–1392.

Perperas, A., Tsantoulas, D., Portmann, B., Eddleston, A.L. and Williams, R. (1981) Auto-immunity to a liver membrane lipoprotein and liver damage in alcoholic liver disease. *Gut* **22**, 149–152.

Persson, J.O., Terelius, Y. and Ingelman-Sundberg, M. (1990) Cytochrome P450-dependent formation of reactive oxygen radicals: isozyme-specific inhibition of P450-mediates reduction of oxygen and carbon tetrachloride. *Xenobiotica* **20**, 887–900.

Pietrangelo, A., Gualdi, R., Casalgrandi, G., Montosi, G. and Ventura, E. (1995a) Molecular and cellular aspects of iron-induced hepatic cirrhosis in rodents. *J Clin Invest* **95**, 1824–1831.

Pietrangelo, A., Borella, F., Casalgrandi, G., Montosi, G. Ceccarelli, D., Gallesi, D., Giovannini, F., Gasparetto, A. and Masini, A. (1995b) Antioxidant activity of silybin *in vivo* during long-term iron overload in rats. *Gastroenterol* **109**, 1941–1949.

Polavarapu, R., Spitz, D.R., Sim, J.E., Follansbee, M.H., Oberley, L.W., Rahemtulla, A. and Nanji, A.A. (1998) Increased lipid peroxidation and impaired antioxidant enzyme function is associated with pathological liver injury in experimental alcoholic liver disease in rats fed diets high in corn oil and fish oil. *Hepatol* **27**, 1317–1323.

Poli, G. and Parola, M. (1996) Oxidative damage and fibrogenesis. *Free Rad Biol Med* **22**, 287–305.

Puntarulo, S. and Cederbaum, A.I. (1989) Chemiluminescence from acetaldehyde oxidation by xanthine oxidase involves generation of and interactions with hydroxyl radicals. *Alcohol Clin Exp Res* **13**, 84–90.

Rabshabe-Step, J. and Cederbaum, A.I. (1994) Generation of reactive oxygen intermediates by human liver microsomes in the presence of NADPH or NADH. *Mol Pharmacol* **45**, 150–157.

Rajagopalan, K.V. and Handler, P. (1964) Hepatic aldehyde oxidase III. The substrate binding side. *J Biol Chem* **239**, 2027–2032.

Rao, D.N.R., Yang, M.X., Lasker, J.M. and Cederbaum, A.I. (1996) 1-hydroxyethyl radical formation during NADPH- and NADH-dependent oxidation of ethanol by human liver microsomes. *Mol Pharmacol* **49**, 814–821.

Reinke, L.A., Lai, E.K., Du, Bose, C.M. and McCay., P.B. (1987) Reactive free radical generation *in vivo* in hearth and liver of ethanol-fed rats: correlation with radical formation *in vitro*. *Proc Natl Acad Sci USA* **84**, 9223–9227.

Reinke, L.A., Rau, J.M. and McCay, P.B. (1990) Possible roles of free radicals in alcohol tissue damage. *Free Rad Res Comms* **9**, 205–211.

Reinke, L.A., Moore, D.R. and McCay, P.B. (1997a) Free radical formation in livers of rats treated acutely and chronically with alcohol. *Alcohol Clin Exp Res* **21**, 642–646.

Reinke, L.A., Moore, D.R. and McCay, P.B. (1997b) Mechanisms for metabolism of ethanol to 1-hydroxyethyl radicals in rat liver microsomes. *Arch Biochem Biophys* **348**, 9–14.

Ribiére, C., Hininger, I., Saffer-Boccara, C., Salbourault, D. and Nordmann, R. (1994) Mitochondrial respiratory activity and superoxide radical generation in the liver, brain and hearth after chronic ethanol intake. *Biochem Pharmacol* **47**, 1827–1833.

Robin, M.-A., Maratrat, M., Le Roy, M., Le Breton, F.-P., Bonierbale, E., Dansett, P., Ballet, F., Mansuy, D. and Pessayre, D. (1996) Antigenic targets in tienilic acid hepatitis. Both cytochrome P450 2C11 and 2C11-tienilic acid adducts are transported to the plasma membrane of rat hepatocytes and recognised by human sera. *J Clin Invest* **98**, 1471–1480.

Rojter, S., Tessler, J., Alvarez, D., Persico, R., Lopez, P., Bandi, J.C., Podesta, A., Terg, R., Gutman, R. and Mastai, R. (1995) Vasodilatatory effects of propylthiouracil in patients with alcoholic cirrhosis. *J Hepatol* **22**, 184–188.

Rolla, R., Vay, D., Mottaran, E., Parodi, M., Sartori, M., Bellomo, G., Klassen, L.W., Thiele, G.M., Tuma, D.J. and Albano, E. (2000) Detection of circulating antibodies against Malondialdehyde-acetaldehyde adducts in patients with alcoholic liver disease. *Hepatol* **31**, 878–884.

Ronis, M.J.J., Lindros, K.O. and Ingelman-Sundberg, M. (1996) The CYP2E family. In *Cytochromes P450: metabolic and toxicological aspects*, edited by C. Ioannides, pp. 211–239. Boca Raton: CRC Press.

Ross, A.D., Dey, I., Janes, N. and Israel, Y. (1998) Effect of antithyroid drugs on hydroxyl radical formation and α-1-proteinase inhibitor inactivation by neutrophils: therapeutical implications. *J Pharmacol Exp Therap* **285**, 1233–1238.

Rouach, H., Houzè, P., Orfanelli, M.T., Gentil, M., Bourdon, R. and Nordmann, R. (1990) Effect of acute ethanol administration of the subcellular distribution of iron in rat liver and cerebellum. *Biochem Pharmacol* **39**, 1095–1100.

Rouach, H., Houzè, P., Gentil, M., Orfanelli, M.-T. and Nordmann, R. (1994) Effect of acute ethanol administration on the uptake of ^{59}Fe-labelled tranferrin by rat liver and cerebellum. *Biochem Pharmacol* **47**, 1835–1841.

Rouach, H., Fattaccioli, V., Gentil, M., French, S.W., Morimoto, M. and Nordmann, R. (1997) Effect of chronic ethanol feeding on lipid peroxidation and protein oxidation in relation to liver pathology. *Hepatol* **25**, 351–355.

Sadrzadeh, S.M.H., Nanji, A.A. and Prince, P.L. (1994a) The oral iron chelator 1,2,-dimethyl-3-hydroxypyrid-4-one reduces hepatic free iron, lipid peroxidation and fat accumulation in chronically ethanol-fed rats. *J Pharmacol Exp Ther* **269**, 632–636.

Sadrzadeh, S.M.H., Nanji, A.A. and Meydani, M. (1994b) Effect of chronic ethanol feeding on plasma and liver α- and γ-tocopherol levels in normal and vitamin E-deficient rats. *Biochem Pharmacol* **47**, 2005–2010.

Sadrzadeh, S.M.H., Meydani, M., Khettry, U. and Nanji, A.A. (1995) High-dose vitamin E supplementation has no effect on ethanol-induced pathological liver injury. *J Pharmacol Exp Ther* **273**, 455–460.

Sadrzadeh, S.M.H., Hallaway, P.E. and Nanji, A.A. (1997) The long-acting parenteral iron chelator hydroxyethylstarch-desferoxamine fails to protect against alcohol-induced liver injury in rats. *J Pharmacol Exp Ther* **280**, 1038–1042.

Sadrzadeh, S.M.H. and Nanji, A.A. (1998) The 21-aminosterolid 16-desmethyl tirilazat mesylate prevents necroinflammatory changes in experimental alcoholic liver desease. *J Pharmacol Exp Ther* **284**, 406–412.

Schuessler, H. (1981) Reaction of ethanol and formate radicals with ribonuclease A and serum albumin in radiolysis. *Int J Radiat Biol* **40**, 483–492.

Schuessler, H., Schmerler-Dremel, G., Danzer, J. and Jung-Kvrner, E. (1992) Ethanol radical-induced protein-DNA crosslinking: a radiolysis study. *Int J Radiat Biol* **62**, 517–526.

Sen, C.K. and Packer, L. (1997) Antioxidant and redox regulation of gene transcription. *FASEB J* **10**, 709–720.

Sergent, O., Griffon, B., Morel, I., Chevanne, M., Dubus, M.P., Cillard, P. and Cillard, J. (1997) Effect of nitric oxide on iron-mediated oxidative stress in primary hepatocyte culture. *Hepatol* **23**, 122–127.

Shaw, S., Jayatilleke, E., Ross, W.A., Gordon, E.R. and Lieber, C.S. (1981) Ethanol induced lipid peroxidation: potentiation by long-term alcohol feeding and attenuation by methionine. *J Lab Clin Med* **98**, 417–425.

Shaw, S., Rubin, K.P. and Lieber, C.S. (1983) Depressed hepatic glutathione and increased diene conjugates in alcoholic liver disease: evidence of lipid peroxidation. *Dig Dis Sci* **28**, 585–589.

Shaw, S. and Jayatilleke, E. (1990a) Ethanol-induced iron mobilization: role of acetaldehyde-aldehyde oxidase generated superoxide. *Free Rad Biol Med* **9**, 11–15.

Shaw, S. and Jayatilleke, E. (1990b) The role of aldehyde oxidase in ethanol-induced hepatic lipid peroxidation in the rat. *Biochem J* **268**, 579–583.

Sheron, N., Bird, G., Koskinas, J., Portmann, B., Ceska, M., Lindsey, I. and Williams, R. (1993) Circulating levels of the neutrophil chemotaxin interleukin-8 are elevated in severe acute alcoholic hepatitis and the tissue levels correlates with neutrophil infiltration. *Hepatol* **18**, 41–46.

Shiratori, Y., Takada, H., Hikiba, G., Nakata, R., Okano, K., Komatsu, Y., Niwa, Y., Matsumura, M., Shiina, S., Omata, M. and Kamii, K. (1993) Production of chemotactic factor interleukin-8 from hepatocytes exposed to ethanol. *Hepatol* **18**, 1477–1482.

Shirley, M.A., Reidhead, C.T. and Murphy, R.C. (1992) Chemotactic LTB4 metabolites produced by hepatocytes in the presence of ethanol. *Biochem Biophys Res Commun* **185**, 604–609.

Sinaceur, J., Ribière, C., Sarburault, D. and Nordmann, R. (1995) Superoxide formation in liver mitochondria during ethanol intoxication: possible role in alcohol hepatotoxicity. In *Free Radicals in Liver Injury*, edited by G. Poli, K.H. Cheeseman, M.U. Dianzani and T.F. Slater, pp. 175–177. Oxford: IRL Press.

Situnayake, R.D., Crump, B.J., Thurnham, D.I., Davies, J.A., Gearty, J. and Davis, M. (1990) Lipid peroxidation and hepatic antioxidants in alcoholic liver disease. *Gut* **31**, 1311–1317.

Slater, A.G.F., Nobel, C.S.I. and Orrenius, S. (1995) The role of intracellular oxidant in apoptosis. *Biochim Biophys Acta* **1271**, 59–62.

Smith, J.A. (1994) Neutrophils, host defence and inflammation: a double-edged sword. *J Leukoc Biol* **56**, 672–686.

Speisky, H., MacDonald, A., Giles, G., Orrego, H. and Israel, Y. (1985) Increased loss and decreased syntheis of hepatic glutathione after acute ethanol administration. *Biochem J* **225**, 565–572.

Speisky, H., Kera, Y., Penttilä, K.E., Israel, Y. and Lindros, K.O. (1988) Depletion of hepatic glutathione by ethanol occurs independently of ethanol metabolism. *Alcohol Clin Exp Res* **12**, 224–228.

Speisky, H., Shackel, N., Vargese, G., Wade, D. and Israel, Y. (1990) Role of hepatic γ-glutamyltransferase in the degradation of circulation glutathione: studies in intact guinea pig perfused liver. *Hepatol* **11**, 843–849.

Stål, P., Johansson, I., Ingelman-Sundberg, M., Hagen, K. and Hultcrantz, R. (1996) Hepatotoxicity induced by iron overload and alcohol: studies on the role of chelatable iron, cytochrome P450 2E1 and lipid peroxidation. *J Hepatol* **25**, 538–546.

Stoyanovsky, D.A., Wu, D. and Cederbaum, A.I. (1998) Interaction of 1-hydroxyethyl radical with glutathione, ascorbic acid and α-tocopherol. *Free Rad Biol Med* **24**, 132–138.

Stoyanovsky, D.A. and Cederbaum, A.I. (1998) ESR and HPLC-EC analysis of ethanol oxidation to 1-hydroxyethyl radical: rapid reduction and quantification of POBN and PBN nitroxides. *Free Rad Biol Med* **25**, 536–545.

Stowel, A., Hillbom, M., Salaspuro, M. and Lindros, K. (1980) Low acetaldehyde levels in blood, breath and cerebrospinal fluid of intoxicated humans assayed by improved methods. *Adv Exp Med Biol* **132**, 635–642.

Strubelt, O., Younes, M. and Pentz, R. (1987) Enhancement by glutathione depletion of ethanol-induced hepatotoxicity *in vitro* and *in vivo*. *Toxicol* **45**, 213–223.

Suematzu, T., Matsumura, T., Sato, N., Miyamoto, T., Ooka, T., Kamada, T. and Abe, H. (1981) Lipid peroxidation in alcoholic disease in humans. *Alchol Clin Exp Res* **5**, 427–430.

Sultatos, L.G. (1988) Effect of acute ethanol administration on the hepatic xanthine dehydrogenese/oxidase system in the rat. *J Pharmacol Exp Ther* **246**, 946–949.

Svegliati-Baroni, G., Marucci, I., Benedetti, A., Mancini, R., Jezequel, A.-M. and Orlandi, F. (1994) Chronic ethanol feeding increases apoptosis and cell proliferation in rat liver. *J Hepatol* **20**, 508–513.

Takase, S., Tsutsumi, M., Kawahara, H., Takada, N. and Takada, A. (1993) The alcohol-altered liver membrane antibody and hepatitis C virus infecion in the progression of alcoholic liver disease. *Hepatol* **17**, 9–13.

Takeshi, H., Kaplowitz, N., Kamimura, T., Tsukamoto, H. and Fernandez-Checa, J.C. (1992) Hepatic mitochondrial GSH depletion and progression of experimental alcoholic liver disease in rats. *Hepatol* **16**, 1423–1428.

Tanner, A.R., Bantock, I., Hinks, L., Lloyd, B., Turner, N.R. and Wright, R. (1986) Depressed selenium and vitamin E levels in an alcoholic population: possible relationship to hepatic injury through increased lipid peroxidation. *Dig Dis Sci* **31**, 1307–1312.

Teare, J.P., Carmichael, A.J., Burnett, F.R. and Reke, M.O. (1993) Detection of antibodies to acetaldehyde-albumin conjugates in alcoholic liver disease. *Alcohol Alcohol* **28**, 11–16.

Thiele, G.M., Tuma, D.J., Willis, M.S., Miller, J.A., McDonalds, T.L., Sorrell, M.F. and Klassen, L.W. (1998) Soluble proteins modified with acetaldehyde and malondialdehyde are immunogenic in the absence of adjuvants. *Alcohol Clin Exp Res* **22**, 1731–1739.

Thome, J., Zhang, J., Davids, E., Foley, E., Weijers, H.G., Weisbeck, G.A., Bönin, J., Riederer, P. and Gerlach, M. (1997) Evidence for increased oxidative stress in alcohol-dependent patients provided by quantification of *in vivo* salicilate hydroxylation products. *Alcohol Clin Exp Res* **21**, 82–85.

Thurman, R.G. (1998) Alcoholic liver injury involves activation of Kupffer cells by endotoxins. *Am J Physiol* **275**, G605–G611.

Tophan, R., Coger, M., Pearce, K. and Schultz, P. (1989) The mobilization of ferritin by liver cytosol: A comparison of xanthine and NADH as reducing substrates. *Biochem J* **261**, 137–142.

Tsukamoto, H., French, S.W., Benson, N., Delgado, G., Rao, G.A., Larkin, E.C. and Largman, C. (1985) Severe and progressive steatosis and focal necrosis in rat liver induced by continuous intragastric infusion of ethanol and low fat diet. *Hepatol* **5**, 224–232.

Tsukamoto, H., Towner, S.J., Ciofalo, L.M. and French, S.W. (1986) Ethanol-induced liver fibrosis in rats fed high fat diet. *Hepatol* **6**, 814–822.

Tsukamoto, H., Horne, W., Kamimura, S., Niemelä, O., Parkkila, S., Ylä-Herttuala, S. and Brittenham, G.M. (1995) Experimental liver cirrhosis induced by alcohol and iron. *J Clin Invest* **96**, 620–630.

Tuma, D.J., Thiele, G.M., Xu, D., Klassen, L.W. and Sorrell, M.F. (1996) Acetaldehyde and malondialdehyde react together to generate distinct protein adducts in the liver during long-term ethanol administration. *Hepatol* **23**, 872–880.

Valenzuela, A., Lagos, C., Schmidt, K. and Videla, L.A. (1985) Silymarin protection against hepatic lipid peroxidation induced by acute ethanol intoxication in the rat. *Biochem Pharmacol* **34**, 2209–2212.

Valenzuela, A. and Guerra, R. (1985) Protective effect of the flavonoid silybin dihemisuccinate on the toxicity of phenylhydrazine on rat liver. *FEBS Lett* **181**, 291–294.

Van Antwerp, D.J., Martin, J.S., Verma, I.M. and Green, D.R. (1998) Inhibition of TNF-induced apoptosis by NFkB. *Trends Cell Biol* **8**, 107–111.

Van Pelt, F.N.A.M., Straub, P. and Manns M.P. (1995) Molecular basis of drug-induced immunological liver injury. *Sem Liver Dis* **15**, 283–300.

Vendemiale, G., Altomare, E., Trizio, T., Grazie, I.E., De Padova, C., Salarno, M.T., Carrieri, V. and Albano, O. (1989) Effects of oral S-adenosyl-L-methionine on hepatic glutathione in patients with liver disease. *Scand J Gastroenterol* **24**, 407–415.

Videla, I.A. and Valenzuela, A. (1982) Alcohol ingestion, liver glutathione and lipoperoxidation metabolic interrelations and pathological implications. *Life Sci* **31**, 2395–2407.

Viitala, K., Israel, Y., Blake, J.E. and Niemela, O. (1997) Serum IgA, IgG and IgM antibodies directed against acetaldehyde-derived epitopes: relationship to liver disease severity and alcohol consumption. *Hepatol* **25**, 1418–1424.

Wang, J.-F. Greenberg, S.S. and Spitzer, J.J. (1995) Chronic alcohol administration stimulates nitric oxide formation in the rat liver with or without pretreatment with lipopolysaccharide. *Alcohol Clin Exp Res* **19**, 387–393.

Wieland, P. and Lauterburg, B.H. (1995) Oxidation of mitochondrial proteins and DNA following administration of ethanol. *Biochem Biophys Res Commun* **213**, 815–819.

Winrow, V.R., Bird, G.R., Koskinas, J., Blake, D.R., Williams, R. and Alexander G.J.M. (1994) Circulating antibodies against a 65 kDa heat shock protein in acute alcoholic hepatitis. *J Hepatol* **20**, 359–363.

Worrall, S., De Jersey, J., Shanley, B.C. and Wilce P.A. (1990) Antibodies against acetaldehyde-modified epitopes: presence in alcoholic, non-alcoholic liver disease and control subjects. *Alcohol Alcohol* **25**, 509–517.

Wu, D. and Cederbaum, A.L. (1996) Ethanol cytotoxicity to transfected HepG2 cell line expressing human cytochrome P4502E1. *J Biol Chem* **271**, 23914–23919.

Wu, D. and Cederbaum, A.L. (1999) Ethanol-induced apoptosis to stable HepG2 cell lines expressing human cytpchrome P-4502E1. *Alcohol Clin Exp Res* **23**, 67–76.

Xu, D., Thiele, G.M., Kearley, M.L., Haugen, M.D., Klassen, L.W., Sorrell, M.F. and Tuma, D.J. (1997) Epitope characterization of malondialdehyde-acetaldehyde adducts using an enzyme-linked immunosorbent assay. *Chem Res Toxicol* **10**, 978–986.

Xu, D., Thiele, G.M., Beckenhauer, J.L., Klassen, L.W., Sorrell, M.F. and Tuma, D.J. (1998a) Detection of circulating antibodies to malondialdehyde-acetaldehyde adducts in ethanol-fed rats. *Gastroenterol* **115**, 686–692.

Xu, J., Jones, B.E., Neufeld, D.S. and Czaja, M.J. (1998b) Glutathione modulates rat and mouse hepatocyte sensitivity to tumor necrosis factor α toxicity. *Gastroenterol* **115**, 1229–1237.

Yacoub, L.K., Fogt, F., Griniuviene, B. and Nanji, A.A. (1995) Apoptosis and bcl-2 protein expression in experimental alcoholic liver disease in the rat. *Alcohol Clin Exp Res* **19**, 854–859.

Zhao, X., Jie, O., Xie, J., Giles, T.D. and Greenberg, S.S. (1997) Ethanol inhibits inducible nitric oxide synthetase transcriptional and post-transcriptional processes *in vivo*. *Alcohol Clin Exp Res* **21**, 1246–1256.

Zindenberg-Cherr, S., Olin, K.L., Villanueva, J., Tang, A., Phinney, S.D., Halstead, C.H. and Keen C.L. (1991) Ethanol-induced changes in hepatic free radical defense mechanism and fatty acid composition in the miniature pig. *Hepatol* **13**, 1185–1192.

Chapter 7

Ethanol and the hepatic microcirculation

Robert S. McCuskey

Significant interactive roles for endotoxin, cytokines, reactive free radicals, nitric oxide (NO), endothelin (ET-1), sinusoidal lining cells, leukocytes and platelets have been demonstrated in the pathophysiology of hepatic microvascular disturbances and parenchymal injury resulting from ethanol alone or in combination with infection or toxicants. Acute ethanol ingestion elicits a dose dependent increase in leukocyte adhesion, endothelial cell swelling and reduced blood flow in hepatic sinusoids during the first few hours following ingestion. Activation of Kupffer cells is initially elicited at low doses while depression occurs at high doses, with daily ingestion for several days, and with chronic exposure. The responses are exacerbated in the presence of endotoxemia or sepsis and are not seen in endotoxin-resistant animals implicating a role for endotoxin in the ethanol-induced inflammatory response. TNFα is a primary mediator of these events. NO derived from sinusoidal endothelial cells initially appears to play an important role in these events by stabilizing the TNFα-mediated hepatic microvascular inflammatory response to acute ethanol ingestion. Chronic ethanol feeding increases the hepatic sinusoidal contractile response to ET-1, presumably due to activation of perisinusoidal stellate cells. Kupffer cells phagocytic activity is significantly decreased, but the blood flow through the sinusoids is relatively normal with little or no leukocyte plugging or sticking in the sinusoids or central venules. Taken together, it is thought that ethanol sensitizes Kupffer cells to stimulation by endotoxin, derived either from increased intestinal absorption or from infection. As a result, the immune status of the liver is altered by modification of the production and release of cytokines and free radicals which affect adjacent endothelial and stellate cells, resulting in a microvascular inflammatory response and altered sinusoidal blood flow mediated by an imbalance in the local release of NO and ET-1. These alterations in the hepatic microcirculation enhance hepatic microvascular and parenchymal injury due to oxidative stress and lipid peroxidation. The responses are exacerbated in the presence of infection or other toxicants.

KEYWORDS: microcirculation, sinusoids, kupffer cells, endothelial cells, stellate cells, endotoxin

INTRODUCTION

Ethanol ingestion produces increased hepatic oxygen consumption, fatty liver, hepatomegaly, hepatocellular damage and with prolonged consumption, ultimately may progress to hepatitis, fibrogenesis and cirrhosis. Alterations in hepatic blood flow and microcirculation have been demonstrated to accompany these responses and are thought to contribute to the hepatic injury elicited by ethanol. The purpose of this chapter is to summarize the current knowledge of the pathophysiology of ethanol on the circulation of blood through the liver and the vascular cells involved.

EFFECT OF ETHANOL ON HEPATIC BLOOD FLOW

Acutely administered ethanol generally increases hepatic blood flow (Castenfors *et al.*, 1960; Shaw *et al.*, 1977). The acute vasodilator effect of ethanol is not thought to be a result of vascular actions of metabolites of ethanol, acetaldehyde or acetate (Altura and Altura, 1982; Altura and Gebrewold, 1981; Carmichael *et al.*, 1988; Orrego *et al.*, 1988) but has been suggested to be due to adenosine and an increase in splanchnic blood flow (Carmichael *et al.*, 1988). However, high doses of ethanol in the perfused liver have been shown to have a vasoconstrictive effect on the intrahepatic vasculature, followed by a slow "escape" phase thought to be initially due to the release of endothelin (ET-1), a potent vasoconstrictor, and the subsequent release of the vasodilator, nitric oxide (NO) (Oshita *et al.*, 1992, 1993). Chronic ingestion of ethanol results in reduced flow and portal hypertension (Mezey, 1982), which has been attributed to hepatocellular swelling since it was seen in the absence of perisinusoidal and perivenular collagen formation (Blendis *et al.*, 1982; Vidins *et al.*, 1985). More recently, it has been suggested that the portal hypertension also may be due to a dominate action of ET-1 over NO (Oshita *et al.*, 1992, 1993).

EFFECT OF ETHANOL ON THE HEPATIC MICROCIRCULATION

At the microcirculatory level, acute, oral administration of ethanol to rats is reported to increase both portal and hepatic arterial blood flow, resulting in an average net increase in the velocity of erythrocyte flow through the sinusoids (Sato *et al.*, 1987a; Sherman and Fisher, 1987). The increased flow in the sinusoids, however, was heterogeneous, with some sinusoids exhibiting dramatic increases in cellular velocity while others had little or no increase and some a decrease (Sherman and Fisher, 1987). As a result, some centrivenular areas became hypoxic while others exhibited an increase in oxygenation (Sato *et al.*, 1987a,b). The reasons for this heterogeneity are not clear but the appearance of "fast" sinusoids suggests "arterialized" vessels due to the dilation of "arterio-sinus twigs" which supply scattered sinusoids at the periphery of the lobule (Sherman and Fisher, 1987). Reduced flow in other sinusoids may have been due to hepatocellular swelling and/or plugging of some sinusoids by formed blood elements. In addition, ethanol may have elicited constriction of some sinusoids through the local release of vasoactive substances or the modification of the action of such substances. Such alterations in vascular responsiveness to agonists in the presence of ethanol has been demonstrated in other microvascular beds (Altura and Altura, 1982, 1983) where ethanol interacts with prostaglandins in bizarre ways which are dose dependent. At low doses of ethanol, vascular responses to agonists can be either potentiated or attenuated while high doses usually are depressive. Similar dose dependent interactions with adrenergic, cholinergic and aminergic substances also have been reported (Altura and Altura, 1982).

Acutely administered ethanol also results in an increase in WBC adhesion and endothelial cell swelling in the sinusoids (Eguchi *et al.*, 1991a; McCuskey, 1991a,b; McCuskey *et al.*, 1991b, 1993b). Some of the dynamics of this hepatic microvascular inflammatory response have been characterized directly using *in vivo* microscopic imaging of the liver following the ingestion of ethanol alone or in combination with endotoxemia and/or sepsis (McCuskey *et al.*, 1990, 1993a,b, 1995a; Eguchi *et al.*, 1991a,b; McCuskey 1991a,b; Nishida *et al.*, 1994a,b, 1995). The basic response includes an increase in the number of leukocytes and platelets adhering to the sinusoidal wall plugging these vessels, swelling of sinusoidal endothelial cells, decreases in the number of sinusoids with blood flow as well as flow velocity, and reduced phagocytic function of Kupffer cells.

Acute ethanol ingestion in mice elicits a dose dependent increase in leukocyte adhesion and endothelial cell swelling in hepatic sinusoids during the first few hours following ingestion (Eguchi *et al.*, 1991a). Activation of Kupffer cells is initially elicited at low doses while depression occurs at high doses (Eguchi *et al.*, 1991a), with daily ingestion for several days and with chronic exposure (McCuskey, 1991b; McCuskcy *et al.*, 1993a). The responses are exacerbated in the presence of endotoxemia or sepsis and are not seen in endotoxin-resistant animals, implicating a role for endotoxin in the ethanol-induced inflammatory response (McCuskey, 1991b; McCuskey *et al.*, 1993b, 1995a; Nishida *et al.*, 1994a). In addition, the responses are abolished with anti-TNFα suggesting that TNFα is a primary mediator of these events (Eguchi *et al.*, 1991b; McCuskey *et al.*, 1993b, 1995a). NO derived from sinusoidal endothelial cells initially appears to play an important role in these events by stabilizing the TNFα-mediated hepatic microvascular inflammatory response to acute ethanol ingestion, thereby helping to protect the liver from ischemia and leukocyte induced oxidative injury (Nishida *et al.*, 1995, 2000; McCuskey *et al.*, 1995a).

While these results are consistent with other reports that chronic ethanol ingestion enhances the production of endotoxin-stimulated TNFα production and hepatic injury (Honchel *et al.*, 1992; Hansen *et al.*, 1994; McClain *et al.*, 1993), they appear at odds with the reported inhibition of TNFα, O_2^- and NOS following acute ethanol infusion (D'Souza *et al.*, 1991; Bautista *et al.*, 1991, 1993; Bautista and Spitzer, 1992; Spolarics *et al.*, 1993). The later studies, however, were evaluating the response to LPS after the rats had been infused for several hours with ethanol by which time their Kupffer cells may have been rendered tolerant to the challenge injection of LPS by the effects of ethanol-induced absorption of gut-derived endotoxin (Nanji *et al.*, 1994c; Enomoto *et al.*, 1998). In this regard, elevated levels of LPS have been measured in the portal blood within 30 minutes after gastric gavage with ethanol (McCuskey *et al.*, 1996) and minute doses of LPS render Kupffer cells, the hepatic microvasculature and animals tolerant to subsequent challenge doses for a period of time followed by enhanced sensitivity (Urbaschek *et al.*, 1984, 1986; Urbaschek, 1987; McCuskey *et al.*, 1982, 1983, 1987; Urbaschek and Urbaschek, 1982).

Taken together, these studies suggest a role for endotoxin in ethanol-induced hepatic microvascular injury (Eguchi *et al.*, 1991a; McCuskey, 1991a; McCuskey *et al.*, 1990, 1995b). Further evidence is provided by the observation that ethanol exacerbates the progression of sepsis by accelerating the elevation of plasma endotoxin levels, the time to achieve lethality as well as the hepatic microvascular inflammatory response as evidenced by increased WBC adhesion and plugging of sinusoids, perhaps due to increased TNFα release from the initially activated Kupffer cells (Nishida *et al.*, 1992b, 1994a; McCuskey *et al.*, 1993b). Ethanol also enhances the hepatotoxic effects of cocaine, both in mice and, to a lesser extent, in rats with an enhanced microvascular inflammatory response, significant reductions in sinusoidal blood flow and a loss of Kupffer cells with assumption of phagocytic function by sinusoidal endothelial cells (McCuskey *et al.*, 1991a,b, 1993a; Earnest *et al.*, 1993). The latter response, as well as WBC adhesion, may be due to IL-1 since this cytokine induces similar changes within 1 hour after administration (McCuskey *et al.*, 1991b; Nishida *et al.*, 1993, 1999). Recently, ethanol has been shown to exacerbate the hepatic microvascular response to acetaminophen resulting in disruption of the sinusoidal endothelium, infiltration of the Space of Disse with blood cells, and severe centrilobular sinusoidal congestion (McCuskey *et al.*, 1999b).

The effects of long-term exposure to ethanol on the hepatic microcirculation also has been studied, but to a lesser extent. Chronic ethanol feeding to rats for 5 weeks increased the hepatic sinusoidal contractile response to ET-1, presumably due to activation of perisinusoidal stellate cells (Bauer *et al.*, 1995). After mice and rats had been maintained on ethanol-containing liquid diets for 24 weeks, Kupffer cell phagocytic activity was significantly decreased, but the blood flow through the sinusoids was relatively normal with little or no leukocyte plugging or sticking in the sinusoids or central venules (McCuskey *et al.*, 1991a, 1993a; Nishida *et al.*, 1992a; Jolley *et al.*, 1991, 1993; Abril *et al.*, 1991; Earnest *et al.*, 1993). These results suggest that long-term exposure to ethanol alters the release and/or production of mediators as well as the functional behavior of sinusoidal lining cells, thereby affecting leukocyte adhesion, sinusoidal diameter and blood flow.

Unfortunately, attempts to provide a small animal model of alcoholic fibrosis and cirrhosis have had only limited success. As a result, most microcirculatory studies of the fibrotic and/or cirrhotic liver have been in chemically-induced models. During fibrosis induced by a choline deficient diet and cirrhosis produced by feeding CCl_4, there is a dilation of central venules (Koo *et al.*, 1976; Koo and Liang, 1976; Sherman and Fisher, 1987). While the average velocity of cellular flow in sinusoids did not increase significantly in livers with moderate fibrosis, there was a marked increase in the average flow velocities in sinusoids and central venules of cirrhotic livers (Koo *et al.*, 1976; Koo and Liang, 1976; Sherman and Fisher, 1987). In large part, this was due to the appearance of "fast" sinusoids which dramatically increased in proportion in cirrhotic livers compared to controls. As with acute ethanol treatment, these "fast" sinusoids may function as intrahepatic shunts (Sherman and Fisher, 1987) since these appeared to represent "arterialized" vessels; further support for this interpretation is that ligation of the hepatic artery abolished the presence of such "fast" sinusoids (Koo *et al.*, 1976). The dilation of central venules, probably is a reflection of increased flow and not the result of downstream distortion or stenosis of hepatic veins since pressures in central venules do not rise significantly under these conditions and the pressure gradient between central venules and the vena cava remains unchanged (Shibayama and Nakata, 1985). This supports the view that alterations in the sinusoids are responsible for a major component of the portal hypertension. However, pressures in terminal portal venules also rise significantly under these conditions, so that attributing increased flow to a hyper-dynamic splanchnic circulation can not be completely discounted.

Taken together, the literature clearly supports an important role for sinusoidal lining cells, cytokines, NO, ET-1, and endotoxin in the pathophysiology of hepatic microvascular disturbances resulting from ethanol alone or in combination with other hepatotoxins or infection. Some of these roles are detailed below.

ALCOHOL, ENDOTOXIN, SINUSOIDAL LINING CELLS AND HEPATIC MICROVASCULAR INJURY

Sinusoidal lining cells (Kupffer cells, endothelial cells and stellate cells) are the principal cells responsible for regulating blood flow through the hepatic sinusoids (McCuskey, 2000). While the pathophysiology associated with ethanol intoxication and alcoholic liver disease is complex, an increasing amount of evidence as suggested above supports important interactive roles for the hepatic microvasculature including both its sinusoidal lining cells as well as leukocytes and platelets with endotoxin, cytokines, reactive free radicals, NO, and ET-1 in the pathophysiology of liver injury resulting from ethanol alone or in combination with infection or toxicants.

Kupffer cells

A variety of clinical and experimental evidence implicates both Kupffer cells and gram-negative bacterial endotoxin in the etiology of alcoholic liver disease (Ali and Nolan, 1967; Nolan and Camara, 1982; Nolan *et al.*, 1980; Liu, 1979; Cooksley *et al.*, 1973; Kaufman *et al.*, 1982; Bode *et al.*, 1987; Fukui *et al.*, 1991; McCuskey *et al.*, 1995a). Clearance of microaggregated albumin and endotoxin is depressed in rats following both acute and chronic administration of alcohol (Nolan and Camara, 1982; Nolan *et al.*, 1980; Ali and Nolan, 1967). Acute human alcoholics with no evidence of liver disease have also demonstrated a depressed RES which returns to normal after several days of alcohol withdrawal (Liu, 1979). Furthermore, RES depression has been demonstrated by reduced clearance of microaggregated albu-min (Cooksley *et al.*, 1973) and the lack of a concentration gradient of immune complexes between portal and hepatic veins (Kaufman *et al.*, 1982). Finally, elevated levels of systemic, circulating endotoxin also have been reported in humans intoxicated with alcohol (Bode *et al.*, 1987) as well as during alcoholic liver disease (Nolan and Camara, 1982; Liu, 1979; Bhagwandeen *et al.*, 1987; Fukui *et al.*, 1991; Urbaschek *et al.*, 1994; McCuskey *et al.*, 1995a; Lumsden *et al.*, 1988), suggesting spill-over of gut-derived endotoxin due to alcohol-depressed clearance by hepatic Kupffer cells (Ali and Nolan, 1967) and/or increased permeability of the intestinal mucosa to endotoxin (Bjarnason *et al.*, 1984). This concept is further supported by animal studies which demonstrated that, in the presence of ethanol, normally innocuous doses of endotoxin become toxic and result in severe liver damage (Bhagwandeen *et al.*, 1987; Shibayama, 1987; Shibayama *et al.*, 1991) which is minimized when Kupffer cells are inactivated (Adachi *et al.*, 1994). Finally, increased levels of endotoxin have been reported in the peripheral blood of rats with experimental alcoholic liver disease. This had a positive correlation both with the severity of the disease as well as with plasma levels of thromboxane B_2 and leukotriene B_4 and a negative correlation with prostaglandin E_2 (Nanji *et al.*, 1993). Alcoholic liver injury was prevented following reduction of bacterial endotoxin production by intestinal sterilization with antibiotics (Adachi *et al.*, 1995). Gut-derived endotoxin has been implicated in the early tolerance and later sensitization of Kupffer cells following ethanol ingestion and its effect on the production of CD-14, the receptor for endotoxin (Enomoto *et al.*, 1998). The role of gut-derived endotoxin and Kupffer cells in the hepatic response to ethanol has been reviewed recently (Thurman *et al.*, 1997, 1998, 1999; Thurman, 1998).

In response to stimulation by ethanol, endotoxin and/or sepsis, Kupffer cells release a variety of toxic, beneficial and vasoactive substances which have been implicated as mediators of hepatic inflammation, injury and subsequent liver disease or organ failure (Nanji *et al.*, 1993; McClain *et al.*, 1993; Hansen *et al.*, 1994; Decker, 1989, 1990; Deaciuc *et al.*, 1994; Bautista and Spitzer, 1992; Bautista *et al.*, 1993, 1994; Bautista, 1998; Nanji *et al.*, 1994a; Nanji, 1993; Oshita *et al.*, 1993; Bone, 1991; Giroir, 1993; Glauser *et al.*, 1991; Luster *et al.*, 1994; Eguchi *et al.*, 1991a,b; McCuskey *et al.*, 1990, 1993a,b, 1995a; McCuskey, 1991a,b; Nishida *et al.*, 1994a,b, 1995; Thurman *et al.*, 1997, 1998, 1999; Thurman, 1998; Vollmar *et al.*, 1994; Zhang *et al.*, 1995). Some of the principal substances released that have been implicated in alcoholic liver disease include: (a) cytokines, especially TNF, IL_1, IL_6 and IL-8 (McClain and Cohen, 1989; McClain *et al.*, 1993; Khoruts *et al.*, 1991; Hansen *et al.*, 1994; D'Souza *et al.*, 1991; Eguchi *et al.*, 1991a,b; Nishida *et al.*, 1995); (b) eicosanoids, especially prostaglandin E_2, thromboxane B_2, and leukotriene B_4 (Nanji *et al.*, 1993, 1994b; Nanji, 1993); and (c) reactive free radicals or their precursors, especially superoxide anion (O_2^-) (Bautista and Spitzer, 1992; Bautista *et al.*, 1993; Bautista, 1998) and nitric oxide (NO) (Spolarics *et al.*, 1993; Greenberg *et al.*, 1994; Nishida *et al.*, 1995) which, through its rapid interaction with O_2^-, forms hepatotoxic peroxynitrite anions (Kurose *et al.*, 1993a,b). All of these substances may directly and/or indirectly affect surrounding parenchymal and sinusoidal lining cells as well as circulating blood elements resulting in an inflammatory response and tissue injury. The initial manifestation of injury is a basic microvascular inflammatory response which is characterized by activation of the endothelium, stimulating these cells from their normal anticoagulant state to a procoagulant state with increased adhesiveness for leukocytes and platelets. Tissue damage subsequently results from oxidative stress and lipid peroxidation, not only due to hypoxia from reduced perfusion of the exchange vessels (sinusoids) but also from injurious substances released from activated, sequestered leukocytes as well as the activated macrophages (Kupffer cells). Such intercellular interactions involve regulated production and interactions of endothelial cell and leukocyte adhesion molecules triggered by a variety of stimuli and resulting in leukocyte-endothelial adhesion, activation and subsequent release of reactive free radicals generated from xanthine oxidase which induce oxidative stress and lipid peroxidation, further exacerbating the injury, and finally transmigration of leukocytes (McMillen *et al.*, 1993; Bone, 1991; Giroir, 1993; Glauser *et al.*, 1991; Albelda *et al.*, 1994). Additional interest has been focused on the role of NO which is produced in the liver by Kupffer cells (Billiar *et al.*, 1989), hepatocytes (Curran *et al.*, 1989) and sinusoidal endothelial cells (Laskin *et al.*, 1993; Spolarics *et al.*, 1993). NO is produced from *L*-arginine by the action of nitric oxide synthase (NOS), which exists in both constitutive (c, endothelial) and inducible (i, macrophage and hepatocyte) forms (Nathan, 1992; Moncada *et al.*, 1991). Beneficial functions attributed to cNO include inhibition of vascular smooth muscle contraction, leukocyte adherence, platelet aggregation and adherence, and maintenance of vascular integrity (Hutcheson *et al.*, 1992; Kubes *et al.*, 1991; Nathan, 1992; Moncada *et al.*, 1991). However, cytotoxic effects including inhibition of hepatic protein synthesis (Billiar *et al.*, 1989) and mitochondrial electron transport (Kurose *et al.*, 1993a,b) have been attributed to iNO through its rapid interaction with O_2^- to form toxic peroxynitrite anions ($OONO^-$) which oxidize tissue sulfhydryls (Radi *et al.*, 1991).

Endothelial cells

Alcohol affects not only the expression of adhesion molecules on sinusoidal endothelial cells (SEC) as indicated above, but also inhibits the ability of these cells to scavenge hyaluonan, elicits increased ET-1 production, and modifies the numbers, size and organization of fenestrae in SEC (Fraser *et al.*, 1980, 1986; Deaciuc and Spitzer, 1996; Horn *et al.*, 1987; Mak and Lieber, 1984; Sarphie *et al.*, 1995, 1996b, 1997). Acute ethanol elicits the loss of some fenestrae and the formation of larger fenestrae and gaps in the sinusoid wall, while chronic ethanol leads to the elimination of the fenestrae being organized as sieve plates. This has implications for trans-sinusoidal transport, particularly for chylomicron remnants (Fraser *et al.*, 1986, 1995). Most evidence suggests that the effects of ethanol on SEC are indirect and mediated in a paracrine fashion by substances released from Kupffer cells which in turn are dependent upon gut-derived endotoxin since the responses of SEC to ethanol are mimicked by endotoxin and eliminated when Kupffer cells are destroyed (Eakes and Olson, 1998; Deaciuc *et al.*, 1994; Deaciuc and Spitzer, 1996; Sarphie *et al.*, 1995, 1996a,b, 1997).

Stellate cells

Both ethanol and endotoxin enhance the hepatic microvascular sensitivity to ET-1 (Pannen *et al.*, 1996; Bauer *et al.*, 1995). ET-1, secreted by sinusoidal endothelial cells, is a potent vasoconstrictor and has been shown dramatically to reduce blood flow though hepatic sinusoids as well as reducing the diameters of these vessels (Bauer *et al.*, 1994a,b). While the latter is thought to be mediated by the constriction of activated perisinusoidal stellate cells (Zhang *et al.*, 1993, 1994; Bauer *et al.*, 1995), a passive response due to reduced sinusoidal blood flow and pressure from subsequent constriction of the portal venules can not be excluded (McCuskey *et al.*, 1999a). The constrictive response of sinusoids may be counteracted by NO derived from sinusoidal endothelial cells (Pannen *et al.*, 1998; Shah *et al.*, 1997) and also by carbon monoxide (CO) derived from hepatocytes (Suematsu *et al.*, 1994, 1995).

A role for CO in regulating blood flow through hepatic sinusoids during health is recently reported to include a "fail safe" mechanism help to maintain flow during endotoxemia (Suematsu and Ishimura, 2000). Whether CO is affected by ethanol has not yet been reported.

CONCLUSION

An increasing amount of literature supports significant interactive roles for endotoxin, cytokines, reactive free radicals, NO, ET-1, sinusoidal lining cells, leukocytes and platelets in the pathophysiology of hepatic microvascular disturbances and parenchymal injury resulting from ethanol alone or in combination with infection or toxicants. Ethanol sensitizes Kupffer cells to stimulation by endotoxin, derived either from increased intestinal absorption or from infection. As a result, the immune status of the liver is altered by modification of the production and release of cytokines and free radicals, which affect adjacent endothelial and stellate cells resulting in a microvascular inflammatory response and altered sinusoidal blood flow mediated by an imbalance in the local release of NO and ET-1. These alterations in the hepatic microcirculation enhance hepatic microvascular and parenchymal injury due to oxidative stress and lipid peroxidation. The responses are exacerbated in the presence of infection or other toxicants.

REFERENCES

Abril, E.R., Jolly, C.S., Krasovich, M.A., McCuskey, R.S. and Earnest, D.L. (1991) Divergent effects of chronic ethanol ingestive on Kupffer cell function: implications for alcoholic liver disease. *Hepatology* **14**, 139A.

Adachi, Y., Bradford, B.U., Gao, W., Bojes, H.K. and Thurman, R.G. (1994) Inactivation of Kupffer cells prevents early alcohol-induced liver injury. *Hepatology* **20**, 453–460.

Adachi, Y., Moore, L.E., Bradford, B.U., Goa, W. and Thurman, R.G. (1995) Antibiotics prevent liver injury in rats following long-term exposure to ethanol. *Gastroenterology* **108**, 218–224.

Albelda, S.M., Smith, C.W. and Ward, P.A. (1994) Adhesion molecules and inflammatory injury. *FASEB Journal* **8**, 504–512.

Ali, M.V. and Nolan, J.P. (1967) Alcohol induced depression in reticuloendothelial function in the rat. *Journal of Laboratory and Clinical Medicine* **70**, 295–301.

Altura, B.M. and Altura, B.T. (1982) Microvascular and vascular smooth muscle actions of ethanol, acetaldehyde, and acetate. *Federation Proceedings* **41**, 2447–2451.

Altura, B.M. and Altura, B.T. (1983) Peripheral vascular actions of ethanol and its interaction with neurohumoral substances. *Neurobehavior, Toxicology and Teratology* **5**, 211–220.

Altura, B.M. and Gebrewold, A. (1981) Failure of acetaldehyde or acetate to mimic the splanchnic arteriolar or venular dilator actions of ethanol: direct *in situ* studies on the microcirculation. *British Journal of Pharmacology* **73**, 580–582.

Bauer, M., Paquette, N.C., Zhang, J.X., Bauer, I., Pannen, B.H.J., Kleeberger, S.R. and Clemens, M.G. (1995) Chronic ethanol consumption increases hepatic sinusoidal contractile response to endothelin-1 in the rat. *Hepatology* 1565–1576.

Bauer, M., Zhang, J.X., Bauer, I. and Clemens, M.G. (1994a) Endothelin-1 as a regulator of hepatic microcirculation: sublobular distribution of effects and impact on hepatocellular secretory function. *Shock* **1**, 457–465.

Bauer, M., Zhang, J.X., Bauer, I. and Clemens, M.G. (1994b) ET-1 induced changes in the hepatic microcirculation: sinusoidal and extrasinusoidal sites of action. *American Journal of Physiology* **267**, G143–G149.

Bautista, A.P. (1998) The role of Kupffer cells and reactive oxygen species in hepatic injury during acute and chronic alcohol intoxication. *Alcoholism: Clinical & Experimental Research* **22**, 255S–259S.

Bautista, A.P., Deaciuc, I.V., Jaeschke, H., Spolarics, Z. and Spitzer, J.J. (1993) Hepatic responses to bacterial endotoxin (LPS). In *Pathophysiology of Shock, Sepsis and Organ Failure*, edited by G. Schlag and H. Redl, pp. 915–934. Berlin: Springer-Verlag.

Bautista, A.P., D'Souza, N.B., Lang, C.H., Bagwell, J. and Spitzer, J.J. (1991) Alcohol-induced downregulation of superoxide anion production by hepatic phagocytes in endotoxemic rats. *American Journal of Physiology* **260**, R969–R976.

Bautista, A.P., Skrepnik, N., Niesman, M.R. and Bagby, G.J. (1994) Elimination of macrophages by liposome-encapsulated dichloromethylene diphosphonate suppresses the endotoxin-induced priming of Kupffer cells. *Journal of Leukocyte Biology* **55**, 321–327.

Bautista, A.P. and Spitzer, J.J. (1992) Acute ethanol intoxication stimulates superoxide anion production by *in situ* perfused rat liver. *Journal of Hepatology* **15**, 892–898.

Bhagwandeen, B.S., Apte, M., Manwarring and Dickenson, J. (1987) Endotoxin induced hepatic necrosis in rats on an alcohol diet. *Journal of Pathology* **152**, 47–53.

Billiar, T.R., Curran, R.D., Stuehr, D.J., West, M.A., Bentz, B.G. and Simmons, R.L. (1989) An L-arginine dependent mechanism mediates Kupffer cell inhibition of hepatocyte protein synthesis *in vitro*. *Journal of Experimental Medicine* **169**, 1467–1472.

Bjarnason, I., Ward, K. and Peters, T. (1984) The leaky gut of alcoholism: possible route of entry for toxic compounds. *Lancet* **ii**, 179–182.

Blendis, L.M., Orrego, H., Crossley, I.R., Blake, J.E., Medline, A. and Israel, Y. (1982) The role of hepatocyte enlargement in hepatic pressure in cirrhotic and noncirrhotic alcoholic liver disease. *Hepatology* **2**, 539–546.

Bode, C., Kugler, V. and Bode, J.C. (1987) Endotoxemia in patients with alcoholic and non-alcoholic cirrhosis and in subjects with no evidence of chronic liver disease following acute alcohol excess. *Journal of Hepatology* **4**, 8–14.

Bone, R.C. (1991) The pathogensis of sepsis. *Annals of Internal Medicine* **115**, 457–469.

Carmichael, F.J., Saldivia, V., Varghese, G.A., Israel, Y. and Orrego, H. (1988) Ethanol-induced increase in portal blood flow: role of acetate and A1- and A2-adenosine receptors. *American Journal of Physiology* **255**, G417-G423.

Castenfors, H., Hultman, E. and Josephson, B. (1960) Effect of intravenous infusions of ethyl alcohol on estimated hepatic blood flow in man. *Journal of Clinical Investigation* **39**, 776–781.

Cooksley, W.G.E., Powell, L.W. and Halliday, J.W. (1973) Reticuloendothelial phagocytic function in human liver disease and its relationship to haemolysis. *British Journal of Haematology* **25**, 147–152.

Curran, R.D., Billiar, T.R., Stuehr, D.J., Hofmann, K. and Simmons, R.L. (1989) Hepatocytes produce nitrogen oxides from L-arginine in response to inflammatory products of Kupffer cells. *Journal of Experimental Medicine* **170**, 1769–1774.

Deaciuc, I.V., Bagby, G.J., Niesman, M.R., Skrepnik, N. and Spitzer, J.J. (1994) Modulation of hepatic sinusoidal endothelial cell function by Kupffer cells: an example of intercellular communication in the liver. *Hepatology* **19**, 464–470.

Deaciuc, I.V. and Spitzer, J.J. (1996) Hepatic sinusoidal endothelial cell in alcoholemia and endotoxemia. *Alcoholism: Clinical & Experimental Research* **20**, 607–614.

Decker, K. (1989) Hepatic mediators of inflammation in cells of the hepatic sinusoids. In *Cells of the Hepatic Sinusoid II*, edited by E. Wisse, D.L. Knook and K. Decker, pp. 171–175. Rijswijk: The Kupffer Cell Foundation.

Decker, K. (1990) Biologically active products of stimulated liver macrophages. *European Journal of Biochemistry* **192**, 245–261.

D'Souza, N.B., Bautista, A.P., Bagby, G.J., Lang, C.H. and Spitzer, J.J. (1991) Acute alcohol intoxication supresses *E. coli* LPS-enhanced glucose utilization by hepatic non-parenchymal cells. *Alcoholism: Clinical and Experimental Research* **15**, 249–254.

Eakes, A.T. and Olson, M.S. (1998) Regulation of endothelin synthesis in hepatic endothelial cells. *American Journal of Physiology* **274**, G1068–G1076.

Earnest, D.L., Abril, E.R., Jolley, C.S., Nishida, J., Krasovich, M.A., McDonnell, D., Watson, R.R. and McCuskey, R.S. (1993) Ethanol feeding significantly potentiates cocaine-induced Kupffer cell dysfunction. In *Cells of the Hepatic Sinusoid*, Vol. 4, edited by E. Wisse and D.L. Knook, pp. 400–402. Leiden: Kupffer Cell Foundation.

Eguchi, H., McCuskey, P.A. and McCuskey, R.S. (1991a) Kupffer cell activity and hepatic microvascular events after acute ethanol ingesion in mice. *Hepatology* **13**, 751–757.

Eguchi, H., McCuskey, P.A., Scuderi, P. and McCuskey, R.S. (1991b) TNFα plays a role in hepatic microvascular events following acute ethanol ingestion in $C_{57}Bl/6$ mice. In *Cells of the Hepatic Sinusoid III*, edited by E. Wisse, D.L. Knook and R.S. McCuskey, pp. 465–468. Leiden: Kupffer Cell Foundation.

Enomoto, N., Ikejima, K., Bradford, B., Rivera, C., Kono, H., Brenner, D.A. and Thurman, R.G. (1998) Alcohol causes both tolerance and sensitization of rat Kupffer cells via mechanisms dependent on endotoxin. *Gastroenterology* **115**, 443–451.

Fraser, R., Bolen, L.M. and Day, W.A. (1980) Damage of rat liver sinusoidal endothelium by ethanol. *Pathology* **12**, 371–376.

Fraser, R., Day, W.A. and Fernando, N.S. (1986) Review: The liver sinusoidal cells. Their role in disorders of the liver, lipoprotein metabolism and atherogenesis. *Pathology* **18**, 5–11.

Fraser, R., Dobbs, B.R. and Rogers, G.W.T. (1995) Lipoproteins and the liver sieve: the role of the fenestrated sinusoidal endothelium in lipoprotein metabolism, atherosclerosis and cirrhosis. *Hepatology* **21**, 863–874.

Fukui, H., Brauner, B., Bode, J.C. and Bode, C. (1991) Plasma endotoxin concentrations in patients with alcoholic and non-alcoholic liver disease: reevaluation with an improved chromogenic assay. *Journal of Hepatology* **12**, 162–169.

Giroir, B.P. (1993) Mediators of septic shock: new approaches for interrupting the endogenous inflammatory cascade. *Critical Care Medicine* **21**, 780–789.

Glauser, M.P., Zanetti, G., Baumgartner, J.-D. and Cohen, J. (1991) Septic shock: pathogenesis. *Lancet* **338**, 732–736.

Greenberg, S.S., Xie, J., Wang, Y., Malinski, T., Summer, W.R. and McDonough, K. (1994) *Escherichia coli*-induced inhibition of endothelium-dependent relaxation and gene expression and release of nitric oxide is attenuated by chronic alcohol ingestion. *Alcohol* **11**, 53–60.

Hansen, J., Cherwitz, D.L. and Allen, J.I. (1994) The role of tumor necrosis factor-α in actue endotoxin-induced hepatotoxicity in ethanol-fed rats. *Hepatology* **20**, 461–474.

Honchel, R., Ray, N.B., Marsano, L., Cohen, D., Lee, E., Shedlofsky, S. and McClain, C.J. (1992) Tumor necrosis factor in alcohol enhanced endotoxin liver injury. *Alcoholism: Clinical and Experimental Research* **16**, 665–669.

Horn, T., Christoffersen, P. and Henriksen, J.H. (1987) Alcoholic liver injury: defenstration in noncirrhotic livers – a scanning electron microscopic study. *Hepatology* **7**, 77–82.

Hutcheson, I.R., Wittle, B.J.R. and Boughton-Smith, N.K. (1992) Role of nitric oxide in maintaining vascular integrity of endotoxin-induced acute intestinal damage in the rat. *British Journal of Pharmacology* **101**, 815–820.

Jolley, C., Zhu, W., Abril, E., Eguchi, H., McCuskey, P., McCuskey, R. and Earnest, D. (1991) High resolution *in vivo* microscopy (HRM) detects subtle changes in Kupffer cell phagocytic function weeks before standard intravenous particle clearance tests. *Gastroenterology* **100**, A757.

Jolley, C.S., Abril, E.R., Olson, G.B., Earnest, D.L., McDonnell, D., Nishida, J. and McCuskey, R.S. (1993) Effects of ethanol on *in vivo* and *in vitro* Kupffer cell function, DNA profile and cytoskeletal staining. In *Cells of the Hepatic Sinusoid*, Vol. 4, edited by E. Wisse and D.L. Knook, pp. 417–420. Leiden: Kupffer Cell Foundation.

Kaufman, R.L., Hoefs, J.C. and Quismorio Jr., F.P. (1982) Immune complexes in the portal and systemic circulation of patients with alcoholic liver disease. *Clinical Immunology and Immunopathology* **22**, 44–54.

Khoruts, A., Stahnke, L., McClain, C.J., Logan, G. and Allen, J.I. (1991) Circulating TNF, IL-1 and IL-6 concentrations in chronic alcoholic patients. *Hepatol* **13**, 267–276.

Koo, A., Liang, I.Y.S. and Cheng, K. (1976) Effect of the ligation of the hepatic artery on the microcirculation in the cirrhotic liver in the rat. *Australian Journal of Experimental Biology and Medical Science* **54**, 287–295.

Koo, A. and Liang, L.Y.S. (1976) Intrahepatic microvascular changes in carbon tetrachloride-induced cirrhotic livers in the rat. *Australian Journal of Experimental Biology and Medical Science* **54**, 277–286.

Kubes, P., Suzuki, M. and Granger, D.N. (1991) Nitric oxide: an endogenous mediator of leukocyte adhesion. *Proceedings of the National Academy of Science* **88**, 4651–4655.

Kurose, I., Kato, S., Ishii, H., Fukumura, D., Miura, S., Suematsu, M. and Tsuchiya, M. (1993a) Nitric oxide mediates lipopolysaccharide-induced alteration of mitochondrial function in cultured hepatocytes and isolated perfused liver. *Hepatology* **18**, 380–388.

Kurose, I., Miura, S., Fukumura, D., Yoni, Y., Saito, H., Tada, S., Suematsu, M. and Tsuchiya, M. (1993b) Nitric oxide mediates Kupffer cell-induced reduction of mitochondrial energization in hepatoma cells: a comparison with oxidative burst. *Cancer Res* **53**, 2676–2682.

Laskin, D.L., Heck, D.E., Feder, L.S., Gardner, C.R. and Laskin, J.D. (1993) Regulation of nitric oxide production by hepatic macrophages and endothelial cells. In *Cells of the Hepatic Sinusoid IV*, edited by D.L. Knook and E. Wisse, pp. 26–28. Leiden: Kupffer Cell Foundation.

Liu, Y.K. (1979) Phagocytic capacity of reticuloendothelial system in alcoholics. *Journal of the Reticuloendothelial Society* **25**, 605–613.

Lumsden, A.B., Henderson, J.M. and Kutner, M.H. (1988) Endotoxin levels measured by chromogenic assay in portal, hepatic and peripheral venous blood in patients with cirrhosis. *Hepatology* **8**, 232–236.

Luster, M.I., Germolec, D.R., Yoshida, T., Kayama, F. and Thompson, M. (1994) Endotoxin-induced cytokine gene expression and excretion in the liver. *Hepatology* **19**, 480–488.

Mak, K.M. and Lieber, C.S. (1984) Alterations in endothelial fenestrations in liver sinusoids of baboons fed alcohol: a scanning electron microscopic study. *Hepatology* **4**, 386–391.

McClain, C., Hill, D., Schmidt, J. and Diehl, A.M. (1993) Cytokines and alcoholic liver disease. *Seminars in Liver Disease* **13**, 170–182.

McClain, C.J. and Cohen, D.A. (1989) Increased tumor necrosis factor production by monocytes in alcoholic hepatitis. *Hepatology* **9**, 349–351.

McCuskey, R.S. (1991a) *In vivo* microscopy of the effects of ethanol on the liver. In *Alcohol and Drug Abuse Reviews: Liver Pathology and Alcohol*, edited by R.R. Watson, pp. 563–574. Clifton, N.J.: Humana Press.

McCuskey, R.S. (1991b) Responses of the hepatic sinusoid lining and microcirculation to combinations of endotoxin, cytokines and ethanol. In *Cells of the Hepatic Sinusoid III*, edited by E. Wisse, D.L. Knook and R.S. McCuskey, pp. 1–5. Leiden: Kupffer Cell Foundation.

McCuskey, R.S. (2000) Morphologic mechanisms for regulating blood flow through hepatic sinusoids. *Liver* **20**, 3–7.

McCuskey, R.S., Eguchi, H., McCuskey, P.A., Krasovich, M.A., Watzl, B. and Watson, R.R. (1991a) Long-term exposure to cocaine in combination with ethanol elicits fibrosis, necrosis and microvascular dysfunction in murine liver. *Gastroenterology* **100**, A773.

McCuskey, R.S., Eguchi, H., McCuskey, P.A., Urbaschek, R. and Urbaschek, B. (1991b) Some effects of ethanol in Kupffer cell function and host defense mechanisms in the liver. In *Frontiers of Mucosal Immunology*, Vol. 2, edited by M. Tsuchiya, H. Nagura, T. Hibi and I. Mono, pp. 187–192. Amsterdam: Excerpta Medica.

McCuskey, R.S., Eguchi, H., Nishida, J., Krasovich, M.A., McDonnell, D., Watzl, B., Jolley, C.S., Abril, E.R., Earnest, D.L. and Watson, R.R. (1993a) Effects of ethanol and cocaine alone or in combination on hepatic sinusoids of mice and rats. In *Cells of the Hepatic Sinusoid IV*, edited by E. Wisse and D.L. Knook, pp. 376–380. Leiden: Kupffer Cell Foundation.

McCuskey, R.S., Eguchi, H., Nishida, J., Urbaschek, R. and Urbaschek, B. (1993b) Effects of ethanol alone or in combination with infection, toxins or drugs of abuse on the hepatic microcirculation. *Advances in Biological-Science* **86**, 227–234.

McCuskey, R.S., Ito, Y., McCuskey, M.K., Ekataksin, W. and Wake, K. (1999a) Morphologic mechanisms for regulating blood flow through hepatic sinusoids: 1998 Update and overview. IX Internat. Symp. Cells of the Hepatic Sinusoid. In *Cells of the Hepatic Sinusoid*, Vol. VII, edited by E. Wisse, D.L. Knook and R. Fraser, pp. 129–134. Leiden: Kupffer Cell Foundation.

McCuskey, R.S., Machen, N.W., Wang, X., McCuskey, M.K. and DeLeve, L.D. (1999b) A single ethanol binge exacerbates early acetaminophen-induced centrilobular injury to the sinusoidal endothelium. *Hepatology* **30**, 335A.

McCuskey, R.S., McCuskey, P.A., Eguchi, H., Crichton, E.G., Urbaschek, R. and Urbaschek, B. (1990) *In vivo* microscopy of the liver following acute administration of ethanol. In *Alcohol, Immunosuppression and AIDS*, edited by A. Pawlowski, D. Seminara and R. Watson, pp. 341–350. New York: Alan R. Liss.

McCuskey, R.S., McCuskey, P.A., Urbaschek, R. and Urbaschek, B. (1987) Kupffer cell function in host defense. *Reviews of Infectious Diseases* **5**, S616–S619.

McCuskey, R.S., Nishida, J., Eguchi, H., McDonnell, D., Baker, G.L., Ekataksin, W., Krasovich, M.A., Rudi, V., Seitz, H.K., Urbaschek, B. and Urbaschek, R. (1995a) Role of endotoxin in the hepatic microvascular inflammmatory response to ethanol. *Journal of Gastroenterology and Hepatology* **10**(Suppl. 1), 518–523.

McCuskey, R.S., Nishida, J., Eguchi, H., McDonnell, D. and Fox, E.S. (1995b) Ethanol acutely sensitizes Kupffer cells to endotoxin exacerbating the hepatic microvascular inflammatory response. *Alcoholism: Clinical and Experimental* **19**(Suppl), 99A.

McCuskey, R.S., Nishida, J., Eguchi, H., McDonnell, D., Urbaschek, B., Baker, G.L. and Urbaschek., R. (1996) Ethanol acutely increases absorption of gut-derived endotoxin stimulating an hepatic microvascular inflammatory response. *Gastroenterology* **110**, 1264A.

McCuskey, R.S., Urbaschek, R., McCuskey, P.A., Sacco, N., Stauber, W., Pinkstaff, C.A. and Urbaschek, B. (1982) Studies of Kupffer cells in mice sensitized or tolerant to endotoxin. In *Sinusoidal Liver Cells*, edited by K.L. Knook and E. Wisse, pp. 387–392. Amsterdam: Elsevier/North-Holland.

McCuskey, R.S., Urbaschek, R., McCuskey, P.A. and Urbaschek, B. (1983) *In vivo* microscopic observations of the responses of Kupffer cells and the hepatic microcirculation to *Mycobacterium bovis* BCG alone and in combination with endotoxin. *Infection and Immunity* **42**, 362–367.

McMillen, M.A., Huribal, M. and Sumpio, B. (1993) Common pathway of endothelial-leukocyte interaction in shock, ischemia, and reperfusion. *Amer. J. Surg* **166**, 557–562.

Mezey, E. (1982) Alcoholic liver disease. *Progress in Liver Disease* **7**, 555–572.

Moncada, S., Palmer, R.M.J. and Higgs, E.A. (1991) Nitric oxide: physiology, pathophysiology and pharmacology. *Pharmacological Reviews* **43**, 103–142.

Nanji, A.A. (1993) Role of eicosanoids in experimental alcoholic liver disease. *Alcohol* **10**, 443–446.

Nanji, A.A., Khettry, U., Sadrzadeh, S.M.H. and Yamanaka, T. (1993) Severity of liver injury in experimental alcoholic liver disease: correlation with plasma endotoxin, prostaglandin E2, leukotriene B4 and thromboxane B2. *Am. J. Pathol* **142**, 367–373.

Nanji, A.A., Khwaja, S., Khettry, U. and Sadrzadeh, S.M.H. (1994a) Plasma endothelin levels in chronic ethanol fed rats: relationship to pathologic liver injury. *Life Sciences* **54**, 423–428.

Nanji, A.A., Khwaja, S. and Sadrzadeh, S.M.H. (1994b) Decreased prostacyclin production by liver non-parenchymal cells precedes liver injury in experimental alcoholic liver disease. *Life Sciences* **54**, 455–461.

Nanji, A.A., Sadrzadeh, S.M.H., Thomas, P. and Yamanaka, T. (1994c) Eicosanoid profile and evidence for endotoxin tolerance in chronic ethanol-fed rats. *Life Sciences* **55**, 611–620.

Nathan, C. (1992) Nitric oxide as a secretory product of mammalian cells. *FASEB Journal* **6**, 3051–3064.

Nishida, J., Abril, E.R., McDonnell, D., Jolley, C.S., Krasovich, M.A., McCuskey, R.S., Earnest, D.L. and Watson, R.R. (1992a) Effects of the combination of ethanol and cocaine on hepatic sinusoids in rats. *Hepatology* **16**, 235A.

Nishida, J., Baker, G.L. and McCuskey, R.S. (1995) Protective role of nitric oxide in the TNFα mediated hepatic microvascular response following acute ethanol ingestion. *Microcirculation* **2**, 108.

Nishida, J., Baker, G.L. and McCuskey, R.S. (2000) TNF-alpha and inhibition of nitric oxide synthesis mediate the hepatic microvascular response induced by acute ethanol ingestion. *Hepatology Research* **16**, 98–111.

Nishida, J., Ekataksin, W., McDonnell, D. and McCuskey, R.S. (1992b) A small dose of ethanol exacerbates hepatic microcirculatory impairment, endotoxemia, and lethality in septic mice. *Hepatology* **16**, 235A.

Nishida, J., Ekataksin, W., McDonnell, D., Urbaschek, R., Urbaschek, B. and McCuskey, R.S. (1994a) Ethanol exacerbates hepatic microvascular dysfunction, endotoxemia and lethality in septic mice. *Shock* **1**, 413–418.

Nishida, J., McCuskey, R.S., McDonnell, D. and Fox, E.S. (1994b) Protective role of nitric oxide in hepatic microcirculatory dysfunction during endotoxemia. *American Journal of Physiology* **30**, G1135–G1141.

Nishida, J., McDonnell, D., Krasovich, M.A., Ekataksin, W. and McCuskey, R.S. (1999) *In vivo* and electron microscopic observations of the responses of the hepatic sinusoid to interleukin-1. *Bulletin of the Tokyo Dental College* **40**, 139–148.

Nishida, J., McDonnell, D., Krasovich, M.A. and McCuskey, R.S. (1993) Effects of IL-1 on Kupffer cells and the hepatic sinusoidal microcirculation. In *Cells of the Hepatic Sinusoid IV*, edited by E. Wisse and D.L. Knook, pp. 148–151. Leiden: Kupffer Cell Foundation.

Nolan, J.P. and Camara, D.S. (1982) Endotoxin, sinusoidal cells, and liver injury. *Progress in Liver Disease* **7**, 361–376.

Nolan, J.P., Leibowitz, A. and Vladutiu, A.L. (1980) Influence of alcohol on Kupffer Cell function and possible significance in liver injury. In *The Reticuloendothelial System and the Pathogenesis of Liver Disease*, edited by H. Liehr and M. Grun, pp. 125–136. Amsterdam: Elsevier/North Holland Press.

Orrego, H., Carmichael, F.J., Saldivia, Giles, H.G., Sandrin, S. and Israel, Y. (1988) Ethanol-induced increase in portal blood flow: role of adenosine. *American Journal of Physiology* **254**, G495–G501.

Oshita, M., Takei, Y., Hijioka, T., Goto, M., Fukui, H., Nishimura, Y., Kawano, S., Fusamoto, H., Kamada, T. and Sato, N. (1992) Ethanol induced vasoconstriction in perfused rat liver. *Microcirc Ann* **8**, 19–22.

Oshita, M., Takei, Y., Kawano, S., Yoshihara, H., Hijioka, T., Fukui, H., Goto, M., Masuda, E., Nishimura, Y., Fusamoto, H. and Kamada, T. (1993) Roles of endothelin-1 and nitric oxide in the mechanism for ethanol-induced vasoconstriction in the rat liver. *Journal of Clinical Investigation* **91**, 1337.

Pannen, B.H.J., Al-Adili, F., Bauer, M., Clemens, M.G. and Geiger, K.K. (1998) Role of endo-thelins and nitric oxide in hepatic reprefusion injury in the rat. *Hepatology* **27**, 755–764.

Pannen, B.H.J., Bauer, M., Zhang, J.X., Robotham, J.L. and Clemens, M.G. (1996) Endotoxin pretreatment enhances the portal venous contractile responses to endothelin-1. *American Journal of Physiology* **270**, H7–H15.

Radi, R., Beckman, J.S., Bush, K.M. and Freeman, B.A. (1991) Peroxynitrite oxidation of sulfhydryls. The cytotoxic potential of superoxide and nitric oxide. *Journal of Biological Chemistry* **266**, 4244–4250.

Sarphie, G., D'Souza, N.B., Thiel, D.H.V., Hill, D., McClain, C.J. and Deaciuc, I.V. (1997) Dose- and time-dependent effects of ethanol on functional and structural aspects of the liver sinusoid in the mouse. *Alcoholism: Clinical and Experimental Research* **21**, 1128–1136.

Sarphie, T.G., Deaciuc, I.V., Spitzer, J.J. and D'Souza, N.B. (1995) Liver sinusoid during chronic alcohol consumption in the rat: an electron microscope study. *Alcoholism: Clinical and Experimental Research* **19**, 291–298.

Sarphie, T.G., D'Souza, N.B. and Deaciuc, I.V. (1996a) Kupffer cell inactivation prevents lipopolysaccharide-induced structural changes in the rat liver sinusoid: an electron-microscope study. *Hepatology* **23**, 788–795.

Sarphie, T.G., D'Souza, N.B., Spitzer, J.J. and Deaciuc, I.V. (1996b) Chronic alcohol feeding in liquid diet or in drinking water has similar effects on electron microscopic appearance of the hepatic sinusoid in the rat. *Alcoholism: Clinical and Experimental Research* **20**, 973–979.

Sato, N., Eguchi, H., Takei, Y., Hijioka, T., Tsuji, S., Matsumura, T., Hayashi, N., Kawano, S. and Kamada, T. (1987a) Microcirculatory aspects of the mechanism of alcoholic liver disease-sinusoidal blood flow and oxygenation at periportal regions of hepatic lobules in rats. In *Microcirculation Vol 2 – An Update*, Vol. 2, edited by M. Tsuchiya, M. Asano, Y. Michima and M. Oda, pp. 357–360. Amsterdam: Excerpta Medica.

Sato, N., Matsumura, T., Kawano, S. and Kamada, T. (1987b) Hepatic microcirculation and hepatic cellular metabolism. In *Microcirculation Vol 2 – An update*, Vol. 2, edited by M. Tsuchiya, M. Asano, Y. Mishima and M. Oda, pp. 309–312. Amsterdam: Excerpta Medica.

Shah, V., Haddad, F.G., Garcia-Cardena, G., Frangos, J.A., Mennone, A., Groszmann, R.J. and Sessa, W.C. (1997) Liver sinusoidal endothelial cells are responsible or nitric oxide modulation of resistance in the hepatic sinusoids. *Journal of Clinical Investigation* **100**, 2923–2930.

Shaw, S., Heller, E.A. and Friedman, H.S. (1977) Increased hepatic oxygenation following ethanol administration in the baboon. *Proceedings of the Society for Experimental Biology and Medicine* **156**, 509–513.

Sherman, I.A. and Fisher, M.M. (1987) Hepatic microvascular patterns in normal and diseased liver. In *Microcirculation Vol 2 – An Update*, Vol. 2, edited by M. Tsuchiya, M. Asano, Y. Mishima and M. Oda, pp. 345–348. Amsterdam: Excerpta Medica.

Shibayama, Y. (1987) Enhanced hepatotoxicity of endotoxin by hypoxia. *Pathology Research and Practice* **182**, 390–395.

Shibayama, Y., Asaka, S. and Nakata, N. (1991) Endotoxin hepatotoxicity augmented by ethanol. *Experimental Molecular Pathology* **55**, 196–202.

Shibayama, Y. and Nakata, K. (1985) Localization of increased hepatic vascular resistance in liver cirrhosis. *Hepatology* **5**, 643–648.

Spolarics, Z., Spitzer, J.J., Wang, J.F., Xie, J., Kolls, J. and Greenberg, S. (1993) Alcohol administration attenuates LPS-induced expression of inducible nitric oxide synthase in Kupffer and hepatic endothelial cells. *Biochemistry and Biophysics Research Communications* **197**, 606–611.

Suematsu, M., Goda, N., Sana, T., Kashiwagi, S., Egawa, T., Shinoda, Y. and Ishimura, Y. (1995) Carbon monoxide: an endogenous modulator of sinusoidal tone in the perfused liver. *Journal of Clinical Investigation* **96**, 2431–2437.

Suematsu, M. and Ishimura, Y. (2000) The heme oxygenase-carbon monoxide system: a regulator of hepatobiliary function. *Hepatology* **31**, 3–6.

Suematsu, M., Kashiwagi, S., Sano, T., Goda, N., Shinoda, Y. and Ishimura, Y. (1994) Carbon monoxide as an endogenous modulator of hepatic vascular perfusion. *Biochemistry and Biophysics Research Communications* **205**, 1333–1337.

Thurman, R.G. (1998) II. Alcoholic liver injury involves activation of Kupffer cells by endotoxin. *American Journal of Physiology* **275**, G605–G611.

Thurman, R.G., Bradford, B.U., Iimuro, Y., Frankenberg, M.V., Knecht, K.T., Connor, H.D., Adachi, Y., Wall, C., Arteel, G.E., Raleigh, J.A., Forman, D.T. and Mason, R.P. (1999) Mechanisms of alcohol-induced hepatotoxicity: studies in rats. *Frontiers in Bioscience* **4**, E42–E46.

Thurman, R.G., Bradford, B.U., Iimuro, Y., Knecht, K.T., Arteel, G.E., Yin, M., Connor, H.D., Wall, C., Raleigh, J.A., Frankenberg, M.V., Adachi, Y., Forman, D.T., Brenner, D., Kadiiska, M. and Mason, R.P. (1998) The role of gut-derived bacterial toxins and free radicals in alcohol-induced liver injury. *Journal of Gastroenterology & Hepatology* **13**(Suppl), S39–S50.

Thurman, R.G., Bradford, B.U., Iimuro, Y., Knecht, K.T., Connor, H.D., Adachi, Y., Wall, C., Arteel, G.E., Raleigh, J.A., Forman, D.T. and Mason, R.P. (1997) Role of Kupffer cells, endotoxin and free radicals in hepatotoxicity due to prolonged alcohol consumption: studies in female and male rats. *Journal of Nutrition* **127**, 903S–906S.

Urbaschek, B. (1987) Perspectives on Bacterial Pathogenesis and Host Defense. *Rev. Infect. Dis* **9**, S431–S659.

Urbaschek, B., Ditter, B., Becker, K.P. and Urbaschek, R. (1984) Protective effects and role of endotoxin on experimental septicemia. *Circulatory Shock* **14**, 209–222.

Urbaschek, R., Seitz, H.K., Rudi, V., Becker, K.P., Urbaschek, B. and McCuskey, R.S. (1994) Endotoxin (ET) and endotoxin-neutralizing capacity (ENC) in plasma of patients with alcoholic and non-alcoholic liver disease. *Hepatology* **20**, 318A.

Urbaschek, R. and Urbaschek, B. (1982) Aspects of beneficial endotoxin-mediated effects. *Klinische Wochenschrift* **60**, 746–748.

Urbaschek, R., Urbaschek, B., McCuskey, P.A. and McCuskey, R.S. (1986) Die Bedeutung des Reticuloendothialen Systems im Endotoxin-Snhock. *Anaesthesist* **35**, 442–443.

Vidins, E.I., Britton, R.S., Medline, A., Blandis, L.J., Israel, Y. and Orrego, H. (1985) Sinusoidal caliber in alcoholic and nonalcoholic liver disease: diagnostic and pathogenic implications. *Hepatology* **5**, 408–414.

Vollmar, B., Glasz, J., Post, S. and Menger, M.D. (1994) Depressed phagocytic activity of Kupffer cells after warm ischemia-reperfusion of the liver. *Journal of Hepatology* **20**, 301–304.

Zhang, J., Pegoli, W. and Clemens, M.G. (1993) Endothelin-1-induced hepatic sinusoidal constriction is mediated by fat storing (Ito) cells. *Circulatory Shock* **2**(Suppl), 44.

Zhang, J.X., Pegoli, W. and Clemens, M.G. (1994) Endothelin-1 induces direct constriction of hepatic sinusoids. *American Journal of Physiology* **266**, G624–G632.

Zhang, P., Xie, M., Zagorski, J. and Spitzer, J.A. (1995) Attenuation of hepatic neutrophil sequestration by anti-CINC antibody in endotoxic rats. *Shock* **4**, 262–268.

Chapter 8

Cytokines and alcohol liver disease

F. Javier Laso, J. Ignacio Madruga and Alberto Orfao

Accumulating evidence exists that chronic alcoholism is associated with an imbalanced immune response. Until now, ethanol intake has been linked to an immunosuppressive state. Nevertheless, in recent years it has been suggested that chronic alcohol consumption is associated with an activation of the immune system, which might contribute to explaining, at least in part, the pathogenesis of alcoholic liver disease. Among different cell-to-cell and soluble signals, cytokines may play an important role in the reported immunological abnormalities detected in these patients. In this chapter, we will review current knowledge on the relationship between ethanol intake, cytokines and alcoholic liver disease. For that purpose we will focus on the pathogenesis of hepatocellular lesions, the hepatic inflammatory changes and the fibrogenesis leading to liver cirrhosis.

KEYWORDS: cytokines, alcohol, alcoholism, ethanol, alcohol liver disease

BACKGROUND

At present, it is well established that chronic alcoholism is associated with important abnormalities involving the immune system which may have several pathological implications. Thus, the existence of an immunosuppressive state contributes to explain both the higher incidence and the severity of infections, usually associated with excessive ethanol (EtOH) consumption (Adams *et al.*, 1984). As an example, previous reports have shown abnormalities in the mechanisms of antigen clearance by both alveolar macrophage (Green and Kass, 1964) and Kupffer cells (Liu, 1979) in chronic alcoholism patients; moreover, in these individuals there is a defective cellular and humoral immune response against different antigens (McGregor, 1986) together with a lower natural killer (NK) cytolitic activity (Laso *et al.*, 1997a). In spite of this, in recent years, it has been suggested that chronic alcoholism is associated with a paradoxal activation of the immune system (Cook *et al.*, 1991, 1995; Kronfol *et al.*, 1993; Laso *et al.*, 1996a,b, 1997b; Santos *et al.*, 1996). A consequence of such activation could be the development of cytotoxic phenomena, which may contribute to the pathogenesis of alcoholic liver disease (ALD). Interestingly, these immunologic changes depend not only on whether or not liver disease is present, but also on the status of EtOH intake (Laso *et al.*, 1996a,b, 1997a,b). In this sense, we have reported that active EtOH intake is associated with an activation of the peripheral blood (PB) T-cells, mainly involving the CD8+ subsets, both in the presence (Laso *et al.*, 1996b, 1997b) or in the absence of

ALD (Laso *et al.*, 1996a). Furthermore, immunohistochemical methods have demonstrated the existence of T-CD8+ lymphocytes which express activation associated antigens infiltrating the liver of patients suffering from both alcoholic hepatitis and alcoholic liver cirrhosis (Si *et al.*, 1983).

In recent years, efforts have been focused on the analysis of potential abnormalities involving cytokines, in order both to understand some of the abnormalities of the immune system described above and to establish their role in the pathogenesis of ALD (McClain *et al.*, 1993; Diehl, 1999). Cytokines are low molecular weight polypeptides (generally <30 kDa), synthesized and released by different immune cells such as monocytes and macrophages, including Kupffer cells (of particular interest in ALD). From the functional point of view, cytokines display a wide range of effects including among others, inflammatory responses, modulation of the T-, B- and NK-cells immune responses, cytotoxic effects, cell growth and differentiation (Nicola, 1994). A particular subset of cytokines, the so-called chemokines, exert chemotactic effects for specific subtypes of inflammatory cells as well as lymphocytes (Luster, 1998). Preliminary studies were published in which the existence of abnormal cytokine levels in ALD were reported. These studies showed that monocytes from ALD produced higher levels of interleukin (IL) 1, IL-6 and tumoral necrosis factor (TNF) α, both spontaneously and after stimulation with lipopolysaccharide (LPS) (McClain and Cohen, 1989; McClain *et al.*, 1993). Furthermore, increased IL-1, TNF-α, IL-6 and IL-8 serum levels have been reported in patients suffering from both alcoholic hepatitis and alcohol liver cirrhosis (Khoruts *et al.*, 1991; Hill *et al.*, 1993), serum levels of IL-6 correlating with the clinical outcome of hepatitis (Hill *et al.*, 1992). Several studies have suggested that TNF-α serum levels are of prognostic value for the identification, among alcoholic hepatitis patients, of those individuals at risk of a shorter period of survival (Felver *et al.*, 1990).

In the present chapter, we will review current knowledge on the relationship between EtOH intake, cytokines and ALD. For that purpose we will focus first on the pathogenesis of hepatocellular lesions; then, we will review the inflammatory changes, present throughout the evolution of ALD, culminating in alcoholic hepatitis; finally, we will discuss the fibrogenesis leading to liver cirrhosis.

THE ROLE OF CYTOKINES ON ALCOHOL-INDUCED HEPATOCELLULAR LESIONS

For a long time, it has been well known that chronic alcoholism is associated with both steatosis and necrosis, this being observed throughout all stages of ALD. More recently, increasing evidence exists that apoptosis occurs in experimental alcoholic liver injury models (Goldin *et al.*, 1993), representing an alternative cell death pathway in human ALD. The role of specific cytokines on these alcohol-induced hepatocellular lesions is currently under study by different groups.

Inflammatory cytokines

Among all inflammatory cytokines, TNF-α has been explored most as regards its role in the mechanisms and pathways of triggering cellular damage both in chronic alcoholism and in ALD. In this sense, accumulating data support the notion that TNF-α is directly involved in inducing liver damage in several different experimental models based on the use of toxic agents (i.e., galactosamine + LPS, Cl₄C, etc.) (Hill *et al.*, 1997). Accordingly, in these models increased TNF-α levels were found both in the serum and in the liver of the treated animals; furthermore, the observed cytotoxic effects decreased, or even disappeared, once TNF-α was blocked (Hill *et al.*, 1997).

TNF-α is a pleiotropic cytokine which may exert inflammatory, cytotoxic and growth effects on a wide range of different cell types (Nicola, 1994). Although TNF-α can be produced by other cells, macrophages and monocytes represent its major source. In chronic alcoholism, liver macrophages (Kupffer cells) are thought to be an important contributor to the overall production of TNF-α, this being especially clear in certain circumstances such as during endotoxemia. TNF-α exerts its effects through two different membrane receptors (p75 and p55) (Tracey, 1997). Binding of TNF-α to these receptors induces transcriptional activity through systems such as Jun *N*-terminal kinases (which are known to activate cell proliferation pathways), caspases (which are involved in apoptosis) or sphingomyelinase (which leads to an increased production of mitochondrial reactive oxygen species -ROS-, involved in cell necrosis/apoptosis) (Diehl, 1999). Therefore, depending on its effects, TNF-α can promote liver cell proliferation as well as hepatocellular death. In spite of this, hepatocytes from normal healthy adults usually do not die once they are exposed *in vitro* to TNF-α (Chapekar *et al.*, 1989); moreover, TNF-α enhances the proliferative activity of hepatocyte growth factor (HGF) and it plays an important role in liver regeneration after partial hepatectomy (Akerman *et al.*, 1992). Interestingly, EtOH *per se* does not induce TNF-α production, but decreases it. Accordingly, decreased TNF-α production, together with a lower secretion of other inflammatory cytokines such as IL-1β, has been shown in experimental models after both *in vitro* and *in vivo* acute EtOH exposure (Szabo *et al.*, 1996; Batey *et al.*, 1998). Thus, in ALD other factors might exist which would eventually contribute to increased TNF-α production and/or induce a greater sensitivity of liver cells to its cytotoxic effects in the absence of protective factors.

Several alcohol-related factors have been shown to stimulate production of TNF-α. LPS, after entering the portal circulation due to increased intestinal permeability during EtOH consumption, would represent a very strong stimulus for TNF-α by Kupffer cells (Bode *et al.*, 1987). Additionally, oxidative stress generated by the EtOH metabolism is an important stimulus for TNF-α production (Tracey, 1997). Oxidative stress is defined by the imbalance between the cellular production of oxidants such as free radicals and ROS, and the antioxidant defense systems such as glutathione. Interestingly, S-adenosylmethionine deficiency *per se* stimulates TNF-α-production (Chawla *et al.*, 1996). Following either of these pathways, it has been shown that in both the hepatocytes and Kupffer cells, an increased activation of nuclear factor κ-B (NF κ-B), a member of the NF κ-B/Rel proteins, exists (Tsukamoto *et al.*, 1997). NF κ-B is formed by a p50 protein and a p65 kDa molecule and it induces expression of genes encoding cell proliferation-associated proteins (i.e., c-myc and p53), cell adhesion molecules, cytokines (i.e., TNF-α, IL-1, IL-2, IL-6, IL-10) and chemokines (Bauerle *et al.*, 1994). In turn, TNF-α together with other cytokines stimulates the NF κ-B pathway, therefore amplifying the response

(Lee *et al.*, 1999). Interestingly, recent studies have shown that activation of NF κ-B may produce opposite effects depending on the type of molecule formed: an homodimer or an heterodimer. Accordingly, LPS would induce the activation of the heterodimer version of NF κ-B, which would lead to inflammatory cytokine gene expression. In contrast, acute EtOH exposure would induce a preferential expression of the NF κ-B homodimer version, which would inhibit TNF production (Mandrekar *et al.*, 1997).

In spite of the fact that TNF-α has been related to the development of liver cell damage, the specific mechanisms involved in this process remain largely unknown. TNF-α regulates lipid homeostasis in both the liver and adipose tissues and it has been suggested that it could be a potential mediator of alcoholic liver steatosis (Lin *et al.*, 1998). Cytotoxicity and hepatocellular death (necrosis/apoptosis) linked to TNFα may be due to either direct or indirect mechanisms. Accordingly, stimulation of TNF-α receptors on the membrane of hepatocytes could induce intracellular signals involved in cell death; TNF-α cell-mediated death could be related either to increased levels of ROS at the intracellular level in mitochondria and/or decreased protective factors such as intramitochondrial glutathion, manganous superoxide dismutase, nitric oxide and bcl-2 (Larrick and Wright, 1990; Hirose *et al.*, 1993; McClain *et al.*, 1993). In addition, TNF-α might act through the stimulation of other cells (i.e., leucocytes) which would release their cytotoxic products (i.e., ROS, nitric oxide, proteases). In summary, it could be hypothesized (McClain *et al.*, 1998) that EtOH consumption induces an overall dysregulation of the TNF-α system. Accordingly, in Kupffer cells, EtOH consumption would induce NF κ-B heterodimers, mainly due to the effect of LPS action, this translating into the expression of genes encoding inflammatory cytokines, including TNF-α. In contrast, a preferential stimulation of NF κ-B homodimers would occur in hepatocytes, making them more sensitive to the cytotoxic effects induced by the TNF-α secreted by Kupffer cells (Figure 8.1).

Secretion of TNF-α is usually associated with the production of other cytokines and chemokines such as IL-1β and IL-12, among others. The stimuli for IL-1 production (i.e., LPS) as well as its effects largely overlap with those of TNF-α, except for the absence of a clear cytotoxic effect on hepatocytes (Nicola, 1994). Regarding IL-12, we have recently reported its increase in serum during active EtOH intake in patients with alcohol liver cirrhosis as well as in alcoholic subjects without ALD (Laso *et al.*, 1998). Increased production of IL-12 could be related to LPS, since high IL-12 serum levels have been found following LPS injection in mice (Heizel *et al.*, 1994); in addition, pretreatment with anti-IL-12 antibodies reduces the effects of endotoxin (Heizel *et al.*, 1994). Increased production of IL-12 could be directly responsible for both the proliferation and functional differentation of the cytolytic compartment of PB lymphocytes and/or for priming secretion of T-helper (Th) -1 cytokines (Hendrzak and Brunda, 1995).

T-cell derived cytokines

For many years, it has been shown that T-cells play an important modulatory role in specific immune responses through the secretion of cytokines. More recently, different patterns of cytokine secretion by T-cells have been described, from which

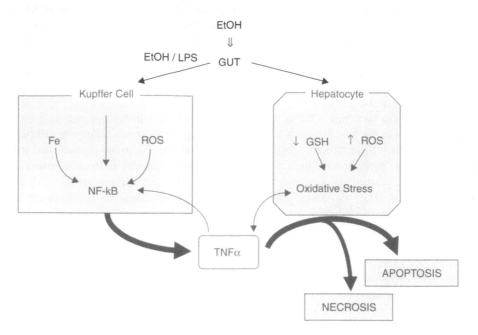

Figure 8.1 The role of TNF-α on alcohol-induced hepatocellular lesions. LPS, lipopolysaccharide; EtOH, ethanol; ROS, reactive oxygen species; GSH, glutathione.

the Th-1 (i.e., IL-2, interferon γ) and Th-2 (i.e., IL-4, IL-5, IL-10, IL-13) would be the most representative ones (Allen and Maizels, 1997). Inconsistent results have been reported in literature regarding the serum levels of Th-1 and Th-2 associated cytokines in chronic alcoholism (Blank *et al.*, 1993; Laso *et al.*, 1998; Means *et al.*, 1996; Vicente *et al.*, 1991; Wang *et al.*, 1994; Watzl *et al.*, 1993). In recent years, methods have been developed which allow the direct assessment of intracellular production of cytokines in specific lymphocyte subsets through the use of multiple stainings in which fluorochrome-conjugated monoclonal antibodies directed against different cytokines and specific lymphoid subsets are combined (Prussin and Metcalfe, 1995). By applying this strategy to the study of cytokine production by PB T-cells from chronic alcoholism patients, it has recently been suggested that active EtOH intake would be associated with a Th-1 pattern of cytokine secretion, both in the presence and in the absence of ALD (Laso *et al.*, 1999). Such observations would be in agreement with previous findings in chronic alcoholism. Firstly, the increased IL-12 serum levels found in the active ethanol consumption phase (Laso *et al.*, 1998; Szabo, 1998), might represent the stimuli responsible for priming a Th-1 response. Secondly, the expansion of NK and activated T-cells, mainly of the CD8+ subset coexpressing the HLA DR and CD11c activation-associated antigens (Laso *et al.*, 1996a,b, 1997a,b). EtOH *per se* (Parent *et al.*, 1987; Singer *et al.*, 1989) or through other mechanisms such as the induction of increased levels of gut-derived toxins (i.e., endotoxin/LPS) (Bode *et al.*, 1987; Presson, 1991) as well as the increased expression of both HLA class I molecules (Chedid *et al.*, 1991)

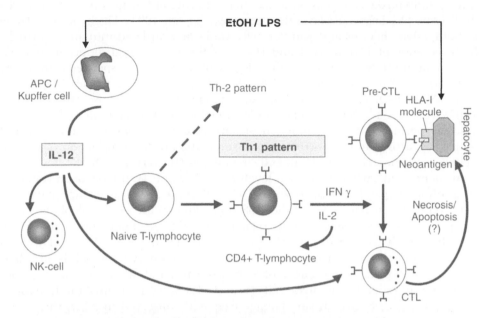

Figure 8.2 Proposed effects of T-cell derived cytokines on alcohol liver disease. Th, T helper; NK, natural killer; IL, interleukin; CTL, cytotoxic T-lymphocyte; APC, antigen-presenting cell; IFN γ, interferon-gamma.

and modified self-antigens on the surface of hepatocytes (Niemelä *et al.*, 1991) could contribute to direct the immune response against the liver. In this sense, self-reactive clones of cytotoxic cells directed against neoantigens presented by the hepatocytes would therefore be responsible, at least in part, for the hepatocellular damage (Figure 8.2). Further studies are necessary to confirm this hypothesis.

INFLAMMATORY CHANGES

Inflammatory changes (infiltrates of neutrophils and mononuclear cells) may occur either during the evolution of ALD or represent the most relevant finding in alcoholic hepatitis. Preliminary reports suggested that EtOH *per se* could be directly responsible for the inflammatory response observed in alcoholic patients; nevertheless, more recent studies have ruled out this possibility (Tsukamoto *et al.*, 1990).

Evidence exists of the important role of cytokines in the inflammatory changes observed in the liver of chronic alcoholism patients; nevertheless, the specific mechanisms underlying their effects remain largely unknown. EtOH-induced hepatocellular damage, apart from apoptosis, is able to trigger an inflammatory response, the cytokines involved in these lesions (i.e., TNF-α) also displaying an important role in the inflammatory response. In this sense, it could be summarized that in ALD, mainly in alcoholic hepatitis, the inflammatory changes observed reflect an excessive response of the immune system to the stimuli usually associated with EtOH intake, as discussed above. Several circumstances such as infection, hypoxia as well as endotoxemia following either massive EtOH intake or digestive bleeding would favor this response (Ishii *et al.*, 1993). The hyperstimulation of both T-lymphocytes and Kupffer cells would be translated into an abnormally high secretion of TNF-α, IL-1 and IL-6 together with several different chemokines including IL-8 as well as a higher degree of lymphocyte associated cytotoxicity (Batey *et al.*, 1998, 1999; Hill *et al.*, 1993; Si *et al.*, 1983). Several studies have shown that TNF-α itself is able to trigger such inflammatory response (Iimuro *et al.*, 1997). It exerts its effects through the production of vasodilatation and increased vascular permeability, the induction of leukocyte and adhesion endothelial cell molecules, activation of neutrophils and stimulation of the production of inflammatory cytokines (IL-1 and IL-6) and chemokines (IL-8) (Figure 8.3).

As mentioned earlier, increased levels of TNF-α and IL-6 have been reported in alcoholic hepatitis (Khoruts *et al.*, 1991). Recently, several groups have also detected high concentrations of the IL-8 chemokine in the sera of alcoholic hepatitis patients, its levels being directly related to the degree of neutrophil infiltration and the severity of the disease (Hill *et al.*, 1993; Huang *et al.*, 1996). The local production of chemoattractants, which favor infiltration by neutrophils and their activation, followed by the release of ROS, proteases and other enzymes together with the infiltration by cytotoxic cells (Si *et al.*, 1983) would contribute to explain the great degree of liver tissue damage frequently observed in ALD; this would represent an additional stimulus for an amplified inflammatory response. The specific role of each chemokine will not be discussed in detail here since it will reviewed in depth elsewhere in this book.

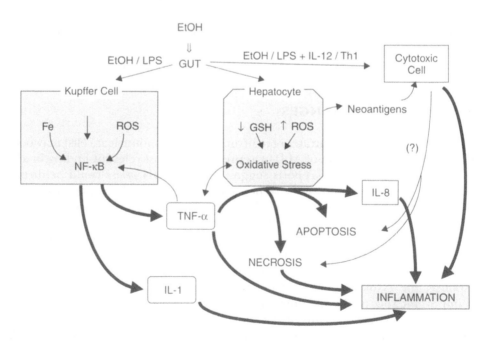

Figure 8.3 Factors promoting liver inflammatory changes in chronic alcoholism.

CYTOKINES AND ALCOHOL-INDUCED HEPATIC FIBROSIS

Liver fibrosis is the end-stage of chronic liver damage. Regardless of the type of injury (i.e., EtOH, viruses, iron or copper overload, etc.), the response of the liver always shows a similar pattern: fibrosis. The key components of the fibrotic response include fibrogenic cells, the extravascular matrix and soluble factors which induce fibrogenesis, among which cytokines play quite a relevant role (Figure 8.4). In ALD, early fibrotic lesions develop around the central vein. From the histopathological point of view, hepatic fibrosis is characterized by the preferential accumulation of extracellular matrix proteins such as the "fibrillar" forms of collagen (type I and III), several types of proteoglycans (i.e., chondroitin sulfate) and specialized glyco-proteins (fibronectin and others). The major fibrogenic cell type is the hepatic stellate cell (HSC), which has also been termed lipocyte and Ito cell. HSCs are resident nonparenchymal cells found in the subendothelial space of Disse, between hepatocytes and sinusoidal endothelial cells. HSCs are the main storage site of vitamin A compounds (retinoids) and they are distributed throughout the liver, specifically accumulating in areas of injury. Chronic exposure of the liver to toxic factors such as EtOH induces activation of HSC. Activation of HSCs develops at least in two different stages: initiation and perpetuation (Friedman, 1999). Initiation refers to the earliest changes in the phenotype that render HSCs more responsive to growth factors such as cytokines, due to the high expression of cytokine receptors on the surface membrane (Friedman, 1999). Afterwards, the transition from a quiescent to a proliferative, fibrogenic and contractile HSC, with

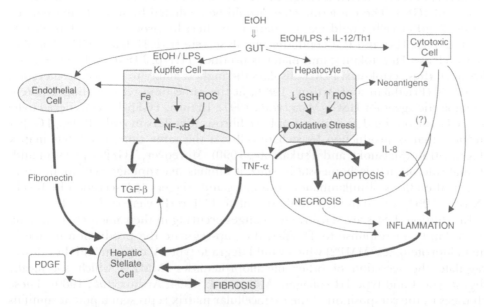

Figure 8.4 Cytokines and alcohol-induced hepatic fibrosis. TGF-β, transforming growth factor-β; PDGF, platelet-derived growth factor.

reduced vitamin A content, is observed, the specific role of vitamin A depletion remaining unknown. Evidence exists supporting the importance of paracrine stimuli from injured hepatocytes, neighbouring endothelium, Kupffer cells, and platelets that trigger the earliest changes observed in HSCs (Friedman, 1999). Accordingly, acetaldhyde, lipid peroxides and ROS generated in the hepatocyte as a consequence of EtOH metabolism, would stimulate HSCs. However, it should be noted that a prerequisite for these factors to exert their effects might be a pre-existing HSC activation state (Maher *et al.*, 1994). Kupffer cells as well as other macrophages that can infiltrate areas of injury before HSC activation, would influence the activation of these latter cells through the secretion of TNF-α, transforming growth factor (TGF) β-1, platelet-derived growth factor (PDGF), IL-1, TGF-α, insulin-like growth factor I (IGF I) and IL-6 (Matsuoka *et al.*, 1989). Endothelial cells from the sinusoid vessels respond to the injury through the secretion of fibronectin, which in turn may also activate HSCs. Endothelial cells also participate in the conversion of TGFβ-1 from the latent profibrogenic protein form to its active form through secretion of plasminogen activating factor (Sato *et al.*, 1990). Platelets may induce a significant paracrine activation of HSCs through secretion of factors involved in fibrogenesis such as PDGF and TGFβ-1 (Tsukamoto, 1999).

Perpetuation of HSC activation is reflected by other effects of soluble factors which induce, on these cells, proliferation, chemotaxis, fibrogenesis, contractility, matrix degradation, cytokine release, etc; the final outcome is an increased production of extracellular matrix. Additionally, the above mentioned factors also act as a stimulus to the already activated HSC, inducing a sustained activation state, even in the absence of the agents initially responsible for the injury. The stimulation of HSCs can be mediated by direct autocrine or paracrine mechanisms. The autocrine effect is exerted through the secretion by HSC of TGF-α, TGF-β, PDGF, IL-6 and IGF I. The paracrine effect would be mediated by several different cell types. Kupffer cells would exert a paracrine effect by producing TGF-β, PDGF, TNF-α, IGF, IL-1 and IL-6; endothelial cells secrete IL-1, IL-6 and HGF; lymphocytes release Th cytokines; and platelets produce TGF-β, PDGF and chemokines. From all these cytokines; PDGF displays the highest ability to induce proliferation of HSCs (Friedman and Arthur, 1989), at the same time representing a potent chemotactic agent for HSCs (Marra *et al.*, 1997). In turn, TGFβ-1 is considered to be a key factor on the development of liver fibrosis (Sanderson *et al.*, 1995). TGFβ-1 induces matrix production by stellate cells. At the same time, it inhibits matrix degradation (Matsuoka and Tsukamoto, 1990). Moreover, TGFβ-1 plays an additional role on matrix homeostasis, since it inhibits macrophage activation, counteracts the effects of inflammatory cytokines and triggers IgA secretion by B-cells (Nicola, 1994), which in turn would stimulate TNF-α (Devière *et al.*, 1991).

In addition, HSCs are sensitive to changes occuring in their microenvironment. Accordingly, in response to TGFβ-1, they up-regulate the production of matrix metalloproteinases (MMP2) which would degrade type IV colagen and they down-regulate the secretion of other metalloproteinases (MMP1) which specifically digest type I and type III collagen (Milani *et al.*, 1994; Arthur *et al.*, 1989). These changes in the composition of the extracellular matrix represent a potent stimulus for a sustained activation of HSCs. Recent studies have suggested the possibility that IL-10, a Th2-associated cytokine, could act on the homeostasis of the extracellular matrix through the induction of secretion of an antifibrogenic factor (Tsukamoto, 1999; Thompson *etal.*, 1997). IL-10 can also be produced by HSCs once stimulated with TNF-α or LPS; these findings demonstrate that the activation of HSCs triggers a negative self-regulatory effect on collagen production by stellate cells. It is possible that the failure of a sustained IL-10 production by the HSC underlies the mechanisms that contribute to the pathological progression to liver cirrhosis. Interestingly, as mentioned above, we have found that in chronic alcoholism, active EtOH consumption is associated with a Th1 pattern of cytokine secretion by PB T-cells, both in patients without liver disease and in alcoholic liver cirrhosis. In contrast, after a withdrawal period of >1 year, cirrhotic patients show a marked increase in intracellular expression of IL-4, a Th2-associated cytokine (Laso *et al.*, 1999). Therefore, it could be speculated that active EtOH intake would amplify the ongoing fibrogenesis in chronic alcoholism patients, while EtOH withdrawal would be associated with a restoration of inhibitory mechanisms of liver fibrogenesis through a higher production of Th2-associated cytokines.

ACKNOWLEDGMENTS

This study was supported by Institutional Grants from both the Fondo de Investigaciones Sanitarias de la Seguridad Social (FIS 91/190201 and 99/1239) and Junta de Castilla y León (SA82/96, SA12/99 and SA071/01).

REFERENCES

Adams, H.G. and Jordan, C. (1984) Infections in the alcoholic. *Med Clin North Am* **68**, 179–200.

Allen, J.E. and Maizels, R.M. (1997) Th1-Th2: reliable paradigm or dangerous dogma? *Immunol Today* **18**, 387–392.

Arthur, M.J.P., Friedman, S.L., Roll, F.J. and Bissell, D.M. (1989) Lipocytes from normal rat liver release a neutral metalloproteinase that degrades basement membrane (type IV) collagen. *J Clin Invest* **84**, 1076–1085.

Batey, R., Cao, Q., Pang, G., Russel, A. and Clancy, R. (1998) Decreased tumor necrosis factor alpha and interleukin-1 production from intrahepatic mononuclear cells in chronic ethanol consumption and upregulation by endotoxin. *Alcohol Clin Exp Res* **22**, 150–156.

Batey, R.G., Clancy, R.L., Pang, G.T. and Cao, Q. (1999) Alcoholic hepatitis as a T-cell mediated disorder: an hypothesis. *Alcohol Clin Exp Res* **23**, 1207–1209.

Bauerle, P.A. and Henkel, T. (1994) Function and activation of NF-κB in the immune system. *Ann Rev Immunol* **12**, 141–179.

Bautista, A.P. (1998) The role of Kupffer cells and reactive oxygen species in hepatic injury during acute and chronic alcohol intoxication. *Alcohol Clin Exp Res* **22**, 255S–259S.

Blank, S.E., Meadows, G.G., Pfister, L.J. and Gallucci, R.M. (1993) Natural killer cells and alcohol. *Adv Bioscience* **86**, 79–90.

Bode, C., Kugler, V. and Bode, J.C. (1987) Endotoxemia in patients with alcoholic and non-alcoholic cirrhosis and in subjects with no evidence of chronic liver disease following acute alcohol excess. *J Hepatol* 8–14.

Cook, R.T., Garvey, M.J., Booth, B.M., Goeken, J.A., Stewart, B. and Noel, M. (1991) Activated CD-8 cells and HLA DR expression in alcoholic without overt liver disease. *J Clin Immunol* **11**, 246–253.

Cook, R.T., Ballas, Z.K., Waldschmidt, T.J., Vandersteen, D., LaBrecque, D.R. and Cook, B.L. (1995) Modulation of T-cell adhesion markers, and the CD45R and CD57 antigens in humans alcoholics. *Alcohol Clin Exp Res* **19**, 555–563.

Chapekar, M.S., Hugget, A.C. and Thorgeirsson, S.S. (1989) Growth modulatory effects of a liver-derived growth inhibitor, transforming growth factor beta 1 and recombinant tumor necrosis factor alpha in normal and neoplastic cells. *Exp Cell Res* **185**, 247–257.

Chawla, R.K., Eastin, C.E., Watson, W.H., Lee, E.Y., Bagby, G.J. and McClain, C.J. (1996) S-adenosylmethionine deficiency and tumor necrosis factor alfa in endotoxin-induced hepatic injury. In *Methionine Metabolism: Molecular Mechanism and Clinical Implications*, edited by J.M. Mato and A. Caballero, pp. 263–270. Madrid: CSIC.

Chedid, A., Mendenhall, C.L. Mortiz, T. and the Veterans Administration Cooperative Study no. 275 (1991) Cell-mediated immune damage in alcoholic liver disease. *Hepatology* **14**, 165 (abstr).

Devière, J., Vaerman, J.P., Content, J., Denys, C., Schandene, L., Vandenbussche, P., Sibille, Y. and Dupont, E. (1991) IgA triggers tumor necrosis factor alfa secretion by monocytes: a study in normal subjects and patients with alcoholic cirrhosis. *Hepatology* **13**, 670–675.

Diehl, A.M. (1999) Cytokines and the molecular mechanisms of alcoholic liver disease. *Alcohol Clin Exp Res* **23**, 1419–1424.

Felver, M.E., Mezey, E., McGuire, M., Mitchell, M.C., Herlong, H.F., Veech, G.A. and Veech, R.L. (1990) Plasma tumor necrosis factor alfa predicts decreased long-term survival in severe alcoholic hepatitis. *Alcohol Clin Exp Res* **14**, 255–259.

Friedman, S.L. and Arthur, M.J.P. (1989) Activation of cultured rat hepatic lipocytes by Kupffer cell conditioned medium: direct enhancement of matrix synthesis and stimulation of cell proliferation via induction of platelet-derived growth factor receptors. *J Clin Invest* **84**, 1780–1785.

Friedman, S.L. (1993) The cellular basis of hepatic fibrosis: mechanisms and treatment strategies. *N Engl J Med* **328**, 1828–1835.

Friedman, S.L. (1999) Stellate cell activation in alcoholic fibrosis – an overview. *Alcohol Clin Exp Res* **23**, 904–910.

Goldin, R.D., Hunt, N.C., Clark, J. and Wickramasinghe, S.N. (1993) Apoptotic bodies in a murine model of alcoholic liver disease: Reversibility of ethanol-induced changes. *J Pathol* **171**, 73–76.

Green, G.M. and Kass, E.H. (1964) Factors influencing the clearance of bacteria by lung. *J Clin Invest* **43**, 769–776.

Heizel, F.P., Berko, R.M., Ling, P., Hakimi, J. and Schoenhaut, D.S. (1994) Interleukin 12 is produced *in vivo* during endotoxemia and stimulates synthesis of gamma interferon. *Infect Immun* **62**, 4244–4249.

Hendrzak, J.A. and Brunda, M.J. (1995) Interleukin-12. Biologic activity, therapeutic utility, and role in disease. *Lab Invest* **72**, 619–637.

Higuchi, H., Kurose, I., Kato, S., Miura, S. and Ishii, H. (1996) Ethanol-induced apoptosis and oxidative stress in hepatocytes. *Alcohol Clin Exp Res* **20**, 340A–346A.

Hill, D.B., Marsano, L.S. and McClain, C.J. (1992) Increased plasma interleukin-6 activity in alcoholic hepatitis. *J Lab Clin Med* **119**, 547–552.

Hill, D.B., Marsano, L.S. and McClain, C.J. (1993) Increased plasma interleukin-8 concentrations in alcoholic hepatitis. *Hepatology* **18**, 576–580.

Hill, D., Shedlofsky, S., McClain, C., Diehl, A.M. and Tsukamoto, H. (1997) Cytokines and liver disease. In *Cytokines in Health and Disease* edited by D.G. Remick and J.S. Friedland, pp. 401–425. New York: Marcel Dekker Inc.

Hirose, K., Longo, D.L., Oppenheim, J.J. and Matsushima, K. (1993) Overexpression of mitochondrial manganese superoxide dismutase promotes the survival of tumor cells exposed to interleukin-1, tumor necrosis factor, selected anticancer drugs and ionizing radiation. *FASEB J* **7**, 361–368.

Huang, Y.S., Chan, C.Y., Wu, J.C., Pai, C.H., Chao, Y. and Lee, S.D. (1996) Serum levels of interleukin-8 in alcoholic liver disease: relationship with disease stage, biochemical parameters and survival. *J Hepatol* **24**, 377–384.

Iimuro, Y., Gallucci, R.M., Luster, M.I., Kono, H. and Thurman, R.G. (1997) Antibodies to tumor necrosis factor alpha attenuate hepatic necrosis and inflammation caused by chronic exposure to ethanol in the rat. *Hepatology* **26**, 1530–1537.

Ishii, K., Furudera, S., Kumashiro, R., Koga, Y., Hamada, T., Sata, M., Abe, H. and Tanikawa, K. (1993) Clinical and pathological features and the mechanism of development in severe alcholic hepatitis, especially in comparison with acute type fulminant hepatitis. *Alcohol Alcohol* (Suppl 1B), 97–103.

Khoruts, A., Stahnke, L., McClain, C.J., Logan, G. and Allen, J.I. (1991) Circulating tumor necrosis factor, interleukin-1 and interleukin-6 concentrations in chronic alcoholic patiens. *Hepatology* **13**, 267–276.

Kronfol, Z., Nair, M., Hill, E., Kroll, P.H., Brower, K. and Greden, J. (1993) Immune function in alcoholism: a controlled study. *Alcohol Clin Exp Res* **17**, 279–283.

Larrick, J.W. and Wright, S.C. (1990) Cytotoxic mechanism of tumor necrosis factor alfa. *FASEB J* **4**, 3215–3223.

Laso, F.J., Madruga, J.I., San Miguel, J.F., Ciudad, J., López, A., Alvarez-Mon, M. and Orfao, A. (1996a) Long lasting immunological effects of ethanol after withdrawal. *Cytometry* **26**, 275–280.

Laso, F.J., Madruga, J.I., López, A., Ciudad, J., Alvarez-Mon, M., San Miguel, J.F. and Orfao, A. (1996b) Distribution of peripheral blood lymphoid subsets in alcoholic liver cirrhosis: Influence of ethanol intake. *Alcohol Clin Exp Res* **20**, 1564–1568.

Laso, F.J., Madruga, J.I., Girón, J.A., López, A., Ciudad, J., San Miguel, J.F., Alvarez-Mon, M. and Orfao, A. (1997a). Decreased natural killer cytotoxic activity in chronic alcoholism is associated with alcohol liver disease but not ethanol consumption. *Hepatology* **25**, 1096–1100.

Laso, F.J., Madruga, J.I., López, A., Ciudad, J., Alvarez-Mon, M., San Miguel, J.F. and Orfao, A. (1997b) Abnormalities of peripheral blood T lymphocytes and natural killer cells in alcoholic hepatitis persist after a 3-month withdrawal period. *Alcohol Clin Exp Res* **21**, 672–676.

Laso, F.J., Iglesias, C., López, A., Ciudad, J., San Miguel, J.F. and Orfao, A. (1998) Increased interleukin-12 serum levels in chronic alcoholism. *J Hepatol* **28**, 771–777.

Laso, F.J., Iglesias, C., López, A., Ciudad, J., Pastor, I. and Orfao, A. (1999) Chronic alcoholism is associated with an imbalanced production of Th1/Th2 cytokines by peripheral blood T cells. *Alcohol Clin Exp Res* **23**, 1306–1311.

Lee, F.Y.J., Li, Y., Zhu, H., Yang, S.Q., Lin, H.Z., Trush, M.A. and Diehl, A.M. (1999) Tumor necrosis factor alpha increases mitochondrial oxidant production and induces expression of uncoupling protein-2 expression in the regenerating mouse liver. *Hepatology* **29**, 677–687.

Lin, H.Z., Yang, S.Q., Zeldin, G. and Diehl, A.M. (1998) Chronic ethanol consumption induces the production of Tumor Necrosis Factor-α and related cytokines in Liver and adipose tissue. *Alcohol Clin Exp Res* **22**, 231S–337S.

Liu, Y.K. (1979) Phagocytic capacity of RES in alcoholics. *J Reticuloendothel Soc* **25**, 605–613.

Luster, A.D. (1998) Chemokines: chemotactic cytokines that mediate inflammation. *N Engl J Med* **338**, 436–445.

Maher, J.J. (1999) Leukocytes as modulator of stellate cell activacion. *Alcohol Clin Exp Res* **23**, 917–921.

Maher, J.J., Tzagarakis, C. and Gimenez, A. (1994) Malondialdehyde stimulates collagen production by hepatic lipocytes only upon activation in primary culture. *Alcohol Alcohol* **29**, 605–610.

Mandrekar, P., Catalano, D. and Szabo, G. (1997) Alcohol-induced regulation of nuclear regulatory Factor-κβ in human monocytes. *Alcohol Clin Exp Res* **21**, 988–994.

Marra, F., Gentilini, A., Pinzani, M., Choudhury, G.G., Parola, M., Herbst, H., Dianzani, M.U., Laffi, G., Abboud, H.E. and Gentilini, P. (1997) Phosphatidylinositol 3-kinase is required for platelet-derived growth factor's actions on hepatic stellate cells. *Gastroenterology* **112**, 1297–1306.

Matsuoka, M., Pham, N.T. and Tsukamoto, H. (1989) Differential effects of interleukin-1 alfa, tumor necrosis factor alpha and transforming growth factor beta-1 on cell prolifer-ation and collagen formation by cultures fat-storin cells. *Liver* **9**, 71–78.

Matsuoka, M. and Tsukamoto, H. (1990) Stimulation of hepatic lipocyte collagen production by Kupffer cell-derived transforming growth factor beta: implication for a pathogenic role in alcoholic liver fibrogenesis. *Hepatology* **11**, 599–605.

McClain, C.J. and Cohen, D.A. (1989) Increased tumor necrosis factor production by mono-cytes in alcoholic hepatitis. *Hepatology* **9**, 349–351.

McClain, C., Hill, D., Schmidt, J. and Diehl, A.M. (1993) Cytokines and alcoholic liver disease. *Semin Liver Dis* **13**, 170–182.

McClain, C.J., Barve, S., Barve, S., Deaciuc, I. and Hill, D.B. (1998) Tumor necrosis factor and alcoholic liver disease. *Alcohol Clin Exp Res* **22**, 248S–252S.

MacGregor, R.R. (1986) Alcohol and immune defense. *JAMA* **256**, 1474–1479.

Means, R.T., Mendenhall, C.L., Worden, B.D., Moritz, T.E. and Chedid, A. (1996) Erythro-poietin and cytokine levels in the anemia of severe liver disease. *Alcohol Clin Exp Res* **20**, 355–358.

Milani, S., Herbst, H., Schuppan, D., Grappone, C., Pellegrini, G., Pinzani, M., Casini, A., Calabro, A., Ciancio, G. and Stefanini, F. (1994) Differential expression of matrix-metallo-proteinase-1 and -2 genes in normal and fibrotic human liver. *Am J Pathol* **144**, 528–537.

Nicola, N.A. (1994). *Guidebook to Cytokines and their receptors.* Oxford: Oxford University Press.

Niemelä, O., Juvonen, T. and Parkkila, S. (1991) Immunohistochemical demonstration of acethaldehyde-modified epitopes in human liver after alcohol consumption. *J Clin Invest* **87**, 1367–1374.

Parent, L.J., Ehrlich, R., Matis, L. and Singer, D. (1987) Ethanol: an enhancer of major histocompatibility complex antigen expression. *FASEB J* **1**, 469–473.

Presson, J. (1991) Alcohol and the small intestine. *Scand J Gastroenterol* **26**, 3–15.

Prussin, C. and Metcalfe, D.D. (1995) Detection of intracytoplasmic cytokine using flow cytometry and directly conjugated anti-cytokine antibodies. *J Immunol Methods* **188**, 117–128.

Sanderson, N., Factor, V., Nagy, P., Kopp, J., Kondaiah, P., Wakefield, L., Roberts, A.B., Sporn, M.B. and Thorgeirsson, S.S. (1995) Hepatic expression of mature transforming growth factor B1 in transgenic mice results in multiple tissue lesion. *Proc Natl Acad Sci USA* **92**, 2572–2576.

Santos, J.L., Díez, A., Luna, L., Soto, J.A., Wachter, H., Fuchs, D. and Gutierrez, F. (1996) T-cell activation, expression of adhesion molecules and response to ethanol in alcoholic cirrhosis. *Immunol Lett* **50**, 179–183.

Sato, Y., Tsuboi, R., Lyons, R., Moses, H. and Rifkin, D.B. (1990) Characterization of the activation of latent TGF-β by co-cultures of endothelial cells and pericytes or smooth muscle cells: a self-regulation system. *J Cell Biol* **111**, 757–763.

Schenker, S. and Martin, R.R. (1999) Treatment of alcoholic liver disease. In *Treatment of Liver Diseases*, edited by V. Arroyo, J. Bosch, M. Bruguera, J. Rodés and J.M. Sánchez Tapias, pp. 207–219. Barcelona: Masson.

Si, L., Whiteside, T.L., Schade, R.R. and Van Thiel, D.H. (1983) Lymphocyte subsets studied with monoclonal antibodies in liver tissues of patients with alcoholic liver disease. *Alcohol Clin Exp Res* **7**, 431–435.

Singer, D.S., Parent, L.J. and Kolber, M.A. (1989) Ethanol: an enhancer of transplantation antigen expression. *Alcohol Clin Exp Res* **13**, 480–484.

Szabo, G., Mandrekar, P., Newman, L. and Catalano, D. (1996) Regulation of human monocyte functions by acute ethanol treatment: Decreased TNF-α, IL-1 β and elevated IL-10, and TGF-β production. *Alcohol Clin Exp Res* **20**, 900–907.

Szabo, G. (1998) Monocytes, alcohol use and altered immunity. *Alcohol Clin Exp Res* **22**, 216S–219S.

Thompson, K.C., Millward-Sadler, G.H., Gentry, J. and Sheron, N. (1997) Transgenic II-10 deleted mice develop increases fibrosis in a carbon tetrachloride-induced model of hepatic cirrhosis. *Hepatology* **26**, 335A (abstr).

Tracey, K.J. (1997) Tumor necrosis factor In *Cytokines in Health and Disease*, edited by D.G. Remick and J.S. Friedland, pp. 223–239. New York: Marcel Dekker Inc.

Tsukamoto, H., Gaal, K. and French, S.W. (1990) Insights into the pathogenesis of alcoholic liver necrosis and fibrosis: Status report. *Hepatology* **12**, 599–608.

Tsukamoto, H., Lin, M., Pham, T.V., Nanji, A. and Fong, T.L. (1997) Role of inflammation in Liver fibrogenesis. In *Therapy in Liver Disease: the pathophysiological Basis of Therapy*, edited by V. Arroyo, J. Bosch, M. Brugera and J. Rodés, pp. 173–178. Barcelona: Masson.

Tsukamoto, H. (1999) Cytokine regulation of hepatic stellate cells in liver fibrosis. *Alcohol Clin Exp Res* **23**, 911–916.

Vicente, M.M., Diez, A., Gil, B., Bermudez, J.M. and Gutierrez, F. (1991) Low serum levels of alpha-interferon, gamma-interferon and interleukin 2 in alcoholic cirrhosis. *Digest Dis Sci* **36**, 1209–1212.

Wang, Y., Huang, D.S., Giger, P.T. and Watson, R.R. (1994) Influence of chronic dietary ethanol on cytokine production by murine splenocytes and thymocytes. *Alcohol Clin Exp Res* **18**, 64–70.

Watzl, B., Lopez, M., Shahbazian, M., Chen, G., Colombo, L.L., Huang, D., Way, D. and Watson, R.R. (1993) Diet and ethanol modulate immune responses in young C57BL/6 mice. *Alcohol Clin Exp Res* **17**, 623–630.

Chapter 9

Adhesion molecules and chemokines in alcoholic liver disease

Neil C. Fisher and David H. Adams

Adhesion molecules promote interactions between cells and provide important signals for cellular activation. As such they play a critical role in regulating cellular growth, differentiation and function. In the immune system, adhesion molecules enable leukocytes to recognize and bind to endothelium, a prerequisite for extravasation into tissue. Once in tissue, adhesion molecules promote interactions between effector cells and their targets and regulate the retention and activation of tissue leukocytes. Adhesion molecules are more than cellular glue because they transmit signals from the environment into the cell (outside-in signaling) and in turn are regulated by inside-out mechanisms. Thus coordinated adhesion is involved in all aspects of inflammation and tissue repair/injury and sophisticated mechanisms have developed to regulate adhesion molecule expression and function. Because much of the liver injury in response to alcohol is mediated by inflammatory mechanisms, it is not surprising that adhesion molecule expression and function is altered in alcoholic liver disease. Increased expression of several molecules on hepatic endothelium in response to the local release of proinflammatory cytokines in alcoholic liver disease (ALD) promotes leukocyte recruitment and increased expression of molecules such as intercellular adhesion molecule 1 (ICAM-1) on hepatocytes promotes leukocyte-mediated tissue injury. A greater understanding of the mechanisms that underlie in this cellular activation will allow new therapeutic strategies to be developed based on blocking or inhibiting the function of specific cell adhesion molecules or factors that regulate their function.

KEYWORDS: inflammation, lymphocyte, leukocyte, endothelium, cytokines, hepatocyte, oxidative stress, ICAM-1, selectins

INTRODUCTION

Adhesion molecules play a critical role in mediating both cell to cell and cell to extracellular matrix interactions throughout in biology systems as diverse as the organization of distinct cell types in embryology, to the regulation of inflammatory responses to invading pathogens (Springer, 1994; Cunningham, 1995; Butcher and Picker, 1996; Gahmberg, 1997). Adhesion molecules not only promote cellular binding but also provide outside-in and inside-out signaling that allows the cells to be aware of and respond to their environment (Gahmberg, 1997; Porter and Hogg, 1997, 1998). The complex processes that regulate immune surveillance and the coordination of inflammatory responses to invading pathogens involve carefully regulated adhesion during both the afferent and efferent/effector arm of

Table 9.1 Some of the functionally important human chemokine receptors and ligands

Receptor	Chemokine
CXCR1	IL-8
CXCR2	IL-8, GRO, ENA-78
CXCR3	IP-10, Mig
CXCR4	SDF-1
CXCR5	BCA-1/BLC
CCR1	RANTES, MIP-1α, MCP-2,3
CCR2	MCP-1,2,3,4
CCR3	Eotaxin, RANTES MCP-2,3,4
CCR4	TARC, RANTES, MCP1, MIP1α
CCR5	RANTES, MIP-1α, MIP-1β
CCR6	LARC/MIP-3α
CCR7	ELC, MIP-3β
CCR8	I-309
CX3CR1	Fractalkine

the immune response. When these processes are dysregulated, they can result in the persistence of inflammatory damage and are thus implicated in the pathogenesis of a wide range of inflammatory and immune mediated diseases.

Much of the liver injury is that a consequence of alcohol-induced liver disease, is the result of the immunological/inflammatory response that alcohol stimulates. Thus, it is not surprising that adhesion molecules play an important part in determining the inflammatory response to alcohol by regulating both leukocyte recruitment and subsequent effector mechanisms that lead to liver damage. In this respect, they are crucial in determining whether patients develop acute inflammation, hepatocyte damage and alcoholic hepatitis or a chronic response and cirrhosis (Adams, 1994; Fisher *et al.*, 1996). In this chapter, we shall outline the characteristics and functional regulation of the major families of adhesion molecules and the chemotactic cytokines (chemokines) that play such a crucial role in regulating leukocyte recruitment and function. We shall then discuss how they are altered in alcoholic liver disease and their role in the pathogenesis of the inflammatory liver damage, that is a consequence of alcoholic liver disease.

The most common abbreviations used for adhesion molecules and chemokines are summarized in Table 9.1.

ADHESION MOLECULES

Categories and characteristics

Adhesion molecules may be broadly divided into four principal structural families that play distinct but complimentary roles in cellular adhesion *in vivo*.

Integrins are transmembrane glycoprotein heterodimers made up of an α and β subunit. They can exist either in an activated or inactivated state, which is dependent upon signals resulting from the engagement of other cell surface molecules or the presence of certain cytokines (Tanaka *et al.*, 1993a,b; Pate and Hogg, 1997). Integrin activation results from a conformational change that rapidly enhances ligand binding and provides a powerful mechanism for the rapid and specific regulation of integrin function (Hynes, 1992). The integrin family of adhesion molecules is subdivided according to the β chain. The most important integrins on leukocytes are the β1 integrins, which are also widely expressed on other cell types, where they mediate interactions with the extracellular matrix and β2 integrins, which are restricted to leukocytes and primarily mediate cell to cell binding via interactions with ligands belonging to the immunoglobulin superfamily (Gahmberg, 1997; Pate and Hogg, 1998). β1 integrins share a common β1 chain (CD29) which is expressed as a heterodimer with distinct α chains (CD49a to CD49f) and are also called Very Late after Activation (VLA) molecules because they were originally described as late markers of activation on T-cells. Most of the β1 integrins bind components of the extracellular matrix and provide important information to the cell about its surrounding microenvironment. In addition, one of the β1 integrins, VLA-4, (CD29/CD49d) can also bind a member of the Ig superfamily, vascular cell adhesion molecule-1 (VCAM-1), that is expressed on activated endothelium and antigen presenting cells and MAdCAM-1 (Bevilacqua, 1993). The expression of β2 integrins is restricted to leukocytes. The common β chain is designated CD18 and can be associated with several α chains including CD11a to form lymphocyte function associated antigen-1 (LFA-1) or CD11b macrophage-1 (Mac-1), which are involved in important adhesive interactions with ICAM-1 and ICAM-2 ligands from the Ig superfamily (Adams and Shaw, 1994) and CD11c which binds fibrinogen. Two β7 integrins have been described on leukocytes, α4β7 which is expressed by intraepithelial lymphocytes in the gut and mediates adhesion of T-cells to epithelium via binding to E-cadherin (Cepek *et al.*, 1994; Ihara *et al.*, 1996) and α4β7 which binds to VCAM-1, the CS-1 fragment of fibronectin or mucosal addressin cell adhesion molecule (MAdCAM-1) (Berlin *et al.*, 1993, 1995) (see below) and is associated with gut homing of T-cells (Schweighoffer *et al.*, 1993).

As well as supporting adhesion, integrins are important signal transducing molecules and their engagement by ligands can lead to diverse responses including the triggering of shape change and migration, cellular activation, proliferation or apoptosis (Ingber, 1991; Damsky and Werb, 1992).

Members of the *immunoglobulin superfamily* of receptors contain immunoglobulin-like domains. These molecules include the definitive T-cell receptors CD2, CD3, CD4 and CD8, ICAM-1 and LFA-3, which are widely expressed, and ICAM-2 and VCAM-1 which are largely restricted to endothelium. These receptors may be involved in binding to other Ig superfamily members (e.g., CD2 and LFA-3) or to integrins (e.g., ICAM-1 and LFA-1) (Adams and Shaw, 1994). The CD4 and CD8 molecules are involved in T-cell recognition of antigen presented by major histocompatibility complex (MHC) class II and MHC class I respectively. CD4 and CD8 mediate weak but crucial adhesive interactions between T-cells and either antigen presenting cells or target cells bearing antigen in association with the appropriate MHC molecules (O'Rourke and Mescher, 1992). Interactions between the T-cell receptor TCR/CD4 or TCR/CD8 on the T-cell and antigen and MHC on apposing cells is enhanced and amplified by other adhesive interactions including CD2 and

LFA-3 and LFA-1/ICAM-1 acting in a cascade of interactions to amplify cell–cell interactions (Schweighoffer and Shaw, 1992).

The ICAM's are ligands for β2 integrins; the most common adhesion molecule of this family, ICAM-1, is widely expressed on many cell types including leukocytes, endothelial and epithelial cells. ICAM-2 is constitutively expressed on endothelium, while ICAM-3 appears to be largely restricted to antigen presenting cells. VCAM-1 is expressed on endothelial cells and some antigen presenting cells and its ligand is the β1 integrin VLA-4. Expression of ICAM-1 and VCAM-1 is up-regulated by cytokine activation consistent with the important role, these receptors play in inflammatory responses (McEver, 1992; Bevilacqua, 1993). CD31 is expressed on endothelium and by a subset of mainly CD8+ T-cells. It mediates homotypic adhesion between endothelial cells and has been proposed as an adhesion trigger for CD31+ T-cells, since engagement of CD31 by antibody or homotypic binding can activate T-cell integrins (Tanaka et al., 1992; Rainger et al., 1997).

MadCAM-1 is a heavily glycosylated member of the immunoglobulin superfamily that is expressed on endothelium in the gut. It can mediate both primary and secondary adhesion of T-cells to endothelium when it engages the T-cell integrin α4β7. This pathway is involved in homing of T-cells to the gut and possibly also to inflamed synovium (Berlin et al., 1993).

Selectins are a family of three long lectin-like molecules that are unusual amongst adhesion molecules in binding not to proteins but to carbohydrate ligands (Lasky, 1992). Expression of these receptors is mainly restricted to leukocytes and endothelial cells and may be up-regulated in response to pro-inflammatory cytokines such as tumor necrosis factor (TNF)-α and interleukin (IL)-1. E-selectin is confined to endothelial cells and mediates binding to several poorly defined oligosaccharide receptors on leukocytes, including a receptor expressed on a subset of CD4 T-cells called cutaneous lymphocyte antigen. L-selectin is expressed on leukocytes and binds to an endothelial oligosaccharide to support lymphocyte binding to lymph node, high endothelial venules (Picker et al., 1993a,b). P-selectin was originally described on platelets, although it is also expressed on endothelium. P-selectin binds a subset of activated T-cells *in vitro* via its ligand PSLG-1 (Alon et al., 1994; Kanwar et al., 1997). Both P- and E-selectin play important roles in the binding of neutrophils and monocytes to inflamed endothelium.

Cadherins are involved in making "zipper"-like junctions between adjacent cell groups such as epithelial or endothelial cells. Homophilic interaction of cadherins is responsible for histogenetic clustering and segregation of embryonic tissues but some cadherins also bind integrins. E-cadherin appears to be an important ligand for the aeb7 integrin that is expressed on intraepitheial lymphocytes (Cepek et al., 1994). Cadherins are not expressed on leukocytes.

Other molecules. Other important adhesion molecules include CD43, CD44, CD73 and vascular adhesion protein-1. CD43 is widely expressed at high levels on all leukocytes including T-cells. It is absent in the Wiskott-Aldrich syndrome of immunodeficiency. CD43 is a sialoglycoprotein with a strong net negative charge-properties that suggest, it might be involved in decreasing adhesion. However, several anti CD43 mAbs can costimulate T-cells and increase homotypic adhesion but its role in the regulation of adhesion remains unclear (Ardman et al., 1992; Mentzer et al., 1987). CD44 is expressed on T- and B-cells, monocytes and granulocytes. It is one of several cell surface molecules with increased expression on memory T-cells compared with naive cells. There are several variants of CD44, produced by variable splicing of at least five different exons, as well as being expressed on leukocytes, some of these variants are also expressed by epithelium and endothelium. CD44 can carry glycosaminoglycan side chains allowing it to act as a proteoglycan. It has been proposed that, in this form, endothelial CD44 can present gycosaminoglycan-binding cytokines at the endothelial surface (Tanaka *et al.*, 1993b). CD44 has structural homology with the cartilage link protein and can act as a receptor for hyaluronate. It has been shown to mediate binding of T-cells to high endothelial venules and to synovial endothelium. Crosslinking CD44 on the cell surface of T-cells enhances their activation (Aruffo *et al.*, 1990; Webb *et al.*, 1990; Uksila *et al.*, 1997).

CD73, otherwise known as ecto-5'-nucleotidase, is a glycosyl-phosphatidylinositol-linked 70-kDa molecule expressed on different cell types, including vascular endothelium and subsets of lymphocytes. CD73 is involved in lymphocyte activation, proliferation and adhesion to endothelium where CD73 probably acts to amplify adhesion via activation of tyrosine phosphorylation dependent pathways (Airas *et al.*, 1995, 1997).

Vascular adhesion protein-1 (VAP-1) is a dimeric 170-kDa endothelial transmembrane molecule that is most strongly expressed on the high endothelial venules of peripheral lymph nodes and on hepatic endothelia under normal conditions, although it can be up-regulated at several sites with inflammation (McNab *et al.*, 1996; Salmi *et al.*, 1993). VAP-1 mediates tissue-selective lymphocyte adhesion in a sialic acid-dependent manner and is also shed in a soluble form, which is elevated in the circulation in liver disease (Salmi *et al.*, 1993). VAP-1 appears to be important for lymphocyte adhesion to hepatic endothelium (Yoong *et al.*, 1998; McNab *et al.*, 1996) (see below).

Regulation of leukocyte adhesion

Adhesion molecules play critical roles at all stages of evolution of an inflammatory response. They are required for antigen presentation and activation of antigen specific T-cells in the instigation of lymphocyte driven responses. We will not discuss these processes at length but direct the interested reader to one of several excellent review articles (Allison *et al.*, 1995; Grewal and Flavell, 1998). The process of leukocyte adhesion to and migration through endothelium, which is critical for recruitment into tissue, is dependent on adhesion; as is the subsequent activation and survival of leukocytes in tissue and their ability to interact with target cells (Adams and Shaw, 1994; Bradley and Watson, 1996; Butcher *et al.*, 1999).

Leukocyte recruitment to tissue

It is important that leukocyte recruitment into tissue is carefully regulated to allow for continuing immune surveillance and the control of unnecessary inflammation (Adams and Shaw, 1994). Recruitment requires that leukocytes first recognize and then adhere to inflamed endothelium before migrating into tissue. Leukocyte adhesion to endothelium is controlled by a sequence of adhesive interactions

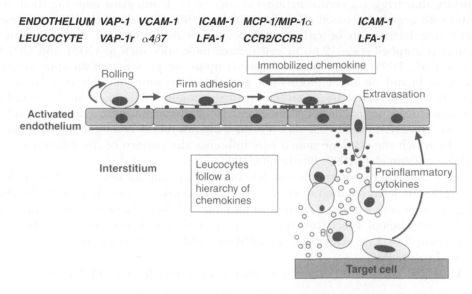

| ENDOTHELIUM | VAP-1 | VCAM-1 | ICAM-1 | MCP-1/MIP-1α | ICAM-1 |
| LEUCOCYTE | VAP-1r | α4β7 | LFA-1 | CCR2/CCR5 | LFA-1 |

Figure 9.1 Leukocyte interactions with endothelium. The molecules involved in mediating the separate adhesive steps between lymphocytes and hepatic endothelium are shown in italics at the top of the figure. Different combinations of molecules will be involved in recruiting different subsets of leukocytes (see text).

acting in a cascade which provides a powerful mechanism for controlling inflammatory responses. The sequence of events involved are illustrated in Figure 9.1 and are dependent upon binding of adhesion molecules and thus in turn other factors that regulate the expression and affinity of adhesion molecule binding (Springer, 1994).

Primary adhesion (tethering). This step involves transient, activation-independent binding of leukocytes to inflamed endothelium and provides the initial point of contact between a circulating leukocyte and endothelium. It is classically mediated by selectins that bind to carbohydrate counter-receptors and induce the leukocyte to roll on the endothelium (Lasky, 1992). The differential expression of selectin receptors on leukocytes may influence the "homing" of those cells to specific tissues. The relatively long length of the selectin molecules extending from the glycocalyx allows them to tether passing leukocytes, which may then either be bound strongly by other endothelial adhesive interactions, or disengage if strong adhesion is not triggered. Under some circumstances other molecules can also mediate tethering including the α4 integrins and their ligands VCAM-1 and MAdCAM-1 (Jones *et al.*, 1994; Berlin *et al.*, 1995; Lalor *et al.*, 1997).

Secondary, strong adhesion. Strong, secondary adhesion is mediated by leukocyte integrins such as LFA-1 and VLA-4 and their respective endothelial ligands, ICAM-1, ICAM-2 and VCAM-1 of the immunoglobulin superfamily. These interactions bring the rolling, tethered leukocyte to a complete halt allowing it to bind strongly to the vascular wall. However, integrin-mediated adhesion requires activation for efficient ligand engagement and an additional step is required after tethering in which leukocytes are exposed to activating factors at the endothelial surface that trigger a conformational change in their integrins allowing them to bind with greatly increased efficiency (Butcher, 1991; Tanaka *et al.*, 1993b). These activating factors can be either cytokines, particularly those of the chemokine family (Campbell *et al.*, 1998) or cell surface molecules such as CD31 and CD73 (Airas *et al.*, 1995). Adhesion also depends upon the presence of an appropriate integrin ligand on the endothelium and the expression of both ICAM-1 and VCAM-1 is increased by pro-inflammatory cytokines. However, under certain circumstances, particular cytokines may have distinct effects on endothelial activation. Thus IL-4 may up-regulate VCAM-1 but not ICAM-1, suggesting a mechanism by which the cytokine milieu may influence the pattern of the inflammatory infiltrate (Chin *et al.*, 1992; Bevilacqua, 1993).

Migration. After strong adhesion, leukocytes may migrate into tissue under the influence of local promigratory factors. Many cytokines may induce leukocyte migration *in vitro*, but the most important family of chemotactic cytokines appears to be the chemokines, structurally related cytokines that share the ability of triggering leukocyte subset-specific adhesion and migration (Adams and Lloyd, 1997; Luster, 1998).

Thus, recruitment of particular leukocytes to specific tissues will depend on:

(i)   The adhesion molecules expressed on the endothelium;
(ii)   The adhesion molecules expressed on the leukocyte;
(iii)   The presence of appropriate proadhesive cytokines and chemotactic factors.

The combination of tethering (primary adhesion), triggering (integrin activation signal), integrin-mediated adhesion (secondary adhesion) and chemotactic factor are all required to fulfill the requirements for leukocyte recruitment (Butcher, 1991) and will determine whether, for instance, a response is characterized by acute inflammation involving neutrophils or chronic inflammation involving monocytes and lymphocytes.

CHEMOKINES

Categories and characteristics

Chemokines are a family of structurally related chemotactic cytokines that are secreted by a wide range of cells including, leukocytes, platelets, fibroblasts, endothelial and epithelial cells (Figure 9.2; Tables 9.1 and 9.2). Around 50 different human chemokines have been demonstrated, which can be divided into 4 groups according to their structure (Baggiolini, 1998; Luster, 1998). The two largest groups are the α or CXC chemokines, in which the first two cysteine residues are separated by an intervening amino acid (hence CXC) and the β or CC chemokines in which the first two cysteines are adjacent (Luster, 1998). Two other chemokines are prototypes of novel structural families; lymphotactin, which exhibits significant homology to both α and β chemokines but contains only two cysteines and fractalkine, a recently described chemokine that contains a mucin-like stalk and a transmembrane domain (Schall, 1997; Bazan *et al.*, 1997). These structural distinctions

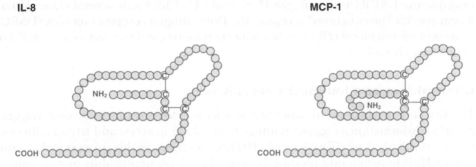

Figure 9.2 Structure of prototypic chemokines. IL-8 with characteristic CXC motif and MCP-I with CC motif.

Table 9.2 Chemokine receptors and leukocyte subset specific recruitment. The expression of various chemokine receptors on different leukocyte subsets is shown

CCR	1	2	3	4	5				
CXCR						1	2	3	4
Neutrophils						+	+		+
Monocytes	+	+			+				+
Eosinophils	+		+						
Basophils	+	+	+						
Rest T-cells									+
Act T-cells	+	+	+		+			+	+

are associated with the ability to act on particular leukocyte subsets. Thus, interleukin-8 (IL-8), the prototype CXC chemokine, is chemotactic for neutrophils predominantly, whilst monocyte chemoattractant protein-1 (MCP-1), the prototype CC chemokine, is chemotactic for mononuclear cells such as monocytes and lymphocytes. Some of the better characterized chemokines and their target cells and actions are shown in Tables 9.1 and 9.2. Chemokines are expressed at low levels in the resting state, but are rapidly up-regulated upon activation, when chemokine mRNA may comprise as much as 1% of total cellular RNA. Secretion is typically induced by pro-inflammatory cytokines such as IL-1, IL-2, TNF-α and the bacterial product lipopolysaccharide (LPS) (Baggiolini, 1998) and may also result from disturbances in the intracellular redox state. Under some circumstances, chemokine secretion may be inhibited by other cytokines such as TGF-β, IL-4 and IL-10 (Morland *et al.*, 1997).

The action of chemokines is mediated via specific cell surface receptors that are members of the rhodopsin superfamily of seven transmembrane-spanning G-protein linked molecules (Sallusto *et al.*, 1997) (Table 9.2) (Baggiolini, 1998). The intracellular domain of these receptors acts as a phosphorylation site for signal transduction. Chemokine-receptor interactions are of variable specificity; for example the CXCR1 is specific for IL-8, whilst CXCR2 binds several chemokines. A non-specific "promiscuous" receptor, the Duffy antigen receptor complex (DARC) is present on red blood cells; this binds all chemokines and may act as a "sump" for circulating chemokines.

Chemokines and leukocyte recruitment

The first step in which chemokines promote leukocyte recruitment involves triggering of a conformational change in integrins resulting in arrest and strong adhesion of tethered leukocytes (Tanaka *et al.*, 1993a). Examples of this process include the role of IL-8 in promoting binding between LFA-1 on neutrophils to its counter-receptor ICAM-1 on endothelial cells and several CC chemokines that can promotes T-cell adhesion via interactions between LFA-1 and ICAM-1 and between VLA-4 and VCAM-1 (Kuijpers *et al.*, 1992; Campbell *et al.*, 1996, 1998).

Chemokines bind to proteoglycans in the endothelial glycocalyx, thus acting as immobilized ligands and exerting their effects locally (Ebnet *et al.*, 1996). The immobilized leukocyte may undergo a sequence of adhesion-separation steps according to local chemotactic factors and cytoskeletal changes, allowing it to traverse a concentration gradient of chemokine immobilized within the extracellular matrix resulting in concentration of leukocytes at the site of chemokine secretion (which would normally correspond to the site of inflammation) (Adams *et al.*, 1994).

Few chemokines show subset-specificity for particular leukocytes and because many chemokines are released at sites of inflammation, the leukocytic infiltrate at most inflammatory sites is mixed and subject to a large number of complementary factors including the local chemokine composition in addition to the adhesion molecules expressed on leukocytes and endothelium (Butcher and Picker, 1996; Baggiolini, 1998). Highly specific chemokines/chemokine receptor interactions are particularly important in some tissues, especially the thymus and lymph node where secondary lymphoid tissue chemokine (SLC) and B lymphocyte chemokine (BLC) direct the compartmentalisation of B and T lymphocytes (Gunn *et al.*, 1998a,b). Because chemokines are secreted by epithelial cells and endothelium in addition to haematopoietic cells, multiple factors are responsible for the make-up of the chemokine milieu at any given inflammatory site and these will determine the patterns of leukocyte recruitment.

Chemokines and leukocyte activation

In addition to promoting leukocyte recruitment via activation of adhesion molecules, chemokines may play further roles in activation of leukocyte function. IL-8, for example, enhances neutrophil phagocytosis, superoxide generation and granule release (Baggiolini *et al.*, 1994) and some CC chemokines have been reported to enhance lymphocyte proliferation, by increasing production of IL-2 (Murphy *et al.*, 1996; Taub *et al.*, 1996).

Thus chemokines, like other cytokines, are likely to play a central role in most acute and chronic inflammatory diseases and evidence is accumulating for the role of chemokines in many diseases (Furie and Randolph, 1995; Luster, 1998). In the case of infectious diseases, leukocyte recruitment is vital for efficient host clearance of the pathogen. However, in uncontrolled inflammation, as occurs in autoimmune disease, graft rejection and alcoholic liver disease (see below), continuing leukocyte recruitment is harmful.

Adhesion and cellular cytotoxicity

Strong adhesion between effector leukocytes and their target cells is required for efficient cytolysis to occur (Makgoba *et al.*, 1989). Antigen independent adhesion of cytotoxic T-cells to target cells requires adhesion by at least two pathways, CD2 interaction with LFA-3 and LFA-1 with ICAM-1, -2 or -3 (Shaw *et al.*, 1986; Makgoba *et al.*, 1989; Springer, 1990). This antigen-independent adhesion promotes and maintains proximity between the two cells, allowing the T-cell receptor complex and CD8 to engage MHC molecules and antigen. This permits several interactions that result either in death of the target cell or in killing of infective agents. Activation of intracellular caspases and the subsequent cascade of molecular events that cause apoptosis can occur as a consequence either of interactions between Fas ligand on the lymphocyte membrane and Fas on the target cell or by the transfer of granules containing perforins from the cytotoxic T-cell (CTL) to the target cell (Figure 9.3) (Henkart, 1985; Anel *et al.*, 1994; Afford *et al.*, 1999). In contrast, secretion of interferon (IFN)γ and TNF-α by CTLs causes death of infecting agents without inducing apoptosis in the target cell (Guidotti and Chisari, 1996).

Antigen-independent NK cell killing also requires an adhesive interaction with the target cell and killing can be inhibited by antibodies to LFA-1 and CD2 (Mami-Chouaib *et al.*, 1990). β-2-integrin-mediated adhesion is also required for

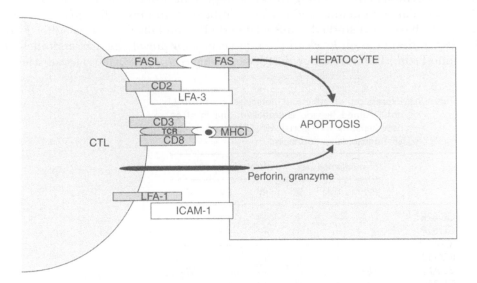

Figure 9.3 Mechanisms of hepatocyte killing by T-cells. The cytotoxic T-cell (CTL) recognises neoantigens on the hepatocyte membrane. Adhesion is provided by LFA-1/ICAM-1 and CD2/LFA-3 allowing the CTL to induce apoptosis via either FasL/Fas or the perforin granzyme pathways.

the efficient effector function of phagocytes. Neutrophils and macrophages require signals from engagement of their β2 integrins by extracellular ligands to enable them to respond to cytokines with a respiratory burst and release of cytotoxic granules (Burnett, 1993).

ADHESION MOLECULES AND CHEMOKINES; FINDINGS IN NORMAL LIVER AND ALCOHOLIC LIVER DISEASE

Inflammation is a characteristic feature of alcoholic liver disease and it is therefore not surprising that it is associated with increased and altered expression of several adhesion molecules and chemokines (Volpes *etal.*, 1991; Sheron *etal.*, 1993; Hill *etal.*, 1993; McClain *etal.*, 1993; Adams *etal.*, 1994; Fisher *etal.*, 1996, 1999; Afford *etal.*, 1998). The patterns of adhesion molecule expression and chemokine induction will determine the inflammatory infiltrate in the liver and are thus crucial in the pathogenesis of ALD.

Adhesion molecule expression

Tissue expression (Table 9.3)

The endothelium in normal liver expresses ICAM-2 and low levels of ICAM-1 but very little of the activation dependent molecules E and P selectin and VCAM-1 (Adams *etal.*, 1989; Volpes *etal.*, 1991, 1992; Steinhoff *etal.*, 1993). Expression of these adhesion molecules is increased on vascular endothelium in the portal tracts in liver inflammation including ALD but important differences are seen between the sinusoidal endothelium and portal endothelium. In most inflammatory conditions that have been studied, sinusoidal endothelium fails to express either E- or P-selectin, despite high levels of these molecules on portal vascular endothelium (Steinhoff *etal.*, 1993; Adams *etal.*, 1996a; Yoong *etal.*, 1998). This lack of selectin

Table 9.3 Expression of adhesion molecules on normal, non-inflamed hepatic endothelium and in alcoholic hepatitis. PV = portal vein, CV = central vein, SE = sinusoidal endothelium

	Non-inflamed liver			Alcoholic hepatitis		
	PV	CV	SE	PV	CV	SE
CD62E	–	–	–	++	++	–
CD62P	–	–	–	++	++	–
ICAM-1	+/–	+/–	+	++	++	+++
ICAM2	+/–	+/–	+	+	+	+
VCAM	+/–	–	+/–	++	+	+/–
CD31	++	++	+/–	++	++	+
LFA3	–	–	+	+	+	++
VAP-1	++	++	++	++	++	++
CD34	+	+	–	++	+	+

inducibility on sinusoidal endothelium has recently been confirmed using intravital microscopy in animal models (Wong et al., 1997) and this has led us to propose that a novel endothelial adhesion molecule, vascular adhesion protein-1 (VAP-1) mediates primary adhesion in the liver. VAP-1 is constitutively expressed on both sinusoidal and vascular endothelium in the liver (Salmi et al., 1993; McNab et al., 1996) and we have demonstrated that it mediates shear dependent adhesion of lymphocytes to hepatic vessels (Yoong et al., 1998). Thus, lymphocyte recruitment into non-inflamed liver appears to be mediated by a VAP-1 (primary adhesion) and LFA-1 and ICAM-2, whereas recruitment into the inflamed liver also involves LFA-1, ICAM-1, VLA-4 and VCAM-1 (Salmi et al., 1998). Although E-selectin is induced on portal vascular endothelium, liver-infiltrating lymphocytes fail to express E-selectin receptors, suggesting that it does not regulate lymphocyte recruitment (Adams, 1996; Adams et al., 1996a). Neutrophils are only recruited into inflamed liver, where it is likely that E-selectin mediates primary adhesion to vascular endothelium with VAP-1 possibly supporting primary adhesion to sinusoidal endothelium (although we have not tested this yet) and ICAM-1 mediating arrest and transendothelial migration.

Alcoholic liver disease is associated with histologically distinct processes including steatosis (parenchymal fat accumulation), alcoholic hepatitis, characterized by parenchymal infiltration by neutrophil polymorphs and alcoholic cirrhosis in which chronic inflammation and fibrosis dominate. Thus, the development of alcohol-induced liver injury is determined, in part, by the immunological/inflammatory response that alcohol stimulates. All three of the manifestations of alcoholic liver disease may be present independently or in combination (International Group, 1981). Although alcoholic hepatitis is frequently associated with cirrhosis, it can present as a distinct clinical syndrome that, in its most extreme form, causes liver failure and has a high mortality (Chedid et al., 1991; French et al., 1993; Lieber, 1994). The factors that regulate leukocyte recruitment to the liver are likely to be crucial in determining whether patients develop acute inflammation, hepatocyte damage and alcoholic hepatitis or a chronic response and cirrhosis.

In pure alcoholic fatty liver, there is no significant increase in adhesion molecule expression but there are distinctive patterns associated with both alcoholic hepatitis and cirrhosis (Volpes et al., 1991; Adams, 1994). Alcoholic hepatitis is characterized by increased expression of E-selectin and ICAM-1 on portal and hepatic venous endothelium in association with inflammatory infiltrates (Adams et al., 1994). VCAM-1 and ICAM-1 expression are increased on sinusoidal endothelium. VAP-1 expression is maintained at high levels throughout the hepatic vascular bed. Thus, the adhesion molecules expressed on hepatic endothelium will potentially promote the recruitment of a wide range of inflammatory cells, including neutrophils, to the liver.

In addition, ICAM-1 is detected on infiltrating inflammatory cells and also around the membrane of ballooned hepatocytes and the ICAM-1 ligand LFA-1 is expressed on inflammatory cells, principally neutrophils infiltrating the parenchyma in alcoholic hepatitis. Increased expression of ICAM-1 on hepatocytes is restricted to alcoholic hepatitis and may be a consequence of high local levels of TNF-α (Afford et al., 1998), a potent inducer of ICAM-1 on epithelial cells (Ayres et al., 1993). This increased expression of ICAM-1 on the hepatocyte membrane will increase susceptibility to cellular cytotoxicity and may be an important factor in the characteristic parenchymal inflammation and damage of alcoholic hepatitis (Burra *et al.*, 1992).

Alcoholic cirrhosis is also associated with increased expression of vascular adhesion molecules but levels tend to be lower than in alcoholic hepatitis and the inflammation is largely restricted to the portal and septal vessels rather than the hepatic parenchyma. ICAM-1 expression is increased, particularly on inflammatory cells in periseptal areas. LFA-1 is also increased on leukocytes but in contrast to alcoholic hepatitis, there is no increased ICAM-1 expression on hepatocytes (Adams *et al.*, 1994).

Circulating levels of soluble adhesion molecules

Many endothelial adhesion molecules are released in soluble forms during inflammation (Gearing and Newman, 1993; Buckley *et al.*, 1999). Levels of E-selectin are increased in subjects with alcoholic hepatitis compared to alcoholic cirrhotics or healthy controls, probably reflecting the intense inflammatory drive from elevated local levels of TNF-α in alcoholic hepatitis (Bird *et al.*, 1990; Ohlinger, 1993; Adams *et al.*, 1994; Afford *et al.*, 1998). In contrast, levels of VCAM-1 are increased in pure alcoholic cirrhosis compared to alcoholic hepatitis suggesting that the alcoholic cirrhosis is associated with a lower grade chronic inflammatory response. Levels of ICAM-1 are increased in both cirrhosis and hepatitis (with little difference between the 2 groups) compared to healthy controls (Adams *et al.*, 1994). We have recently reported that VAP-1 is also released in a soluble form and that levels of this molecule are elevated in liver disease but not in other inflammatory diseases such as rheumatoid arthritis and inflammatory bowel disease (Kurkijarvi *et al.*, 1998). A further analysis, as yet unpublished, suggests that VAP-1 is particularly elevated in alcoholic liver disease with the highest levels being detected in alcoholic hepatitis (Shimada, 1993).

The finding of increased tissue and circulating levels of the vascular adhesion molecules, E-selectin and VCAM-1 in alcoholic liver disease suggest endothelial activation. The presence of E-selectin and ICAM-1 should promote the tethering and subsequent arrest of neutrophils in alcoholic hepatitis whereas the higher levels of VCAM-1 in alcoholic cirrhosis would promote lymphocyte recruitment and chronic inflammation. The factors that induce lymphocyte tethering remain unclear; in contrast to lymphocyte recruitment to cutaneous tissue, E-selectin does not appear to play a significant role in lymphocyte recruitment to the liver. However, VCAM-1 may play a part both in primary tethering and in strong adhesion of lymphocytes and the presence of VAP-1 might be sufficient to provide initial tethering (Adams *et al.*, 1996a; Lalor *et al.*, 1997; Wong *et al.*, 1997).

It is likely that the increased expression of adhesion molecules in alcoholic liver disease is a consequence of local cytokine release. Increased levels of the cytokines IL-1, IL-6 and TNF-α are detected in alcoholic hepatitis (Bird *et al.*, 1990; Khoruts, 1991) and these are associated with increased tissue levels (Afford *et al.*, 1998). TNF-α has been shown to increase expression of ICAM-1 on primary human epithelial cells (Ayres *et al.*, 1993) and endothelial cells (Bevilacqua, 1993) and to stimulate Mac-1 expression on neutrophils *in vitro* (Pichyangkul, 1988). Immunohistochemical studies of tissue sections in alcoholic hepatitis show co-localization of

TNF-α with ICAM-1 and CD11b (the β chain of Mac-1) (Khoruts, 1991). Additionally, circulating endotoxin, which is increased in alcoholic liver disease (Bode, 1987), may stimulate increased hepatocyte expression of ICAM-1 (Satoh et al., 1994) and oxidative stress, which occurs during alcoholic injury, can also increase expression of adhesion molecules on endothelium and hepatocytes. IL-4, which is released in chronic, Th2 inflammatory responses can lead to increased expression of VCAM-1 (Swerlick et al., 1992), which would promote the recruitment of lymphocytes in chronic alcoholic cirrhosis.

Chemokine expression

Tissue expression (Tables 9.4 and 9.5)

Many chemokines can be detected in normal liver tissue by immunohistochemistry and in situ hybridization (Adams et al., 1996b; Afford et al., 1998; Marra et al., 1998). IL-8, MCP-1 and regulated on activation normal T-cell expressed and secreted (RANTES) are present on leukocytes, vascular endothelium and biliary epithelium, whilst the CC chemokines, macrophage inflammatory protein (MIP)-1α and MIP-1β are restricted to leukocytes and vascular endothelial cells. Many cell types contribute to chemokine synthesis. Although leukocytes and vascular endothelial cells account for the majority of the production, hepatocytes and biliary epithelial cells can also secrete chemokines and may be responsible for some of the constitutive expression (Morland et al., 1997). The expression of chemokines in normal liver is probably a consequence of the constitutive inflammation that is responsible for leukocyte trafficking during immune surveillance and may arise as a consequence of

Table 9.4 Chemokine expression in alcoholic liver disease. Immunohistochemistry staining patterns for three chemokines are shown for different structures within the liver. (For more detailed analysis see Afford et al., 1998)

Chemokine		Normal	Alc hep	Alc cirr
MIP-1α	Leukocytes	+	+++	+++
	Sinusoids	−	++	−
	Vascular Ec	+	+++	+++
	Hepatocytes	−	+	−
	Fibrous septa	np	+++	+++
MCP-1	Leukocytes	+	+++	+++
	Sinusoids	−	++	−
	Vascular Ec	+	+++	+++
	Hepatocytes	−	++	++
	Fibrous septa	np	+++	+++
IL-8	Leukocytes	+/−	+++	++
	Sinusoids	−	++	+/−
	Vascular Ec	++	+++	+++
	Hepatocytes	−	+++	−
	Fibrous septa	np	+++	+/−

Table 9.5 Comparison between protein and mRNA expression for the CC chemokine MIP-1β in alcoholic hepatitis; similar results were seen with MIP-1α and MCP-1. Chemokine mRNA was confined to infiltrating inflammatory cells (IC) and sinusoidal cells in the parenchyma and vascular endothelium in portal tracts

| | Portal tracts | | | Parenchyma | | |
	BD	VE	IC	SC	Hep	IC
mRNA	–	+	+	++	–	++
Protein	++	+++	++	+	+++	++

low grade endotoxinaemia from the gut (Salmi *et al.*, 1998). In alcoholic liver disease, increased expression of many chemokines is seen with distinctive patterns that reflect the severity and nature of the inflammatory infiltrate (Sheron *et al.*, 1993; Maltby *et al.*, 1996; Afford *et al.*, 1998; Fisher *et al.*, 1999).

Alcoholic Hepatitis is characterized by an increased hepatic expression of several CXC and CC chemokines including IL-8, MCP-1, MIP-1α and MIP-1β, RANTES and ENA-78 (Maltby *et al.*, 1996). Expression of all these chemokines is increased, particularly in inflamed portal tracts where they can be detected on infiltrating leukocytes and endothelium. In the parenchyma, a distinct pattern of expression is seen with intense staining for IL-8, MCP-1 and the MIPs in areas of ballooning degeneration and leucocytic infiltration. The chemokines are detected within sinusoids and also on and within inflamed hepatocytes (Afford *et al.*, 1998). *In situ* hybridization shows intense expression of mRNA within portal tracts (principally vascular endothelium and inflammatory cells) and in the parenchyma where it is mainly localized to sinusoidal lining cells and inflammatory cells, with only a small amount of mRNA within hepatocytes (Table 9.5). The pattern of hybridization in sinusoidal lining cells corresponds to the pattern of pericellular fibrosis and stellate cell activation. Thus stellate cells, which are responsible for fibrous tissue deposition, may be either intimately linked with cells secreting chemokines or indeed may themselves be an important source (Marra *et al.*, 1997, 1998; Sprenger *et al.*, 1997; Pinzani *et al.*, 1998). Furthermore, the levels and tissue expression of MCP-1 correlate closely with the degree of fibrotic activity in chronic hepatitis (Marra *et al.*, 1997, 1998).

In *alcoholic cirrhosis*, up-regulation of chemokines is largely restricted to portal tracts and fibrous septa and parallels the degree of inflammatory infiltration. Clear distinctions in chemokine distribution between alcoholic hepatitis and cirrhosis are difficult to define since at the time of presentation, alcoholic hepatitis and cirrhosis often coexist. Nevertheless, the presence of a neutrophil infiltrate in alcoholic hepatitis is associated with increased expression and circulating levels of the CXC chemokines gro-α and IL-8 (Bird *et al.*, 1990; Sheron *et al.*, 1993; Maltby *et al.*, 1996). In the chronic inflammatory response of alcoholic cirrhosis, however, CC chemokines such as MCP-1, MIP-1α and MIP-1β predominate. The role of IL-8 in neutrophil recruitment is further supported by animal studies in which some of the histological features of alcoholic hepatitis can be reproduced by transfecting hepatocytes *in vivo* with α chemokines (Maher, 1995; Maher *et al.*, 1996). Although hepatocytes themselves can secrete chemokines, including IL-8 and MCP-1, it seems likely that local secretion with the parenchyma will be a result of interactions between different cell types including stellate cells, kupffer cells and hepatocytes.

Circulating chemokines

Several groups have found raised circulating levels of IL-8 in alcoholic liver disease with serum levels, reflecting the degree of active inflammation (Hill *et al.*, 1993; McClain *et al.*, 1993; Sheron *et al.*, 1993). Serum levels correlate with other laboratory indicators of disease severity such as serum bilirubin, creatinine, prothrombin time, peripheral white blood cell count, tumor necrosis factor and soluble tumor necrosis factor receptor, whilst the serum levels of IL-8 in alcoholic hepatitis slowly fall over a period of months following recovery from the acute illness. Subjects with alcohol dependency but without overt liver disease also have raised levels although to a lesser degree, and interestingly IL-8 levels have been shown to rise in the period following hospitalization for detoxification (Masumoto, 1993).

Serum levels of MCP-1 are also raised in alcoholic liver disease; levels correlate with histological features of inflammation and biochemical indices of liver injury including serum AST and bilirubin. Higher levels of MCP-1 were found in the hepatic vein compared to peripheral veins in subjects with histologically severe hepatitis (but not in those with mild or quiescent alcoholic liver disease), suggesting that the liver is the primary source of MCP-1 synthesis in alcoholic hepatitis (Fisher *et al.*, 1999). However, evidence was also found for chemokine synthesis in peripheral mononuclear cells (predominantly monocytes) using *in situ* hybridization analysis (Fisher *et al.*, 1999). This finding may reflect activation of circulating monocytes within the liver, but may also result from the increased circulating levels of endotoxin that characterize alcoholic liver disease (Bode, 1987).

Cellular sources of chemokines within the liver

As the principal site of metabolism of alcohol within the body, the hepatocyte is the main target of cellular damage from reactive intermediaries in ALD. However, evidence from *in situ* hybridization studies and *in vitro* experiments with cultured liver cell isolates suggests that, although hepatocytes can secrete chemokines after exposure to alcohol or alcohol metabolites, other cells are the principal sources during hepatic inflammation (Shiratori, 1993; Fisher *et al.*, 1999). Several liver cell types have been shown to produce chemokines under appropriate conditions, including hepatocytes (Maher, 1995) sinusoidal endothelial cells (McNab *et al.*, 1997; Sheilds *et al.*, 1999), cholangiocytes (Morland *et al.*, 1997), Kupffer cells (Maher, 1995; Bautista, 1995) and stellate (fat-storing or Ito) cells (Pinzani *et al.*, 1998). Of these cell types, the latter two are probably the most significant sources during hepatic inflammation. Kupffer cells have been shown to be potent sources of TNF-α, TGF-β and chemotactic intermediaries after experimental liver injury and in alcohol-fed rats (Armendariz-Borunda, 1991; Maher, 1995). Stellate cells have also been shown to be the principal source of MCP-1 after carbon tetrachloride-induced liver injury in rats (Czaja, 1994). In contrast, sinusoidal lining cells have been shown to be more potent sources of IL-8 compared to Kupffer cells and primary hepatocytes in cultured rat cells (Ohkubo et al., 1998).

The mechanisms that regulate chemokine secretion from the liver in alcoholic liver disease are not known. Hypoxia is a potent stimulus for chemokine release and alteration of the redox state occurs in hepatocytes exposed to alcohol. However, evidence that alcohol or acetaldehyde directly trigger chemokine release from cultured hepatocytes is not conclusive. In fact, several studies suggest that alcohol down-regulates chemokine secretion, in the same way that it down-regulates cytokine secretion (Nelson, 1989; Fisher et al., 1999). What do appear to be important are interactions between different liver cell types in modulating chemokine release (Maher, 1995). It is possible that the presence of acetaldehyde or hydroxyethyl-modified proteins on the membrane of hepatocytes may, in the presence of other co-stimulatory factors, engage Kupffer cells and trigger release of chemokines and other cytokines (Bautista, 1995). Alternatively, the presence of increased circulating lipopolysaccharide resulting from enhanced gut permeability induced by alcohol may be a direct trigger to Kupffer cells (Bautista, 1997).

THERAPEUTIC IMPLICATIONS

A greater understanding of the molecular regulation of the inflammatory processes that result in fibrosis after alcohol exposure should allow novel approaches to therapy. Anti-adhesion molecule therapy has been developed and tested in several animal models and a few limited clinical settings (Adams, 1995). The problems with this approach lie partly in the reliance on antibody-based therapy, which is complicated by human anti-mouse responses and the need to give antibodies intravenously. However, the development of humanized, chimeric antibodies and perhaps more realistically small peptide inhibitors might make this a more practical treatment in future (Vedder et al., 1988, 1989; Winn et al., 1995). This still leaves the problem of which adhesion pathway to target. Treatment aimed at inhibiting widely used molecules such as ICAM-1 or CD18 is frequently associated with toxicity, particularly infections, and it may be that inhibiting molecules with a more restricted, potentially tissue selective role, such as VAP-1 will prove more effective. With regard to anti-chemokine therapy, one problem is determining which of the many chemokines is crucial for disease pathogenesis. This will be assisted by the recent development of antibodies against specific chemokine receptors that will allow one to determine which receptors are expressed by leukocyte subsets infiltrating the liver (Mackay, 1996; Yoong et al., 1999; Sheilds et al., 1999). The development of genetically modified mice that fail to express particular chemokines or chemokine receptors may prove useful in determining which pathways to target. One attractive target would appear to be MCP-1 because expression of this chemokine correlates well with fibrosis, an important prognostic factor in alcoholic liver disease (Marra et al., 1998). The development of anti-sense strategies and peptide inhibitors for chemokine receptors is likely to result in a large number of potentially novel treatments for inflammation in the next few years (Mackay, 1997). It will be interesting to see if such approaches provide the tools for inhibiting liver inflammation and fibrosis in alcoholic liver disease.

REFERENCES

Adams, D.H. (1994) Leukocyte adhesion and alcoholic liver disease. *Alcohol and Alcoholism* **29**, 249–260.

Adams, D.H. (1995) Adhesion molecules and liver transplantation: new strategies for therapeutic intervention. *J Hepatol* **23**, 225–231.

Adams, D.H. (1996) Lymphocyte-endothelial interactions in hepatic inflammation. *Hepatogastroenterology* **43**, 32–43.

Adams, D.H., Burra, P., Hubscher, S.G., Elias, E. and Newman, W. (1994) Endothelial activation and circulating vascular adhesion molecules in alcoholic liver disease. *Hepatology* **19**, 588–594.

Adams, D.H., Fear, J., Shaw, S., Hubscher, S.G. and Afford, S. (1996b) Hepatic expression of macrophage inflammatory protein-1α and macrophage inflammatory protein-1β after liver transplantation. *Transplantation* **61**, 817–825.

Adams, D.H., Harvath, L., Bottaro, D.P., Interrante, R., Catalano, G., Tanaka, Y., Strain, A., Hubscher, S.G. and Shaw, S. (1994) Hepatocyte growth factor and macrophage inflammatory protein-1β: structurally distinct cytokines that induce rapid cytoskeletal changes and subset-preferential migration in T-cell. *Proc Natl Acad Sci USA* **91**, 7144–7148.

Adams, D.H., Hubscher, S.G., Fisher, N.C., Williams, A. and Robinson, M. (1996a) Expression of E-selectin (CD62E) and E-selectin ligands in human liver inflammation. *Hepatology* **24**, 533–538.

Adams, D.H., Hubscher, S.G., Shaw, J., Rothlein, R. and Neuberger, J.M. (1989) Intercellular adhesion molecule 1 on liver allografts during rejection. *Lancet* **2**, 1122–1125.

Adams, D.H. and Lloyd, A.R. (1997) Chemokines: leukocyte recruitment and activation cytokines. *Lancet* **349**, 490–495.

Adams, D.H. and Shaw, S. (1994) Leukocyte endothelial interactions and regulation of leukocyte migration. *Lancet* **343**, 831–836.

Afford, S.C., Fisher, N.C., Neil, D.A.H., Fear, J., Brun, P., Hubscher, S.G. and Adams, D.H. (1998) Distinct patterns of chemokine expression are associated with leukocyte recruitment in alcoholic hepatitis & alcoholic cirrhosis. *Journal of Pathology* **186**, 82–89.

Afford, S.C., Rhandawa, S., Eliopoulos, A.G., Hubscher, S.G., Young, L.S. and Adams, D.H. (1999). CD40 activation induces apoptosis in cultured human hepatocytes via induction of cell surface FasL expression and amplifies Fas mediated hepatocyte death during allograft rejection. *The Journal of Experimental Medicine* **189**, 441–446.

Airas, L., Hellman, J., Salmi, M., Bono, P., Puurunen, T., Smith, D.J. and Jalkanen, S. (1995) Cd73 is involved in lymphocyte binding to the endothelium – characterization of lymphocyte vascular adhesion protein-2 identifies it as cd73. *Journal of Experimental Medicine* **182**, 1603–1608.

Airas, L., Niemela, J., Salmi, M., Puurunen, T., Smith, D.J. and Jalkanen, S. (1997) Differential regulation and function of cd73, a glycosyl-phosphatidylinositol-linked 70-kd adhesion molecule, on lymphocytes and endothelial cells. *Journal of Cell Biology* **136**, 421–431.

Allison, J.P., Hurwitz, A.A. and Leach, D.R. (1995) Manipulation of costimulatory signals to enhance antitumor T-cell responses. *Current Opinion in Immunology* **7**, 682–686.

Alon, R., Rossiter, H., Wang, X., Springer, T.A. and Kupper, T.S. (1994) Distinct cell surface ligands mediate T-lymphocyte attachment and rolling on P and E selectin under physiological flow. *J Cell Biol* **127**, 1485–1495.

Anel, A., Buferne, M., Boyer, C., Schmittverhulst, A.M. and Golstein, P. (1994) T-cell receptor-induced fas ligand expression in cytotoxic T-lymphocyte clones is blocked by protein-tyrosine kinase inhibitors and cyclosporine-α. *European Journal of Immunology* **24**, 2469–2476.

Ardman, Sikorski, M.A. and Staunton, D.E. (1992) CD43 interferes with T-lymphocyte adhesion. *Proc Natl Acad Sci USA* **89**, 5001–5005.

Armendariz-Borunda, J.S.J.M.P.A.E.A.K.A.H. (1991) Kupffer cells from carbon tetrachloride-injured rat liver produce chemotactic factors for fibroblasts and monocytes: the role of tumour necrosis factor-α. *Hepatology* **14**, 895–900.

Aruffo, A., Stamenkovic, I., Melnick, M., Underhill, C.B. and Seed, B. (1990) CD44 is the principal cell surface receptor for hyaluronate. *Cell* **61**, 1303–1313.

Ayres, R., Neuberger, J.M., Shaw, J. and Adams, D.H. (1993) Intercellular adhesion molecule-1 and MHC antigens on human intrahepatic bile duct cells: effect of proinflammatory cytokines. *Gut* **34**, 1245–1249.

Baggiolini, M. (1998) Chemokines and leukocyte traffic. *Nature* **392**, 565–568.

Baggiolini, M., Dewald, D. and Moser, B. (1994) Interleukin-8 and related chemotactic cytokines: CXC and CC chemokines. *Adv Immunol* **55**, 97–179.

Bautista, A.P. (1997) Chronic alcohol intoxication induces hepatic injury through enhanced macrophage inflammatory protein-2 production and intercellular adhesion molecule-1 expression in the liver. *Hepatology* **25**, 342.

Bautista, A.P. (1995) Chronic alcohol-intoxication enhances the expression of cd18 adhesion molecules on rat neutrophils and release of a chemotactic factor by kupffer cells. *Alcoholism Clinical and Experimental Research* **19**, 285–290.

Bazan, J.F., Bacon, K.B., Hardiman, G., Wang, W., Soo, K., Rossi, D., Greaves, D.R., Zlotnik, A. and Schall, T.J. (1997) A new class of membrane-bound chemokine with a CX3C motif. *Nature* **385**, 640–644.

Berlin, C., Bargatze, R.F., Campbell, J.J., Vonandrian, U.H., Szabo, M.C., Hasslen, S.R., Nelson, R.D., Berg, E.L., Erlandsen, S.L. and Butcher, E.C. (1995) Alpha-4 integrins mediate lymphocyte attachment and rolling under physiological flow. *Cell* **80**, 413–422.

Berlin, C., Berg, E.L., Briskin, M.J., Andrew, D.P., Kilshaw, P.J., Holzmann, B., Weissman, I.L., Hamman, A. and Butcher, E.C. (1993) Alpha 4 beta 7 integrin mediates binding to the mucosal vascular addressin MAdCAM-1. *Cell* **74**, 185–195.

Bevilacqua, M.P. (1993) Endothelial-leukocyte adhesion molecules. *Annu Rev Immunol* **11**, 767–784.

Bird, G.L.A., Sheron, N., Goka, A.K.J., Alexander, G.J.M. and Williams, R. (1990) Increased plasma tumour necrosis factor in severe alcoholic hepatitis. *Ann Intern Med* **112**, 917–920.

Bode, C.K.V.a.B.J.C. (1987) Endotoxemia in patients with alcoholic and non-alcoholic cirrhosis and in subjects with no evidence of chronic liver disease following acute alcohol excess. *J Hepatol* **4**, 14.

Bradley, L.M. and Watson, S.R. (1996) Lymphocyte migration into tissue – the paradigm derived from cd4 subsets. *Current Opinion in Immunology* **8**, 312–320.

Buckley, C.D., Adams, D.H. and Simmons, D. (1999) Soluble Leukocyte-endothelial adhesion molecules. In *Physiology of Inflammation*, edited by K. Ley.

Burnett, D. (1993) Other effector cells. In *Immunology of Liver Transplantation*, edited by J. Neuberger and D.H. Adams, pp. 34–57. Boston: Edward Arnold.

Burra, P., Hubscher, S.G., Shaw, J., Elias, E. and Adams, D.H. (1992) Is the ICAM-1/LFA-1 pathway of leukocyte adherence involved in the hepatocyte damage of alcoholic hepatitis? *Gut* **33**, 268–271.

Butcher, E.C. (1991) Leukocyte-endothelial cell recognition: three (or more) steps to specificity and diversity. *Cell* **67**, 1033–1036.

Butcher, E.C. and Picker, L.J. (1996) Lymphocyte homing and homeostasis. *Science* **272**, 60–66.

Butcher, E.C., Williams, M., Youngman, K., Rott, L. and Briskin, M. (1999) Lymphocyte trafficking and regional immunity. *Adv Immunol* **72**, 209–253.

Campbell, J.J., Hedrick, J., Zlotnick, A., Siani, M.A., Thompson, D.A. and Butcher, E.C. (1998) Chemokines and the arrest of lymphocytes rolling under flow. *Science* **279**, 381–384.

Campbell, J.J., Qin, S.X., Bacon, K.B., Mackay, C.R. and Butcher, E.C. (1996) Biology of chemokine and classical chemoattractant receptors – differential requirements for adhesion-triggering versus chemotactic responses in lymphoid-cells. *Journal of Cell Biology* **134**, 255–266.

Cepek, K.L., Shaw, S.K., Parker, C.M., Russell, G.J., Morrow, J.S., Rimm, D.L. and Brenner, M.B. (1994) Adhesion between epithelial-cells and T-lymphocytes mediated by E-cadherin and the alpha(e)beta(7) integrin. *Nature* **372**, 190–193.

Chedid, A., Mendenhall, C.L., Garside, P., French, S.W., Chen, T., Rabin, L. and the VA Cooperative Group (1991) Prognostic factors in alcoholic liver disease. *Am J Gastroenterol* **82**, 210–216.

Chin, Y.H., Cai, J.P. and Xu, X.M. (1992) Transforming growth factor-β1 and IL-4 regulate the adhesiveness of Peyer's patch high endothelial venule cells for lymphocytes. *Journal of Immunology* **148**, 1106–1112.

Cunningham, B.A. (1995) Cell adhesion molecules as morphoregulators. *Curr Opin Cell Biol* **7(5)**, 628–633.

Czaja, M.J.G.A.X.J.S.P.A.J.Y. (1994) Monocyte Chemoattractant Protein-1 expression occurs in toxic rat liver injury and human liver disease. *Journal of Leukocyte Biology* **55**, 120–126.

Damsky, C.H. and Werb, Z. (1992) Signal transduction by integrin receptors for extra-cellular matrix: cooperative processing of extracellular information. *Curr Opin Cell Biol* **4**, 772–781.

Ebnet, K., Kaldjian, E.P., Anderson, A.O. and Shaw, S. (1996) Orchestrated information-transfer underlying leukocyte-endothelial interactions. *Annual Review of Immunology* **14**, 155–177.

Fisher, N.C., Afford, S.C. and Adams, D.H. (1996) Adhesion molecules and alcoholic liver disease. *Hepatogastroenterology* **43**, 1113–1116.

Fisher, N.C., Neil, D.A., Williams, A. and Adams, D.H. (1999) Serum concentrations and peripheral secretion of the beta chemokines monocyte chemoattractant protein 1 and macrophage inflammatory protein 1alpha in alcoholic liver disease. *Gut* **45**, 416–420.

French, S.W., Nash, J., Shitabata, P., Kachi, K., Hara, C., Chedid, A., Mendenhall, C.L. and The VA Cooperative Group (1993) Pathology of alcoholic liver disease. *Seminars in Liver Disease* **13**, 154–169.

Furie, M.B. and Randolph, G.J. (1995) Chemokines and tissue injury. *Am J Pathol* **146**, 1287–1301.

Gahmberg, C.G. (1997) Leukocyte adhesion: CD11/CD18 integrins and intercellular adhesion molecules. *Curr Opin Cell Biol* **9**, 500–643.

Gearing, A.J.H. and Newman, W. (1993) Circulating adhesion molecules in disease. *Immunol Today* **14(10)**, 506–512.

Grewal, I.S. and Flavell, R.A. (1998) CD40 and CD154 in cell-mediated immunity. *Annu Rev Immunol* **16**, 111–135.

Guidotti, L.G. and Chisari, F.V. (1996) To kill or to cure – options in host-defense against viral-infection. *Current Opinion in Immunology* **8**, 478–483.

Gunn, M.D., Ngo, V.N., Ansel, K.M., Ekland, E.H., Cyster, J.G. and Williams, L.T. (1998a) A B-cell-homing chemokine made in lymphoid follicles activates Burkitt's lymphoma receptor-1. *Nature* **19**, 799–803.

Gunn, M.D., Tangemann, K., Tam, C., Cyster, J.G., Rosen, S.D. and Williams, L.T. (1998b) A chemokine expressed in lymphoid high endothelial venules promotes the adhesion and chemotaxis of naive T lymphocytes. *Proc Natl Acad Sci USA* **95**, 258–633.

Henkart, P.A. (1985) Mechanism of lymphocyte-mediated cytotoxicity. *Annu Rev Immunol* **3**, 31–30.

Hill, D.B., Marsano, L.S. and McClain, C.J. (1993) Increased plasma interleukin-8 concen-trations in alcoholic hepatitis. *Hepatology* **18**, 576–580.

Hynes, R.O. (1992) Integrins: versatility, modulation, and signaling in cell adhesion. *Cell* **69**, 11–25.

Ihara, A., Koizumi, H., Hashizume, R. and Uchikoshi, T. (1996) Expression of epithelial cadherin and alpha-catenins and beta-catenins in nontumoral livers and hepatocellular carcinomas. *Hepatology* **23**, 1441–1447.

Ingber, D. (1991) Integrins as mechanochemical transducers. *Curr Opin Cell Biol* **3**, 841–848.

International Group (1981) Alcoholic liver disease: morphological manifestations. *Lancet* **1**, 707–771.

Jones, D.A., McIntire, L.V., Smith, C.W. and Picker, L.J. (1994) A 2-step adhesion cascade for T-cell endothelial-cell interactions under flow conditions. *Journal of Clinical Investigation* **94**, 2443–2450.

Kanwar, S., Bullard, D.C., Hickey, M.J., Smith, C.W., Beaudet, A.L., Wolitzky, B.A. and Kubes, P. (1997) The association between alpha(4)-integrin, p-selectin, and e-selectin in an allergic model of inflammation. *Journal of Experimental Medicine* **185**, 1077–1087.

Khoruts, A.S.L.M.C.J.L.G.A.A.J.I. (1991) Circulating tumor necrosis factor, interleukin-1 and interleukin-6 concentrations in chronic alcoholic patients. *Hepatology* **13**, 267–276.

Kuijpers, T.W., Hoogerwerf, M. and Roos, D. (1992) Neutrophil migration across monolayers of resting or cytokine activated endothelial cells: role of intracellular calcium and fusion of specific granules with the plasma membrane. *Journal of Immunology* **148**, 72–77.

Kurkijarvi, R., Adams, D.H., Leino, R., Mottonen, T., Jalkanen, S. and Salmi, M. (1998) Circulating form of human vascular adhesion protein-1 (VAP-1): increased serum levels in inflammatory liver diseases. *Journal of Immunology* **161**, 1549–1557.

Lalor, P.E., Clements, J.M., Pigott, R., Humphries, M.J., Spragg, J.H. and Nash, G.B. (1997) Association between receptor density, cellular activation, and transformation of adhesive behavior of flowing lymphocytes binding to VCAM-1. *European Journal of Immunology* **27**, 1422–1426.

Lasky, L.A. (1992) Selectins: interpreters of cell-specific carbohydrate information during inflammation. *Science* **258**, 964–969.

Lieber, C.S. (1994) Alcohol and the liver: 1994 update. *Gastroenterology* **106**, 1085–1105.

Luster, A.D. (1998) Chemokines-chemotactic cytokines that mediate inflammation. *New England Journal of Medicine* **338**, 436–445.

Mackay, C.R. (1997) Chemokines: what chemokine is that? *Curr Biol* **7**, 384–386.

Mackay, C.R. (1996) Chemokine receptors and T-cell chemotaxis. *Journal of Experimental Medicine* **184**, 799–802.

Maher, J.J. (1995) Rat hepatocytes and kupffer cells interact to produce interleukin-8 (cinc) in the setting of ethanol. *American Journal of Physiology-Gastrointestinal and Liver Physiology* **32**, G518–G523.

Maher, J.J., Scott, M.K., Saito, J.M. and Burton, M.C. (1996) Adenovirus-mediated expression of cinc/gro (IL-8) in rat-liver induces a neutrophilic hepatitis. *FASEB J* **10**, 22.

Makgoba, M.W., Sanders, M.E. and Shaw, S. (1989) The CD2-LFA-3 and LFA-1-ICAM-1 pathways: relevance to T-cell recognition. *Immunol Today* **10**, 417–422.

Maltby, J., Wright, S., Bird, G. and Sheron, N. (1996) Chemokine levels in human liver homogenates – associations between gro alpha and histopathological evidence of alcoholic hepatitis. *Hepatology* **24**, 1156–1160.

Mami-Chouaib, F., Miossec, C., Del Porto, P., Flament, C., Triebel, F. and Hercend, T. (1990) T cell target 1 (TCT-1): a novel target molecule for human non-major histocompatibility complex-restricted T lymphocytes. *J Exp Med* **172**, 1071–1082.

Marra, F., DeFranco, R., Grappone, C., Milani, S., Pastacaldi, S., Pinzani, M., Romanelli, R.G., Laffi, G. and Gentilini, P. (1998) Increased expression of monocyte chemotactic protein-1 during active hepatic fibrogenesis: correlation with monocyte infiltration. *Am J Pathol* **152**, 423–430.

Marra, F., Pastacaldi, S., Romanelli, R.G., Pinzani, M., Ticali, P., Carloni, V., Laffi, G. and Gentilini, P. (1997) Integrin-mediated stimulation of monocyte chemotactic protein-1 expression. *FEBS Lett* **414**, 221–255.

Masumoto, T.O.M.H.N.A.O.Y. (1993) Assay of serum interleukin-8 levels in patients with alcoholic hepatitis. *Alcohol and alcoholism* **28**, 99–102.

McClain, C., Hill, D., Schmidt, J. and Diehl, A.M. (1993) Cytokines and alcoholic liver disease. *Seminars in Liver Disease* **13**, 170–182.

McEver, R.P. (1992) Leukocyte-endothelial interactions. *Curr Opin Cell Biol* **4**, 840–849.

McNab, G., Afford, S.C., Morland, C.M., Strain, A.J., Joplin, R. and Adams, D.H. (1997) Cultured human hepatic sinusoidal endothelial cells express and secrete adhesion molecules and chemokines that are important for leukocyte recruitment to the liver. In *Cells of the Hepatic Sinusoid*, edited by E. Wisse, D.L. Knook and C. Balabaud, pp. 123–127. Leiden: The Kupffer Cell Foundation.

McNab, G., Reeves, J.L., Salmi, M., Hubscher, S.G., Jalkanen, S. and Adams, D.H. (1996) Vascular adhesion protein-1 supports adhesion of T-lymphocytes to hepatic endothelium. A mechanism for T-cell recirculation to the liver? *Gastroenterology* **110**, 522–528.

Mentzer, S., Remold-O'Donnell, E., Crimmins, M., Bierer, B., Rosen, F. and Burakoff, S. (1987) Sialophorin, a surface sialoglycoprotein defective in the Wiskott-Aldrich Syndrome, is involved in human T-lymphocyte proliferation. *J Exp Med* **165**, 1383.

Morland, C.M., Fear, J., McNab, G., Joplin, R. and Adams, D.H. (1997) Promotion of leukocyte transendothelial cell migration by chemokines derived from human biliary epithelial cells *in vitro*. *Proceedings of the Association of American Physicians* **109**, 372–382.

Murphy, W.J., Tian, Z.G., Asai, O., Funakoshi, S., Rotter, P., Henry, M., Strieter, R.M., Kunkel, S.L., Longo, D.L. and Taub, D.D. (1996) Chemokines and T-lymphocyte activation 2: facilitation of human T-cell trafficking in severe combined immunodeficiency mice. *Journal of Immunology* **156**, 2104–2111.

Nelson, S.B.G.J.B.B.G.A.S.W.R. (1989) The effects of acute and chronic alcoholism on tumor necrosis factor and the inflammatory response. *Journal of Infectious Diseases* **160**, 422–429.

O'Rourke, A.M. and Mescher, M.F. (1992) Cytotoxic T-lymphocyte activation involves a cascade of signalling and adhesion events. *Nature* **358**, 253–255.

Ohkubo, K., Masumoto, T., Horiike, N. and Onji, M. (1998) Induction of CINC (interleukin-8) production in rat liver by non-parenchymal cells. *J Gastroenterol Hepatol* **13**, 696–702.

Ohlinger, W.D. (1993) Immunohistochemical detection of tumour necrosis factor-alpha, other cytokines and adhesion molecules in human livers with alcoholic hepatitis. *Virchows Archiv A* **423**, 169–176.

Pichyangkul, S.S. (1988) Increaed Expression of Adhesive Proteins on Leukocytes by TNF-α. *Experimental Haematology* **16**, 588–593.

Picker, L.J., Treer, J.R., Ferguson-Darnell, B., Collins, P.A., Bergstresser, P.R. and Terstappen, L.W. (1993b) Control of lymphocyte recirculation in man. II. Differential regulation of the cutaneous lymphocyte-associated antigen, a tissue-selective homing receptor for skin-homing T-cells. *Journal of Immunology* **1500**, 1122–1136.

Picker, L.J., Treer, J.R., Ferguson-Darnell, B., Collins, P.A., Buck, D. and Terstappen, L.W. (1993a) Control of lymphocyte recirculation in man: I. Differential regulation of the peripheral lymph node homing receptor L-selectin on T-cells during the virgin to memory cell transition. *Journal of Immunology* **150**, 1105–1121.

Pinzani, M., Marra, F. and Carloni, V. (1998) Signal transduction in hepatic stellate cells. *Liver* **18**, 2–13.

Pate, J.C. and Hogg, N. (1997) Integrin cross talk: activation of lymphocyte function-associated antigen-1 on human T-cells alters $\alpha 4 \beta 1$- and $\alpha 5 \beta 1$-mediated function. *J Cell Biol* **138**, 1437–1477.

Pate, J.C. and Hogg, N. (1998) Integrins take partners: cross-talk between integrins and other membrane receptors [In Process Citation]. *Trends Cell Biol* **8**, 390–396.

Rainger, G.E., Buckley, C., Simmons, D.L. and Nash, G.B. (1997) Cross-talk between cell adhesion molecules regulates the migration velocity of neutrophils. *Curr Biol* **7**, 316–325.

Sallusto, F., Mackay, C.R. and Lanzavecchia, A. (1997) Selective expression of the eotaxin receptor CCR3 by human T helper 2 cells. *Science* **277**, 2005–2008.

Salmi, M., Adams, D.H. and Jalkanen, S. (1998) Lymphocyte trafficking in the intestine and liver. *Am J Physiol* **274**, G1–G6.

Salmi, M., Kalimo, K. and Jalkanen, S. (1993) Induction and function of vascular adhesion protein 1 at sites of inflammation. *Journal of Experimental Medicine* **178**, 2255–2260.

Satoh, S., Nussler, A.K., Liu, Z.Z. and Thomson, A.W. (1994) Proinflammatory cytokines and endotoxin stimulate ICAM-1 gene-expression and secretion by normal human hepatocytes. *Immunology* **82**, 571–576.

Schall, T. (1997) Fractalkine – a strange attractor in the chemokine landscape. *Immunol Today* **18(4)**, 147–177.

Schweighoffer, T. and Shaw, S. (1992) Adhesion cascades: Diversity through combinatorial strategies. *Curr Opin Cell Biol* **4**, 824–829.

Schweighoffer, T., Tanaka, Y., Tidswell, M., Erle, D.J., Horgan, K.J., Luce, G.E., Lazarovits, A.I., Buck, D. and Shaw, S. (1993) Selective expression of integrin $\alpha 4\beta 7$ on a subset of human CD4+ memory T-cells with hallmarks of gut-trophism. *Journal of Immunology* **151**, 717–729.

Shaw, S., Luce, G.E.G., Quinones, R., Gress, R.E., Springer, T.A. and Sanders, M.E. (1986) Two antigen-independent adhesion pathways used by human cytotoxic T-cell clones. *Nature* **323**, 262–264.

Sheilds, P.L., Morland, C.M., Salmon, M., Qin, S., Hubscher, S.G. and Adams, D.H. (1999) Chemokine and chemokine receptor interactions provide a mechanism for selective T cell recruitment to specific liver compartments within hepatitis C-infected liver. *Journal of Immunology* **163**, 6236–6243.

Sheron, N., Bird, G., Koskinas, J., Portmann, B., Ceska, M., Lindley, I. and Williams, R. (1993) Circulating and tissue-levels of the neutrophil chemotaxin interleukin-8 are elevated in severe acute alcoholic hepatitis, and tissue-levels correlate with neutrophil infiltration. *Hepatology* **18**, 41–46.

Shimada, S.Y. M.A. T.G. (1993) Serum levels of intercellular adhesion molecule-1 in patients with alcoholic liver disease. *Alcohol and Alcoholism* 47–51.

Shiratori, Y. (1993) Production of chemotactic factor, interleukin-8, from hepatocytes exposed to ethanol. *Hepatology* **18**, 1477–1482.

Sprenger, H., Kaufmann, A., Garn, H., Lahme, B., Gemsa, D. and Gressner, A.M. (1997) Induction of neutrophil-attracting chemokines in transforming rat hepatic stellate cells. *Gastroenterology* **113**, 277–285.

Springer, T.A. (1990) Adhesion receptors of the immune system. *Nature* **346**, 425–434.

Springer, T.A. (1994) Traffic signals for lymphocyte recirculation and leukocyte emigration: the multistep paradigm. *Cell* **76**, 301–314.

Steinhoff, G., Behrend, M., Schrader, B., Duijvestijn, A.M. and Wonigeit, K. (1993) Expression patterns of leukocyte adhesion ligand molecules on human liver endothelia – lack of ELAM-1 and CD62 inducibility on sinusoidal endothelia and distinct distribution of VCAM-1, ICAM-1, ICAM-2 and LFA-3. *American Journal of Pathology* **142**, 481–488.

Swerlick, R.A., Lee, K.H. and Lawley, T.J. (1992) Regulation of VCAM-1 on human dermal microvascular endothelial cells. *J Cell Biochem* **16A**, 54.

Tanaka, Y., Adams, D.H. and Shaw, S. (1993a) Proteoglycan on endothelial cells present adhesion-inducing cytokines to leukocytes. *Immunol Today* **14**, 111–114.

Tanaka, Y., Adams, D.H., Hubscher, S., Hirano, H., Siebenlist, U. and Shaw, S. (1993b) T-cell adhesion induced by proteoglycan-immobilized cytokine MIP-1β. *Nature* **361**, 79–82.

Tanaka, Y., Albelda, S.M., Horgan, K.J., van Seventer, G.A., Shimizu, Y., Newman, W., Hallam, J., Newman, P.J., Buck, C.A. and Shaw, S. (1992) CD31 expressed on distinctive T-cell subsets is a preferential amplifier of β1 integrin-mediated adhesion. *J Exp Med* **176**, 245–253.

Taub, D.D., Turcovskicorrales, S.M., Key, M.L., Longo, D.L. and Murphy, W.J. (1996) Chemokines and T-lymphocyte activation. 1. Beta chemokines costimulate human T-lymphocyte activation *in vitro*. *Journal of Immunology* **156**, 2095–2103.

Uksila, J., Salmi, M., Butcher, E.C., Tarkkanen, J. and Jalkanen, S. (1997) Function of lymphocyte homing-associated adhesion molecules on human natural killer and lymphokine-activated killer cells. *Journal of Immunology* **158**, 1610–1617.

Vedder, N.B., Winn, R.K., Rice, C.L., Chi, E.Y., Arfors, K.E. and Harlan, J.M. (1988) A monoclonal antibody to the adherence-promoting leukocyte glycoprotein, CD18, reduces organ injury and improves survival from hemorrhagic shock and resuscitation in rabbits. *J Clin Invest* **81**, 939–944.

Vedder, N.B., Winn, R.K., Rice, C.L. and Harlan, J.M. (1989) Neutrophil-mediated vascular injury in shock and multiple organ failure. *Prog Clin Biol Res* **299**, 181–191.

Volpes, R., van den Oord, J.J. and Desmet, V.J. (1991) Distribution of the VLA family of integrins in normal and pathological human tissue. *Gastroenterology* **101**, 200–206.

Volpes, R., van den Oord, J.J. and Desmet, V.J. (1992) Vascular adhesion molecules in acute and chronic liver disease. *Hepatology* **15**, 269–275.

Webb, D.S., Shimizu, Y., van Seventer, G.A., Shaw, S. and Gerrard, T.L. (1990) LFA-3, CD44, and CD45: Physiologic triggers of human monocyte TNF and IL-1 release. *Science* **249**, 1295–1297.

Winn, R.K., Sharar, S.R., Vedder, N.B. and Harlan, J.M. (1995) The contribution of adherent leukocytes to septic shock. In *Physiology and Pathophysiology of Leukocyte Adhesion*, edited by D.N. Granger and G.W. Schmid-Schonbein, pp. 381–392. New York: Oxford University Press.

Wong, J., Johnston, B., Lee, S.S., Bullard, D.C., Smith, C.W., Beaudet, A.L. and Kubes, P. (1997) A minimal role for selectins in the recruitment of leukocytes into the inflamed liver microvasculature. *Journal of Clinical Investigation* **99**, 2782–2790.

Yoong, K.F., Afford, S.C., Adujla, P., Qin, S., Price, K., Hubscher, S.G. and Adams, D.H. (1999) Expression and function of CXC and CC chemokines in human malignant liver tumors: A role for HuMIG in lymphocyte recruitment to hepatocellular carcinoma. *Hepatology* **30**, 100–111.

Yoong, K.F., McNab, G., Hubscher, S.G. and Adams, D.H. (1998) Vascular adhesion protein-1 and ICAM-1 support the adhesion of tumor infiltrating lymphocytes to tumor endothelium in human hepatocellular carcinoma. *Journal of Immunology* **160**, 3978–3988.

Chapter 10

Role of endotoxin and Kupffer cells as triggers of hypoxia-reoxygenation in alcoholic liver injury

R.G. Thurman*, B.U. Bradford, K.T. Knecht, Y. Iimuro,
G.E. Arteel, M. Yin, H.D. Connor, C. Rivera,
J.A. Raleigh, M.v. Frankenberg, Y. Adachi, D.T. Forman,
D. Brenner, M. Kadiiska and R.P. Mason

Research from this laboratory using a continuous enteral alcohol administration model has demonstrated that Kupffer cells are pivotal in the development of alcohol-induced liver injury. Destruction of Kupffer cells with gadolinium chloride (GdCl$_3$) or sterilization of the gut with neomycin and polymixin B blocked early inflammation due to alcohol. Anti-TNF-α antibody markedly decreased alcohol-induced liver injury and increased TNF mRNA. These data led to the hypothesis that alcohol-induced liver injury involves increases in circulating endotoxin leading to activation of Kupffer cells. Pimonidazole, a nitroimidazole marker, was used to quantitate hypoxia in downstream pericentral regions of the lobule. Following acute alcohol or chronic enteral alcohol, pimonidazole binding was increased significantly in pericentral regions of the liver lobule and was reduced after GdCl$_3$. Enteral alcohol increased free radical generation detected with ESR. These radical species had coupling constants matching α-hydroxyethyl radical and were shown conclusively to arise from alcohol, based on a doubling of the ESR lines when ^{13}C-ethyl alcohol was given. α-Hydroxyethyl radical production was decreased by destruction of Kupffer cells with GdCl$_3$.

Female alcoholics develop more severe alcohol-induced liver injury faster and with less alcohol than males. Female rats on the enteral protocol exhibited injury more quickly with widespread fatty changes over a larger portion of the liver lobule than males. Plasma endotoxin, ICAM-1, free radical adducts, infiltrating neutrophils and NF κ-B were about 2-fold greater in livers from females than males after one month of enteral alcohol treatment. Furthermore, estrogen treatment increased the sensitivity of Kupffer cells to endotoxin. These data are consistent with the hypothesis that Kupffer cells participate in important gender differences in liver injury caused by alcohol.

KEYWORDS: Kupffer cells, endotoxin, alcohol, hepatic injury, hypoxia-reoxygenation, gender, rats

INTRODUCTION

The toxic effects of alcohol on the liver have been described in detail (Lieber, 1991); however, factors responsible for its hepatotoxicity have not been fully

---

*Dr Thurman died suddenly on July 14, 2001. His contribution to Science and Mentorship are immeasurable.

characterized. It is known that chronic alcohol ingestion stimulates hepatic oxygen consumption and causes atty liver, hepatomegaly, inflammation, fibrosis, and cirrhosis. Now Kupffer cells appear to be involved in several aspects of this pathology.

Since alcoholics are prone to infection, interest in the effect of alcohol on the reticuloendothelial system (RES) has increased (Adams and Jordan, 1984). After consumption of alcohol, significant alterations in host defense mechanisms occur, including changes in reticuloendothelial function as well as modified immune, lymphocyte, granulocyte and platelet functions (McCuskey, 1991; Tabakoff *et al.*, 1988). Recently, attention has turned toward the effect of alcohol on Kupffer cell function, which is activated by gut endotoxin (LPS), and its possible relationship to alcohol-induced liver damage (Nolan *et al.*, 1980). Conversely, the hepatocyte has been the chief focus of most studies on the effects of alcohol on liver function.

The ability of Kupffer cells to eliminate and detoxify various exogenous and endogenous substances (e.g., endotoxin) is an important physiologic regulatory function. Recent experiments have shown that Kupffer cell function modulates metabolism of alcohol in rats (Bradford *et al.*, 1993), supporting the hypothesis that Kupffer cells produce mediators (e.g., prostaglandins or cytokines) necessary for oxidation of alcohol (McCuskey *et al.*, 1987).

It has been suggested that the cascade of events leading to hepatotoxicity by alcohol is initiated by increasing the delivery of endotoxin. We hypothesize that endotoxin stimulates Kupffer cells initially, a critical step in producing a hypermetabolic state (e.g., the Swift Increase in Alcohol Metabolism; SIAM) in parenchymal cells (see Figure 10.1). Subsequently, hypoxia develops in pericentral regions of the liver lobule where toxic free radicals are formed upon reintroduction of oxygen, resulting in cell death. This chapter will review new evidence for the proposal that Kupffer cells play a pivotal role in hepatotoxicity following alcohol exposure, focusing predominantly on new information obtained with an enteral alcohol delivery system.

GUT INVOLVEMENT IN ALCOHOL-INDUCED LIVER DAMAGE

Much evidence suggests that the gut and endotoxin participate in alcoholic liver injury. Elevated levels of circulating endotoxin delivered to the liver via portal blood could cause hepatic tissue injury (Figure 10.1). One hypothesis is that ethanol alters gut microflora, resulting in increased gram-negative bacteria, which is the source of gut-derived endotoxin. Alternatively, ethanol could alter the permeability of the gut to macromolecules, thus increasing the release of endotoxin from the gut into the portal circulation. What evidence supports these ideas?

THE EFFECT OF ETHANOL ON THE GUT FLORA

Since malnutrition is frequently a complication of alcoholism, the effect of diet and ethanol on the gut flora is an important consideration (Rao *et al.*, 1987; French, 1993). French demonstrated that a diet rich in unsaturated fatty acids (linoleic or

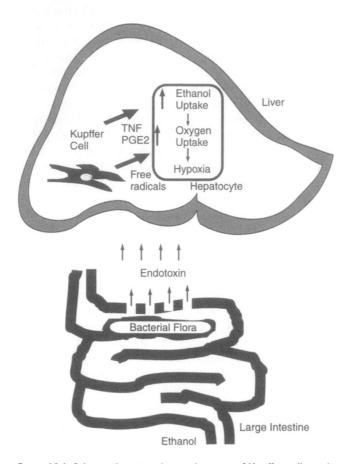

Figure 10.1 Scheme depicting the involvement of Kupffer cells, endotoxin, hypoxia, and free radicals in the mechanism of ethanol-induced liver injury. Ethanol consumption alters gut permeability, and levels of endotoxin in the blood increase. Endotoxin activates Kupffer cells, which release many chemicals including cytokines and eicosanoids. We hypothesize that these substances stimulate oxygen and ethanol uptake leading to hypoxic conditions, free radical generation, and ultimately liver injury.

linolenic) was an absolute requirement for ethanol-induced liver damage in an enteral ethanol delivery model (French, 1993). Rats fed a beef tallow diet showed minimal hepatic injury after chronic ethanol exposure (Nanji *et al.*, 1989; French, 1993) and had normal gut bacterial flora (Hentges *et al.*, 1977). In contrast, several studies demonstrated that the gut microflora was relatively insensitive to diet (Rowland *et al.*, 1985). Despite these reports, jejunal microflora was increased in alcoholics, and the rise occurred principally in gram-negative species, a major source of endotoxin (Bode *et al.*, 1984). A key variable in the latter study appeared to be gut pH. A shift of the pH of gastric juice to more basic values observed in alcoholics, may explain the increase of bacteria in the jejunum (Ruddell *et al.*, 1980). Furthermore, ethanol-induced liver injury was diminished when gut microflora was reduced after lactobacillus or antibiotic administration in an enteral ethanol feeding model (Tsukamoto-French) (Nanji *et al.*, 1994). Lactobacillus can suppress the growth of a broad range of gram-negative bacteria due to the production of low molecular weight substances. Taken together, these studies demonstrate that the gut microflora could become more virulent (i.e., produce and/or release more endotoxin) when exposed to ethanol; however, a causal relation to the disease process has not been proved.

ENDOTOXIN PARTICIPATES IN ETHANOL-INDUCED INJURY

Under normal conditions, the gut mucosal layer is an imperfect barrier, allowing small amounts of antigens and other macromolecules to pass through the intestinal wall into the blood. Gut permeability to macromolecules is increased by exposure to ethanol (Bode, 1980). Both acute and chronic contact with ethanol increases gut permeability to hemoglobin, horseradish peroxidase and polyvinyl pyrolidon-macromolecules (Bode, 1980). Furthermore, acute *in vitro* exposure to ethanol increases permeability of the isolated small intestine to labeled endotoxin in a dose-dependent fashion (Arai, 1986). In alcoholics, permeability to labeled EDTA was elevated about 2-fold in the small intestine as compared to healthy controls (Bjarnason *et al.*, 1984). Physical and chemical studies employing electron spin resonance (ESR) of interactions of lipids with membranes have demonstrated that ethanol increases membrane fluidity due to alterations in the lipid and lipoprotein composition of the cell membrane (Chin and Goldstein, 1977). This modification of membrane fluidity due to ethanol could result in increased transport and absorption of macromolecules. Changes in membrane fluidity due to ethanol were observed almost 20 years prior to significant experiments using the Tsukamoto-French model, which demonstrated that dietary requirements were involved in ethanol toxicity. At this point, it is not clear whether dietary effects that prevent hepatic injury can be explained at the level of the gut mucosal barrier.

THE EFFECT OF ENDOTOXIN ON KUPFFER AND PARENCHYMAL CELLS

Acute exposure to endotoxin causes hepatic injury, and it has been reported that Kupffer cells participate in this mechanism since they are the principal site of removal of circulating endotoxin from blood (Nolan and Camara, 1988). Endotoxin activates Kupffer cells and triggers the release of a variety of potent effectors and cytokines. The majority of the biologic effects of endotoxin are likely to be mediated by these chemical factors, including chemoattractants (e.g., tumor necrosis factor), procoagulants, cytotoxic factors (lysosomal enzymes, reactive oxygen free radicals), and vasoactive eicosanoids (prostaglandins, leukotrienes). Hepatic Kupffer cells scavenge 90% of endotoxin injected intravenously (Arii *et al.*, 1988). Moreover, it is possible that the production of mediators from activated Kupffer cells leads directly to parenchymal cell injury (Monden *et al.*, 1991a,b). Two key cytokines which can produce a shock-like state induced by endotoxin treatment are tumor necrosis factor-alpha (TNF-α) and platelet activating factor (PAF) (Tracy *et al.*, 1986; Wallace *et al.*, 1987). TNF-α increases PAF release, and perhaps both participate in a cytokine cascade that precipitates the toxic response of LPS. Indeed, it was recently demonstrated that glycine, a simple amino acid which prevented mortality due to LPS (Ikejima *et al.*, 1996), decreased TNF-α release by about 80%.

Several studies have reported the direct effect of LPS on hepatocytes (DePalma *et al.*, 1970; Utili *et al.*, 1979; Ramadori *et al.*, 1990). Hepatocytes have membrane receptors for both endotoxin and the lipid A component of LPS. Since LPS impairs the uptake and excretion of dyes into the bile (DePalma *et al.*, 1970; Utili *et al.*, 1979), a direct effect of LPS on hepatocytes could lead to hepatic injury. On the other hand, LPS causes glycogenolysis in hepatocytes by stimulating Kupffer cells to release prostaglandins (Kuiper *et al.*, 1989), suggesting an indirect regulatory effect of Kupffer cells on hepatocytes. Therefore, Kupffer cells are not only the main site of removal of LPS, but also the cell type responsible for mediating the metabolic effects of LPS. Although endotoxin activates neutrophils and induces their accumulation in the liver very rapidly, inactivation of Kupffer cells by $GdCl_3$ treatment attenuates this effect. These results indicate that Kupffer cells may participate in the mechanism of neutrophil-mediated hepatic injury, most likely via production of chemoattractants.

Not much evidence has been reported on pathological changes or tissue injury induced by chronic treatment with LPS. However, a series of studies showed a toxic effect of chronic endotoxin exposure. When rats received a choline-deficient diet for a year, 70% of the animals developed cirrhosis; but when the antibiotic neomycin was administered in the drinking water, fibrosis was averted (Rutenburg *et al.*, 1957). However, when purified *E. coli* LPS was added with neomycin, the protective effect of the antibiotic was not observed (Broitman *et al.*, 1964). These results led to the conclusion that LPS is a crucial factor in the development of cirrhosis due to choline deficiency.

Carbon tetrachloride (CCl_4) also enhanced the toxicity of LPS. When CCl_4 was administered in small doses, the LD_{50} for endotoxin decreased 600-fold (Formal *et al.*, 1960), and treatment with antibiotics diminished the intestinal microflora and prevented toxicity due to CCl_4 (Leach and Forbes, 1941). Similarly, various experimental animal models of toxic liver injury have demonstrated the toxic effects of CCl_4 occurred by limiting the intestinal production of endotoxin.

D-galactosamine causes hepatic injury by inhibiting the synthesis of uracil nucleotides; however, when LPS production was blocked by colectomy, damage did not occur even when the hepatocyte was unable to synthesize protein (Liehr *et al.*, 1978). Recent studies have demonstrated that glycine and gadolinium chloride, which act on the Kupffer cell, prevent *D*-galactosamine toxicity in rats (Stachlewitz and Thurman, 1997). Interestingly, in all of these studies, LPS produced midzonal and pericentral lesions similar to those observed in chronic ethanol-induced liver disease.

ETHANOL AGGRAVATES THE EFFECT OF ENDOTOXIN

Previously, it has been reported that blood endotoxin is often elevated in alcoholics (Bode *et al.*, 1987; Fukui *et al.*, 1991). In exciting experiments using the

Tsukamoto-French model, levels of endotoxin in the blood began to rise after approximately 2 weeks of continuous intragastric administration of ethanol in the diet (Nanji *et al.*, 1993). Endotoxin values increased nearly 5-fold in the systemic circulation and levels of endotoxin in the portal circulation were most likely even higher. Interestingly, a good correlation ($r = 0.84$) between blood endotoxin and pathology (necrosis, steatosis, infiltration, etc.) was observed (Nanji *et al.*, 1993). The Bodes (Bode, 1980; Bode *et al.*, 1987) as well as Herbert Remmer (Remmer, 1981) have consistently been the proponents of the theory that endotoxin plays a role in alcoholic liver injury.

Adachi *et al.* (1995) demonstrated that administration of antibiotics protected rats maintained on the Tsukamoto-French model from ethanol-induced liver injury. In this study, rats received diets, supplemented with Polymixin B, neomycin (150 mg/kg/day and 450 mg/kg/day respectively) and ethanol. Serum AST levels were decreased significantly about 50% by antibiotics (Figure 10.2). Moreover, a summary pathology score which quantitates necrosis, steatosis and inflammation was reduced from 4.5 to 1 by destruction of endotoxin-producing bacteria. These data are consistent with the hypothesis that removal of endotoxin from the gut protects against ethanol-induced liver injury.

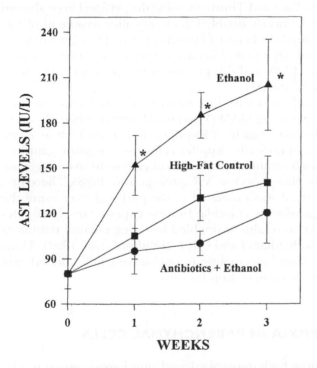

Figure 10.2 The effect of ethanol and antibiotic treatment on serum AST levels in the rat. Blood was collected from the tail vein weekly and AST was determined colorimetrically. Control rats were fed a high-fat corn oil-based liquid diet. Results are expressed as mean $\pm$ SEM; $n = 5$–10. *, $p < 0.05$ compared with other values.

Acute exposure to ethanol activates Kupffer cells (D'Souza *et al.*, 1992, 1993). During acute exposure to ethanol, carbon uptake by the perfused liver due to phagocytosis of particles by Kupffer cells increased about 25% (D'Souza *et al.*, 1993). Further, carbon uptake in the perfused liver was also elevated significantly by about 35% in rats treated with 5.0 g/kg ethanol, 2.5 hours prior to perfusion. Similar results have been obtained *in vivo* (Earnest *et al.*, 1990).

Little data linking Kupffer cell function to chronic ethanol exposure have been reported (Yamada *et al.*, 1991). In a recent study, however, oxygen radical production by Kupffer cells was increased following chronic ethanol treatment (Yamada *et al.*, 1991). Others have reported that TNF release and the mRNA of TNF expression were increased by ethanol (Earnest *et al.*, 1993), supporting findings that TNF increases in alcoholics (Martinez *et al.*, 1992). However, a number of studies have shown that ethanol suppresses Kupffer cell function (Nelson *et al.*, 1989; D'Souza *et al.*, 1993). Reasons for these discrepancies remain unclear.

KUPFFER CELLS AND PARENCHYMAL CELLS PLAY A ROLE IN HYPERMETABOLISM

Israel and colleagues (1975) were the first to describe a hypermetabolic state due to ethanol exposure. Moreover, Yuki and Thurman, using the perfused liver, showed that oxygen and ethanol uptake nearly doubled 2.5 hours after treatment of rats with a single large dose of ethanol (Yuki and Thurman, 1980). They later demonstrated that hormone-mediated depletion of hepatic carbohydrate reserves a play role in this process (Yuki *et al.*, 1980) and this phenomenon was named the "Swift Increase in Alcohol Metabolism" (SIAM).

Elevation of ethanol metabolism occurs in concert with a reduction in both glycolysis and glycogen reserves during SIAM (Yuki and Thurman, 1980). Recently, studies have demonstrated the involvement of Kupffer cells in carbohydrate metabolism (Casteleijn *et al.*, 1988). Specifically, Kupffer cells produce prostaglandins, primarily PGD_2 and PGE_2, which stimulate production of glucose from endogenous hepatic glycogen by activating phosphorylase A (Casteleijn *et al.*, 1988). Therefore, the role of Kupffer cells in SIAM was evaluated in the perfused liver using the selective Kupffer cell toxin, gadolinium chloride. In these experiments, basal rates of oxygen and ethanol uptake were almost doubled following ethanol treatment and blocked after treatment with ethanol and $GdCl_3$ (Bradford *et al.*, 1993). Thus, increases in respiration and ethanol metabolism were observed, following ethanol treatment were blocked by inactivation of Kupffer cells.

ETHANOL CAUSES HYPOXIA IN PARENCHYMAL CELLS

In addition to hypermetabolism, high doses of ethanol alter hepatic microcirculation (Hijioka *et al.*, 1991) by stimulating endothelin-1 production (Oshita *et al.*, 1993). Furthermore, hypoxia increases pathological changes in the Tsukamoto-French model (French *et al.*, 1984). Substantial evidence indicates that hypoxia contributes to ethanol-induced liver injury. Since ethanol also causes a compensatory increase in hepatic blood flow and thus elevates hepatic oxygen concentration, it has been proposed that this increase negates any effect of hypoxia due to hypermetabolism or microcirculatory disturbances (Shaw *et al.*, 1977). Pimonidazole, a 2-nitroimidazole hypoxia marker, was used to address this question (Arteel *et al.*, 1995). Pimonidazole, which is reductively activated by nitroreductases, binds to thiol residues on proteins and macromolecules in the cell in the absence of oxygen. Marker adducts can be detected immunochemically (e.g., with ELISA or immunohistochemical analysis). The results of these experiments confirmed that downstream (i.e., pericentral) hypoxia occurs after induction of SIAM which was blocked when Kupffer cells were destroyed with $GdCl_3$ (Bradford *et al.*, 1993).

Previous studies using miniature oxygen electrodes and microfiber optics have demonstrated that oxygen uptake by the liver is dependent on local oxygen tension (Matsumura and Thurman, 1983). Indeed, when livers were perfused in the retrograde direction, oxygen uptake was shifted predominantly from periportal to pericentral areas of the liver lobule (Thurman and Kauffman, 1985). This phenomenon was the first clue that an oxygen sensing system is present in the liver. Rapid metabolic functions of the liver, such as urea and glucose synthesis, follow the oxygen concentration gradient; in contrast, very slow enzyme-limited processes, such as cytochrome P-450-dependent metabolism of drugs, predominate in pericentral regions irrespective of the local oxygen tension (Thurman and Kauffman, 1985). Hypermetabolism associated with a local elevation of phosphorylase A, a calcium-sensitive enzyme (Matsumura *et al.*, 1992), and the effect of oxygen supply on oxygen uptake, was blocked by W-7, an inhibitor of calcium-calmodulin (Hoek and Rubin, 1990). It is well known that ethanol activates polyphosphoinositide-specific phospholipase C in hepatocytes (Hoek and Rubin, 1990). Therefore, calcium is likely involved in oxygen-dependent metabolism, but its precise role remains unclear.

It was recently demonstrated that chronic ethanol treatment using the Tsukamoto-French protocol also causes hypoxia (Adachi *et al.*, 1994). These data provide direct evidence that ethanol *in vivo* increases tissue hypoxia (Arteel *et al.*, 1996). Miniature oxygen electrodes were used to measure oxygen tension on the surface of livers from Tsukamoto-French rats. This methodology is based on the fact that the terminal portal venule ends about 200 microns from the liver surface. Lower values reflect relative hypoxia regardless of its mechanisms (e.g., hypermetabolism or microcirculatory disturbances). Surface hepatic oxygen tension determined with this technique was decreased over 30% by ethanol treatment (Adachi *et al.*, 1995) and hypoxia was blocked when Kupffer cells were inactivated with $GdCl_3$. By employing the hypoxia marker pimonidazole, hypoxia could be quantitated in Tsukamoto-French rats following 4 weeks of ethanol feeding. Image analysis techniques demonstrated that ethanol treatment for 1 or 4 weeks increased pimonidazole binding from 18% (control) to 32–35% (ethanol) in the liver (Figure 10.3) (Arteel *et al.*, 1997). Thus, direct evidence has been obtained demonstrating that hypoxia caused by ethanol treatment occurs downstream in the clinically relevant Tsukamoto-French model or after acute ethanol treatment.

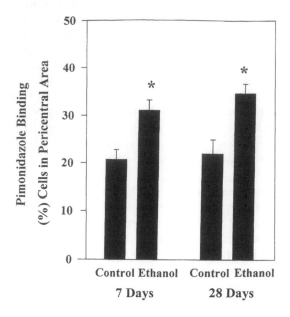

Figure 10.3 Effect of ethanol on pimonidazole binding quantitated by immunohistochemistry. Controls received a high-fat enteral diet for 7 or 28 days as indicated. Image-analysis was performed to determine the percentage of cells stained in pericentral regions. Results are means ± SEM; $n = 4$. *, $p < .05$ compared with controls using one-way ANOVA.

KUPFFER CELLS IN ETHANOL-INDUCED LIVER INJURY *IN VIVO*

Several observations support the hypothesis that Kupffer cells are involved in hepatic injury caused by ethanol. First, ethanol affects Kupffer cell functions such as phagocytosis, bactericidal activity and cytokine production (Martinez *et al.*, 1992; Yamada *et al.*, 1991). Second, increased serum TNF-α concentrations in alcoholics (Stahnke *et al.*, 1991) support the idea that Kupffer cells are activated in patients with alcoholic liver disease. TNF is produced exclusively by the monocyte-macrophage lineage and Kupffer cells are the major population of this lineage (Decker *et al.*, 1989). Third, Kupffer cells, which contain Ca^{2+} channels (Hijioka *et al.*, 1992), are activated by Ca^{2+} (Decker, 1990) and chronic ethanol treatment facilitates activation of Ca^{2+} channels in Kupffer cells (Goto *et al.*, 1994). Iimuro and colleagues recently demonstrated that nimodipine, a calcium channel blocker, reduced ethanol-induced injury in the Tsukamoto-French model, suggesting that calcium channels play a crucial role in Kupffer cell activation (Iimuro *et al.*, 1996). Collectively, these observations support the hypothesis that chronic exposure to ethanol leads to stimulation of Kupffer cells.

The lack of appropriate experimental models hampered studies on the mechanism of ethanol-induced liver injury in laboratory animals until Tsukamoto and French introduced the *in vivo* rat model of continuous intragastric ethanol administration (Tsukamoto *et al.*, 1984, 1985). In addition to steatosis present in other models of ethanol injury, this model exhibits significant characteristics of human alcoholic liver disease, including inflammation, pericentral necrosis and ultimately fibrosis (French *et al.*, 1986).

Adachi *et al.* (1994) demonstrated that when Kupffer cells in rats on the Tsukamoto-French protocol were inactivated by twice weekly treatment with gadolinium chloride ($GdCl_3$), serum enzyme levels were decreased significantly. Moreover, fatty changes, inflammation and necrosis were all reduced by $GdCl_3$ treatment (Adachi *et al.*, 1994). The hepatic pathological score of rats treated with ethanol for 4 weeks of 4.3 ± 0.6 was decreased significantly in ethanol- and $GdCl_3$-treated rats to 1.8 ± 0.5 (Figure 10.4). In addition, oxygen tension on the surface of the liver was similar in controls and rats treated with $GdCl_3$ and ethanol. These results demonstrated that inactivation of Kupffer cells by $GdCl_3$ treatment prevents early

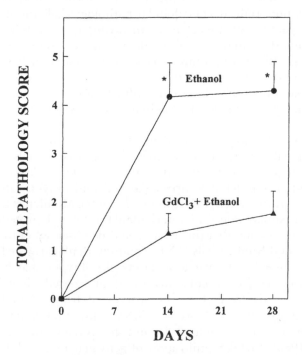

Figure 10.4 Effect of $GdCl_3$ on pathology of livers from rats treated chronically with ethanol using the Tsukamoto-French model. Liver pathology was scored as described by Nanji *et al.* (1989) as follows: steatosis (the percentage of liver cells containing fat): <25% = 1+; <50% = 2+; <75% = 3+; >75% = 4+; inflammation and necrosis: 1 focus per low power field = 1 +; 2 or more = 2 +. One point was given for each grade of severity of histological abnormality as described, and a total score was calculated for each liver. *, $p < 0.05$ vs control value. $n = 4$–6, mean $\pm$ SEM.

hepatic injury. A logical conclusion is that Kupffer cells play a pivotal role in the early changes that lead ultimately to alcohol-induced liver disease.

HOW DO KUPFFER CELLS, ACTIVATED BY ETHANOL TREATMENT, PARTICIPATE IN LIVER INJURY?

As described above, a possible mechanism of ethanol-induced liver injury involves hypoxia. Israel and colleagues reported that chronic ethanol treatment increased hepatic oxygen uptake (Videla *et al.*, 1973; Bernstein *et al.*, 1973), while Ji *et al.* (1982) demonstrated that the increased tissue respiration induced by chronic treatment with ethanol, enhanced the intralobular oxygen gradient. This increase in oxygen uptake is caused by an ethanol-induced hypermetabolic state (Yuki and Thurman, 1980). Consequent centrilobular hypoxia may be responsible for pericentral liver damage induced by ethanol, and inactivation of Kupffer cells with GdCl$_3$ treatment prevented the increases in oxygen uptake (Bradford *et al.*, 1993). In the Tsukamoto-French model, rates of metabolism of ethanol, which require oxygen, were elevated 2- to 3-fold in rats exposed to ethanol for 2–4 weeks. As expected from previous findings, inactivation of Kupffer cells with GdCl$_3$ blocked the elevation in ethanol elimination. Indeed, centrilobular pathological alterations observed in this study are compatible with a mechanism involving hypoxia. When O$_2$ tension in the liver was diminished, injury in this model was increased (French *et al.*, 1984; Tsukamoto and Xi, 1989). Importantly, conditioned medium from isolated Kupffer cells of ethanol-treated rats stimulated parenchymal cell oxygen consumption and contained elevated levels of prostaglandin E$_2$ (Qu *et al.*, 1996). Moreover, when prostaglandin E$_2$ was added to parenchymal cells, oxygen uptake was also stimulated.

An alternative explanation for the involvement of the Kupffer cell in hepatic injury is that activated Kupffer cells release mediators that are toxic to liver cells or serve as chemoattractants for cytotoxic neutrophils that invade the liver. Various toxic mediators including TNF-α, interleukins, prostaglandins and oxygen radicals are released from activated Kupffer cells (Martinez *et al.*, 1992). Monden *et al.* (1991a) reported that TNF-α, superoxide and interleukin-1 inhibited protein synthesis in cultured rat hepatocytes and that this effect could be observed in the supernatant of cultures of activated Kupffer cells. TNF-α and interleukin-1, which have been demonstrated to be directly cytotoxic to a variety of cell types, may be direct mediators of hepatocyte injury. In a recent study, rats administered ethanol enterally and injected with antibody to TNF-α were protected from ethanol-induced hepatic injury (Iimuro *et al.*, 1997b). Moreover, TNF-α and interleukin-1 stimulate neutrophil migration and activation and also induce protease and oxygen radical release (Thiele, 1989). Cellular infiltration of activated neutrophils, which produce oxygen radicals and secrete other toxic mediators, may increase the inflammatory response, leading to cell injury and death. Indeed, inflammatory cell infiltration due to ethanol was blocked by GdCl$_3$ treatment (see Figure 10.4). Microcirculatory disturbances caused by vasoconstrictive mediators released from Kupffer cells and neutrophils could enhance hypoxia and lead to a vicious cycle of pathophysiology.

ROLE OF GENDER

Evaluation of 1600 alcoholic patients demonstrated that the two independent risk factors for development of cirrhosis are being overweight for at least 10 years and being female (Naveau *et al.*, 1997). A recent study using the Tsukamoto-French model of enteral ethanol feeding has established that ethanol causes more hepatic injury in female than male rats (Iimuro *et al.*, 1997a). In this study, parameters including serum AST, pathological score, neutrophil infiltration levels of circulating endotoxin and intracellular adhesion molecule-1 expression were measured. Interestingly, all parameters assessed were increased significantly in females as compared to males. The most impressive histological change was the overall deposition of fat in livers from female rats at 2 and 4 weeks of ethanol feeding. The distribution of fat was panlobular in females, whereas it was localized in the pericentral region of the livers from male rats. Plasma endotoxin levels were significantly higher in female rats after 4 weeks of ethanol (Figure 10.5). Furthermore, infiltration of inflammatory cells was not different between males and females (Figure 10.6); however, significant increases were observed after 4 weeks of ethanol administration in both genders, and a 2-fold greater increase was observed in the female liver (Figure 10.6). These data collectively demonstrate that females are more susceptible to ethanol-induced liver injury. The mechanism of this phenomenon should be carefully evaluated.

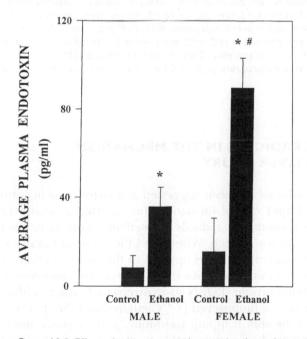

Figure 10.5 Effect of ethanol on endotoxin levels in plasma. Plasma endotoxin levels in control and ethanol-fed male and female rats were determined with the limulus amebocyte lysate assay. Data represent mean ± SEM, $n = 4$–7. *, $p < 0.05$ compared with control rats. #, $p < 0.05$ compared with male ethanol-fed rats by ANOVA.

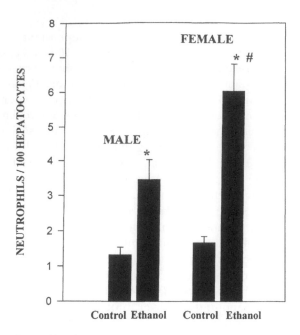

Figure 10.6 The effect of ethanol treatment on the number of inflammatory cells in the liver. Numbers of inflammatory cells observed in hematoxylin and eosin sections of the liver in control and ethanol-fed rats are depicted. Values were determined by counting polymorphonuclear cells in 5 high-power fields (×400) per slide. The number of hepatocytes was also counted in each field, and the number of inflammatory cells was expressed per 100 hepatocytes. Data represent mean ± SEM, $n = 5$–6. *, $p < 0.05$ compared with control rats. #, $p < 0.05$ compared with male ethanol-fed rats by ANOVA.

INVOLVEMENT OF FREE RADICALS IN THE MECHANISM OF ETHANOL-INDUCED LIVER INJURY

Production of free radicals by ethanol has been suggested as a factor in its hepato-toxicity. Although evidence of lipid radical formation due to ethanol treatment *in vivo* has been reported, only recently free radicals from ethanol alone have been detected in living animals (Knecht *et al.*, 1990). When the EPR (electron paramag-netic resonance) technique of spin trapping was applied to the study of ethanol-treated alcohol dehydrogenase-deficient deer mice (ADH⁻, *Peromyscus maniculatus*), the α-(4-pyridyl-1-oxide)-*N*-*t*-butylnitrone (POBN)/α-hydroxyethyl radical adduct was detected in bile from deer mice administered [1-^{13}C]ethanol and the spin trap POBN (Knecht *et al.*, 1990). In the spin trapping technique, a diamagnetic mole-cule reacts with a free radical to produce a more stable species or a radical adduct which can be readily detected by EPR. Radical adducts are substituted by nitroxide free radicals, which tend to be relatively long-lived compared to most free radicals, which are extremely transient. Nitroxides produced by other biological radicals are sufficiently stable to survive extraction into an organic solvent. Therefore, with spin trapping techniques, a very short-lived free radical is replaced by the comparatively long-lived radical adduct.

When a solution containing the free radical adduct is placed in a typical EPR spectrometer's magnetic field, unpaired electrons will occupy one of two energy states. These states are due to the interaction of the unpaired electron's spin angular momentum with the magnetic field and they exist only when the sample is subjected to a magnetic field. Detection of an electron resonance spectrum involves increasing the magnetic field while simultaneously exposing the sample to microwave radiation. Absorption of microwave energy, which causes electrons in the lower energy state to be excited to higher energy states, occurs only when the energy difference between the two states matches the microwave frequency precisely. The absorption of microwave energy at that particular magnetic field strength is rectified and detected by a microwave diode and then recorded as the first derivative of the absorption peak. A six-line EPR spectrum is characteristically exhibited by POBN radical adducts (Figure 10.7). ^{13}C substitution on the α-carbon of a spin-trapped species creates an additional hyperfine coupling as a result of the

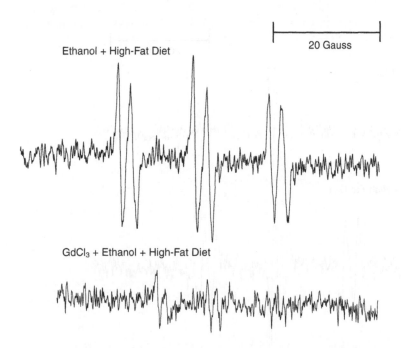

Figure 10.7 Enteral ethanol produces free radicals in the liver. Representative EPR spectra of radical adducts in bile from rats treated for at least two weeks with continuous intragastric infusion of diet: (Upper) ethanol + high-fat diet; (Lower) GdCl$_3$ + ethanol + high-fat diet. Bile ducts were cannulated under Nembutal anesthesia and 100 mg/kg of the spin trap POBN was administered i.p. Bile samples were collected into vials containing 50 mM desferal to prevent *ex vivo* free radical formation for 3–4 hours, frozen on dry ice, and analyzed for free radical adducts with EPR spectroscopy.

magnetic interaction of the ^{13}C nucleus with the free electron. The subsequent production of a 12-line spectrum confirms that the trapped radical arises from the labeled parent compound (Knecht *et al.*, 1990). Therefore, the radical detected is derived from ethanol and the unpaired electron density is centered at the α-carbon of ethanol.

Free radical formation most likely participates in the progression of early events in alcoholic liver disease. Recently, we detected a free radical in bile from rats exposed to ethanol on the Tsukamoto-French model (Figure 10.7; Adachi *et al.*, 1994). This free radical signal was diminished by over 50% when Kupffer cells were destroyed by treatment with GdCl$_3$. A six-line radical adduct spectrum was also detected in bile of Tsukamoto-French rats treated with an ethanol-containing, high-fat diet but not in bile from normal chow-fed rats. Furthermore, bile from animals fed with the control corn oil diet contained low concentrations of radical adducts. The free radical was identified as α-hydroxyethyl on the basis of the 12-line spectrum obtained when ^{13}C ethanol was used (Knecht *et al.*, 1995). Thus, ethanol-derived free radical formation was detected in the bile of Tsukamoto-French rats treated intragastrically with a high-fat, ethanol-containing diet.

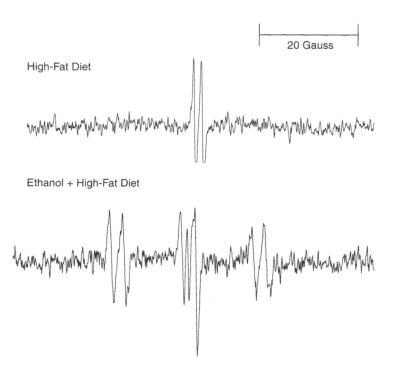

Figure 10.8 Radical adducts in pancreatic secretions. Rats were maintained on continuous enteral feeding of high-fat control (Upper) or ethanol + high fat-containing (Lower) diet for 4 weeks. Pancreatic secretions were collected by cannulation of the common bile duct after ligation of the bile duct near the liver and at the end of the duct near the Sphincter of Oddi. Samples were collected and analyzed by EPR. Representative experiments were repeated three times.

Antioxidant-insensitive free radicals have also been detected in livers of ethanol-treated rats after transplantation (Gao *et al*., 1995). Although the precise pathways responsible for formation of free radicals in ethanol-treated rats remain unclear, a likely candidate is oxygen radical production by the NADPH oxidase system in resident Kupffer cells and neutrophils, since the EPR signal was reduced by GdCl$_3$ treatment. However, a reperfusion injury involving hypoxia and free radical formation via the xanthine-xanthine oxidase system cannot be excluded, especially since radicals in bile would be expected to originate from parenchymal cells.

In a recently developed model of pancreatitis employing the Tsukamoto-French model of enteral ethanol delivery, radical adducts were analyzed in pancreatic secretions (Knecht *et al*., 1995) (Figure 10.8). In rats fed control diet, only a semiquinone ascorbate signal was detected in pancreatic secretions, whereas a robust six-line signal was observed in samples obtained from ethanol-fed rats. This signal was indicative of a carbon-centered radical adduct. Therefore, this study demonstrated that early oxidative stress occurs in the pancreas during ethanol exposure. Elucidating the source of these radicals could lead to understanding the clinical pathology.

CONCLUSION

Ethanol most likely either enhances production of gram-negative bacteria, thereby increasing endotoxin production, or increases membrane permeability of the gut to endotoxin (see Figure 10.1). Elevated levels of endotoxin activate Kupffer cells leading to the release of substances such as eicosanoids, TNF, cytokines, prostaglandins and free radicals. Prostaglandins increase oxygen uptake and most likely participate in a hypermetabolic state. Increased oxygen demand leads to hypoxia in the liver and on reperfusion, free radicals are formed which cause tissue damage in pericentral areas of the liver lobule.

ACKNOWLEDGMENTS

The authors wish to thank NIAAA for partial support of this work (AA-09156 and AA-03626).

REFERENCES

Adachi, Y., Bradford, B.U., Gao, W., Bojes, H.K. and Thurman, R.G. (1994) Inactivation of Kupffer cells prevents early alcohol-induced liver injury. *Hepatology* **20**, 453–460.

Adachi, Y., Moore, L.E., Bradford, B.U., Gao, W. and Thurman, R.G. (1995) Antibiotics prevent liver injury in rats following long-term exposure to ethanol. *Gastroenterology* **108**, 218–224.

Adams, H.G. and Jordan, C. (1984) Infections in the alcoholic. *Med Clin North Am* **68**, 179–200.

Arai, M. (1986) Effect of ethanol on the intestinal uptake of endotoxin. *Nippon Shokakibyo Gakkai Zasshi* **83**, 1060.

Arii, S., Monden, K., Itai, S., Sasaoki, T., Shibagaki, M. and Tobe, T. (1988) The three different phases of reticuloendothelial system phagocytic function in rats with liver injury. *J Surg Res* **45**, 314–319.

Arteel, G.E., Thurman, R.G., Yates, J.M. and Raleigh, J.A. (1995) Evidence that hypoxia markers detect oxygen gradients in liver: Pimonidazole and retrograde perfusion of rat liver. *Br J Cancer* **72**, 889–895.

Arteel, G.E., Raleigh, J.A., Bradford, B.U. and Thurman, R.G. (1996) Acute alcohol produces hypoxia directly in rat liver tissue *in vivo*: Role of Kupffer cells. *Am J Physiol* **271**, G494–G500.

Arteel, G.E., Iimuro, Y., Yin, M., Raleigh, J.A. and Thurman, R.G. (1997) Chronic enteral ethanol treatment causes hypoxia in rat liver tissue *in vivo*. *Hepatology* **25**, 920–926.

Bernstein, J., Videla, L. and Israel, Y. (1973) Metabolic alterations produced in the liver by chronic ethanol administration. Changes related to energetic parameters of the cell. *Biochem J* **134**, 515–521.

Bjarnason, I., Ward, K. and Peters, T.J. (1984) The leaky gut of alcoholism: Possible route of entry for toxic compounds. *Lancet* **1**, 179–182.

Bode, C., Kugler, V. and Bode, J.C. (1987) Endotoxemia in patients with alcoholic and non-alcoholic cirrhosis and in subjects with no evidence of chronic liver disease following acute alcohol excess. *J Hepatol* **4**, 8–14.

Bode, J.C., Bode, C., Heidelbach, R., Durr, H.-K. and Martini, G.A. (1984) Jejunal microflora in patients with chronic alcohol abuse. *Hepatogastroenterology* **31**, 30–34.

Bode, J.C. (1980) Alcohol and the gastrointestinal tract. In *Advances in Internal Medicine and Pediatrics*, edited by H.P. Frick, G.A. Harnack, G.A. Martini and A. Prader, pp. 1–75. Heidelberg: Springer-Verlag.

Bradford, B.U., Misra, U.K. and Thurman, R.G. (1993) Kupffer cells are required for the swift increase in alcohol metabolism. *Res Commun Subst Abuse* **14**, 1–6.

Broitman, S.A., Gottlieb, L.S. and Zamcheck, N. (1964) Influence of neomycin and ingested endotoxin in the pathogenesis of choline deficiency cirrhosis in the adult rat. *J Exp Med* **119**, 633–647.

Casteleijn, E., Kuiper, J., Van Rooij, H.C.J., Kamps, J.A.A.M., Koster, J.F. and Van Berkel, T.J.C. (1988) Hormonal control of glycogenolysis in parenchymal liver cells by Kupffer and endothelial liver cells. *J Biol Chem* **263**, 2699–2703.

Chin, J.H. and Goldstein, D.B. (1977) Effects of low concentration of ethanol on the fluidity of spin-labeled erythrocyte and brain membranes. *Mol Pharmacol* **13**, 435–441.

D'Souza, N.B., Baustista, A.P., Lang, C.H. and Spitzer, J.J. (1992) Acute ethanol intoxication prevents lipopolysaccharide-induced down regulation of protein kinase C in rat Kupffer cells. *Alcohol Clin Exp Res* **16**, 64–67.

D'Souza, N.B., Bagby, G.J., Lang, C.H., Deaciuc, I.V. and Spitzer, J.J. (1993) Ethanol alters the metabolic response of isolated, perfused rat liver to a phagocytic stimulus. *Alcohol Clin Exp Res* **17**, 147–154.

Decker, K. (1990) Biologically active products of stimulated liver macrophages (Kupffer cells). *Eur J Biochem* **192**, 245–261.

Decker, T., Lohmann-Matthes, M.L., Karck, U., Peters, T. and Decker, K. (1989) Comparative study of cytotoxicity, tumor necrosis factor, and prostaglandin release after stimulation of rat Kupffer cells, murine Kupffer cells, and murine inflammatory liver macrophages. *J Leukoc Biol* **45**, 139–146.

DePalma, R.G., Harano, Y. and Robinson, A.V. (1970) Stucture and function of hepatic mitochondria in hemorrage and endotoxemia. *Surg Forum* **21**, 3–10.

Earnest, D.L., Sim, W.W., Smith, T.L. and Eskelson, C.D. (1990) Ethanol, acetaldehyde and Kupffer cell function: potential role for Kupffer cells in alcohol induced liver injury. *Prog Clin Biol Res* **325**, 255–265.

Earnest, D.L., Abril, E.R., Jolley, C.S. and Martinez, F. (1993) Ethanol and diet-induced alterations in Kupffer cell function. *Alcohol and Alcoholism* **28**, 73–83.

Formal, S.B., Noyes, H.E. and Schneider, H. (1960) Experimental shigella infections. III. Sensitivity of normal, starved, and carbon tetrachloride treated guinea pigs to endotoxin. *Proc Soc Exp Biol Med* **103**, 415–418.

French, S.W., Benson, N.C. and Sun, P.S. (1984) Centrilobular liver necrosis induced by hypoxia in chronic ethanol-fed rats. *Hepatology* **4**, 912–917.

French, S.W., Miyamoto, K. and Tsukamoto, H. (1986) Ethanol-induced hepatic fibrosis in the rat: role of the amount of dietary fat. *Alcohol Clin Exp Res* **10**, 13S–19S.

French, S.W. (1993) Nutrition in the pathogenesis of alcoholic liver disease. *Alcohol and Alcoholism* **28**, 97–109.

Fukui, H., Brauner, B., Bode, J.C. and Bode, C. (1991) Plasma endotoxin concentrations in patients with alcoholic and non-alcoholic liver disease: re-evaluation with an improved chromogenic assay. *J Hepatology* **12**, 162–169.

Gao, W., Connor, H.D., Lemasters, J.J., Mason, R.P. and Thurman, R.G. (1995) Primary nonfunction of fatty livers produced by alcohol is associated with a new, antioxidant-insensitive free radical species. *Transplantation* **59**, 674–679.

Goto, M., Lemasters, J.J. and Thurman, R.G. (1994) Activation of voltage-dependent calcium channels in Kupffer cells by chronic treatment with alcohol in the rat. *J Pharmacol Exp Therapeut* **267**, 1264–1268.

Hentges, D.A., Maier, B.R., Burton, G.C., Flynn, M.A. and Tsutakawa, R.K. (1977) Effect of a high-beef diet on the fecal bacterial flora of humans. *Cancer Res* **37**, 568–571.

Hijioka, T., Sato, N., Matsumura, T., Yoshihara, H., Takei, Y., Fukui, H., Oshita, M., Kawano, S. and Kamada, T. (1991) Ethanol-induced disturbance of hepatic microcirculation and hepatic hypoxia. *Biochem Pharmacol* **11**, 1551–1557.

Hijioka, T., Rosenberg, R.L., Lemasters, J.J. and Thurman, R.G. (1992) Kupffer cells contain voltage-dependent calcium channels. *Mol Pharmacol* **41**, 435–440.

Hoek, J.B. and Rubin, E. (1990) Alcohol and membrane-associated signal transduction. *Alcohol and Alcoholism* **25**, 143–156.

Iimuro, Y., Ikejima, K., Rose, M.L., Bradford, B.U. and Thurman, R.G. (1996) Nimodipine, a dihydropyridine-type calcium channel blocker, prevents alcoholic hepatitis due to chronic intragastric ethanol exposure in the rat. *Hepatology* **24**, 391–397.

Iimuro, Y., Frankenberg, M.v., Arteel, G.E., Bradford, B.U., Wall, C.A. and Thurman, R.G. (1997a) Female rats exhibit greater susceptibility to early alcohol-induced injury than males. *Am J Physiol* **272**, G1186–G1194.

Iimuro, Y., Gallucci, R.M., Luster, M.I., Kono, H. and Thurman, R.G. (1997b) Antibodies to tumor necrosis factor-α attenuate hepatic necrosis and inflammation due to chronic exposure to ethanol in the rat. *Hepatology* **26**, 1530–1537.

Ikejima, K., Iimuro, Y., Forman, D.T. and Thurman, R.G. (1996) A diet containing glycine improves survival in endotoxin shock in the rat. *Am J Physiol* **271**, G97–G103.

Israel, Y., Videla, L. and Bernstein, J. (1975) Liver hypermetabolic state after chronic ethanol consumption: hormonal interrelations and pathogenic implications. *Fed Proc* **34**, 2052–2059.

Ji, S., Lemasters, J.J. and Thurman, R.G. (1982) Intralobular hepatic pyridine nucleotide fluorescence: Evaluation of the hypothesis that chronic treatment with ethanol produces pericentral hypoxia. *Proc Natl Acad Sci* **80**, 5415–5419.

Knecht, K.T., Bradford, B.U., Mason, R.P. and Thurman, R.G. (1990) *In vivo* formation of a free radical metabolite of ethanol. *Mol Pharmacol* **38**, 26–30.

Knecht, K.T., Adachi, Y., Bradford, B.U., Iimuro, Y., Kadiiska, M., Qun-Hui, X. and Thurman, R.G. (1995) Free radical adducts in the bile of rats treated chronically with intragastric alcohol: inhibition by destruction of Kupffer cells. *Mol Pharmacol* **47**, 1028–1034.

Kuiper, J., Casteleyn, E. and van Berkel, T.J. (1989) The role of prostaglandins in endotoxin-stimulated glycogenolysis in the liver. *Agents Actions* **26**, 201–202.

Leach, B.E. and Forbes, J.C. (1941) Sulfonamide drugs as protective agents against carbon tetrachloride poisoning. *Proc Soc Exp Biol Med* **48**, 361.

Lieber, C.S. (1991) Hepatic, metabolic and toxic effects of ethanol: 1991 update. *Alcohol Clin Exp Res* **15**, 573–592.

Liehr, H., Grun, M. and Seeling, H. (1978) On the pathogenesis of galactosamine hepatitis. *Virchows Arch B Cell Pathol* **26**, 331–335.

Martinez, F., Abril, E.R., Earnest, D.L. and Watson, R.R. (1992) Ethanol and cytokine secretion. *Alcohol* **9**, 455–458.

Matsumura, T., Yoshihara, H., Jeffs, R., Takei, Y., Nukina, S., Hijioka, T., Evans, R.K., Kauffman, F.C. and Thurman, R.G. (1992) Hormones increase oxygen uptake in peri-portal and pericentral regions of the liver lobule. *Am J Physiol* **262**, G645–G650.

Matsumura, T. and Thurman, R.G. (1983) Measuring rates of O_2 uptake in periportal and pericentral regions of liver lobule: Stop-flow experiments with perfused liver. *Am J Physiol* **244**, G656–G659.

McCuskey, R.D., McCuskey, P.A., Urbaschek, R. and Urbaschek, B. (1987) Kupffer cell function in host defense. *Rev Infect Dis* **9**, S616–S619.

McCuskey, R.S. (1991) *In vivo* microscopy of the effects of ethanol on the liver. In *Liver Pathology and Alcohol*, edited by R.R. Watson, pp. 563–570. Totowa, N.J: Humana Press.

Monden, K., Arii, S., Itai, S., Sasaoki, T., Adachi, Y., Funaki, N., Higashitsuji, H. and Tobe, T. (1991a) Enhancement and hepatocyte-modulating effect of chemical mediators and monokines produced by hepatic macrophages in rats with induced sepsis. *Res Exp Med* **191**, 177–187.

Monden, K., Arii, S., Itai, S., Sasaoki, T., Adachi, Y., Funaki, N. and Tobe, T. (1991b) Enhancement of hepatic macrophages in septic rats and their inhibitory effect on hepato-cyte function. *J Surg Res* **50**, 72–76.

Nanji, A.A., Mendenhall, C.L. and French, S.W. (1989) Beef fat prevents alcoholic liver disease in the rat. *Alcohol Clin Exp Res* **13**, 15–19.

Nanji, A.A., Khettry, U., Sadrzadeh, S.M. and Yamanaka, T. (1993) Severity of liver injury in experimental alcoholic liver disease. Correlation with plasma endotoxin, prostaglandin E_2, leukotriene B_4 and thromboxane B_2. *Am J Pathol* **142**, 367–373.

Nanji, A.A., Khettry, U. and Sadrzadeh, S.M.H. (1994) Lactobacillus feeding reduces endotox-emia and severity of experimental alcoholic liver disease. *Proc Soc Exp Biol Med* **205**, 243–247.

Naveau, S., Giraud, V., Borotto, E., Aubert, A., Capron, F. and Chaput, J.C. (1997) Excess weight risk factor for alcoholic liver disease. *Hepatology* **25**, 108–111.

Nelson, S., Bagby, G.J., Bainton, B.G. and Summer, W.R. (1989) The effects of acute and chronic alcoholism on tumor necrosis factor and the inflammatory response. *J Infect Dis* **160**, 422–429.

Nolan, J.P., Leibowitz, A. and Vladatin, A.L. (1980) Influence of alcohol on Kupffer cell function and possible significance in liver injury. In *The Reticuloendothelial System and Patho-genesis of Liver Disease*, edited by H. Liehr and M. Green, pp. 125–136. Amsterdam: Elsevier.

Nolan, J.P. and Camara, D.S. (1988) Intestinal endotoxins and macrophages as mediators of liver injury. *Trans Am Clin Climatol Assoc* **100**, 115–125.

Oshita, M., Takei, Y., Kawano, S., Yoshihara, H., Hijioka, T., Fukui, H., Goto, M., Masuda, E., Nishimura, Y., Fusamoto, H. and Kamada, T. (1993) Roles of endothelin-1 and nitric oxide in the mechanism for ethanol-induced vasoconstriction in rat liver. *J Clin Invest* **91**, 1337–1342.

Qu, W., Zhong, Z., Goto, M. and Thurman, R.G. (1996) Kupffer cell prostaglandin E_2 stimu-lates parenchymal cell O_2 consumption: alcohol and cell-cell communication. *Am J Physiol* **270**, G574–G580.

Ramadori, G., Hopf, F. and Galanos, C. (1990) *In vitro* and *in vivo* reactivity of lipopolysaccharides and lipid A with parenchymal and non parenchymal liver cells in mice. In *The Reticuloendothelial System and the Pathogenesis of Liver Disease*, edited by H. Leihr and M. Grun, pp. 285–290. Amsterdam: Elsevier-North Holland Biomedical Press.

Rao, G.A., Larkin, E.C. and Derr, R.F. (1987) Inadequate nutrition in the model for alcoholic liver damage using an ethanol +4-methylpyrazole liquid diet. *Biochemical Archives* **3**, 325–330.

Remmer, H. (1981) Die Wirkungen des Alkohols. *Alkoholwirkungen* **17**, 1–11.

Rowland, I.R., Mallett, A.K. and Wise, A. (1985) The effect of diet on the mammalian gut flora and its metabolic activities. *Crit Rev Toxicol* **16**, 31–103.

Ruddell, W.S., Axon, A.T.R. and Findlay, J.M. (1980) Effect of cimetidine on the gastric bacterial flora. *Lancet* **1**, 672–674.

Rutenburg, A.M., Sonnenblick, E., Koven, I., Aprahamian, H.A., Reiner, L. and Fine, J. (1957) The role of intestinal bacteria in the development of dietary cirrhosis in rats. *J Exp Med* **106**, 1–14.

Shaw, S., Heller, E.A., Friedman, H.S. and Lieber, C.S. (1977) Increased hepatic oxygenation following ethanol administration in the baboon. *Proc Soc Exp Biol Med* **156**, 509–513.

Stachlewitz, R.F. and Thurman, R.G. (1997) Dietary glycine prevents acute D-galactosamine hepatotoxicity. *Fund Appl Toxicol* **36**, 229.

Stahnke, L.L., Hill, D.B. and Allen, J.I. (1991) TNF-α and IL-6 in alcoholic liver disease. In *Cells of the Hepatic Sinusoid*, edited by E. Wisse, D.L. Knook and R.S. McCuskey, pp. 472–475. Leiden: Kupffer Cell Foundation.

Tabakoff, B., Hoffman, P.L., Lee, J.M., Saito, T., Willard, B. and Leon-Jones, F.D. (1988) Differences in platelet enzyme activity between alcoholics and nonalcoholics. *N Engl J Med* **318**, 134–139.

Thiele, D.L. (1989) Tumor necrosis factor, the acute phase response and the pathogenesis of alcoholic liver disease. *Hepatology* **9**, 497–499.

Thurman, R.G. and Kauffman, F.C. (1985) SCOPE: metabolic fluxes in periportal and pericentral regions of the liver lobule. *Hepatology* **5**, 144–151.

Tracy, K., Beutler, B. and Lowry, S. (1986) Shock and tissue injury induced by recombinant human cachectin. *Science* **234**, 470–472.

Tsukamoto, H., Reiderberger, R.D., French, S.W. and Largman, C. (1984) Long-term cannulation model for blood sampling and intragastric infusion in the rat. *Am J Physiol* **247**, R595–R599.

Tsukamoto, H., French, S.W., Reidelberger, R.D. and Largman, C. (1985) Cyclical pattern of blood alcohol levels during continuous intragastric ethanol infusion in rats. *Alcohol Clin Exp Res* **9**, 31–37.

Tsukamoto, H. and Xi, X.P. (1989) Incomplete compensation of enhanced hepatic oxygen consumption in rats with alcoholic centrilobular liver necrosis. *Hepatology* **9**, 302–306.

Utili, R., Abernathy, C.O. and Zimmerman, H.J. (1979) Hepatic excretory function in the endotoxin tolerant rat. *Proc Soc Exp Biol Med* **161**, 554–560.

Videla, L., Bernstein, J. and Israel, Y. (1973) Metabolic alteration produced in the liver by chronic alcohol administration. Increased oxidative capacity. *Biochem J* **134**, 507–514.

Wallace, J.L., Steel, G. and Whittle, B.J. (1987) Evidence for platelet-activating factor as a mediator of endotoxin-induced gastrointestinal damage in the rat: effects of three platelet-activating factor antagonists. *Gastroenterology* **93**, 765–773.

Yamada, S., Mochida, S., Ohno, A., Hirata, K., Ogata, I., Ohta, Y. and Fujiwara, K. (1991) Evidence for enhanced secretory function of hepatic macrophages after long-term ethanol feeding in rats. *Liver* **11**, 220–224.

Yuki, T., Bradford, B.U. and Thurman, R.G. (1980) Role of hormones in the mechanism of the swift increase in alcohol metabolism in the rat. *Pharmacol Biochem Behav* **13**, 67–71.

Yuki, T. and Thurman, R.G. (1980) The swift increase in alcohol metabolism: Time course for the increase in hepatic oxygen uptake and the involvement of glycolysis. *Biochem J* **186**, 119–126.

Chapter 11

Ethanol and protein turnover

Elena Volpi

Protein turnover can be profoundly influenced by ethanol intake in humans. The effects of ethanol are mostly due to its oxidation and oxidative by-products, are dose related and dependent upon the drinking pattern.

Acute alcohol drinking in non-habitual ethanol users induces a shift in liver redox state that appears to be responsible for a reduction in liver export protein synthesis and/or secretion. The production of reducing equivalents combined with increased acetate availability in the peripheral tissues are likely to be responsible for the reduced protein oxidation rate observed in these circumstances.

Chronic ethanol abuse induces loss of nitrogen and muscle wasting with different mechanisms. Despite several discrepancies between studies performed to assess the mechanisms of protein loss in chronic ethanol abuse, it is reasonable to hypothesize that tissue-specific imbalances between protein synthesis and protein catabolism are probably responsible for the loss of nitrogen in habitual alcohol abusers. A number of studies have shown that skeletal muscle protein synthesis is reduced with chronic alcohol abuse, whereas indirect evidence suggests that increased intestinal protein breakdown might be responsible for the reduction in intestinal protein content.

In conclusion, there is the need for new studies focusing on the effects of ethanol on the turnover rate of specific tissues and proteins. Given the recent evidence of a protective effect of moderate alcohol intake on the cardiovascular system, particular attention should be paid to dose-response studies in habitual drinkers of low to moderate doses of alcohol.

KEYWORDS: protein metabolism, synthesis, oxidation, tracers, liver, muscle

INTRODUCTION

Proteins play a central role in all physiological and pathological processes, as they are the direct translation of genomic information into biologically active molecules. In the 1930s, Shoenheimer and colleagues (1939), using stable isotopes of amino acids, discovered that body proteins are not static, but on the contrary they are continuously hydrolyzed and re-synthesized. Subsequent studies have shown that the rate of protein turnover is very high. It has been estimated that only ~20% of daily protein synthesis is due to protein intake during meals, whereas most protein synthesis, ~80%, is due to recycling of amino acids deriving from endogenous proteolysis. It has also been estimated that a significant portion of the basal energy expenditure, ~20%, is used for protein synthesis (Wolfe, 1992b). The cycling of protein turnover at a high rate is important to ensure rapid amplification of the signals that control protein synthesis (Newsholme and Crabtree, 1976). Higher protein turnover rates are found in all those conditions that require high protein synthesis rates, for example, physiologically, in growing children, and pathologic-ally, in severe injuries, such as trauma, sepsis and burns (Ferrando *et al.*, 1999), when a high protein synthesis rate is necessary for tissue and wound repair. A high protein turnover rate also ensures a continuous protein remodeling, so that older or altered proteins are degraded to be replaced with newly synthesized ones. This is particularly important for proteins involved in cell function such as enzymes, receptors and contractile proteins, that always need to function well in order for the cell itself to remain healthy and functional. Therefore, the high protein turnover rate is one of the major determinants of cell survival, despite the repeated alter-ations from exposure to exogenous noxious agents.

Ethanol (ethyl-alcohol; ethanol and alcohol will be used as synonyms in this chapter) is one of the most commonly used substances that may exert toxic effects on protein turnover. Evidence of dietary, social and therapeutic use of ethanol by humans can be dated back 4,000 years (Lucia, 1972). At present, in Western countries ethanol accounts for approximately 5–10% of the energy intake in the adult diet (Mitchell and Herlong, 1986) and the percentage of adults who drink alcohol, at least occasionally, has been reported to be somewhere between 50 and 90% (Kannel and Ellison, 1996), depending on age and gender. The prevalence of chronic alcohol abuse is estimated to be between 3 and 16%, depending upon age, gender, ethnicity, geographic region and social status (Hill *et al.*, 1998; Lamberts and Okkes, 1999; Reid *et al.*, 1999; Steele *et al.*, 1999), and the incidence of alcoholic liver disease among alcohol abusers is quite high (Diehl, 1989) (the epidemiology of alcoholic liver disease is discussed in Chapters 16 and 17).

The mechanisms by which ethanol affects protein turnover are multiple, and they are essentially due to ethanol oxidative by-products. Since most ethanol oxidation takes place in the liver (Lieber, 1997), the initial and most evident effects of ethanol intake involve liver protein metabolism. However, protein metabolism of all the major organs and systems are affected by ethanol intake, especially in chronic ethanol abuse. For example, the function of skeletal and heart muscle is impaired by chronic ethanol abuse (Preedy and Peters, 1989c, 1990d; Pacy *et al.*, 1991). It is important to note that the effects of ethanol on different aspects of protein turn-over and other metabolic functions are dose dependent and that some of these effects may be beneficial at low to moderate intakes. In fact, there is growing evid-ence that moderate ethanol intake protects from coronary artery disease (Kannel and Ellison, 1996; Marques-Vidal *et al.*, 1996; Muntwyler *et al.*, 1998; Valmadrid *et al.*, 1999; Yang *et al.*, 1999; Menotti *et al.*, 1999), stroke (Camargo *et al.*, 1997a; Berger *et al.*, 1999; Sacco *et al.*, 1999) and peripheral arterial disease (Camargo *et al.*, 1997b) by virtue of several mechanisms. These include increased plasma HDL concentrations, higher levels of apolipoprotein A-I and A-II (Frohlich, 1996; Goldberg *et al.*, 1996; Dardevet *et al.*, 1998) and reduced fibrinogen concentration (Krobot *et al.*, 1992; Mattiasson and Lindgarde, 1993). However, the debate regard-ing the definition of "low to moderate" ethanol intake, i.e., on the threshold dose of ethanol that positively affects the cardiovascular outcomes while not exerting toxic effects, is still open. Therefore, it is extremely important to understand fully the mechanisms of ethanol toxicity on intermediary metabolism, the dose-related changes in ethanol toxicity and the effects of intake patterns. Knowledge of such mechanisms will help to prevent ethanol addiction and alcoholic liver disease and, at the same time, make possible the utilization of the protective effects of moderate ethanol intake against the development of cardiovascular diseases.

This chapter will focus initially on the methods used to measure the effect of ethanol on protein turnover and subsequently on the acute and chronic effects of ethanol on liver and whole body protein turnover.

METHODS FOR *IN VIVO* MEASUREMENT OF PROTEIN TURNOVER

There are several methods available for measuring protein turnover of variable difficulty and cost. The simplest one is the measurement of nitrogen balance, which is fairly inexpensive although it requires relatively long periods of observation. Other methods rely on isotope dilution techniques, are more expensive, but allow a detailed observation of the protein turnover phenomena and can be used in acute conditions, over a period of few hours. Isotopic techniques can also be used to measure the synthesis and/or breakdown rate of specific proteins. Finally, arterio-venous catheterization methods allow the measurement of amino acid and/or protein net balance across specific organs or anatomical regions (i.e., the splanch-nic region, the leg, the forearm). When combined with isotope dilution methods, they allow the estimation of the relative contribution of protein synthesis and break-down to the chemical net balance of amino acids and/or proteins across the region studied. However, since no studies on the effect of ethanol on human protein metabolism have been performed using the arteriovenous balance methods, they will be omitted from the discussion below.

Nitrogen balance

The measurement of nitrogen balance has been used for more than 100 years (Hegsted, 1978) to assess the net balance between nitrogen intake and nitrogen loss. The nitrogen balance technique is still widely used to estimate the recommended dietary protein allowances in humans of all ages (Matthews, 1999).

Nitrogen balance is theoretically a very simple method (Figure 11.1) based on the concept that body nitrogen comes from proteins and amino acids contained in food and is lost through urine, feces, skin and other sources (i.e., nasal secretion, hair, etc.). Thus, the simple subtraction of the daily nitrogen losses from the daily nitrogen intake would give the net amount of nitrogen retained or lost in that given day. An adult and healthy individual eating the daily protein requirements should therefore have a nitrogen balance equal to zero, indicating that there is no net gain or loss of nitrogen.

However, despite its apparent simplicity, the nitrogen balance method has several limitations and drawbacks. First, the subjects undergoing nitrogen balance studies need to be placed on a diet containing a specific amount of nitrogen for several days up to a few weeks and the nitrogen content of food and leftovers needs to be measured. The subjects are required to collect all urine and feces over 24-hour periods in

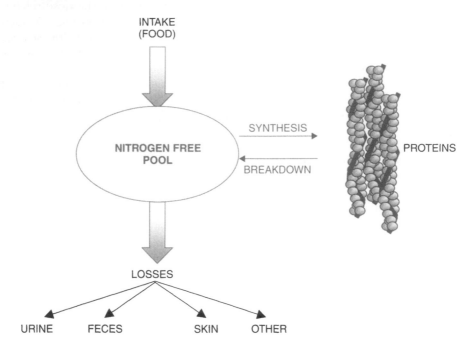

Figure 11.1 Nitrogen balance technique. The balance between the nitrogen coming from alimentary proteins and amino acids, and the nitrogen lost through urine, feces, skin and other sources determines the body nitrogen pool size. Intake and losses as well as protein breakdown and synthesis add nitrogen to or subtract nitrogen from the free pool. The measurement of the difference between nitrogen intake and losses represents the net amount of nitrogen that is retained or lost in a given day. This method, however, does not provide any insight on the mechanism(s) leading to the net effect on nitrogen balance, i.e., it is not possible to measure protein synthesis and breakdown.

order to measure nitrogen excretion. In some studies, dermal nitrogen loss is measured on samples of laundry and bath water (Sirbu *et al.*, 1967). The long periods of collection are quite inconvenient for the subjects and they do not allow the measurement of acute changes in nitrogen balance. In addition, besides the possibility that the subjects may not compliant with the collection of urine and feces, the estimation of nitrogen losses other than urine and feces, especially at low nitrogen intakes, may be another possible source of error (Munro, 1972). Second, normal individuals can adapt to a wide variety of nitrogen intakes (Scrimshaw *et al.*, 1972). This is extremely important when nitrogen balance is used to assess the nutritional requirements or recommended dietary protein allowances, as it may underestimate the actual needs. Third, nitrogen balance is systematically overestimated at high nitrogen intakes due to inherent and unexplained errors. In fact, Hegsted (1978) showed that when nitrogen intake is above the basal requirement there seems to be a significant retention of nitrogen of ~20%. In case, the retention of the extra nitrogen was true, over the long-term it would lead to non-physiological changes in body composition. Other concerns regard the quality of the proteins fed, as differences in nitrogen balance have been observed when the same amount of nitrogen was given in the form of different types of proteins (i.e., lactalbumin vs. gluten) (Hegsted, 1978).

Given these limitations, the use of nitrogen balance as a reference method for the measurement of the net balance between protein synthesis and breakdown is questionable. Furthermore, the measurement of nitrogen balance does not provide any insight on the mechanism(s) that leads to changes in balance. In other words, it is not possible to assess if the observed changes are due to changes in protein synthesis, or in protein breakdown, or both. Therefore, although still useful for specific study designs, the nitrogen balance technique has been used less frequently in the recent past due to the emergence of new methodologies.

Measurement of whole body protein turnover

Since the nitrogen balance technique, although useful, is insufficient to describe the phenomena that characterize protein turnover, other methods have been developed that enable us to assess the general physiological mechanisms that regulate whole body protein turnover. The use of isotopes of amino acids (radioactive or stable) as tracers allows the distinction between protein synthesis and protein breakdown and, under certain circumstances, it permits the measurement of amino acid oxidation.

However, the data regarding whole body protein turnover need to be carefully interpreted, as the so-called "whole body protein turnover" is the integrated sum of the different turnover rates of each single protein in every tissue of the body (Waterlow *et al.*, 1978). Therefore, in order to obtain meaningful data, it is necessary to choose carefully the tracer, the sampling site and the model for the calculation of the pertinent protein turnover parameters. In addition, exact reference values would be necessary to validate the method, but despite the progress in the field of protein metabolism and tracer methodologies, no method can be considered the gold standard (Arends *et al.*, 1992).

Single pool model

The development of modern tracer methodologies for the study of protein metabolism is due to the initial work of Waterlow and Stephen (Waterlow, 1967; Waterlow and Stephen, 1967) who described the general model of protein metabolism (Figure 11.2). At steady state, protein turnover (Q) can be defined with a simple mass balance equation:

$$Q = I + B = S + C \tag{1}$$

I is the intake of amino-nitrogen, B is protein breakdown, S is protein synthesis and C is amino acid catabolism.

Keeping in mind, this simple model that focuses on the overall process, it is possible to calculate the parameters of protein metabolism using isotopically labeled amino acids. The tracers are identical to the naturally occurring molecule with the exception that one or more atoms are substituted with an isotope that can be either radioactive or stable. The tracer, by definition, is given in "trace"

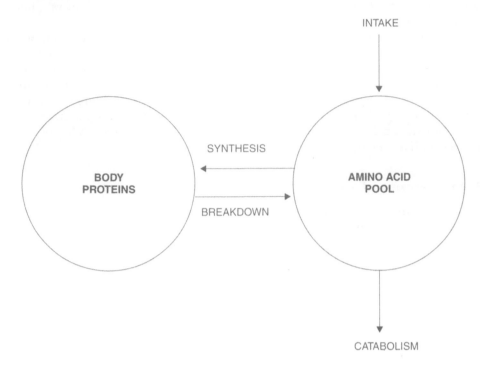

Figure 11.2 Single pool model. The different amino acid compartments of the body are assumed to be in instantaneous equilibrium so that a single pool can describe the kinetics of the amino acids. The amino acids enter the free pool from protein breakdown and food intake, and leave the pool via protein synthesis and amino acid catabolism. The injection of an adequate tracer allows the measurement of all the pertinent parameters (see text).

amounts, meaning that the quantity of isotope administered is negligible compared to the pool of the traced compound that is called "tracee". This is true for radioactive tracers, whereas for stable isotope tracers, the amount given cannot be considered negligible because the tracer has to be given in such a quantity in order to exceed the naturally occurring abundance of stable isotopes (Wolfe, 1992a). Therefore, the contribution of a stable isotope tracer to whole body protein turnover needs to be taken into account. The tracer is administered either orally or intravenously and its dilution is measured. The sampling site for measurement of isotope dilution can be urine or blood, according to the method used, i.e., the end product method or methods based on the kinetics of individual amino acids. Also, the tracer can be given as a bolus or as a constant infusion. The tracer dilution depends on the turnover rate of the tracee and the tracer dose (for bolus injection) or infusion rate (for constant infusion). The general equation that describes this relationship is the following:

$$\text{Dilution of the tracer} = \frac{\text{Tracer infusion rate or dose}}{\text{Tracee turnover rate}} \tag{2}$$

If the tracer is given as a bolus, the dilution of the tracer will be the area under the isotope decay curve, whereas if a constant infusion is utilized, the dilution of the tracer will be measured at isotopic equilibrium, i.e., when the dilution of the tracer has reached a steady state. From (2) it is possible to calculate the protein turnover rate described in (1):

$$\text{Tracee turnovern rate } = \frac{\text{Tracer infusion rate or dose}}{\text{Dilution of the tracer}} = Q = I + B = S + C \tag{3}$$

The turnover rate Q is equal to protein breakdown in the fasting state, when the intake I is zero. Otherwise it is always possible to measure the intake I and subtract it from Q to obtain B. The synthesis rate S can be estimated only indirectly if catabolism C is measured. The measurement of catabolism depends on the method used (see below).

Whole body nitrogen kinetics

Whole body nitrogen kinetics can be measured with the end product method that is based on infusion or oral administration of an amino acid labeled with a stable isotope of nitrogen (^{15}N). The labeled nitrogen will be exchanged by transamination so that after an adequate equilibration period, the labeled nitrogen will be evenly distributed in the endogenous amino-nitrogen pool. On the basis of the measurement of ^{15}N dilution (called enrichment) in the urinary urea or ammonia (end product), it will be possible to calculate the turnover rate of whole body amino-nitrogen (Picou and Taylor-Roberts, 1969; Picou et al., 1969). The assumptions of this method are that the size of the amino-nitrogen pool is constant during the infusion, there is no recycling of the ^{15}N tracer or isotopic discrimination, dietary amino acids and the amino acids coming from protein breakdown are handled in the same way and the tracer used is valid to trace the amino-nitrogen pool. ^{15}N-glycine is generally used, although it has been suggested that ^{15}N-alanine might be preferable (Wolfe, 1992b). When ^{15}N-glycine is used, it takes a long time for urea to reach the isotopic steady state, whereas the plateau value for ammonia is achieved much earlier. In addition, when both end products were used, the synthesis rate calculated with ammonia as *end product* was 66% of that calculated with urea. Thus, with ^{15}N-glycine the choice of the end product may be problematic. On the contrary, when ^{15}N-alanine is used, the enrichments of urea and ammonia are comparable (Waterlow et al., 1978). Overall, this method can be useful, but particular attention needs to be paid to the limitations. Especially important for the study of liver diseases is the observation that the end product method overestimates whole body protein synthesis in liver failure patients (Stein et al., 1983).

Amino acid kinetics

Another approach used to measure whole body protein turnover is measurement of the whole body kinetics of individual amino acids (Waterlow et al., 1978; Cobelli et al., 1992; Bier, 1992; Wolfe, 1992b). When the kinetics of an essential amino acid is measured, it is possible to extrapolate the results to whole body protein turnover since essential amino acids are not produced in the body (Matthews, 1999). If non-essential amino acids are used, their *de novo* synthesis would lead to an overestimation of protein breakdown due to the fact that the newly synthesized amino acids cannot be distinguished from those released from proteolysis.

The measurement of the kinetics of an individual amino acid is performed using the general single pool model described previously (Waterlow, 1967; Waterlow and Stephen, 1967). The isotopic tracer of an essential amino acid is infused intravenously and the dilution measured in blood samples. Most of the studies performed with this technique have used the constant tracer infusion that allows the measurement of amino acid turnover rate at isotopic steady state. Using the general model depicted in Figure 11.2 and described by (3), it is possible to calculate the turnover rate, which is also called rate of appearance (Ra), as it represents the rate at which the unlabeled amino acid appears in the blood.

$$\text{Ra} = \frac{\text{Tracer infusion rate}}{\text{Dilution of the tracer in blood}} \tag{4}$$

The Ra of an essential amino acid in the fasting state is usually referred to as the rate at which the essential amino acid is released from endogenous proteolysis, whereas in the fed state it is the sum of endogenous proteolysis and exogenous amino acid appearing in the blood from the intestine. The latter can be measured using the double tracer technique, which requires the infusion of a second tracer of the amino acid through the gastrointestinal route (Matthews *et al.*, 1993).

The constant infusion method implies that the amino acid pool size is constant throughout the experimental period. In this case, the Ra is equal to the rate of disappearance (Rd), which is the sum of amino acid utilization for protein synthesis and catabolism. In order to distinguish between these two components of Rd, it is necessary to measure at least one of the two. The use of a carbon-labeled (^{13}C or ^{14}C) amino acid as tracer and the measurement of the labeled CO_2 excretion rate enable the measurement of the amino acid oxidation rate. The labeled CO_2 ($*CO_2$) excretion rate depends upon the oxidation rate and the dilution of the tracer in the pool of the amino acid that is used as a precursor for the oxidative process:

$$*CO_2 \text{ excretion rate} = \text{Oxidation rate} \cdot \text{Tracer dilution in the precursor} \tag{5}$$

Assuming that the dilution of the tracer in the blood represents the dilution of the tracer in the precursor pool for the oxidation of the amino acid, the oxidation of the amino acid can be calculated as follows:

$$\text{Oxidation rate} = \frac{*CO_2 \text{ excretion rate}}{\text{Blood tracer dilution}} \tag{6}$$

At steady state, it is possible to calculate the rate at which the amino acid is used for protein synthesis by subtracting the oxidation rate from the Ra. However, the choice of the tracer to measure oxidation is extremely important. Some amino acids, such as leucine, lose one specific carbon as CO_2 in the first step of the oxidative process, whereas others are initially converted to other products before being oxidized and/or may be oxidized by several different pathways so that no specific carbon is lost first (Newsholme and Leech, 1983a). Leucine is the amino acid most widely used for measurement of whole body protein turnover, since the carboxylic carbon is quantitatively released as CO_2 in the first step of its oxidation, which is irreversible

(Newsholme and Leech, 1983a). Most of the released CO_2 is then expired, so that if leucine is labeled on the 1-carbon (carboxylic), the measurement of the isotope dilution in expired CO_2 will allow a reliable estimation of leucine oxidation. Part of the CO_2 released from leucine oxidation, approximately 10–20%, is retained in the body due to metabolic pathways that utilize blood bicarbonate (Hoerr *et al.*, 1989), so that metabolic conditions that change bicarbonate retention may lead to errors in the estimation of leucine oxidation. In those cases, the measurement of bicarbonate retention with a bicarbonate tracer is necessary in order to obtain a reliable estimation of leucine oxidation (Hoerr *et al.*, 1989).

The model used to calculate amino acid turnover requires several assumptions (Cobelli *et al.*, 1992; Bier, 1992). First, the tracer is uniformly distributed throughout the whole tracee pool, so that the tracer dilution found in the blood is similar to that of all tissues where the metabolic processes take place. Second, the size of the metabolic pool does not change in the experimental period, i.e., the pool is at steady state. Third, tracer and tracee are metabolized in an identical fashion, i.e., there is no isotopic discrimination. Fourth, the amino acid tracer is not recycled back into the free amino acid pool once it is incorporated into proteins.

The assumption that the tracer incorporated into proteins is not recycled back into the free pool is not correct. It has been calculated that, due to the rapid turnover of proteins, the recycling rate of an amino acid tracer is approximately 1.5% per hour (Schwenk *et al.*, 1985b; Volpi *et al.*, 1996). This means that there is a second, unaccounted "source" of tracer infusion. Thus, for experiments longer than a few hours, the recycling of the tracer leads to a significant overestimation of its dilution with consequent underestimation of the Ra. However, the major limitation of the single pool model for the measurement of amino acid kinetics is the assumption that the dilution of the tracer in the blood is a good reflection of its dilution in the tissues, where amino acid metabolism takes place. This is not true since the tissue dilution of an amino acid tracer is always lower than that found in the blood due to the fact that protein breakdown continuously dilutes the tracer intracellularly, whereas the equilibrium between the intracellular and blood compartments is not instantaneous, leading to a systematic error (Waterlow *et al.*, 1978).

Reciprocal pool model

The problem of the differences in the dilution of an amino acid tracer between blood and tissues has been solved at least partially by the use of a metabolic characteristic of leucine. When leucine enters a cell, it reaches an equilibrium with its keto acid, α-ketoisocaproate (KIC) (Nissen and Haymond, 1981), due to a transamination reaction that is exclusively intracellular and rapidly reversible (Matthews *et al.*, 1981). Thus, when carbon or hydrogen labeled leucine is infused, its intracellular dilution (enrichment in the case of stable isotopes, ^{13}C or ^2H; specific activity in the case of a radioactive isotope, ^{14}C or ^3H) will be rapidly similar to that of intracellular KIC. Since intracellular KIC is in rapid equilibrium with plasma KIC, the measurement of plasma KIC enrichment allows the estimation of the intracellular leucine enrichment or specific activity (Figure 11.3) (Schwenk *et al.*, 1985a). Due to these characteristics it has been termed "reciprocal pool model," as opposed to the "primary pool model" that refers to the use of leucine plasma enrichment or specific activity as an

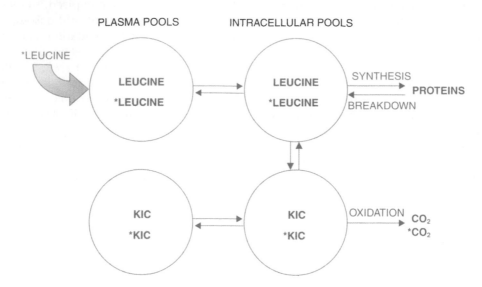

Figure 11.3 Reciprocal pool model. Leucine is in equilibrium with its ketoacid KIC due to a trans-amination reaction that is exclusively intracellular and rapidly reversible. Intracellular KIC is in equilibrium with plasma KIC, so that if a leucine tracer is injected in the blood, the isotope dilution in plasma KIC will reflect the isotope dilution of the intracellular leucine pool. In addition, the first irreversible step of leucine oxidation is the oxidative decarboxylation of KIC, so that plasma KIC is also the most appropriate precursor for the calculation of leucine oxidation (see text for further details).

index of intracellular leucine enrichment or specific activity (Schwenk *et al.*, 1985a). During the infusion of a stable isotope of leucine, such as 1-^{13}C-leucine, leucine turnover (Ra) will be calculated by modifying (3) as follows:

$$\text{Leucine Ra} = \frac{\text{1-}^{13}\text{C-leucine infusion rate}}{\text{Plasma }^{13}\text{C-KIC enrichment}} \qquad (7)$$

In this circumstance leucine oxidation will be calculated by dividing the $^{13}CO_2$ excretion rate by the plasma ^{13}C-KIC enrichment.

$$\text{Leucine oxidation} = \frac{^{13}CO_2 \text{ excretion rate}}{\text{Plasma }^{13}\text{C-KIC enrichment}} \qquad (8)$$

The non-oxidative leucine disposal for protein synthesis (NOLD) will be calculated by subtracting the oxidation rate from the Ra (see also (3)):

$$\text{NOLD} = \text{Ra} - \text{Oxidation} \qquad (9)$$

The assumptions of the model are identical to those described for the single pool model of amino acid kinetics. In addition, another assumption is necessary for the application of this model: the enrichment (or specific activity) of plasma KIC during labeled leucine infusion accurately reflects the enrichment (or specific activity) of intracellular leucine. Several studies using compartmental modeling have shown that the reciprocal pool model overestimates intracellular leucine enrichment (or specific activity), and for this reason it underestimates the parameters of protein oxidation and proteolysis (Cobelli *et al.*, 1991; Carraro *et al.*, 1991). However, the difficulty in the application of complicated compartmental models to routine metabolic studies prevents their current use. Furthermore, studies where tissue isotope dilution was directly measured with multiple tissue biopsies have shown that the extent of the error in the estimation of the intracellular leucine enrichment (or specific activity) with the reciprocal pool model does not exceed 10% of the true value. On the contrary, it has been shown that the primary pool model overestimates the intra cellular value by 20–40% (Layman and Wolfe, 1987; Horber *et al.*, 1989; Watt *et al.*, 1991; Bennet *et al.*, 1993). Thus, although the results obtained with this method should not be considered in quantitative terms, the reciprocal pool approach works quite well when used to detect the direction of changes in whole body protein metabolism.

Measurement of the synthesis of individual proteins

The synthesis of individual plasma or tissue proteins can be measured with the precursor-product approach by measuring the incorporation of a precursor for protein synthesis (amino acid) into the product (protein).

Constant tracer infusion

The traditional method for measurement of protein synthesis rate with the precursor-product model requires the primed-continuous infusion of an isotope of an amino acid and the measurement of the tracer incorporation into the protein, as well as of its dilution in the precursor pool (D_{AA}). The rate of variation of the tracer content into the protein (ΔP) in a given time frame (Δt) depends upon the difference between the rate at which the tracer is incorporated into the protein from the precursor and the rate at which the tracer exits from the protein due to break-down. The rate of entry of the tracer into the protein is given by the protein synthesis rate k_1 and the dilution of the tracer in the precursor pool D_{AA} (*tracer entry* = $k_1 \cdot D_{AA}$). The rate of exit of the tracer from the protein is given by the protein breakdown rate k_2 and the dilution of the tracer in the protein D_P (*tracer exit* = $k_2 \cdot D_P$). Thus, the change in protein tracer content over time is described by the following equation:

$$\frac{\Delta P}{\Delta t} = k_1 \cdot D_{AA} - k_2 \cdot D_P \tag{10}$$

If the experimental time frame Δt is short compared to the half-life of the protein, the dilution of the tracer in the protein (D_P) will be negligible compared to the dilution of the tracer in the precursor pool (D_{AA}) so that (10) can be simplified as follows:

$$\frac{\Delta P}{\Delta t} = k_1 \cdot D_{AA} \tag{11}$$

Rearranging (11), the fractional synthesis rate (FSR) or k_1 can be calculated as follows:

$$k_1 = FSR = \frac{\Delta P / \Delta t}{D_{AA}} \tag{12}$$

This model requires several assumptions (Wolfe, 1992b; Toffolo *et al.*, 1993). First, the precursor pool and the protein pool are accessible to sampling. Second, the incorporation of the precursor into the product is linear in the experimental period. Third, the precursor pool can be embedded in a larger system, but knowledge of the structure of that system is not necessary. Fourth, the measured precursor is the immediate precursor for protein synthesis, i.e., there are no intermediate steps between the precursor and the product, and the measured precursor is the only precursor for the product. Fifth, the dilution of the tracer in the precursor is at steady state in the experimental period. Sixth, none of the tracer incorporated into the protein is lost via proteolysis.

The major concerns when using this method regard the validity of the fourth assumption. Specifically, the true precursor for protein synthesis is the charged tRNA of the tissue where the protein is produced. The measurement of tracer dilution on isolated aminoacyl-tRNA cannot be used routinely in humans because it requires relatively large amounts of tissue (Watt *et al.*, 1989, 1991). Thus, if the measurement of the dilution of the tracer on the isolated aminoacyl-tRNA is not performed, surrogate measures of the dilution of the tracer in the precursor pool need to be used. The most common solution to this problem is the use of KIC enrichment or specific activity as dilution of the tracer in the precursor pool during the infusion of labeled leucine. Another method for assessing the validity of a precursor for protein synthesis in a tissue, if the dilution of the tracer on the charged tRNA cannot be measured, consists of infusing an amino acid tracer at a constant rate and following the incorporation of the tracer up to plateau into a fast turnover protein produced by the tissue. The tracer dilution into the protein at plateau is equal to that of the precursor pool, so by simple comparison it is possible to establish which one of the surrogate measures better estimates the precursor pool tracer dilution value. This technique has been applied in humans to assess the validity of plasma KIC specific activity as a surrogate measure of the specific activity of the precursor pool for liver protein synthesis during the infusion of ^{14}C-leucine (De Feo *et al.*, 1995; Volpi *et al.*, 1996). The incorporation of labeled leucine into VLDL apoB-100 was followed to plateau and compared to the specific activity of plasma leucine and KIC specific activity. These studies show that in humans, plasma KIC specific activity closely approximates that of the true precursor for liver protein synthesis in the fasting state (De Feo *et al.*, 1995; Volpi *et al.*, 1996), in the fed state (De Feo *et al.*, 1995; Volpi *et al.*, 1996) and during acute ethanol intake (De Feo *et al.*, 1995). Another study performed with multiple tracers, leg arteriovenous catheterization and muscle biopsies from the vastus lateralis has shown that the precursor pool for muscle protein synthesis is better estimated by sampling blood leucine during the infusion of labeled KIC, instead of by sampling blood KIC during labeled leucine infusion (Chinkes *et al.*, 1996). This indicates that the characteristics of the precursor pool for protein synthesis are variable according to the tissue studied, and this needs to be taken into account when planning experiments. It is important to stress that the validity of a method in one tissue is unaffected by the fact that the same method is not valid in any other tissue. Another problem may arise when measuring the synthesis of plasma proteins, especially liver export proteins, in conditions that reduce the secretion of the proteins from the cells into the plasma. Specifically, if a stimulus reduces only the secretion rate of plasma proteins, the measured plasma FSR will appear reduced although the protein synthesis rate is unaffected due to a slower appearance in the blood of the newly synthesized proteins. For this reason some authors prefer to define the plasma protein FSR "fractional secretory rate" (De Feo *et al.*, 1995; Volpi *et al.*, 1997, 1998).

Flooding dose technique

An alternative approach that could yield better estimates of the precursor pool for protein synthesis is the use of the flooding dose technique (Garlick *et al.*, 1980, 1989). The rationale of this method is that by injecting a bolus of both unlabeled amino acid and its tracer in excess of its total body free pool, the entire amino acid pool will be "flooded" and uniform enrichments in any compartment of the pool obtained, including in the precursor for protein synthesis. The advantages of this method are the theoretical elimination of the uncertainty of the precursor since all the compartments should reach the same value of tracer dilution. In this case, the tracer dilution in the blood should be an adequate measure of the dilution of the tracer in the precursor pool for protein synthesis. Further, it is possible to deliver the tracer at a high dose enabling the measurement of protein synthesis over a short time frame.

However, several problems derive from the basic assumptions of this technique. The first assumption is that a flooding dose of one amino acid will not stimulate protein synthesis (Wolfe, 1992b). Although older data indicated that flooding doses of phenylalanine (Manchester and Tyobeka, 1980; McNurlan *et al.*, 1982) or leucine (McNurlan *et al.*, 1982) did not stimulate protein synthesis either *in vitro* (Manchester and Tyobeka, 1980) or *in vivo* (McNurlan *et al.*, 1982), more recent studies have shown that flooding doses of essential amino acids such as leucine (Garlick *et al.*, 1989; Jahoor *et al.*, 1992; Smith *et al.*, 1992, 1994), phenylalanine (Smith *et al.*, 1998), and threonine (Smith *et al.*, 1998) stimulate albumin (Smith *et al.*, 1994) and muscle protein (Garlick *et al.*, 1989; Jahoor *et al.*, 1992; Smith *et al.*, 1992, 1998) synthesis *in vivo*. On the other hand, non-essential amino acids do not stimulate muscle protein synthesis when given in a flooding dose (Smith *et al.*, 1998), meaning that non-essential amino acids seem to be the ideal tracers when using the flooding dose technique.

Another less important assumption of the flooding dose technique is that the process of protein synthesis is instantaneous (Wolfe, 1992b). This is not necessarily true especially for export proteins such as albumin, which shows a delay of approximately 30 minutes between the time of tracer injection and the appearance of the tracer in the secreted protein (Patterson *et al.*, 1993).

EFFECTS OF ETHANOL ON PROTEIN TURNOVER IN HUMANS

The effects of ethanol on protein turnover, as well as its effects on fat, glucose and drug metabolism, are essentially due to its oxidation. These effects differ between acute and chronic alcohol intake, due to the diverse pathways involved in ethanol oxidation, and are dose related because of the different K_m of the enzymes involved in ethanol oxidation. Thus, a brief summary of the ethanol oxidative pathways is provided below. An in depth discussion of this topic can be found elsewhere in this book.

Ethanol oxidation

Soon after ingestion, the gastrointestinal tract promptly absorbs ethanol, and less than 10% of the absorbed ethanol is eliminated by the lung and kidneys, whereas the majority is oxidized mainly by the liver (Lieber, 1997). The stomach is the most important site of extrahepatic ethanol oxidation (Lieber, 1997) and contributes significantly to ethanol first pass metabolism, thus reducing its availability since it is the first organ to be exposed to high ethanol concentrations (Julkunen *et al.*, 1985a,b).

The three major pathways of ethanol oxidation are the alcohol dehydrogenase (ADH) pathway located in the cell cytoplasm, the microsomal ethanol oxidizing system (MEOS) localized in the endoplasmic reticulum and the peroxisomal catalase. Utilizing different mechanisms, all these pathways produce acetaldehyde (Lieber, 1997). Since the peroxisomal catalase pathway does not appear to play a major role in ethanol oxidation *in vivo* (Lieber, 1997), only ADH and MEOS will be reviewed below.

Alcohol dehydrogenase (ADH)

The ADH pathway oxidizes alcohol to acetaldehyde by reducing NAD^+, with consequent formation of NADH (French, 1989). The resulting increase in the $NADH/NAD^+$ ratio results in a shift of the redox state towards the reduced state, which is responsible for numerous metabolic changes in the cell including inhibition of gluconeogenesis (Madison *et al.*, 1967) with consequent hypoglycemia, inhibition of glycolysis (Berry *et al.*, 1994), fatty acid oxidation (Lieber and Schmid, 1961), citric acid cycle (French, 1989), increased fatty acid synthesis (Lieber and Schmid, 1961) and lactic acid production (French, 1989). The inhibition of the major oxidative pathways and the preferential utilization of the α-glycerol phosphate as a shuttle for the reducing equivalents induces sequestration of phosphate with depletion of ATP (Desmoulin *et al.*, 1990). The plasma lactate/pyruvate ratio can be used to monitor changes in whole body redox state that, in the case of ethanol intake, mostly reflects changes in the hepatic redox state. ADH is present in different forms and allelic variants with widely different K_m, the prevalence of each isozyme and variant depending upon the ethnicity. The most common form of liver ADH has a low K_m (0.2–5 mM; 1–10 mg/dl), and for this reason it is responsible for ethanol oxidation at low concentrations (Lieber, 1988, 1997; French, 1989). In the stomach, ADH is present in three forms with either high or low K_m, which during alcohol consumption are usually all active given the high ethanol concentrations achieved in the stomach (Julkunen *et al.*, 1985a,b). Gastric ADH is less active in chronic alcoholics (DiPadova *et al.*, 1987), young women (Frezza *et al.*, 1990) and in subjects taking aspirin (Roine *et al.*, 1990) and H_2-blockers (Caballeria *et al.*, 1989, 1991).

Microsomal ethanol oxidizing system (MEOS)

The MEOS like other microsomal drug-metabolizing enzymes requires the utilization of cytochrome P-450 in order to oxidize ethanol to acetaldehyde with utilization of oxygen and NADPH, and production of $NADP^+$ and water (French, 1989). Thus, unlike the ADH pathway, ethanol oxidation by MEOS is energy inefficient, i.e., does not produce energy (ATP), so that the energy provided by ethanol is wasted in the form of heat (Lieber, 1988). Furthermore, the MEOS pathway depletes oxygen in the cell (hypoxia), and favors lipid oxidation and free radical formation (French, 1989). The MEOS pathway has a high K_m (10–15 mM; 50–80 mg/dl) and high capacity as the V_{max} is reached at concentrations as high as 30 mM (150 mg/dl), so that it is responsible for alcohol oxidation at high blood concentrations (Teschke et al., 1974). In addition, chronic ethanol consumption induces the expression of an ethanol specific cytochrome P-450 (2E1) that increases overall MEOS activity. Thus, in chronic ethanol abusers, MEOS is the primary ethanol oxidative pathway.

Acetaldehyde oxidation

Acetaldehyde is oxidized in mitochondria to acetate by aldehyde dehydrogenase (ALDH), an enzyme with a low K_m, that reduces NAD^+ to NADH. At low to moderate ethanol intake, acetaldehyde is completely oxidized in the cell and does not appear in the blood (Lieber, 1997). However, in chronic ethanol abusers ALDH is down-regulated (Hasumura et al., 1975) and unable to dispose all the produced acetaldehyde due to the increased capacity of the MEOS pathway (Lieber, 1997). Thus, alcohol abusers usually have detectable blood concentrations of acetaldehyde.

Acetaldehyde is the most toxic by-product of ethanol oxidation as it is highly reactive so that it can form protein adducts that will inactivate metabolic enzymes, DNA repair and tubulin polymerization (Espina et al., 1988). Since tubulin is involved in the secretive processes of cells, the reduced ability of tubulin to polymerize reduces the ability to secrete export proteins (Baraona et al., 1977, 1980; Sorrell et al., 1983). This is extremely important for liver synthesized plasma proteins (see below). In addition, acetaldehyde is responsible for the depletion of reduced glutathione and consequent reduced ability to withstand the stresses that cause lipid peroxidation (Lieber, 1997).

Acute ethanol intake

The acute intake of ethanol exerts numerous effects on whole body protein turnover and the metabolism of liver and other tissues.

Whole body

Several studies have shown that during acute intravenous or oral administration of ethanol, protein oxidation is reduced regardless of the dose and experimental method used (Shelmet et al., 1988; De Feo et al., 1995; Volpi et al., 1997, 1998).

In fact, both urinary nitrogen excretion (Shelmet *et al.*, 1988) and leucine oxidation were significantly reduced by ethanol (De Feo *et al.*, 1995; Volpi *et al.*, 1997, 1998). The reduction of amino acid oxidation during acute ethanol intake is accompanied by a concomitant reduction in carbohydrate and lipid oxidation rates measured by indirect calorimetry with correction for the contribution of ethanol oxidation to the respiratory quotient (Shelmet *et al.*, 1988). The significant effects of ethanol on the major oxidative pathways are likely not only due to the generation of excess reducing equivalents in the liver that selectively inhibit the hepatic oxidative processes (see Ethanol Oxidation section), but also to the production of an oxidative substrate, specifically acetate, that can be released from the liver and utilized in the peripheral tissues. This hypothesis is corroborated by the observation that the large reduction of protein oxidation, approximately 25–40% (Shelmet *et al.*, 1988; De Feo *et al.*, 1995; Volpi *et al.*, 1997, 1998), and lipid oxidation (Shelmet *et al.*, 1988), approximately 79%, can be explained not only by an isolated effect of ethanol on the liver, but rather, by an additional effect on other tissues. It should be pointed out that in these studies the suppressive effect of ethanol on protein oxidation might have been overestimated because ethanol was added, and not isocalorically substituted, to the other nutrients (Shelmet *et al.*, 1988; De Feo *et al.*, 1995; Volpi *et al.*, 1997; Volpi *et al.*, 1998). Therefore it is still uncertain whether the greater caloric content contributed to the reduction of the oxidative rates.

The reduction of leucine oxidation was the only significant effect of ethanol intake during a meal (De Feo *et al.*, 1995; Volpi *et al.*, 1997, 1998). In fact, neither whole body proteolysis nor whole body protein synthesis changed during ethanol administration. However, the plasma concentrations of leucine and KIC were significantly higher during ethanol administration. Overall these data suggest that the amino acids saved from oxidation during ethanol intake were most likely stored in the body free pool, since they were not used for protein synthesis. In the hours following ethanol consumption, the amino acids accumulated in the free pool were probably oxidized rather then utilized for protein synthesis. In fact, it has been shown that the night following acute ethanol consumption nitrogen excretion increases, so that overall acute ethanol intake does not affect protein balance (Suter *et al.*, 1992). These authors also showed that the absence of an effect of acute ethanol intake on 24-hour nitrogen excretion does not depend on the modality of ethanol administration, since the results were similar both when ethanol was added to the diet or isocalorically substituted for some of the carbohydrate and fat of the diet.

Liver

The most striking effects of acute high-dose ethanol intake are those exerted on liver protein synthesis and/or secretion. In healthy humans, when ethanol was added to a mixed meal, albumin and fibrinogen FSR were significantly reduced (De Feo *et al.*, 1995; Volpi *et al.*, 1997, 1998) (Figure 11.4). This effect was observed even though the estimates of whole body protein synthesis were not significantly affected by ethanol (De Feo *et al.*, 1995; Volpi *et al.*, 1997, 1998). It is interesting to note that albumin FSR is normally stimulated by meal absorption (De Feo *et al.*, 1992, 1995; Volpi *et al.*, 1996, 1997, 1998) due to both increased insulin concentration

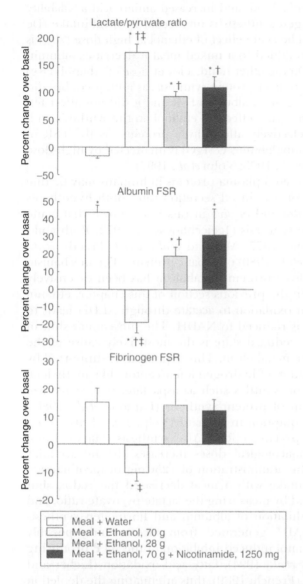

Figure 11.4 Acute effects of ethanol on the response of albumin and fibrinogen FSR to a meal in healthy non-habitual alcohol users. The administration of a meal in healthy individuals stimulates albumin FSR and does not affect fibrinogen FSR. The administration of a high dose of ethanol (70 g) increases the lactate/pyruvate from the normal value of ~10 to ~30 and inhibits albumin and fibrinogen FSRs below the fasting values. A moderate dose of ethanol (28 g) doubles lactate/pyruvate ratio, but only marginally affects liver protein metabolism as it only slightly blunts the meal-induced increase in albumin FSR, whereas does not affect fibrinogen FSR. The administration of 1250 mg of nicotinamide, the precursor of NAD^+, with a high dose of ethanol (70 g) reduces the effect of ethanol on the lactate/pyruvate ratio to values comparable to those obtained with a moderate dose of ethanol, and restores the normal response of albumin and fibrinogen to the meal. *$P < 0.05$ meal vs. fasting, †$P < 0.05$ vs. meal+water, ‡$P < 0.05$ vs. others.

(De Feo *et al.*, 1992, 1993; Volpi *et al.*, 1996) and increased amino acid availability (Volpi *et al.*, 1996), whereas fibrinogen synthesis is unaffected by meal intake (De Feo *et al.*, 1992; Volpi *et al.*, 1996). The acute effect of ethanol at high dose (70 g) is extremely potent so that when it is added to a mixed meal it decreases albumin FSR well below the fasting values. On the other hand, a lower dose of ethanol (28 g) induced only minimal disturbances to liver protein synthesis, as it blunted, but did not suppress, the meal induced increase of albumin FSR and it did not affect fibrinogen FSR (Volpi *et al.*, 1998). The acute effects of ethanol on the synthesis and/ or secretion of plasma proteins selectively affects liver proteins, as the FSR of extrahepatic proteins such as immunoglobulins G (IgG) is unaffected by high-dose ethanol intake in humans (De Feo *et al.*, 1995; Volpi *et al.*, 1997).

The reduction in FSR of liver-secreted plasma proteins in humans may be due to either a reduced synthesis rate or a reduced secretion rate. Both hypotheses may be valid, as experiments *in vitro* and *in vivo* in rats have shown that acute ethanol administration inhibits the synthesis (Jeejeebhoy *et al.*, 1972; Rothschild *et al.*, 1974; Mørland and Bessesen, 1977; Mørland *et al.*, 1979; Preedy *et al.*, 1988b) and the secretion (Baraona *et al.*, 1980) of hepatic proteins. The mechanism by which alcohol acutely impairs liver protein metabolism has been extensively investigated *in vitro*. As described in the previous section of this chapter, ethanol oxidation via ADH and subsequent oxidation to acetate through ALDH leads to the consumption of NAD^+, which is reduced to NADH. The subsequent shift in the redox equilibrium toward the reduced state is the most likely cause of the impairment in hepatic intermediate metabolism. This hypothesis is supported by the observation that the administration of hydrogen ion acceptors like methylene blue or high doses of hydrogen ion shuttles such as aspartate, that re-oxidize NADH, prevents ethanol inhibition of protein synthesis (Baraona *et al.*, 1980). A recent study has addressed this question in humans (Volpi *et al.*, 1997) using nicotinamide, which is the direct precursor for NAD^+ synthesis (Mayes, 1996) and when administered at pharmacological doses increases the intracellular NAD^+ pool (Lewis *et al.*, 1993). The administration of 1250 mg of nicotinamide during acute high-dose ethanol intake with a meal decreased the redox shift towards the reduced state, estimated by measuring the lactate/pyruvate ratio, and prevented the ethanol-induced inhibition of albumin and fibrinogen synthesis (Figure 11.4). The increased NAD^+ generated from nicotinamide possibly removed, at least partially, the ethanol induced inhibition of the ATP producing pathways such as glycolysis (Berry *et al.*, 1994), fatty acid oxidation (Lieber and Schmid, 1961) and citric acid cycle (French, 1989), thus attenuating the depletion of ATP, which has been shown to be responsible for the ethanol-induced inhibition of protein synthesis (Masson *et al.*, 1993). Furthermore, NAD^+ is the coenzyme of aldehyde dehydrogenase, so that nicotinamide administration could have also accelerated acetaldehyde oxidation by increasing intracellular NAD^+ availability and, thus, maintained the secretory process of newly synthesized hepatic proteins. Although the latter mechanism cannot be excluded, it is less likely to take place, as very high concentrations of ethanol and acetaldehyde are required to demonstrate an effect on tubulin polymerization. It is also interesting to note that the lactate/pyruvate ratio, which was ~30 during ethanol alone, decreased to ~20 with nicotinamide, but was not completely normalized (normal value: ~10). Yet the negative effect on liver protein synthesis was completely reversed. Similarly, the values of lactate/pyruvate ratio observed with low- and high-dose ethanol intake were approximately 20 and 30, respectively (Volpi *et al.*, 1998) (Figure 11.4). Combining these data, it is possible to conclude that the shift of the redox state is the major cause of acute ethanol toxicity on liver protein metabolism. Finally, these data suggest that the plasma lactate/pyruvate ratio can be used as an indicator of the effect of ethanol on liver protein synthesis, with a value of approximately 20 to be considered borderline for ethanol toxicity.

Other tissues

The acute administration of ethanol has been shown to decrease skeletal muscle (Preedy *et al.*, 1992), intestinal smooth muscle (Preedy *et al.*, 1988a), heart (Preedy and Peters, 1990d), bone and skin (Preedy *et al.*, 1990b) protein synthesis in rats, but no data on specific tissues other than liver are available in humans. The reduction of protein synthesis in the rat's major body organs and tissues should significantly affect whole body protein metabolism, since those tissues and organs comprise most body proteins. On the other hand, studies in humans have shown that only liver protein synthesis appears to be reduced whereas whole body protein synthesis and breakdown are unaffected by acute ethanol intake (see Acute Ethanol Intake – *Whole Body* section). Thus, it is unlikely that acute ethanol intake reduces the synthesis rate of most of the proteins in humans in the absence of a measurable effect at the whole body level. Most of the effects of acutely administered ethanol on rat protein synthesis have been attributed to its oxidative by-product acetaldehyde (Preedy *et al.*, 1992; Siddiq *et al.*, 1993). Acetaldehyde is usually undetectable in healthy humans given an acute ethanol challenge due to the high capacity and low K_m of ALDH (Newsholme and Leech, 1983b; Lieber, 1997). Thus, a generalized negative effect on protein synthesis in tissues other than liver is unlikely. However, studies in humans are necessary to clarify this issue.

Chronic ethanol abuse

The chronic consumption of high-dose ethanol leads to numerous anatomical and functional alterations of almost all the major organs and tissues. In fact, ethanol abuse leads not only to an impairment of liver (Lieber, 1997) and nervous system (Lyons *et al.*, 1998) functions, but also to muscle wasting (Preedy and Peters, 1990a), malabsorption (Lindenbaum and Lieber, 1975), cardiomyopathy (Preedy and Richardson, 1994), osteoporosis and osteopenia (Gonzalez-Calvin *et al.*, 1993). These alcohol-related changes, at least in part, are due to alterations in protein turnover, which may be attributed to a combination of the direct effects of ethanol and/or its metabolites and malnutrition. The latter was initially thought to be the major cause of alcohol-related diseases (Korsten and Lieber, 1979), but at present it is believed that the major pathogenetic factors are related to ethanol oxidation (Lieber, 1993). However, protein-calorie malnutrition in chronic alcohol abusers should not be underestimated as a contributing factor to the pathogenesis of alcohol related diseases considering that in these patients ethanol can supply over 50% of the daily caloric intake.

Whole body

Several studies have shown that chronic ethanol intake profoundly affects whole body protein turnover. The isocaloric replacement of glucose and lipids with ethanol for 3–6 weeks resulted in negative nitrogen balance and weight loss both in healthy volunteers (McDonald and Margen, 1986) and in chronic alcohol abusers (Bunout *et al.*, 1987; Reinus *et al.*, 1989). The presence of adequate amounts of amino acids in the diet allowed the exclusion of protein malnutrition as a factor responsible for the negative nitrogen balance (McDonald and Margen, 1986; Reinus *et al.*, 1989). Furthermore, in chronic ethanol abusers nitrogen balance remained negative for up to one week after alcohol withdrawal, and a positive nitrogen balance was observed only after two weeks of abstinence (Bunout *et al.*, 1987).

The mechanisms of nitrogen loss during chronic ethanol abuse are still unclear. Whole body protein turnover studies have been performed in order to assess whether a reduction of protein synthesis and/or an increase in proteolysis are responsible for the negative nitrogen balance. However, conflicting results have been obtained. A study carried out in chronic alcohol abusers in the absence of elevated blood ethanol concentrations showed that, when compared to healthy controls, chronic ethanol abusers had a lower rate of leucine oxidation, but no differences were found with regard to estimates of protein breakdown and synthesis (Pacy *et al.*, 1991). Unfortunately, a reduction in leucine oxidation would lead to a reduction in nitrogen excretion, which is in contrast with the nitrogen balance studies. This study was also in contrast with a study in rats showing an increase in leucine oxidation after chronic ethanol feeding (Bernal *et al.*, 1993). However, Pacy *et al.* (1991) studied the chronic ethanol abusers only in the fasting state and in the absence of ethanol so that it is not possible to extrapolate their data to a 24-hour protein balance.

In contrast to Pacy's study, another paper showed that ethanol abusers during early abstinence had higher rates of leucine Ra and non-oxidative leucine disposal compared to healthy controls, suggesting that chronic alcohol abusers have a higher protein turnover rate, whereas no differences in leucine oxidation were found (Petermann *et al.*, 1993). When these two groups of subjects were acutely administered ethanol as a bolus injection, the leucine turnover and oxidation rates remained unaffected in the healthy volunteers, whereas leucine Ra and non-oxidative leucine disposal decreased in ethanol abusers to values similar to those observed in the healthy volunteers. The lack of an effect of ethanol on leucine oxidation in chronic alcohol abusers is, again, in contrast with the nitrogen balance studies reported above, showing an increased nitrogen excretion with chronic alcohol intake. Further, the observation that ethanol does not affect protein oxidation in healthy subjects discords with the observations of Shelmet *et al.* (1988), obtained with nitrogen balance, and with those of De Feo *et al.* (1995) and Volpi *et al.* (1997, 1998), obtained measuring leucine kinetics.

A possible explanation for these differences is that although Petermann *et al.* (1993) used labeled leucine to measure protein kinetics, they employed the primary pool approach instead of the reciprocal pool model used by De Feo *et al.* (1995) and Volpi *et al.* (1997, 1998). The choice of the model used is critical in these circumstances, since specific alterations of leucine-KIC kinetics are observed during ethanol intake. These include a steady expansion of the free amino acid pool observed in humans (Shaw and Lieber, 1978; Avogaro *et al.*, 1986) or chronically ethanol fed rats (Stanko *et al.*, 1979; Bernal *et al.*, 1993), which results in increased concentrations of branched chain amino acids in plasma and tissues, and mitochodrial abnormalities that may reduce KIC oxidation (Lauterburg *et al.*, 1993). Since KIC is the direct precursor of labeled CO_2 production during the infusion of labeled leucine, the use of plasma KIC dilution appears to be more appropriate than leucine dilution for the calculation of leucine oxidation. The fact that Petermann *et al.* (1993) employed the primary pool model may also be responsible for the differences between their results and those of Pacy *et al.* (1991) who used the reciprocal pool model.

Thus, methodological problems (Petermann *et al.*, 1993) and incomplete study design (Pacy *et al.*, 1991) are probably responsible for the inconsistencies between these studies and the nitrogen balance experiments. However, the clinically evident muscle wasting in chronic alcohol abusers, the observation that despite no difference in whole body protein turnover muscle protein FSR is reduced in chronic alcohol abusers (Pacy *et al.*, 1991) and data from animal studies showing reduced rates of protein synthesis in skeletal muscle (Preedy and Peters, 1989d, 1990b) all suggest that body proteins are lost with chronic ethanol abuse.

Regarding the possible mechanisms responsible for the alterations of protein turnover with chronic alcohol abuse, several theories have been proposed. Obviously, if ethanol intake is accompanied by a reduced protein intake, as often observed in the clinical setting, the protein malnutrition will result in a reduction of body protein mass over time. However, the observation that nitrogen balance is negative even when protein intake is adequate (McDonald and Margen, 1986; Reinus *et al.*, 1989) has led to the exploration of other hypotheses. The first focuses on the energetic value of ethanol. In chronic ethanol intake, when ethanol is isocalorically substituted to carbohydrate and fat, the alcohol may be a less efficient source of energy due to the induction of MEOS that does not produce ATP, but generates heat (Lieber, 1988). However, Reinus *et al.* (1989) showed that when chronic alcohol abusers were fed a diet in which ethanol was isocalorically substituted to carbohydrate (up to 60% of the total daily calories) there was no increase in heat production. In addition, this study showed that the isocaloric substitution of carbohydrate with ethanol did not affect nitrogen balance unless the amount of ethanol administered was above the liver clearance capacity. When ethanol was delivered at a rate above the liver oxidative capacity nitrogen balance became negative, although the calories from ethanol were not used for heat generation, but regularly utilized (Reinus *et al.*, 1989). The authors hypothesized that the negative effect of high ethanol intake on nitrogen balance in chronic ethanol abusers is possibly due to either the decrease in insulin response induced by the reduced carbohydrate intake, or the direct toxicity of ethanol or its metabolites on protein turnover. Preedy *et al.* (1999) favor the latter hypothesis and have recently theorized that ethanol itself, and/or through acetaldehyde, impairs protein synthesis, thus triggering a cascade of metabolic consequences including loss of water, minerals and electrolytes, which in turn reduces lean body mass (Preedy *et al.*, 1999).

Liver

Alcohol-induced liver disease is a very common complication of chronic ethanol abuse, the clinical characteristics ranging from fatty liver to alcoholic hepatitis to liver cirrhosis (Diehl, 1989). Several features of chronic alcohol-induced liver disease indicate that alterations of liver protein turnover are involved in the pathogenesis and clinical history of this disease, specifically, hypoalbuminemia (Lindholm *et al.*, 1991), collagen deposition in the liver (Friedman, 1993), swelling of hepatocytes due to the accumulation of lipids and, possibly, also of proteins (Lieber, 1988). Unfortunately, only very few studies have been performed in humans to assess the effects of chronic alcohol abuse on liver protein turnover. Most of the studies have focused on animal and *in vitro* models of chronic ethanol intake. However, despite the clinical and pathological evidence, the experimental studies assessing the effects of chronic ethanol intake on liver protein metabolism have yielded somewhat contradictory results.

A study in chronic alcohol abusers has shown some evidence of an increased synthesis of type III procollagen (Leblond-Francillard *et al.*, 1989) and *in vitro* data have confirmed that liver stellate cells (or lipocytes) are transformed by acetaldehyde into collagen producing cells (Friedman, 1993). Thus, an imbalance between collagen synthesis and degradation is a possible mechanism for alcohol-induced liver fibrosis and cirrhosis (Lieber, 1995). However, it is still debated whether chronic ethanol intake affects hepatic protein content. Some authors have reported that chronic ethanol exposure in rats increases protein content (Baraona *et al.*, 1975, 1977; Pignon *et al.*, 1987) whereas others have not been able to reproduce these results (Preedy and Peters, 1989b). It is possible that differences in the units used to report the results, i.e., protein content relative to body weight or relative to liver wet weight, may explain these data.

A further problem concerns the assessment of liver protein synthesis after chronic ethanol feeding. Studies in animals and *in vitro* have shown that chronic ethanol intake is associated with increased (Baraona *et al.*, 1977), reduced (Sorrell *et al.*, 1983; Smith-Kielland *et al.*, 1983; Preedy and Peters, 1989b) or unchanged (Smith-Kielland *et al.*, 1983) rates of liver protein synthesis. These inconsistencies may be due to the different methods used to measure protein synthesis and to the different study designs. For example, Baraona *et al.* (1977) used fed anesthetized rats and measured liver protein synthesis by bolus injection of ^{14}C-leucine using the leucyl-t-RNA specific activity as precursor pool, Preedy *et al.* (1989) used fed conscious rats and the flooding dose technique with phenylalanine and Smith-Kielland *et al.* (1983) used fasted rats and the continuous infusion of labeled valine. Whereas the other authors measured liver protein synthesis after 4–6 weeks, Smith-Kielland *et al.* (1983) performed the measurements two and eight weeks after the start of the ethanol diet and found the rate of liver protein synthesis unchanged at two weeks and reduced at eight weeks. A reduced protein synthesis rate during chronic ethanol intake would not justify the increased liver protein content found by some authors (Baraona *et al.*, 1977; Pignon *et al.*, 1987).

However, several papers have shown that one of the possible mechanisms that may increase liver protein content is the reduction of export protein secretion (Baraona *et al.*, 1977; Sorrell *et al.*, 1983), including albumin and transferrin, and a reduction of liver protein catabolism (Donohue *et al.*, 1989). These two problems either alone or combined could justify an increased liver protein content even in the absence of changes in protein synthesis. Furthermore, the reduced secretion of albumin may be important for long-term nitrogen economy of chronic alcohol abusers, even when well nourished. Several studies have shown that albumin synthesis and secretion is specifically stimulated by a meal and that this stimulation is responsible for subtracting a significant part of the dietary amino acids from the oxidative processes and for storing them for future utilization (De Feo *et al.*, 1992; Volpi *et al.*, 1996). The amino acids contained in albumin are subsequently made available for usage by virtually all the tissues of the body where albumin hydrolysis takes place. It is evident that any stimulus that can interrupt this mechanism may be responsible for a loss of amino-nitrogen in the long-term.

Acetaldehyde, which is not immediately degraded because of the down-regulation of ALDH in chronic alcohol abuse, is probably the major factor responsible for abnormal liver protein turnover (see Ethanol Oxidation – *Acetaldehyde oxidation* section). The formation of protein adducts can impair the function of hepatic enzymes, export proteins and proteins of the cytoskeleton, such as tubulin, with consequent reduction in secretive capacity (Baraona *et al.*, 1977, 1980; Sorrell *et al.*, 1983). However, one study has shown that one of the major contributors to increased liver protein content is the cytosolic fatty-acid binding protein, which can account for up to one third of the increase in cytosolic proteins (Pignon *et al.*, 1987).

Other tissues

The protein turnover of any organ and tissue is affected by chronic ethanol abuse. Unfortunately, little data are available on humans. Several studies have shown that skeletal muscle protein synthesis is decreased by chronic ethanol intake in humans (Pacy *et al.*, 1991) and animals (Preedy and Peters, 1989d, 1990b; Preedy *et al.*, 1990a). On the other hand, the synthesis rate of heart proteins in rats appears unaffected by chronic ethanol feeding (Preedy and Peters, 1990b,d), or only marginally impaired when the synthesis of specific proteins is measured (Preedy and Peters, 1989c). Similarly, protein synthesis rate in the rat's small intestine is not significantly influenced by chronic ethanol feeding (Preedy and Peters, 1989a, 1990b,c). However, since the protein content of small intestine is decreased by chronic alcohol consumption in rats, the lack of an effect of ethanol on protein synthesis suggests that an increase in proteolysis is likely to be promoted by ethanol (Preedy and Peters, 1989a, 1990c).

Interestingly, protein synthesis in the pancreas was stimulated by ethanol intake in rats receiving a diet containing adequate amounts of proteins, whereas a diet deficient in proteins resulted in lower rates of pancreas protein synthesis, which were similar to those observed in rats given an ethanol-free protein-adequate diet (Korsten *et al.*, 1990). Although no data are at present available on humans, the results from Korsten *et al.* (1990) might help to explain the reason why well-nourished alcohol abusers are at higher risk of pancreatitis than their malnourished counterparts.

CONCLUSION

Ethanol influences the protein turnover rates of almost any tissue and organ in many different ways, according to the pattern of intake (i.e., acute or chronic) and the dose. It may reduce the synthesis of certain proteins, such as skeletal muscle proteins, increase the synthesis of others such as collagen and reduce the synthesis and/or secretion of liver export proteins, thus influencing whole body protein turnover and nitrogen balance. The understanding of the effects of ethanol on protein metabolism is extremely important as it helps shed light on the mechanisms of ethanol toxicity. Whereas at present there is scientific consensus regarding certain effects of ethanol on protein turnover, such as the well established induction of a loss of nitrogen and lean body mass in chronic alcoholics, other areas still need to be explored. For example, almost no data are available on hepatic protein turnover in humans who chronically drink high amounts of alcohol. Little is known about the effects of habitual drinking of ethanol on liver, muscle and whole body protein turnover, at low to moderate doses (<30 g/day), which are known to reduce the risk of coronary artery disease, stroke and peripheral artery disease. Other possible investigations may focus on the effects of alcohol on regional or tissue protein synthesis and breakdown in humans with the help of new methods that allow a better estimation of these important parameters of protein turnover (Biolo et al., 1995; Zhang et al., 1996). Finally, an in depth analysis of the biochemical and molecular mechanisms involved in the alterations of protein metabolism with the contemporaneous assessment of protein synthesis and degradation, enzyme activity, activation/deactivation of specific signaling pathways and gene expression is warranted.

REFERENCES

Arends, J., Ostlund, R.E. and Bier, D.M. (1992) Measurement of in-vivo protein synthesis using stable isotopes: comparison of four different amino acid tracers. In *Protein Metabolism in Diabetes Mellitus*, edited by K.S. Nair, pp. 277. London: Eldred Smith-Gordon.

Avogaro, A., Cibin, M., Croatto, T., Rizzo, A., Galimberti, L. and Tiengo, A. (1986) Alcohol intake and withdrawal: effects of branched chain amino acids and alanine. *Alcoholism (Zagreb)* **10**, 300–304.

Baraona, E., Leo, M.A., Borowsky, S.A. and Lieber, C.S. (1977) Pathogenesis of alcohol-induced accumulation of protein in the liver. *Journal of Clinical Investigation* **60**, 546–554.

Baraona, E., Leo, M.A., Borowsky, S.A. and Lieber, C.S. (1975) Alcoholic hepatomegaly: accumulation of protein in the liver. *Science* **190**, 794–795.

Baraona, E., Pikkarainen, P., Salaspuro, M., Finkelman, F. and Lieber, C.S. (1980) Acute effects of ethanol on hepatic protein synthesis and secretion in the rat. *Gastroenterology* **79**, 104–111.

Bennet, W.M., O'Keefe, S.J. and Haymond, M.W. (1993) Comparison of precursor pools with leucine, alpha-ketoisocaproate, and phenylalanine tracers used to measure splanchnic protein synthesis in man. *Metabolism: Clinical & Experimental* **42**, 691–695.

Berger, K., Ajani, U.A., Kase, C.S., Gaziano, J.M., Buring, J.E., Glynn, R.J. and Hennekens C.H. (1999) Light-to-moderate alcohol consumption and risk of stroke among U.S. male physicians. *New England Journal of Medicine* **341**, 1557–1564.

Bernal, C.A., Vazquez, J.A. and Adibi, S.A. (1993) Leucine metabolism during chronic ethanol consumption. *Metabolism: Clinical & Experimental* **42**, 1084–1086.

Berry, M.N., Gregory, R.B., Grivell, A.R., Phillips, J.W. and Schon, A. (1994) The capacity of reducing-equivalent shuttles limits glycolysis during ethanol oxidation. *European Journal of Biochemistry* **225**, 557–564.

Bier, D.M. (1992) Whole body protein kinetic measurements. In *Protein Metabolism in Diabetes Mellitus*, edited by K.S. Nair, pp. 61–68. London: Eldred Smith-Gordon.

Biolo, G., Fleming, R.Y., Maggi, S.P. and Wolfe, R.R. (1995) Transmembrane transport and intracellular kinetics of amino acids in human skeletal muscle. *American Journal of Physiology, Endocrinology and Metabolism* **268**, E75–E84.

Bunout, D., Petermann, M., Ugarte, G., Barrera, G. and Iturriaga, H. (1987) Nitrogen economy in alcoholic patients without liver disease. *Metabolism: Clinical & Experimental* **36**, 651–653.

Caballeria, J., Baraona, E., Deulofeu, R., Hernandez-Munoz, R., Rodes, J. and Lieber, C.S. (1991) Effects of H$_2$-receptor antagonists on gastric alcohol dehydrogenase activity. *Digestive Diseases & Sciences* **36**, 1673–1679.

Caballeria, J., Baraona, E., Rodamilans, M. and Lieber, C.S. (1989) Effects of cimetidine on gastric alcohol dehydrogenase activity and blood ethanol levels. *Gastroenterology* **96**, 388–392.

Camargo, C.A.J., Hennekens, C.H., Gaziano, J.M., Glynn, R.J., Manson, J.E. and Stampfer M.J. (1997a) Prospective study of moderate alcohol consumption and mortality in US male physicians. *Archives of Internal Medicine* **157**, 79–85.

Camargo, C.A.J., Stampfer, M.J., Glynn, R.J., Gaziano, J.M., Manson, J.E., Goldhaber, S.Z. and Hennekens, C.H. (1997b) Prospective study of moderate alcohol consumption and risk of peripheral arterial disease in US male physicians. *Circulation* **95**, 577–580.

Carraro, F., Rosenblatt, J. and Wolfe, R.R. (1991) Isotopic determination of fibronectin synthesis in humans. *Metabolism: Clinical & Experimental* **40**, 553–561.

Chinkes, D., Klein, S., Zhang, X.J. and Wolfe, R.R. (1996) Infusion of labeled KIC is more accurate than labeled leucine to determine human muscle protein synthesis. *American Journal of Physiology, Endocrinology and Metabolism* **270**, E67–E71.

Cobelli, C., Saccomani, M.P. and Matthews, D.E. (1992) Evolution of models of leucine kinetics for measuring protein turnover. In *Protein Metabolism in Diabetes Mellitus*, edited by K.S. Nair, pp. 69–77. London: Eldred Smith-Gordon.

Cobelli, C., Saccomani, M.P., Tessari, P., Biolo, G., Luzi, L. and Matthews, D.E. (1991) A compartmental model of leucine kinetics in humans. *American Journal of Physiology, Endocrinology and Metabolism* **261**, E538–E550.

Dardevet, D., Sornet, C., Savary, I., Debras, F., Patureau-Mirand, P. and Grizard, J. (1998) Glucocorticoid effects on insulin- and IGF-I-regulated muscle protein metabolism during aging. *Journal of Endocrinology* **156**, 83–89.

De Feo, P., Horber, F.F. and Haymond, M.W. (1992) Meal stimulation of albumin synthesis: a significant contributor to whole body protein synthesis in humans. *American Journal of Physiology, Endocrinology and Metabolism* **263**, E794–E799.

De Feo, P., Volpi, E., Lucidi, P., Cruciani, G., Monacchia, F., Reboldi, G., Santeusanio, F., Bolli, G.B. and Brunetti, P. (1995) Ethanol impairs post-prandial hepatic protein metabolism. *Journal of Clinical Investigation* **95**, 1472–1479.

De Feo, P., Volpi, E., Lucidi, P., Cruciani, G., Reboldi, G., Siepi, D., Mannarino, E., Santeusanio, F., Brunetti, P. and Bolli, G.B. (1993) Physiological increments in plasma insulin concentrations have selective and different effects on synthesis of hepatic proteins in normal humans. *Diabetes* **42**, 995–1002.

Desmoulin, F., Canioni, P., Masson, S., Gerolami, A. and Cozzone, P.J. (1990) Effect of ethanol on hepatic energy metabolism and intracellular pH in chronically ethanol-treated rats. A 31P NMR study of normoxic or hypoxic perfused liver. *NMR in Biomedicine* **3**, 132–138.

Diehl, A.M. (1989) Alcoholic liver disease. *Medical Clinics of North America* **73**, 815–830.

DiPadova, C., Worner, T.M., Julkunen, R.J. and Lieber, C.S. (1987) Effects of fasting and chronic alcohol consumption on the first-pass metabolism of ethanol. *Gastroenterology* **92**, 1169–1173.

Donohue, T.M.J., Zetterman, R.K. and Tuma, D.J. (1989) Effect of chronic ethanol administration on protein catabolism in rat liver. *Alcoholism: Clinical & Experimental Research* **13**, 49–57.

Espina, N., Lima, V., Lieber, C.S. and Garro, A.J. (1988) *In vitro* and *in vivo* inhibitory effect of ethanol and acetaldehyde on O6-methylguanine transferase. *Carcinogenesis* **9**, 761–766.

Ferrando, A.A., Chinkes, D.L., Wolf, S.E., Matin, S., Herndon, D.N. and Wolfe, R.R. (1999) A submaximal dose of insulin promotes net skeletal muscle protein synthesis in patients with severe burns. *Annals of Surgery* **229**, 11–18.

French, S.W. (1989) Biochemical basis for alcohol-induced liver injury. *Clinical Biochemistry* **22**, 41–49.

Frezza, M., Di Padova, C., Pozzato, G., Terpin, M., Baraona, E. and Lieber, C.S. (1990) High blood alcohol levels in women. The role of decreased gastric alcohol dehydrogenase activity and first-pass metabolism. *New England Journal of Medicine* **322**, 95–99.

Friedman, S.L. (1993) Seminars in medicine of the Beth Israel Hospital, Boston. The cellular basis of hepatic fibrosis. Mechanisms and treatment strategies. *New England Journal of Medicine* **328**, 1828–1835.

Frohlich, J.J. (1996) Effects of alcohol on plasma lipoprotein metabolism. *Clinica Chimica Acta* **246**, 39–49.

Garlick, P.J., McNurlan, M.A. and Preedy, V.R. (1980) A rapid and convenient technique for measuring the rate of protein synthesis in tissues by injection of [^{3}H]phenylalanine. *Biochemical Journal* **192**, 719–723.

Garlick, P.J., Wernerman, J., McNurlan, M.A., Essen, P., Lobley, G.E., Milne, E., Calder, G.A. and Vinnars, E. (1989) Measurement of the rate of protein synthesis in muscle of postabsorptive young men by injection of a 'flooding dose' of [1-^{13}C]leucine. *Clinical Science* **77**, 329–336.

Goldberg, D.M., Garovic-Kocic, V., Diamandis, E.P. and Pace-Asciak, C.R. (1996) Wine: does the colour count? *Clinica Chimica Acta* **246**, 183–193.

Gonzalez-Calvin, J.L., Garcia-Sanchez, A., Bellot, V., Munoz-Torres, M., Raya-Alvarez, E. and Salvatierra-Rios, D. (1993) Mineral metabolism, osteoblastic function and bone mass in chronic alcoholism. *Alcohol & Alcoholism* **28**, 571–579.

Hasumura, Y., Teschke, R. and Lieber, C.S. (1975) Acetaldehyde oxidation by hepatic mitochondria: decrease after chronic ethanol consumption. *Science* **189**, 727–729.

Hegsted, D.M. (1978) Assessment of nitrogen requirements. *American Journal of Clinical Nutrition* **31**, 1669–1677.

Hill, A., Rumpf, H.J., Hapke, U., Driessen, M. and John, U. (1998) Prevalence of alcohol dependence and abuse in general practice. *Alcoholism: Clinical & Experimental Research* **22**, 935–940.

Hoerr, R.A., Yu, Y.M., Wagner, D.A., Burke, J.F. and Young, V.R. (1989) Recovery of ^{13}C in breath from NaH^{13}CO$_3$ infused by gut and vein: effect of feeding. *American Journal of Physiology, Endocrinology and Metabolism* **257**, E426–E438.

Horber, F.F., Horber-Feyder, C.M., Krayer, S., Schwenk, W.F. and Haymond, M.W. (1989) Plasma reciprocal pool specific activity predicts that of intracellular free leucine for protein synthesis. *American Journal of Physiology, Endocrinology and Metabolism* **257**, E385–E399.

Jahoor, F., Zhang, X.J., Baba, H., Sakurai, Y. and Wolfe, R.R. (1992) Comparison of constant infusion and flooding dose techniques to measure muscle protein synthesis rate in dogs. *Journal of Nutrition* **122**, 878–887.

Jeejeebhoy, K.N., Phillips, M.J., Bruce-Robertson, A., Ho, J. and Sodtke, U. (1972) The acute effect of ethanol on albumin, fibrinogen and transferrin synthesis in the rat. *Biochemistry Journal* **126**, 1111–1126.

Julkunen, R.J., Di Padova, C. and Lieber, C.S. (1985a) First pass metabolism of ethanol – a astrointestinal barrier against the systemic toxicity of ethanol. *Life Sciences* **37**, 567–573.

Julkunen, R.J., Tannenbaum, L., Baraona, E. and Lieber, C.S. (1985b) First pass metabolism of ethanol: an important determinant of blood levels after alcohol consumption. *Alcohol* **2**, 437–441.

Kannel, W.B. and Ellison, R.C. (1996) Alcohol and coronary heart disease: the evidence for a protective effect. *Clinica Chimica Acta* **246**, 59–76.

Korsten, M.A. and Lieber, C.S. (1979) Nutrition in the alcoholic. *Medical Clinics of North America* **63**, 963–972.

Korsten, M.A., Wilson, J.S. and Lieber, C.S. (1990) Interactive effects of dietary protein and ethanol on rat pancreas. Protein synthesis and enzyme secretion. *Gastroenterology* **99**, 229–236.

Krobot, K., Hense, H.W., Cremer, P., Eberle, E. and Keil, U. (1992) Determinants of plasma fibrinogen: relation to body weight, waist-to-hip ratio, smoking, alcohol, age and sex: results from the second MONICA Augsburg survey 1989–1990. *Arteriosclerosis & Thrombosis* **12**, 780–788.

Lamberts, H. and Okkes, I. (1999) Patients with chronic alcohol abuse in Dutch family practices. *Alcohol & Alcoholism* **34**, 337–345.

Lauterburg, B., Liang, D., Schwarzenbach, F. and Breen, K. (1993) Mitochondrial dysfunction in alcoholic patients as assessed by breath analysis. *Hepatology* **17**, 418–422.

Layman, D.K. and Wolfe, R.R. (1987) Sample site selection for tracer studies applying a unidirectional circulatory approach. *American Journal of Physiology, Endocrinology and Metabolism* **253**, E173–E178.

Leblond-Francillard, M., Augereau, C., Nalpas, Trinchet, J.C., Hartmann, D.J., Berthelot, P., Beaugrand, M. and Brechot, C. (1989) Liver collagen mRNA and serum amino-terminal peptide of type III procollagen (PIIINP) levels in patients with alcoholic liver disease. *Journal of Hepatology* **9**, 351–358.

Lewis, G.F., Uffelman, K.D., Szeto, L.W. and Steiner, G. (1993) Effects of acute hyperinsulinaemia on VLDL triglyceride and VLDL apoB production in normal weight and obese individuals. *Diabetes* **42**, 833–842.

Lieber, C.S. (1988) Biochemical and molecular basis of alcohol-induced injury to liver and other tissues. *New England Journal of Medicine* **319**, 1639–1650.

Lieber, C.S. (1993) Herman Award Lecture, 1993: a personal perspective on alcohol, nutrition, and the liver. *American Journal of Clinical Nutrition* **58**, 430–442.

Lieber, C.S. (1995) Medical disorders of alcoholism. *New England Journal of Medicine* **333**, 1058–1065.

Lieber, C.S. (1997) Ethanol metabolism, cirrhosis and alcoholism. *Clinica Chimica Acta* **257**, 59–84.

Lieber, C.S. and Schmid, R. (1961) The effect of ethanol on fatty acid metabolism: stimulation of hepatic fatty acid synthesis *in vitro*. *Journal of Clinical Investigation* **40**, 394–399.

Lindenbaum, J. and Lieber, C.S. (1975) Effects of chronic ethanol administration on intestinal absorption in man in the absence of nutritional deficiency. *Annals of the New York Academy of Sciences* **252**, 228–234.

Lindholm, J., Steiniche, T., Rasmussen, E., Thamsborg, G., Nielsen, I.O., Brockstedt Rasmussen, H., Storm, T., Hyldstrup, L. and Schou, C. (1991) Bone disorder in men with chronic alcoholism: a reversible disease? *Journal of Clinical Endocrinology & Metabolism* **73**, 118–124.

Lucia, S.P. (1972) Wine: a food throughout the ages. *American Journal of Clinical Nutrition* **25**, 361–362.

Lyons, D., Whitlow, C.T., Smith, H.R. and Porrino, L.J. (1998) Brain imaging: functional consequences of ethanol in the central nervous system. *Recent Developments in Alcoholism* **14**, 253–284.

Madison, L.L., Lochner, A. and Wulff, J. (1967) Ethanol induced hypoglycemia: mechanism of suppression of hepatic gluconeogenesis. *Diabetes* **16**, 252–258.

Manchester, K.L. and Tyobeka, E.M. (1980) Influence of individual amino acids on incorporation of [^{14}C]leucine by rat liver ribosomes. *Journal of Nutrition* **110**, 241–247.

Marques-Vidal, P., Ducimetiere, P., Evans, A., Cambou, J.P. and Arveiler, D. (1996) Alcohol consumption and myocardial infarction: a case-control study in France and Northern Ireland. *American Journal of Epidemiology* **143**, 1089–1093.

Masson, S., Desmoulin, F., Sciaky, M. and Cozzone, P.J. (1993) Catabolism of adenine nucleotides and its relation with intracellular phosphorylated metabolite concentration during ethanol oxidation in perfused rat liver. *Biochemistry* **32**, 1025–1031.

Matthews, D.E. (1999) Proteins and amino acids. In *Modern Nutrition in Health and Disease*, 9th edn., edited by M.E. Shils, J.A. Olson, M. Shike and A.C. Ross, pp. 11–48. Baltimore: Williams & Wilkins.

Matthews, D.E., Bier, D.M., Rennie, M.J., Edwards, R.H.T., Halliday, D., Millward, D.J. and Clugston, G.A. (1981) Regulation of leucine metabolism in man: a stable isotope study. *Science* **214**, 1129–1131.

Matthews, D.E., Marano, M.A. and Campbell, R.G. (1993) Splanchnic bed utilization of leucine and phenylalanine in humans. *American Journal of Physiology, Endocrinology and Metabolism* **264**, E109–E118.

Mattiasson, I. and Lindgarde, F. (1993) The effect of psychosocial stress and risk factors for ischaemic heart disease on the plasma fibrinogen concentration. *Journal of Internal Medicine* **234**, 45–51.

Mayes, P.A. (1996) Structure and functions of the water-soluble vitamins. In *Harper's Biochemistry*, 24th edn., edited by R.K. Murray, D.K. Granner, P.A. Mayes and V.W. Rodwell, pp. 601–603. Stamford, CT: Appleton & Lange.

McDonald, J.T. and Margen, S. (1986) Wine versus ethanol in human nutrition.I. Nitrogen and calorie balance. *American Journal of Clinical Nutrition* **29**, 1093–1103.

McNurlan, M.A., Fern, E.B. and Garlick, P.J. (1982) Failure of leucine to stimulate protein synthesis *in vivo*. *Biochemistry Journal* **204**, 831–838.

Menotti, A., Kromhout, D., Blackburn, H., Fidanza, F., Buzina, R. and Nissinen, A. (1999) Food intake patterns and 25-year mortality from coronary heart disease: cross-cultural correlations in the Seven Countries Study. The Seven Countries Study Research Group. *European Journal of Epidemiology* **15**, 507–515.

Mitchell, M.C. and Herlong, H.F. (1986) Alcohol and nutrition: caloric value, bioenergetics, and relationship to liver damage. *Annual Review of Nutrition* **6**, 457–474.

Mørland, J. and Bessesen, A. (1977) Inhibition of protein synthesis by ethanol in isolated rat liver parenchymal cells. *Biochimica et Biophysica Acta* **474**, 312–320.

Mørland, J., Bessesen, A. and Svendsen, L. (1979) Incorporation of labelled amino acids into proteins of isolated parenchymal and nonparenchymal rat liver cells in the absence and presence of ethanol. *Biochimica et Biophysica Acta* **561**, 464–474.

Munro, H.N. (1972) Amino acid requirements and metabolism and their relevance to parenteral nutrition. In *Parenteral Nutrition*, edited by A.W. Wilkinson, pp. 34–67. London: Churchill-Livingstone.

Muntwyler, J., Hennekens, C.H., Buring, J.E. and Gaziano, J.M. (1998) Mortality and light to moderate alcohol consumption after myocardial infarction. *Lancet* **352**, 1882–1885.

Newsholme, E.A. and Crabtree, B. (1976) Substrate cycles in metabolic regulation and heat generation. *Biochemical Society Symposia* **41**, 61–109.

Newsholme, E.A. and Leech, A.R. (1983a) Amino acid metabolism. In *Biochemistry for the Medical Sciences*, edited by E.A. Newsholme and A.R. Leech, pp. 382–441. Chichester: John Wiley & Sons.

Newsholme, E.A. and Leech, A.R. (1983b) Carbohydrate metabolism in the liver. In *Biochemistry for the Medical Sciences*, edited by E.A. Newsholme and A.R. Leech, pp. 442–480. Chichester: John Wiley & Sons.

Nissen, S.L. and Haymond, M.W. (1981) Effects of fasting on flux and interconvertion of leucine and a-keto-isocaproate *in vivo*. *American Journal of Physiology, Endocrinology and Metabolism* **241**, E72–E75.

Pacy, P.J., Preedy, V.R., Peters, T.J., Read, M. and Halliday, D. (1991) The effect of chronic alcohol ingestion on whole body and muscle protein synthesis. A stable isotope study. *Alcohol and Alcoholism* **26**, 505–513.

Patterson, B.W., Carraro, F. and Wolfe, R.R. (1993) Measurement of 15N enrichment in multiple amino acids and urea in a single analysis by gas chromatography/mass spectrometry. *Biological Mass Spectrometry* **22**, 518–523.

Petermann, M., Gonzalez, C., Hirsch, S., Pia, d.l.M. and Bunout, D. (1993) Leucine and glucose turnover in chronic alcoholics during early abstinence and after an ethanol load. *Alcoholism: Clinical & Experimental Research* **17**, 1295–1300.

Picou, D. and Taylor-Roberts, T. (1969) The measurement of total protein synthesis and catabolism and nitrogen turnover in infants in different nutritional states and receiving different amounts of dietary protein. *Clinical Science* **36**, 283–296.

Picou, D., Taylor-Roberts, T. and Waterlow, J.C. (1969) The measurement of total protein synthesis and nitrogen flux in man by constant infusion of 15N-glycine. *Journal of Physiology* **200**, 52P–53P.

Pignon, J.P., Bailey, N.C., Baraona, E. and Lieber, C.S. (1987) Fatty acid-binding protein: a major contributor to the ethanol-induced increase in liver cytosolic proteins in the rat. *Hepatology* **7**, 865–871.

Preedy, V.R., Duane, P. and Peters, T.J. (1988a) Acute ethanol dosage reduces the synthesis of smooth muscle contractile proteins in the small intestine of the rat. *Gut* **29**, 1244–1248.

Preedy, V.R., Duane, P. and Peters, T.J. (1988b) Comparison of the acute effects of ethanol on liver and skeletal muscle protein synthesis in the rat. *Alcohol & Alcoholism* **23**, 155–162.

Preedy, V.R., Keating, J.W. and Peters, T.J. (1992) The acute effects of ethanol and acetaldehyde on rates of protein synthesis in type I and type II fiber-rich skeletal muscles of the rat. *Alcohol & Alcoholism* **27**, 241–251.

Preedy, V.R., Marway, J.S., Macpherson, A.J. and Peters, T.J. (1990a) Ethanol-induced smooth and skeletal muscle myopathy: use of animal studies. *Drug & Alcohol Dependence* **26**, 1–8.

Preedy, V.R., Marway, J.S., Salisbury, J.R. and Peters, T.J. (1990b) Protein synthesis in bone and skin of the rat are inhibited by ethanol: implications for whole body metabolism. *Alcoholism: Clinical & Experimental Research* **14**, 165–168.

Preedy, V.R. and Peters, T. (1989a) Protein metabolism in the small intestine of the ethanol-fed rat. *Cell Biochemistry & Function* **7**, 235–242.

Preedy, V.R. and Peters, T.J. (1989b) An investigation into the effects of chronic ethanol feeding on hepatic mixed protein synthesis in immature and mature rats. *Alcohol & Alcoholism* **24**, 311–318.

Preedy, V.R. and Peters, T.J. (1989c) Synthesis of subcellular protein fractions in the rat heart *in vivo* in response to chronic ethanol feeding. *Cardiovascular Research* **23**, 730–736.

Preedy, V.R. and Peters, T.J. (1989d) The effect of chronic ethanol ingestion on synthesis and degradation of soluble, contractile and stromal protein fractions of skeletal muscles from immature and mature rats. *Biochemical Journal* **259**, 261–266.

Preedy, V.R. and Peters, T.J. (1990a) Alcohol and skeletal muscle disease. *Alcohol & Alcoholism* **25**, 177–187.

Preedy, V.R. and Peters, T.J. (1990b) Changes in protein, RNA and DNA and rates of protein synthesis in muscle-containing tissues of the mature rat in response to ethanol feeding: a comparative study of heart, small intestine and gastrocnemius muscle. *Alcohol & Alcoholism* **25**, 489–498.

Preedy, V.R. and Peters, T.J. (1990c) Protein synthesis of muscle fractions from the small intestine in alcohol fed rats. *Gut* **31**, 305–310.

Preedy, V.R. and Peters, T.J. (1990d) The acute and chronic effects of ethanol on cardiac muscle protein synthesis in the rat *in vivo*. *Alcohol* **7**, 97–102.

Preedy, V.R., Reilly, M.E., Patel, V.B., Richardson, P.J. and Peters, T.J. (1999) Protein metabolism in alcoholism: effects on specific tissues and the whole body. *Nutrition* **15**, 604–608.

Preedy, V.R. and Richardson, P.J. (1994) Ethanol induced cardiovascular disease. *British Medical Bulletin* **50**, 152–163.

Reid, M.C., Fiellin, D.A. and O'Connor, P.G. (1999) Hazardous and harmful alcohol consumption in primary care. *Archives of Internal Medicine* **159**, 1681–1689.

Reinus, J.F., Heymsfield, S.B., Wiskind, R., Casper, K. and Galambos, J.T. (1989) Ethanol: relative fuel value and metabolic effects *in vivo. Metabolism: Clinical & Experimental* **38**, 125–135.

Roine, R., Gentry, R.T., Hernandez-Munoz, R., Baraona, E. and Lieber C.S. (1990) Aspirin increases blood alcohol concentrations in humans after ingestion of ethanol. *JAMA* **264**, 2406–2408.

Rothschild, M.A., Oratz, M. and Schreiber, S.S. (1974) Alcohol, amino acids, and albumin synthesis. *Gastroenterology* **67**, 1200–1213.

Sacco, R.L., Elkind, M., Boden-Albala, B., Lin, I.F., Kargman, D.E., Hauser, W.A., Shea and Paik, M.C. (1999) The protective effect of moderate alcohol consumption on ischemic stroke. *JAMA* **281**, 53–60.

Schwenk, W.F., Beaufrere, B. and Haymond, M.W. (1985a) Use of reciprocal pool specific activities to model leucine metabolism in humans. *American Journal of Physiology, Endocrinology and Metabolism* **249**, E646–E650.

Schwenk, W.F., Tsalikian, E., Beaufrere, B. and Haymond, M.W. (1985b) Recycling of an amino acid label with prolonged isotope infusion: implications for kinetic studies. *American Journal of Physiology, Endocrinology and Metabolism* **248**, E482–E487.

Scrimshaw, N.S., Hussein, M.A., Murray, E., Rand, W.M. and Young, V.R. (1972) Protein requirements of man: variations in obligatory urinary and fecal nitrogen losses in young men. *Journal of Nutrition* **102**, 1595–1604.

Shaw, S. and Lieber, C.S. (1978) Plasma amino acids abnormalities in the alcoholic: respective role of alcohol, nutrition and liver injury. *Gastroenterology* **74**, 677–683.

Shelmet, J.J., Reichard, G.A., Skutches, C.L., Hoeldtke, R.D., Owen, O.E. and Boden, G. (1988) Ethanol causes acute inhibition of carbohydrate, fat, and protein oxidation and insulin resistance. *Journal of Clinical Investigation* **81**, 1137–1145.

Shoenheimer, R., Rutner, S. and Rittenberg, D. (1939) Studies in protein metabolism; metabolic activity of body proteins investigated with 1-leucine containing 2 isotopes. *Journal of Biological Chemistry* **130**, 730–732.

Siddiq, T., Richardson, P.J., Mitchell, W.D., Teare, J. and Preedy, V.R. (1993) Ethanol-induced inhibition of ventricular protein synthesis *in vivo* and the possible role of acetaldehyde. *Cell Biochemistry & Function* **11**, 45–54.

Sirbu, E.R., Margen, S. and Calloway, D.H. (1967) Effect of reduced protein intake on nitrogen loss from the human integument. *American Journal of Clinical Nutrition* **20**, 1158–1165.

Smith-Kielland, A., Blom, G.P., Svendsen, L., Bessesen, A. and Morland, J. (1983) A study of hepatic protein synthesis, three subcellular enzymes, and liver morphology in chronically ethanol fed rats. *Acta Pharmacologica et Toxicologica* **53**, 113–120.

Smith, K., Barua, J.M., Watt, P.W., Scrimgeour, C.M. and Rennie, M.J. (1992) Flooding with [1-^{13}C]leucine stimulates human muscle protein incorporation of continuously infused L-[1-^{13}C]valine. *American Journal of Physiology, Endocrinology and Metabolism* **262**, E372–E376.

Smith, K., Downie, S., Barua, J.M., Watt, P.W., Scrimgeour, C.M. and Rennie, M.J. (1994) Effect of a flooding dose of leucine in stimulating incorporation of constantly infused valine into albumin. *American Journal of Physiology, Endocrinology and Metabolism* **266**, E640–E644.

Smith, K., Reynolds, N., Downie, S., Patel, A. and Rennie, M.J. (1998) Effects of flooding amino acids on incorporation of labeled amino acids into human muscle protein. *American Journal of Physiology, Endocrinology and Metabolism* **275**, E73–E78.

Sorrell, M.F., Nauss, J.M., Donohue, T.M. and Tuma, D.J. (1983) Effects of chronic ethanol administration on hepatic glycoprotein secretion in the rat. *Gastroenterology* **84**, 580–586.

Stanko, R.T., Morse, E.L. and Adibi, S.A. (1979) Prevention of effects of ethanol on amino acid concentrations in plasma and tissues by hepatic lipotropic factors in rats. *Gastroenterology* **76**, 132–138.

Steele, R.S., Sesney, J.W. and Kreher, N.E. (1999) The prevalence of alcohol abuse and dependence in two geographically distinct regions in Michigan: an UPRNet study. *WMJ* **98**, 54–57.

Stein, T.P., Ang, S.D., Schluter, M.D., Leskiw, M.J. and Nusbaum, M. (1983) Whole-body protein turnover in metabolically stressed patients and patients with cancer as measured with [^{15}N] glycine. *Biochemical Medicine* **30**, 59–77.

Suter, P.M., Schutz, Y. and Jequier, E. (1992) The effect of ethanol on fat storage in healhty subjects. *New England Journal of Medicine* **326**, 983–987.

Teschke, R., Hasumura, Y. and Lieber, C.S. (1974) Hepatic microsomal ethanol-oxidizing system: solubilization, isolation, and characterization. *Archives of Biochemistry & Biophysics* **163**, 404–415.

Toffolo, G., Foster, D.M. and Cobelli, C. (1993) Estimation of protein fractional synthetic rate from tracer data. *American Journal of Physiology, Endocrinology and Metabolism* **264**, E128–E135.

Valmadrid, C.T., Klein, R., Moss, S.E., Klein, B.E. and Cruickshanks, K.J. (1999) Alcohol intake and the risk of coronary heart disease mortality in persons with older-onset diabetes mellitus. *JAMA* **282**, 239–246.

Volpi, E., Lucidi, P., Cruciani, G., Monacchia, F., Reboldi, G., Brunetti, P., Bolli, G.B. and De Feo, P. (1997) Nicotinamide counteracts alcohol-induced impairment of hepatic protein metabolism in humans. *Journal of Nutrition* **127**, 2199–2204.

Volpi, E., Lucidi, P., Cruciani, G., Monacchia, F., Santoni, S., Reboldi, G., Brunetti, P., Bolli, G.B. and De Feo, P. (1998) Moderate and large doses of ethanol differentially affect hepatic protein metabolism in humans. *Journal of Nutrition* **128**, 198–203.

Volpi, E., Lucidi, P., Monacchia, F., Cruciani, G., Reboldi, G., Santeusanio, F., Brunetti, P., Bolli, G.B. and De Feo, P. (1996) Contribution of amino acids and insulin to protein anabolism during meal absorption. *Diabetes* **45**, 1245–1252.

Waterlow, J.C. (1967) Lysine turnover in man measured by intravenous infusion of L-[U-^{14}C]lysine. *Clin Sci* **33**, 507–515.

Waterlow, J.C., Garlick, P.J. and Millward, D.J. (1978) *Protein Turnover in Mammalian Tissues and in the Whole Body*, pp. 687–687. Amsterdam: North-Holland.

Waterlow, J.C. and Stephen, J.M.L. (1967) The measurement of total lysine turnover in the rat by intravenous infusion of L-[U-^{14}C]lysine. *Clinical Science* **33**, 489–506.

Watt, P.W., Lindsay, Y., Scrimgeour, C.M., Chien, P.A.F., Gibson, J.N.A., Taylor, D.J. and Rennie, M.J. (1991) Isolation of aminoacyl-tRNA and its labeling with stable isotope tracers: use in studies of human tissue protein synthesis. *Proceedings of the National Academy of Science of the United States of America* **88**, 5892–5896.

Watt, P.W., Stenhouse, M.G., Corbett, M.E. and Rennie, M.J. (1989) tRNA charging in pig muscle measured by [1-^{13}C]leucine during fasting and infusion of amino acids. *Clinical Nutrition* 8 (Suppl), 47.

Wolfe, R.R. (1992a) Calculation of substrate kinetics: single pool model. In *Radioactive and Stable Isotope Tracers in Biomedicine: principle and Practice of Kinetic Analysis*, 1st edn, edited by R.R. Wolfe, pp. 119–144. New York: Wiley-Liss.

Wolfe, R.R. (1992b) Protein synthesis and breakdown. In *Radioactive and Stable Isotope Tracers in Biomedicine: principle and Practice of Kinetic Analysis*, 1st edn, edited by R.R. Wolfe, pp. 377–416. New York: Wiley-Liss.

Yang, T., Doherty, T.M., Wong, N.D. and Detrano, R.C. (1999) Alcohol consumption, coronary calcium, and coronary heart disease events. *American Journal of Cardiology* **84**, 802–806.

Zhang, X.J., Chinkes, D.L., Sakurai, Y. and Wolfe, R.R. (1996) An isotopic method for measurement of muscle protein fractional breakdown rate *in vivo*. *American Journal of Physiology, Endocrinology and Metabolism* **270**, E759–E767.

Chapter 12

Insulin-like growth factors: clinical and experimental

Anthony J. Donaghy

Alcohol exerts multiple influences on the endocrine GH:IGF axis predominantly resulting in decreased IGF bioavailability and adverse influences on growth. Alcohol has been shown to have direct toxic effects on GH and IGF-I production and also to exert indirect influences through nutritional effects and those associated with the pathological lesion of cirrhosis. *In vitro* studies have shown effects at multiple levels of the complex GH:IGF axis and to also demonstrate impairment of IGF-I receptor signal transduction, compounding the adverse effects on growth of low IGF bioavailability. Although not conclusive, recent studies have suggested a role for IGF deficiency in the pathogenesis of ALD and many studies have strongly suggested that low IGF bioavailability may be an important factor in the complications of cirrhosis such as starvation metabolism, insulin resistance, malnutrition and immune dysfunction. Further studies have shown that measurements of IGF-I and IGFBP-3 give important prognostic information and may prove helpful in the assessment and timing of liver transplantation. Treatment of alcoholic cirrhotics with GH has been shown to increase IGF-I and IGFBP-3 levels with associated improvements in nitrogen balance and body composition. Therapeutic manipulation of the GH:IGF axis holds significant promise in the battle to reverse the catabolic state which so adversely affects outcome in this patient group.

KEYWORDS: growth hormone (GH), insulin-like growth factors (IGFs), insulin-like growth factor binding protein 1, insulin-like growth factor binding protein 3, malnutrition

INTRODUCTION

The pathogenesis of alcoholic liver disease (ALD) is multifactorial with toxic, metabolic, inflammatory and immune derangements shown to interreact with nutritional and genetic factors to effect liver injury. Alcohol is a potent inhibitor of DNA, RNA and protein synthesis at the cellular level and decreases growth at the whole body level. Insulin-like growth factor-I (IGF-I) is a growth factor essential to the growth and function of almost every organ of the body and an increasing body of literature has defined the role of decreased IGF-I levels in the pathophysiology of catabolic disease.

Two important factors point to potential indirect relationships between alcohol and the IGFs in the pathogenesis of ALD and its complications: firstly, that the liver is the major site of production of the IGFs and their binding proteins (Figure 12.1) in addition to being the major target organ of ethanol induced toxicity. Secondly, liver production of IGF-I is tightly regulated by nutritional factors

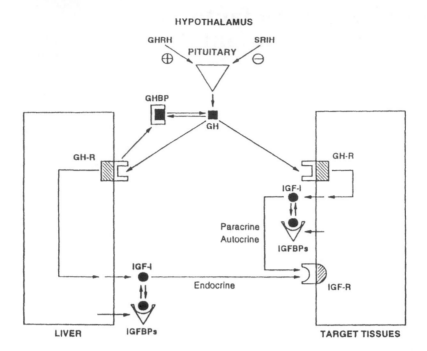

Figure 12.1 Overview of the GH:IGF axis. Reproduced with permission from Thissen, J.P. *et al.* (1994) Nutritional regulation of the IGFs. *Endocrine Reviews* **15**, 80–101.

(Figure 12.2) and it is well established that nutrition plays an essential role in the pathogenesis of alcoholic liver injury.

A direct link between alcohol exposure, the GH:IGF-I axis and liver damage has been more difficult to define. However, two recent interesting studies have important possible implications for direct relationships. Brenzel and Gressner (1996) showed, in a study of IGF-I receptor numbers in stellate cells, that hepatocyte generated IGF-I or IGFBPs which might mediate stellate cell activation during the initial transformation to myofibroblasts. Castilla *et al.* (1997b) showed that IGF-I had hepatoprotective effects by improving liver function and reducing oxidative liver damage and fibrosis in rats with compensated or advanced cirrhosis. This particular decrease in pro-oxidant liver injury and resulting fibrogenesis might be extremely important as this is a major pathogenic mechanism in ALD.

This chapter will review the reported relationships of the GH:IGF axis to alcohol exposure and to alcoholic liver disease. It will focus on four major areas of research:

1   the potential role of the IGFs in the pathogenesis of ALD;
2   the potential pathogenic role of IGF deficiency in the complications of ALD;
3   the role of growth hormone and IGF-I as therapy in ALD;
4   the efficacy of serum levels of the IGFs as prognostic markers in ALD.

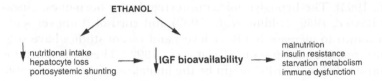

Figure 12.2 The relationships of ethanol to IGF bioavailability and to alcoholic liver disease and its complications. Ethanol decreases IGF bioavailability directly as exhibited by *in vitro* studies and also indirectly through its pathogenic role in the development of cirrhosis.

OVERVIEW OF THE GROWTH HORMONE (GH): INSULIN-LIKE GROWTH FACTOR (IGF) AXIS (FIGURE 12.1)

The somatomedin hypothesis of Salmon and Daughaday (1957) established that the majority of growth-producing effects of pituitary derived growth hormone (GH) were produced by the somatomedins, later termed as the insulin-like growth factors (IGFs). IGF-I is an anabolic peptide that is vital to cell proliferation and differentiation in virtually every organ (Jones and Clemmons, 1995). IGF-I plays a critical role in the regulation of whole body growth and in the maintenance of body composition in later life. The biologic role of IGF-II remains uncertain, although roles in fetal and tumor development have been defined. In addition to their functions as endocrine growth factors, the IGFs are thought to exert growth-promoting effects at the local tissue level through paracrine and autocrine mechanisms.

The IGFs are not secreted and stored in a specific organ but circulate bound to IGFBPs (insulin-like growth factor binding proteins), of which six have been characterized and cloned (IGFBP-1 to -6) (Baxter, 1993). The IGFBPs bind greater than 90% of circulating IGFs with less than 5% existing free in the circulation. The IGFBPs have a major influence on the bioactivity of the IGFs at the level of their tissue receptors by prolonging IGF half-life in the circulation, controlling release of IGFs from the vascular to the extracellular space and modulating the presentation of IGF to its receptor (Jones and Clemmons, 1995).

IGFBP-3 binds the majority of circulating IGFs (Martin and Baxter, 1992) and in association with IGF and an acid labile protein subunit (ALS) (Baxter, 1988) forms a stable ternary complex which prolongs IGF half-life, functions as a reservoir for IGFs and limits their extravascular transit (Bar *et al.*, 1990). IGFBP-3 has also been shown to both stimulate and inhibit IGF-I activity at the cell surface although exact mechanisms remain unclear (Conover, 1992). The stability of the ternary complex, which appears to have a half-life of 16–24 hours, is probably determined by the stability of ALS itself, since binary IGF-IGFBP-3 complexes leave the circulation rapidly. For this reason, IGF and IGFBP-3 levels do not show acute changes in response to metabolic disturbances.

IGFBP-1 is present at much lower concentration in serum, and may provide most of the freely available IGF binding sites. Levels fluctuate acutely in response to metabolic variables, with a half-life of about 30 minutes. Insulin is a principal regulator of hepatic IGFBP-1 production through inhibition of gene transcription

(Powell *et al.*, 1991), with an inverse relationship reported in most patient groups studied (Lee *et al.*, 1993). The hypoglycemic counterregulatory hormones, glucagon (Lewitt and Baxter, 1989; Hilding *et al.*, 1993) and cortisol (Conover *et al.*, 1993), have been shown to increase IGFBP-1 levels and recent studies have suggested a regulatory role for somatostatin (Ezzat *et al.*, 1992). These relationships suggest that a central role for IGFBP-1 might be the limitation of the considerable hypoglycemic and growth-promoting potential of free IGF-I during periods of low substrate availability.

IGFBP-2 appears to occupy an intermediate role in IGF regulation. In conditions where the capacity of the IGFBP-3 complex is insufficient to carry the available IGFs – for example, following IGF-I administration, in the presence of an IGF-II secreting tumor, or in conditions such as fasting where IGFBP-3 and IGF-I levels, but not IGF-II, are decreased – IGFBP-2 increases in the circulation and appears to act as an alternative carrier of IGFs (Jones and Clemmons, 1995).

EXPERIMENTAL STUDIES

Studies at the cell culture and whole body *in vitro* levels have demonstrated the deleterious effects of ethanol at multiple levels of the GH:IGF axis.

Animal studies

Hypothalamic and pituitary regulation

Soszynski and Frohman (1992) showed that ethanol inhibited GH secretion primarily at the hypothalamic level resulting in a 90% reduction in hypothalamic GHRH mRNA levels. While starvation has been shown to effect similar changes (Bruno *et al.*, 1990), the direct influence of ethanol was demonstrated in the finding that the suppression of GHRH and GH levels was significantly greater in the ethanol fed than control pair fed animals (Soszynski and Frohman, 1992) (Figure 12.3). However, a later study by the same authors showed that chronic ethanol exposure decreases pituitary GH mRNA levels, indicating possible additional influences of ethanol at the pituitary level. The study of Emanuele *et al.* (1992) supported this finding by demonstrating that acute or binge ethanol decreases serum GH levels and pituitary GH mRNA levels in a rat model.

Hepatic production of IGF-I

A number of animal studies have shown that both acute and chronic ethanol administration decrease circulating IGF-I levels. Sonntag and Boyd (1989) showed that chronic ethanol exposure decreased plasma IGF-I concentrations compared to either pair fed or ad libitum fed animals but this effect was not caused by a further reduction in overall GH secretory dynamics. In a later study, Xu *et al.* (1995) showed that ethanol inhibited GH-induced protein synthesis and IGF-I gene expression in rat liver slices but did so without changing GH receptor number or the affinity of GH for its receptor. These findings suggested that ethanol directly suppressed GH-induced signal transduction. Srivastava *et al.* (1995) showed that

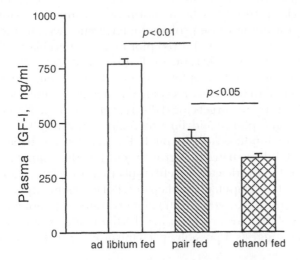

Figure 12.3 Plasma ethanol levels in ethanol (5%) liquid diet fed, pair fed, and *ad libitum* fed rats. Values are shown as the mean ± SEM ($n = 6$ for each group). Reproduced with permission from Soszynski, P.A. and Frohman, L.A. (1992) Inhibitory effects of ethanol on the growth hormone (GH)-releasing hormone-GH-insulin-like growth factor-I axis in the rat. *Endocrinology* **131**, 2603–2608.

chronic ethanol fed rats showed a significant decrease in serum IGF-I levels with a parallel decrease in the expression of hepatic IGF-I mRNA.

Insulin-like growth factor binding proteins

The IGFBPs influence IGF bioavailability by regulating the delivery and binding of the IGFs to tissue IGF receptors. Few animal studies have examined the impact of ethanol on IGFBP production and secretion. Flyvberg showed that acute oral ethanol administration increased liver IGFBP-I gene expression by 218% with a concomitant rise in circulating levels of IGFBP-I, identified by immunoprecipitation and Western ligand blotting (Flyvberg *et al.*, 1997). High levels of IGFBP-I are thought to limit short-term IGF bioavailability by binding circulating free IGF-I and these findings suggest a further mechanism whereby acute ethanol decreases IGF action.

Block *et al.* (1997) demonstrated that levels of a 39–42 kDa IGFBP, likely IGFBP-3, were decreased in a chronic ethanol model suggesting the possible impact of ethanol on longer-term IGF bioavailability through decreased levels of the ternary complex and therefore decreased IGF-I half-life.

Cell culture studies

The IGF-I receptor and IGF-I signal transduction

Many studies have demonstrated important effects of ethanol on the IGF-I receptor, through which IGF-I exerts its cellular mitogenic and proliferative properties.

Most cells in primary culture require the interaction of IGF-I with the IGF-I receptor to enter S phase of the cell cycle. Ethanol has been shown not to interfere with the binding of IGF-I to its receptor but to cause profound interference with ligand mediated tyrosine autophosphorylation of the IGF-I receptor in a 3T3 fibroblast cell line (Resnicoff *et al.*, 1993) and in C6 rat glioblastoma cells (Resnicoff *et al.*, 1994). Tyrosine autophosphorylation of the IGF-I receptor is essential for its mitogenic function and the targeting of ethanol to the IGF-I receptor was further emphasized by the findings of inhibition of downstream targets for IGF-I receptor tyrosine kinase such as insulin-related substrate-1 and phosphatidylinositol 3-kinase (Resnicoff *et al.*, 1994). In these studies, the ethanol-induced effects on IGF-I signal transduction effected profound decreases in IGF-I mediated cell growth and together imply an important interactive role for IGF-I in the deleterious effects of ethanol on important physiological processes such as fetal development and hepatocellular regeneration.

A recent study from the same group (Cui *et al.*, 1997) demonstrated that ethanol inhibited the antiapoptotic action of the IGF-I receptor in a TNF-α model of apoptosis. This exciting finding further suggests a possible mechanism relating IGF-I to ethanol-induced cytotoxicity.

However, the inhibitory effects of ethanol on IGF-I mediated cell growth have not been a universal finding. Tomono and Kiss (1995) reported that ethanol in concentrations that were pathophysiologically relevant (50–100 mM) significantly enhanced the stimulatory effects of both IGF-I and insulin on DNA synthesis in 3T3 fibroblasts. Smith *et al.* (1992) had earlier shown, in a whole body model, that ethanol fed rats were able to maintain normal levels of IGF-I compared to pair fed controls. This study stressed the important influence of fasting with decreased hepatic IGF-I mRNA levels seen in control fed animals who had a significant fasting period.

Effects on ethanol metabolism, tolerance and sensitivity

Mezey *et al.* (1990) demonstrated that IGF-I treatment of hepatocytes resulted in increased alcohol dehydrogenase activity, preceded by increased mRNA expression suggesting an interrelationship between the GH:IGF-I axis and alcohol metabolic pathways. Pucilowski *et al.* (1996) showed that chronically, increased exposure to IGF-I in IGF-I transgenic mice attenuated some of the central depressant effects of alcohol. Mice overexpressing IGFBP-1, and therefore likely to have lower free levels of IGF-I, showed the opposite effects, with the effect of IGF-I thought possibly to relate to IGF-I induced increases in intracellular calcium being neuroprotective.

Effects on the immune system

Multiple studies have demonstrated that acute and chronic ethanol exposure directly decrease IGF bioavailability, and while not proven, it is possible that low IGF-I levels may play a role in the increased susceptibility to infection which accounts for much of the morbidity and mortality seen in ALD. Auernhammer and Strasburger (1995) reviewed studies which demonstrate that GH and IGF-I stimulate the proliferation of immunocompetent cells and modulate humoral and cellular immune functions. Bjerknes and Aarskog (1995) showed that IGF-I can selectively stimulate mature neutrophil functions such as phagocytic capacity, complement receptor expression, degranulation and oxidative burst.

The relationship between nutrition and hepatic IGF-I gene expression and protein production has been stressed in many studies. Casafont *et al.* (1997) demonstrated that bacterial translocation across the intestine and the risk of spontaneous bacterial peritonitis was significantly higher in malnourished rats. Sugiura *et al.* (1997) noted that IGF-I improved nitrogen balance, promoted the proliferation of intestinal mucosa and reduced the translocation of endotoxin in burned rats receiving parenteral nutrition. These studies point to a possible critically important link between low IGF-I bioavailability, intestinal permeability and the pathophysiology of the gram negative infections which are so common in ALD.

THE FETAL ALCOHOL SYNDROME

Maternal abuse of alcohol during pregnancy may have severely deleterious effects on the fetus, the fulminant manifestation of which is called the fetal alcohol syndrome (FAS). The classical features of this syndrome include pre- and postnatal growth retardation, central nervous system dysfunction, facial abnormalities and cardiac valvular abnormalities. Many studies including gene knockouts have suggested that the IGFs are key regulators of fetal growth and development and a number of studies in the FAS have shed light on the relationships between alcohol, the GH:IGF axis and somatic growth.

FAS in humans

Halmesmaki *et al.* (1989) demonstrated higher levels of GH and lower levels of somatomedin C (IGF-I) in human infants with fetal alcohol effects compared to healthy infants of drinking and nondrinking mothers. Alcohol has been shown to decrease placental transport of nutrients to the fetus and these authors suggested that placental malnutrition as a cause of low IGF-I levels may have been an important mechanism in FAS.

Experimental studies of FAS

Animal studies have shed further light on the possible role of the IGFs in the pathogenesis of FAS. While studies have demonstrated that maternal serum and placental levels of IGF-I are reduced in alcohol consuming pregnant mothers (Breese and Sonntag, 1995; Fatayerji *et al.*, 1996) it is important to recognize that maternal IGFs and IGFBPs do not cross the placenta. Breese and Sonntag (1995) showed that ethanol exposure reduced plasma IGF-I levels by 40% in fetal offspring compared to either *ad libitum* or pair fed animals. This group also found that IGF-I mRNA levels in fetal liver of the same animals were not reduced suggesting that low serum IGF-I levels may result from diminished translation of hepatic IGF-I mRNA. In contrast, Singh *et al.* (1994) demonstrated low serum levels and low hepatic IGF-I mRNA levels of IGF-I in fetal offspring of ethanol fed rats. This study suggested a possible direct effect of ethanol on IGF-I gene transcription.

The bioavailability of the IGFs is significantly influenced by the levels of IGF binding proteins in serum and a number of studies have reported changes that might contribute to the somatic changes of the FAS. Breese *et al*. (1993) noted, by Western ligand blotting, that levels of the 30 kDa band, likely to correspond to IGFBPs 1 and 2, were not different in rats exposed to alcohol at up to 20 days after birth. In contrast, Singh *et al*. (1994) showed significant increases in this 30 kDa band in the alcohol-exposed offspring. Importantly, in this study, the high serum IGFBP levels induced by maternal ethanol ingestion showed a significant inverse correlation with fetal body weight. This possible regulatory function for IGFBP-1 is consistent with the study of Unterman *et al*. (1993), which reported high IGFBP-1 levels in the serum of offspring that were growth retarded because of bilateral uterine ligation. High IGFBP-1 levels, related to either undernutrition or low insulin levels, may bind free IGFs in serum and therefore limit growth.

The higher molecular weight circulating ternary complex becomes the dominant IGFBP species only after 40 days in rodents. Only one study reported to date has examined IGFBP levels this late into neonatal life: Breese *et al*. (1993) showed that a 40 kDa species, possibly an IGFBP-3 – IGF complex, was decreased in ethanol-exposed offspring. This is potentially an important finding suggesting a direct influence of alcohol on the dominant IGFBP of adult life.

In many studies, it has been difficult to disentangle the probable coeffects of maternal nutritional factors and the direct influence of alcohol, particularly on the growth retardation component of the FAS. Decreased maternal food intake has been shown to cause decreased fetal expression of IGF-I (Davenport *et al*., 1990). Two of the studies discussed above specifically addressed this problem by showing that levels of IGF-I (Breese *et al*., 1993; Singh *et al*., 1994), IGFBPs and IGF-I gene expression (Singh *et al*., 1994) were decreased in the offspring of ethanol fed animals compared to pair fed animals. These findings point to a direct interaction of alcohol with the GH:IGF axis that is independent of the effects of alcohol-induced maternal malnutrition (Krishna and Phillips, 1994).

While the liver is the major source of circulating levels of the IGFs and IGFBPs, IGF-I is expressed and produced by many tissues and thought to exert additional growth promoting actions by paracrine and autocrine mechanisms. Snyder showed that ethanol inhibited the stimulatory effects of IGF-I on DNA, RNA and protein synthesis in fetal rat astrocyte cultures (Snyder *et al*., 1992). Singh *et al*. (1996) demonstrated decreased IGF-I mRNA levels in fetal brain tissue of ethanol ingesting mothers. The further relationship of brain IGF-I level to brain weight strongly suggested a pathogenic role for low IGF levels in the brain growth retardation associated with FAS.

CLINICAL STUDIES I: PREVALENCE STUDIES OF THE GH:IGF AXIS IN HUMAN ALCOHOLIC LIVER DISEASE (ALD)

The impact of alcohol at multiple levels of the GH:IGF axis has been reported in many studies of ALD in humans. However, in many of these studies it has been difficult to clearly differentiate the relative contributions of the toxic effects of ongoing alcohol intake and altered dietary intake, related to alcoholism, metabolic and body composition changes related to malnutrition and the impact of the pathological lesion of cirrhosis on the regulation of the GH:IGF axis. Indeed, in many alcoholic patients a combination of some or all of these mechanisms may interact to effect profound changes at many levels of the GH:IGF axis. Further difficulties arise in examining the specific influences of these individual factors as only the toxic effect of alcohol can be regarded as a separate pathogenic influence that is unrelated to the pathological lesion of cirrhosis.

Alcohol toxicity

The impact of alcohol toxicity on the regulation of GH secretion has been largely studied in animal models with few studies reported in humans without cirrhosis and malnutrition. In acutely intoxicated males, Valimaki *et al.* (1990) demonstrated decreased GH secretion. However, studies of chronic ethanol intoxication have shown both decreased and normal GH secretion (Muller *et al.* 1989).

In a study of acute alcohol ingestion in nine healthy volunteers, Knip *et al.* (1995) demonstrated a dose dependent increase in serum levels of IGFBP-1 despite simultaneous hyperinsulinemia. Insulin is usually a potent inhibitor of IGFBP-1 gene transcription (Powell *et al.*, 1991), with these findings implying that ethanol has a direct stimulatory effect on hepatic IGFBP-1 synthesis. High levels of IGFBP-1 may bind increasing quantities of free or bioavailable IGF-I, thereby inhibiting tissue growth and anabolism.

In the discussion of the following aetiological factors, it must be stressed that ongoing alcohol intake may be exerting additional effects on the GH:IGF axis to those described that more directly relate to the pathological lesion of cirrhosis.

Hepatocyte loss

Hypothalamic and pituitary regulation

Abnormalities at the hypothalamic-pituitary level of the GH:IGF axis in ALD have been suggested by studies demonstrating abnormal GH responses to growth hormone releasing hormone (GHRH) (Salerno *et al.*, 1987) and thyrotrophin releasing hormone (TRH) (Zanobi *et al.*, 1983). Santolaria *et al.* (1995) demonstrated raised serum GH levels in 24 hospitalized alcoholic cirrhotics, but noted that GHRH levels were not significantly altered. Stewart *et al.* (1983) showed that GH levels were increased in alcoholic cirrhosis but not in alcoholic hepatitis, suggesting that the development of cirrhosis was central to the development of GH resistance in these patients. Cuneo *et al.* (1995) documented increased frequency of GH secretory bursts, increased total daily GH secretion rates and markedly impaired endogenous GH clearance in adult cirrhotic patients.

Earlier studies had demonstrated low serum GHBP levels in cirrhosis with decrements correlating with the degree of hepatocellular dysfunction (Baruch, 1991, #5989; Hattori *et al.*, 1992). In contrast, Cuneo *et al.* (1995) demonstrated only a slight decrease in serum GHBP levels in their cirrhotic cohort. An explanation for this apparent discrepancy might be found in our recent study showing that serum levels of GHBP were only significantly decreased in the most severe disease (Child's group C) (Donaghy, manuscript in preparation). The high affinity circulating GHBP is thought to be derived from the extramembranous domain of the GH receptor in humans (Barnard *et al.*, 1989) and it has been speculated that decreased GHBP levels might indicate influences of liver disease directly on the GH receptor. An early study by Chang *et al.* (1990) demonstrated decreased GH binding to cirrhotic liver by radioreceptor assay and a recent study by Holt *et al.* (1997) in children with cirrhosis complicating biliary atresia showed decreased GH receptor gene expression by the semiquantitative RT-PCR technique. These findings suggest a direct effect of the cirrhotic lesion on hepatic GH receptor gene expression.

Hepatic production of IGF-I and IGFBPs

The liver is thought to be the major source of circulating levels of IGF-I, and many historical studies have documented low levels of both alcoholic and nonalcoholic aetiology in patients with liver disease (Russell, 1985). The lack of negative feedback of low IGF-I levels is thought to contribute to the high GH levels in this state of acquired GH resistance (Jenkins and Ross, 1996). The critical importance of the functional hepatocyte mass to the hepatic production of IGF-I has been most dramatically demonstrated in studies showing that low serum levels of IGF-I and IGFBP-3 return to control levels after successful orthotopic liver transplantation (Holt *et al.*, 1996).

Moller *et al.* (1993) showed markedly reduced serum IGF-I levels, in alcoholic cirrhotics with IGF-I levels, reflecting the degree of hepatic insufficiency. Our group has demonstrated low serum levels of IGF-I and its dominant binding protein IGFBP-3 (Donaghy *et al.*, 1995) in a cirrhotic group which included patients with ALD (Figure 12.4). Recently we have also shown decreased levels of the acid labile subunit (ALS) which is the third protein of the circulating ternary complex

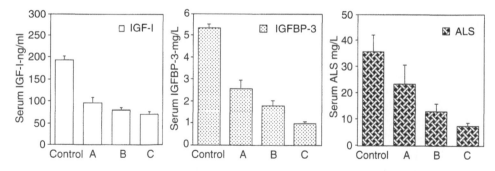

Figure 12.4 Serum levels (mean ± SEM) of the three components of the circulating ternary complex (A) IGF-I, (B) IGFBP-3 and (C) the ALS in controls and in a group of cirrhotic patients of widespread aetiology including alcohol. Patients with cirrhosis are graded in the three Child's Pugh prognostic groups. Levels of all components of the ternary complex are reduced significantly likely decreasing IGF bioavailability.

(Donaghy, manuscript in preparation) (Figure 12.4). We also noted strong correlations of IGFBP-3 and ALS levels with disease severity as measured by the Child's Pugh score indicating the possible further impact of cirrhosis on the bioavailability of low IGF-I levels. In a later study, Scharf *et al.* (1996) confirmed low IGF-I and IGFBP-3 levels in adult cirrhotics but importantly also showed that proteolysis of IGFBP-3 was not seen in this group. This finding supports decreased IGFBP-3 production from cirrhotic liver rather than increased clearance from the circulation. This group also demonstrated that levels of the 140 kD circulating complex were decreased possibly due to the lower circulating levels of ALS.

Hepatic IGF-I gene expression

Gene expression studies in human cirrhotic liver have yielded somewhat conflicting results. Ross *et al.* (1996) found that IGF-I mRNA levels were highly variable in adult cirrhotic liver, but not significantly different from that of normal liver. In contrast, in a more recent study of paediatric cirrhotic patients, Holt *et al.* (1997) showed markedly reduced IGF-I gene expression. Further studies are required to determine the impact of cirrhosis on the regulation of IGF-I gene expression in this patient group.

Portosystemic shunting

The finding of low levels of serum IGF-I in hepatic schistosomiasis (portal hypertension but normal hepatocyte function) (Assaad *et al.*, 1990) suggested that portosystemic shunting might be a significant pathogenic factor. In an elegant study, Moller *et al.* (1995) found strong correlations between the wedged hepatic venous pressure and high GH, low IGF-I and low IGFBP-3 levels in a group of alcoholic cirrhotics. These findings suggested that the shunting of nutrient-rich blood from the portal vasculature away from the hepatic sinusoids had at least an additional effect to the hepatocyte loss of cirrhosis. A possible explanation for these findings may come from the early work of Baxter and Turtle (1978) demonstrating, in a rat model, that significant concentrations of insulin are required for optimal binding of GH to hepatocyte GH receptors.

Nutritional intake

The pattern of dietary intake in alcoholic patients is often substantially altered. With increasing alcohol intake, the percentage of energy derived from protein, fat and carbohydrate decreases and the nutritional quality of the diet declines. Mendenhall *et al.* (1984) observed a direct correlation between the prevalence of malnutrition and daily total energy intakes in patients with ALD.

The recent study of Sarin *et al.* (1997) showed that intakes of protein and carbohydrate, estimated by dietary recall, were significantly lower in patients with ALD than controls, although they were not significantly lower than the intakes of non-alcoholic cirrhotics or alcoholics without liver disease. This study also demonstrated that patients with severe alcoholic hepatitis had the lowest intakes of protein, carbohydrate and fat.

Jackson Smith *et al.* (1995) showed that short-term caloric or protein restriction in normal humans resulted in decreased levels of IGF-I and IGFBP-3 in association with a deterioration in nitrogen balance. We have recently studied, weighed dietary substrate intakes in hospitalized cirrhotic patients of varying aetiologies including alcohol, and demonstrated decremental protein and total energy intakes with increasing disease severity (Donaghy, unpublished observations). In this group, low fasting serum IGF-I levels correlated with intakes of fat, protein and total energy and predicted nitrogen balances on following days. This data suggests that IGF-I bioavailability may be an important intermediary link between substrate intake and protein economy in cirrhotic patients.

CLINICAL STUDIES II: IGFS AND THE COMPLICATIONS OF CIRRHOSIS

A number of studies have suggested that low levels of IGF-I, particularly in association with changes in the profiles of the IGFBPs which further reduce IGF-I bioavailability, may play an important role in the pathogenesis of the complications of cirrhosis.

Abnormal metabolism

The impaired capacity of the cirrhotic liver to store glycogen contributes to a metabolic state in cirrhosis resembling starvation with early recruitment of alternative fuel stores during periods of fasting. Indeed the glycogen stores of the cirrhotic liver may be depleted in less than 6 hours of fasting compared to 36–48 hours in normal livers, necessitating breakdown of tissue, fat and protein stores to provide fuel substrates for gluconeogenesis (Owen *et al.*, 1983). Resistance to the actions of the anabolic growth factors GH and insulin is central to the pathogenesis of this altered metabolism in starvation.

Recent studies (Frystyk *et al.*, 1997a) have shown that the short-term regulation of free IGF-I levels, and probably IGF bioavailability, in response to metabolic variables may be effected by changes in the serum levels of IGFBP-1. We have demonstrated high fasting levels of IGFBP-1 in cirrhotic patients in the setting of high fasting insulin levels with loss of the usual inverse relationship (Donaghy *et al.*, 1995). However, the provision of a glucose load (standard glucose tolerance test) with subsequent increases in insulin levels effected a fall in serum IGFBP-1 levels in all patients (Figure 12.5), suggesting that substrate availability might be a more potent regulator of IGFBP-1 than insulin during periods of fasting. Scharf *et al.* (1996) also described high fasting IGFBP-1 levels in association with low levels of free IGF-I, but interestingly did not find any relationship with free IGF-I levels, as has been reported in normals (Frystyk *et al.*, 1997b).

Insulin resistance

The insulin resistance of alcoholic cirrhosis is of multifactorial pathogenesis and remains incompletely understood. While the current major deficit is thought to be

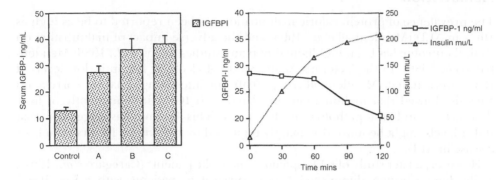

Figure 12.5 (A) Fasted serum levels of IGFBP-1 in the same group of cirrhotic patients described in Figure 12.4. Serum IGFBP-1 levels are higher in the cirrhotic patients than the normal controls and may reflect the state of low substrate availability consequent upon the impaired glycogen storage capacity of the cirrhotic liver. (B) During a standard oral glucose tolerance test serum IGFBP-1 levels fell in all patients of a group of Child's C cirrhotics in association with rising insulin levels.

of nonoxidative glucose disposal, i.e., impaired glycogen synthesis in skeletal muscle, there are many other suggested contributing factors including high circulating levels of the counterregulatory hormones glucagon, cortisol and GH (Petrides *et al.*, 1992). Recent studies have suggested a pathogenic role for the GH:IGF axis both directly and indirectly through relationships of malnutrition to insulin resistance.

Shankar *et al.* (1988) showed that suppression of GH with somatostatin in euglycemic clamp studies resulted in significantly improved insulin sensitivity. This study of alcoholic cirrhotic patients suggested a direct pathogenic role of high GH levels in the insulin resistance of these patients. In a later study, however, Shmueli *et al.* (1994) could not show any significant effect of GH suppression on whole body glucose uptake, forearm glucose uptake or insulin sensitivity. The differences in these study findings may have been at least partially explained by the ongoing alcohol intake of the patients in the earlier study.

Shmueli's group also showed that high serum IGFBP-1 levels seen in their alcoholic cirrhotic group showed a strong inverse correlation with insulin sensitivity (Shmueli *et al.*, 1996). Serum levels of IGFBP-1 fluctuate in response to metabolic variables, predominantly insulin and substrate availability (Lee *et al.*, 1993; Donaghy *et al.*, 1995), with high IGFBP-1 levels believed to decrease IGF-I bioavailability. This finding further strongly suggests the potential significance of low IGF-I bioavailability in the insulin resistance of cirrhosis.

Wahl *et al.* (1992) showed strong correlations of serum markers of protein energy malnutrition (PEM) to insulin sensitivity as measured by euglycemic insulin clamping. The finding that nutritional support improved insulin sensitivity in these alcoholic cirrhotic patients gives further evidence of a relationship of PEM to insulin resistance in this patient group. The close relationship of low IGF-I bioavailability to PEM suggests a possible additional indirect role for low IGF-I in the insulin resistance of cirrhosis.

Malnutrition

The prevalence of protein calorie malnutrition has been reported to be as high as 100% in ALD (Mendenhall *et al.*, 1995) and the adverse impact of malnutrition on clinical outcome has been highlighted in many studies (Shaw *et al.*, 1985; Mendenhall *et al.*, 1986). In the Veterans Affairs Study of alcoholic hepatitis, low levels of IGF-I were noted (Mendenhall *et al.*, 1989) but interestingly partial correlation analysis showed that malnutrition correlated with IGF-I independently of liver dysfunction and histopathological alterations. This finding has suggested that IGF-I levels might be more dominantly regulated by nutritional factors than liver disease in ALD.

However, a later study of 64 hospitalized alcoholic patients (Caregaro *et al.*, 1997), while demonstrating diminished 2 year survival in patients with a low IGF-I z score, did not note any significant correlation of IGF-I with anthropometric indices. These findings might be explained by the increased disease severity seen in hospitalized alcoholics but probably highlight the multipathogenesis of the low IGF-I levels seen in advanced cirrhosis.

CLINICAL STUDIES III: IGFS AS PROGNOSTIC MARKERS IN ALD

An early indication of the possible prognostic relevance of serum levels of IGF-I came from the study of hospitalized alcoholic cirrhotics by Caufriez *et al.* (1991). The authors demonstrated that serum IGF-I levels correlated most strongly with amino-pyrine breath test values ($r = 0.68$; $p < 0.001$) followed by the Childs Pugh score ($r = -0.57$; $p < 0.01$), with weaker correlations observed with serum levels of hepatic export proteins such as albumin. These findings strongly suggest that in alcoholic cirrhosis IGF-I may be a sensitive marker of functional hepatocellular capacity.

The first longitudinal data relating survival to serum IGF-I levels came from a study of 36 hospitalized alcoholic cirrhotics reported by Moller *et al.* (1993). The authors noted that 2 year survival as plotted by Kaplan Meier curves was significantly lower in patients with a serum IGF level below 3.1 nmol/L. The same group (Moller *et al.*, 1996) studied a much larger group of 352 alcoholic cirrhotics and noted that serum levels of both IGF-I and its major binding protein IGFBP-3 had significant prognostic survival value. Using a time dependent Cox regression model the authors showed that these markers provided prognostic information that was independent of other prognostic factors such as alcohol intake, coagulation factors, creatinine or serum IgM levels. However, a surprising finding was that with the concurrence of alcoholic hepatitis and cirrhosis, usually portending a worse prognosis, a trend but no statistical significance was noted for both IGF-I and IGFBP-3 as prognostic markers.

In a study of 64 hospitalized alcoholic patients, Caregaro *et al.* (1997) showed significantly diminished 2 year survival in patients with a low IGF-I z score. They did not note any significant correlation of IGF-I with anthropometric indices of nutritional status which contrasted to the findings of Mendenhall *et al.* which has been discussed previously. The authors concluded that low levels of IGF-I in alcoholic cirrhosis may be effected by a number of factors acting synergistically: liver function impairment; portal hypertension; hyperestrogenism; abnormalities of glucose and insulin metabolism; and malnutrition.

The identification of factors accurately predicting survival in ALD has proven extremely difficult. Liver transplantation now has an established role as definitive therapy for endstage liver disease and the identification of its optimal timing is of paramount importance. Further studies of serial measurements of IGF-I and its major binding protein IGFBP-3 in patients with advanced cirrhosis are required to assess their efficacy as predictors of clinical outcome. Serum levels of these proteins are influenced by hepatocyte dysfunction, insulin resistance and nutritional factors: factors that have been shown to adversely influence survival. It is extremely tempting to speculate that IGF-I and IGFBP-3 may find a role in the indication of critical liver dysfunction and malnutrition in these patients.

CLINICAL STUDIES IV: GH AND IGF-I AS THERAPY IN ALD

Human studies

In severe catabolic illness, including cirrhosis, a number of studies have demonstrated that aggressive nutritional support alone does not prevent significant loss of lean body mass (Streat et al., 1987), and much recent research has examined the role of exogenous growth factor therapy in this setting. Recombinant human GH therapy has been shown to improve protein anabolism and to impact on short-term morbidity after abdominal surgery (Ward et al., 1987), major trauma and severe sepsis (Douglas et al., 1990) and severe burns (Herndon et al., 1990). In growth retarded children with chronic renal failure, GH effected striking improvement in height velocity (Hokken et al., 1991). This study importantly demonstrated that GH-induced improvements in short-term nitrogen economy can effect significant changes in body composition with longer term therapy.

In the first reported study of GH therapy in human liver disease Moller et al. (1994) showed significant increases in serum levels of IGF-I in a group of male alcoholic cirrhotics treated with rh GH for six weeks. Serum IGFBP-3 levels increased in both treatment and placebo groups, whereas no changes in serum IGFBP-1 levels were seen. No change in biochemical liver function tests was noted and no significant side effects were seen.

We studied the impact of high dose GH therapy on both the IGF:IGFBP axis and on nitrogen balance in a group of cirrhotic patients of varying aetiologies including alcohol (Donaghy et al., 1997). In the GH treated group, a significant rise in IGF-I levels was seen but this was markedly attenuated in comparison to that seen in a group of normal subjects we had previously treated, probably reflecting the severity of the GH resistance of cirrhosis (Figure 12.6). In contrast to the Moller study serum IGFBP-3 levels improved significantly only in those patients treated with GH. Importantly we also demonstrated that improvement in serum IGF-I levels was associated with a significant improvement in cumulative nitrogen balance, likely to be due to improved nitrogen retention.

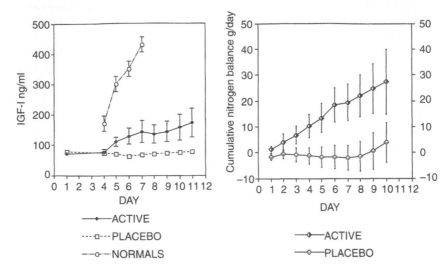

Figure 12.6 (A) A significant rise in serum IGF-I levels was observed in cirrhotic patients treated with recombinant human GH. (B) The rise in serum IGF-I levels accompanied a significant improvement in cumulative nitrogen balance only in the GH treated patients. GH induced a significant improvement in nitrogen retention in this group of cirrhotic patients of multiple aetiologies including alcohol.

A later study by Wallace *et al.* (1997) confirmed the GH-induced increases in IGF-I and IGFBP-3 shown in previous studies but also demonstrated that GH effected improvement in lean body mass as measured by total body potassium counting. This study of predominantly alcoholic cirrhotics also showed that hepatocyte function as measured by the MEGX test was not altered by GH therapy.

Experimental studies

Studies of IGF-I therapy in human cirrhosis have not been reported, perhaps because of the risks of IGF-I induced hypoglycemia in patients predisposed to this problem because of impaired glycogen storage. Picardi *et al.* (1997) demonstrated that low doses of IGF-I improved nitrogen retention and food efficiency in rats with early stage cirrhosis. In this study, possible mechanisms of IGF-I action included enhancement of appetite and improvements in substrate utilization for energy generation and muscle protein metabolism.

Two recent studies have suggested that IGF-I therapy might affect nonnutritional complications of cirrhosis. In addition to showing that both GH and IGF-I partially reversed the weight loss seen in severely dietary restricted rats, Mendenhall *et al.* (1997) demonstrated that IGF-I but not GH produced significant improvements in immune parameters such as thymus and splenic T lymphocyte counts. A provocative study by Castilla *et al.* (1997a) reported that low doses of IGF-I were able to revert the testicular atrophy seen in rats with advanced cirrhosis.

While the number of reported studies remains small, the demonstration that GH-induced improvements in nitrogen balance in the short-term can lead to improved nutritional status with prolonged therapy holds significant promise. Further studies of longer duration are required to assess the impact on clinical outcome in severely malnourished cirrhotics, many of whom succumb while awaiting liver transplantation.

FUTURE RESEARCH AND THERAPEUTIC INITIATIVES

While much is now understood of the toxic effects of ethanol on the GH:IGF axis and of relationships to pathogenic cofactors such as nutritional factors and cirrhosis, the recent studies linking the IGFs to pathogenesis are extremely provocative. The role of the IGFs in stellate cell activation will be increasingly explored and the finding that IGF-I may be hepatoprotective and reverse oxidative liver damage may have great significance as the search continues for effective therapies in ALD. Longitudinal studies are urgently required to assess the prognostic value of serum measurements of components of the GH:IGF axis as these protein markers may accurately reflect both the liver dysfunction and the malnutrition which so adversely influence clinical outcome in this patient group.

REFERENCES

Assaad, S.N., Cunningham, G.R. and Samaan, N.A. (1990) Abnormal growth hormone dynamics in chronic liver disease do not depend on severe parenchymal disease. *Metabolism* **39**, 349–356.

Auernhammer, C.J. and Strasburger, C.J. (1995) Effects of growth hormone and insulin-like growth factor I on the immune system. *Eur J Endocrinol* **133**, 635–645.

Bar, R.S., Boes, M., Clemmons, D.R., Busby, W.H., Sandra, A., Dake, B.L. and Booth, B.A. (1990) Insulin differentially alters transcapillary movement of intravascular IGFBP-1, IGFBP-2 and endothelial cell IGF-binding proteins in the rat heart. *Endocrinology* **127**, 497–499.

Barnard, R., Quirk, P. and Waters, M.J. (1989) Characterization of the growth hormone-binding protein of human serum using a panel of monoclonal antibodies. *J Endocrinol* **123**, 327–332.

Baxter, R. (1993) Circulating binding proteins for the insulin-like growth factors. *Trends in Endocrinology and Metabolism* **4**, 91–96.

Baxter, R. and Turtle, J. (1978) Regulation of hepatic growth hormone receptors by insulin. *Biochemical and Biophysical Research Communications* **84**, 350–357.

Baxter, R.C. (1988) Characterization of the acid-labile subunit of the growth hormone-dependent insulin-like growth factor binding protein complex. *J Clin Endocrinol Metab* **67**, 265–272.

Bjerknes, R. and Aarskog, D. (1995) Priming of human polymorphonuclear neutrophilic leukocytes by insulin-like growth factor I: increased phagocytic capacity, complement receptor expression, degranulation, and oxidative burst. *J Clin Endocrinol Metab* **80**, 1948–1955.

Block, G., Styche, A., Barsic, N. and Eagon, P. (1997) Effects of ethanol on Insulin-like growth factor binding proteins in rats. *Gastroenterology* **104**, A878.

Breese, C.R., D'Costa, A., Ingram, R.L., Lenham, J. and Sonntag, W.E. (1993) Long-term suppression of insulin-like growth factor-1 in rats after *in utero* ethanol exposure: relationship to somatic growth. *J Pharmacol Exp Ther* **264**, 448–456.

Breese, C.R. and Sonntag, W.E. (1995) Effect of ethanol on plasma and hepatic insulin-like growth factor regulation in pregnant rats. *Alcohol Clin Exp Res* **19**, 867–873.

Brenzel, A. and Gressner, A.M. (1996) Characterization of insulin-like growth factor (IGF)-I-receptor binding sites during *in vitro* transformation of rat hepatic stellate cells to myofibroblasts. *Eur J Clin Chem Clin Biochem* **34**, 401–409.

Bruno, J.F., Olchovsky, D., White, J.D., Leidy, J.W., Song, J. and Berelowitz, M. (1990) Influence of food deprivation in the rat on hypothalamic expression of growth hormone-releasing factor and somatostatin. *Endocrinology* **127**, 2111–2116.

Caregaro, L., Alberino, F., Amodio, P., Merkel, C., Angeli, P., Plebani, M., Bolognesi, M. and Gatta, A. (1997) Nutritional and prognostic significance of insulin-like growth factor 1 in patients with liver cirrhosis. *Nutrition* **13**, 185–190.

Casafont, F., Sanchez, E., Martin, L., Aguero, J. and Romero, F.P. (1997) Influence of malnutrition on the prevalence of bacterial translocation and spontaneous bacterial peritonitis in experimental cirrhosis in rats. *Hepatology* **25**, 1334–1337.

Castilla, C.I., Garcia, M., Calvo, A., Diez, N., Pascual, M., Perez, R., Quiroga, J., Prieto, J. and Santidrian, S. (1997a) In *European Association for the Study of the Liver London*, England.

Castilla, C.I., Garcia, M., Muguerza, B., Quiroga, J., Perez, R., Santidrian, S. and Prieto, J. (1997b) Hepatoprotective effects of insulin-like growth factor I in rats with carbon tetrachloride-induced cirrhosis. *Gastroenterology* **113**, 1682–1691.

Caufriez, A., Reding, P., Urbain, D., Golstein, J. and Copinschi, G. (1991) Insulin-like growth factor I: a good indicator of functional hepatocellular capacity in alcoholic liver cirrhosis. *J Endocrinol Invest* **14**, 317–321.

Chang, T.C., Lin, J.J., Yu, S.C. and Chang, T.J. (1990) Absence of growth-hormone receptor in hepatocellular carcinoma and cirrhotic liver. *Hepatology* **11**, 123–126.

Conover, C.A. (1992) Potentiation of insulin-like growth factor (IGF) action by IGF-binding protein-3: studies of underlying mechanism. *Endocrinology* **130**, 3191–3199.

Conover, C.A., Divertie, G.D. and Lee, P.D. (1993) Cortisol increases plasma insulin-like growth factor binding protein-1 in humans. *Acta Endocrinol Copenh* **128**, 140–143.

Cui, S.J., Tewari, M., Schneider, T. and Rubin, R. (1997) Ethanol promotes cell death by inhibition of the insulin-like growth factor I receptor. *Alcohol Clin Exp Res* **21**, 1121–1127.

Cuneo, R.C., Hickman, P.E., Wallace, J.D., Teh, B.T., Ward, G., Veldhuis, J.D. and Waters, M.J. (1995) Altered endogenous growth hormone secretory kinetics and diurnal GH-binding protein profiles in adults with chronic liver disease. *Clin Endocrinol Oxf* **43**, 265–275.

Davenport, M.L., Clemmons, D.R., Miles, M.V., Camacho, H.C., D'Ercole, A.J. and Underwood, L.E. (1990) Regulation of serum insulin-like growth factor-I (IGF-I) and IGF binding proteins during rat pregnancy. *Endocrinology* **127**, 1278–1286.

Donaghy, A., Ross, R., Gimson, A., Hughes, S.C., Holly, J. and Williams, R. (1995) Growth hormone, insulin like growth factor-1, and insulin like growth factor binding proteins 1 and 3 in chronic liver disease. *Hepatology* **21**, 680–688.

Donaghy, A., Ross, R., Wicks, C., Hughes, S.C., Holly, J., Gimson, A. and Williams, R. (1997) Growth hormone therapy in patients with cirrhosis: a pilot study of efficacy and safety. *Gastroenterology* **113**, 1617–1622.

Douglas, R., Humberstone, D., Haystead, A. and Shaw, J. (1990) Metabolic effects of recombinant human growth hormone: studies in the postabsorptive state and during total parenteral nutrition. *Br J Surg* **77**, 787–790.

Emanuele, M.A., Tentler, J.J., Kirsteins, L., Emanuele, N.V., Lawrence, A. and Kelley, M.R. (1992) The effect of "binge" ethanol exposure on growth hormone and prolactin gene expression and secretion. *Endocrinology* **131**, 2077–2082.

Ezzat, S., Ren, S.G., Braunstein, G.D. and Melmed, S. (1992) Octreotide stimulates insulin-like growth factor-binding protein-1: a potential pituitary-independent mechanism for drug action. *J Clin Endocrinol Metab* **75**, 1459–1463.

Fatayerji, N., Engelmann, G.L., Myers, T. and Handa, R.J. (1996) *In utero* exposure to ethanol alters mRNA for insulin-like growth factors and insulin-like growth factor-binding proteins in placenta and lung of fetal rats. *Alcohol Clin Exp Res* **20**, 94–100.

Flyvberg, A., van Neck, J., van Kleffens, M., Groffen, C. and Drop, S. (1997) In *Fourth International Symposium on the IGFs*, p. 108, Tokyo.

Frystyk, J., Grofte, T., Skjaerbaek, C. and Orskov, H. (1997a) The effect of oral glucose on serum free insulin-like growth factor-I and -II in health adults. *J Clin Endocrinol Metab* **82**, 3124–3127.

Frystyk, J., Hussain, M., Skjaerbaek, C., Schmitz, O., Christiansen, J.S., Froesch, E.R. and Orskov, H. (1997b) Serum free IGF-I during a hyperinsulinemic clamp following 3 days of administration of IGF-I vs. saline. *Am J Physiol*.

Halmesmaki, E., Valimaki, M., Karonen, S.L. and Ylikorkala, O. (1989) Low somatomedin C and high growth hormone levels in newborns damaged by maternal alcohol abuse. *Obstet Gynecol*.

Hattori, N., Kurahachi, H., Ikekubo, K., Ishihara, T., Moridera, K., Hino, M., Saiki, Y. and Imura, H. (1992) Serum growth hormone-binding protein, insulin-like growth factor-I, and growth hormone in patients with liver cirrhosis. *Metabolism* **41**, 377–381.

Herndon, D.N., Barrow, R.E., Kunkel, K.R., Broemling, L. and Rutan, R.L. (1990) Effects of recombinant human growth hormone on donor site healing in severely burned children. *Ann Surg* **212**, 424–431.

Hilding, A., Brismar, K., Thoren, T. and Hall, K. (1993) Glucagon stimulates insulin-like growth factor binding protein-1 secretion in healthy subjects, patients with pituitary insufficiency, and patients with insulin-dependent diabetes mellitus. *J Clin Endocrinol Metab* **77**, 1142–1147.

Hokken, K.A., Stijnen, T., de, M.K.S.S., Wit, J.M., Wolff, E.D., de, J.M., Donckerwolcke, R.A., Abbad, N.C., Bot, A., Blum, W.F. *et al.* (1991) Placebo-controlled, double-blind, cross-over trial of growth hormone treatment in prepubertal children with chronic renal failure. *Lancet* **338**, 585–590.

Holt, R.I., Crossey, P., Jones, J.S., Baker, A.J., Portmann, B. and Miell, J.P. (1997) Hepatic growth hormone receptor, insulin-like growth factor I and insulin-like growth factor binding protein messenger RNA expression in paediatric liver disease. *Hepatology* **26**, 1600–1606.

Holt, R.I., Jones, J.S., Stone, N.M., Baker, A.J. and Miell, J.P. (1996) Sequential changes in insulin-like growth factor I (IGF-I) and IGF-binding proteins in children with end-stage liver disease before and after successful orthotopic liver transplantation. *J Clin Endocrinol Metab* **81**, 160–168.

Jackson Smith, W., Underwood, L. and Clemmons, D. (1995) Effects of caloric or protein restriction on insulin-like growth factor-I (IGF-I) and IGF-binding proteins in children and adults. *J Clin Endocrinol Metab* **53**, 1247–1250.

Jenkins, R. and Ross, R. (Eds) (1996) Acquired growth hormone resistance in catabolic states. In *Bailliere's Clinical Endocrinology and Metabolism*. London: Bailliere Tindall.

Jones, I. and Clemmons, D. (1995) Insulin-like growth factors and their binding proteins: biological actions. *Endocrine Reviews* **16**, 3–34.

Knip, M., Ekman, A.C., Ekman, M., Leppaluoto, J. and Vakkuri, O. (1995) Ethanol induces a paradoxical simultaneous increase in circulating concentrations of insulin-like growth factor binding protein-1 and insulin. *Metabolism* **44**, 1356–1359.

Krishna, A. and Phillips, L.S. (1994) Fetal alcohol syndrome and insulin-like growth factors [editorial; comment]. *J Lab Clin Med* **124**, 149–151.

Lee, P.D., Conover, C.A. and Powell, D.R. (1993) Regulation and function of insulin-like growth factor-binding protein-1. *Proc Soc Exp Biol Med* **204**, 4–29.

Lewitt, M.S. and Baxter, R.C. (1989) Regulation of growth hormone-independent insulin-like growth factor-binding protein (BP-28) in cultured human fetal liver explants. *J Clin Endocrinol Metab* **69**, 246–252.

Martin, J.L. and Baxter, R.C. (1992) Insulin-like growth factor binding protein-3: biochemistry and physiology. *Growth Regul* **2**, 88–99.

Mendenhall, C.L., Anderson, S., Weesner, R.E., Goldberg, S.J. and Crolic, K.A. (1984) Protein calorie malnutrition associated with alcoholic hepatitis. *Am J Med* **76**, 211–222.

Mendenhall, C.L., Chernhausek, S.D., Ray, M.B., Gartside, P.S., Roselle, G.A., Grossman, C.J., Chedid, A. and Group, a. t. V.A.C.S. (1989) The interactions of Insulin-like Growth Factor-1 (IGF-1) with protein-calorie malnutrition in patients with alcoholic liver disease: V.A. Cooperative study on Alcoholic Hepatitis V1. *Alcohol and Alcoholism* **24**, 319–329.

Mendenhall, C.L., Moritz, T.E., Roselle, G.A., Morgan, T.R., Nemchausky, B.A., Tamburro, C.H., Schiff, E.R., McClain, C.J., Marsano, L.S., Allen, J.I. *et al.* (1995) Protein energy malnutrition in severe alcoholic hepatitis: diagnosis and response to treatment. The VA Cooperative Study Group #275. *Jpen J Parenter Enteral Nutr* **19**, 258–265.

Mendenhall, C.L., Roselle, G.A., Gartside, P. and Grossman, C.J. (1997) Effects of recombinant human insulin-like growth factor-1 and recombinant human growth hormone on anabolism and immunity in calorie-restricted alcoholic rats. *Alcohol Clin Exp Res* **21**, 1–10.

Mendenhall, C.L., Tosch, T. and Weesner, M.D. (1986) VA cooperative study on alcoholic hepatitis 11: prognostic significance of protein calorie malnutrition. *American Journal of Clinical Nutrition* **43**, 213–218.

Mezey, E., Potter, J.J., Mishra, L., Sharma, S. and Janicot, M. (1990) Effect of insulin-like growth factor I on rat alcohol dehydrogenase in primary hepatocyte culture. *Arch Biochem Biophys* **280**, 390–396.

Moller, S., Becker, U., Gronbaek, M., Juul, A., Winkler, K. and Skakkebaek, N.E. (1994) Short-term effect of recombinant human growth hormone in patients with alcoholic cirrhosis. *J Hepatol* **21**, 710–717.

Moller, S., Becker, U., Juul, A., Skakkebaek, N.E. and Christensen, E. (1996) Prognostic value of insulin like growth factor I and its binding protein in patients with alcohol-induced liver disease. EMALD group. *Hepatology* **23**, 1073–1078.

Moller, S., Gronbaek, M., Main, K., Becker, U. and Skakkebaek, N.E. (1993) Urinary growth hormone (U-GH) excretion and serum insulin-like growth factor 1 (IGF-1) in patients with alcoholic cirrhosis. *J Hepatol* **17**, 315–320.

Moller, S., Juul, A., Becker, U., Flyvbjerg, A., Skakkebaek, N.E. and Henriksen, J.H. (1995) Concentrations, release, and disposal of insulin-like growth factor (IGF)-binding proteins (IGFBP), IGF-I, and growth hormone in different vascular beds in patients with cirrhosis. *J Clin Endocrinol Metab* **80**, 1148–1157.

Muller, N., Hoeche, M., Klein, H., Nieberle, G., Kapfhammer, H., May, F., Muller, O. and Fichter, M. (1989) Endocrinological studies in alcoholics during withdrawal and after abstinence. *Psychoneuroendocrinology* **14**, 13–123.

Owen, O.E., Trapp, V.E., Reichard, G.J., Mozzoli, M.A., Moctezuma, J., Paul, P., Skutches, C.L. and Boden, G. (1983) Nature and quantity of fuels consumed in patients with alcoholic cirrhosis. *J Clin Invest* **72**, 1821–1832.

Petrides, A.S., Strohmeyer, G. and DeFronzo, R.A. (1992) Insulin resistance in liver disease and portal hypertension. *Prog Liver Dis* **10**, 311–328.

Picardi, A., de, O.A., Muguerza, B., Tosar, A., Quiroga, J., Castilla, C.I., Santidrian, S. and Prieto, J. (1997) Low doses of insulin-like growth factor-I improve nitrogen retention and food efficiency in rats with early cirrhosis. *J Hepatol* **26**, 191–202.

Powell, D.R., Suwanichkul, A., Cubbage, M.L., DePaolis, L.A., Snuggs, M.B. and Lee, P.D. (1991) Insulin inhibits transcription of the human gene for insulin-like growth factor-binding protein-1. *J Biol Chem* **266**, 18868–18876.

Pucilowski, O., Ayensu, W.K. and D'Ercole, A.J. (1996) Insulin-like growth factor I expression alters acute sensitivity and tolerance to ethanol in transgenic mice. *Eur J Pharmacol* **305**, 57–62.

Resnicoff, M., Rubini, M., Baserga, R. and Rubin, R. (1994) Ethanol inhibits insulin-like growth factor-1-mediated signalling and proliferation of C6 rat glioblastoma cells. *Lab Invest* **71**, 657–662.

Resnicoff, M., Sell, C., Ambrose, D., Baserga, R. and Rubin, R. (1993) Ethanol inhibits the autophosphorylation of the insulin-like growth factor 1 (IGF-1) receptor and IGF-1-mediated proliferation of 3T3 cells. *J Biol Chem* **268**, 21777–21782.

Ross, R.J., Chew, S.L., D'Souza, L.L., Yateman, M., Rodriguez, A.J., Gimson, A., Holly, J. and Camacho, H.C. (1996) Expression of IGF-I and IGF-binding protein genes in cirrhotic liver. *J Endocrinol* **149**, 209–216.

Russell, W.E. (1985) Growth hormone, somatomedins, and the liver. *Semin Liver Dis* **5**, 46–58.

Salerno, F., Locatelli, V. and Muller, E.E. (1987) Growth hormone hyperresponsiveness to growth hormone-releasing hormone in patients with severe liver cirrhosis. *Clin Endocrinol Oxf* **27**, 183–190.

Salmon, W.D. and Daughaday, W.H. (1957) A hormonally controlled serum factor which stimulates sulphate incorporation *in vitro*. *Journal of Laboratory and Clinical Medicine* **49**, 825–836.

Santolaria, F., Gonzalez, G.G., Gonzalez, R.E., Martinez, R.A., Milena, A., Rodgiguez, M.F. and Gonzalez, G.C. (1995) Effects of alcohol and liver cirrhosis on the GH-IGF-I axis. *Alcohol Alcohol* **30**, 703–708.

Sarin, S.K., Dhingra, N., Bansal, A., Malhotra, S. and Guptan, R.C. (1997) Dietary and nutritional abnormalities in alcoholic liver disease: a comparison with chronic alcoholics without liver disease. *Am J Gastroenterol* **92**, 777–783.

Scharf, J., Schmitz, F., Frystyk, J., Skjaerbaek, C., Moesus, H., Blum, W., Ramadori, G. and Hartmann, H. (1996) Insulin-like growth factor-I serum concentrations and patterns of Insulin-like growth factor binding proteins in patients with chronic liver disease. *Journal of Hepatology* **25**, 689–699.

Shankar, T.P., Solomon, S.S., Duckworth, W.C., Jerkins, T., Iyer, R.S. and Bobal, M.A. (1988) Growth hormone and carbohydrate intolerance in cirrhosis. *Horm Metab Res* **20**, 579–583.

Shaw, B.W., Wood, W.P. and Gordon, R.D. (1985) Influence of selected patient variables and operative blood loss on six month survival following liver transplantation. *Semin Liver Dis* **5**, 385–393.

Shmueli, E., Miell, J.P., Stewart, M., Alberti, K.G. and Record, C.O. (1996) High insulin-like growth factor binding protein 1 levels in cirrhosis: link with insulin resistance. *Hepatology* **24**, 127–133.

Shmueli, E., Stewart, M., Alberti, K.G. and Record, C.O. (1994) Growth hormone, insulin-like growth factor-1 and insulin resistance in cirrhosis. *Hepatology* **19**, 322–328.

Singh, S.P., Ehmann, S. and Snyder, A.K. (1996) Ethanol-induced changes in insulin-like growth factors and IGF gene expression in the fetal brain. *Proc Soc Exp Biol Med* **212**, 349–354.

Singh, S.P., Srivenugopal, K.S., Ehmann, S., Yuan, X.H. and Snyder, A.K. (1994) Insulin-like growth factors (IGF-I and IGF-II), IGF-binding proteins, and IGF gene expression in the offspring of ethanol-fed rats. *J Lab Clin Med* **124**, 183–192.

Smith, D.J., Yang, H., Scheff, A.J., Ploch, S.A. and Schalch, D.S. (1992) Ethanol-fed Sprague-Dawley rats maintain normal levels of insulin-like growth factor I. *J Nutr* **122**, 229–233.

Snyder, A.K., Singh, S.P. and Ehmann, S. (1992) Effects of ethanol on DNA, RNA, and protein synthesis in rat astrocyte cultures. *Alcohol Clin Exp Res* **16**, 295–300.

Sonntag, W.E. and Boyd, R.L. (1989) Diminished insulin-like growth factor-1 levels after chronic ethanol: relationship to pulsatile growth hormone release. *Alcohol Clin Exp Res* **13**, 3–7.

Soszynski, P.A. and Frohman, L.A. (1992) Inhibitory effects of ethanol on the growth hormone (GH)-releasing hormone-GH-insulin-like growth factor-I axis in the rat. *Endocrinology* **131**, 2603–2608.

Srivastava, V., Hiney, J.K., Nyberg, C.L. and Dees, W.L. (1995) Effect of ethanol on the synthesis of insulin-like growth factor 1 (IGF-1) and the IGF-1 receptor in late prepubertal female rats: a correlation with serum IGF-1. *Alcohol Clin Exp Res* **19**, 1467–1473.

Stewart, A., Johnston, D.G., Alberti, K.G., Nattrass, M. and Wright, R. (1983) Hormone and metabolite profiles in alcoholic liver disease. *Eur J Clin Invest* **13**, 397–403.

Streat, S., Beddoe, A. and Hill, G.L. (1987) Aggressive nutritional support does not prevent protein loss despite fat gain in septic intensive care patients. *J Trauma* **27**, 262–266.

Sugiura, T., Tashiro, T., Yamamori, H., Morishima, Y., Otsubo, Y., Hayashi, N., Furukawa, K., Nitta, H., Nakajima, N., Ishizuka, T., Tatibana, M., Ino, H. and Ito, I. (1997) Effects of insulin-like growth factor-1 on endotoxin translocation in burned rats receiving total parenteral nutrition. *Nutrition* **13**, 783–787.

Tomono, M. and Kiss, Z. (1995) Ethanol enhances the stimulatory effects of insulin and insulin-like growth factor-1 on DNA synthesis in NIH 3T3 fibroblasts. *Biochem Biophys Res Commun* **208**, 63–67.

Unterman, T.G., Simmons, R.A., Glick, R.P. and Ogata, E.S. (1993) Circulating levels of insulin, insulin-like growth factor-I (IGF-I), IGF-II, and IGF-binding proteins in the small for gestational age fetal rat. *Endocrinology* **132**, 327–336.

Valimaki, M., Tuominen, J.A., Huhtaniemi, I. and Ylikahri, R. (1990) The pulsatile secretion of gonadotropins and growth hormone, and the biological activity of luteinizing hormone in men acutely intoxicated with ethanol. *Alcohol Clin Exp Res* **14**, 928–931.

Wahl, D.G., Dollet, J.M., Kreher, M., Champigneulle, B., Bigard, M.A. and Gaucher, P. (1992) Relationship of insulin resistance to protein-energy malnutrition in patients with alcoholic liver cirrhosis: effect of short-term nutritional support. *Alcohol Clin Exp Res* **16**, 971–978.

Wallace, J., Cuneo, R. and Abbott, W. (1997) In *International Congress of Endocrinology*, San Francisco, p. 116.

Ward, H.C., Halliday, D. and Sim, A.J.W. (1987) Protein and energy metabolism with biosynthetic human growth hormone after gastrointestinal surgery. *Ann Surg* **206**, 56–61.

Xu, X., Ingram, R.L. and Sonntag, W.E. (1995) Ethanol suppresses growth hormone-mediated cellular responses in liver slices. *Alcohol Clin Exp Res* **19**, 1246–1251.

Zanobi, A., Zecca, L. and Zanoboni-Muciaccia, W. (1983) Failure of inhibition by TRH of L-dopa stimulated GH secretion in patients with alcoholic cirrhosis of the liver. *Clin Endocrinol* **18**, 233–239.

Chapter 13

Cellular mechanisms of liver regeneration and the effect of alcohol

Martin Phillips, Elika Kashef and Robin Hughes

Progress in the understanding of the complex phenomenon of hepatic regeneration has been accomplished by extensive study of the partial hepatectomy animal model. Hepatocytes are normally relatively resistant to hepatotrophic signals and need priming before proliferation can commence. Growth factors (mitogens and co-mitogens) and growth inhibitors are involved. Priming activates a number of transcription factors that activate the genes necessary for mitosis. Tumor necrosis factor-α (TNF-α) appears to play a central role in hepatic regeneration. TNF-α is also important in the pathogenesis of alcoholic liver disease (ALD). Study of hepatic regeneration is a much more difficult problem in clinical chronic liver disease than after partial hepatectomy, but it appears to be impaired in ALD. Ethanol impairs hepatic regeneration by interfering with post-translational processing of transcription factors. TNF-α can also propagate apoptosis, though what determines whether the hepatocyte follows the pathway of regeneration or apoptosis remains unanswered. Early reports suggest that intracellular oxidative stress may be important in deciding the fate of the hepatocyte. These processes need to be understood better before they can be manipulated in the setting of clinical ALD.

KEYWORDS: liver growth factors, cytokines, transcription factors, signal transduction, apoptosis, alcohol

MOLECULAR MECHANISMS OF HEPATIC REGENERATION

The process of hepatic regeneration is complex and although modern molecular biology techniques have helped define the intracellular mechanisms involved, the question as to "what exactly triggers regeneration?" remains unanswered. Research currently suggests that a variety of factors/pathways work together to initiate regeneration and lead to cell division. The first part of this chapter has drawn heavily on the excellent reviews of this field of Fausto (1997, 1999) and Michalpopoulos and De Frances (1997) together with the excellent book edited by Strain and Diehl (1998) with its distinguished contributors.

Hepatic regeneration can be separated into two major phases: priming (or competence), and progression (Figure 13.1). Priming corresponds to the G_0–G_1 phase of the cell cycle. It consists of three stages: transcription factor activation, primary gene response and the secondary gene response. Progression is the development of the cell cycle into replication, DNA synthesis and ultimately cell division.

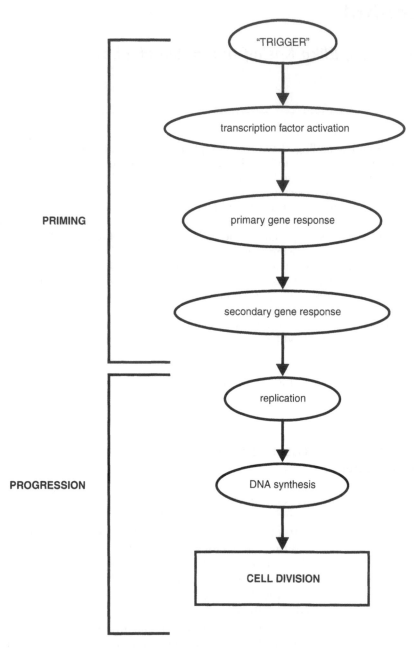

Figure 13.1 Phases of hepatic regeneration.

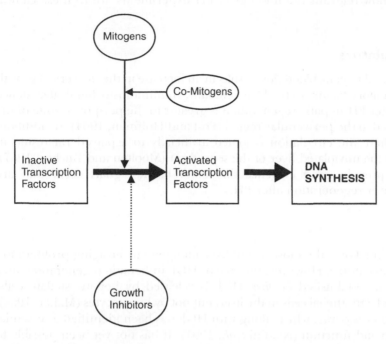

Figure 13.2 Growth regulation during hepatic regeneration (——▶ = augmentation, ······▶ = inhibition).

There are three types of growth regulators of hepatocytes: mitogens, co-mitogens and growth inhibitors (Figure 13.2). Mitogens such as hepatocyte growth factor (HGF), transforming growth factor-α (TGF-α) and epidermal growth factor (EGF) directly increase the rate of DNA synthesis in hepatocytes. Mitogens are not cell specific and can induce proliferation in different types of epithelial cells and are usually not produced by hepatocytes (Diehl and Rai, 1996b). Co-mitogens promote the action of mitogens, but have no effect on the rate of DNA synthesis on their own (e.g., insulin and glucagon). Together, mitogens and co-mitogens initiate a cascade of events that leads to hepatic regeneration. They activate a number of transcription factors, which play an important role in switching on DNA synthesis. The growth inhibitors such as transforming growth factor-β1 (TGF-β1) and hepatocyte growth inhibitory factor block the hepatotrophic effects of mitogens and are important in the switching-off of DNA synthesis.

Partial hepatectomy (PH) is the most used experimental model for these studies, usually involving the removal of 70% of a rat liver. Regeneration of the liver to original size after PH occurs within 14 days in rodents but may take 2–3 months in humans (Fausto, 1997). DNA synthesis in non-parenchymal cells begins within 24-hours of PH. PH in animals is a useful model for investigating the factors that may be important in triggering and controlling hepatic regeneration. In humans, similar events may occur after surgical liver resection, usually in the context of malignant disease. However, in the much more common scenario of acute toxic liver damage or chronic liver disease, there are even more complex interactions to consider.

It is unknown how relevant the findings in PH experiments are to these clinical situations.

Growth regulators

After PH, increased hepatic blood flow results in an increase in the delivery of growth factors and inhibitory factors to the liver remnant. Immunohistochemical evidence suggests that after PH hepatic regeneration is greater in the periportal zone of the liver as compared to the perivenular region (Post and Hoffman, 1964). In addition, PH in a rat where the circulation is joined artificially to a paired rat results in regeneration of the unviolated liver of the second rat (Moolten and Bucher, 1967). These studies provide good evidence that blood-borne signals occur and are important for liver regeneration after PH.

HGF

The glycoprotein HGF is the most potent liver mitogen encouraging proliferation of hepatocytes in culture. However, the role of HGF in hepatic regeneration after PH has yet to be established *in vivo*. HGF is released by hepatic stellate cells, Kupffer cells and endothelial cells in the liver, but not by hepatocytes (Maher, 1993). The HGF receptor is c-*Met*, which along with HGF has been identified as essential for liver growth and function (Naldini *et al.*, 1991). It has not yet been possible to study whether hepatic regeneration can occur in the absence of HGF, as mice that lack the HGF gene die during embryonic development (Uehara *et al.*, 1995). HGF plasma levels increase rapidly after PH in the rat, rising to 20 times normal within the first hour. This time period correlates well with the known rapid changes in gene expression which occur in hepatic regeneration. However, the cause for this early rise in HGF is not clear, as stellate cell expression of HGF mRNA only occurs 3–6 hours after PH. Within 5 minutes of PH plasminogen activator activity increases markedly, resulting in breakdown of some of the hepatic biomatrix, which is rich in HGF. This allows rapid release of HGF and could explain the sudden increase in HGF levels after liver injury. Further studies have also shown that plasminogen activator converts HGF from its inactive form into its active receptor binding state (Naldini *et al.*, 1992). The other problem with the theory that HGF is the major initiator of regeneration is that it is not specific for the liver. HGF mRNA is also elevated after PH in other tissues such as spleen and lung for reasons that are not understood.

Injection of HGF into the portal vein of normal rats caused moderate numbers of hepatocytes to undergo DNA synthesis. EGF and TGF-α injections also demonstrated similar but less marked effects (Webber *et al.*, 1994). Normal resting adult hepatocytes seem to be relatively insensitive to the mitogenic effects of growth factors *in vivo*. This suggested that hepatocytes require "sensitizing" in order to undergo regeneration. This could involve activation of the HGF receptor c-*Met* and the EGF receptor. Fausto (1999) suggested that part of the priming process could be the binding of transcription factors Nuclear Factor for κ-chain in B cells (NF-κB) and Signal Transducer and Activator of Transcription-3 (STAT-3) to their specific receptors.

EGF

EGF and TGF-α are also believed to be important in initiating regeneration. EGF is released by Brunner's glands in the duodenum and transported to the liver through the portal system (Olsen *et al.*, 1988). The secretion of EGF is increased by norepinephrine, plasma concentrations of which are markedly elevated after PH (Olsen *et al.*, 1985). Eight hours after PH in mice, both the EGF receptor mRNA and receptor binding activity increased (Noguchi *et al.*, 1991), suggesting that EGF is involved in the early stages of regeneration after PH. In rats large reductions in plasma EGF levels decrease regeneration after PH.

TGF-α

TGF-α is produced by hepatocytes and acts in an autocrine manner stimulating further synthesis and release of TGF-α both in tissue culture and *in vivo*. TGF-α shares 35% homology with EGF such that they share the same cell surface receptor. TGF-α mRNA levels increase within 4 hours of PH (Webber *et al.*, 1993). However, Russell *et al.* (1996) found that deletion of the TGF-α gene did not disrupt hepatic regeneration, which progressed as normal. This is probably due to the compensatory up-regulation of EGF receptors.

Tumor necrosis factor-α (TNF-α)

TNF-α appears to be the most important cytokine involved in hepatic regeneration. It is a weak mitogen released predominantly by Kupffer cells and non-parenchymal cells which is stimulated by endotoxin delivered via the portal venous blood inflow to the liver. There has been significant recent progress in the understanding of TNF-α-mediated signal transduction. There are two TNF-α receptors (TNFR-I and TNFR-II). Activation of these receptors by TNF-α results in aggregation of receptors and activation of kinases, proteases and lipases that are responsible for the intracellular actions of TNF-α. Activation of Jun *N*-terminal kinases (JNK) is vital to liver regeneration as deletion of c-*jun* (the substrate of JNK) results in embryonic death due to hepatic agenesis (Hilberg *et al.*, 1993). TNF-α-induced activation of the lipase sphingomyelinase increases intracellular ceramide, which inhibits mitochondrial function and increased mitochondrial oxidative stress via increased mitochondrial reactive oxygen species production. This increased oxidative stress activates NF-κB and helps binding of this transcription factor which is important in hepatic regeneration (Fitzgerald *et al.*, 1995). However, JNK activation of the protease caspase-8 initiates the cascade of events leading to activation of caspase-3 and the phenomenon of apoptosis. Therefore, TNF-α signal transduction is capable of promoting both proliferation and cell death. The factors determining the final outcome are not well understood.

In vitro and *in vivo* TNF-α potentiates the effects of growth factors on hepatocytes (Akerman *et al.*, 1992). In landmark studies, infusion of anti-TNF-α antibodies inhibited hepatocyte DNA synthesis after PH (Akerman *et al.*, 1992). JNK, c-*jun* mRNA binding and nuclear Activating Protein-1 (AP-1) activities were also suppressed (Diehl *et al.*, 1994). This suggested that TNF-α is important in the regeneration process. Recent data showed that TNFR-I deficiency in mice resulted in impaired binding of STAT-3 and NF-κB and disrupted DNA synthesis after PH (Yamada *et al.*, 1997). This receptor also contains a Fas-like domain (the so-called "death domain") which induces apoptosis. Injection of interleukin-6 (IL-6) into these mice prior to the PH, rectified the disruption, although there was no change in NF-κB binding. This illustrates that there are probably several parallel signaling pathways involved in the regenerative response.

When PH in mice was accompanied by gut decontamination, it was found that hepatic regenerative capabilities were diminished (Cornell, 1985). It is known that bacterial factors such as endotoxin can stimulate TNF-α release by Kupffer cells. It is possible that after PH, increased blood flow to the remaining liver delivers higher doses of endotoxin to the remaining Kupffer cells, stimulating enhanced TNF-α release. Recent studies, however, have demonstrated that Kupffer cells are not the sole source of TNF-α production after PH. After the removal of Kupffer cells, elevation of TNF-α mRNA levels still occurred. The other sources of TNF-α have not yet been identified. It is probable that cells such as sinusoidal endothelial cells, biliary epithelial cells and immature tissue macrophages also release TNF-α (Diehl and Rai, 1996a).

Current data suggest that TNF-α is involved in one of the most important pathways of hepatic regeneration which involves TNFR-I, NF-κB, IL-6, and STAT-3 (Figure 13.3).

Interleukin-6 (IL-6)

IL-6 is also a pro-inflammatory cytokine with important roles in the acute inflammatory response, the sepsis syndrome, and a variety of other areas. The release of IL-6 is stimulated by TNF-α produced by Kupffer cells, biliary endothelial cells and hepatocytes. IL-6 concentration increases after PH and within 24-hours reaches a maximum level. Deletion of the IL-6 gene in mice decreased STAT-3 and AP-1 activation and prevented hepatocyte DNA synthesis. These mice had severely impaired hepatic regeneration after PH and developed massive liver necrosis and liver failure. Injection of IL-6 prior to PH corrected these observations (Cressman *et al.*, 1996). This study suggests that IL-6 is an essential part of the signaling pathway of hepatic regeneration.

It is important to note that both TNF-α and IL-6 have other metabolic effects on the liver and systemically as both are part of the acute phase response, which takes place in order to maintain homeostasis after injury (including PH) or infection. During regeneration acute phase proteins act in a defensive role and compensate for the limited phagocytic abilities of Kupffer cells (Moshage, 1997). They can also regulate proteolytic activity during regeneration. This is important as the acute phase response could divert hepatocytes away from the pathways involved in hepatic regeneration.

Therefore, it would appear that TNF-α is very important to hepatic regeneration but the pathway involved also has the potential to induce cell death. TNF-α-stimulated IL-6 production also appears vital to the process of regeneration although this is less well characterized.

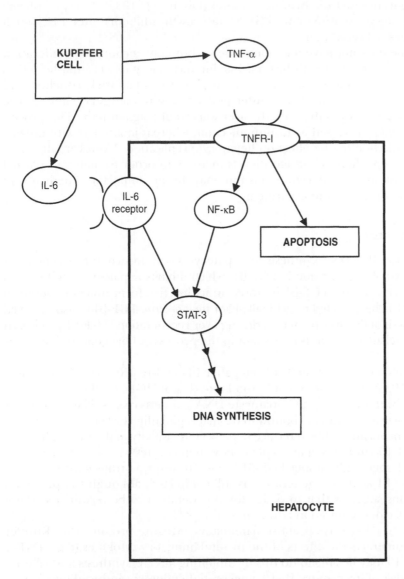

Figure 13.3 The TNF-α signal transduction pathway in hepatic regeneration. (IL-6 = interleukin-6, NF-κB = Nuclear Factor for κ-chain in B cells, TNF-α = Tumour necrosis factor-α, TNFR-I = Tumour necrosis factor-α receptor-I, STAT-3 = Signal Transducer and Activator of Transcription-3).

Co-mitogens

Plasma norepinephrine levels are elevated within an hour of PH (Cruise *et al.*, 1987), which enhances the mitogenic signals of EGF and HGF by binding to α_1-adrenoceptors (Cruise *et al.*, 1985). Norepinephrine also enhances EGF activity by stimulating its release from Brunner's glands (Olsen *et al.*, 1985). Norepinephrine decreases hepatocyte sensitivity to TGF-β1 (a growth inhibitor) after PH, which also encourages cell replication.

Insulin alone does not have mitogenic effects, but may encourage proliferation in the presence of other growth factors. Insulin and glucagon were implicated as important hepatotrophic substances in early experimental work (Bucher and Swaffield, 1975; Farivar *et al.*, 1976). After portocaval shunt surgery where portal blood is diverted away from the liver, the liver will atrophy significantly. This process can be prevented or reversed by insulin injection, whereas in animals with normal livers insulin injection has no effect on hepatocyte replication. However, after PH, insulin levels drop whereas glucagon levels increase in order to maintain plasma glucose concentrations. Therefore, insulin may be an important mediator of regeneration but is not a primary trigger.

Inhibitory factors

By 72 hours after PH, DNA synthesis in hepatocytes is almost complete. The most studied inhibitor of regeneration is TGF-β1, which inhibits hepatocyte proliferation *in vitro* (Carr *et al.*, 1986). TGF-β1 is stored in its inactive form unless exposed to proteases and can be activated by acid, alkali, or heat *in vitro*. TGF-β1 is also involved with the synthesis of the liver biomatrix during liver regeneration. TGF-β1 is released from hepatic stellate cells and is important in the process of fibrogenesis in chronic liver disease.

TGF-β1 levels increase within 3–4 hours after PH and reach a peak by 72 hours (Braun *et al.*, 1988). This time course is similar to that of HGF and the peak plasma levels coincide with the time that hepatocyte DNA synthesis ceases. Plasma TGF-β1 is probably inactivated by being bound to α2-macroglobulin (LaMarre *et al.*, 1991). Plasma norepinephrine is able to reduce hepatocyte sensitivity to the mito-inhibitory effects of TGF-β1 and this may explain how hepatocytes are able to continue proliferation despite high plasma TGF-β1 levels. However, in transgenic mice with enhanced TGF-β1 activity regeneration is still completed, although the process is prolonged. This suggests that in order for regeneration to be terminated there may be other factors required in addition to TGF-β1.

Interleukin-10 (IL-10) is an anti-inflammatory cytokine produced by Kupffer cells which counteracts the effects of the pro-inflammatory cytokines (e.g., TNF-α and IL-6). IL-10 may be able to do this by inhibiting TNF-α synthesis and release. In animal models of liver injury IL-10 ameliorated endotoxin-induced liver injury (Santucci *et al.*, 1996). If PH is performed after gadolinium chloride administration (which depletes Kupffer cells) hepatic regeneration is enhanced and accompanied by elevated TNF-α levels (Rai *et al.*, 1996). These early data suggest that IL-10 may well be an important factor in addition to TGF-β1 in the switching-off of hepatic regeneration.

Activation pathways

Growth factors such as EGF, TNF-α and HGF bind to receptor ligands with tyrosine kinase activity causing auto-phosphorylation of tyrosine amino acids residues in the cytoplasmic domain of the receptor (Brenner, 1998). These phosphorylated tyrosine residues bind to a variety of signal transducing proteins including phospholipase C-γ, phosphotidylinositol 3-kinase, Src-related tyrosine kinase, p59 fyn, GRB2 and rasGAP. The complex GRB2-SOS binds with Ras and helps the substitution of GDP for GTP. This process results in the activation of Ras followed by the activation of Raf. The activated form of Raf in turn leads to the phosphorylation of MAPK kinase (MEK), which resides in the cytosol. MEK activates mitogen-activated protein kinase (MAPK) through phosphorylation, which permits the activated kinases to migrate to the nucleus where they activate transcription factors (Marshall, 1995; Heldin, 1995). EGF and HGF increase MAPK phosphorylation in cultures of hepatocytes (Stolz and Michalopoulos, 1994). Activation of these transcription factors is further enhanced through the stress-activated protein kinase (SAPK) pathway, which runs parallel to and interacts with the MAPK pathway. Stress inducers such as ultraviolet radiation and TNF-α can activate SAPK via the binding of TNF to its receptors (Sluss *et al.*, 1994). During hepatic regeneration, there are increases in phosphoinositide hydrolysis and calcium intermediates, suggesting that these cascades are involved in regeneration as well as normal cell activities (Baffy *et al.*, 1992).

Hepatocyte mitogens bind to different tyrosine kinase receptors activating different signaling pathways (including the MAPK cascade), but all lead to transcription factor activation. For example, the HGF receptor c-*Met* and the EGF receptor bind to different signal transduction components. HGF and EGF are both inducers of MAPK pathway and both phosphorylate cytoskeletal-associated F-actin (Stolz and Michalopoulos, 1994). However, HGF phosphorylates two cytoskeletal-associated proteins, which are not affected by EGF, suggesting that they function through different cascades.

Transcription factors

Transcription factors induce the primary and secondary gene response in hepatocytes and their function is essential for regeneration. Activation of transcription factors such as NF-κB, STAT-3, AP-1 and CAAT enhancer binding protein (C/EBP) occurs shortly after PH and is important in binding of DNA which precedes DNA synthesis.

NF-κB

NF-κB consists of a group of proteins that are present in many cell types and are involved in gene activation, immune reactions and cell proliferation. Activation of NF-κB may occur via one of many stimuli such as endotoxin, cytokines (e.g., TNF-α, IL-1, IL-2), ultraviolet light and oxidant stress (Grilli *et al.*, 1993; Liou and Baltimore, 1993). NF-κB binds to immunoglobulin, adhesion molecule, cytokine and acute-phase response genes and c-*myc* proto-oncogene. These genes have recognition sequences specific to NF-κB and are activated by the binding of NF-κB. NF-κB exists in an inactive form in the cytoplasm. It consists of two subunits, p50 and p65. These two subunits are bound to IκB (inhibitor of κB) and in order for NF-κB to be activated, IκB must be degraded and separated from the complex.

IκB is phosphorylated by an enzyme catalyzed by reactive oxygen species. The phosphorylated IκB is then digested by proteasomes present in the cytosol activating NF-κB which then enters the nucleus (Anderson *et al.*, 1994).

The protein complex post-hepatectomy factor (PHF) has been reported to bind to DNA (in its activated form) almost immediately after PH (Tewari *et al.*, 1992). PHF was found to be associated with NF-κB. Tewari *et al.* (1992) also identified regenerating liver inhibitor factor-1, a gene which was later recognized as IκB-α. NF-κB plays an important role in the early stages of regeneration (i.e., the initial gene response), but this is not sufficient alone to trigger DNA synthesis. This was demonstrated in PH studies in animals that were unable to undergo DNA synthesis, yet still responded to growth and transcription factors (Webber *et al.*, 1994).

Studies in mice have shown that the p65 component of NF-κB is vital for hepatic development. Elimination of p65 in mice resulted in cell apoptosis after 16 days of normal development (Beg *et al.*, 1995). However, elimination of p50 did not disrupt the normal development of the hepatocytes. It is not yet clear whether or not p65 acts to induce cell proliferation or to prevent cell apoptosis.

NF-κB activation can be induced by intra-peritoneal injection of TNF-α in rats. Extensive studies have shown that TNF-α causes an increase in levels of c-*jun*, *jun* kinase and AP-1 after PH and that inhibition of TNF-α limits liver regeneration. TNF-α stimulates NF-κB and AP-1 activation via reactive oxygen species generation and increased oxidative stress, as discussed earlier (Diehl and Rai, 1996b). After PH, increased metabolic activity in the remaining liver also leads to excessive production of oxygen free radicals by mitochondria as a result of oxidative phosphorylation (Goossens *et al.*, 1995). This also enhances NF-κB activation. In summary, NF-κB activation may occur through stimulation by TNF-α, IκB phosphorylation, IκB degradation (i.e., proteolytic activation) or by oxidative stress.

STAT-3

STAT is a group of transcription factors which includes STAT-3. It exists in an inactive form in the cytosol and requires phosphorylation to become activated. Stimuli such as EGF, endotoxin and IL-6 can activate STAT-3 in the liver. These stimuli activate the enzyme c-*jun* amino-terminal kinase (JAK), which dimerizes and phosphorylates STAT-3 at tyrosine residues. Phosphorylated STAT-3 then relocates to the nucleus of the hepatocyte where it undergoes a second phosphorylation at serine residues by the enzyme MAPK (Figure 13.4). STAT-3 activation is slower than NF-κB and it remains at a high level for six or more hours after PH, suggesting that this transcription factor is involved in both the early and the secondary gene response (Fausto, 1999).

AP-1

Activating protein-1 is a transcription factor consisting of heterodimers of c-*fos* and a member of the Jun family (e.g., c-*jun*, *jun*-B, *jun*-D) or of dimers of the *jun* family. Liver regeneration factor-1 (LRF-1) is a heterodimeric complex composed of a member of the *fos* family, combined with *jun*-B and c-*jun*. This and other

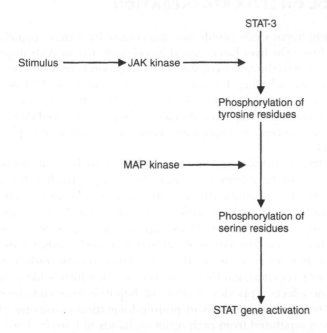

Figure 13.4 Activation of STAT-3 (JAK = c-*jun* amino-terminal kinase, MAP = Mitogen-Activated Protein, STAT-3 = Signal Transducer and Activator of Transcription-3).

growth factors are important AP-1 activators. AP-1 activation is a rapid process. Within 30 minutes of the PH, c-*fos* mRNA levels become elevated returning to normal levels by 2 hours.

Jun nuclear kinase increases the binding activity of AP-1 within 1 hour of the PH. It is believed that different complexes of AP-1 (e.g., c-*fos*/c-*jun*, c-*jun*/c-*jun*) are activated by different genes, although most overlap with each other (Fausto, 1999). It is probable that AP-1 proteins can be activated by MAPK and the SAPK pathways. MAPK activation results in the phosphorylation of transcription factors, which leads to the activation of c-*fos* (Brenner, 1998).

CAAT enhancer binding protein (C/EBP)

C/EBP is also a transcription factor and is expressed in normal liver. C/EBP and AP-1 are members of the leucine zipper protein transcription family. C/EBP is responsible for activating genes specific to the liver. C/EBP is present in two isoforms in the liver, C/EBPα and C/EBPβ. After PH, the ratio of C/EBPα to C/EBPβ changes so that C/EBPα levels drop and C/EBPβ levels rise. C/EBPα is thought to have an inhibitory effect on proliferation. Therefore, after PH the relative decrease in C/EBPα encourages replication and differentiation (Fausto, 1999).

In summary, HGF, EGF, TNF-α, IL-6, NF-κB and STAT-3 are the most important factors so far identified and seem to be vital for hepatic regeneration to occur after PH. However, much more remains to be uncovered about this complex process and its interaction with other cellular processes such as apoptosis.

EFFECTS OF ALCOHOL ON LIVER REGENERATION

Following PH, the remaining hepatocytes proliferate and restore liver mass, usually without residual scarring. Once the liver has reached its original size, growth stops and proliferative activity returns to the quiescent state. The situation is very different in clinical chronic liver disease, including that due to chronic alcohol use. Chronic liver injury usually occurs over a number of years, and involves many factors in addition to hepatic regeneration including toxic damage to hepatocytes, cell death, an inflammatory response, fibrogenesis and apoptosis. This is a much more complex situation than that after PH.

ALD comprises three different pathological entities: alcoholic fatty liver, alcoholic hepatitis and cirrhosis. Alcoholic fatty liver is thought to be a relatively benign condition. Alcoholic hepatitis is predominantly an inflammatory condition. The most severe form of alcoholic hepatitis is a clinical syndrome which has many similarities with acute liver failure and is associated with high mortality rates. Standard therapy for alcoholic hepatitis is based on administration of corticosteroids, on the basis of reducing the inflammatory response in the liver. However, steroids also have inhibitory effects on liver regeneration (Nagasue et al., 1979) which is likely to be due to their anti-cytokine effects. Episodes of alcoholic hepatitis invariably heal leaving areas of fibrosis. Over time this results in nodule formation consisting of areas of hepatic regeneration separated from each other by bands of fibrosis. Eventually the histological appearance of cirrhosis develops.

The pathogenesis of ALD remains elusive although there has been much progress in recent years (reviewed in Lieber, 2000). Endotoxin levels are raised in ALD. Endotoxin activates Kupffer cells to produce pro-inflammatory cytokines (e.g., TNF-α, IL-1, IL-6). These cytokines induce the production of IL-8 from hepatocytes and adhesion molecules, which are chemoattractant for neutrophils, resulting in the characteristic neutrophilic infiltrate of alcoholic hepatitis. More recently, attention has focused on the role of oxidant stress in the liver in ALD (reviewed in Nordmann, 1994). Not only do alcoholics without liver disease (Lecomte, 1994) and patients with ALD have lower levels of natural antioxidants in the liver (e.g., glutathione, vitamin C, vitamin E, selenium) (Bell et al., 1992), ethanol metabolism and pro-inflammatory cytokines induce the production of copious reactive oxygen species, thereby inducing further oxidant stress on the hepatocyte. Oxidant stress is known to disrupt many important cellular activities and is currently thought to play a major role in the pathogenesis of ALD (Bjorneboe and Bjorneboe, 1993). Non-parenchymal cells play an important part in ALD. Activated Kupffer cells (cytokine production) and hepatic stellate cells (fibrogenesis) are instrumental in orchestrating the fate of hepatocytes in ALD (Spitzer and Bautista, 1998).

The process of hepatic regeneration may be different in alcohol-induced liver injury compared to that after PH for a number of reasons (Czaja, 1998). Cell membrane structure is altered by reactive oxygen species formed in ALD by the process of lipid peroxidation. This could disrupt growth factor interaction with their receptors. The characteristic inflammatory infiltrate in the liver in ALD due to oxidative stress and elevated pro-inflammatory cytokines may alter the rate of hepatic regeneration. Activation of hepatic stellate cells, which occurs early in ALD, produces TGF-β1 and IL-10 which inhibit hepatic regeneration. Ethanol directly inhibits RNA and protein synthesis in the liver (Poso and Poso, 1981), which could be due to inhibition of transcription factors involved in liver regeneration or switching to other metabolic processes such as the acute phase response at the expense of cell proliferation. The obvious difference between PH and alcohol-induced liver injury is that of dose and timing. While liver injury occurs at a specific time point after PH, in ALD hepatotoxicity from ethanol is a chronic issue over a period of years or decades. The implications of repeated lower level toxic insults to the liver remain largely unknown.

There is a widely held view that alcohol has inhibitory effects on the process of liver regeneration. However, the evidence for this is not conclusive. In fact, there have been both positive and negative experimental studies on the effects of ethanol on cell proliferation. In experimental toxic liver injury after carbon tetrachloride or D-galactosamine, there is a marked delay in hepatocyte proliferation compared to PH (Schmiedeberg et al., 1993). Others have found similar results suggesting that after toxic liver injury hepatocytes may be relatively resistant to entering the cell cycle or that growth factors or other promotors of regeneration are reduced or impaired.

Experimental studies investigating the effects of ethanol on hepatic regeneration have been ongoing for more than 20 years (Leevy and Chen, 1979). Administration of ethanol to rats resulted in unchanged (Frank et al., 1979; Orrego et al., 1981) or reduced (Wands et al., 1979; Diehl et al., 1988, 1990a; Akerman et al., 1993) incorporation of ^{3}H-thymidine into hepatic DNA after PH. These results may have been influenced by methodology in that negative studies used a much shorter period of ethanol feeding compared to studies demonstrating reduced regeneration. Chronic administration of ethanol caused a significant inhibition of liver regeneration in rats after toxic liver injury due to galactosamine (MacIntosh et al., 1992). The latter is perhaps a more appropriate model of the clinical situation where there is diffused hepatocellular injury in the liver.

Baskin et al. (1988) reviewed the evidence for effects of ethanol on hepatic regeneration. It had been reported that chronic dosing with ethanol inhibited liver regeneration in rats, but this was not due to suppression of ornithine decarboxylase (ODC) activity (Diehl et al., 1988), a key enzyme in DNA synthesis as had been reported earlier for acute exposure to ethanol (Orrego et al., 1981). The review highlighted possible methodological aspects, particularly in the use of ^{3}H-thymidine incorporation into DNA, which was one of the most popular techniques. Results could be influenced by changes in hepatocyte size induced by ethanol and by intracellular derangement caused by ^{3}H-thymidine uptake and metabolism. It was also important to clarify whether DNA synthesis/cell proliferation was reduced rather than just delayed.

Studies on hepatocyte proliferation using mRNA expression of proliferating cell nuclear antigen (PCNA) and human histone (H3) as markers of proliferation in acute alcoholic hepatitis showed a good correlation with outcome (Fang et al., 1994). Therefore, in this form of ALD in particular, delay or reduction in the amount of hepatic regeneration may be a major determinant of survival.

Alcohol and HGF

HGF is the most potent stimulator of liver growth and has been investigated extensively in clinical liver disease, including that due to alcohol. Serum HGF levels were increased in patients with alcoholic hepatitis and/or cirrhosis (Mendenhall *et al.*, 1996). As in acute liver failure (Hughes *et al.*, 1994), higher levels of HGF in alcoholic hepatitis were associated with a worse outcome. However, the level of HGF is less in ALD than that found in acute liver failure. It is not known whether excess alcohol affects HGF production. HGF was detected in hepatic sinusoidal cells in only 7/19 patients with alcoholic hepatitis, but 6 of them survived. Expression of HGF was associated with greater expression of PCNA suggesting a role for HGF in cell proliferation (Fang *et al.*, 1994). Experimental studies in rat hepatocytes have shown that ethanol has an inhibitory effect on HGF stimulated DNA synthesis *in vitro* (Saso *et al.*, 1996). These observations suggest that although HGF levels are elevated in ALD the ability of the hepatocyte to respond is impaired.

Alcohol and EGF

Ethanol treatment of rat hepatocytes inhibits the proliferative response to EGF *in vitro* (Carter and Wands, 1985). Acute ethanol treatment of hepatocytes was found to increase EGF receptor numbers and therefore increase EGF receptor binding. However, internalization of the ligand-bound receptor was inhibited (Henderson *et al.*, 1989).

In fetal rat hepatocytes ethanol inhibited EGF-dependent DNA synthesis, which was associated with intracellular glutathione depletion. Glutathione repletion prior to EGF stimulation normalized the proliferative response (Devi *et al.*, 1993). Thus, chronic effects of ethanol on the hepatocyte may impair response to growth factors due to membrane dysfunction, dysregulation of the process of receptor-mediated endocytosis, or problems with signal transduction.

Alcohol and TGF-β1

The development of cirrhosis in ALD is related to the fibrogenic effects of TGF-β1 (Czaja *et al.*, 1989). TGF-β1 produced as a result of the anti-inflammatory response to alcoholic liver injury may reduce liver regeneration, particularly in alcoholic hepatitis. Production of TGF-β1 by hepatic stellate cells and Kupffer cells can also trigger apoptosis. Inhibition of liver regeneration may be an important factor in outcome from acute liver failure where there is massive hepatic necrosis and survival is dependent on adequate liver regeneration. Increased plasma levels and hepatic mRNA expression of TGF-β1 were detected in acute liver failure (Miwa *et al.*, 1997) and it is possible that there are parallels with severe alcoholic hepatitis.

Insulin and glucagon

In vitro, ethanol inhibits the proliferative response to insulin and glucagon in rats (Carter and Wands, 1985). Insulin and glucagon combination therapy has been used to promote hepatic regeneration in patients with severe alcoholic hepatitis. In a randomized double-blind placebo controlled clinical trial involving 50 patients with alcoholic hepatitis, patients were treated for 3 weeks (Baker *et al.*, 1981). Mortality rates were not significantly different between the groups, though serum biochemistry and prothrombin time improved significantly faster in the treated group. However, there was one death as a result of hypoglycemia. A similar study from Hungary showed significantly improved biochemistry and survival in 66 patients with alcoholic hepatitis treated for 3 weeks (Feher *et al.*, 1987). There was no clear evidence, however, that this treatment specifically enhanced liver regeneration. Trinchet *et al.* (1992) reported no significant benefit from insulin and glucagon therapy in 72 patients with biopsy proven severe alcoholic hepatitis. In a study of 83 patients with severe alcoholic hepatitis from King's College Hospital, there was also no observed benefit from treatment (Bird *et al.*, 1991). Largely as a result of these last two studies, and the inherent risk of severe hypoglycemia induced by this form of treatment, the use of insulin and glucagon therapy for severe alcoholic hepatitis has fallen out of favor.

Polyamines

Polyamine biosynthesis is vital for cell growth and also appears important for hepatic regeneration. ODC is the rate-limiting enzyme in polyamine synthesis. It catalyzes the formation of putrescine from ornithine. Putrescine is further metabolized to spermidine and then spermine. Acute administration of ethanol reduces the rise in ODC activity and putrescine in rats after PH (Tanaka *et al.*, 1991). However, ODC mRNA levels were not inhibited and ODC half-life was increased. This suggests that ethanol affected ODC translation.

Chronic administration of ethanol for 6 weeks also reduced the rise in hepatic putrescine levels after PH and, unlike the acute ethanol studies, also lowered spermidine and spermine levels (Diehl *et al.*, 1990b). Administration of putrescine reversed the inhibitory effects of ethanol on liver regeneration, confirming the importance of this polyamine. These studies suggest that relative deficiency of putrescine after chronic ethanol feeding is an important factor in the poor regenerative response after PH. It is also of interest that endotoxin, IL-1 and TNF, all factors implicated in the pathogenesis of ALD, have been reported to induce ODC activity.

Alcohol and cytokines

Research into the pathogenesis of ALD over the last 30 years has demonstrated that cytokines are intimately involved. Another consistent finding has been that ethanol appears to increase gut permeability, which returns to normal on ethanol withdrawal and results in elevated endotoxin levels in ALD. Endotoxin is an effective inducer of cytokine production. Kupffer cells are now known to be activated by alcohol (Spitzer and Bautista, 1998), which then release the pro-inflammatory cytokines IL-1 and TNF-α. Inactivation of Kupffer cells has also been shown to inhibit alcohol-induced injury. Antibiotic treatment of the gut (i.e., gut decontamination) also demonstrated the same result. This is due to the inhibition of endotoxin absorption.

The levels of cytokines have been best studied in severe alcoholic hepatitis. Several studies have shown that TNF-α, IL-1, IL-6 and IL-8 levels are elevated in the plasma of patients with severe alcoholic hepatitis (Bird *et al.*, 1990; Khoruts *et al.*, 1991; Sheron *et al.*, 1991; Hill *et al.*, 1992). Indeed, these plasma levels have been shown to be prognostic. For example, IL-6 levels were shown to correlate with mortality in severe alcoholic hepatitis (Sheron *et al.*, 1991). IL-6 is also involved in the acute phase response in alcoholic hepatitis and it is not clear if its actions are related to hepatic damage or regeneration. IL-8 is a chemokine, the main function of which is to attract neutrophils to the liver in alcoholic hepatitis. Further studies have shown that IL-8 levels in the plasma correlate well with tissue levels and with the degree of tissue neutrophil infiltration (Sheron *et al.*, 1993). It may be difficult to differentiate between cytokines produced as part of the inflammatory response in the liver to alcohol-induced injury involving non-parenchymal cells and infiltrating neutrophils and those produced as part of the regenerative response.

Treatment of rats after PH with anti-TNF antibodies inhibited DNA synthesis but with more marked effects observed in animals also chronically fed ethanol for 5 weeks (Akerman *et al.*, 1993). This suggested that alcohol increased the dependence of hepatocytes on TNF-α for proliferation. Chronic ethanol also up-regulated expression of the TNFR-I. This would suggest augmented TNF-α responses in ethanol fed rats after PH. Zeldin *et al.* (1996) demonstrated that acute exposure of rats to alcohol resulted in a further 5-fold increase in TNF-α gene expression than one would have expected after PH of a normal liver. However, induction of JNK after PH was impaired. JNK is required for the mitogenic action of EGF and for MAPK activation. NF-κB activation was also inhibited after PH in ethanol-fed rats (Zeldin *et al.*, 1996).

Although there is an overproduction of TNF-α (and other pro-inflammatory cytokines) in alcoholic hepatitis, chronic ethanol use may inhibit regenerative mechanisms in the liver. Neutralization of TNF-α has been considered as a therapy for alcoholic hepatitis, but could likewise prove deleterious to liver regeneration. On the other hand, if it is assumed that regeneration has already been initiated, removal of excess TNF associated with liver injury/apoptosis may be beneficial. These deliberations have most clinical relevance to patients with severe alcoholic hepatitis, where treatment which promotes regeneration may well be life saving. In a recent study thus far only reported in abstract, 96 patients with clinically severe alcoholic hepatitis were randomized to 4 weeks treatment with pentoxifylline, a TNF-α inhibitor, or placebo (Akriviadis *et al.*, 1997). The 4 week mortality rate was 41.7% in the placebo group compared to 22.9% in the treatment group. Deaths as a result of hepatorenal syndrome were significantly reduced by pentoxifylline. Although this is preliminary data, these results suggest that ongoing clinical research in this area is warranted.

Cell signaling

Stimulation of hepatocytes by growth factors leads to rapid expression of genes involved in cell proliferation. The proto-oncogenes c-*fos*, c-*myc*, and the *jun* family are an important part of this early gene response. When rats were fed with ethanol for 6 weeks before PH, liver regeneration was delayed but there were no changes in expression of c-*fos*, c-*myc*, or other proto-oncogenes as compared to pair fed controls (Diehl *et al.*, 1990a). Silverman *et al.* (1994) investigated the expression of pro-thymosin α, a protein regulated by c-*myc*, after PH. They found increases in pro-thymosin α mRNA of similar magnitude in ethanol-fed and control rats, but pro-thymosin α protein production was delayed in the ethanol-fed rats. This suggests that ethanol affects post-transcriptional or later events in the growth related genes.

Alcohol and apoptosis

Another possible mechanism for the apparent lack of liver regeneration in alcoholic hepatitis could be the presence of apoptosis affecting both mature and/or newly produced cells. Apoptosis occurs in normal liver as part of the cell renewal process and is involved in liver damage associated with viral hepatitis B and C (Galle *et al.*, 1995). There are studies suggesting that apoptosis might be involved in alcoholic hepatitis (Kuwahara *et al.*, 1994; Tagami *et al.*, in press).

There are a number of possible mechanisms by which alcohol could promote apoptosis. Ethanol causes oxidative stress through two possible mechanisms: increased production of reactive oxygen species, or reduction in endogenous anti-oxidants (Ishii *et al.*, 1997). CYP2E1, a member of the cytochrome P450 family, is the most abundant cytochrome in the liver and is induced by ethanol. CYP2E1 oxidizes ethanol via the 1-hydroxyethyl radical, which results in lipid peroxidation and hepatic apoptosis. Thirty percent of chronic alcoholics have evidence of hemosiderosis on liver histology. Studies in rats demonstrated that apoptosis occurred in hepatocytes where there was iron overload (Amin, 1998). Kato *et al.* (1996) suggested that iron induces apoptosis by promoting free radical formation.

Glutathione is important in protecting cells from oxidant stress. Acute ethanol exposure also inhibits glutathione-S-transferase activity and reduces glutathione levels in the liver (Vina *et al.*, 1980). Lipid peroxidation is further promoted by a decrease in glutathione levels (Ishii *et al.*, 1997). Kurose *et al.* (1996) however, claimed that glutathione levels were unaffected by alcohol. The discrepancies found in different studies with respect to glutathione could be due to the length of ethanol exposure and other factors such as dietary intake. On the other hand in chronic alcohol exposure, glutathione-S-transferase activity is elevated which can be seen as a protective adaptation against lipid peroxidation (Ishii *et al.*, 1997).

Recently, considerable interest has focused on apoptotic injury induced by TNF-α and Fas ligand. These two cell death factors bind to their respective receptors, TNFR-I or Fas, inducing apoptosis, with cell death occurring within hours. Much effort has been made to characterize the intracellular pathways responsible for apoptosis by TNF-α or Fas-ligand. TNFR-I and Fas contain cytoplasmic "death domains" that activate apoptotic machinery of the cell. A family of cysteine-aspartate proteases termed "caspases" are involved as TNF-α and Fas-ligand signaling molecules downstream that lead to cell death (Enari *et al.*, 1996).

Taieb *et al.* (1998) have reported that plasma concentrations of both soluble Fas and Fas ligand are raised in ALD, particularly in severe acute alcoholic hepatitis. In recent preliminary experiments, we found that plasma soluble Fas levels measured by ELISA in alcoholic hepatitis patients were significantly higher than in normal controls (Tagami *et al.*, in press). In these studies, the hepatic expression of Fas, Fas ligand, the cytoplasmic "death domain" FADD and caspases ICE and CPP32 detected by immunoblot analysis in liver tissue from patients with alcoholic hepatitis ($n = 11$) were significantly increased compared to patients with alcoholic cirrhosis ($n = 8$). This is further evidence for activation of the Fas system. Thus,

Table 13.1 The effect of chronic alcohol ingestion on mediators of hepatic regeneration

Factor	Effect of alcohol
MITOGENS	
HGF	levels increased in ALD but proliferative response to HGF reduced
EGF	increased receptor binding but proliferative response to EGF reduced
TNF-α	levels increased and up-regulation of TNF receptors with enhanced proliferation but can also initiate apoptosis
IL-6	levels increased and proliferation stimulated
CO-MITOGENS	
Insulin	proliferative response inhibited
Glucagon	proliferative response inhibited
GROWTH INHIBITORS	
TGF-β1	levels increased and proliferative response inhibited
IL-10	levels increased and proliferative response inhibited
TRANSCRIPTION FACTORS	
NF-κB	activation inhibited

Fas-mediated apoptosis may be an important factor in liver cell loss in acute alcoholic hepatitis and could be a mechanism for the apparent reduced liver regeneration in patients with alcoholic hepatitis. Agents which modulate apoptosis, such as caspase inhibitors, could have therapeutic use.

As mentioned above, TNF-α mediates apoptosis via mechanisms, which parallel those of Fas. Chronic alcohol intake increases the sensitivity of the hepatocytes to TNF-α (Akerman *et al.*, 1993) and could result in impairment of liver regeneration or apoptosis. Ethanol also inhibits protein synthesis, which further promotes apoptosis in the liver. It has also been suggested that alcohol can directly cause apoptosis.

SUMMARY

Experimental studies have demonstrated a reduction in hepatic DNA synthesis after PH with both acute and chronic alcohol intake and that ethanol affects some of the main mediators of hepatic regeneration (Table 13.1). Alcohol increases cytokine release, specifically TNF, IL-1 and IL-6, though it must be noted that hepatocyte damage *per se* has similar effects. Growth factors such as HGF and inhibitory factors such as TGF-β1 may be important. Chronic ethanol feeding in animal studies suggest that increased levels of TNF-α may impair post-translational processing of transcription factors and thereby interfere with hepatic regeneration. Tumor formation is also a consequence of long-term alcoholic liver injury and it may be that the mechanisms discussed in this chapter are also relevant to this.

The data from human studies as to the impact of alcohol abuse on regenerative pathways is far less clear. There are many reasons why PH may not be particularly a good model for studying regeneration in the context of chronic ethanol-induced liver injury. Current work suggests that TNF-α plays a central role in the pathogenesis of ALD, hepatic regeneration and apoptosis. It is unknown how the cell determines which pathway to follow when it is stimulated by TNF-α although early reports suggest that oxidative stress and endogenous glutathione levels may be important (Fausto, 2000). Once we have understood that how regeneration takes place in the presence of alcohol and if it is abnormal, then research can be carried out on how to prevent this defective regeneration.

REFERENCES

Akerman, P., Cote, P., Yang, S.Q., McClain, C., Nelson, S., Bagby, G.J. and Diehl, A.M. (1992) Antibodies to tumor necrosis factor-alpha inhibit liver regeneration after partial hepatectomy. *American Journal of Physiology* **263**, G579–G585.

Akerman, P.A., Cote, P.M., Yang, S.Q., McClain, C., Nelson, S., Bagby, G. and Diehl, A.M. (1993) Long-term ethanol consumption alters the hepatic response to the regenerative effects of tumor nerosis factor-α. *Hepatology* **17**, 1066–1073.

Akriviadis, F., Botla, R., Briggs, W., Han, S., Reynolds, T. and Shakil, O. (1997) Improved short-term survival with pentoxifylline treatment in severe acute alcoholic hepatitis. *Hepatology* **26**, 250A.

Amin, A.N. (1998) Apoptosis and alcoholic liver disease. *Seminars in Liver Disease* **18**, 187–190.

Anderson, M.T., Staal, F.J., Gitler, C. and Herzenberg, L.A. (1994) Separation of oxidant-mediated and redox regulated steps in the NF-kappa B signal transduction pathway. *Proceedings of the National Academy of Sciences of the United States of America* **91**, 11527–11531.

Baffy, G., Yang, L., Michalopoulos, G.K. and Williamson, L.R. (1992) Hepatocyte growth factor induces calcium mobilization and inositol phosphate production in rat hepatocytes. *Journal of Cellular Physiology* **153**, 332–339.

Baker, A.L., Jaspan, B., Haines, N.W., Hatfield, G.E., Krager, P.S. and Schneider, J.F. (1981) A randomized clinical trial of insulin and glucagon infusion for treatment of alcoholic hepatitis: A progress report in 50 patients. *Gastroenterology* **80**, 1410–1414.

Baskin, G., Henderson, G.I. and Schenker, S. (1988) Ethanol and hepatic regeneration. *Hepatology* **8**, 408–411.

Beg, A.A., Sha, W.C., Bronson, R.T., Ghosh, S. and Baltimore, D. (1995) Embryonic lethality and liver degeneration in mice lacking the RelA component of NF-κB. *Nature* **376**, 167–170.

Bell, H., Bjorneboe, A., Eidsvoll, B., Norum, K.R., Raknerud, N., Try, K., Thomassen, Y. and Drevon, C.A. (1992) Reduced concentrations of hepatic α-tocopherol in patients with alcoholic liver cirrhosis. *Alcohol and Alcoholism* **27**, 39–46.

Bird, G.L.A., Sheron, N., Goka, J., Alexander, G.J. and Williams, R.S. (1990) Increased plasma tumor necrosis factor in severe alcoholic hepatitis. *Annals of Internal Medicine* **112**, 917–920.

Bird, G., Lau, J.Y., Koskinas, J., Wicks, C. and Williams, R. (1991) Insulin and glucagon infusion in acute alcoholic hepatitis: a prospective randomized controlled trial. *Hepatology* 1097–1101.

Bjorneboe, A. and Bjorneboe, G.-E. (1993) Antioxidant status and alcohol-related diseases. *Alcohol and Alcoholism* **28**, 111–116.

Braun, L., Mead, J.E., Panzica, M., Mikumo, R., Bell, G.I. and Fausto, N. (1988) Transforming growth factor beta mRNA increases during liver regeneration: a possible paracrine mechanism of growth regulation. *Proceedings of the National Academy of Sciences of the United States of America* **85**, 1539–1543.

Brenner, D.A. (1998) Signal transduction during liver regeneration. *Journal of Gastroenterology and Hepatology* **13**, S93–S95.

Bucher, N.L.R. and Swaffield, M.N. (1975) Regulation of hepatic regeneration in rats by synergistic action of insulin and glucagon. *Proceedings of the National Academy of Sciences of the United States of America* **72**, 1157–1160.

Carr, B.I., Hayashi, I., Branum, E.L. and Moses, H.L. (1986) Inhibition of DNA synthesis in rat hepatocytes by platelet-derived type beta transforming growth factor. *Cancer Research* **46**, 2330–2334.

Carter, E.A. and Wands, J.R. (1985) Ethanol inhibits hormone stimulated hepatocyte DNA synthesis. *Biochemical and Biophysical Research Communications* **128**, 767–774.

Cornell, R.P. (1985) Restriction of gut derived endotoxins impairs DNA synthesis for liver regeneration. *American Journal of Physiology* **249**, R563–R569.

Cressman, D.E., Greenbaum, L.E., DeAngelis, R.A., Ciliberto, G., Furth, E.E., Poli, V. and Taub, R. (1996) Liver failure and defective hepatocyte regeneration in interleukin-6 deficient mice. *Science* **274**, 1379–1383.

Cruise, J.L., Houck, K.A. and Michalopoulos, G. (1985) Induction of DNA synthesis in cultured rat hepatocytes through stimulation of alpha 1 adrenoreceptor by norepinephrine. *Science* **227**, 749–751.

Cruise, J.L., Knechtle, S.J., Bollinger, R.R., Kuhn, C. and Michalopoulos, G. (1987) Alpha 1-adrenergic effects and liver regeneration. *Hepatology* **7**, 1189–1194.

Czaja, M.J., Weiner, F.R., Flanders, K.C., Giambrone, M.A., Wind, R., Biempica, L. and Zern, M.A. (1989) The *in vitro* and *in vivo* association of transforming growth factor-β with hepatic fibrosis. *Journal of Cell Biology* **108**, 2477–2482.

Czaja, M.J. (1998) Liver regeneration following hepatic injury. In *Liver Growth and Repair*, edited by A. Strain and A.M. Diehl, pp. 28–49. London: Chapman and Hall.

Devi, B.G., Henderson, G.I., Frosto, T.A. and Schenker, S. (1993) Effect of ethanol on rat fetal hepatocytes: studies on cell replication, lipid peroxidation and glutathione. *Hepatology* **18**, 648–659.

Diehl, A.M., Chacon, M. and Wagner, P. (1988) The effect of chronic ethanol feeding on ornithine decarboxylase activity and liver regeneration. *Hepatology* **8**, 237–242.

Diehl, A.M., Thorgeirsson, S.S. and Steer, C.J. (1990a) Ethanol inhibits liver regeneration in rats without reducing transcripts of key protooncogenes. *Gastroenterology* **99**, 1105–1112.

Diehl, A.M., Wells, M., Brown, N.D., Thorgeirsson, S.S. and Steer, C.J. (1990b) Effect of ethanol on polyamine synthesis during liver regeneration in rats. *Journal of Clinical Investigation* **85**, 385–390.

Diehl, A.M., Yin, M., Fleckenstein, J., Yang, S.Q., Lin, H.Z., Brenner, D.A., Westwick, J., Bagby, G. and Nelson, S. (1994) Tumor necrosis factor-α induces c-*jun* during the regenerative response to liver injury. *American Journal of Physiology* G552–G561.

Diehl, A.M. and Rai, R.M. (1996a) Regulation of signal transduction during liver regeneration. *FASEB Journal* **10**, 215–227.

Diehl, A.M. and Rai, R. (1996b) Regulation of liver regeneration by pro-inflammatory cytokines. *Journal of Gastroenterology and Hepatology* **11**, 466–470.

Enari, M., Talanian, R.V., Wong, W.W. and Nagata, S. (1996) Sequential activation of ICE-ike and CPP32-like proteases during Fas-mediated apoptosis. *Nature* **380**, 723–726.

Fang, J.W.S., Bird, G.L.A., Nakamura, T., Davis, G.L. and Lau J.Y.N. (1994) Hepatocyte proliferation as an indicator of outcome in acute alcoholic hepatitis. *Lancet* **343**, 820–823.

Farivar, M., Wands, J.R., Isselbacher, K.J. and Bucher, N.L. (1976) Effect of insulin and glucagon on fulminant murine hepatitis. *New England Journal of Medicine* **295**, 1517–1519.

Fausto, N. (1997) Hepatic replication and liver regeneration. In *Acute Liver Failure*, edited by W.M. Lee, pp. 93–113. Cambridge: Cambridge University Press.

Fausto, N. (1999) Regulation of liver cell mass. In *Oxford Textbook of Clinical Hepatology*, 2nd edn, edited by J. Bircher, J.P. Benhamou, N. McIntyre, M. Rizzetto and J. Rodes, pp. 189–201. UK: Oxford Medical Publications.

Fausto, N. (2000) Liver regeneration. *Journal of Hepatology* **32**(suppl 1), 19–31.

Feher, J., Cornides, A., Romany, A., Karteszi, M., Szalay, L., Gogl, A. and Picazo, J. (1987) A prospective multicenter study of insulin and glucagon infusion therapy in acute alcoholic hepatitis. *Journal of Hepatology* **5**, 224–231.

Fitzgerald, M.J., Webber, E.M., Donovan, J.R. and Fausto, N. (1995) Rapid DNA binding by nuclear factor kappa B in hepatocytes at the start of liver regeneration. *Cell Growth & Differentiation* **6**, 417–427.

Frank, W.O., Rayyes, A.N., Washington, A. and Holt, P.R. (1979) Effect of ethanol administration upon liver regeneration. *Journal of Laboratory and Clinical Medicine* **93**, 402–413.

Galle, P.R., Hoffman, W.J., Walczak, H., Schaller, H., Otto, C., Stremmel, W., Krammer, P.H. and Runkel, L. (1995) Involvement of the CD95 (APO-1/Fas) receptor and ligand in liver damage. *Journal of Experimental Medicine* **182**, 1223–1230.

Goossens, V., Grooten, J., Devos, K. and Fiers, W. (1995) Direct evidence for tumor necrosis factor-induced mitochondrial reactive oxygen intermediates and their involvement in cytotoxicity. *Proceedings of the National Academy of Sciences of the United States of America* **92**, 8115–8119.

Grilli, M., Chui, J.-S. and Lenardo, M. (1993) NF-κB and Rel: participants in a multiform transcriptional regulatory system. *International Review of Cytology* **143**, 1–62.

Heldin, C.H. (1995) Dimerization of cell surface receptors in signal transduction. *Cell* **80**, 213–224.

Henderson, G.I., Baskin, G.S., Horbach, J., Porter, P. and Schenker, S. (1993) Arrest of epidermal growth factor-dependent growth in fetal hepatocytes after ethanol exposure. *Journal of Clinical Investigation* **84**, 1287–1294.

Hilberg, F., Aguzzi, A., Howells, N. and Wagner, E.F. (1993) c-*jun* is essential for normal mouse development and hepatogenesis. *Nature* **365**, 179–181.

Hill, D.B., Marsano, L., Cohen, D., Allen, J. and Shedlofsky, S. (1992) Increased plasma IL-6 concentration in alcoholic hepatitis. *Journal of Laboratory and Clinical Medicine* **119**, 547–552.

Hughes, R.D., Zhang, L., Tsubouchi, H., Daikuhara, Y. and Williams, R. (1994) Plasma hepatocyte growth factor and biliprotein levels and outcome in fulminant hepatic failure. *Journal of Hepatology* **20**, 106–111.

Ishii, H., Kurose, I. and Shinzo, K. (1997) Pathogenesis of alcoholic liver disease with particular emphasis on oxidative stress. *Journal of Gastroenterology and Hepatology* **12**, S272–S282.

Kato, J., Kobune, M., Kohgo, Y., Sugawara, N., Hisai, H., Nakamura, T., Sakamaki, S., Sawada, N. and Niitsu, Y. (1996) Hepatic iron deprivation prevents spontaneous development of fulminant hepatitis and liver cancer in Long-Evans Cinnamon rats. *Journal of Clinical Investigation* **98**, 923–929.

Khoruts, A., Stahnke, L., MacClain, C.J., Logan, G. and Allen, J.L. (1991) Circulating tumor necrosis factor, interleukin-1 and interleukin-6 concentrations in chronic alcoholic patients. *Hepatology* **13**, 267–276.

Kurose, I., Higuchi, H., Kato, S., Miura, S. and Ishii, H. (1996) Ethanol induced oxidative stress in the liver. *Alcoholism, Clinical and Experimental Research* **20**, 77A–85A.

Kuwahara, H., Matsuda, Y. and Takase, S. (1994) Expression of Ley antigen as a phenotypic marker of apoptosis in alcoholic hepatitis. *International Hepatology Communications* **2**, 321–327.

LaMarre, J., Hayes, M.A., Wollenberg, G.K., Hussaini, I., Hall, S.W. and Gonias, S.L. (1991) An alpha 2-macroglobulin receptor-dependent mechanism for the plasma clearance of transforming growth factor-beta 1 in mice. *Journal of Clinical Investigation* **87**, 39–44.

Lecomte, E., Herbeth, B., Pirollet, P., Chancerelle, Y., Arnaud, J., Musse, N., Paille, F., Siest, G. and Artur, Y. (1994) Effect of alcohol consumption on blood antioxidant nutrients and oxidative stress indicators. *American Journal of Clinical Nutrition* **60**, 255–261.

Leevy, C.M. and Chen, T. (1979) Ethanol inhibition of liver regeneration. *Gastroenterology* **77**, 1151–1153.

Lieber, C.S. (2000) Alcohol liver disease: new insights in pathogenesis lead to new treatments. *Journal of Hepatology* **32** (Suppl l), 113–128.

Liou, H.-C. and Baltimore, D. (1993) Regulation of the NF-κB transcription factor and I κB inhibitor system. *Current Opinion in Biology* **5**, 477–487.

MacIntosh, E., Gauthier, T., Pettigrew, N. and Minuk, G. (1992) Liver regeneration and the effect of exogenous putrescine on regenerative activity after partial hepatectomy in cirrhotic rats. *Hepatology* **16**, 1428–1433.

Maher, J.J. (1993) Cell-specific expression of hepatocyte growth factor in liver. Upregulation in sinusoidal endothelial cells after carbon tetrachloride. *Journal of Clinical Investigation* **91**, 2242–2252.

Marshall, C.J. (1995) Specificity of receptor tyrosine kinase signaling: transient versus sustained extracellular signals-regulated kinase activation. *Cell* **80**, 179–185.

Mendenhall, C.L., Roo, F., Moritz, T.E., Roselle, G.A., Cledid, A. and Grossman, C.J. (1996) Human hepatocyte growth factor in alcoholic liver disease: a comparison with change in α-fetoprotein. *Alcoholism, Clinical and Experimental Research* **20**, 1625–1630.

Michalopoulos, G.K. and De Frances, M.C. (1997) Liver regeneration. *Science* **276**, 60–66.

Miwa, Y., Harrison, P.M., Farzaneh, F., Langley, P.G., Williams, R. and Hughes, R.D. (1997) Plasma levels and hepatic mRNA expression of transforming growth factor-β_1 in patients with fulminant hepatic failure. *Journal of Hepatology* **27**, 780–788.

Moolten, F.L. and Bucher, N.L. (1967) Regeneration of rat liver: transfer of humoral agent by cross circulation. *Science* **158**, 272–274.

Moshage, H. (1997) Cytokines and the hepatic acute phase response. *Journal of Pathology* **181**, 257–266.

Nagasue, N., Kanashima, R. and Inokuchi, K. (1979) Deleterious effect of pharmacological doses of corticosteroids after partial hepatectomy in rats. *Annales Chirurgiae et Gynaecologiae* **68**, 137–142.

Naldini, L., Vigna, E., Narsimhan, R.P., Gaudino, G., Zarnegar, R., Michalopoulos, G.K. and Comoglio, P.M. (1991) Hepatocyte growth factor (HGF) stimulates the tyrosine kinase activity of the receptor encoded by the proto-oncogene c-*met*. *Oncogene* **6**, 501–504.

Naldini, L., Tamagnone, L., Vigna, E., Sachs, M., Hartmann, G., Birchmeier, W., Daikuhara, Y., Tsubouchi, H., Blasi, F., and Comoglio, P.M. (1992) Extracellular proteo-lytic cleavage by urokinase is required for activation of hepatocyte growth factor/scatter factor. *EMBO Journal* **11**, 4825–4833.

Noguchi, S., Ohba, Y. and Oka, T. (1991) Influence of epidermal growth factor on liver regeneration after partial hepatectomy in mice. *Journal of Endocrinology* **128**, 425–431.

Nordmann, R. (1994) Alcohol and antioxidant systems. *Alcohol and Alcoholism* **29**, 513–522.

Olsen, P.S., Poulsen, S.S. and Kirkegaard, P. (1985) Adrenergic effects on secretion of epidermal growth factor from Brunner's glands. *Gut* **26**, 920–927.

Olsen, P.S., Boesby, S., Kirkegaard, P., Therkelsen, K., Almdal, T., Poulsen, S.S. and Nexo, E. (1988) Influence of epidermal growth factor on liver regeneration after partial hepatectomy in rats. *Hepatology* **8**, 992–996.

Orrego, H., Crossley, I.R., Saldivia, V., Medline, A., Varghese, G. and Israel, Y. (1981) Long-term ethanol administration and short- and long-term liver regeneration after partial hepatectomy. *Journal of Laboratory and Clinical Medicine* **97**, 221–230.

Poso, H. and Poso, A.R. (1981) Inhibition of RNA and protein synthesis by ethanol in the regenerating rat liver: evidence for transcriptional inhibtion of protein synthesis. *Acta Pharmacologica et Toxicologica* **49**, 125–129.

Post, J. and Hoffman, J. (1964) Changes in the replication times and patterns of the liver cell during the life of the rat. *Experimental Cell Research* **36**, 11–21.

Rai, R.M., Yang, S.Q., McClain, C., Karp, C.L., Klein, A.S. and Diehl, A.M. (1996) Kupffer cell depletion by gadolinium chloride enhances liver regeneration after partial hepatectomy in rats. *American Journal of Physiology* **270**, G909–G918.

Russell, W.E., Kaufmann, W.K., Sitaric, S., Luetteke, N.C. and Lee, D.C. (1996) Liver regeneration and hepatocarcinogenesis in transforming growth factor-alpha-targeted mice. *Molecular Carcinogenesis* **15**, 183–189.

Santucci, L., Fiorucci, S., Chiorean, M., Brunori, P.M., Di Matteo, F.M., Sidoni, A., Migliorati, G. and Morelli, A. (1996) Interleukin 10 reduces lethality and hepatic injury induced by lipopolysaccaride in galactosamine-sensitized mice. *Gastroenterology* **111**, 736–744.

Saso, K., Higashi, K., Nomura, T., Hoshino, M., Ito, M., Moehren, G. and Hoek, J.B. (1996) Inhibitory effect of ethanol on hepatocyte growth factor-induced DNA synthesis and Ca^{2+} mobilisation in rat hepatocytes. *Alcoholism: Clinical and Experimental Research* **20**, 330A–334A.

Schmiedeberg, P., Biempica, L. and Czaja, M.J. (1993) Timing of protooncogene expression varies in toxin-induced liver regeneration. *Journal of Cellular Physiology* **154**, 294–300.

Sheron, N., Bird, G., Goka, J., Alexander, G. and Williams, R. (1991) Elevated plasma interleukin-6 and increased severity and mortality in alcoholic hepatitis. *Clinical and Experimental Immunology* **84**, 449–453.

Sheron, N., Bird, G., Koskinas, J., Portmann, B., Ceska, M., Lindley, I. and Williams, R. (1993) Circulating and tissue levels of the neutrophil chemotaxin interleukin-8 are elevated in severe acute alcoholic hepatitis, and tissue levels correlate with neutrophil infiltration. *Hepatology* **18**, 41–46.

Silverman, A.L., Smith, M.R., Sasaki, D., Mutchnick, M.G. and Diehl, A.M. (1994) Altered levels of prothymosin immunoreactive peptides, a growth-related gene product, during liver regeneration after chronic ethanol feeding. *Alcoholism, Clinical and Experimental Research* **18**, 616–619.

Sluss, H., Barrett, T., Derijard, B. and Davis, R.J. (1994) Signal transduction by tumor necrosis factor is mediated by JNK kinases. *Molecular and Cell Biology* **14**, 8376–8384.

Spitzer, J.J. and Bautista, A.P. (1998) Tolerance and sensitivity: ethanol and Kupffer cells. *Gastroenterology* **115**, 494–495.

Stoltz, D.B. and Michalopoulos, G.K. (1994) Comparative effects of hepatocyte growth factor and EGF on motility, morphology, mitogenesis and signal transduction of primary rat hepatocytes. *Journal of Cellular Biochemistry* **55**, 445–469.

Strain, A.J. and Diehl, A.M. (1998) *Liver Growth and Repair*. London: Chapman and Hall.

Tagami, A., Ohnishi, H., Moriwaki, H., Phillips, M. and Hughes, R.D. Fas-mediated apoptosis in acute alcoholic hepatitis. *Hepato-Gastroenterology* (in press).

Taieb, J., Mathurin, P., Poynard, T., Gougerot-Pocidalo, M.A. and Chollet-Martin, S. (1998) Raised plasma soluble Fas and fas-ligand in alcoholic liver disease. *Lancet* **351**, 1930–1931.

Tanaka, T., Nishiguchi, S., Kuroki, T., Kobayashi, K., Matsui-Yuasa, I., Otani, S., Toda, T., Monna, T. and Sukegawa, Y. (1991) Effects of single ethanol administration on hepatic ornithine decarboxylase induction and polyamine metabolism. *Hepatology* **14**, 696–700.

Tewari, M., Dobrzanski, P., Mohn, K.L., Cressman, D.E., Hsu, J.C., Bravo, R. and Taub, R. (1992) Rapid induction in regenerating liver of RL/IF-1 and PHF a novel κB site-binding complex. *Molecular and Cell Biology* **12**, 2898–2908.

Trinchet, J.C., Balkau, B., Poupon, R.E., Heintzmann, F., Callard, P., Gotheil, C., Grange, J.D., Vetter, D., Pauwels, A., Labadie, H., Chazouilleres, O., Mavier, P., Desmorat, H., Zarski, J.P., Barbare, J.P., Chambre, J.F., Pariente, E.A., Roulot, D. and Beaugrand, M. (1992) Treatment of severe alcoholic hepatitis by infusion of insulin and glucagon: a multicenter sequential trial. *Hepatology* **15**, 76–81.

Uehara, Y., Minowa, O., Mori, C., Shiota, K., Kuno, J., Noda, T. and Kitamura, N. (1995) Placental defect and embryonic lethality in mice lacking hepatocyte growth factor/scatter factor. *Nature* **373**, 702–705.

Vina, J., Estrela, J.M., Guerri, C. and Romero, F.J. (1980) Effect of ethanol on glutathione concentration in isolated hepatocytes. *Biochemistry Journal* **188**, 549–552.

Wands, J.R., Carter, E.A., Bucher, N.L.R. and Isselbacher, K.J. (1979) Inhibition of hepatic regeneration in rats by acute and chronic ethanol intoxication. *Gastroenterology* **77**, 528–531.

Webber, E.M., Fitzgerald, M.J., Brown, P.I., Bartlett, M.H. and Fausto, N. (1993) Transforming growth factor-alpha expression during liver regeneration after partial hepatectomy and toxic injury, and potential interactions between transforming growth factor-alpha and hepatocyte growth factor. *Hepatology* **18**, 1422–1431.

Webber, E.M., Godowski, P.J. and Fausto, N. (1994) *In vivo* response of hepatocytes to growth factors requires an initial priming stimulus. *Hepatology* **19**, 489–497.

Yamada, Y., Kirillova, I., Peshon, J.J. and Fausto, N. (1997) Initiation of liver growth by tumor necrosis factor: deficient liver regeneration in mice lacking type I tumor necrosis factor receptor. *Proceedings of the National Academy of Sciences of the United States of America* **94**, 1441–1446.

Zeldin, G., Yang, S.Q., Lin, H.Z., Rai, R. and Diehl, A.M. (1996) Alcohol and cytokine-inducible transcription factors. *Alcoholism, Clinical and Experimental Research* **20**, 1639.

Chapter 14

Alcohol and hepatocellular carcinoma

Stephen D. Ryder

Alcohol is a recognized cause of hepatic cirrhosis and hepatocellular carcinoma. The risk of HCC in populations correlates well with per capita alcohol consumption in low risk areas for viral hepatitis. The risk of developing HCC is probably 1% per year in male alcoholic cirrhotics and there is no convincing evidence that abstinence reduces the risk. The risk in non-cirrhotic individuals is very low. The risks of HCC development in alcoholic cirrhosis is probably similar to viral infections and screening of appropriate groups for HCC development is probably justified.

The epidemiology of alcohol associated HCC suggests cirrhosis is not essential for the development of HCC. Despite this evidence, there is no clear mechanism by which alcohol can be shown to have a direct carcinogenic effect. Alcohol is an established co-carcinogen in the presence of other factors known to induce liver carcinogenesis such as hepatitis C and haemochromatosis. The molecular changes in alcohol associated HCC show no characteristic patterns of mutations in genes common in the cancer pathway in the liver. Hyperproliferation of hepatocytes and non-genotoxic damage are the most likely mechanisms explaining the enhanced cancer risks in alcoholic cirrhosis.

KEYWORDS: carcinogenesis, hepatocyte, ethanol, toxin, proliferation oncogenes

INTRODUCTION

There is a strong epidemiological link between per capita alcohol consumption and the development of primary liver cell cancer. Despite this, the mechanism or mechanisms by which alcohol contributes to this increased cancer risk remain(s) obscure. This is primarily because of a lack of any direct effect of alcohol as a carcinogen in laboratory experiments and a substantial number of confounding clinical entities which tend to obscure the real risk associated with excessive ethanol intake.

EPIDEMIOLOGY OF HEPATOCELLULAR CARCINOMA IN ALCOHOL RELATED LIVER DISEASE

Alcohol intake has long been recognized to be associated with an increased risk of cancers in humans. This overall excess risk of cancer death is primarily explained by a strong association with cancers of the oropharynx and oesophagus. On the basis of this epidemiological link, the World Health Organization recognizes

Table 14.1 Risk of hepatocellular carcinoma development in a cohort of Swedish patients with alcoholism, alcoholic cirrhosis and cirrhosis of other causes

	Number of patients	Number of cancers	Median follow-up (years)	Standardised incidence ratio	95% CI
Alcoholism	8517	14	7.6	3.1	1.6–5.3
Cirrhosis	3589	139	4.1	35.1	26.7–45.3
Alcoholism plus cirrhosis	836	17	5.7	34.5	17.1–61.3

Adami et al. (1992).

ethanol as a class 2 carcinogen. Primary liver cell cancer in individuals who abuse alcohol is well described (Kew, 1984).

There is relatively little data defining the absolute risk to an individual with alcoholic liver disease for the development of primary liver cell cancer. Probably the best data comes from Sweden, in a very large cohort study comparing patients with alcoholic cirrhosis to cirrhosis of other causes. The study also included a large group of patients where a diagnosis of alcoholism was made without apparent liver cirrhosis. This showed an increased risk of hepatocellular carcinoma for alcoholism *per se* but a markedly increased risk in patients with alcohol related cirrhosis (Table 14.1).

There is a strong relationship between population alcohol consumption and the risk of hepatocellular carcinoma development, seen most clearly in geographical areas with a relatively low incidence of hepatocellular carcinoma development due to viral infections, such as the United States and Northern Europe. A study in 30 countries showed alcohol consumption contributed significantly and independently of hepatitis B surface antigen positivity to the risk of death from hepatocellular carcinoma (Qiao et al., 1988). This appears to be a robust finding replicated in other smaller studies. Some authors have shown a dose-response relationship with risk of hepatocellular carcinoma and rising per capita alcohol intake (Sternhagen, 1983). Hepatocellular carcinoma is much more common in men than women. The epidemiological link between alcohol and cancer of all causes is much stronger for males than females. This relationship and the gender difference appears constant in diverse populations from Japan (Tsugane et al., 1999; Makimoto and Higuchi, 1999) Europe (Benhamiche, 1998) and North America (Seitz, 1998).

Role of hepatic cirrhosis in the development of primary liver cell cancer

Cirrhosis of the liver is an important risk factor for the development of hepatocellular carcinoma in alcoholic liver disease. Data from Sweden (Table 14.1) shows that the risk attributable for alcohol excess in the absence of cirrhosis is significant, but is enhanced greatly in the presence of cirrhosis. This increase in risk was of comparable magnitude to cirrhosis of other types, such as hepatitis B. This data gives an approximate risk of developing primary liver cell cancer in alcoholic cirrhosis of 2% per year. Other studies have suggested a lower risk for the development of hepatocellular carcinoma in alcohol related cirrhosis than in viral cirrhosis

(La Vecchia, 1998). It is very difficult to reach firm conclusions about the relative magnitude of risk attributable to each factor in populations with different levels of viral carriage and retrospective estimates of ethanol intake.

Hepatoma usually occurs on a background of hepatic cirrhosis but cirrhosis is not a prerequisite for hepatoma development as hepatocellular carcinoma in alcoholics without cirrhosis, is well described (Lieber et al., 1981). The evidence suggests that less than 10% of all hepatocarcinomas occurring in patients with alcohol excess do so on the background of a non-cirrhotic liver (Shikata, 1971). This is in contrast to other agents such as hepatitis B virus infection, where a direct carcinogenic effect, probably mediated by direct DNA integration of hepatitis B virus genes, produces a relatively high risk of non-cirrhotic hepatocarcinomas. In a large study from France, alcohol was the etiological factor in less than 10% of non-cirrhotic hepatomas (Grando-Lemaire, 1999). This evidence suggests that alcohol is either a very weak carcinogen as far as its effect on the liver or that it acts as a co-carcinogen, only able to promote the development of liver cancer where another factor also exists. Once cirrhosis is established cessation of alcohol consumption, does not abolish the risk of developing primary liver cell cancer (Lee, 1996). It is difficult to establish the relative incidence of hepatocellular carcinoma in abstinent versus non-abstinent patients with alcoholic cirrhosis because of the high mortality, up to 35% in the first year, of the continued drinkers from both liver failure and other "lifestyle associated" diseases. Most published data suggests that stopping alcohol consumption reduces risk (Lee, 1996). A small study from Japan, however, showed an 18% risk of hepatocellular carcinoma development in cirrhotic alcoholics who continue to drink over a six year follow-up period whereas 32% of abstinent alcoholic cirrhotics developed hepatocellular carcinoma (Nishiuchi and Shinji, 1990). While the numbers included in this study are small, it certainly confirms that a significant risk of cancer development persists in abstinent patients with established cirrhosis and is supported by other studies from Japan showing an increased mortality from hepatocellular carcinoma in abstinent alcoholic cirrhotics (Kato et al., 1990).

IMPACT OF ALCOHOL EXCESS ON LIVER CANCER RISK IN OTHER LIVER DISEASES

There is a strong evidence that alcohol enhances the risk of development of primary liver cell cancer in many other conditions; probably the best evidence is in hepatitis C infection. An excess risk of hepatoma is seen in patients with hepatitis C cirrhosis who continue to drink large quantities of alcohol (Table 14.2). This increased risk is important, as many patients with alcohol excess are also at high risk of hepatitis virus infections. Hepatitis C infection is found in up to 15% of patients with alcoholism (15). Miyakawa et al. (Table 14.2) showed an increased incidence of hepatoma development in patients with hepatitis C who consumed more than 80g of alcohol per day. This relationship has not been seen in all studies reporting, but in larger study groups at least a trend toward increased tumor risk with increased alcohol consumption is seen. An example from Europe, showed an attributable risk of hepatocellular carcinoma of 45% for heavy alcohol

Table 14.2 Incidence of hepatocellular carcinoma in patients with hepatitis C or alcohol related cirrhosis or both risk factors

	Cumulative incidence of hepatocellular carcinoma (%)		
Years of follow-up	1	2	3
Cirrhosis due to:			
Hepatitis C	9	14	23
Hepatitis C and alcohol excess	13	17	28
Alcohol	0	0.5	1

Miyakawa et al. (1996).

users compared to 36% for hepatitis C infection alone. The increase in risk of cancer development with both risk factors was more than additive, the relative risk rising from 29.8 for hepatitis C patients to 66.3 for those with both hepatitis C and alcohol excess, suggesting a synergistic effect (Donato, 1997).

Other data support the relationship, Suzuki *et al*. showed not only a higher risk of hepatoma development in hepatitis C infected alcohol abusers but showed an earlier age of tumor development, 58 versus 64 years (Suzuki, 1993).

Hepatitis B virus infection is a major risk factor for hepatocellular cancer development and the interaction of hepatitis B virus and exposure to the environmental chemical carcinogen aflatoxin B is well described (Ozturk *et al*., 1991). There has been considerable debate with much conflicting evidence about the risk posed to hepatitis B positive individuals who consume alcohol. A large case control study from Japan (Oshima *et al*., 1984) showed doubling of the risk of hepatoma development with alcohol consumption over 100g per day (relative risk for hepatitis B alone 26 vs. 61 for alcohol plus hepatitis B). A large cohort study, including hepatitis B surface antigen positive patients with and without cirrhosis who were followed for up to 8 years showed both an increased progression to cirrhosis and increased liver cell cancer incidence with alcohol consumption in excess of 80g per day (Ohnishi *et al*., 1991).

Even in low incidence areas, 3–4% of patients with alcoholism may have a positive test of some sort for hepatitis B virus infection (Gludd *et al*., 1992). Such data provoked a search for "occult" hepatitis B infection in patients with alcoholic liver disease complicated by hepatocellular carcinoma, on the basis that the etiology of some or all of such patients' cancers was integration of hepatitis B virus DNA sequences into the host genome with disruption of genetic control sequences vital for maintaining normal proliferation. Many patients, even in the absence of traditional serological markers of past hepatitis B infection were shown to have hepatitis B virus DNA detectable in tumor and non-tumor liver cells (Brechot *et al*., 1982). Subsequent studies in patients without traditional markers of hepatitis B virus infection (surface antigen or anti-core antibodies) suggest that hepatitis B virus does not appear to have a pathogenic role in the vast majority of alcoholic hepatocellular carcinomas. Hepatitis B virus DNA could not be detected in liver or tumor tissue by Southern blotting (Walter, 1988).

Hereditary hemochromatosis is a condition which carries a very high risk of hepatocellular carcinoma development, up to 200 times that of the normal population (Bradbear *et al.*, 1985; Deugnier *et al.*, 1993). Alcohol excess (greater than 100 g per day) doubles the risk of hepatoma in hemochromatosis (Deugnier *et al.*, 1993; Fargion *et al.*, 1994).

These observations confirm that excess alcohol consumption enhances the risk of developing primary liver cell cancer in patients with an alternative liver pathology. The magnitude of risk is debatable and there is no data to provide much insight into potential thresholds of alcohol consumption where this risk becomes of an appreciable magnitude. All such data relate to groups who have an alcohol intake which would be described as a high risk activity in its own right (80 g/day or more). In clinical practice, most clinicians advise patients with any other liver disease that they should either abstain totally or consume alcohol at very modest levels to minimize this risk.

PRESENTATION OF HEPATOCELLULAR CARCINOMA IN ALCOHOLIC LIVER DISEASE

The development of primary liver cell cancer is frequently the cause of initial presentation in patients with underlying alcoholic liver disease in the United Kingdom. In the Trent Region of the UK, more than half of primary liver cell cancers due to alcohol excess occurred in patients who were not previously known to have liver disease (Figure 14.1). In the group presenting with primary liver cell cancer, almost all had advanced disease with weight loss, ascites or jaundice. A similar pattern of presentation to this is generally the norm in the developed world. A large study from Japan shows a similar high rate of symptomatic presentations in this patient group (Table 14.3).

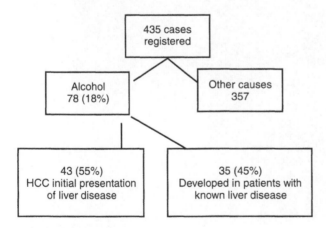

Figure 14.1 Hepatocellular carcinoma and alcohol in Trent region 1990–1995. Data from Trent Cancer Registry.

Table 14.3 Presenting features of hepatocellular
carcinoma

Symptom	% present at presentation
Abdominal pain	46%
Anorexia	45%
Weight loss	29%
Ascites	27%
Jaundice	17%
Oedema	17%
Variceal heamorrhage	8%

Okuda *et al.* (1979).

PATTERN OF HEPATOCELLULAR CARCINOMA IN ALCOHOLIC CIRRHOSIS

Primary liver cell cancer complicating ALD not only tends to present at an advanced stage but is also very frequently multifocal (Figure 14.2). Within the

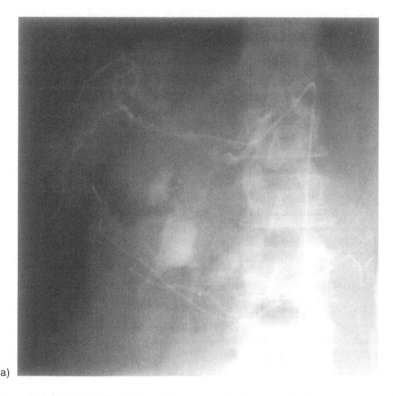

(a)

Figure 14.2a Hepatic arteriography showing multiple tumor blushes in a patient with alcoholic cirrhosis.

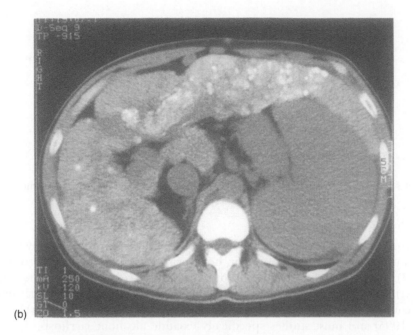

Figure 14.2b Follow-up CT scan 7 days after hepatic arteriography and lipiodol injection. Multiple areas of lipiodol retention are seen throughout the liver confirming a diagnosis of multifocal hepatocellular carcinoma.

Trent Cancer Registry data, of the 78 tumors complicating ALD 52 (67%) were multifocal tumors at the time of presentation as compared to hepatitis B where only 13% were obviously multifocal at initial assessment. Other groups have shown that multifocal tumors are more likely in patients with more than one potential cause for liver disease, usually viral infections and alcohol excess (Fasani *et al.*, 1991). This relationship is a difficult one to disentangle. In the above Italian study, detected tumors were screened for in a population under follow-up for their chronic liver disease. In this screened group of patients with alcohol as the only risk factor, 32% were multifocal at detection, similar to the figure for those with viral hepatitis (38%). It is certainly possible that many liver cancers develop multiple lesions over time and the difference in the two studies may be that over half of UK patients with alcohol related hepatocellular carcinomas present initially with cancer without knowledge of pre-existing liver disease. Further analysis of the Trent Cancer Registry data do not suggest this to be the case, the 35 screening detected cancers were just as likely to be multifocal as the *de-novo* presentations. This suggests that alcohol predisposes to multiple liver tumor development. This difference in pattern has two major implications. The first is that treatment options are often extremely limited as neither liver transplantation or resection is possible in these patients. The second is that this pattern of presentation suggests, there may be specific molecular mechanisms leading to a higher probability of "field change" with disruption of oncogenes or tumor suppressive genes occurring in alcoholic cirrhosis.

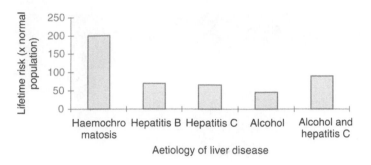

Figure 14.3 Estimated lifetime increase in risk of Hepatocellular carcinoma development in cirrhosis of different aetiologies compared to general population risk.

These factors and the relative risks associated with other liver diseases may have important implications for screening for hepatocarcinoma in high risk groups (Figure 14.3). There is no data at present to suggest that screening of patients with alcoholic cirrhosis is effective at improving survival. Most data on hepatoma screening comes from areas with a high frequency of virally induced cirrhosis (Colombo, 1995) and most studies specifically exclude alcoholic cirrhosis. There are arguments for and against screening in this group. The only curative therapy is liver transplantation (and possibly in highly selected patients liver resection) and alcoholic patients have a high incidence of cardiac disease which reduces applicability of this technique. The frequent multifocal nature of hepatocelluar carcinoma in alcoholics and its potential to be the presenting feature of the underlying cirrhosis also cast doubt on its likely cost-effectiveness. There is, however, little doubt that early detection of hepatocellular carcinoma represents the only possible chance of cure and most clinicians would undertake screening by ultrasound scanning and alpha-fetoprotein estimation in abstinent male alcoholics who would be surgical candidates.

POTENTIAL CARCINOGENIC MECHANISMS IN ALCOHOL RELATED LIVER DISEASE

There have been considerable difficulties in understanding the scientific basis by which alcohol either causes or potentiates hepatocarcinogenesis. There is no good animal model of alcoholic cirrhosis, few animals will consume alcohol as a part of their diet and those which do, do not have a parallel process of liver injury.

There is no direct evidence to suggest that alcohol itself is directly carcinogenic; its effects seem to be to promote cancer development in cancer prone states. A number of theories have been produced, these include a co-carcinogenic effect via the increased solubility of other specific carcinogens in ethanol, hence promoting absorption (Kuratsune *et al.*, 1965).

Alcoholic drinks contain substances other than alcohol and there is potential for other carcinogens to be present. Cancer causing chemicals have been shown to be present in some alcoholic drinks (Walker *et al.*, 1979) and even asbestos and other fibers have been detected and potentially implicated (Biles and Emerson, 1968).

Many individuals who consume alcohol to excess, gain the majority of their caloric intake from ethanol and nutritional deficiencies are common (Leo and Lieber, 1982). Nutritional status is known to play a role in "resistance" to cancer development in other disease states and lack of antioxidant vitamins, for example, may potentiate any DNA damage induced in the liver (Lieber *et al.*, 1986).

Immune suppression is a major feature of alcohol related liver disease. Alcohol intake is associated with a change in lymphocyte and mononuclear cell function and this effect is often profound in patients with alcohol related liver disease (Berenyi *et al.*, 1974). Immune surveillance is therefore reduced which could result in lack of identification of pre-neoplastic or neoplastic foci in the damaged liver.

Alcohol has direct effects on the metabolic pathways in the liver and this effect suggests further mechanisms by which alcohol may potentiate carcinogenesis. Alcohol is a potent inducer of the cytochrome p450 system and this enhanced activity may produce a higher level of toxic metabolites, hence increasing cancer risk. This is documented with nitrosamines (Garro *et al.*, 1981), classic carcinogens with chronic ethanol ingestion. This finding is, however, of uncertain significance as DMN liver cancers are not increased by ethanol feeding (Teschke *et al.*, 1983). An alternative theory to explain a potential effect of cytochrome p450 of tumor development is that polymorphisms of certain p450 genes produce altered ability to degrade toxic compounds but initial studies pointing to a relationship have not been confirmed (Lee *et al.*, 1997).

Liver cell injury, hepatocyte proliferation and cell death are major histological features of alcohol related liver disease. There are three basic processes associated with alcohol related hepatocyte damage which may contribute to carcinogenesis. Increases in proliferation will allow carcinogenic molecules, a greater opportunity to act on DNA in an active stage of the cell cycle. Changes in the rates of cell death, such as inhibitors of the apoptotic cell pathway, which will allow survival of DNA damaged cells form the best described mechanisms in many tumor types. Genotoxic damage can, however, occur independently from cell proliferation, this is seen with free radical induced DNA strand breakage or damage to mitochondrial DNA.

Ethanol has been reported to affect the proliferation of hepatocytes both *in vitro* and *in vivo*. The results of various studies, however, produce considerable conflict as to the overall positive or negative influence of ethanol on cell division. Ethanol augmented mitogen stimulated embryonic hepatocyte proliferation (Reddy and Shukla, 1996), but has been shown consistently to inhibit proliferation in the setting of hepatic regeneration after hepatectomy (Frank *et al.*, 1982). There is no doubt that ethanol interacts with a number of enzyme and signaling peptide systems in the liver, such as adenylyl cyclase, protein kinase C and Tyrosine-kinases (Hoek, 1992). The effects *in vitro* are frequently highly dependent on the system used, the presence of other mitogenic stimuli and the timing of ethanol challenge. A recent observation has raised the possibility that ethanol may directly affect expression and activity of inhibitory guanine nucleotide regulatory proteins (Gi-proteins) (McKillop *et al.*, 1999). These molecules act on mitogen activated protein kinases (MAPK), which in turn have an integral role in control of proliferation (Pelech *et al.*, 1993). Increased MAPK expression (Schmidt *et al.*, 1997) and Gi-protein expression (McKillop *et al.*, 1999b) have both been described in hepatocellular carcinoma. Experimental data suggest that chronic ethanol exposure produces selective increases in Gi-proteins with consequent hyperproliferation on stimulation, possibly acting via MAPK (McKillop *et al.*, 1999b).

Retinoic acid is well known to modulate growth and differentiation in a number of cell types (Jetten, 1985) and has a variety of effects on growth receptors in the liver. Its action may, at least in part, involve modulation of the hepatic synthesized receptors for insulin-like growth factor-I and II, IGF-binding proteins 1 and 3. Down-regulation of these receptors by retinoic acid has been shown to induce differentiation and reduce proliferation in hepatoma cell lines (Kim *et al.*, 1999). Such alterations may have profound implications for cell signaling and retinoids are known to play a key role in cell homeostasis. There are a significant number of studies showing that low retinol levels predispose to cancer development in many organs including the liver. The Vitamin A metabolic pathway, involving retinoic acid and its receptors in the liver, is altered in the presence of alcohol excess (Wang, 1999). It is therefore possible that nutritional deficiency of retinoids or alterations to retinoic acid receptors on the hepatocyte in alcoholic liver disease may predispose to hyperproliferation and de-differentiation of hepatocytes and be involved in the carcinogenic pathway.

Endotoxin appears to play a major role in the pathogenesis of liver cell injury in alcohol related liver disease (Nanji *et al.*, 1993). There is no evidence to suggest that such bacterial products are themselves involved in the process of carcinogenesis, although mutagenesis occurring with bacterial infection is well described. It seems most likely that any role for endotoxin is to initiate or propagate cell damage via a number of potential mechanisms which may in turn lead to DNA damage.

Many cytokines have been shown to be significantly elevated in alcoholic liver injury, including tumor necrosis factor alpha (TNF-α), and interleukins-1, 6 and 8. While there is no doubt that the TNF-α pathway is intimately involved in the cell death process, and altered expression of TNF-α has been described in hepatocellular carcinoma, there is no data to suggest a specific mechanism for TNF or other cytokines to produce genotoxic damage.

Activation of pro-inflammatory eicosanoids occurs in alcoholic liver injury, which is dependent on increased cyclooxygenase activity (Cox). Cox is a membrane bound enzyme which catalyzes the conversion of arachadonic acid to prostaglandin G2 by cyclooxygenase activity and then to G2 to prostaglandin H2 by peroxidase activity. There are two isoforms of Cox: Cox-1 is consitutively expressed in most human tissues whereas Cox-2 is expressed only after induction by cytokines and mitogenic factors. Cox-2 may play a role in modulation of liver cell injury in the liver, acting via a TNF-α independent pathway (Dinchuk *et al.*, 1995). Cox-2 expression has been shown to be increased in alcoholic liver injury (Nanji *et al.*, 1997). Cox-2, but not Cox-1, appears to play a significant role in colorectal carcinogenesis (Eberhart *et al.*, 1994) and Cox-2 inhibitors, non-steroidal anti-inflammatory drugs, have been shown to inhibit colorectal adenoma development (Rao *et al.*, 1995). The mechanism by which Cox-2 has its anti-tumor action is unknown, but Cox-2 does act on both adhesion molecules and the apoptotic pathway (Tsuji and DuBois, 1995). Cox-2 expression has been shown to be elevated in human hepatocellular carcinomas (Koga *et al.*, 1999) suggesting that Cox-2 alterations seen in alcoholic liver injury may play a part in the carcinogenic process. Cyclooxygenase actions on proliferation and cell death may be modulated by peroxisome proliferators and there is emerging evidence that these molecules may be altered in hepatocarcino-genesis (Roberts, 1996).

Free radicals and oxidative stress are clearly involved in liver cell injury in alcoholic liver disease (Nanji et al., 1995). Free radicals and oxidative stress produce DNA damage, usually by strand breakage. This remains a possible mechanism of carcinogenesis in the liver, particularly as iron is known to increase free radical injury (Tsukamoto et al., 1995) and there is a clear increase in hepatocellular carcinoma development in patients with genetic hemochromatosis who drink excess alcohol. The increase in free radical dam-age seen in alcohol related liver disease may in part be modulated by alter-ations in fat metabolism (Zhou et al., 1998) and there is a substantial body of data to show that lipid peroxidation and dietary fat are important in colorectal carcinogenesis. There is no convincing data to support this in alcohol related hepatocarcinogenesis.

There is circumstantial evidence of genotoxic damage occurring in alcoholic patients, usually by measurement of DNA adducts in blood or urine, which can be shown to decrease markedly with abstinence (Castelli et al., 1999). Acetaldehyde and its DNA adducts may play a major role in the pathogenesis of alcohol-induced liver injury. There is also evidence that these compounds may contribute to genotoxic damage (Kunitoh et al., 1997). Any compound with high reactivity with DNA bases which forms a stable molecule has the potential to interact with synthesis of correct DNA sequences, although there is no direct experimental evidence to support this in the case of acetaldehyde adducts.

It remains a possibility that alcohol may have a carcinogenic effect via an effect on other cell types within the liver. As a response to alcohol related toxic liver cell injury, not only is hyperproliferation of hepatocytes a feature but proliferation of oval cells has been shown to occur (Smith et al., 1996). Oval cells are thought to be a multipotent "stem cell" within the liver with the potential to differentiate into either biliary or hepatocyte lineages. Hyperproliferation of these cells is a marked feature of acute liver injury and hepatic regeneration; their potential role in car-cinogenesis is much less well established. It seems clear that such cells could form an alternative population with oncogenic potential.

Despite the acceptance of all the above mechanisms as potential inducers of DNA damage in patients with alcoholic cirrhosis, there is no significant evidence of a specific molecular pathway in alcohol related hepatocarcinomas. It is well recog-nized that certain chemical carcinogens leave a "genetic hallmark" of exposure by the production of specific base changes in oncogenes or tumor suppressor genes. The best described is that seen with aflatoxin exposure in hepatitis B virus infec-tion, where a specific mutation, codon 249 G to T substitution, is seen in the p53 tumor suppressor gene (Ozturk et al., 1991). This observation led to a search for other agents which may produce specific DNA lesions. A similar mutational "hot spot" was described in hereditary hemochromatosis and the same authors studied a group of hepatocellular carcinomas where alcohol was the only etiology (Vautier et al., 1999). They found that p53 mutations occur in 29% of alcohol related hep-atocellular carcinomas but there was no clustering of mutations to suggest a direct molecular mechanism. Other groups have found changes in oncogenes such as Kirsten *ras* in hepatocellular carcinoma, but there is no specific relationship with an alcoholic etiology.

The role of alcohol in cancer development in other organs is better understood, but appears to have a very different molecular basis. Tumors of the esophagus and oropharynx have a high incidence of p53 mutations, which do cluster at specific mutational sites (particularly codon 176). It may be, however, that these changes reflect the influence of other strong risk factors for the development of such cancers, mainly cigarette smoking (Gray *et al.*, 1993).

In general, there are few clues as to a defined molecular etiology for alcohol related carcinogenesis in any organ. The role and significance of alcohol in the process of cancer development is now well established. There remains, however, considerable uncertainty as to how this increased risk is modulated. This will be the focus of considerable research effort in the future.

REFERENCES

Adami, H.-O., Hsing, A.W., McLauglin, J.K., Trichopoulos, D., Hacker, D. and Ekbom, A. (1992) Alcoholism and liver cirrhosis in the aetiology of primary liver cancer. *Int J Cancer* **51**, 898–902.

Benhamiche, A.M., Faivre, C., Minello, A., Clinard, F., Mitry, E., Hillon, P. and Faivre, J. (1998) Time trends and age-period-cohort effects on the incidence of primary liver cancer in a well-defined French population: 1976–1995. *J Hepatol* **29**, 802–806.

Berenyi, M.R., Staus, B. and Cruz, D. (1974) *In vitro* and *in vivo* studies of cellular immunity in alcoholic cirrhosis. *Am J Dig Dis* **19**, 199–205.

Biles, B. and Emerson, T.R. (1968) Examination of fibres in beer. *Nature* **219**, 93–94.

Bradbear, R., Bain, C., Suskind, V. *et al.* (1985) Cohort study of internal malignancy in genetic haemochromatosis and other chronic non-alcoholic liver disease. *J Natl Cancer Inst* **75**, 81–84.

Brechot, C., Nalpas, B., Courouce, A.M., Duhamael, G., Gallard, P., Carnot, F., Tiollais, P. and Berthloth, P. (1982) Evidence that hepatitis B virus has a role in liver cell carcinoma in alcoholic liver disease. *N Engl J Med* **36**, 1384–1387.

Castelli, E., Hrelia, P., Maffei, F., Fimognari, C., Foschi, F.G., Caputo F., Cantelli-Forti G., Stefanini G.F. and Gasbarrini G. (1999) Indicators of genetic damage in alcoholics: reversibility after alcohol abstinence. *Hepatogastroenterology* **46**, 1664–1668.

Colombo, M. (1995) Debates in hepatitis. Should patients with chronic viral hepatitis be screened for hepatocellular carcinoma? *Viral Hep Reviews* **1**, 67–75.

Deugnier, Y., Guyader, D., Crantock, T. *et al.* (1993) Primary liver cancer in genetic haemochromatosis: a clinical and pathogenetic study of 54 cases. *Gastroenterology* **104**, 228–234.

Dinchuk, J.E., Lar, B.D. and Focht, R.J. (1995) Renal abnormalities and an altered inflammatory response in mice lacking cycooxygenase II. *Nature* **378**, 406–409.

Donato, F., Tagger, F., Chiesa, R., Ribero, M.L., Tomasoni, V., Fasola, M., Gelati, U., Portera, G., Boffetta, P. and Nardi, G. (1997) Hepatitis B and C virus infection, alcohol drinking and hepatocellular carcinoma: a case control study in Italy. *Hepatology* **26**, 579–584.

Fargion, S., Fracanzani, A., Piperno, A. *et al.* (1994) Prognostic factors for hepatocellular carcinoma in genetic haemochromatosis. *Hepatology* 1426–1431.

Fasani, P., Sangiovanni, A., De Fazio, C., Borzio, M., Bruno, S., Ronchi, G., Del Ninno, E. and Colombo, M. (1999) High prevalence of multinodular hepatocellular carcinoma in patients with cirrhosis attributable to multiple risk factors. *Hepatology* **29**, 1704–1707.

Frank, W.O., Rayes, A.N., Washinton, A. and Holt, P.R. (1982) Effect of acute ethanol administration on hepatic regeneration. *J Lab Clin Med* **93**, 402–413.

Garro, A.J., Seitz, H.K. and Lieber, C.S. (1981) Enhancement of dimethylnitrosamine metabolism and activation to a mutagen following chronic ethanol consumption. *Cancer Res* **41**, 120–124.

Gludd, C., Aldershville, T., Henriksen, J., Kryger, P. and Mathieson, L. (1982) Hepatitis B and A virus antibodies in alcoholic hepatitis and cirrhosis. *J Clin Pathol* **35**, 693–697.

Grando-Lemaire, V., Guettier, C., Chevret, S., Beaugrand, M. and Trinchet, J.C. (1999) Hepatocellular carcinoma without cirrhosis in the West: epidemiological factors and histopathology of the non-tumorous liver. Groupe d'Etude et de Traitement du Carcinome Hepatocellulaire. *J Hepatol* **31**, 508–513.

Gray, M.R., Donnelly, R.J. and Kingsnorth, A.N. (1993) The role of smoking and alcohol in metaplasia and cancer risk in Barrett's columnar lined oesophagus. *Gut* **34**, 727–731.

Hoek, J.B., Thomas, A.P., Rooney, T.A., Higashi, K. and Rubin, E. (1992) Ethanol and signal transduction in the liver. *FASEB J* **6**, 2386–2396.

Jetten, A.M. (1985) Retinoids and their modulation of cell growth. In *Growth and Maturation Factors*, edited by G. Guroff, Vol 3, pp. 252–293. New York: Wiley.

Kato, K., Nishimura, D., Sano, H., Katada, N., Sugimoto, Y., Noba, H., Yoshino, M., Samori, T., Mitani, Y. and Takeichi, M. (1990) Long-term follow-up study of alcoholic liver disease. *Nippon Shokakibyo Gakkai Zasshi – Japanese Journal of Gastroenterology* **87**, 1829–1836.

Kew, M.C. (1984) The relationship between HCC and cirrhosis. *Seminars in Liver Disease* **4**, 136–149.

Kunitoh, S., Imaoka, S., Hiroi, T., Yabusaki, Y., Monna, T. and Funae, Y. (1997) Acetaldehyde as well as ethanol is metabolized by human CYP2E1. *J Pharmacol Exp Ther* **280**, 527–532.

Kuratsune, M., Kohohi, S., Horie, A. and Nishizumi, M. (1965) Test of alcoholic beverages and ethanol solutions for carcinogencity and tumor promoting activity. *Gann* **62**, 395–405.

La Vecchia, C., Negri, E., Cavalieri d'Oro, L. and Franceschi, S. (1998) Liver cirrhosis and the risk of primary liver cancer. *Eur J Cancer Prev* **7**, 315–320.

Lee, F. (1996) Cirrhosis and hepatoma in alcoholics. *Gut* **7**, 77–85.

Lee, H.S., Yoon, J.H., Kamimura, S., Iwata, K., Watanabe, H. and Kim, C.Y. (1997) Lack of association of cytochrome P450 2E1 genetic polymorphisms with the risk of human hepatocellular carcinoma. *Int J Cancer* **71**, 737–740.

Leo, M.A. and Lieber, C.S. (1982) Hepatic vitamin A depletion in alcoholic liver injury in man. *N Eng J Med* **307**, 597–607.

Kim, D.-E., Lee, D.-Y., Cho, B.-H., You, K.-R., Kim, M.-Y. and Ahn, D.-S. (1999) Down regulation of insulin-like growth factor binding proteins and growth modulation in hepatoma cells by retinoic acid. *Hepatology* **29**, 1091–1098.

Koga, H., Sakisaka, S., Ohishi, M., Kawaguch, T., Taniguchi, E., Satsumoto, K., Harada, M., Kusaba, T., Tanaka, M., Kimura, R., Nakashima, Y., Kakashima, O., Kojiro, M., Kurohiji, T. and Sata, M. (1999) Expression of cyclooxygenase-2 in human hepatocellular carcinoma: relevance to tumor differentiation. *Hepatology* **29**, 688–696.

Lieber, C.S., Garro, A.J., Leo, M.A., Mak, K.M. and Worner, T. (1986) Alcohol and cancer. *Hepatology* **6**, 1005–1019.

Lieber, C.S., Seitz, H.K., Garrow, A.J. and Worner, T.N. (1981) Alcohol as a co-carcinogen. In *Frontiers of Liver Disease*, edited by P.D. Berk and T.C. Charmers, pp. 320–335. Stuttgart: Thieme.

Makimoto, K. and Higuchi, S. (1999) Alcohol consumption as a major risk factor for the rise in liver cancer mortality rates in Japanese men. *Int J Epidemiol* **28**, 30–34.

McKillop, I.H., Vyas, N., Schmidt, C.M., Cahill, P.A. and Sitzmann, J.V. (1999a) Enhanced Gi-protein-mediated mitogenesis following chronic ethanol exposure in a rat model of experimental hepatocellular carcinoma. *Hepatology* **29**, 412–420.

McKillop, I.H., Schmidt, C.M., Cahill, P.A. and Sitzmann, J.V. (1999b) Altered Gq/G11 guanine nucleotide regulatory protein expression in a rat model of hepatocellular carcinoma: role in mitogenesis. *Hepatology* **29**, 371–378.

Miyakawa, H., Izumi, N., Mazumo, F. and Sato, C. (1996) Roles of alcohol, hepatitis virus infection and gender in the development of hepatocellular carcinoma in patients with liver cirrhosis. *Alcoholism, Clinical and Experimental Research* **20** (suppl 1), 91A–94A.

Nanji, A.A., Griniuviene, B., Sadrzadeh, S.M.H., Levitsky, S. and McCully, J.D. (1995) Effect of type of dietary fat and ethanol on antioxidant enzyme mRNA induction in rat liver. *J Lipid Res* **36**, 736–744.

Nanji, A.A., Miao, L. and Thomas, P. (1997) Enhanced cyclooxgenase-2 gene expression in alcoholic liver disease in the rat. *Gastroenterology* **112**, 943–951.

Nanji, A.A., Khettry, U., Sadrzaheh, S.M.H. and Yamanaka, T. (1993) Severity of liver injury in experimental alcoholic liver disease: correlation with plasma endotoxin, prostaglandin E2, leukotriene B4 and thromboxane B2. *Am J Pathol* **142**, 367–373.

Nishiuchi, M. and Shinji, Y. (1990) Increased incidence of hepatocellular carcinoma in abstinent patients with alcoholic cirrhosis. Gan to Kagaku Ryoho *Japanese Journal of Cancer & Chemotherapy* **17**, 1–6.

Ohnishi, K., Lida, S., Iwana, S., Gato, N., Nomura, F., Takahashi, M., Mishima, A., Kono, K., Kimura, K., Muska, H., Kotata, K. and Okuda, K. (1982) The effect of chronic habitual alcohol intake on the development of liver cirrhosis and hepatocellular carcinoma. *Cancer* **49**, 672–677.

Okuda, K., Suzuki, N., Kubo, Y. and Obata, H. (1979) Clinical aspects of hepatocellular carcinoma. In *Advances in Medical Oncology, Research and Education*, edited by N. Thatcher, pp. 133–140. London: Churchill Livingstone.

Oshima, A., Tsukuma, H., Hiyama, T., Fujimoto, I., Yamano, H. and Tanaka, M. (1984) Follow-up study of hepatitis B surface antigen positive blood donors with special reference to the effect of drinking and smoking on development of liver cancer. *Int J Cancer* **34**, 775–779.

Ozturk, M., Bressac, B., Puisieux, A., Kew, M., Volkmann, M., Bozcall, S., Mura, J.B., De La Monte, S., Carlson, R., Blum, H. and Takahashi H. (1991) p53 mutations and HCC after aflatoxin exposure. *Lancet* **388**, 1356–1359.

Pelech, S.L., Charest, D.L., Mordet, G.P., Siow, Y.L., Palaty, C., Campbell, D., Charlton, L. *et al.* (1993) Networking with mitogen protein kinases. *Mol Cell Biochem* **127/128**, 157–169.

Qiao, Z.K., Halliday, M.L., Rankin, J.G. and Coates, R.A. (1988) Relationship between hepatitis B surface antigen prevalence, per capita alcohol consumption and primary liver cancer death rates in 30 countries. *J Clin Epidemiol* **41**, 787–792.

Rao, C.V., Rivenson, A., Simi, B., Zang, E., Kelloff, G., Steele, V. and Reddy, B.S. (1995) Chemoprevention of colon carcinogenesis by sulindac, a non-steroidal anti-inflammatory agent. *Cancer Res* **55**, 1464–1472.

Reddy, M.A. and Shukla, S.D. (1996) Potentiation of mitogen-activated protein kinase by ethanol in embryonic liver cells. *Biochem Pharmacol* **51**, 661–668.

Roberts, R.A. (1996) Non-genotoxic hepatocarcinogenesis: suppression of apoptosis by peroxisome proliferators. *Ann N Y Acad Sci* **804**, 588–611.

Schmidt, C.M., McKillop, I.H., Cahill, P.A. and Sitzmann, J.V. (1997) Increased MAPK expression and activity in primary human hepatocellular carcinoma. *Biochem Biophys Res Commun* **236**, 54–58.

Seitz, H.K., Poschl, G. and Simanowski, U.A. (1998) Alcohol and cancer. *Recent Dev Alcohol* **14**, 67–95.

Shikata, T. (1976) Primary liver cell cancer and liver cirrhosis. Edited by K. Okuda and R.L. Peters, pp. 53–72. Wiley: New York.

Smith, P.G., Tee, L.B. and Yeoh, G.C. (1996) Appearance of oval cells in the liver of rats after long term exposure to ethanol. *Hepatology* **23**, 145–154.

Sternhagen, A., Slade, J., Altman, R. and Bill, J. (1983) Occupational risk factors and liver cancer in New Jersey. A retrospective, case control study of primary liver cell cancer. *Am J Epidemiol* **1167**, 443–454.

Suzuki, M., Suzuki, H., Mizuno, H., Tominaga, T., Kono, M., Kato, Y., Sato, A. and Okabe, K. (1993) Studies on the incidence of hepatocellular carcinoma in heavy drinkers with liver cirrhosis. *Alcohol and Alcoholism* **28**, 109–114.

Teschke, R., Minzlaff, M., Oldiges, H. and Frenzel, H. (1983) Effect of chronic alcohol consumption on tumour incidence due to DMN administration. *J Cancer Res Clin Oncol* **106**, 58–64.

Tsugane, S., Fahey, M.T., Sasaki, S. and Baba, S. (1999) Alcohol consumption and all-cause and cancer mortality among middle-aged Japanese men: seven-year follow-up of the JPHC study Cohort I. Japan Public Health Center. *Am J Epidemiol* 1; **150**, 1201–1207.

Tsuji, M. and DuBois, R.N. (1995) Alterations in cellular adhesion and apoptosis in epithelial cells overexpressing prostaglandin endoperoxidase synthase 2. *Cell* **83**, 493–501.

Tsukamoto, H., Horne, W. and Kamimura, S. (1995) Experimental liver cirrhosis induced by alcohol and iron. *J Clin Invest* **96**, 620–630.

Vautier, G., Bomford, A., Portmann, B., Metivier, E., Williams, R. and Ryder, S. (1999) p53 mutations in British patients with hepatocellular carcinoma: clustering in genetic hemochromatosis. *Gastroenterology* **117**, 154–160.

von Weizsacker, F., Maedi, E. and Brown, N.V. (1995) Hepatitis B and C virus infection in HBsAg negative alcoholics without IV drug use or previous drug transfusions. *Int Hepatol Commun* **4**, 80–87.

Walker, E.A., Castegnaro, M., Garren, L., Touissant, G. and Kowalski, B. (1979) Intake of volatile nitrosamines from consumption of alcohol. *J Natl Cancer Inst* **63**, 947–951.

Walter, E., Blum, H.E., Meier, P., Huonker, M., Schmid, M., Maier, K.P., Offensperger, W.B., Offensperger, S. and Gerok, W. (1988) Hepatocellular carcinoma in alcoholic liver disease: no evidence for a pathogenetic role of hepatitis B virus infection. *Hepatology* **8**, 745–748.

Wang, X.D. (1999) Chronic alcohol intake interferes with retinoid metabolism and signaling. *Nutr Rev* **57**, 51–59.

Zhou, S.L., Gordon, R.E., Bradbury, M., Stump, D., Kiang, C.L. and Berk, P.D. (1998) Ethanol up-regulates fatty acid uptake and plasma membrane expression and export of mitochondrial aspartate aminotransferase in HepG2 cells. *Hepatology* **27**, 1064–1074.

Chapter 15

Animal models of ethanol-induced liver damage

Harri A. Järveläinen and Kai O. Lindros

Animals have been administered in ethanol chronically by various methods in order to develop liver lesions resembling those seen in human alcoholics. For lesions to develop, the daily intake of ethanol must result in sustained high blood alcohol levels. In rats this has been achieved by administration of ethanol as a component of a nutritionally adequate liquid diet, either orally or by forced intragastric infusion. To cause liver lesions beyond steatosis, the content of carbohydrates in the ethanol liquid diet must be low and the fat rich in polyunsatured fatty acids. Fibrotic changes are difficult to produce in rats, but are observed in micropigs and baboons, that can be kept on ethanol liquid diet for many months. Even cirrhosis is produced in baboons kept for several years on ethanol diet. Much of our rapidly expanded knowledge on the contribution of different factors in the development of injury is based on these animal models, but many questions remain. Most recently, ethanol treatment models have been applied to knock-out mice to study the involvement of specific gene products in the disease process. In the further development of these models, more emphasis should be put on long-term models, that better mimic the slow progression of human liver damage. In the continued efforts to understand this disease, current and future animal models clearly will remain important tools. Once the basic mechanisms are delineated in more detail, this knowledge can be used in the development of new therapeutic strategies.

KEYWORDS: animal models, liquid ethanol diet, nutritional requirements, fatty liver, inflammation, cytokines, experimental liver cirrhosis

INTRODUCTION

Animal models have been of invaluable help in elucidating mechanisms of human diseases. During the last decades various models have also been applied to study the pathogenesis of alcohol-associated liver injury. In spite of much progress, the role of different factors contributing to the development and aggravation of alcoholic liver disease (ALD) remain poorly defined. Alcoholic liver damage is commonly regarded as a diffuse multifactorial disease and ethanol as an idiosynchratic hepatotoxin. Although the risk of developing cirrhosis increases with the duration and extent of alcohol abuse, only 15–25% of alcoholics ever develop serious ALD (Savolainen *et al.*, 1993; Becker *et al.*, 1996). Accepting the fact that there are confounding factors interacting with ethanol may explain why there is no animal model that would replicate all the pathological features of human ALD.

Regardless of what aspect of ALD is studied, a successful model should be reproducible and have a minimum of complicating side effects. For practical reasons it should also be technically and economically feasible. Most experimental ALD studies have been performed with rats. The biology of the laboratory rat is well known, the handling is easy and the costs are moderate. Consequently, this review will deal mainly with this species. The baboon model, successfully developed in the early seventies (Lieber and DeCarli, 1975), should be superior to other animal models, since extrapolation to human ALD can be expected to be more straightforward. Indeed, much valuable and relevant information has been obtained with primates, but the model is very expensive. In addition to rats and primates, promising data based on micropigs and mice have been obtained. These models will also be briefly presented. A survey of animal models currently in use is presented in Table 15.1.

To overcome the natural aversion of most animals to ethanol, it is administered as a component of a totally liquid diet, that provides a maximum of 30–50% of total calories from alcohol. This situation resembles that of many alcoholics, who often receive up to 50% of their total energy as ethanol (Patek *et al.*, 1975; Salaspuro and Lieber, 1980). To maximize ethanol intake without compromising the nutritional balance poses a problem. Consequently, the role of nutritional factors remains an important and somewhat controversial issue.

Several excellent reviews describing the earlier use of animal models in ALD have been published (Lieber *et al.*, 1989; Lieber and DeCarli, 1989a; Tsukamoto, 1990; Goldin, 1994; French *et al.*, 1995; Thurman, 1998). The reader is referred to these texts for more background information.

STAGES OF ALCOHOL LIVER DISEASE IN MAN AND ANIMALS

Chronic ethanol administration to rodents has been demonstrated to lead to a number of hepatic changes including steatosis, hepatocellular necrosis, inflammatory cell infiltration, terminal hepatic venular sclerosis, proliferation of the smooth endoplasmic reticulum and mitochondrial abberrations (Iseri *et al.*, 1966; Lieber and DeCarli, 1976; Tsukamoto *et al.*, 1985a). All these changes also occur in the early phase of human alcoholic liver disease, demonstrating the relevance of the experimental models (MacSween and Burt, 1986; Hall, 1995).

On the other hand, lesions beyond these changes, such as alcoholic hepatitis, Mallory bodies and full blown cirrhosis are seen only exceptionally in animal models. These lesions are only produced in the presence of additional factors or in combination with some type of nutritional deficiency. General conclusions based on the results obtained by such models therefore must be made judiciously. Furthermore, a clear distinction must be made between the experimental production of steatosis and more severe damage. Steatosis is considered to be a rapid and direct result of alcohol ingestion, but the evidence that inflammation and necrosis can develop as a result of alcohol toxicity alone is less convincing.

Alcoholic fatty liver

Steatosis is considered mainly as a direct consequence of the metabolism of ethanol. It encompasses reduced fatty acid oxidation, increased triglyceride synthesis,

Table 15.1 Survey of animal models in experimental alcohol liver disease

Alcohol administration model	Duration, species and gender	Daily ethanol consumption (g/kg body wt.)	Blood alcohol levels (BAL; mg/dl)	Fold-elevation of ALAT (/ASAT)	Fatty liver	Focal inflammation	Focal necrosis	Fibrosis	Cirrhosis	Comments
Oral Lieber-DeCarli liquid diet (Lieber et al., 1989)	4–6 weeks male rats	12–18	~0–150	–	X	–	–	–	–	Modest BALs, only steatosis.
Oral 4-MP–liquid diet model (Lindros et al., 1983)	3 months male rats	12	100–350	N.D.	X	X	X	–	–	Sustained elevation of BALs. Effect of 4-methylpyrazole (4-MP) on CYP2E1? Sustained high BALs.
Oral LOC model (low-carbohydrate liquid diet, Lindros and Järveläinen, 1998)	6 weeks male rats	12–18	150–250	2–3x	X	X	X	–	–	Sustained high BALs.
Oral LOC model (Järveläinen et al., 2001)	6 weeks female rats	12–18	150–350	7x	X	X	X	–	–	Sustained high BAL, advanced liver injury.
Oral alcohol (→40%) in drinking water (Keegan et al., 1995)	29 weeks male rats	11–15	~100	–	X	X	X	–	–	Locally bred Wistar rats. Restricted diet intake!
Intragastric alcohol feeding model (Tsukamoto et al., 1985a)	6 weeks male rats	11–13	~0–500	2–3x	X	X	X	–	–	BAL cycling phenomenon. Technical complications?
Intragastric alcohol feeding, prolonged treatment (Tsukamoto et al., 1986)	3–6 months male rats	11–13	~0–500	2–10x	X	X	X	X	–	In addition to above: fibrotic changes in rat.
Intragastric intubation daily (Enomoto et al., 1999)	6 weeks female rats	5	~0–350	2–3x	X	X	X	–	–	–
Ethanol vapour inhalation (Goldin et al., 1987)	3 weeks female mice	?	40–160	(2.5x)	X	X	X	–	–	Requires individual BAL monitoring.
Knock-out mice, intragastric alcohol feeding model (Kono et al., 1999)	4 weeks male mice	28	0–400	2–3	X	X	X	–	–	Risk of high mortality.
Micropig model (Halsted et al., 1993)	1 year male micropigs	5–6	~180	2x	X	X	X	X	–	Fibrosis with a high-fat diet.
Baboon model (Lieber et al., 1975)	2–4 years male baboons	3–5	~380	2–3x	X	X	X	X	X	Fibrosis in most animals, cirrhosis in some.

reduced fat export and mobilization of extrahepatic fat stores (Lindros, 1995). Fatty infiltration is usually macrovacuolar, with one large fat droplet per hepatocyte and lateral displacement of the nucleus (Ishak *etal.*, 1991). Microvesicular steatosis, characterized by many small fat droplets in an enlarged liver cell, is also common (Fromenty and Pessayre, 1995). A mixture of macro- and microvesicular steatosis is frequently observed. It was long considered that steatosis was a rather benign condition, due to its rapid disappearance upon ethanol withdrawal (Lieber and Rubin, 1968). However, more recent studies confirm earlier suspicions that the cellular changes taking place during the fatty infiltration, particularly the microvesicular form, may sensitize the cells to further injury. In fact, both experimental and clinical data suggest an association between the severity of fatty accumulation and the development of damage (Sorensen *etal.*, 1984; Nanji *etal.*, 1989c; Day and James, 1998).

Experimental studies have clearly shown that the amount and type of fat affects the development of fatty liver. Thus, steatosis increases with the long-chain fatty acid content of the diet and the composition of the dietary fat is reflected in that of the lipids accumulating in the liver of ethanol-fed animals (Lieber and Decarli, 1970a). Aggravation of alcohol-induced fatty liver is also seen if diet is low in protein or carbohydrates (Yonekura *etal.*, 1989; Nanji *etal.*, 1989a; Sankaran *etal.*, 1994). In man, early alcohol-induced fatty infiltration predominates in the centrilobular zone (MacSween and Burt, 1986), but this is not consistently seen in animals. In rats either centrilobular, periportal or panlobular fat accumulation is observed, depending on dietary factors, and also on gender (Lindros and Järveläinen, 1998; Thurman, 1998).

Inflammation and necrosis

Our knowledge on how inflammation develops and on the immunological response has expanded rapidly. Kupffer cell activation and release of pro-inflammatory cytokines have been shown to be crucial events in the development of ALD (Schenker and Bay, 1995; Zeldin *etal.*, 1996). Acute hepatitis in man is characterized by infiltration of polymorphonuclear leukocytes, hepatocyte degeneration and necrosis. Appearance of Mallory bodies is common, but not considered an obligatory diagnostic sign (MacSween and Burt, 1986; Hall, 1995). The inflammatory lesions seen in animals are somewhat different. In rodents the corresponding lesion is best described as inflammatory cell infiltration rather than hepatitis. In most studies no more than 1–2 mononuclear inflammatory foci per liver lobulus are seen, occasionally even in livers of controls (Nanji *etal.*, 1989a).

Animal experiments do not provide direct evidence that ethanol *per se* would cause inflammation. There is evidence for an involvement of bacterial endotoxins and viral hepatitis (Sata *etal.*, 1996; Thurman, 1998). Furthermore, oxidative stress induced either by dietary polyunsatured fatty acids or by iron supplementation may aggravate inflammation (Nanji *etal.*, 1994; Tsukamoto *etal.*, 1995). A more pronounced inflammatory response seen in livers from female rats as compared to males suggests an immunomodulatory effect of estrogen (Thurman, 1998; Yin *etal.*, 2000).

Only restricted hepatocyte necrosis, either single cell or focal, has been observed in rodents (Tsukamoto *etal.*, 1985a; Järveläinen *etal.*, 2001) and baboons (Popper and Lieber, 1980). Extensive liver cell necrosis, characterized by polymorpho-nuclear neutrophil infiltration, is not ordinarily observed in animal experiments, but can be precipitated by an acute endotoxin challenge to chronically ethanol fed rats with steatotic hepatocytes (Bhagwandeen *et al.*, 1987; Pennington *et al.*, 1997). In contrast, chronic intravenous endotoxin produces no such lesions in ethanol treated rats, in spite of sinusoidal polymorphonuclear infiltration. This suggests that in the rat, marked tolerance develops to the continuous presence of endotoxin (Järveläinen *et al.*, 1999).

Fibrosis and cirrhosis

Centrilobular fibrosis is considered the first irreversible step progressing into severe fibrotic changes and eventually to cirrhosis (Worner and Lieber, 1985; MacSween and Burt, 1986). The hepatic stellate cells (HSCs) are responsible for the production of collagens and other extracellular matrix proteins involved in hepatic fibrosis (Friedman, 1997). The mechanisms of HSC activation are still partly unknown. Increased inflammatory activity, oxygen-derived free radicals, ethanol itself and its metabolite acetaldehyde have been invoked (Lieber, 1991a; Niemelä *et al.*, 1995).

Fibrotic changes seldom appear in rats fed ethanol and a normal diet, but can be provoked with dietary manipulations. A high-fat ethanol diet marginal in choline, proteins and vitamins caused centrilobular fibrosis in 3 months (French *et al.*, 1988a; French *et al.*, 1988b). This was also achieved by oversupplementation of ethanol liquid diet with vitamin A (Leo and Lieber, 1983) and in studies with baboons and micropigs (Porto *et al.*, 1989; Lieber *et al.*, 1990; Niemelä *et al.*, 1999).

Cirrhosis seldom develops in alcoholics until after at least 10–20 years of heavy drinking. It is commonly micronodular, with uniformly sized regenerating small nodules surrounded by fibrotic tissue (MacSween and Burt, 1986). To replicate such severe changes by ethanol exposure alone in animal models has proven difficult. In rodents cirrhosis only develops if ethanol is combined with a nutritionally defi-cient diet, by dietary supplementation with carbonyl-iron, or by inclusion of another hepatotoxin such as carbon tetrachloride (Hall *et al.*, 1991; Bosma *et al.*, 1994; Tsukamoto *et al.*, 1995). In baboon experiments lasting 1–8 years, one out of five animals developed cirrhosis (Lieber and DeCarli, 1975; Popper and Lieber, 1980; Lieber *et al.*, 1990). It is of interest that this resembles the unpredictable precipitation of cirrhosis in humans, although the possibility of a nutritional con-founding factor cannot be excluded (Ainley *et al.*, 1988).

EVALUATION OF PATHOLOGICAL CHANGES IN ANIMALS

Results based on the histopathological analysis can be supported by assay from plasma of liver specific enzymes and metabolites. The histopathological score usu-ally encompasses steatotic, inflammatory, necrotic and fibrotic changes. The way of expression of the frequency of inflammatory and necrotic changes in experi-mental ALD is not well standardized. It would appear advisable to express the number of necrotic hepatocytes and polymorphonuclear cells per square mm liver tissue (Iimuro et al., 1997) and to examine different lobes. Animal studies have the advantage that they allow sequential sampling and analysis of liver biopsies during the course of the ethanol treatment (French et al., 1988b; Cmielewski et al., 1997), so that temporal changes can be followed (Nanji et al., 1995a).

Valuable additional information can now be obtained from analysis of the activation of various signal molecules, such as the pro-inflammatory cytokines TNF-α, IL-1 and IL-6 (McClain et al., 1993; Lands, 1995), mediators of leukocyte adhesion in the endothelium (i.e., ICAM-1) (Nanji et al., 1995b) and of molecules indicating endotoxin-induced Kupffer cell activation, such as the lipopolysaccharide binding protein LBP and the endotoxin receptor CD14 (Järveläinen et al., 1997, 1999). Immunological analysis of these proteins appear to have great promise as additional diagnostic and prognostic indicators of alcoholic liver disease (Burra et al., 1992; Oesterreicher et al., 1995; McClain et al., 1999).

METHODS OF CHRONIC ETHANOL ADMINISTRATION TO RODENTS

Ethanol is a drug and also a rich source of energy. One gram ethanol contains about 7 kilocalories, as compared to about 9 for fats and 4.5 for carbohydrates and proteins. Accordingly, alcoholics frequently obtain 30–50% of their daily calories from ethanol. Much work has been done to develop animal models mimicking this situation without severely compromising the general health or the nutritional balance of the animals. In most cases animals do not voluntarily consume enough ethanol if it is added to their drinking fluid. To overcome this, ethanol has been administered by gavage, by inhalation, by forced intragastric infusion or as a component of an orally consumed totally liquid diet.

Oral alcohol feeding models

Alcohol in drinking water

Simple inclusion of ethanol in the drinking fluid does not ordinarily cause sustained elevation of blood ethanol levels. Liver triglycerides may be moderately elevated, but no other histologically observable changes are observed. If the ethanol concentration is increased, the total fluid intake commonly is reduced, resulting in dehydration, reduced food intake and ceased growth rate. A 15% ethanol solution providing 18% of total calories does not even produce fatty liver when given with a nutritionally adequate diet (Best et al., 1949). The aversive taste of ethanol can be partly overcome by adding sucrose or artificial sweeteners, such as aspartame and cyclamate (Plummer et al., 1997). The ethanol content can also be substantially elevated after appropriate initiation procedures (Slawecki and Samson, 1996). Locally bred Wistar male rats on 40% ethanol/2% sucrose fluid and fed a low fat/ high-carbohydrate chow diet were reported to develop macrovacuolar steatosis, inflammation, hepatocyte necrosis and pericentral sclerosis in 29 weeks (Keegan *et al.*, 1995). In this study daily ethanol consumption (11–15 g/kg) resulted in moderately elevated blood ethanol levels throughout the day. This is an interesting study that needs to be replicated in other laboratories.

Additional supplementation of ethanol in agar gels has been reported (Landrigan *et al.*, 1989). In spite of the surprisingly high daily ethanol intake reported in these rats (30 g/kg), a 16 week treatment only resulted in micro/macrovesicular fatty changes.

The presence of ethanol has also been maximized by using specific inhibitors of alcohol dehydrogenase, the main ethanol metabolizing enzyme of the liver. The consistent presence of ethanol in rats given 4-methylpyrazole to attenuate ethanol metabolism by approximately 20%, resulted in more severe lesions as compared to pair-fed rats metabolizing identical amounts of ethanol in the 17.5% drinking fluid (15–17 g/kg/d) (Lindros *et al.*, 1984).

Alcohol administration by liquid diet

The method to force rats to consume high amounts of ethanol by its inclusion in a balanced liquid diet, that contains sufficient water and all necessary nutrients, was developed almost four decades ago (Lieber *et al.*, 1963) and proved very useful in studies of the pathogenesis of early ethanol-induced changes. Controls were pair-fed an equicaloric amount of diet with ethanol replaced by carbohydrates (Lieber *et al.*, 1989). The original diet was a mixture of sucrose, amino acids and an oil suspension. The improved formula consisted of casein (providing 18% of calories) supplemented with methionine and cystine, a mixture of dextrin and maltose (providing 11% and 47% of calories for ethanol and control diet respectively) and fat (35% of calories, mainly olive oil, corn oil and safflower oil). All essential vitamins (A, D, E, K, Bs), minerals and fiber were present (Lieber and DeCarli, 1986; Lieber *et al.*, 1989). The amount of ethanol in the diet was gradually increased during the first week to provide 36% of total calories. This proportion was found to be crucial. Little steatosis developed if ethanol provided 30% of total calories, while increasing ethanol calories to 40% led to reduced diet intake (Lieber and Decarli, 1970a, 1989a).

The Lieber-DeCarli formula has been extensively used in rodent studies. The average daily ethanol intake, 12–15 g/kg, resulted in fatty liver and in metabolic tolerance, i.e., their ethanol elimination rate was increased (Lieber and DeCarli, 1970b). A 6-fold increase in hepatic triglycerides was observed after 1 month of feeding, an effect that persisted for 22 weeks (Lieber and DeCarli, 1970a). For proper fatty liver to develop, at least 21% of the calories had to be derived from fat (Lieber and DeCarli, 1970a), although even a low-fat (13%) ethanol diet causes some steatosis (Di Luzio and Hartman, 1969). The incorporation pattern of dietary fatty acids in liver triglycerides indicated that most fat comes from the diet (Lieber *et al.*, 1966) and much less from hepatic lipogenesis (Tsukamoto *et al.*, 1984a). Lesions beyond steatosis are rare in this model. For example, rats fed for up to 9 months had no fibrotic changes (Leo and Lieber, 1983). This probably is a consequence of the rather modest blood ethanol levels achieved with this regimen (Lieber *et al.*, 1989). The levels fluctuate between 0–1.5‰ with the circadian rhythm.

Sustained high blood alcohol concentration indeed seems to be a prerequisite for the progression of alcoholic liver disease process beyond steatosis (Lieber and DeCarli, 1976; French *et al.*, 1995; Lindros and Järveläinen, 1998). Evidence for this was first obtained by adding a low dose of 4-methyl pyrazole (4-MP) to the diet to decelerate alcohol metabolism by about 20%. Rats on this diet had elevated ethanol levels and developed steatosis, inflammation and mild necrosis in 12 weeks (Lindros *et al.*, 1983). A later study demonstrated exacerbated damage with an increased fat content (Takada *et al.*, 1986). However, it cannot be excluded that 4-MP, even at low doses, may have had side effects (Lieber and DeCarli, 1970a), including additional induction of CYP2E1, which may be pathogenic (Koop *et al.*, 1985; Dicker *et al.*, 1991).

Recently, a modified Lieber-DeCarli low-carbohydrate (5% of calories)/high fat (44% of calories) liquid diet model was presented (Lindros and Järveläinen, 1998). Rats on this regimen had continuously elevated blood ethanol levels (1.5–3‰), with only moderate diurnal fluctuation. A low carbohydrate content of the diet may reduce the rate of ethanol metabolism (Rao *et al.*, 1987). In 6 weeks, this liquid diet regimen resulted in the appearance of mixed macro- and microvesicular steatosis and inflammatory foci (Figure 15.1). In addition, increased levels of endotoxin and cytokine activation was observed (Järveläinen *et al.*, 1999), further supporting the pathogenic role of persistently elevated blood ethanol levels.

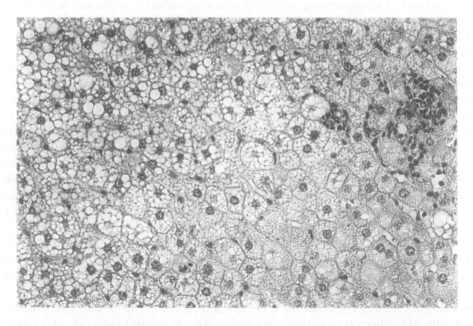

Figure 15.1 Marked steatosis and an inflammatory spot in a liver of a rat after consuming low-carbohydrate/high-fat ethanol liquid diet for 6 weeks. Note the high incidence of microvesicular steatosis. Details of the alcohol treatment are given in Lindros and Järveläinen (1998). (see *Color Plate 7*)

Considering the natural aversion to ethanol of rats, induction of maximal ethanol acceptance is critical. Consequently, animals have been started on ethanol soon after weanling (Landrigan *et al.*, 1989). However, to avoid a possible nutritional imbalance in growing animals with a high metabolic turnover, ethanol treatment is usually initiated in adult rats, in spite of their lower relative ethanol intake (Miller *et al.*, 1980).

Since the presence of ethanol in the diet reduces total intake, controls are pair-fed an equicaloric amount of control diet. Ethanol diet is consumed in small portions, but pair-fed controls consume their daily ration in a few hours and can be considered to be starved the rest of the day. This has to be kept in mind if parameters that are influenced by starvation, such as the expression of CYP2E1 and deposition of glycogen, are investigated (Hu *et al.*, 1995). To account for this, a system that provided control diet by "continuous pair-feeding" was developed (Israel *et al.*, 1984). This rather complicated method has not been generally accepted and may not be needed in most studies investigating pathogenic mechanisms.

Clearly, an oral ethanol liquid diet feeding model has several advantages. Many animals can be treated in parallel, which enables comparison of several different regimens in the same experiment. The technique is relatively inexpensive and the rate of mortality is low. Most importantly, the amount of daily ethanol intake is high and sufficient for production of many of the pathological changes in ALD.

Forced intragastric infusion of liquid ethanol diet

The method of administering drugs via an intragastrically implanted gastrostomy tube (Lukas and Moreton, 1979) was first applied in ethanol studies by Forssell (1981). Intragastric infusion of ethanol solution for 3 weeks was found to result in accumulation of liver triglycerides and elevated serum liver enzymes. French and Tsukamoto combined this method with the Lieber-DeCarli liquid diet model (French *et al.*, 1984; Tsukamoto *et al.*, 1984b). A nutritionally adequate liquid diet with up to 47% of total calories as ethanol was infused into the stomach. By regular monitoring of blood ethanol levels, the ethanol infusion rate could be titrated (to an average of 12–13 g/kg/d) and high blood ethanol levels achieved. As in the oral feeding model, controls were infused isocaloric amounts of ethanol-free diet, with carbohydrates replacing ethanol. This model is currently used by a handful laboratories in the US and has for a long time been considered the best rodent model and has been an invaluable tool for investigating pathogenic mechanisms of ALD (Tsukamoto *et al.*, 1990). Steatosis, focal inflammation and necrotic cells appear in 6 weeks (Figure 15.2) (French *et al.*, 1995).

The gastrostomy tube is usually implanted on adult rats weighing 300–400 g (Tsukamoto *et al.*, 1985a), but growing rats weighing 200–250 g have also been used (French, 1993). In younger animals the liver injury was found to be more severe and the fibrotic activity stronger (Takahashi *et al.*, 1990). Either single or double gastrostomy cannulas have been inserted via the neck into the stomach. The tube is connected to spring coils and swivels to protect cannulas and permit free movement of the infused animal (Tsukamoto *et al.*, 1985a). Daily monitoring of alcohol intoxication is necessary, since the rate of ethanol infusion needs to be adjusted to achieve consistently high, yet tolerable ethanol levels. Monitoring of

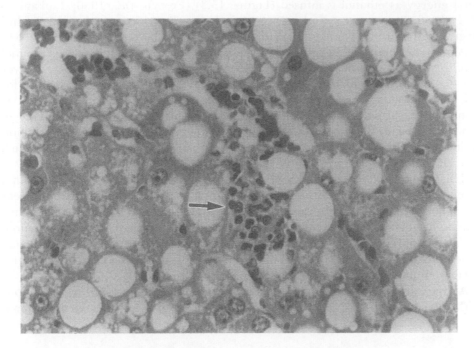

Figure 15.2 Focal necrosis (arrow) and associated pericentral inflammation in a liver of a rat after six weeks of intragastric feeding. Note that the fatty changes are mainly macrovacuolar. HE staining. (Figures 15.2 and 15.3 are courtesy of Dr Samuel French, Harbor-UCLA Medical Center, Department of Pathology, Torrance, CA.) (see *Color Plate 8*)

ethanol inebriation is by jugular blood or urine sampling and also by visual inspection of the animals (Badger *et al.*, 1993; Yin *et al.*, 1999).

The intragastric feeding technique was recently applied to mice (Zhang-Gouillon *et al.*, 1998). Knock-out mice were treated to investigate the role of specific gene products in ALD (Yin *et al.*, 1999). This is a promising but demanding avenue. Even with high surgical skill the rate of mortality may be high (Zhang-Gouillon *et al.*, 1998). Moreover, since mice metabolize ethanol extremely rapidly, it is difficult to maintain high blood ethanol levels without compromising the nutritional balance.

As for the oral liquid diet model, the macrocomposition of the intragastrically fed diet is crucial. A high-fat/low-carbohydrate diet causes more severe damage, while an ethanol diet with 21% carbohydrate only results in steatosis (French, 1993; Korourian *et al.*, 1999). Also, few lesions develop unless the diet contains oils rich in unsaturated fatty acids, such as corn oil (Nanji *et al.*, 1989b). Indeed, the most severe lesions after ethanol are observed with fish oil, which has a very high content of polyunsaturated fatty acids (Nanji *et al.*, 1994). All rats on a low-carbohydrate/high-fat ethanol diet developed macro- and microvesicular steatosis and focal necrosis and mononuclear inflammation in 30–50% of the animals (Tsukamoto *et al.*, 1985a; Tsukamoto *et al.*, 1986; French *et al.*, 1988b). Early perivenous fibrogenesis starts to develop in 3–6 months, provided that a high-fat diet with 42% to 49% of total energy as ethanol is infused (Figure 15.3) (French *et al.*, 1986; Tsukamoto *et al.*, 1986; Kamimura *et al.*, 1992). Addition of carbonyl iron to the diet further aggravates injurious changes (Tsukamoto *et al.*, 1995).

A peculiar feature of the intragastric feeding procedure is that the blood ethanol levels cycle between maximal levels as high as 5‰ and levels close to zero over a 5–6 day period (Tsukamoto *et al.*, 1985b; Badger *et al.*, 1993). The mechanism for this phenomenon, which occurs in spite of a constant rate of ethanol diet delivery, is not fully clarified. It has been suggested to relate to changes in the rate of ethanol clearance (Tsukamoto *et al.*, 1990; Badger *et al.*, 1993) or to an ethanol-induced cycling in thyroid hormone levels controlled by the hypothalamus (French *et al.*, 1999).

The cycling phenomenon may be of pathogenic relevance. Oscillating ethanol levels may cause artificially recurring inflammatory activation of Kupffer cells (Enomoto *et al.*, 1998; Bautista and Spitzer, 1999). Indeed, the extent of ethanol fluctuation has been found to correlate to the degree of hepatic damage (Tsukamoto *et al.*, 1985c). If the cycling phenomenon is mimicked by intubating a large ethanol dose daily for two months, liver lesions similar to those obtained by chronic intragastric ethanol liquid diet infusion develop (Enomoto *et al.*, 1999).

A disadvantage with the intragastric infusion model is the risk of complications with fatal outcome. In addition to infections or postsurgical problems, ethanol

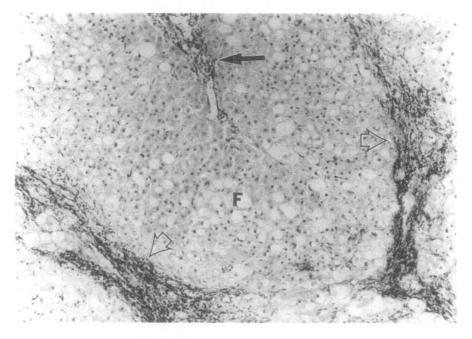

Figure 15.3 Central fibrotic changes (open arrows) and fat accumulation (F) in a liver of a rat after two months on intragastric ethanol liquid diet administration. The black arrow depicts a portal tract. The fibrotic changes are depicted by staining stellate cells for actin. (see *Color Plate 9*)

overdosing may lead to convulsions or death and cannulas may malfunction or get plugged (French *et al.*, 1988b; French *et al.*, 1995). Expert surgical expertise and careful daily monitoring is therefore required. This makes the technique labor-intensive and thus expensive. In addition, the intragastric diet model must be considered stressful to the animals, since the chronic cannula restricts their movements and they are deprived of a fundamental behavioral function of rodents: oral intake of food.

Chronic ethanol administration by gavage

Chronic ethanol organ damage effects were earlier studied by daily intubations (Majchrowicz and Hunt, 1976). High blood ethanol levels are achieved, but only transiently for a few hours. Although one single large dose already increases liver triglycerides (Ylikahri *et al.*, 1972), several daily intubations are needed for sustained intoxication and more severe lesions. Fatty liver was obtained by intubating liquid diet with 25% of the energy as alcohol (Carrol and Williams, 1971) or by combining gavage with ethanol in the drinking fluid (Ashworth *et al.*, 1947). However, animals on free diet access that are intubated with high doses of ethanol eat little and lose weight. This most probably contributes to the development of organ damage and complicates the interpretation. The recent finding that female rats intubated one intoxicating dose of ethanol (5 g/kg) per day for 2 months developed steatosis, inflammation and necrosis nevertheless suggests that pathogenic mechanisms can be studied by this "binge"-type alcohol exposure (Enomoto *et al.*, 1999). However, damage may be more attributed to a recurring alcohol-induced burst of inflammatory activity than to a steady cumulative alcohol effect (Abril *et al.*, 1997; Enomoto *et al.*, 1998).

Ethanol inhalation

Induction of ethanol intoxication via the breath was originally developed to study alcohol tolerance and behavioral changes (Goldstein *et al.*, 1971). This alternative forced-administration model also requires regular monitoring of circulating ethanol levels of each animal, to achieve maximal, yet non-lethal ethanol exposure. Care must be taken to feed control animals with similar amounts of diet. Thus also chronic inhalation experiments are laborious. The presence of ethanol vapor can lead to respiratory tract irritation and reduced fluid intake, which may cause dehydration and reduced body weight (Freund, 1980). On the other hand, normal solid animal food can be used, many animals can be exposed simultaneously and individual cages are not needed.

Only a few studies have addressed liver changes using this model. In one study mice developed steatosis and polymorphonuclear inflammation in 19 days (Goldin and Wickramasinghe, 1987). However, in another study rats exposed to ethanol vapor only developed fatty changes (DiLuzio and Stege, 1979). It is unclear whether the different outcomes of these studies reflect a difference between species or in the ethanol exposure regimen. It appears that in spite of its restrictions, it would be worthwhile to further explore the use of chronic ethanol inhalation to induce experimental ALD.

COMBINED TOXICITY MODELS

Drugs and chemicals

Animal models focusing on specific confounding factors in the pathogenesis of ALD are getting increased attention, since these factors may be responsible for the full blown liver disease of some alcoholics. These factors include nutritional and antioxidant deficiencies (for example choline, vitamin E and vitamin A), oxidants (carbonyl iron) and inflammatory agents (gut-derived endotoxin, viral hepatitis). As expected, most hepatotoxic compounds aggravate ethanol damage. This may tell more about the hepatotoxin than about actions of ethanol. As one example, alcoholics frequently develop acute liver failure after an overdose of paracetamol (Schiodt *et al.*, 1997). Animal experiments have shown that paracetamol (acetaminophen) is activated to the highly toxic intermediate *N*-acetyl-*p*-benzoquinoneimine (NAPQI), mainly by ethanol-inducible CYP2E1. Thus the accelerated formation of the quinone (Anundi *et al.*, 1993) may deplete glutathione, especially in the mitochondria (Fernandez-Checa *et al.*, 1998), and this may contribute to the enhanced hepatotoxicity.

Carbon tetrachloride is also activated by CYP2E1. Rats exposed to a low dose of carbon tetrachloride and 5% alcohol in the drinking water developed nearly full blown liver cirrhosis within 4 weeks, in contrast to animals treated with either compound (Siegers *et al.*, 1986). Likewise, exposure of rats to carbon tetrachloride vapour caused extensive hepatic fibrosis at 5 weeks and micronodular cirrhosis at 10 weeks, but only in animals receiving ethanol by liquid diet (Hall *et al.*, 1991, 1994). Although, as stated above, these studies cannot be regarded as models of alcoholic liver disease, they enlighten mechanisms of fibrogenesis and pathogenesis of alcohol-associated liver damage.

Iron

Several studies have addressed the interaction of iron overload and ethanol. Pretreatment with carbonyl iron was shown to accentuate effects of chronic ethanol liquid diet feeding (Stål *et al.*, 1993). Intragastric alcohol diet feeding together with carbonyl iron caused enhanced lipid peroxidation, promoted liver fibrogenesis and even cirrhotic changes were observed after 4 months (Tsukamoto *et al.*, 1995). Feeding an oral iron chelator reduced hepatic non-haem iron and lipid peroxidation (Sadrzadeh *et al.*, 1994a).

Endotoxin

Based on clinical evidence of elevated endotoxins in alcoholics, and on the concept that endotoxin may trigger the fatty liver to episodes of alcoholic hepatitis, many animal studies on the interaction of endotoxin and ethanol have been undertaken. Most of these are based on the effect of one acute dose of endotoxin. In one rat study, a bolus of endotoxin after 6 weeks on Lieber-DeCarli ethanol liquid diet precipitated in the steatotic livers coagulative necrosis and polymorphonuclear infiltration (Bhagwandeen *et al.*, 1987). This is interesting from the clinical point of view, since neutrophil infiltrates are prominent in alcoholic hepatitis, but may not necessarily reflect the situation of the alcoholics with a continuous moderate endotoxemia. To simulate this, an animal model was developed, in which animals that received alcohol orally by liquid diet also were infused endotoxin for 4 weeks from subcutaneously implanted minipumps (Järveläinen *et al.*, 1999). In this model the circulating endotoxin levels were 20–50 times higher than in rats only receiving ethanol and enhanced expression of liver pro-inflammatory cytokines was observed. Yet little additional damage was seen, indicating marked tolerance to the continuous presence of endotoxin, possibly as a consequence of a counter-acting increase in anti-inflammatory cytokines.

Viruses

The prevalence of viral hepatitis, especially hepatitis B (HBV) and C (HCV), in ALD is high (Brechot *et al.*, 1996; Sata *et al.*, 1996). From a clinical point of view, experimental studies of the interaction of chronic alcohol abuse and viral infection therefore would be of great interest. However, relevant chronic viral infection of rodents has not so far been successful. Consequently an animal model to study this aspect does not yet exist.

A model mimicking ALDH2-deficiency in Oriental alcoholics

About every second Oriental possesses a mutant inactive form of the mitochondrial aldehyde dehydrogenase (ALDH2*2). They avoid alcohol drinking, since this results in high blood acetaldehyde levels and unpleasant symptoms. In spite of this, some ALDH2*2 positive Orientals continue drinking and eventually become alcoholic. During drinking, the hepatic acetaldehyde levels of these individuals would be expected to be highly elevated. Many *in vitro* studies have suggested that acetaldehyde at these concentrations is cytotoxic (Lieber, 1991b), suggesting that the incidence of ALD among ALDH2*2 positive Japanese should be high. However, published data do not support this notion (Yamauchi *et al.*, 1995). To investigate this pathogenically relevant issue, an animal model to mimic these oriental alcoholics was established. Rats received ethanol intragastrically in a fish oil-based liquid diet for 6 weeks. Acetaldehyde levels were elevated by using two different ALDH inhibitors, disulfiram and benzcoprine. Contrary to expectations, the ALDH inhibitors, which resulted in high acetaldehyde levels, protected rather than promoted ALD (Lindros *et al.*, 1999). This study exemplifies the usefulness of an animal model to investigate a specific proposed pathogenic component.

PRIMATE MODELS

A primate model for experimental ALD based on baboons was developed by Rubin and Lieber (1973). The baboons received up to 50% of their calories as ethanol and could be kept on ethanol liquid diet for years. This made it possible to mimic the slow progression of damage in alcoholics. The baboons developed more damage than seen in rodent studies. Peak blood alcohol levels of baboons kept on a regimen with 11% carbohydrates approached 4‰. After 3–8 years on a diet with approximately 50% of the calories as ethanol, fatty liver, increased mononuclear inflammatory activity and perivenular fibrosis was seen in most of the animals. Importantly, in one or two out of five animals fibrosis eventually progressed to cirrhosis (Figure 15.4) (Lieber and DeCarli, 1974; Lieber *et al.*, 1975; Popper and Lieber, 1980; Lieber *et al.*, 1990). This prevalence is of the same magnitude among human alcoholics (Morgan, 1984). On the other hand, some of the histological features typically seen in human alcoholic hepatitis, such as heavy infiltration of neutrophil polymorphs and formation Mallory bodies, were not observed (Popper and Lieber, 1980). Alcoholic hepatitis is generally considered an essential step in the transition to cirrhosis, although in some populations, particularly in Japan, fibrosis and cirrhosis may develop without preceding hepatitis (Takada *et al.*, 1982; Takada *et al.*, 1993).

The baboon data were not replicated in a study by Ainley *et al.* (1988), who failed to observe cirrhosis or even fibrosis in spite of treating baboons for up to 60 months with a nutritionally different diet, the Mazuri primate diet supplemented with lipotropes, vitamins and minerals. The authors suggested that the diet used by Lieber *et al.* was nutritionally inadequate. However, in a follow-up study, Lieber and DeCarli (1994) demonstrated fibrotic injury in spite of supplementation with massive amounts of choline and methionine. Contradictory results have also been obtained with rhesus monkeys. Ethanol given with a high-fat low-choline diet produced cirrhosis in 8 months, but damage was avoided by choline supplementation

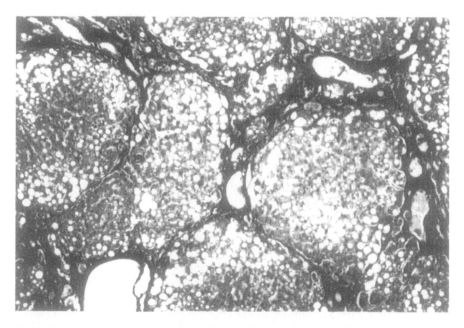

Figure 15.4 Cirrhosis in a baboon fed alcohol for four years. Chromotrope-aniline blue staining. Reproduced with permission from Lieber and DeCarli (1974). (*see Color Plate 10*)

(Cueto *et al.*, 1967). Several negative results have been reported, in spite of high alcohol consumption (up to 50% of calories) and extended study periods of 1–4.5 years (Rogers *et al.*, 1981; Mezey *et al.*, 1983). In a recent rhesus monkey study, a diet marginal in antioxidants and containing 24% of calories as ethanol resulted in macro- and microvesicular steatosis and mild fibrotic changes after 18–36 months (Pawlosky *et al.*, 1997; Pawlosky and Salem, 1999).

It is unfortunate that the data based on primate experiments so far are not unequivocal, since the mechanisms of ALD should resemble that of human alcoholics. More extensive studies on primates seem warranted, although such experiments require years of exposure and specially trained personnel, which make them extremely expensive and out of reach for most laboratories.

OTHER ANIMALS

Mice

Surprisingly few studies on ALD in mice have been undertaken. One problem is that their metabolism of alcohol is so rapid (i.e., 25 g/kg/d) that it is difficult to feed them enough ethanol without compromising their nutritional balance. This may explain the loss of animals reported during intragastric ethanol feeding to mice (Zhang-Gouillon *et al.*, 1998). In one liquid diet study with 30% of calories as ethanol, only moderate steatosis appeared in 4–10 weeks (Smith and Hoy, 1990). Steatosis, inflammation and a 2-fold elevation of liver enzymes was reported in female mice that inhaled ethanol vapor for up to 19 days. Blood alcohol levels were between 40 mg/dl–160 mg/dl (Goldin and Wickramasinghe, 1987). Mice have also been used in a binge-drinking model to study immunological effects of ethanol (Carson and Pruett, 1996).

Micropigs

Since pigs seem to tolerate ethanol better than most animals and their metabolism is considered to resemble humans closer than rats, they should be very useful for ALD studies. Minipigs given alcohol in a slurry-type low-fat diet consumed 6.0 g ethanol/kg per day, exhibited somewhat elevated hepatic triglyceride levels but only minimal histological changes after 8 weeks (Kusewitt *et al.*, 1977). However, when the fat content was increased (to 35–40% of calories) and the treatment time prolonged to 12 months, steatonecrosis developed and in some animals interstitial and perivenous fibrosis was observed (Halsted *et al.*, 1993; Niemelä *et al.*, 1995, 1999). Thus the micropig may provide a manageable model to study ALD.

Other animals

Occasional ALD studies using other mammals have been published. Ferrets given ethanol in a liquid diet consumed approximately 3.4 g/kg per day and developed steatosis and cell degeneration in 11 weeks, but bone marrow toxicity was also found (Roselle *et al.*, 1986). Guinea pigs given 40% calories as ethanol in a low-fat liquid diet for 8 months developed fatty liver (Wallerstedt *et al.*, 1975). Livers of guinea pigs kept on 15% (v/v) ethanol drinking water for 90 days were normal, but inflammation and fibrosis was reported to have developed if the animals were immunized with acetaldehyde adducts (Yokoyama *et al.*, 1995).

NUTRITIONAL ASPECTS

The role of malnutrition in experimental ALD was long controversial and became almost an academic question (Bunout *et al.*, 1983; Lieber *et al.*, 1986; Rao *et al.*, 1997). After all, mild nutritional deficiency certainly is common among alcoholics, who cover a major proportion of their energy intake by "empty" ethanol calories, consume a poor diet and may encounter deficient intestinal uptake of vitamins and minerals (Nazer and Wright, 1983). Indeed, the risk of developing cirrhosis seems to be higher in alcoholics covering more than 50% of their total energy as ethanol (Patek *et al.*, 1975; Salaspuro and Lieber, 1980). Thus mild nutritional deficiency is a clinically relevant state and experimental studies focusing on their role in aggravating ALD are warranted.

Animals diets are usually based on the recommendations of the American Institute of Nutrition (AIN, 1977; Reeves *et al.*, 1993). The nutritional adequacy of the Lieber-DeCarli diet is indicated from experiments showing that neither reduced diet intake, nor supplementation with extra proteins, essential minerals and vitamins affects ethanol-related hepatic changes (Lieber and DeCarli, 1989b).

Many investigators have noticed an apparent "ethanol energy wastage" phenomenon. Both in oral liquid diet and intragastric pair feeding protocols, ethanol-fed animals often gain weight less than their isocaloric controls (Morimoto *et al.*, 1994; Korourian *et al.*, 1999). Interestingly, a similar effect has been demonstrated in a human ward experiment (Pirola and Lieber, 1972). Whether this is due to malnutrition, changed growth regulation or energy wastage is still open (Pirola and Lieber, 1976; Rao *et al.*, 1997).

Excess calories generating obesity must also be considered. For instance, the incidence of steatosis and steatohepatitis correlates with the degree of obesity (Sheth *et al.*, 1997) and genetically obese mice are sensitive to endotoxin-induced liver injury (Yang *et al.*, 1997).

Carbohydrates

The protocol to isocalorically replace ethanol with carbohydrates in the pair-fed control diet was developed by Lieber *et al.* (1963). The lower carbohydrate content of the ethanol diet is important to keep in mind. Thus the carbohydrate content rather than the fat content seems to affect the deposition of triacylglycerides in the liver and increasing the dietary carbohydrate content prevents alcohol-induced steatosis (Yonekura *et al.*, 1993).

The carbohydrate restriction also seems to have a secondary effect on the inflammatory activity of the liver, possibly because fatty liver is more vulnerable to insults triggering inflammation (Day and Jones, 1998; Colell *et al.*, 1998). A recent intragastric ethanol feeding study exemplifies this. Ethanol diet with 21% carbohydrates only produced steatosis. However, a 2.5% carbohydrate diet produced necrotic changes and elevated ALT levels (Korourian *et al.*, 1999). In consonance, lowering the carbohydrate content of oral liquid diet, that by itself only led to steatosis, produced aggravated hepatic changes (Lindros and Järveläinen, 1998), but feeding a low-carbohydrate control diet has no effect on liver morphology or fat content (Lieber *et al.*, 1965).

Sucrose should be avoided, because high dietary concentrations of sucrose cause several complications in rodents, including hepatic steatosis (Bacon *et al.*, 1984).

Fat

The degree of hepatic injury induced by ethanol also depends on the amount and the type of fat in the diet. Thus increasing the amount of fat leads to more severe changes, including abnormalities of mitochondrial function and enhanced microsomal ethanol oxidizing capacity (Lieber *et al.*, 1970; Wahid *et al.*, 1980; Lindros, 1995). Consequently, the diet protocols used in experimental ALD models include a high amount of calories as fat. This high fat diet resembles that consumed by some alcoholics in the US (Mitchell and Herlong, 1986).

The type of fat also proved to be essential. It was found that the proportion of unsaturated fat correlates with damage. Thus a diet low in corn oil produced less damage than a diet high in corn oil and virtually no damage was seen if corresponding amounts of saturated fats (tallow oil or lard) were given (Nanji *et al.*, 1989b). Furthermore, experimental alcoholic liver injury was shown to be reversed by switching to a diet with saturated fatty acids (Nanji *et al.*, 1995a). Even more extensive damage, particularly inflammation and necrosis, was seen by giving fish oil, which is unusually rich in polyunsaturated fatty acids (Nanji *et al.*, 1994). This suggests that the combined presence of ethanol and unsaturated fatty acids provokes damage via a high rate of lipid peroxidation. Combined exposure of ethanol and unsaturated fatty acids, which aggravates ALD, also leads to unusually high induction of the ethanol-metabolizing CYP2E1 enzyme, supporting the notion of a pathogenic role of CYP2E1 in ALD (Takahashi *et al.*, 1992; Morimoto *et al.*, 1993).

Protein

Most liquid diets are based on casein, that should be supplemented with sulphur containing amino acids. A range of different dietary contents of protein have been used, from protein deficiency (4% of calories), to excess (25%) (Lieber and DeCarli, 1982). A protein content of 13% is considered to be nutritionally adequate for adult rats, while young growing rats require 17–20% (AIN, 1977; McDonald, 1997; Reeves, 1997). A low-protein diet aggravates experimental alcohol-induced liver injury (Nanji *et al.*, 1989a).

Micronutrients

Over the years the composition of the ethanol liquid diet with respect to various vitamins (e.g., vitamin A, Bs, D, E, K), minerals and trace elements has been improved (Lieber, 1989). Currently, all commercial diets should contain adequate amounts of these elements. For example, the Lieber and DeCarli (1989) diet formula follows closely the AIN 1977 formulation with vitamins and minerals. An exception to this is vitamin A, which is in 6-fold excess to compensate for the reduced bioavailability in the presence of alcohol. It is, on the other hand, important to keep in mind that the therapeutic window for vitamin A is relatively narrow (Leo and Lieber, 1983; Lieber and Leo, 1986; Lieber and DeCarli, 1989a). In general, although vitamin deficiency has often been found to aggravate alcoholic liver injury, massive supplementation with vitamin E and other vitamins to an adequate diet has failed to prevent the development of injury rodents (Lieber *et al.*, 1989; Sadrzadeh *et al.*, 1994b, 1995).

Choline has received special attention in the pathogenesis of ALD, because its deficiency in itself causes fatty liver and fibrosis in rodents and alcohol enhances its requirement (Rogers *et al.*, 1981). Liver injuries of several etiologies, including alcohol, are augmented, with a diet poor in choline. The content of choline (as bitartrate) in the Lieber-DeCarli control diet (0.53 g/l) is considered adequate (Lieber and DeCarli, 1994).

Nutritional aspects have been central issues in attempts to develop more specific treatment methods for ALD. For example, S-adenosyl-L-methionine (SAM) enhances the synthesis of glutathione, a non-protein thiol crucial in antioxidant defence (Lu, 1998). Ethanol-induced depletion of glutathione is reversed by administration of SAM in baboons, and recent findings suggest that it may affect survival in patients with liver disease (Lieber, 1999; Mato *et al.*, 1999). Promising results in counteracting the fibrotic process have been reported based on the baboon model. Administration of fatty acid lecithin or its main component phosphatidylcholine may afford protection against alcoholic fibrosis and cirrhosis (Lieber *et al.*, 1990, 1994).

CONCLUSIONS AND FUTURE DIRECTIONS

Alcoholic liver damage develops slowly and commonly involves one or several confounding factors, in addition to the constant burden of alcohol. It is therefore not surprising that our picture of this disease still is rather diffuse. Nevertheless, much of our present knowledge comes from experimental animal studies. Two rodent models and one primate model have been instrumental. The first working rodent model was based on oral administration of ethanol by a standardized nutritionally adequate liquid diet. This procedure only resulted in low or moderate blood ethanol levels, but was extremely useful in elucidating the role of various nutritional factors in the development of alcohol-induced steatosis. A major step forward was made by developing the forced intragastric feeding of ethanol liquid diet. This technically demanding technique results in high blood ethanol levels and inflammatory changes, opening new possibilities for study of factors interacting with this process. To study mechanisms involved in the slowly evolving fibrotic process requires extended intragastric ethanol feeding, which frequently results in loss of animals. For severe lesions to develop, the ethanol diet needed to be rich in unsaturated fatty acids and low in carbohydrates. Similar lesions were observed in rats continuously intoxicated by consuming this diet, suggesting that this oral model affords a convenient alternative to the intragastric technique. However, conclusions drawn on the basis of these diets should be drawn judiciously, since the role of lipid peroxidation as a confounding factor in ALD may be overemphasized.

The fibrotic process and even cirrhosis can be successfully studied by long-term ethanol liquid diet feeding to primates. However, the experiments are slow, labor-intensive and expensive and this has restricted research progress in this area. Emphasis should be put on developing affordable and working models to study the fibrotic process. Promising data on minipigs have been obtained. In addition, long-term rodent models, including the method to adapt rodents to a high content of ethanol in their drinking fluid, need to be developed further.

More work is also needed in developing nutritionally controlled ethanol models, that produce proper liver lesions in mice. Promising data treating knock-out mice with ethanol have already been obtained and should have great promise in further studies on the role of specific gene products in ALD. Viral hepatitis is the major complicating factor in human ALD. Once stable viral transfection of mice is mastered, the interaction of chronic ethanol and relevant viral infections can be subject to experimental studies. In the future new animal models tailored to answer specific questions, also in the field of ALD, will be needed. However, in order to understand the disease process as a whole, the development of ALD models encompassing all stages will continue to be an important goal for a long time. Once the picture of the disease process gets sharper, new avenues will open for studies focusing on the development of efficient therapeutic compounds to stop, relieve and cure alcoholic liver disease in its various stages.

ACKNOWLEDGMENTS

We thank Dr J. Christian Bode for valuable comments on the manuscript.

REFERENCES

Abril, E.R., Jones, J., Jolley, C.S., Holubec, H., Waite, S. and Sipes, I.G. (1997) Binge-type alcohol intake recruits immune cells into rat liver and stimulates Kupffer cell release of cytokines and superoxide prior to any evidence of overt liver injury. In *Cells of the Hepatic Sinusoid*, edited by E. Wisse, D.L. Knook and C. Balabaud, pp. 303–305. CE Leiden: Kupffer Cell Foundation.

Ainley, C.C., Senapati, A., Brown, I.M., Iles, C.A., Slavin, B.M., Mitchell, W.D., Davies, D.R., Keeling, P.W. and Thompson, R.P. (1988) Is alcohol hepatotoxic in the baboon? *Journal of Hepatology* **7**, 85–92.

AIN (1977) Report of the American institute of nutrition ad hoc committee on standards for nutritional studies. *Journal of Nutrition* **107**, 1340–1348.

Anundi, I., Lähteenmäki, T., Rundgren, M., Moldeus, P. and Lindros, K.O. (1993) Zonation of acetaminophen metabolism and cytochrome P450 2E1-mediated toxicity studied in isolated periportal and perivenous hepatocytes. *Biochemical Pharmacology* **45**, 1251–1259.

Ashworth, C.T. (1947) Production of fatty infiltration of liver in rats by alcohol in spite of adequate diet. *Proceedings of the Society for Experimental Biology and Medicine* **66**, 382–285.

Bacon, B.R., Park, C.H., Fowell, E.M. and McLaren, C.E. (1984) Hepatic steatosis in rats fed diets with varying concentrations of sucrose. *Fundamental & Applied Toxicology* **4**, 819–826.

Badger, T.M., Ronis, M.J., Ingelman-Sundberg, M. and Hakkak, R. (1993) Pulsatile blood alcohol and CYP2E1 induction during chronic alcohol infusions in rats. *Alcohol* **10**, 453–457.

Bautista, A.P. and Spitzer, J.J. (1999) Role of Kupffer cells in the ethanol-induced oxidative stress in the liver. *Frontiers in Bioscience* **15**, D589–D595.

Becker, U., Deis, A., Sorensen, T.I., Gronbaek, M., Borch-Johnsen, K., Muller, C.F., Schnohr, P. and Jensen G. (1996) Prediction of risk of liver disease by alcohol intake, sex, and age: a prospective population study. *Hepatology* **23**, 1025–1029.

Best, C.H., Hartroft, W.S., Lucas, C.C. and Ridout, J.H. (1949) Liver damage produced by feeding alcohol or sugar and its prevention by choline. *British Medical Journal* **2**, 1001–1006.

Bhagwandeen, B.S., Apte, M., Manwarring, L. and Dickeson, J. (1987) Endotoxin induced hepatic necrosis in rats on an alcohol diet. *Journal of Pathology* **152**, 147–153.

Bosma, A., Seifert, W.F., van Thiel-de Ruiter, G.C., van Leeuwen, R.E., Blauw, B., Roholl, P., Knook, D.L. and Brouwer, A. (1994) Alcohol in combination with malnutrition causes increased liver fibrosis in rats. *Journal of Hepatology* **21**, 394–402.

Brechot, C., Nalpas, B. and Feitelson, M.A. (1996) Interactions between alcohol and hepatitis viruses in the liver. *Clinics in Laboratory Medicine* **16**, 273–287.

Bunout, D., Gattas, V., Iturriaga, H., Perez, C., Pereda, T. and Ugarte, G. (1983) Nutritional status of alcoholic patients: it's possible relationship to alcoholic liver damage. *American Journal of Clinical Nutrition* **38**, 469–473.

Burra, P., Hubscher, S.G., Shaw, J., Elias, E. and Adams, D.H. (1992) Is the intercellular adhesion molecule-1/leukocyte function associated antigen 1 pathway of leukocyte adhesion involved in the tissue damage of alcoholic hepatitis? *Gut* **33**, 268–271.

Carroll, C. and Williams, L. (1971) Modification of ethanol-induced changes in rat liver composition by the carbohydrate-fat component of the diet. *Journal of Nutrition* **101**, 997–1012.

Carson, E.J. and Pruett, S.B. (1996) Development and characterization of a binge drinking model in mice for evaluation of the immunological effects of ethanol. *Alcoholism, Clinical and Experimental Research* **20**, 132–138.

Cmielewski, P.L., Plummer, J.L., Ahern, M.J., Ilsley, A.H. and Hall, P.M. (1997) A technique for obtaining repeated liver biopsies from rats. *Pathology* **29**, 286–288.

Colell, A., Garcia-Ruiz, C., Miranda, M., Ardite, E., Mari, M., Morales, A., Corrales, F., Kaplowitz, N. and Fernandez-Checa, J.C. (1998) Selective glutathione depletion of mitochondria by ethanol sensitizes hepatocytes to tumor necrosis factor. *Gastroenterology* **115**, 1541–1551.

Cueto, J., Tajen, N., Gilbert, E. and Currie, R.A. (1967) Experimental liver injury in the rhesus monkey. I. Effects of cirrhogenic diet and ethanol. *Annals of Surgery* **166**, 19–28.

Day, C.P. and James, O.F. (1998) Hepatic steatosis: innocent bystander or guilty party? *Hepatology* **27**, 1463–1466.

Di Luzio, N.R. and Hartman, A.D. (1969) Modification of acute and chronic ethanol-induced hepatic injury and the role of lipid peroxidation in the pathogenesis of the ethanol-induced fatty liver. In *Biochemical and Clinical Aspects of Alcohol Metabolism*, edited by V.M. Sardesai, pp.133–153. Springfield: Charles C. Thomas.

Di Luzio, N.R. and Stege, T.E. (1979) Influence of chronic ethanol vapor inhalation on hepatic parenchymal and Kupffer cell function. *Alcoholism, Clinical and Experimental Research* **3**, 240–247.

Dicker, E., McHugh, T. and Cederbaum, A.I. (1991) Increased catalytic activity of cytochrome P-450IIE1 in pericentral hepatocytes compared to periportal hepatocytes isolated from pyrazole-treated rats. *Biochimica et Biophysica Acta* **1073**, 316–323.

Enomoto, N., Ikejima, K., Bradford, B., Rivera, C., Kono, H., Brenner, D.A. and Thurman, R.G. (1998) Alcohol causes both tolerance and sensitization of rat Kupffer cells via mechanisms dependent on endotoxin. *Gastroenterology* **115**, 443–451.

Enomoto, N., Yamashina, S., Kono, H., Schemmer, P., Rivera, C.A., Enomoto, A., Nishiura, T., Nishimura, T., Brenner, D.A. and Thurman, R.G. (1999) Development of a new, simple rat model of early alcohol-induced liver injury based on sensitization of Kupffer cells. *Hepatology* **29**, 1680–1689.

Fernandez-Checa, J.C., Kaplowitz, N., Garcia-Ruiz, C. and Colell, A. (1998) Mitochondrial glutathione: importance and transport. *Seminars in Liver Disease* **18**, 389–401.

Forssell, L. (1981) Metabolic effects of ethanol in rats as studied with an intragastric infusion technique. *Substance and Alcohol Actions/Misuse* **2**, 25–30.

French, S.W., Benson, N.C. and Sun, P.S. (1984) Centrilobular liver necrosis induced by hypoxia in chronic ethanol-fed rats. *Hepatology* **4**, 912–917.

French, S.W., Miyamoto, K. and Tsukamoto, H. (1986) Ethanol-induced hepatic fibrosis in the rat: role of the amount of dietary fat. *Alcoholism, Clinical and Experimental Research* **10**, 13S–19S.

French, S.W., Miyamoto, K., Wong, K., Jui, L. and Briere, L. (1988a) Role of the Ito cell in liver parenchymal fibrosis in rats fed alcohol and a high fat-low protein diet. *American Journal of Pathology* **132**, 73–85.

French, S.W., Miyamoto, K., Ohta, Y. and Geoffrion, Y. (1988b) Pathogenesis of experimental alcoholic liver disease in the rat. *Methods and Achievement in Experimental Pathology* **13**, 181–207.

French, S.W. (1993) Nutrition in the pathogenesis of alcoholic liver disease. *Alcohol and Alcoholism* **28**, 97–109.

French, S.W., Morimoto, M. and Tsukamoto, H. (1995) Animal models of alcohol-associated liver injury. In *Alcoholic liver disease* edited by P. Hall, pp. 279–296. London: Edward Arnold.

French, S.W., Fu, P., Li, J., Yuan, Q.X. and French, B.A. (1999) Mechanism of the cyclic oscillation of the urinary alcohol levels in rats fed ethanol: role of the hypothalamic-pituitary thyroid axis. *Hepatology* **30**, 337A.

Freund, G. (1980) Comparison of alcohol dependence, withdrawal and hangover in humans and animals. In *Animal Models in Alcoholic Research*, edited by K. Eriksson, J.D. Sinclair and K. Kiianmaa, pp. 293–308. New York: Academic Press.

Friedman, S.L. (1997) Molecular mechanisms of hepatic fibrosis and principles of therapy. *Journal of Gastroenterology* **32**, 424–430.

Fromenty, B. and Pessayre, D. (1995) Inhibition of mitochondrial beta-oxidation as a mechanism of hepatotoxicity. *Pharmacology & Therapeutics* **67**, 101–154.

Goldstein, D.B. and Pal, N. (1971) Alcohol dependence produced in mice by inhalation of ethanol: grading the withdrawal reaction. *Science* **172**, 288–290.

Goldin, R.D. and Wickramasinghe, S.N. (1987) Hepatotoxicity of ethanol in mice. *British Journal of Experimental Pathology* **68**, 815–824.

Goldin, R. (1994) Rodent models of alcoholic liver disease. *International Journal of Experimental Pathology* **75**, 1–7.

Hall, P.D., Plummer, J.L., Ilsley, A.H. and Cousins, M.J. (1991) Hepatic fibrosis and cirrhosis after chronic administration of alcohol and "low-dose" carbon tetrachloride vapor in the rat. *Hepatology* **13**, 815–819.

Hall, P.M., Plummer, J.L., Ilsley, A.H., Ahern, M.J., Cmielewski, P.L. and Williams, R.A. (1994) The pathology of liver injury induced by the chronic administration of alcohol and 'low-dose' carbon tetrachloride in Porton rats. *Journal of Gastroenterology and Hepatology* **9**, 250–256.

Hall, P.M. (1995) Pathological spectrum of alcoholic liver disease. In *Alcoholic liver disease*, edited by P. Hall, pp. 41–70. London: Edward Arnold.

Halsted, C.H., Villanueva, J., Chandler, C.J., Ruebner, B., Munn, R.J., Parkkila, S. and Niemelä, O. (1993) Centrilobular distribution of acetaldehyde and collagen in the ethanol-fed micropig. *Hepatology* **18**, 954–960.

Hu, Y., Ingelman-Sundberg, M. and Lindros, K.O. (1995) Induction mechanisms of cytochrome P450 2E1 in liver: interplay between ethanol treatment and starvation. *Biochemical Pharmacology* **17**, 155–161.

Iimuro, Y., Frankenberg, M.V., Arteel, G.E., Bradford, B.U., Wall, C.A. and Thurman, R.G. (1997) Female rats exhibit greater susceptibility to early alcohol-induced liver injury than males. *American Journal of Physiology* **272**, G1186–G1194.

Iseri, O.A., Lieber, C.S. and Gottlieb, L.S. (1966) The ultrastructure of fatty liver induced by prolonged ethanol ingestion. *American Journal of Pathology* **48**, 535–555.

Ishak, K.G., Zimmerman, H.J. and Ray, M.B. (1991) Alcoholic liver disease: pathologic, pathogenetic and clinical aspects. *Alcoholism, Clinical and Experimental Research* **15**, 45–66.

Israel, Y., Oporto, B. and MacDonald, A.D. (1984) Simultaneous pair-feeding system for the administration of alcohol-containing liquid diets. *Alcoholism, Clinical and Experimental Research* **8**, 505–508.

Järveläinen, H.A., Oinonen, T. and Lindros, K.O. (1997) Alcohol-induced expression of the CD14 endotoxin receptor protein in rat Kupffer cells. *Alcoholism, Clinical and Experimental Research* **21**, 1547–1551.

Järveläinen, H.A., Fang, C., Ingelman-Sundberg, M. and Lindros, K.O. (1999) Effect of chronic co-administration of endotoxin and ethanol on rat liver pathology and pro- and anti-inflammatory cytokines. *Hepatology* **29**, 1503–1510.

Järveläinen, H.A., Lukkari, T.A., Heinaro, S., Sippel, H. and Lindros, K.O. (2001) The anti-estrogen toremifene protects against alcoholic liver injury in female rats. *Journal of Hepatology* **35**, 46–52.

Kamimura, S., Gaal, K., Britton, R.S., Bacon, B.R., Triadafilopoulos, G. and Tsukamoto, H. (1992) Increased 4-hydroxynonenal levels in experimental alcoholic liver disease: association of lipid peroxidation with liver fibrogenesis. *Hepatology* **16**, 448–453.

Keegan, A., Martini, R. and Batey, R. (1995) Ethanol-related liver injury in the rat: a model of steatosis, inflammation and pericentral fibrosis. *Journal of Hepatology* **23**, 591–600.

Koop, D.R., Crump, B.L., Nordblom, G.D. and Coon, M.J. (1985) Immunochemical evidence for induction of the alcohol-oxidizing cytochrome P-450 of rabbit liver microsomes by diverse agents: ethanol, imidazole, trichloroethylene, acetone, pyrazole, and isoniazid. *Proceedings of the National Academy of Sciences of the United States of America* **82**, 4065–4069.

Korourian, S., Hakkak, R., Ronis, M.J., Shelnutt, S.R., Waldron, J., Ingelman-Sundberg, M. and Badger, T.M. (1999) Diet and risk of ethanol-induced hepatotoxicity: carbohydrate-fat relationships in rats. *Toxicological Sciences* **47**, 110–117.

Kusewitt, D.F., Burke, J.P. and Tumbleson, M.E. (1977) Effect of chronic ethanol consumption on liver metabolites in Sinclair (S-1) miniature swine. *General Pharmacology* **8**, 335–339.

Landrigan, J., Patterson, F. and Batey, R. (1989) A histological study of the use of agar as a delivery vehicle for alcohol or iron to rats. *Alcohol* **6**, 173–178.

Lands, W.E. (1995) Cellular signals in alcohol-induced liver injury: a review. *Alcoholism, Clinical and Experimental Research* **19**, 928–938.

Leo, M.A. and Lieber, C. (1983) Hepatic fibrosis after long-term administration of ethanol and moderate vitamin A supplementation in the rat. *Hepatology* **3**, 1–11.

Lieber, C.S., Jones, D.P., Mendelson, J. and DeCarli, L.M. (1963) Fatty liver, hyperlipemia and hyperuricemia produced by prolonged alcohol consumption despite adequate dietary intake. *Transactions of the Association of American Physicians* **76**, 289–300.

Lieber, C.S., Jones, D.P. and DeCarli, L.M. (1965) Effects of prolonged ethanol intake. *Journal of Clinical Investigation* **44**, 1009–1021.

Lieber, C.S., Spritz, N. and DeCarli, L.M. (1966) Role of dietary, adipose, and endogenously synthesized fatty acids in the pathogenesis of the alcoholic fatty liver. *Journal of Clinical Investigation* **45**, 51–62.

Lieber, C.S. and Rubin, E. (1968) Ethanol – a hepatotoxic drug. *Gastroenterology* **54**, 642–646.

Lieber, C.S. and DeCarli, L.M. (1970a) Quantitative relationship between amount of dietary fat and severity of alcoholic fatty liver. *American Journal of Clinical Nutrition* **23**, 474–478.

Lieber, C.S. and DeCarli, L.M. (1970b) Hepatic microsomal ethanol-oxidizing system. *In vitro* characteristics and adaptive properties *in vivo*. *Journal of Biological Chemistry* **245**, 2505–2512.

Lieber, C.S., Rubin, E., DeCarli, L.M., Misra, P. and Gang, H. (1970) Effects of pyrazole on hepatic function and structure. *Laboratory Investigation* **22**, 615–621.

Lieber, C.S. and DeCarli, L.M. (1974) An experimental model of alcohol feeding and liver injury in the baboon. *Journal of Medical Primatology* **3**, 153–163.

Lieber, C.S. and DeCarli, L.M. (1975) Alcoholic liver injury: experimental models in rats and baboons. *Adv Exp Med Biol* **59**, 379–393.

Lieber, C.S., DeCarli, L. and Rubin, E. (1975) Sequential production of fatty liver, hepatitis and cirrhosis in sub-human primates fed ethanol with adequate diets. *Proceedings of the National Academy of Sciences of the United States of America* **72**, 437–441.

Lieber C.S. and Decarli, L.M. (1976) Animal models of ethanol dependence and liver injury in rats and baboons. *Federation Proceedings* **35**, 1232–1236.

Lieber, C.S. and DeCarli, L.M. (1982) The feeding of alcohol in liquid diets: two decades of applications and 1982 update. *Alcoholism, Clinical and Experimental Research* **6**, 523–531.

Lieber, C.S. and DeCarli, L.M. (1986) The feeding of ethanol in liquid diets. *Alcoholism, Clinical and Experimental Research* **10**, 550–553.

Lieber, C.S. and Leo, M.A. (1986) Interaction of alcohol and nutritional factors with hepatic fibrosis. *Progress in Liver Diseases* **8**, 253–272.

Lieber, C.S. and DeCarli, L.M. (1989a) Liquid diet technique of ethanol administration: 1989 update. *Alcohol and Alcoholism* **24**, 197–211.

Lieber, C.S. and DeCarli, L.M. (1989b) Effects of mineral and vitamin supplementation on the alcohol-induced fatty liver and microsomal induction. *Alcoholism, Clinical and Experimental Research* **13**, 142–143.

Lieber, C.S., DeCarli, L.M. and Sorrell, M.F. (1989) Experimental methods of ethanol administration. *Hepatology* **10**, 501–510.

Lieber, C.S., DeCarli, L.M., Mak, K.M., Kim, C.I. and Leo, M.A. (1990) Attenuation of alcohol-induced hepatic fibrosis by polyunsaturated lecithin. *Hepatology* **12**, 1390–1398.

Lieber, C.S. (1991a) Alcohol and fibrogenesis. *Alcohol and Alcoholism* **1** (Suppl), 339–344.

Lieber, C.S. (1991b) Biochemical mechanisms of alcohol-induced hepatic injury. *Alcohol and Alcoholism* **1** (Suppl), 283–290.

Lieber, C.S., Robins, S.J., Li, J., DeCarli, L.M., Mak, K.M., Fasulo, J.M. and Leo, M.A. (1994) Phosphatidylcholine protects against fibrosis and cirrhosis in the baboon. *Gastroenterology* **106**, 152–159.

Lieber, C.S. and DeCarli, L.M. (1994) Animal models of chronic ethanol toxicity. *Methods in Enzymology* **233**, 585–594.

Lieber, C.S. (1999) Role of *S*-adenosyl-*L*-methionine in the treatment of liver diseases. *Journal of Hepatology* **30**, 1155–1159.

Lindros, K.O., Stowell, L., Väänänen, H., Sipponen, P., Lamminsivu, U., Pikkarainen, P. and Salaspuro, M. (1983) Uninterrupted prolonged ethanol oxidation as a main pathogenetic factor of alcoholic liver damage: evidence from a new liquid diet animal model. *Liver* **3**, 79–91.

Lindros, K.O., Väänänen, H., Sarviharju, M. and Haataja, H. (1984) A simple procedure using 4-methylpyrazole for developing tolerance and other chronic alcohol effects. *Alcohol* **1**, 145–150.

Lindros, K.O. (1995) Alcoholic liver disease: pathobiological aspects. *Journal of Hepatology* **23** (Suppl), 7–15.

Lindros, K.O. and Järveläinen, H.A. (1998) A new oral low-carbohydrate alcohol liquid diet producing liver lesions: a preliminary account. *Alcohol and Alcoholism* **33**, 347–353.

Lindros, K.O., Jokelainen, K. and Nanji, A.A. (1999) Acetaldehyde prevents nuclear factor-kappa B activation and hepatic inflammation in ethanol-fed rats. *Laboratory Investigation* **79**, 799–806.

Lu, S.C. (1998) Regulation of hepatic glutathione synthesis. *Semin Liver Dis* **18**, 331–343.

Lukas, S.E. and Moreton, J.E. (1979) A technique for chronic intragastric drug administration in the rat. *Life Sciences* **25**, 593–600.

MacSween, R.N. and Burt, A.D. (1986) Histologic spectrum of alcoholic liver disease. *Seminars in Liver Diseases* **6**, 221–232.

Majchrowicz, E. and Hunt, W.A. (1976) Temporal relationship of the induction of tolerance and physical dependence after continuous intoxication with maximum tolerable doses of ethanol in rats. *Psychopharmacology* **10**, 107–112.

Mato, J.M., Camara, J., Fernandez de Paz, J., Caballeria, L., Coll, S., Caballero, A. *et al.* (1999) S-adenosylmethionine in alcoholic liver cirrhosis: a randomized, placebo-controlled, double-blind, multicenter clinical trial. *Journal of Hepatology* **30**, 1081–1089.

McClain, C., Hill, D., Schmidt, J. and Diehl, A.M. (1993) Cytokines and alcoholic liver disease. *Seminars in Liver Diseases* **13**, 170–182.

McClain, C.J., Barve, S., Deaciuc, I., Kugelmas, M. and Hill, D. (1999) Cytokines in alcoholic liver disease. *Seminars in Liver Diseases* **19**, 205–219.

McDonald, R.B. (1997) Some considerations for the development of diets for mature rodents used in long-term investigations. *Journal of Nutrition* **127**, 847S–850S.

Mezey, E., Potter, J.J., French, S.W., Tamura, T. and Halsted, C.H. (1983) Effect of chronic ethanol feeding on hepatic collagen in the monkey. *Hepatology* **3**, 41–44.

Miller, S.S., Goldman, M.E., Erickson, C.K. and Shorey, R.L. (1980) Induction of physical dependence on and tolerance to ethanol in rats fed a new nutritionally complete and balanced liquid diet. *Psychopharmacology* **68**, 55–59.

Mitchell, M.C. and Herlong, H.F. (1986) Alcohol and nutrition: caloric value, bioenergetics and relationship to liver damage. *Annual Review of Nutrition* **6**, 457–474.

Morgan, M.Y. (1994) The prognosis and outcome of alcoholic liver disease. *Alcohol and Alcoholism* **2** (Suppl), 335–343.

Morimoto, M., Hagbjörk, A-L., Nanji, A.A., Ingelman-Sundberg, M., Lindros, K.O., Fu, P.C., Albano, E. and French S.W. (1993) Role of cytochrome P4502E1 in alcohol liver disease pathogenesis. *Alcohol* **10**, 459–464.

Morimoto, M., Zern, M.A., Hagbjork, A.L., Ingelman-Sundberg, M. and French, S.W. (1994) Fish oil, alcohol, and liver pathology: role of cytochrome P450 2E1. *Proceedings of the National Academy of Sciences of the United States of America* **207**, 197–205.

Nanji, A.A., Tsukamoto, H. and French, S.W. (1989a) Relationship between fatty liver and subsequent development of necrosis, inflammation and fibrosis in experimental alcoholic liver disease. *Experimental and Molecular Pathology* **51**, 141–148.

Nanji, A.A., Mendenhall, C.L. and French, S.W. (1989b) Beef fat prevents alcoholic liver disease in the rat. *Alcoholism, Clinical and Experimental Research* **13**, 15–19.

Nanji, A.A., Zhao, S., Sadrzadeh, S.M., Dannenberg, A.J., Tahan, S.R. and Waxman, D.J. (1994) Markedly enhanced cytochrome P450 2E1 induction and lipid peroxidation is associated with severe liver injury in fish oil-ethanol-fed rats. *Alcoholism, Clinical and Experimental Research* **18**, 1280–1285.

Nanji, A.A., Sadrzadeh, S.M., Yang, E.K., Fogt, F., Meydani, M. and Dannenberg, A.J. (1995a) Dietary saturated fatty acids: a novel treatment for alcoholic liver disease. *Gastroenterology* **109**, 547–554.

Nanji, A.A., Griniuviene, B., Yacoub, L.K., Fogt, F. and Tahan, S.R. (1995b) Intercellular adhesion molecule-1 expression in experimental alcoholic liver disease: relationship to endotoxemia and TNF alpha messenger RNA. *Experimental and Molecular Pathology* **62**, 42–51.

Nazer, H. and Wright, R.A. (1983) The effect of alcohol on the human alimentary tract: a review. *Journal of Clinical Gastroenterology* **5**, 361–365.

Niemelä, O., Parkkila, S., Ylä-Herttuala, S., Villanueva, J., Ruebner, B. and Halsted, C.H. (1995) Sequential acetaldehyde production, lipid peroxidation, and fibrogenesis in micropig model of alcohol-induced liver disease. *Hepatology* **22**, 1208–1214.

Niemelä, O., Parkkila, S., Pasanen, M., Viitala, K., Villanueva, J.A. and Halsted, C.H. (1999) Induction of cytochrome P450 enzymes and generation of protein-aldehyde adducts are associated with sex-dependent sensitivity to alcohol-induced liver disease in micropigs. *Hepatology* **30**, 1011–1017.

Oesterreicher, C., Pfeffel, F., Petermann, D. and Muller, C. (1995) Increased *in vitro* production and serum levels of the soluble lipopolysaccharide receptor CD14 in liver disease. *Journal of Hepatology* **23**, 396–402.

Patek, A.J., Toth, I.G., Saunders, M.G., Castro, G.A. and Engel, J.J. (1975) Alcohol and dietary factors in cirrhosis. An epidemiological study of 304 alcoholic patients. *Archives of Internal Medicine* **135**, 1053–1057.

Pawlosky, R.J., Flynn, B.M. and Salem Jr., N. (1997) The effects of low dietary levels of polyunsaturates on alcohol-induced liver disease in rhesus monkeys. *Hepatology* **26**, 1386–1392.

Pawlosky, R.J. and Salem Jr., N. (1999) A chronic ethanol-feeding study in rhesus monkeys. *Lipids* **34**, S131–S132.

Pennington, H.L., Hall, P.M., Wilce, P.A. and Worrall, S. (1997) Ethanol feeding enhances inflammatory cytokine expression in lipopolysaccharide-induced hepatitis. *Journal of Gastroenterology and Hepatology* **12**, 305–313.

Pirola, R.C. and Lieber, C.S. (1972) The energy cost of the metabolism of drugs, including ethanol. *Pharmacology* **7**, 185–196.

Pirola, R.C. and Lieber, C.S. (1976) Hypothesis: energy wastage in alcoholism and drug abuse: possible role of hepatic microsomal enzymes. *American Journal of Clinical Nutrition* **29**, 90–93.

Plummer, J.L., Hall, P.M., Cmielewski, P.L., Ilsley, A.H. and Ahern, M.J. (1997) Use of artificial sweeteners to promote alcohol consumption by rats. *Pathology* **29**, 57–59.

Popper, H. and Lieber, C.S. (1980) Histogenesis of alcoholic fibrosis and cirrhosis in the baboon. *American Journal of Pathology* **98**, 695–716.

Porto, L.C., Chevallier, M. and Grimaud, J.A. (1989) Morphometry of terminal hepatic veins. 2. Follow up in chronically alcohol-fed baboons. *Virchows Archiv A Pathological Anatomy and Histopathology* **414**, 299–307.

Rao, G.A., Riley, D.E. and Larkin, E.C. (1987) Dietary carbohydrates stimulates alcohol diet ingestion, promotes growth and prevents fatty liver in rats. *Nutrition Research* **7**, 81–87.

Rao, G.A. and Larkin, E.C. (1997) Nutritional factors required for alcoholic liver disease in rats. *Journal of Nutrition* **127**, 896S–898S.

Reeves, P.G. (1997) Components of the AIN-93 diets as improvements in the AIN-76A diet. *Journal of Nutrition* **127**, 838S–841S.

Rogers, A.E., Fox, J.G. and Murphy, J.C. (1981) Ethanol and diet interactions in male rhesus monkeys. *Drug Nutrient Interactions* **1**, 3–14.

Roselle, G.A., Mendenhall, C.L., Muhleman, A.F. and Chedid, A. (1986) The ferret: a new model of oral ethanol injury involving the liver, bone marrow and peripheral blood lymphocytes. *Alcoholism, Clinical and Experimental Research* **10**, 279–284.

Rubin, E. and Lieber, C.S. (1973) Experimental alcoholic hepatitis: a new primate model. *Science* **182**, 712–713.

Sadrzadeh, S.M., Nanji, A.A. and Price, P.L. (1994a) The oral iron chelator, 1,2-dimethyl-3-hydroxypyrid-4-one reduces hepatic-free iron, lipid peroxidation and fat accumulation in chronically ethanol-fed rats. *Journal of Pharmacology and Experimental Therapeutics* **269**, 632–636.

Sadrzadeh, S.M., Nanji, A.A. and Meydani, M. (1994b) Effect of chronic ethanol feeding on plasma and liver alpha- and gamma-tocopherol levels in normal and vitamin E-deficient rats. Relationship to lipid peroxidation. *Biochemical Pharmacology* **47**, 2005–2010.

Sadrzadeh, S.M., Meydani, M., Khettry, U. and Nanji, A.A. (1995) High-dose vitamin E supplementation has no effect on ethanol-induced pathological liver injury. *Journal of Pharmacology and Experimental Therapeutics* **273**, 455–460.

Salaspuro, M.P. and Lieber, C.S. (1980) Comparison of the detrimental effects of chronic ethanol intake on humans and animals. In *Animal Models in Alcoholic Research*, edited by K. Eriksson, J.D. Sinclair and K. Kiianmaa, pp. 359–375. New York: Academic Press.

Sankaran, H., Baba, G.C., Deveney, C.W. and Rao, G.A. (1991) Enteral macronutrients abolish high blood alcohol levels in chronic alcoholic rats. *Nutrition Research* **11**, 217–222.

Sata, M., Fukuizumi, K., Uchimura, Y., Nakano, H., Ishii, K., Kumashiro, R., Mizokami, M., Lau, J.Y. and Tanikawa, K. (1996) Hepatitis C virus infection in patients with clinically diagnosed alcoholic liver diseases. *Journal of Viral Hepatitis* **3**, 143–148.

Savolainen, V.T., Liesto, K., Mannikko, A., Penttilä, A. and Karhunen, P.J. (1993) Alcohol consumption and alcoholic liver disease: evidence of a threshold level of effects of ethanol. *Alcoholism, Clinical and Experimental Research* **17**, 1112–1117.

Schenker, S. and Bay, M.K. (1995) Alcohol and endotoxin: another path to alcoholic liver injury? *Alcoholism, Clinical and Experimental Research* **19**, 1364–1366.

Schiodt, F.V., Rochling, F.A., Casey, D.L. and Lee, W.M. (1997) Acetaminophen toxicity in an urban county hospital. *New England Journal of Medicine* **16**, 1112–1117.

Sheth, S.G., Gordon, F.D. and Chopra, S. (1997) Nonalcoholic steatohepatitis. *Annals of Internal Medicine* **126**, 137–145.

Siegers, C.P., Pauli, V., Korb, G. and Younes, M. (1986) Hepatoprotection by malotilate against carbon tetrachloride-alcohol-induced liver fibrosis. *Agents and Actions* **18**, 600–603.

Slawecki, C.J. and Samson, H.H. (1997) Changes in oral ethanol self-administration patterns resulting from ethanol concentration manipulations. *Alcoholism, Clinical and Experimental Research* **6**, 1144–1149.

Smith, S.M. and Hoy, W.E. (1990) Ad libitum alcohol ingestion does not induce renal IgA deposition in mice. *Alcoholism, Clinical and Experimental Research* **14**, 184–186.

Sorensen, T.I., Orholm, M., Bentsen, K.D., Hoybye, G., Eghoje, K. and Christoffersen, P. (1984) Prospective evaluation of alcohol abuse and alcoholic liver injury in men as predictors of development of cirrhosis. *Lancet* **2**, 241–244.

Stål, P. and Hultcrantz, R. (1993) Iron increases ethanol toxicity in rat liver. *Journal of Hepatology* **17**, 108–115.

Takada, A., Nei, J., Matsuda, Y. and Kanayama, R. (1982) Clinicopathological study of alcoholic fibrosis. *American Journal of Gastroenterology* **77**, 660–666.

Takada, A., Matsuda, Y. and Takase, S. (1986) Effects of dietary fat on alcohol-pyrazole hepatitis in rats: the pathogenetic role of the nonalcohol dehydrogenase pathway in alcohol-induced hepatic cell injury. *Alcoholism, Clinical and Experimental Research* **10**, 403–411.

Takada, A., Takase, S. and Tsutsumi, M. (1993) Characteristic features of alcoholic liver disease in Japan: a review. *Gastroenterologia Japonica* **28**, 137–148.

Takahashi, H., Geoffrion, Y., Butler, K.W. and French, S.W. (1990) *In vivo* hepatic energy metabolism during the progression of alcoholic liver disease: a noninvasive 31P nuclear magnetic resonance study in rats. *Hepatology* **11**, 65–73.

Takahashi, H., Johansson, I., French, S.W. and Ingelman-Sundberg, M. (1992) Effects of dietary fat composition on activities of the microsomal ethanol oxidizing system and ethanol-inducible cytochrome P450 (CYP2E1) in the liver of rats chronically fed ethanol. *Pharmacology and Toxicology* **70**, 347–351

Thurman, R.G. (1998) Alcoholic liver injury involves activation of Kupffer cells by endotoxin. *American Journal of Physiology* **275**, G605–G611.

Tsukamoto, H., Lew, G., Larkin, E.C., Largman, C. and Rao, G.A. (1984a) Hepatic origin of triglycerides in fatty livers produced by the continuous intragastric infusion of an ethanol diet. *Lipids* **19**, 419–422.

Tsukamoto, H., Reidelberger, R.D., French, S.W. and Largman, C. (1984b) Long-term cannulation model for blood sampling and intragastric infusion in the rat. *American Journal of Physiology* **247**, R595–R599.

Tsukamoto, H., French, S.W., Benson, N., Delgado, G., Rao, G.A., Larkin, E.C. and Largman, C. (1985a) Severe and progressive steatosis and focal necrosis in rat liver induced by continuous intragastric infusion of ethanol and low fat diet. *Hepatology* **5**, 224–232.

Tsukamoto, H., French, S.W., Reidelberger, R.D. and Largman, C. (1985b) Cyclical pattern of blood alcohol levels during continuous intragastric ethanol infusion in rats. *Alcoholism, Clinical and Experimental Research* **9**, 31–37.

Tsukamoto, H., French, S.W. and Largman, C. (1985c) Correlation of cyclical blood alcohol levels with progression of alcoholic liver injury. *Biochemical Archives* **1**, 215–220.

Tsukamoto, H., Towner, S.J., Ciofalo, L.M. and French, S.W. (1986) Ethanol-induced liver fibrosis in rats fed high fat diet. *Hepatology* **6**, 814–822.

Tsukamoto, H., Gaal, K. and French, S.W. (1990) Insights into the pathogenesis of alcoholic liver necrosis and fibrosis: status report. *Hepatology* **12**, 599–608.

Tsukamoto, H., Horne, W., Kamimura, S., Niemelä, O., Parkkila, S., Ylä-Herttuala, S. and Brittenham, G.M. (1995) Experimental liver cirrhosis induced by alcohol and iron. *Journal of Clinical Investigations* **96**, 620–630.

Wallerstedt, S., Olsson, R. and Korsan-Bengtsen, K. (1975) Effects on lipids, coagulation factors and liver histology of long-term ethanol administration to guinea-pigs. *Acta Hepatogastroenterologica* (Stuttgart) **22**, 236–241.

Wahid, S., Khanna, J.M., Carmichael, F.J. and Israel, Y. (1980) Mitochondrial function following chronic ethanol treatment: effect of diet. *Research Communications in Chemical Pathology & Pharmacology* **30**, 477–491.

Worner, T.M. and Lieber, C.S. (1985) Perivenular fibrosis as precursor lesion of cirrhosis. *JAMA* **254**, 627–630.

Yamauchi, M., Maezawa, Y., Mizuhara, Y., Ohata, M., Hirakawa, J., Nakajima, H. and Toda, G. (1995) Polymorphisms in alcohol metabolizing enzyme genes and alcoholic cirrhosis in Japanese patients: a multivariate analysis. *Hepatology* **22**, 1136–1142.

Yang, S.Q., Lin, H.Z., Lane, M.D., Clemens, M. and Diehl, A.M. (1997) Obesity increases sensitivity to endotoxin liver injury: implications for the pathogenesis of steatohepatitis. *Proceedings of the National Academy of Sciences of the United States of America* **94**, 2557–2562.

Yin, M., Wheeler, M.D., Kono, H., Bradford, B.U., Gallucci, R.M., Luster, M.I. and Thurman, R.G. (1999) Essential role of tumor necrosis factor alpha in alcohol-induced liver injury in mice. *Gastroenterology* **117**, 942–952.

Yin, M., Ikejima, K., Wheeler, M.D., Bradford, B.U., Seabra, V., Forman, D.T., Sato, N. and Thurman, R.G. (2000) Estrogen is Involved in Early Alcohol-Induced Liver Injury in a Rat Enteral Feeding Model. *Hepatology* **31**, 117–123.

Ylikahri, R.H., Kahonen, M.T. and Hassinen, I. (1972) Modification of metabolic effects of ethanol by fructose. *Acta Medica Scandinavica* **542** (Suppl), 141–150.

Yokoyama, H., Nagata, S., Moriya, S., Kato, S., Ito, T., Kamegaya, K. and Ishii, H. (1995) Hepatic fibrosis produced in guinea pigs by chronic ethanol administration and immunization with acetaldehyde adducts. *Hepatology* **21**, 1438–1442.

Yonekura, I., Nakano, M. and Sato, A. (1993) Effects of carbohydrate intake on the blood ethanol level and alcoholic fatty liver damage in rats. *Journal of Hepatology* **17**, 97–101.

Zeldin, G., Yang, S.Q., Yin, M., Lin, H.Z., Rai, R. and Diehl, A.M. (1996) Alcohol and cytokine-inducible transcription factors. *Alcoholism, Clinical and Experimental Research* **20**, 1639–1645.

Zhang-Gouillon, Z.Q., Yuan, Q.X., Hu, B., Marceau, N., French, B.A., Gaal, K., Nagao, Y., Wan, Y.J. and French, S.W. (1998) Mallory body formation by ethanol feeding in drug-primed mice. *Hepatology* **27**, 116–122.

Part IV

Epidemiology and diagnosis

Chapter 16

Epidemiology and comparative incidence of alcohol-induced liver disease

John B. Saunders and Benedict M. Devereaux

Alcoholic liver disease is the most common type of chronic liver disease in many countries. Its incidence has fluctuated considerably over recent decades, mainly due to the changes in the level of consumption of alcohol in the population. The risk of chronic alcoholic liver disease increases when daily consumption exceeds 60 g in men and 20–40 g in women. Average daily consumption in the range of 80–160 g for women and 160–240 g for men, a relatively unvarying pattern of drinking and long duration confers the highest risk. Even so, there is considerable variation in susceptibility to alcohol-related liver disease, which remains largely unexplained. Alcohol can interact with several other risk factors for liver disease, most notably hepatitis C infection, but also hepatotoxic drugs such as paracetamol, nutritional deficiency and disorders of iron metabolism, to result in more severe disease than occurs when alcohol is the only risk factor present. Such interactions may explain some of this variation. Alcohol probably now accounts for around 50% of cases of chronic liver disease. Although alcohol-related liver disease is less common in some countries than it was 20 and more years ago, it could rapidly increase in prevalence again if the consumption of alcohol by the population returned to its former levels.

KEYWORDS: cirrhosis, liver diseases, alcoholic, epidemiology, alcohol abuse

INTRODUCTION

The association between chronic liver disease and heavy alcohol consumption has been recognized for centuries. By the late 18th century, the link was well established (Baillie, 1793). There is a spectrum of alcohol-induced hepatic injury, which ranges from minor biochemical and clinically insignificant damage, to fatty liver, alcoholic hepatitis and on to cirrhosis. The latter two conditions have a high morbidity and mortality. With the increase in prevalence and rate of diagnosis of various forms of viral hepatitis, in particular hepatitis C, alcoholic liver disease (ALD) has become somewhat overshadowed in general hepatology practice. However, it remains one of the ten most common causes of death in many developed countries (Grant *et al.*, 1988; Lieber, 1993; Saunders and Latt, 1993) and is the second most frequent indication for orthotopic liver transplantation in several cases.

For many years, cirrhosis in the alcoholic was thought to be secondary to nutritional deficiency. Indeed it was thought that progression of liver disease could be arrested with a nutritionally replete diet. Even today the exact role of diet and nutrition remains the subject of debate. It is now generally accepted, however, that alcohol is the fundamental cause of a spectrum of liver diseases through its direct and indirect hepatotoxic effects.

Several factors have been implicated in the pathogenesis of alcoholic liver damage. The quantity and pattern of alcohol consumption is important. Other factors, for which there is a varying degree of evidence, include the formation of toxic metabolites from oxidation of alcohol, immune responsiveness to alcohol-induced neo-antigens and concomitant infection with hepatitis viruses. In addition, gender and genetic influences are thought to play a role. One of the most enduring mysteries is why only a proportion of patients who consume excessive amounts of alcohol over long periods of time develop cirrhosis. It is acknowledged that liver disease can progress even following cessation of alcohol consumption. Clearly the pathogenesis of ALD is more complex than just direct hepatotoxicity.

In this chapter we shall examine the relationship between the level and pattern of alcohol consumption and the risk of liver disease, both in clinical series and in populations, and identify the contribution made by alcohol to the occurrence of liver disease. The evidence suggesting that alcohol is a sufficient cause *per se* of liver disease will be reviewed and the interaction between alcohol and other risk factors for liver disease explored. Synergy between alcohol and the hepatitis viruses, nutritional deficiencies, hepatotoxic drugs and inherited metabolic disorders such as hereditary haemochromatosis is increasingly recognized. In particular, we shall examine the interaction between excessive alcohol consumption and hepatitis C, consistent with the magnitude of both of these entities.

POPULATION ALCOHOL CONSUMPTION AND LIVER DISEASE

Over the past 200 years the etiological model of ALD has fluctuated. Initially alcohol was considered directly toxic to the liver (Blair, 1888). This concept was supported by the finding that cirrhosis mortality declined during periods of reduced alcohol consumption, as during prohibition in the United States, following an increase in liquor taxes in England, and rationing of alcohol in Europe between 1914 and 1950 (Ledermann, 1956; Stone *et al.*, 1968).

Per capita consumption

Epidemiological studies over the past 50 years have demonstrated a strong association between population alcohol consumption (calculated as *per capita* intake) and cirrhosis morbidity and mortality. This has been seen most clearly when there have been interruptions to the sale of alcoholic drinks, as for example in the First and Second World Wars. In several countries in Europe, official or *de facto* rationing of alcohol was in force during these periods and also during the prohibition era (1919–1932) in the USA. When restrictions on the availability of alcohol were introduced, there was an abrupt decline in cirrhosis mortality, as experienced in France during the Second World War when cirrhosis mortality declined to 10% of the pre-war rates within four years of rationing being introduced. When alcohol was made freely available, at the cessation of rationing, cirrhosis mortality returned to previous levels (Ledermann, 1956; Péquignot, 1960; Thaler, 1990; Seeley, 1960; Smart, 1974).

Per capita alcohol consumption increased steadily in most Western countries from the late 1940s to the late 1970s and this was associated with a considerably increased mortality rate from cirrhosis. In the UK, Australia, Canada, New Zealand, Sweden and the United States, *per capita* consumption doubled, reaching a peak by the late 1970s, and either leveled off or slightly declined thereafter (Hilton, 1988; Smart, 1989; Roizen *et al.*, 1999). The post-war rise in alcohol consumption was associated with proportionately greater rises in cirrhosis mortality in men than in women (Saunders *et al.*, 1981a; Royal College of Physicians, 1987).

In the United Kingdom, *per capita* consumption of alcohol roughly doubled between 1950 and 1980, following which it plateaued and has since then declined slightly. Cirrhosis mortality has in general followed these trends. A long-term, prospective UK study in a defined geographical area in the West Midlands demonstrated a 4-fold increase in the incidence of alcoholic cirrhosis from 1959–1961 to 1974–1976 (Saunders *et al.*, 1981a). In the latter period, alcohol accounted for 66% of cases of cirrhosis. This study was unique in that consistent diagnostic criteria were applied throughout 20 years so that it was possible to distinguish alcoholic cirrhosis from other causes, and not use total cirrhosis morbidity as a proxy measure. The increase in alcoholic cirrhosis correlated with an increase in *per capita* alcohol consumption of 70–80% over this period (Saunders and Latt, 1993).

Analysis of USA population data indicates that *per capita* alcohol consumption rose steadily from 1964 through the mid-1970s, leveled off and fell slightly after the mid 1980s to the present time (Roizen *et al.*, 1999). The prevalence of heavy drinking increased particularly in the younger age group (21–34 years) in both sexes (Hilton, 1988). The total cirrhosis mortality rate reached a peak at 15.0 per 100,000 population in 1973. During the period from 1964 to 1973 there was a 4-fold increase in cirrhosis death rates among non-white males, which was 1.7 times the corresponding death rate in white males (Grant *et al.*, 1991). From the early 1980s onwards there has been an increase in abstention and a decrease in heavier drinking among both sexes, although there are considerable geographical variations (Williams and DeBakey, 1992). This correlates with a decline in overall alcohol-related mortality from 1979 to 1988 (Stinson and DeBakey, 1992). Cirrhosis death rates decreased steadily to 9.1 per 100,000 population by 1988 and to 7.9 per 100,000 by 1993 (Roizen *et al.*, 1999). Nevertheless, cirrhosis of the liver is still ranked in the top ten causes of death in the USA, and is the sixth leading cause of death in the 45–64 year age group (Grant *et al.*, 1991). Blue-collar workers and those working in jobs where alcohol is easily available have the highest cirrhosis mortality rates (Harford and Brooks, 1992).

In Canada, from the late 1940s onwards annual *per capita* alcohol consumption rose from 7.1 liters in 1958 to 11 liters between 1975 and 1981 and has subsequently slightly declined. There was a significant correlation between alcoholic cirrhosis mortality and annual *per capita* alcohol consumption (Mao *et al.*, 1992), with rapid increases in morbidity and mortality from cirrhosis until the mid-1970s (Schmidt, 1977), and then a decline of approximately 25%, particularly in the younger age group (Smart, 1988; Hunter *et al.*, 1988). There was no time lag between changes in consumption and cirrhosis mortality, which led to the conclusion that cirrhosis mortality rates were related to changes in recent alcohol consumption (Halliday *et al.*, 1991).

As in many Western countries, alcohol consumption and total cirrhosis mortality in Australia gradually increased from 1945 to reach a peak in the mid-1970s. Both *per capita* intake and cirrhosis mortality then leveled off and have since declined. *Per capita* consumption fell from 9.6 liters in 1976–1997 to 7.7 liters presently. As in Canada, no lag period in changes in cirrhosis mortality was evident. Among various states in Australia, hospital morbidity rates from ALD were highest in the Northern Territory which has the highest *per capita* consumption in the country (Department of Community Services and Health, 1988).

In contrast to Australia and Canada, in Finland a marked lag period was evident when *per capita* alcohol consumption increased from 4.2 liters to 6.5 liters during the period 1969–1974, coinciding with removal of restrictions and introduction of low alcohol beer. Results of over 800 autopsies from 1968 to 1988 revealed a highly significant increase in liver cirrhosis (particularly in males in the younger age group) in this period. This rise in cirrhosis morbidity and mortality after a lag period of 10 years following increases in *per capita* alcohol consumption was thought to represent development of liver disease in a new and younger group of consumers (Savolainen *et al.*, 1993).

In Sweden, increases in both alcohol consumption and cirrhosis mortality were described following abolition of the Swedish rationing system in 1955. Between 1950 and 1980, *per capita* alcohol consumption increased by approximately 50%, while male cirrhosis mortality quadrupled. The sharper increase in mortality than would be expected from the rise in *per capita* consumption was attributed to a "redistributive impact" of the reform. It was found that the greater an individual's consumption of alcohol during rationing, the larger the relative increase in that consumption after abolition of rationing (Norstrom, 1987). In the follow-up period 1979–1982, there was a 17% reduction in sales of alcohol and this was associated with a significant decline in mortality from cirrhosis of the liver (by approximately 28%) in both men and women (Romelsjo and Agren, 1985).

In some Asian countries, alcohol intake has increased greatly. In Japan there was a 5-fold increase in *per capita* consumption of alcohol from 1.1 liters in 1950 to 5.5 liters in 1975; it increased further to 11.9 liters by 1984. This correlated with rises in cirrhosis morbidity and mortality from 1969 to 1985, particularly among men in the 45–55 year age group. There was no increase in incidence of cirrhosis among women, 80% of whom are abstainers or light drinkers (Parrish *et al.*, 1991). Cirrhosis now ranks as the fourth leading cause of death in Japan (Ohnishi and Okuda, 1986; Parrish *et al.*, 1991). Alcohol accounts for an estimated two-thirds of cirrhosis deaths among men in the 24–85 year age group and half of all cirrhosis deaths. Concurrent infection with hepatitis B or C is thought to have contributed to the increased mortality from cirrhosis (Parrish *et al.*, 1991).

In summary, cirrhosis mortality rose steadily from the 1950s onwards in many Western countries and has now declined for the past 10–15 years. In Canada and the USA, this reduction has been disproportionate to the reduction in *per capita* alcohol consumption. This might be explained by changes in the pattern of drinking. In some countries there have been substantial changes in the ethnic make-up of the population and/or its age structure. Other reasons for the disproportionate decrease in ALD might be an increase in the proportion of persons receiving treatment for alcohol misuse, earlier diagnosis and more effective treatment of liver disease (National Institute on Alcohol Abuse and Alcoholism, 1990).

Beverage type and pattern of drinking

Population-level research on alcohol consumption and cirrhosis has concentrated almost exclusively on the relationship with *per capita* consumption, such is the intellectual appeal of having a single summary measure of consumption. The influence of beverage type and the pattern of drinking has been little explored at this level.

When the high death rates from cirrhosis in the wine-producing countries of Southern Europe were first quantified, there was an assumption that wine was more hepatotoxic than other beverages. It was difficult to disentangle the effect of wine consumption from total consumption because of the high proportion of the total that was consumed as wine. The most compelling evidence to date of a differential effect of beverage type comes from a recent analysis of USA consumption data (Roizen *et al.*, 1999). These authors explored the disparity in the USA between the fall in cirrhosis mortality over the decade from 1973 onwards and the continuing increase in *per capita* consumption of alcohol until the early 1980s. Analysis by beverage type revealed that the closest correlation between cirrhosis deaths and consumption over the entire period from 1949 was with spirits consumption. There was no significant correlation with wine or beer consumption.

The authors speculate that their findings may not be related to drinking spirits as such, but that spirit drinkers have a higher overall consumption and that they may be less well nourished. This is a valid point, and it may well be that a beverage favored by a particular socio-economic group or in a particular country will be consumed in larger quantities and perhaps more regularly than other drinks.

The influence of the pattern of drinking has also been relatively neglected in population-level studies. European wine-producing countries have a tradition of regular daily consumption. In North America and the Nordic countries, binge drinking is more usual. It has been difficult to dissect out the influence of various patterns of drinking by comparing national data. The effect of different patterns of drinking on the development of liver disease has been explored, albeit in an embryonic way, in studies of individual alcohol consumption, as described in the following section.

Conclusions from population studies

The strong overall correlation between alcohol intake and cirrhosis morbidity and mortality suggests that alcohol has been the predominant cause of cirrhosis in most Western societies over the past half century. When there is a divergence, as has been evident since the mid-1970s, it suggests that particularly hepatotoxic patterns of drinking may have declined, the treatment of ALD may have improved, or other forms of cirrhosis have changed in incidence. In the latter case, the most obvious etiological suspect is hepatitis C.

INDIVIDUAL ALCOHOL CONSUMPTION AND LIVER DISEASE

In this section we shall examine the relationship between individual alcohol intake and the risk and severity of liver disease. Findings from clinical series, case-control studies and longitudinal studies will be considered in turn. The main purpose of these studies has been to define levels and patterns of consumption that may result in liver disease, and whether there are individuals who are particularly susceptible to this.

Findings from clinical studies

In clinical series, ALD has been defined typically on the basis of three criteria. The first is that on clinical, biochemical and histological grounds, the liver damage is compatible with an alcoholic etiology. Second, there is a history of excessive alcohol intake (variably defined but usually exceeding 60 or 80 g per day). Third, no other cause of liver disease has been identified.

Several studies have reported detailed information on alcohol intake. This is usually expressed as the mean daily intake and the duration of excessive drinking, and less commonly the pattern of drinking (its regularity and variability), or summary measures such as the cumulative lifetime alcohol intake. Men with ALD have typically reported intakes averaging 140–210 g per day, and women between 80 and 160 g per day. Duration of excessive drinking exceeds 5 years in nearly all cases, with average periods of 15.7 years reported for men and 9.8 years for women (Saunders *et al.*, 1981b).

Because of the restricted spectrum of disease in many series, attempts to correlate consumption measures with damage have often not been illuminating. In some series, patients with lesser damage (for example, fatty liver or steatofibrosis) have had lower intakes than cirrhotic patients, but in others intake levels have been no different (Saunders *et al.*, 1985).

Intriguingly, many patients with ALD have not experienced psychosocial consequences of excessive drinking or been referred for treatment for an alcohol problem (Saunders *et al.*, 1985). Alcohol intake, although undeniably high, has seemingly been an unremarkable feature of the person's daily life and physical dependence has not been prominent. Patients with alcoholic cirrhosis may have lower daily consumption and less dependence than those with lesser degrees of damage (Wodak *et al.*, 1983).

Persons with other recognized causes of liver disease may also have a high alcohol intake, though it appears that those in this category have been excluded from some series. Approximately one-third of patients with hereditary haemochromatosis have an excessive alcohol intake. In contrast, only 10% of patients with autoimmune hepatitis were reported to have an alcohol intake exceeding 20 g per day, a finding which is compatible with the known prevalence of consumption in the general population in developed countries. In most studies of non-alcoholic steato-hepatitis, an alcohol consumption above 20 or 40 g per day has been an exclusion criterion for this diagnosis (George *et al.*, 1998). Selection criteria such as these mean that it is difficult to gauge from clinical series the contribution of excessive alcohol consumption to the totality of chronic liver damage.

Case-control studies

Clinical series cannot provide evidence that a certain level or pattern of alcohol consumption is the cause of the liver damage, even when no other etiological factor can be identified. To demonstrate causation, analytical studies must be undertaken in which the alcohol intake of patients with liver disease is compared with that of a control group of subjects without liver disease.

The pioneer of such case-control studies was the French epidemiologist Péquignot. Beginning in the mid-1950s, he and his colleagues in the French National Institute for Health and Medical Research (INSERM) investigated the alcohol intake of patients with cirrhosis, irrespective of supposed etiology, and compared it with that of age-sex matched control subjects. In the first study, men admitted to hospital with cirrhosis, defined on clinical grounds by the presence of signs of hepatic decompensation, were compared with hospitalized patients without liver disease. Of those with cirrhosis, 55% had a daily alcohol intake of 160 g or more, 44% had an intake of between 80 and 160 g per day, while only one had an intake under 80 g. This compares with only 6% of control subjects who drank 160 g or more per day, 22% between 80 g and 160 g, and 72% under 80 g (Péquignot, 1960). The intake range below 80 g was described as the "zone d'innocuité" for the development of cirrhosis.

Because of the disadvantages of using hospitalized controls, Péquignot and his colleagues in a subsequent study recruited patients with decompensated cirrhosis from a defined geographical area, whether they were hospitalized or remained at home, and compared their intake with control subjects without liver disease who were drawn at random from the electoral register, after matching for age and sex.

The "differential cirrhosis morbidity quotient" was 9 per 100,000 for men drinking 20 g alcohol per day, 6 per 100,000 for those with an intake 21–40 g per day, and 7 per 100,000 for those with intakes of 41–60 g per day. For men drinking 61–80 g per day the morbidity quotient was 15 per 100,000 (described by Péquignot *et al.* as "slightly above the baseline," but apparently not significantly so). For those whose intake exceeded 80 g per day the risk was significant, and increased exponentially as daily consumption rose (Péquignot *et al.*, 1974). For women drinking 0–20 g per day the cirrhosis morbidity quotient was 5 per 100,000. The risk was somewhat above baseline for women drinking 21–40 g per day (at 14 per 100,000, not apparently a statistically significant difference), and was significantly increased, at 58 per 100,000 for those drinking 41–60 g per day. At all intakes above this, the risk was significantly greater than baseline, with the relationship being an exponential one, as seen in men.

In subsequent studies the risk of cirrhosis was found to increase above a mean daily intake of 60 g for men, and above an intake of between 20 and 40 g per day for women (Péquignot *et al.*, 1974). These studies were extended to other areas of France, with similar findings, although in one no clear threshold of alcohol intake was identified (Péquignot *et al.*, 1978). Instead, the risk seemed to increase at any level of consumption above zero intake.

This approach was later adopted by Australian investigators. Norton and her colleagues recruited cirrhotic patients admitted to eight hospitals in Sydney and compared their alcohol and nutritional intakes with hospitalized controls.

Patients with liver disease of "known non-alcoholic cause" were excluded. The risk of cirrhosis in women was found to increase when daily alcohol intake exceeded 40 g (Norton *et al.*, 1987). An identical study was conducted among males admitted with cirrhosis, again with exclusion of those with known non-alcoholic forms of liver disease. The risk of liver disease among men was found to increase when intake exceeded 60 g per day (Batey *et al.*, 1992).

Liver disease in excessive drinkers

There are numerous reports extending back over 30 years of liver enzyme abnormalities in alcoholics and in more heterogeneous groups of problem drinkers. However, the information that can be gleaned from such studies is extremely limited. Neither liver enzyme abnormalities nor non-invasive imaging procedures such as liver scan and ultrasound have sufficient specificity for the diagnosis of alcohol-related liver disease, in its various forms.

Two studies have been reported when liver biopsies were taken routinely in problem drinkers admitted to hospital for detoxification. The first was conducted by Lelbach in Germany. He undertook a detailed assessment of lifetime alcohol consumption in 320 alcoholic patients who underwent liver biopsy. Subjects were rank ordered according to their cumulative lifetime alcohol intake, and the percentage of those in each group who had (1) cirrhosis and (2) any form of chronic liver disease, namely cirrhosis, steatofibrosis, and alcoholic hepatitis, was calculated. Of those in the highest intake category (men who had consumed an average of 240 g alcohol per day for 20 years), 50% had an established cirrhosis, and 80% had some form of chronic liver disease (Lelbach, 1975).

This approach was employed by Saunders (1986) who recruited 160 patients admitted to a general hospital with various alcohol-related problems. A detailed history of alcohol intake was obtained from each, using a time-line, follow-back technique. Each patient underwent liver biopsy. The average cumulative alcohol intake of those with cirrhosis was 1250 kg, those with alcoholic hepatitis or steatofibrosis was 1127 kg, those with fatty liver was 740 kg, and those with normal liver histology 665 kg (Table 16.1). Of men in the highest cumulative intake category, 52% had developed cirrhosis, and 83% some form of chronic liver damage. Importantly, 91% of those with cirrhosis drank excessively 6–7 days per week compared

Table 16.1 Cumulative alcohol intake in relation to severity of liver disease

Severity of liver disease	Cumulative lifetime alcohol intake (kg)		
	Men (n = 106)	Women (n = 42)	Both sexes (n = 148)
Normal histology/minimal changes	736 ± 115	468 ± 152	665 ± 96
Fatty liver	952 ± 114	318 ± 53	740 ± 89
Steatofibrosis/alcoholic hepatitis	1318 ± 120	365 ± 101	1127 ± 117
Cirrhosis	1493 ± 158	707 ± 90	1250 ± 124

Data reproduced from Saunders (1986).

Table 16.2 Pattern of drinking in relation to severity of liver disease

Severity of liver disease	Days per week when consumption exceeded 80 g			
	1–3	4–5	6	7
Normal histology/minimal changes (n = 19)	42%	37%	16%	5%
Fatty liver (n = 48)	15%	25%	25%	27%
Steatofibrosis/alcoholic hepatitis (n = 36)	0%	20%	20%	47%
Cirrhosis (n = 45)	2%	7%	7%	51%

Figures are row percentages. Overall χ^2 = 45.4 (9 d.f.); $p < 0.001$.
Data reproduced from Saunders (1986).

with 60% of those who had fatty liver only and 21% of those with normal histology (Table 16.2) (Saunders, 1986). On logistic regression analysis, the pattern of consumption (on a week to week basis) was a stronger predictor of the severity of liver damage than was the average daily intake, the duration of excessive drinking, or the cumulative alcohol intake.

The extent to which low or medium levels of alcohol consumption cause liver disease was assessed by Savolainen and colleagues (1993), who analyzed a consecutive autopsy series of 210 men. Their average daily intake and the duration of alcohol consumption was determined by an interview with the spouse or a close acquaintance, and compared with semi-quantitative histological scores for stage of liver disease. The frequency of fatty liver increased significantly in the group consuming 40–80 g of alcohol daily. Similarly there was a significantly increased rate of alcoholic hepatitis in the 40–80 g group. An increase in cirrhosis or bridging fibrosis in the absence of cirrhosis was observed in the group consuming greater than 80 g of alcohol daily. Intriguingly, above a daily alcohol consumption of 80 g there was no dose-response relationship. It was concluded that the rate of occurrence of ALD abruptly increased with a daily intake between 40 and 80 g, and that progression of liver fibrosis to cirrhosis required long-term consumption in excess of 80 g per day. The absence of a dose-response relationship in the higher intake ranges raises the possibility that additional factors influence which excessive drinkers develop cirrhosis.

Longitudinal studies

Serial studies with repeat liver biopsy samples have demonstrated that fatty liver develops within 10–14 days of a person consuming in excess of 80 g alcohol per day. No longitudinal studies exist where biopsy samples have been taken in persons with a range of intakes over a period of years, for obvious ethical reasons. However, there are some studies where excessive drinkers or persons with existing ALD have undergone repeat biopsies. The most relevant to our discussion are those of Sørensen and colleagues.

In a prospective study, 258 alcohol-abusing men, free from cirrhosis on primary liver biopsy, were followed for 10–13 years. Over this time cirrhosis developed in 38, corresponding to a rate of 2% per year (Sørensen *et al.*, 1984). Neither the duration of the preceding alcohol abuse nor the average daily consumption between initial assessment and follow-up was significantly related to the subsequent occurrence of cirrhosis. The presence of steatosis or hepatitis on the first biopsy was found to be a good indicator of the risk of developing cirrhosis. These authors concluded that beyond a daily intake of 50–80 g of alcohol per day, further consumption did not enhance the risk of ALD (Sørensen *et al.*, 1984). Furthermore, a liver biopsy provided more information than an alcohol history about the likelihood of future cirrhosis in an alcohol-abusing person. This work provided support for a contrasting hypothesis to that of a dose-response relationship, namely that there is a hepatotoxic range of alcohol consumption, with a lower boundary and an upper level above which the risk of liver disease is permissive rather than dose-related: alcohol consumption establishes conditions for the development of cirrhosis (Sørensen, 1989).

In a more recent study, however, Becker and colleagues from Sørensen's group reported that self-reported current alcohol intake was a good predictor of the future risk of alcohol-induced liver disease (Becker *et al.*, 1996). A dose-dependent relationship between self-reported alcohol intake and the risk of developing alcohol-induced liver disease during the subsequent 12 years was observed in both men and women. This increased risk was significant from 7 to 13 beverages per week for women and 14–27 beverages for men. The relative risk increased more sharply for women than for men with increasing intake.

ALCOHOL AS A DIRECT HEPATOTOXIN

Alcoholic fatty liver, alcoholic hepatitis and characteristic forms of cirrhosis are found in persons whose only known risk factor for liver disease is their alcohol consumption. Fatty liver is very common in heavy drinkers; indeed it is estimated that approximately 80% of heavy drinkers show some features of it. The other lesions are more idiosyncratic; only 10–35% develop alcoholic hepatitis and approximately 10% develop cirrhosis (Grant *et al.*, 1988; Ishak *et al.*, 1991).

It was previously thought that these entities represented a pathological continuum, with cirrhosis being preceded by alcoholic hepatitis and earlier steatosis. It is now acknowledged that cirrhosis can develop in the alcoholic without alcoholic hepatitis as a precursor. In addition it is generally accepted that both steatosis and hepatitis regress following abstinence from alcohol. An important caveat is that hepatocellular damage related to severe alcoholic hepatitis can actually progress for a period after cessation of alcohol intake.

Comparatively little is known as to why a particular individual is predisposed to the development of liver disease in the face of excessive consumption. Many alcohol dependent persons tolerate decades of excessive alcohol consumption without developing chronic liver disease; however others develop cirrhosis after only a few years. It is clear that, despite copious research into the pathogenesis of ALD, much remains unexplained.

Alcohol could be directly hepatotoxic, or indirectly so, due to the formation of toxic metabolites or via other pathways. Alcohol is metabolized by both oxidative and non-oxidative mechanisms. The prominent mechanism is oxidative and is facilitated by three enzyme systems – alcohol dehydrogenase, the microsomal ethanol oxidizing system (MEOS), and catalase. The primary product of each of these systems is acetaldehyde.

The most important pathway of alcohol metabolism in the non-alcoholic is alcohol dehydrogenase. This enzyme converts alcohol to acetaldehyde which is subsequently metabolized to acetate by acetaldehyde dehydrogenase. Acetaldehyde can exert a number of pathologic effects on the hepatocyte. By contributing to lipid peroxidation, acetaldehyde can result in damage to the cell membrane. It does this by producing increased amounts of reduced nicotinamide adenine dinucleotide (NADH) and hydroxy radicals, inducing xanthine oxidase activity, increasing hepatic iron levels, and by inhibiting the cell's ability to inactivate reactive oxygen intermediates (Goldin, 1994). A further mechanism includes the formation of acetaldehyde adducts as a result of covalent bonding of acetaldehyde to amino groups, nucleotides, collagen, albumin and phospholipids (Lieber, 1994). These adducts may constitute neo-antigens and incite an immune response with subsequent hepatic inflammation.

The microsomal ethanol oxidizing system is induced by continued exposure to alcohol and therefore is of increased importance in the metabolism of alcohol in the alcohol dependent person. The cytochrome, P450IIE1 is of particular importance in the metabolism of ethanol. MEOS generates oxygen free radicals which can contribute to lipid peroxidation. Catalase contributes to less than 5% of alcohol consumption. Non-oxidative mechanisms like fatty acid ethyl synthase also contribute minimally to alcohol metabolism in the human.

Clearly, there are several metabolic pathways through which excessive alcohol consumption could lead to liver disease. Multiple molecular forms of both alcohol dehydrogenase and aldehyde dehydrogenase exist, and there are significant differences in the kinetic properties of several of them. It has been suggested that individuals who possess an allelic variant of the mitochondrial form of aldehyde dehydrogenase (ALDH$_2$), which is biologically inactive, are more susceptible to alcoholic liver injury. However, biochemical studies have so far provided minimal evidence as to why there is such a variation in susceptibility to liver damage.

WHY THE VARIATION IN SUSCEPTIBILITY?

From epidemiological, clinical and laboratory studies, we can conclude that excessive alcohol consumption is a cause of a spectrum of acute and chronic liver disease. In general, the higher the average daily intake, the more regular the consumption and the longer the duration of drinking, the more likely liver disease is to develop and the more likely it is to be severe. Animal models have demonstrated the successive development of alcoholic fatty liver, steatofibrosis, alcoholic hepatitis and, albeit in a small percentage of cases, an established cirrhosis.

Variation in susceptibility to liver damage is evident in the range of disease seen in persons consuming seemingly similar quantities of alcohol, and also from epidemiological studies that show that the risk of liver disease increases from a relatively low threshold, of the order of 20–60 g per day depending on gender. At these levels some individuals develop chronic liver damage, but the great majority do not. The reasons for this variation could be as follows:

1 There is considerable individual biological variation in susceptibility to the hepatotoxic effects of alcohol;
2 There are errors in reporting, classifying or summating alcohol intake;
3 Alcohol interacts with a range of other risk factors, resulting in disease at levels of consumption that would normally be innocuous.

Biological variation in response to alcohol

That the difference in risk is related primarily to differences in the biological response to repeated alcohol consumption is a plausible one. Wide variation is seen in the pharmacokinetics of alcohol and its acute effects. In studies conducted to determine whether various amounts of alcohol would result in blood alcohol concentrations exceeding the legal limit, persons given 30 g of alcohol (3 standard drinks) had blood alcohol concentrations after 1 hour ranging between 10 mg/100 ml and 90 mg/100 ml. Psychomotor performance showed a similar range of response. Reaction time varied from a 20% improvement to an 80% worsening. Equivalent variation is seen in the response to alcohol consumption of certain liver function tests, such as gamma glutamyltransferase and carbohydrate-deficient transferrin. Allelic variation in several forms of alcohol dehydrogenase and aldehyde dehydrogenase, with consequent variations in the metabolism of alcohol, may be a partial explanation for the pharmacokinetic and pharmacodynamic differences.

Measurement errors

Consumption data based on self-report are clearly vulnerable to errors in recall, dissembling, recording errors and lack of precision in their categorization. As judged by importation and sales figures determined by customs and excise departments and the licensed trade, only 40–60% of the alcohol consumed in a country is accounted for by that reported in general population surveys. There is evidence for systematic under-reporting of consumption, failure to sample the heaviest drinkers in general population surveys and errors of recall and recording. It is therefore possible that the supposed increase in risk of liver disease at low to moderate levels of consumption is a spurious one.

Let us suppose that a certain percentage of persons drinking 150 g alcohol per day report their consumption as 100 g per day. It seems likely that another percentage, presumably a smaller one, would report their consumption as 50 g per day. It is not inconceivable that a further percentage, presumably smaller still, will report their consumption as 25 g per day. The risk of liver disease due to consumption of 150 g alcohol per day would, therefore, be ascribed erroneously to a consumption range of 25–150 g. In this scenario, the relative risk of developing liver disease would increase progressively from 25 g per day up to 150 g per day, yet the basis for this relationship would be entirely false.

Synergism with other etiological factors

Clearly there is potential for synergism between alcohol and other risk factors when both are common in a population. Of the other causes of liver disease the following would fall within this category – hepatitis B, hepatitis C, possibly hepatitis G, disorders of iron metabolism, alpha$_1$ antitrypsin deficiency and certain commonly used hepatotoxic drugs such as paracetamol (acetaminophen). The autoimmune forms of liver disease, other inherited metabolic disorders and miscellaneous conditions such as hepatic venous thrombosis do not occur with sufficient frequency in the general population to act as co-factors to a meaningful extent. The same argument would apply to most drugs with hepatotoxic properties.

INTERACTION OF ALCOHOL AND OTHER CAUSES OF LIVER DISEASE

Given the high prevalence of excessive alcohol consumption, and the high prevalence of certain other causes of liver disease, for example infection with HCV or HBV or disorders of iron metabolism, it would not be uncommon for an individual's liver disease to have more than one etiology. Whether such an interaction is simply additive, or synergistic, is significant for the likelihood of liver disease developing and its natural history. In this section, we shall examine the evidence for an interaction between alcohol consumption and other causes of liver disease.

Alcohol and hepatitis C

Since the development of sensitive serological assays for hepatitis C infection in 1990, it has become evident that chronic hepatitis C represents a major public health problem. Hepatitis C constitutes an ever increasing proportion of hepatological practice. The prevalence of hepatitis C in the general population from different countries is reported to range from 0.15–2.5%. The commonest means of transmission in Western countries is now through injecting drug use, with sharing of contaminated injecting equipment. In Asian countries, vertical transmission is the more usual route of infection. Excessive alcohol consumption is only a modest risk factor for the acquisition of the hepatitis C virus.

Hepatitis C in alcoholic liver disease

Several studies have reported an increased prevalence of hepatitis C infection amongst patients with ALD. Mendenhall and colleagues (1993) reported that of 288 patients with ALD, 18.4% were positive for serological markers of hepatitis C. In this group of male veterans, 43.4% of HCV positive patients acquired their disease without an obvious mode of transmission. This increased prevalence of hepatitis C in patients with ALD without an obvious recognized risk-factor has been reported elsewhere (Befrits et al., 1995). The explanation for this observation remains unclear. The immunosuppression secondary to alcohol excess and pre-existing liver disease has been postulated to increase the susceptibility of such patients to infection with HCV. However, this correlation has also been otherwise ascribed to a high background prevalence of HCV in the population from which the studied group was drawn. In a cohort of 60 consecutive patients admitted for investigation of ALD in the west of Scotland, Bird and colleagues (1995) did not find serological evidence of HCV infection in any patient. The background population prevalence of HCV infection in this population was 0.07%.

In their USA multicenter study of patients with ALD, Mendenhall and colleagues (1993) reported that the presence of hepatitis C infection correlated with the clinical severity of liver disease and the presence of cirrhosis. Among 55 patients with alcohol-related liver disease, Kyriacou and colleagues (1995) found 15% were positive for HCV RNA using the polymerase chain reaction technique. All of the biopsy specimens showed features consistent with ALD. The histological features of hepatitis C could be distinguished in a liver already showing evidence of alcohol-induced damage. The presence of lymphoid aggregates in the triads and in the lobules, the pattern of fibrosis being periportal spurring rather than diffuse pericellular or venular fibrosis, and single apoptotic bodies were features of biopsies from HCV positive patients. However, in those patients with cirrhosis, it was not possible to determine the relative contribution of alcohol or hepatitis C (Kyriacou et al., 1995). Liver biopsy is a useful investigation in the alcoholic patient with chronic hepatitis C, but currently our capacity to define the relative contribution of either factor to the presence of cirrhosis is limited on histological evidence alone.

Hepatitis C and alcohol consumption

There have been several studies of persons with hepatitis C infection that have examined the influence of concomitant alcohol consumption. Seeff and colleagues (1992) studied the long-term mortality after transfusion-associated non-A, non-B hepatitis after an average follow-up of 18 years. In this study there was no significant difference in the proportion of patients with non-A, non-B hepatitis who were heavy drinkers and control subjects without hepatitis. In Australia, among 102 patients seen in an hepatology clinic, in whom the duration of hepatitis C infection was known, 21% of patients with high alcohol consumption had cirrhosis compared with 15% who had nil, low or moderate intake (Selvey et al., 1994). In the subset of 50 patients in whom the duration of infection was greater than 10 years, cirrhosis was present in 27% of those with a high intake of alcohol consumption compared with 17% of those with nil, low or moderate alcohol consumption.

More recently, Roudot-Thoraval and colleagues (1997) studied a large cohort of patients with hepatitis C to determine the role of the route of transmission of hepatitis C in the onset of cirrhosis. Six thousand, six hundred and sixty-four patients were enrolled in a nationwide survey of chronic hepatitis C in France. Of these, 21.4% had biopsy proven cirrhosis. The patient's alcohol consumption was determined. In this cohort, cirrhosis was more frequent in patients with excessive alcohol intake (34.9% vs. 18.2%; $p < 0.001$). This risk was independent of the route of transmission of hepatitis C. These data certainly suggest that excessive alcohol consumption in patients with hepatitis C results in more severe hepatic injury with a greater risk of the development of cirrhosis.

Two cross-sectional studies of patients being investigated for hepatitis C associated liver disease have found further evidence of exacerbation due to concomitant alcohol consumption. Hepatitis C positive patients with cirrhosis had a greater total lifetime alcohol consumption than those with chronic hepatitis (Ostapowicz *et al.*, 1998). Cumulative intake had also been greater during the known period of infection with hepatitis C. Total consumption was independent of age as a risk factor. Similarly, Pessione and colleagues (1998) reported that age and alcohol intake were independent risk factors for the development of fibrosis in patients with chronic hepatitis C infection. In this study there was a highly significant correlation between alcohol intake and HCV RNA levels, which is not the general experience.

Wiley and colleagues (1998) investigated 176 patients with hepatitis C infection, and subdivided them according to their history of alcohol consumption. Those in the higher intake range (average intake >40 g per day for women and >60 g per day for men, for more than 5 years) had a 2- to 3-fold higher risk of having cirrhosis and features of decompensated liver disease, than the lower intake group. In the former group, 58% had developed cirrhosis in the second decade after diagnosis compared with 10% of the lower range drinker. The effect of alcohol was independent of age, sex or mode of exposure.

The most persuasive evidence for the interaction between excessive alcohol consumption and hepatitis C derives from Corrao and Arico (1998), who adopted a case-control design among hospitalized patients. A careful history of alcohol intake throughout various phases of life was taken from each patient. Average daily consumption was calculated and patients ranked according to their intake. Among those in the lowest intake range (with a mean intake of zero), the odds ratio for cirrhosis rose from 1.0 in those who were HCV seronegative (the reference group) to 9.2 in those who were HCV scropositive. In those with the highest intakes, averaging 175 g per day, the odds ratio for cirrhosis was 15.0. This increased nearly 10-fold (to 147.2) in the hepatitis C seropositive group. The interaction between alcohol and hepatitis C appeared to be additive at intakes less than 50 g per day and multiplicative when consumption exceeded 125 g per day (Corrao and Arico, 1998).

Further studies are required to delineate the significance of this interaction. In particular, the interaction between chronic hepatitis C and ALD in predisposing to hepatocellular carcinoma remains to be explored (Cooksley, 1996). Importantly, the impact of concomitant alcoholic liver disease on the treatment of chronic hepatitis C with interferon and other agents remains undefined.

Alcohol and hepatitis B

Since the development of methods for detecting hepatitis B virus infection in the early-mid 1970s, there have been many studies examining possible synergy between alcohol and hepatitis B infection. Mills and his colleagues (1981) showed a significant difference in the prevalence of markers of hepatitis B between patients diagnosed as having alcoholic cirrhosis and a control group of alcoholic patients without significant liver disease.

Also in Scotland, Hislop and colleagues (1983) found evidence that prior hepatitis B infection (as demonstrated by anti-HBs) was significantly more common in patients with cirrhosis than those with alcoholic hepatitis or alcoholic fatty liver. Saunders and his colleagues (1983) found, in a series from King's College Hospital, London, no significant difference in the prevalence of hepatitis B markers between cirrhotic patients and those with alcoholic fatty liver. Occurrence of hepatitis B markers was linked to previous blood transfusions and residence in early life in a country with a high rate of endemic hepatitis B infection. In more recent studies the evidence continues to be inconsistent, but generally argues against a prominent interaction between alcohol use and hepatitis B, unlike the compelling evidence described above for hepatitis C.

Alcohol and other viruses

Little information is available about any interaction between alcohol and hepatitis G virus. Indeed, although this is an hepatotropic virus there is no consistent evidence that it is hepatotoxic to a significant extent. Patients with hepatitis G infection have only mild elevations of transaminase levels and there is no significant difference in these levels between those patients who are regular consumers of alcohol and those who are not.

Alcohol and nutrition

The relationship between ALD and nutrition has been the subject of debate throughout this century. Malnutrition is common in alcohol dependent individuals. This is generally ascribed to poor nutritional intake, but malabsorption and a hypercatabolic state may be contributing factors.

For many years ALD was thought to be predominantly a nutritional deficiency disorder. In an extensive series of studies, Lieber and colleagues have demonstrated that malnutrition is not obligatory for ALD to occur. Electron microscopic abnormalities and steatosis developed in human volunteers while on nutritionally adequate diets consisting in part of alcohol (Rubin and Lieber, 1968). In adolescent baboons fed a nutritionally adequate diet, with 50% of their calories from alcohol, Lieber and his colleagues showed that all developed fatty change, four developed hepatitis and two developed cirrhosis.

Notwithstanding these findings, there is evidence that malnutrition may lead to more severe alcoholic liver disease than would otherwise be expected. Mendenhall et al. (1984) reported that of 363 patients with alcoholic hepatitis, over half were substantially malnourished and none was completely free of malnutrition. The degree of nutritional deficiency correlated with clinical severity of liver disease (Mendenhall et al., 1984) and with mortality (Mendenhall et al., 1986).

The percentage of total energy intake consumed in the form of alcohol is strongly associated with mortality from cirrhosis. While it is known that correction of malnutrition, vitamin deficiencies and electrolyte disturbances improves the prognosis in ALD, there are no universally accepted guidelines for daily nutritional vitamin and mineral requirements in chronic heavy drinkers.

Alcohol and drugs

Numerous chemicals and pharmacological agents are associated with liver injury. The causative mechanisms are varied. Many adverse hepatic reactions are idiosyncratic and are immune-mediated. Most forms of drug-induced hepatitis do not occur with sufficient frequency to contribute to liver disease morbidity at a population level. Paracetamol (acetaminophen) may, however, be an exception. This analgesic is freely available. It exhibits a dose-dependent effect in producing hepatic toxicity. Acute hepatotoxicity is likely to result with ingestion of greater than 10 g of paracetamol. However, consumption of "safe" doses of paracetamol can result in hepatotoxicity in the presence of pre-existing liver disease, when ingested in combination with other enzyme-inducing drugs or in combination with other hepatotoxic agents. The total dose of paracetamol required to induce hepatic injury is significantly reduced in the alcohol-dependent person; doses as low as 3–4 g per day may be injurious.

The metabolism of paracetamol in the hepatocyte results in the formation of N-acetyl-p-benzoquinonimine (NAPBQI). This toxic metabolite is subsequently conjugated with glutathione and excreted in the urine. In paracetamol overdose this mechanism is saturated. When the level of glutathione falls to below 70% of normal, NAPBQI conjugates with hepatoproteins resulting in hepatocyte injury (Collins and Starmer, 1995).

Collins and Starmer (1995) summarized the findings in 58 alcohol-dependent patients who sustained severe hepatic injury following ingestion of therapeutic doses of paracetamol. The enhanced susceptibility of alcohol-dependent patients to paracetamol-induced hepatotoxicity may be explained by an enhanced rate of formation of the toxic metabolite, NAPBQI or by a reduction in the amount of glutathione available for its detoxification. Conceivably chronic ingestion of therapeutic doses of paracetamol in combination with excessive alcohol consumption may result in chronic, progressive liver disease.

Alcohol and iron metabolism

Hereditary hemochromatosis is a well characterized inherited metabolic disorder in which there is excessive storage of iron secondary to unregulated and excessive iron absorption. The excess iron is deposited in the liver, pancreas, skin, myocardium, and pituitary in addition to other organs, resulting in well described clinical manifestations. One of the major manifestations of iron overload in hereditary hemochromatosis is hepatic injury with the development of fibrosis and subsequent cirrhosis.

Approximately one-third of patients with hereditary hemochromatosis are excessive drinkers. Excessive iron stores are also detected in liver biopsies of patients with ALD (termed alcoholic siderosis). The distinction between hereditary hemochromatosis and alcoholic siderosis has been enhanced by the use of hepatic iron concentration and hepatic iron index. A pivotal finding in 1996 was the description by Feder and colleagues (1996) of a strong candidate gene for hereditary hemochromatosis on the short arm of chromosome 6. Eighty-three per cent of cases of hereditary hemochromatosis were associated with homozygosity for a cysteine to arginine point mutation at codon 282 (C282Y). Several other cases were compound heterozygotes for the C2827 mutation and a H63D mutation.

To clarify the relationship between hereditary hemochromatosis and ALD and siderosis, Adams and Agnew (1996) retrospectively analyzed the clinical features, iron status, alcohol history, liver histology and long-term survival in 105 homozygotes for hemochromatosis. Only subjects with a HLA identical sibling with iron overload were included. Heavy alcohol consumption was found in 15% of subjects. Despite heavy alcohol consumption, histological features associated with ALD were absent from most biopsies. Importantly, those hemochromatosis patients with heavy alcohol consumption had a higher prevalence of cirrhosis at the time of diagnosis. There was no difference in iron load, which suggests a synergistic, direct toxic effect of alcohol rather than a secondary effect on iron absorption or metabolism. Survival was significantly reduced in hemochromatosis patients with heavy alcohol consumption; however, the cause of death was not directly related to alcohol abuse in most cases.

There is also evidence that iron loading acts as a hepatotoxin that aggravates liver damage from other causes (George *et al.*, 1999). Thus there is now support for the concept that iron overload and alcohol excess are independent hepatotoxins and act synergistically to cause liver disease. It emphasizes the advisability for persons with hemochromatosis to restrict alcohol consumption severely.

COMPARATIVE INCIDENCE OF ALCOHOL-INDUCED LIVER DISEASE

The incidence of ALD is closely related to the *per capita* consumption of alcohol in the population. At the peak of alcohol consumption in modern times, during the 1960s and 1970s, it was estimated that 80–90% of all cases of chronic liver disease in some countries was due to alcohol. With the decline in overall consumption over the past two decades in most Western countries and the rise in incidence of (and our awareness of) hepatitis C infection, it is likely that this percentage has fallen, but to what? The question is made more difficult because of the evidence now that alcohol consumption has a synergistic effect with other risk factors for liver disease. A level of consumption that would be innocuous in itself may cause disease in the presence of a hepatotropic virus or hepatotoxin. Because of the biases inherent in clinical series, the answer must await population-level studies in which all cases of chronic liver disease are identified and the effects of changing consumption on its incidence can be determined. Perhaps a best estimate is that approximately 50% of the burden of chronic liver disease in most Western countries is due to excessive alcohol consumption. This percentage inevitably fluctuates with changes in levels and patterns of consumption. We need to be mindful that ALD could rapidly assume its former status as the overwhelmingly dominant form of chronic liver disease, if excessive alcohol consumption were to become as prevalent as it was 20 years ago.

REFERENCES

Adams, P.C. and Agnew, S. (1996) Alcoholism in hereditary haemochromatosis revisited: prevalence and clinical consequences among homozygous siblings. *Hepatology* **23**, 724–727.

Baillie, M. (1793) *The Morbid Anatomy of the Most Important Parts of the Human Body*, edited by J. Johnson and G. Nicol, London: St Paul's Churchyard and Pall Mall.

Batey, R.G., Burns, T., Benson, R.J. and Blyth, K. (1992) Alcohol consumption and the risk of cirrhosis. *Medical Journal of Australia* **156**, 413–416.

Becker, U., Deis, A., Sørensen, T.I.A., Grønbæk, M., Borch-Johnsen, K., Müller, C.F., Schnohr, P. and Jensen, G. (1996) Prediction of risk of liver disease by alcohol intake, sex and age: a prospective population study. *Hepatology* **23**, 1025–1029.

Befrits, R., Hedman, M., Blomquist, L., Allander, T., Grillner, L., Kinnman, N., Rubio, C. and Hultcrantz, R. (1995) Chronic hepatitis C in alcoholic patients: prevalence, genotypes and correlation to liver disease. *Scandinavian Journal of Gastroenterology* **30**, 1113–1118.

Bird, G.L.A., Tibbs, C.J., Orton, D., Hillan, K.J., MacSween, R.N.M., Williams, R. and Mills, P.R. (1995) Does hepatitis C contribute to liver injury in alcohol abusers in the west of Scotland? *European Journal of Gastroenterology and Hepatology* **7**, 161–163.

Blair, H.W. (1888) *The Temperance Movement or Conflict between Man and Alcohol*, edited by William E. Smythe, Boston.

Collins, C. and Starmer, G.A. (1995) A review of the hepatotoxicity of paracetamol at therapeutic or near-therapeutic dose levels, with particular reference to alcohol abusers. *Drug Alcohol Review* **14**, 63–79.

Cooksley, W.G.E. (1996) Chronic liver disease: Do alcohol and hepatitis C interact? *Journal of Gastroenterology and Hepatology* **11**, 187–192.

Corrao, G. and Arico, S. (1998) Independent and combined action of hepatitis C virus infection and alcohol consumption on the risk of symptomatic liver cirrhosis. *Hepatology* **27**, 914–919.

Department of Community Services and Health (1988) *Alcohol: The Facts*. Canberra: Australian Government Publishing Service.

Feder, J.N., Gnirke, A., Thomas, W., Tsuchihashi, Z., Ruddy, D.A., Basava, A. *et al.* (1996) A novel MHC class 1-like gene is responsible in patients with hereditary haemochromatosis. *Nature Genetics* **13**, 399–408.

George, D.K., Goldwurm, S., MacDonald, G.A. *et al.* (1998) Increased hepatic iron concentration in non-alcoholic steatohepatitis is associated with increased fibrosis. *Gastroenterology* **114**, 311–318.

George, D.K., Powell, L.W. and Losowsky, M.S. (1999) The haemochromatosis gene: a co-factor for chronic liver diseases? *Journal of Gastroenterology and Hepatology* **14**, 745–749.

Goldin, R. (1994) The pathogenesis of alcoholic liver disease. *International Journal of Experimental Pathology* **75**, 71–78.

Grant, B.F., Dufour, M.C. and Harford, T.C. (1988) Epidemiology of alcoholic liver disease. *Seminars in Liver Disease* **8**, 12–25.

Grant, B.G., DeBakey, S. and Zobeck, T.S. (1991) Liver cirrhosis mortality in the United States, 1973–1988. *National Institute of Alcohol Abuse and Alcoholism Surveillance Report* **18**, 1–44.

Halliday, M.L., Coates, R.A. and Rankin, J.G. (1991) Changing trends in cirrhosis mortality in Ontario, Canada 1911–1986. *International Journal of Epidemiology* **20**, 199–208.

Harford, T.C. and Brooks, S.D. (1992) Cirrhosis mortality and occupation. *Journal of Studies on Alcohol* **53**, 463–468.

Hilton, M.E. (1988) Trends in US drinking patterns: further evidence from the past 20 years. *British Journal of Addiction* **83**, 269–278.

Hislop, W.S., Bouchier, I.A.D., Allan, J.G., Brunt, P.W., Eastwood, M., Finlayson, N.D.C., James, O., Russell, R.I. and Watkinson, G. (1983) Alcoholic liver disease in Scotland and North-eastern England: presenting features in 510 patients. *Quarterly Journal of Medicine* **206**, 232–242.

Hunter, D.J.W., Halliday, M.L., Coates, T.A. and Rankin, J.G. (1988) Hospital morbidity from cirrhosis of the liver and per capita consumption of absolute alcohol in Ontario 1978–1982: a descriptive analysis. *Canadian Journal of Public Health* **79**, 243–248.

Ishak, K.G., Zimmerman, H.J. and Ray, M.B. (1991) Alcoholic liver disease: pathologic, pathogenic and clinical aspects. *Alcoholism: Clinical and Experimental Research* **15**, 45–66.

Kyriacou, E., Simmonds, P., Miller, E.K., Bouchier, I.A.D., Hayes, P.C. and Harrison, D.J. (1995) Liver biopsy findings in patients with alcoholic liver disease complicated by chronic hepatitis C infection. *European Journal of Gastroenterology and Hepatology* **7**, 331–334.

Ledermann, S. (1956) *Alcool, Alcoolisme, Alcoolisation. Donnés Scientifiques de Caractère Physiologique, Economique et Socials,* pp. 124–128. Paris: Presses Universitaires de France.

Lelbach, W.K. (1975) Cirrhosis in the alcoholic and its relation to volume of alcohol abuse. *Annals of the New York Academy of Science* **252**, 85–105.

Lieber, C.S. (1993) Alcoholic liver disease: a public health issue in need of a public health approach. *Seminars in Liver Disease* **13**, i–iii.

Lieber, C.S. (1994) Alcohol and the liver: 1994 update. *Gastroenterology* **106**, 1085–1105.

Mao, Y., Morrison, H., Johnson, R.J. and Semenciw, R. (1992) Liver cirrhosis mortality and per capita alcohol consumption in Canada. *Revue Canadienne de Santé Publique* **83**, 80–81.

Mendenhall, C.L., Anderson, S., Weesner, R.E., Goldberg, S.J. and Crolic, K.A. (1984) Protein-calorie malnutrition associated with alcoholic hepatitis. *American Journal of Medicine* **76**, 211–222.

Mendenhall, C.L., Tosch, T., Weesner, R.E., Garcia-Pont, P., Goldberg, S.J., Kiernan, T., Seeff, M.D., Sorrell, M., Tamburro, C., Zetterman, R., Chedid, A., Chen, T. and Rabin, L. (1986) VA co-operative study on alcoholic hepatitis II: prognostic significance of protein-calorie malnutrition. *American Journal of Clinical Nutrition* **43**, 213–218.

Mendenhall, C.L., Moritz, T., Rouster, S., Roselle, G., Polito, A., Quan, S., DiNelle, R.K. and the VA Cooperative Study Group 275 (1993) Epidemiology of hepatitis C among veterans with alcoholic liver disease. *American Journal of Gastroenterology* **88**, 1022–1026.

Mills, P.R., Follett, E.A.C., Urquhart, G.E.D., Clements, G., Watkinson, G. and MacSween, R.N. (1981) Evidence for previous hepatitis B virus infection in alcoholic cirrhosis. *British Medical Journal* **282**, 437–438.

National Institute on Alcohol Abuse and Alcoholism. (1990) *Alcohol and Health.* Washington, DC: US Department of Health and Human Services.

Norstrom, T. (1987) The abolition of the Swedish alcohol rationing system: effects on consumption distribution and cirrhosis mortality. *British Journal of Addiction* **82**, 633–641.

Norton, R., Batey, R., Dwyer, T. and MacMahon, S. (1987) Alcohol consumption and risk of alcohol related cirrhosis in women. *British Medical Journal* **295**, 80–82.

Ohnishi, K. and Okuda, K. (1986) Alcoholic liver disease in Japan. *Journal of Clinical Gastroenterology* **8**, 503–508.

Ostapowicz, G., Watson, K.J.R., Locarnini, S.A. and Desmond, P.V. (1998) Role of alcohol in the progression of liver disease caused by hepatitis C virus infection. *Hepatology* **27**, 1730–1735.

Parrish, K.M., Higuchi, S., Muramatsu, T., Stinson, F.S. and Harford, T.C. (1991) A method for estimating alcohol related liver cirrhosis mortality in Japan. *International Journal of Epidemiology* **20**, 921–926.

Péquignot, G. (1960) Enquête par interrogatoire sur les circonstances diététiques de la cirrhose alcoolique en France. *Annales Medico Chirurgicales du Centre* **17**, 1–21.

Péquignot, G., Chabert, C., Eydoux H. *et al.* (1974) Augmentation du risque de cirrhose en fonction de la ration d'alcool. *Revue de l'Alcoolisme* **20**, 191–202.

Péquignot, G., Tuyns, A.J. and Berta, J.L. (1978) Ascitic cirrhosis in relation to alcohol consumption. *International Journal of Epidemiology* **7**, 113–120.

Pessione, F., Degos, F., Marcellin, P., Duchatelle, V., Njapoum, C., Martinot-Peignoux, M., Degott, C., Valla, D., Erlinger, S. and Rueff, R. (1998) Effect of Alcohol Consumption on Serum Hepatitis C Virus RNA and Histological Lesions in Chronic Hepatitis C. *Hepatology* **27**, 1717–1722.

Roizen, R., Kerr, W.C. and Fillmore, K.M. (1999) Cirrhosis mortality and per capita consumption of distilled spirits, United States, 1949–1994: trend analysis. *British Medical Journal* **319**, 666–670.

Romelsjo, A. and Agren, G. (1985) Has mortality related to alcohol decreased in Sweden? *British Medical Journal* **291**, 167–170.

Roudot-Thoraval, F., Bastic, A., Pawlotsky, J.-M., Dhumeaux, D. and the Study Group for the Prevalence and Epidemiology of Hepatitis C Virus (1997) Epidemological factors affecting the severity of hepatitis C virus-related liver disease: a French survey of 6,664 patients. *Hepatology* **26**, 485–490.

Royal College of Physicians (1987) *The Medical Consequences of Alcohol Abuse: a Great and Growing Evil*. London: Tavistock.

Rubin, E. and Lieber, C.S. (1968) Alcohol induced hepatic injury in non-alcoholic volunteers. *New England Journal of Medicine* **278**, 869–876.

Saunders, J.B. (1986) *Studies in Alcoholic Liver Disease: its Natural History, Detection and Pathogenesis*. MD Thesis, University of Cambridge.

Saunders, J.B., Walters, J.R.F., Davies, P. and Paton, A. (1981a) A 20-year prospective study of cirrhosis. *British Medical Journal* **282**, 263–266.

Saunders, J.B., Davis, M. and Williams, R. (1981b) Do women develop alcoholic liver disease more readily than men? *British Medical Journal* **282**, 1140–1143.

Saunders, J.B., Wodak, A.D., Morgan-Capner, P., White, Y.S., Portmann, B., Davis, M. and Williams, R. (1983) Importance of markers of hepatitis B virus in alcoholic liver disease. *British Medical Journal* **286**, 1851–1854.

Saunders, J.B., Wodak, A.D. and Williams, R. (1985) Past experience of advice and treatment for drinking problems of patients with alcoholic liver disease. *British Journal of Addiction* **80**, 51–56.

Saunders, J.B. and Latt, N. (1993) Epidemiology of alcoholic liver disease. *Ballière's Clinical Gastroenterology* **7**, 555–579.

Savolainen, V.T., Liesto, K., Mannikko, A., Penttila, A. and Karhunen, P.J. (1993) Alcohol consumption and alcoholic liver disease: evidence of a threshold level of effects of ethanol. *Alcoholism: Clinical and Experimental Research* **17**, 1112–1117.

Schmidt, W. (1977) The epidemiology of cirrhosis of the liver: a statistical analysis of mortality data with special reference to Canada. In *Alcohol and the Liver*, edited by M.N. Fisher and J.G. Rankin, pp. 1–26. New York: Plenum.

Seeff, L.B., Buskell-Bales, Z., Wright, E.C., Durako, S.J., Alter, H.J., Iber, F.L., Hollinger, F.B., Gitnick, G., Knodell, R.G., Perrillo, R.P., Stevens, C.E., Hollingsworth, C.G. and the National Heart, Lung and Blood Institute Study Group (1992) Long-term mortality after transfusion-associated non-A, non-B hepatitis. *New England Journal of Medicine* **327**, 1906–1911.

Seeley, J.R. (1960) Death by liver cirrhosis and the price of beverage alcohol. *Canadian Medical Association Journal* **83**, 1361–1366.

Selvey, L., Srirajalingam, M., Crawford, D. and Cooksley, W.G.E. (1994) Alcohol does not play a significant role in promoting cirrhosis in chronic hepatitis C: analysis of 202 patients. In *Round Table Conference: Alcohol and Viruses*. Surfers Paradise, Australia: International Society for Biomedical Research in Alcoholism.

Smart, R.G. (1974) The effect of licensing restrictions during 1914–1918 on drunkenness and liver cirrhosis deaths in Britain. *British Journal of Addiction* **69**, 109–121.

Smart, R.G. (1988) Recent international reductions and increases in liver cirrhosis deaths. *Alcoholism: Clinical and Experimental Research* **12**, 239–242.

Smart, R.G. (1989) Is the post-war drinking binge ending? Cross-national trends in per capita alcohol consumption. *British Journal of Addiction* **84**, 743–748.

Sørensen, T.I.A. (1989) Alcohol and liver injury: Dose-related or permissive effect? *Liver* **9**, 189–197.

Sørensen, T.I.A., Orholm, M., Bentsen, K.D., Høybye, G., Eghøje, K. and Christoffersen, P. (1984) Prospective evaluation of alcohol abuse and alcoholic liver injury in men as predictors of development of cirrhosis. *Lancet* **ii**, 241–244.

Stinson, F.S. and DeBakey, S.M. (1992) Alcohol related mortality in the United States 1979–1988. *British Journal of Addiction* **87**, 777–783.

Stone, W.D., Islam, N.R.K. and Paton, A. (1968) The natural history of cirrhosis. *Quarterly Journal of Medicine* **37**, 119–132.

Thaler, H. (1990) Alcoholic cirrhosis: what do we really know about its aetiology? *Tokai Journal of Experimental and Clinical Medicine* **15**, 275–284.

Wiley, T.E., McCarthy, M., Breidi, L. and Loyden, T.J. (1998) Impact of alcohol on the histological and clinical progression of hepatitis C infection. *Hepatology* **28**, 805–809.

Williams, G.D. and DeBakey, S.F. (1992) Changes in levels of alcohol consumption: United States, 1983–1988. *British Journal of Addiction* **87**, 643–648.

Wodak, A.D., Saunders, J.B., Ewusi-Mensah, I., Davis, M. and Williams, R. (1983) Severity of alcohol dependence in patients with alcoholic liver disease. *British Medical Journal* **287**, 1420–1422.

Chapter 17

Serum diagnosis of alcoholic liver disease and markers of ethanol intake

Onni Niemelä

Although excessive ethanol intake is known to be a common reason for hospital admissions, the diagnosis of problem drinking in its early phase usually fails. Health problems due to ethanol intake are known to arise at a level of 5–6 daily standard drinks (men) or 3–4 drinks (women). Therefore, diagnostic tests to screen for alcohol abuse should be highly sensitive. They should also be very specific to achieve positive predictive power. However, to date such methods have not been available and far too many alcohol consuming patients enter the stage of severe dependence and tissue injury, including alcoholic liver disease, before being referred for treatment. Questionnaires for alcohol consumption are unreliable because they depend on self-reports. Currently recommended laboratory markers of alcohol abuse, such as γ-glutamyltransferase (GGT) or mean corpuscular volume of erythrocytes (MCV), are often altered due to reasons unrelated to alcohol abuse. Carbohydrate-deficient transferrin (CDT) has shown promise as a more specific indicator of ethanol consumption and alcohol-related liver disease, but unfortunately this marker lacks sensitivity, identifying only about one third of the problem drinkers without liver disease.

Preliminary measurements of protein-acetaldehyde adducts have indicated elevated concentrations from erythrocytes of alcohol abusers and of healthy volunteers after ethanol intake. However, no routine applications of adduct measurements are available. Autoimmune responses towards proteins modified with ethanol metabolites have been demonstrated from patients with alcoholic liver disease, which may prove to be useful in the differential diagnosis of alcoholic versus non-alcoholic liver diseases. In patients with liver disease, serum collagen-derived peptides, primarily the aminoterminal propeptide of type III procollagen (PIIINP), should be measured to assess the activity of fibrogenesis.

KEYWORDS: alcohol markers, acetaldehyde adducts, desialotransferrin, connective tissue metabolism

INTRODUCTION

Alcohol-related diseases are currently one of the leading causes of morbidity and mortality throughout the world (Lieber, 1995). The detrimental effects of alcohol abuse also continue to grow. Surveys in many general hospitals have revealed that 15–30% of all hospital admissions are related to excessive drinking (Scheig, 1991; Bonkovsky, 1992). However, hazardous drinking practices usually remain unrecognized by the clinicians. Therefore, such patients also tend to escape specific treatment (Rosman and Lieber, 1994).

The methods available for identifying problem drinking include various structural questionnaires and laboratory tests for biological variables that are known to be altered as a result of heavy alcohol intake (Salaspuro, 1986; Skinner *et al.*, 1986; Watson *et al.*, 1986; Crabb, 1990; Rosman and Lieber, 1992; Rosman and Lieber, 1994; Sillanaukee, 1996; Allen *et al.*, 1997; Helander *et al.*, 1997; Allen and Litten, 2001). Questionnaires (such as CAGE, MAST, or AUDIT) have been considered unreliable for a variety of reasons, such as the prevailing attitudes towards drinking both among patients and healthcare personnel. They are, however, useful to obtain information from the pattern of drinking, which is important since many adverse consequences of ethanol intake are related to heavy drinking on occasions whereas others are found from individuals with continuous consumption (Seppä *et al.*, 1990; MacKenzie *et al.*, 1996; Allen *et al.*, 1997).

Laboratory markers for ethanol consumption and alcoholic liver disease are important to help the clinicians to raise the issue of excessive drinking as the underlying cause for health problems. They are also needed in the follow-up of patients who are willing to reduce their ethanol intake (Rosman and Lieber, 1994). Analogously, studies in patients with diabetes have indicated that the patient's knowledge of blood test results on glucose balance markedly improves compliance and treatment outcome (Larsen *et al.*, 1990). Assessment of ethanol consumption by laboratory methods has, however, not been satisfactory, since all the markers available continue to lack both sensitivity and specificity (Salaspuro, 1986; Skinner *et al.*, 1986; Allen *et al.*, 1997; Helander *et al.*, 1997). Ideally, the following types of markers should be available:

1   Specific markers for the amount of ethanol consumed;
2   Specific markers for ethanol-induced damage in any given tissue;
3   Genetic markers to examine the predisposition and risk for alcohol dependence.

This contribution will focus on the current knowledge on laboratory markers of ethanol intake and alcoholic liver disease. Although an extensive amount of literature in this field is available, the information on the sensitivities and specificities of even the most commonly used markers has remained controversial (Allen *et al.*, 1997). Many marker studies have also contrasted extreme populations such as obvious alcoholics to teetotalers. Not surprisingly, studies have also usually failed to clearly distinguish between the amount of alcohol consumed and the secondary effects of liver disease. In addition, striking gender differences on the development of alcohol-induced diseases and on the clinical performance of alcohol markers should be emphasized (Iimuro *et al.*, 1997; Schenker, 1997).

THE RELATIONSHIP OF ALCOHOL CONSUMPTION AND HEALTH PROBLEMS

Assessment of the actual amount of ethanol consumption is important since it is known to determine the risk for subsequent medical problems (Lieber, 1988a; Crabb, 1990; Lieber, 1995). At the population level, alcohol use is usually expressed as *per capita* consumption, which is obtained by dividing the total quantity of alcohol sold by the total population aged 14 years or older. At the individual level, assessment of alcohol consumption is more difficult since it is based on self-reports, which are known to usually account for only about half of the alcohol sold (Poikolainen, 1985).

It should be pointed out that most people who drink alcohol are able to limit their intake to amounts that produce no apparent health problems. Those who drink no alcohol are *teetotalers*, whereas *moderate drinkers* are individuals who are able to control their drinking and who consume amounts that are so small that no adverse consequences are to be expected. Interestingly, several population studies have indicated that the rate of mortality in individuals who consume one to three drinks daily (10–30 g ethanol/day) is lower than that in teetotalers. However, at higher levels of consumption the risk of morbidity and mortality starts to increase rapidly. *Heavy drinkers* drink large amounts on any single occasion or frequently consume moderate amounts. Although there is no clear threshold for heavy drinking, epidemiological studies have suggested that exceeding the level of approximately 300 grams for men or 200 grams for women of ethanol per week creates health problems. Quantities exceeding 5–6 drinks (men), or 3–4 drinks (women) on any single drinking occasion are also harmful. *Alcohol abuse* refers to problem drinking that results in health consequences, social problems or both. In such patients, alcohol has caused mental or physical complications, although the criteria for alcoholism may not be fulfilled. *Alcoholism* is the most severe problem related to alcohol consumption involving severe dependency and increased tolerance. In alcoholics, withdrawal symptoms appear after cessation of drinking.

MAIN FEATURES OF ALCOHOLIC LIVER DISEASE

The liver is the primary site for alcohol metabolism and therefore it is also subject to a variety of adverse effects of excessive ethanol intake. Ethanol-induced liver pathology in turn is known to result in striking alterations in a variety of laboratory parameters which reflect liver status. In fact, many currently available alcohol markers rather mark liver damage than alcohol consumption *per se*.

The wide spectrum of alcoholic liver disease (ALD) includes fatty liver, alcoholic hepatitis, fibrosis, and cirrhosis (Diehl, 1989; Rubin and Farber, 1994; Lieber, 1995). These lesions usually develop sequentially, although they may coexist in combinations (Rubin and Farber, 1994). *Alcoholic fatty liver* may appear even after a few days of excess alcohol and is usually reversible. In cases of uncomplicated fatty liver, the patients usually lack clinical symptoms of liver disease. *Alcoholic hepatitis* is a clinically severe condition, which is histologically characterized by necrosis of hepatocytes, cytoplasmic hyaline inclusions within hepatocytes, neutrophilic inflammatory response and perivenular fibrosis (Rubin and Farber, 1994). The typical clinical symptoms include malaise, right upper quadrant abdominal pain and jaundice. There may also be fever and mild leukocytosis. *Fibrosis* showing a pericellular distribution can be seen as an early feature of ALD. With continuing inflammation there is usually progressive fibrosis. In about 15% of alcoholics, this leads to the formation of fibrous septa surrounding hepatocellular nodules, which are characteristic of *liver cirrhosis*. Such patients present distinct systemic effects of altered metabolism, changes in hormone levels, protein abnormalities and defective coagulation.

CONVENTIONAL MARKERS OF ETHANOL CONSUMPTION AND ALCOHOLIC LIVER DISEASE

Ethanol measurements

Measurements of ethanol concentrations from blood, breath, or urine samples are normally used to diagnose ethanol intoxication. However, such measurements can also be used as an aid to reach conclusions on long-term alcohol consumption (Salaspuro, 1986; Sillanaukee, 1996). When combined with the clinical observations, the demonstration of high blood ethanol concentrations may reveal increased tolerance towards alcohol. According to the National Council on Alcoholism (NCA, USA), blood or breath alcohol levels exceeding 150 mg/L (33 mmol/L) without obvious evidence of intoxication or 300 mg/L (65 mmol/L) at any time indicate alcoholism (Table 17.1). These criteria may also help to distinguish between acute intoxication and chronic alcohol consumption (Salaspuro, 1986). Ethanol measurements are simple to perform and therefore suitable for screening both by law enforcement agencies or by hospitals. They are also useful in follow-up studies to examine non-compliance for abstinence. Unfortunately, the short half-life of ethanol limits the use of this marker. It should also be noted that ethanol elimination rate is influenced by drinking practice, e.g., heavy drinkers typically show 1.5-times faster elimination rates than non-drinkers.

Gamma-glutamyl transferase (GGT)

Gamma-glutamyl transferase (GGT) is a membrane-bound glycoprotein enzyme that catalyzes the transfer of the gamma-glutamyl moiety of glutathione to the various peptide acceptors. Chronic ethanol consumption is known to induce a rise in serum GGT (Table 17.1). The increased concentrations of the enzyme usually return to normal if the patient abstains from alcohol. Serum GGT is currently the most widely used laboratory parameter of problem drinking (Salaspuro, 1986; Watson *et al.*, 1986; Rosman and Lieber, 1992). In most studies, the sensitivity of GGT has been reported to be higher than those of other commonly used markers. Results from a recent WHO/ISBRA collaborative project on state and trait markers of alcoholism (Helander *et al.*, 1997) indicated that serum GGT concentrations are increased in 52% of alcohol-dependent subjects, in 28% of heavy drinkers, in 15% of light/moderate drinkers, although also in 10% of non-drinkers (Table 17.2).

Monitoring serum GGT concentrations may also help to distinguish chronic alcoholics with or without liver disease (Moussavian *et al.*, 1985; Rosman and Lieber, 1994). Persistently abnormal values in the absence of continuing exposure to ethanol suggest the presence of liver disease. Liver disease may be present if GGT is initially 8–10 times normal and if the elevation persists after 6–8 weeks of abstention from alcohol. On the other hand, if initial GGT levels are only 2–3 times normal and return to normal after abstention, the patient is likely to be devoid of liver disease (see Balisteri and Rej, 1994). Due to the lack of specificity, GGT is a poor marker when alcohol consumption needs to be screened in patients with non-alcoholic liver diseases or in hospitalized patients in general (Table 17.1). Serum GGT is increased in all forms of liver disease, particularly in cases of intra- or

Table 17.1 Characteristics of blood alcohol markers

	Half-life, elimination rate	Characteristics
Conventional markers		
B-Ethanol	1 g/1 hour/10 kg	Blood or breath alcohol levels exceeding 150 mg/L (33 mmol/L) without obvious evidence of intoxication or 300 mg/L (65 mmol/L) at any time indicate excessive alcohol consumption.
S-GGT	2–4 weeks	GGT is elevated in 10–20% of middle-aged men, of which 75% are due to alcohol consumption (Salaspuro, 1986). False positive values are found in non-alcoholic liver diseases, liver malignancies, diabetes (in 57% of those with arterial complications), obesity, pancreatitis, hyperlipidemia, cardiac insufficiency, severe trauma, medications (barbiturates, drugs for epilepsy, anticoagulants), nephrotic syndrome, renal rejection, advanced age.
E-MCV	2–4 months	More sensitive in women. Specificity is decreased by B$_{12}$-vitamin or folic acid deficiency, liver diseases, haematological diseases, hypothyroidism, reticulocytosis, smoking. Note! Elevated red cell distribution width, RDW, may indicate alcohol abuse even if MCV is normal (alcoholics with iron deficiency).
S-CDT	2–3 weeks	Most specific of the currently available methods. Specificity is decreased by high serum transferrin (CDTect method) for instance in patients with iron deficiency, some liver diseases, especially primary biliary cirrhosis, chronic hepatitis, liver malignancies, genetic D-variants of transferrin (rare).
S-AST	2–3 weeks	Specificity is decreased by non-alcoholic liver disease, muscle injury. S-AST/S-ALT ratio of >1.0 is suggestive of alcoholic liver disease.
Other markers		
fS-HDL		Increases even after relatively moderate doses of ethanol (3–5 drinks per day regularly) and decreases within a week upon abstinence.
fS-Trigly		Even acute excessive doses of ethanol may increase serum triglyseride levels for about a week.
B-Thromb		Thrombocytopenia (low platelet count) is common in alcoholics (present in about one third of those admitted to hospitals). Upon abstinence, the levels normalise rapidly and may turn to reactive thrombocytopenia for a period of few days.
S-IgA		Is increased in chronic alcoholic liver disease. In ALD, specific IgA antibodies directed towards protein modifications induced by ethanol are also seen. An increased ratio of IgA/IgG is indicative of ALD.
S-ALB		Low in severe liver disease. Albumin levels below 25 g/L are associated with poor prognosis.
S-BIL		Bilirubin levels above 136 µmol/L are associated with poor prognosis.
S-PIIINP		High values suggest fibrogenesis. Follow-up of liver fibrogenesis.

Abbreviations: B, Blood; S, Serum; GGT, Gamma-Glutamyltransferase; E-MCV, Mean Corpuscular Volume of Erythrocytes, CDT, Carbohydrate Deficient Transferrin; AST/ALT, Aspartate Aminotransferase/Alanine Aminotransferase Ratio; fS, Fasting Serum; HDL, High-Density Lipoprotein; Trigly, Triglycerides; Thromb, Thrombocytes; Ferrit, Ferritin; IgA, Immunoglobulin A; ALB, Albumin; BIL, Bilirubin; PIIINP, Aminoterminal Propeptide of Type III Procollagen. For ethanol, 1 g/L = 21.7 mmol/L.

Table 17.2 Sensitivities and specificities of commonly used markers of ethanol intake

	n	GGT	CDT	AST
Sensitivity				
Light/Moderate drinkers	26	15%	11%	15%
Heavy drinkers	25	28%	27%	32%
Alcoholics	23	52%	39%	39%
Specificity	21	90%	100%	86%

Source: Helander *et al.*, 1997 (WHO/ISBRA collaborative project on state and trait markers of alcoholism).

posthepatic biliary obstruction. Small increases (2–5 times normal) are observed in patients with fatty liver. Transient increases also occur in patients with drug intoxication.

Mean corpuscular volume (MCV)

Red blood cell size (MCV, mean corpuscular volume) is often used as a part of the screening procedure for the detection of alcohol abuse. It is known to increase as a result of ethanol consumption, particularly in women (Table 17.1). Most studies have indicated 40–80% sensitivities for this marker. Morgan and co-workers (1981) have reported a 86% incidence of macrocytosis in female alcoholics as compared to 63% in males. In studies comparing the sensitivities of GGT and MCV, the former has usually reached higher sensitivities at least in males. In some studies, MCV has shown a stronger correlation with the reported drinking than GGT (see Sillanaukee, 1996). MCV responds slowly to abstinence which hampers its use as a tool for follow-up. Although MCV returns to normal upon abstinence, this may require 2 to 4 months.

Morphological examination of blood films from patients with alcohol abuse and high MCV (macrocytosis) show several characteristic abnormalities (Lindenbaum, 1977, 1987). Macrocytes from alcohol abusers are typically round rather than oval. Erythrocyte morphology may also reveal excessive stomatocytosis or knizocytosis. Macrocytosis in heavy drinkers is normally found without anemia, whereas anemia is common in patients with severe dependence and liver disease. Such patients may also suffer from folate deficiency and megaloblastic alterations in bone marrow. When there is simultaneous iron-deficiency, an increased red cell distribution width (RDW) and dimorphic blood film are typical findings (Seppä *et al.*, 1991). Alcoholic liver disease may also be associated with spur-cell (acanthoid cells, irregularly spiculated cells) hemolytic anemia. Pathological ring sideroblasts have been reported to occur even in 25–30% of anemic alcoholic patients, particularly in the presence of malnutrition and folate deficiency (see Lindenbaum, 1987).

MCV has limited specificity as an alcohol marker in patients with vitamin B_{12} or folic acid deficiency, liver diseases, several hematological diseases, hypothyroidism, or reticulocytosis (Table 17.1).

Platelet count

Low platelet count (thrombocytopenia) is one of the most common laboratory abnormalities in patients with recent excessive alcohol consumption (Lindenbaum, 1987). Studies have shown that ethanol can suppress platelet production. As a result of experimental administration of ethanol, thrombocytopenia occurs in almost half of normal subjects. Over 50% of patients admitted to hospitals with a history of recent drinking show thrombocytopenia. A 5–10 day period of excessive ethanol ingestion appears to be required to produce thrombocytopenia, which may occur even without accompanying vitamin deficiency or anemia. However, low platelet count has not been widely used as a marker of alcohol abuse. When ethanol is withdrawn, the platelet count returns to normal or supernormal levels (rebound thrombocytosis) in 1–3 weeks. Thrombocytosis may also occur following withdrawal of alcohol in patients who are not thrombocytopenic at the time of admission.

Serum aminotransferases

Serum concentrations of liver-derived enzymes, aspartate aminotransferase (AST) and alanine aminotransferase (ALT), are frequently elevated in patients with chronic alcohol consumption (Salaspuro, 1989). Liver tissue contains abundant amounts of aminotransferases and increase in serum AST actually marks hepatocyte injury rather than alcohol consumption *per se*. Elevated AST levels have been reported in 39% of alcohol-dependent individuals, in 32% of heavy drinkers, in 15% of light/moderate drinkers, and in 14% of non-drinkers (Helander *et al.*, 1997) (Table 17.2). Serum AST (as well as GGT and MCV) can be increased in abstinent alcoholics with chronic liver disease. AST values may give more specific information on alcoholic liver disease when interpreted together with ALT values (Table 17.1). It has been demonstrated that the ratio of AST to ALT over two is suggestive for alcoholic etiology (Rosman and Lieber, 1992, 1994). Most patients with non-alcoholic liver disease have ratios below one. ALT is relatively specific for the liver, whereas in chronic alcoholics the increase in serum AST may be potentiated owing to skeletal muscle injury (alcoholic myopathy) or alcoholic cardiomyopathy (Salaspuro, 1986; Balisteri and Rej, 1994).

Total hepatic AST consists of two isoenzymes: mitochondrial aminotransferase (mAST) and cytosolic aminotransferase. Alcohol-related liver damage has been suggested to selectively injure mitochondria and therefore abundant amounts of mAST may be released into the serum. Nalpas and co-workers (1986) have reported that 84% of alcoholic patients have elevated serum mAST levels. The specificity of mAST measurements may further improve, when the ratio of mAST to total AST is calculated.

Blood lipid profile

High density lipoprotein (HDL) cholesterol increases as a consequence of prolonged alcohol consumption (Table 17.1). Several studies have suggested that this phenomenon may be related to the reduced incidence of cardiovascular mortality in individuals consuming moderate amounts of ethanol. Since increased HDL concentrations are found as a result of drinking rather low amounts of alcohol

(≤5drinks per day) it can be used to examine early phase drinking problems in individual patients. It is also useful in the follow-up of patients without significant liver injury. In addition, alcohol abusers frequently show increased serum trigly-seride concentrations; approximately 80% may have hypertriglyseridemia following recent heavy drinking.

CDT (CARBOHYDRATE-DEFICIENT TRANSFERRIN, DESIALOTRANSFERRIN)

Carbohydrate-deficient transferrin (CDT) is one of the most promising new markers of alcohol abuse (Stibler, 1991; Allen *et al.*, 1994; Helander, 1999; Allen and Litten, 2001). Stibler and co-workers (Stibler and Kjellin, 1976; Stibler and Borg, 1986) originally reported that the amount of desialylated isoforms of transferrin in bio-logical fluids increases as a result of alcohol consumption. The mechanisms by which altered sialylation is brought about have, however, remained obscure (van Eijk *et al.*, 1987; de Jong *et al.*, 1990; Stibler, 1991; Sillanaukee *et al.*, 2001). Transferrin is synthesized in the liver and it has a half-life of 7–10 days (Bonford and Munro, 1985). Transferrin desialylation appears, however, to require very high concentra-tion of ethanol *in vivo* (Löf *et al.*, 1996). It has been postulated that the synthesis of the carbohydrate chain of transferrin may be disturbed by ethanol metabolites interfering with the transferase enzymes required in this process (Stibler and Borg, 1991; Ghosh *et al.*, 1993; Xin *et al.*, 1995). Disturbed function of various liver cell receptors (Miller *et al.*, 1996; Thiele *et al.*, 1996) could possibly also influence the serum concentrations of the desialylated fractions.

CDT methods

Several different methods for CDT measurements have been introduced. So far, these have been rather laborious and expensive for routine use. During the past years, the most widely used method has been ion-exchange separation of the desialylated transferrin fraction followed by transferrin radioimmunoassay for quantification (CDTect). In this procedure, values above 20 U/L for men or 26 U/L for women have been used to suggest alcohol abuse. Recent modifications of CDT assays report results more conveniently as relative amounts to total transferrin (%CDT RIA or %CDT TIA, Axis Biochemicals AS, Norway) (Bean *et al.*, 1997; Viitala *et al.*, 1998; Helander, 1999). The %CDT TIA employs a partly automatized tur-bidimetric procedure, which is also more cost-effective. It detects transferrin isoforms with 0–3 terminal sialic acid residues, whereas the %CDT RIA detects primarily disialo- and asialotransferrin isoforms (transferrin variants with 0–2 terminal sialic acid residues) (Heggli *et al.*, 1996). Accordingly, the suggested cut-off limits have been different (2.5% for %CDT RIA versus 6% for %CDT TIA). The CDTect method detects transferrin isoforms, which have isoelectric points (pI values) at 5.7 (disialo-transferrin) and above 5.7 (mono- and asialotransferrin) (Stibler, 1991). Trans-ferrin isoforms have also been measured by isoelectric focusing/immunoblotting and by HPLC (Xin *et al.*, 1991; Bean and Peter, 1993; Jeppsson *et al.*, 1993; Bean and Peter, 1994). Currently, further standardization, method comparisons and the development of external quality control programs for CDT measurements are under extensive investigation, which is expected to lead to a more widespread clinical use of CDT in the near future.

CDT as a marker of ethanol consumption and ALD

All the different CDT methods have previously shown excellent sensitivities (>80%) in detecting heavy drinking (Stibler *et al.*, 1986; Storey *et al.*, 1987; Behrens *et al.*, 1988a; Kapur *et al.*, 1989; Kwoh-Gain *et al.*, 1990; Stibler, 1991; Nyström *et al.*, 1992; Stowell *et al.*, 1997). However, Helander and co-workers (1997) in the WHO/ISBRA collaborative study found a sensitivity of only 39% for alcohol-dependent subjects, 27% for heavy drinkers and 11% for light/moderate drinkers – for a 100% specificity (Table 17.2). In a recent study on 200 problem drinkers with no apparent liver pathology, the sensitivity of the CDTect method was 34% (for 100% specificity) in problem drinkers reporting a mean of 710±80 (mean±2SE) grams of ethanol per week, as compared to the sensitivities of 47% and 34% for GGT and MCV, respectively (Niemelä *et al.*, 1995a). In patients drinking a mean of 1160±180 grams of ethanol per week, the sensitivity of CDTect increased to 64% as compared to 55% for GGT and 39% for MCV (Figure 17.1). CDT concentrations seem to be significantly affected by liver injury (Tsutsumi *et al.*, 1994; Yamauchi *et al.*, 1994; Niemelä *et al.*, 1995a). The CDTect values were found to be significantly higher in ALD patients than those in the alcoholics without liver pathology. Interestingly, when ALD patients are further classified according to the clinical, laboratory and morphological severity of liver disease, CDT, as measured with the CDTect method, appears to be primarily elevated in patients with the early stages of ALD (Fletcher *et al.*, 1991; Niemelä *et al.*, 1995a). This may in part be due to the fact that the patients with an early stage of ALD have an active synthesis of transferrin protein (Potter *et al.*, 1985). Apparently, such patients also consume the most abundant amounts of alcohol.

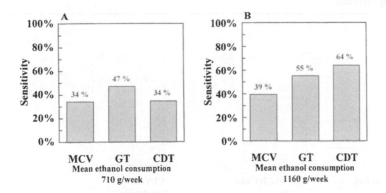

Figure 17.1 Sensitivities of MCV, GGT and CDT as markers of excessive ethanol consumption in alcohol abusers with a mean (± 2SE) ethanol intake of 710 ± 80 grams (A) and, as separated from the former group, in patients reporting a mean of 1160 ± 180 grams (B) during the past one week. The sensitivities of CDT are expressed for 100% specificity based on reference values obtained from 42 healthy non-drinking individuals (Modified from Niemelä *et al.*, 1995a, with permission).

Comparisons of the clinical performance of the various CDT methods

Comparisons of the CDTect method to isoelectric focusing/immunoblotting or to HPLC methods have revealed essentially similar clinical sensitivities and specificities (Anton and Bean, 1994; Helander, 1999). However, the %CDT and the CDTect methods seem to be different with respect to their clinical value as alcohol markers (Table 17.3) (Viitala *et al.*, 1998). CDTect has usually shown better sensitivities than the %CDT methods (Figure 17.2). In patients with ALD, the sensitivities of CDTect and %CDT RIA were 90% and 70%, respectively (Bell *et al.*, 1993, 1994; Niemelä *et al.*, 1995a). In heavy drinkers without liver disease, sensitivities of 49% and 22% were found, respectively (Sorvajärvi *et al.*, 1996). The correlation between the results obtained by these methods is also rather weak (in the order of 0.6–0.7)

Table 17.3 Summary of the practical characteristics of the %CDT TIA and the CDTect methods as markers of alcohol abuse. (Adapted from Viitala *et al.*, 1998 with permission)

%CDT TIA	CDTect
+ Economical, partly automated sample processing	+ Diagnostic performance is higher than that of %CDT TIA in men (higher ROC area in comparisons of alcohol abusers and healthy controls)
+ Minor interference by serum transferrin concentration	
+ Immunoturbidimetric method is convenient for personnel and environment	+ Eluted samples are stable and may be analysed after more than a week (if stored refrigerated)
− Low sensitivity in patients with early-phase drinking problems	− Expensive, manual sample processing
− Eluted samples are not stable and must be analysed immediately	− Significant interference by serum transferrin
− Because CDT fraction and total transferrin are determined separately, risk for errors in sample handling increases	

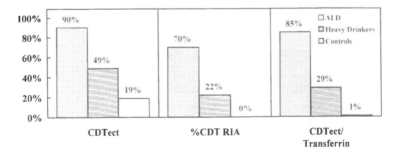

Figure 17.2 Percentages of values exceeding the upper normal limits for CDTect, %CDT RIA, and CDTect/total transferrin ratio in alcoholics with liver disease (ALD), heavy drinkers without liver disease, in NALD patients, and in controls. The thresholds recommended by the manufacturers were used for CDTect and %CDT RIA measurements (Modified from Sorvajärvi *et al.*, 1996, with permission).

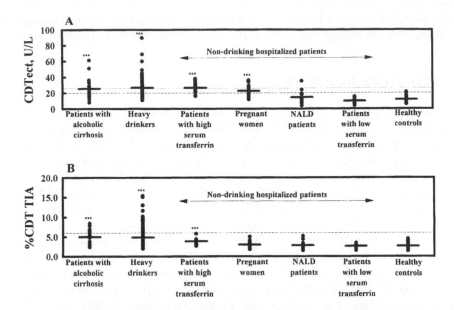

Figure 17.3 CDTect (A) and %CDT TIA (B) values in alcohol consumers and control individuals. The significant differences (as compared to the healthy controls) are illustrated by asterisks: *** $p < 0.001$, ** $p < 0.01$, * $p < 0.05$. The solid bars (—) indicate the means of the groups. (A) upper normal limits of the CDTect values for women (...) and for men (- - -); (B) upper normal limit of the %CDT TIA values (- - -) (Modified from Viitala *et al.*, 1998, with permission).

and therefore these assays are not easily replaceable by each other in routine laboratory work (Table 17.3). There is also a significant effect of gender on the performance of these assays. The overall sensitivity for CDT is higher for males (Sillanaukee *et al.*, 1993, 2000; Anton and Bean, 1994; Löf *et al.*, 1994; Niemelä *et al.*, 1995a; Sorvajärvi *et al.*, 1996; Viitala *et al.*, 1998). While the sensitivity of %CDT is lower than that of CDTect in males, there appears to be less difference in females.

The above variations in the analytical characteristics are largely due to the fact that conditions associated with alterations in serum transferrin concentration influence the specificity of CDT (Figure 17.3). CDTect results correlate positively with serum transferrin in non-drinkers with a wide range of transferrin levels ($r = 0.727$). For instance, in hospitalized non-drinking patients with high serum transferrin, the specificity of CDTect for detecting alcohol abuse is less than 50% (Viitala *et al.*, 1998). Therefore, in patients with iron deficiency who typically show high serum transferrin concentrations, the interpretation of CDTect results is complicated. It is likely that the high incidence of iron deficiency in women has also been a major reason for the need of higher cut-off limits for CDTect in females (Anton and Moak, 1994; Löf *et al.*, 1994; Sillanaukee *et al.*, 1994; Grønbæk *et al.*, 1995; Niemelä *et al.*, 1995a). Specificity problems with CDTect have also been encountered when interpreting the assay results in pregnant women, or in patients with liver diseases (Potter *et al.*, 1985; Sorvajärvi *et al.*, 1996). In the %CDT methods, high serum transferrin concentration does not create similar problems with specificity. However, it remains to be established whether conditions associated with abnormally low transferrin levels could decrease specificity in these methods.

ACETALDEHYDE ADDUCTS

Adducts of proteins with acetaldehyde, the first metabolite of ethanol, have been described in a number of studies. Acetaldehyde forms adducts primarily to reactive lysine residues of preferred target proteins (Gaines *et al.*, 1977; Stevens *et al.*, 1981; Donohue *et al.*, 1983; Wehr *et al.*, 1993; Israel *et al.*, 1986; San George and Hoberman, 1986; Jennett *et al.*, 1989; Smith *et al.*, 1989; Jukkola and Niemelä, 1989; Braun *et al.*, 1995; Lin *et al.*, 1995a; Tuma and Sorrell, 1995; Zhu *et al.*, 1996; Niemelä, 1999). Under appropriate reducing conditions, proteins with abundant amounts of reactive lysine residues appear to become modified at relatively low concentrations of acetaldehyde (Sorrell and Tuma, 1985, 1987; Tuma *et al.*, 1987; Jennett *et al.*, 1989; Lin *et al.*, 1993; Klassen *et al.*, 1994). In the absence of reducing agents stable cyclic imidazolidinone structures have also been shown to be formed between acetaldehyde and the free alpha-amino group of the aminoterminal valine of hemoglobin (San George and Hoberman, 1986; Fowles *et al.*, 1996; Braun *et al.*, 1997).

In theory, acetaldehyde adducts would be ideal markers for alcohol consumption since they represent specific metabolites of ethanol forming an integral part of the analyte. However, as yet no routine applications of adduct measurements have been developed.

Adduct measurements from erythrocytes

The first experiments on acetaldehyde adduct measurements from erythrocytes have been carried out using immunological and HPLC techniques. Antibodies which recognize acetaldehyde-protein condensates independently of the nature of the carrier protein have been generated by immunization of experimental animals with acetaldehyde-protein condensates (Israel *et al.*, 1986, 1992; Niemelä *et al.*, 1991; Lin *et al.*, 1993, 1995a). Such antibodies are able to recognize acetaldehyde adducts prepared at 20–100 μM concentrations of acetaldehyde, which may also occur in the blood of alcohol consuming individuals (Nuutinen *et al.*, 1983; Eriksson and Fukunaga, 1993). On the other hand, Yokoyama *et al.* (1993) have also reported protein adducts, which can be measured with antibodies recognizing adducts prepared with high acetaldehyde concentrations.

Preliminary studies have indicated that protein–acetaldehyde adducts are generated in erythrocytes of heavy drinkers (Gross *et al.*, 1992; Niemelä and Israel, 1992; Sillanaukee *et al.*, 1992; Lin *et al.*, 1993; Hurme *et al.*, 1998). Lin and co-workers reported a sensitivity of 71% and a specificity of 96% for adduct measurements in comparisons contrasting chronic alcoholics and teetotalers (Lin *et al.*, 1993). In larger materials, approximately 50% of alcohol abusers were shown to have elevated values (Figure 17.4) (Niemelä and Israel, 1992). Peterson and coworkers also reported elevated concentrations of hemoglobin-acetaldehyde adducts from chronic

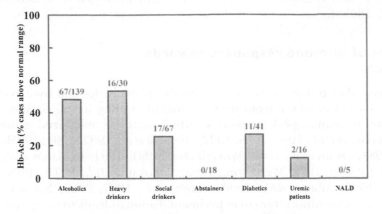

Figure 17.4 Percentages of patients exceeding the reference interval in immunoassays for haemoglobin-acetaldehyde (Hb-Ach) adducts. NALD, non-alcoholic liver disease. (Modified from Niemelä and Israel, 1992, with permission).

alcoholics using a fluorigenic labeling with 1,3-cyclohexanedione for aldehyde quantitation (Peterson and Polizzi, 1987; Peterson and Scott, 1989; Chen *et al.*, 1995; Hui-Min *et al.*, 1995). Acetaldehyde adducts appear to accumulate in the erythrocytes of non-alcoholic volunteers even after single heavy drinking bouts, whereas GGT or MCV do not show any change (Niemelä *et al.*, 1990a; Sillanaukee *et al.*, 1992). Experiments on acute ethanol intake and on hospitalized alcoholics have indicated that the adducts in the erythrocytes remain elevated after blood ethanol reaches zero. In chronic alcoholics, the values returned to normal levels after 1–3 weeks of abstinence (Niemelä and Israel, 1992). Acetaldehyde adducts were also previously found from erythrocytes of women who continued to drink during pregnancy and subsequently gave birth to children with fetal alcohol effects (Niemelä *et al.*, 1991). Comparisons between the sensitivities of adduct measurements and the conventional markers have, however, been limited.

Adduct measurements from plasma proteins

In addition to erythrocytes, protein adducts can also be assayed from serum proteins, particularly from those which are synthesized in the liver and thereby exposed to high concentrations of acetaldehyde. Some studies have reported, increased adduct concentrations from plasma proteins (Wickramasinghe *et al.*, 1986; Peterson and Polizzi, 1987; Lin *et al.*, 1990; French *et al.*, 1993). *In vitro*, acetaldehyde binds to albumin more efficiently than to erythrocyte proteins (Israel *et al.*, 1986). Acetaldehyde binding to lipoproteins has also been described in a number of *in vitro* studies (Steinbrecher *et al.*, 1984; Savolainen *et al.*, 1987). Such binding may also occur *in vivo* and create immunogenic epitopes (Wehr *et al.*, 1993; Melkko *et al.*, 1996). Therefore, it is possible that quantitation of acetaldehyde binding to specific lipoproteins could be utilized in the development of diagnostic tools for alcohol abuse. Interestingly, it has also been suggested that lipoprotein modification *in vivo* may cause activation of apolipoprotein E synthesis in macrophages and thereby contribute to the promotion of atherogenesis in alcohol abusers (Lin *et al.*, 1995b).

Measurements of immune responses towards protein adducts

Several studies have shown that adducts of proteins with aldehydes and hydroxyl radicals (reactive species resulting from protein-ethanol binding in the presence of iron) stimulate immunological responses, which can be measured from serum specimens (Israel *et al.*, 1986, 1988, 1992; Niemelä *et al.*, 1987, 1994, 1995b; Hoerner *et al.*, 1988; Izumi *et al.*, 1989; Worrall *et al.*, 1991, 1994; Koskinas *et al.*, 1992; Tuma and Klassen, 1992; Wehr *et al.*, 1993; Yokoyama *et al.*, 1993, 1995b; Clot *et al.*, 1995, 1996; Albano *et al.*, 1996; Viitala *et al.*, 1997, 2000; Xu *et al.*, 1998). Chronic ethanol administration to experimental animals leads to the generation of circulating immunoglobulins with anti-acetaldehyde adduct specificity (Israel *et al.*, 1986; Worrall *et al.*, 1994). Both IgA and IgG responses appear to occur in human alcoholics (Worrall *et al.*, 1991; Clot *et al.*, 1995; Viitala *et al.*, 1997). Viitala and co-workers (1997) showed that IgA titers are elevated in 69% of patients with ALD, these titers being significantly higher than those from patients with non-alcoholic liver disease, non-drinking controls, or heavy drinkers without clinical and biochemical signs of liver disease (Figure 17.5). Anti-adduct IgGs have been found both from some ALD patients and from heavy drinkers without liver disease. The anti-adduct IgA and IgG antibodies also show an association with the severity of ALD, as measured with the combined clinical and laboratory index (Viitala *et al.*, 1997). The antibody titers also correlate with the presence of inflammation and necrosis in the biopsy specimens. In follow-up studies, parallel changes were observed in the anti-adduct IgG titers, disease severity, and serum markers of fibrogenesis, suggesting an association between the immune responses and aggravation of liver disease (Marshall *et al.*, 1983; Viitala *et al.*, 1997).

Autoantibodies against cytochrome P450IIE1 hydroxyethyl radical adducts (Clot *et al.*, 1995, 1996) and against malondialdehyde-acetaldehyde hybrid adducts (MAA adducts) (Xu *et al.*, 1998; Rolla *et al.*, 2000) have also been found from the blood of human alcoholics and from ethanol-fed experimental animals. The highest titers of such antibodies are found from patients with severe liver disease (Clot *et al.*, 1995; Rolla *et al.*, 2000).

Protein adducts in tissue specimens as diagnostic markers

The specific diagnosis of ALD based on conventional serum parameters and liver histology is very difficult (Diehl, 1989). It is tempting to speculate that detection of specific ethanol-induced protein adducts from tissue samples could serve as markers to aid in the differential diagnosis of liver diseases of alcoholic versus non-alcoholic origin.

Aldehydic products capable of adduct formation originate both from ethanol metabolism and ethanol-induced oxidative stress (Lieber, 1988b; Cederbaum, 1989; French, 1989; Nordmann *et al.*, 1992; Tuma and Sorrell, 1995; Niemelä 1999).

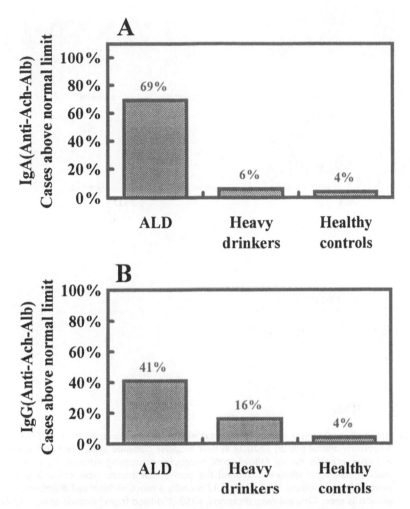

Figure 17.5 Incidence of elevated anti-albumin adduct IgA (anti-Ach-Alb IgA) (A) and IgG (anti-Ach-Alb IgG) (B) titers in ALD, in heavy drinkers, in NALD and in healthy controls. The upper normal limits were obtained by calculating the mean +2SD from the values from healthy controls (Modified from Viitala *et al.*, 1997, with permission).

In vivo, there seem to be selective target proteins for adduct formation (Mauch *et al.*, 1986; Behrens *et al.*, 1988b; Yokoyama *et al.*, 1993), such as Δ^4-3-ketosteroid-5-β-reductase (Zhu *et al.*, 1996; Lin *et al.*, 1998). Acetaldehyde-modified epitopes have also been detected from the surface of hepatocytes by flow-cytometry (Trudell *et al.*, 1990, 1991; Lin *et al.*, 1992).

Immunohistochemical studies have revealed acetaldehyde-protein adducts in the centrilobular region of the liver in the early phase of liver disease both in human alcohol abusers and in experimental animals (Niemelä *et al.*, 1991, 1994). Protein adducts in zone 3 hepatocytes occurred in heavy drinkers with no obvious

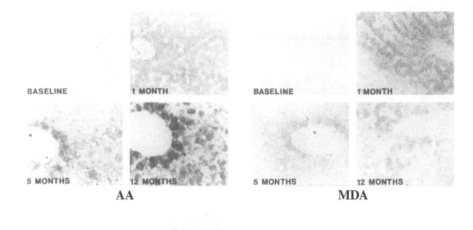

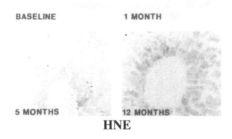

BASELINE   1 MONTH

5 MONTHS   12 MONTHS

HNE

Figure 17.6 Immunohistochemical staining for acetaldehyde (AA) malondialdehyde (MDA) and 4-hydroxynonenal (HNE) adducts in liver biopsies obtained at baseline and at various time intervals during follow-up of micropigs consuming ethanol. At 1 month, positive staining is observed around the perivenular hepatocytes coinciding with elevated transaminases. At 5, and at 12 months a more widespread distribution of adducts is seen. Original magnifications, x250 (Modified from Niemelä *et al.*, 1995b, with permission).

clinical, biochemical or histological signs of ALD (Niemelä *et al.*, 1991, 1994, 1995b; Halsted *et al.*, 1993; Holstege *et al.*, 1994). With progression of ALD the staining becomes more irregular and widespread. Studies by Holstege *et al.* (1994) have further indicated that the presence of sinusoidal acetaldehyde adducts in human alcohol consumers also contributes to the prognosis of the patients.

Aldehydic products of lipid peroxidation, malondialdehyde (MDA) and 4-hydroxynonenal (4-HNE) also form Schiff's base adducts with proteins. MDA is generated in non-enzymatic lipid peroxidation of unsaturated fatty acids, in lipid peroxidation that occurs during phagocytosis by monocytes and in arachidonic acid catabolism in thrombocytes (Palinski *et al.*, 1990; Esterbauer *et al.*, 1991). The free radical-mediated oxidation of long-chain polyunsaturated fatty acids generates 4-HNE, which can react with the sulfhydryl groups of proteins through a Michael addition type of mechanism (Palinski *et al.*, 1990; Stadtman, 1992). Oxidative modification of proteins with MDA and 4-HNE have been demonstrated both from arterial vessel walls of atherosclerotic lesions (Haberland *et al.*, 1988; Palinski *et al.*, 1989; Steinberg *et al.*, 1989) and from hepatic tissue in alcoholic liver disease and in iron overload (Houglum *et al.*, 1990; Niemelä *et al.*, 1994, 1999; Parkkila *et al.*, 1996; Paradis *et al.*, 1997). Double immunofluorescence stainings for acetaldehyde and malondialdehyde adducts have revealed a significant colocalization between these two types of adducts and histological tissue damage. In a micropig model of alcohol-induced liver disease progressive accumulation of adducts with acetaldehyde, MDA and 4-HNE have been demonstrated upon continuous ethanol intake (Figure 17.6). After 1 month on ethanol-containing diet, acetaldehyde (AA) and MDA adducts were observed in the perivenous regions co-localizing with each other and appearing together with increased serum concentrations of AST and ALT (Niemelä *et al.*, 1995b). The co-occurrence of acetaldehyde adducts and collagen deposition in the early phase of liver disease has also been demonstrated (Halsted *et al.*, 1993; Niemelä *et al.*, 1994). High fat diet may stimulate the formation of protein adducts. However, when the diet is further supplemented with iron, an enhancer of oxidative stress, a further potentiation of adduct formation is seen coinciding with elevated levels of serum liver-derived enzymes and progressive histopathology (Tsukamoto *et al.*, 1995; Houglum, 1996).

Hybrid adducts with malondialdehyde and acetaldehyde (MAA adducts) are also generated in the liver *in vivo* as a result of ethanol consumption (Tuma *et al.*, 1996). In addition, hydroxyethyl radical adducts may be formed in liver microsomes of ethanol-fed animals (Moncada *et al.*, 1994; Clot *et al.*, 1995).

OTHER MARKERS OF ALCOHOL CONSUMPTION

Blood acetate

The induction of ethanol metabolism as a consequence of chronic alcohol abuse leads to the elevation of blood concentration of ethanol metabolites, acetaldehyde and acetate (Salaspuro, 1986). Blood acetate concentration is influenced by hepatic ethanol oxidation and by its rate of use by peripheral tissues. During ethanol metabolism, blood acetate concentration increases correlating with the rate of ethanol elimination. Thus, it increases with the development of metabolic tolerance to alcohol. In some studies, the sensitivity of blood acetate as a marker of heavy drinking (65%) has been shown to exceed that of GGT (Salaspuro, 1986). However, blood acetate determinations are useful only in situations when there is ethanol in the blood.

β-hexosaminidase

Ethanol consumption increases serum β-hexosaminidase, which is a hepatic lysosomal enzyme. Studies have reported that serum β-hexosaminidase is elevated in

85% of alcoholics. Unfortunately, these measurements lack specificity since patients with non-alcoholic liver disease also show elevated values (Rosman and Lieber, 1992).

Urinary dolichols

Dolichols are long-chain 2,3-dihydro-polyprenols, which serve as carrier lipids in the biosynthesis of glycoproteins. Dolichol levels are significantly higher in chronic alcoholics than in controls (Pullarkat and Raguthu, 1985; Roine *et al.*, 1987). The clinical utility of dolichols is, however, limited because of their short biological half-life and lack of specificity (Rosman and Lieber, 1992).

5-hydroxytryptophol

The ratio of the serotonin metabolite 5-hydroxytryptophol (5-HTOL) to creatinine or to 5-hydroxyindol-3-acetic acid (5-HIAA) in urine has been proposed to be a specific marker for alcohol consumption. 5-HTOL stays elevated for 6–20 hours after ethanol disappearance. This marker seems to have a high diagnostic accuracy for detecting recent alcohol consumption (Helander *et al.*, 1997).

Other commonly observed laboratory abnormalities in alcohol abusers

Alcoholic patients present several other typical laboratory abnormalities after a period of heavy drinking, such as increased osmolal and anion gap, hypoglycemia, lactic acidosis, ketoacidosis, hypophosphatemia, hypomagnesemia and hyper-uricemia. Alcoholic ketosis, which is characterized by a high ratio of β-hydroxy-butyrate to acetoacetate, may be related to starvation. A diabetic type of glucose tolerance may occur in patients with liver disease probably due to endogenous insulin resistance. Hypomagnesemia may be seen as a result of dietary deficiencies (nutritional reasons, vomiting, diarrhea) and increased urinary losses. Severe magnesium deficiency can also lead to hypocalcemia and hypokalemia. Dilutional hyponatremia and hypokalemia from excessive urinary loss are frequent in patients with severe liver disease. Hyperuricemia is due to increased production and decreased renal excretion as a consequence of circulating lactate and ketones which diminish renal tubular urate secretion. Alcohol abuse may also result in clinical features of Cushing's syndrome. Non-dexamethasone suppressible-hypercortisolemia is common in alcohol abusers.

Combinations of markers

Since no single marker is ideal for reliable detection of alcohol abuse, several combinations of markers have been introduced to improve diagnostic accuracy. The most popular of these are various combinations of GGT, MCV, AST and CDT (Watson *et al.*, 1986; Sillanaukee *et al.*, 2000). Obviously, such combinations increase sensitivity but specificity may simultaneously be sacrificed. The costs of analyses also increase.

LABORATORY EVALUATION OF LIVER DISEASE
IN ALCOHOL CONSUMERS

Although several laboratory tests for the assessment of liver function are available, too few of them are disease-specific (for review see Balisteri and Rej, 1994). A single test is rarely sufficient. Therefore, selected groups of tests have been used to examine whether liver disease is present or not and how severe it is. Unfortunately, many alcohol abusing patients continue to enter the stage of severe liver disease before being correctly diagnosed.

Markers of liver disease

The most frequently used laboratory parameters for confirming the presence of liver disease are serum bilirubin, AST, ALT, GGT, and alkaline phosphatase (ALP). These tests complement each other and reflect certain morphological alterations in tissue, such as cell damage or cholestasis. Although liver disease can exist in patients with normal marker values, normal values on all of the above screening tests can, with substantial certainty, rule out significant liver or biliary tract disease (Balisteri and Rej, 1994).

Acute liver cell injury (parenchymal disease) is typical of alcoholic liver disease, although it may also be seen in viral hepatitis, drug- or toxin-induced liver disease, hypoxemia, shock, or metabolic liver damage (Balisteri and Rej, 1994; Rosman and Lieber, 1994). In all of the above conditions, except for alcoholic hepatitis, the cell injury is reflected by a marked increase in serum aminotransferase concentrations showing a relationship to the degree of hepatocyte injury. However, in alcoholics the activities of GGT or AST do not clearly correlate with the magnitude of liver injury. In alcohol abusing patients with mild liver disease (fatty liver), the serum aminotransferase levels may be slightly elevated – up to twice normal or less. The bilirubin level is normal except for the combination of fatty liver and cholestasis. Serum AST is moderately elevated, but not to the levels often noted in viral hepatitis. In alcoholic hepatitis, the characteristic abnormalities are usually severe. Anemia occurs in 50–70% of patients. Serum AST and ALT are elevated in all cases. ALP is elevated in 80% of cases and serum bilirubin in 90% of cases. The characteristic biochemical feature of acute alcoholic hepatitis is a markedly elevated serum GGT and AST/ALT ratio of >1.0 when AST is <300 U/L. Serum albumin is usually decreased and prothrombin time is abnormal. In severe cases the prothrombin time may be prolonged to such an extent that liver biopsy is not feasible. Depending upon the severity of the liver disease and the nutritional status, hypoalbuminemia or hypergammaglobulinemia or both may be present. Hypoalbuminemia is also an important factor in the pathogenesis of edema. Blood ammonia levels are increased in the blood and brain of patients with hepatic encephalopathy.

Cholestasis is characterized by an accumulation of bile components in serum. ALP and, to a greater degree, GGT activities are increased in most forms of cholestasis (GGT/ALP ratio of more than 5 is common in ALD). Hyperbilirubinemia and other manifestations of cholestasis may complicate ALD and there may be bile duct obstruction secondary to pancreatitis. Increased serum bilirubin is indicative of liver/bile duct affision or increased erythrocyte destruction. In alcoholic fatty liver, hyperbilirubinemia is observed in about 25% of cases.

The abnormalities in laboratory markers in cirrhosis are less pronounced than those in alcoholic hepatitis. In compensated cirrhosis, most tests are normal. Mild increases in AST, ALT, and ALP may be seen. Measurements of ALT and AST concentrations are usually not helpful in monitoring the course of cirrhosis. Depression of serum albumin, elevated serum globulins, prolonged prothrombin time, leukopenia, thrombocytopenia, and anemia are common. In some cases, acute hemolysis accompanied by marked elevation of serum lipids may be found (Zieve's syndrome).

Prognostic markers of alcoholic liver disease

Laboratory parameters can also be used to assess liver disease severity and prognosis in alcoholics (Blake and Orrego, 1991; Chedid *et al.*, 1991). For such purposes, histological variables, although important, have several practical problems. For instance, liver biopsies cannot be repeated frequently enough to assess changes in liver pathology. In alcoholics, the presence of necrosis, Mallory's hyalin and inflammation in biopsy specimens are the histological variables which have been shown to be significantly related to the risk for mortality (Orrego *et al.*, 1987).

The laboratory variables of liver disease severity are used as parts of well-established global combinations, such as the Combined Clinical and Laboratory Index (CCLI), the Child-Turcotte-Pugh Index, or the Cox model. During the development of the CCLI index, analysis of the laboratory variables revealed that the most important prognostic abnormalities of ALD are albumin <25 g/L and bilirubin >136 µmol/L. Hemoglobin <75% of normal and prothrombin time >8 s longer than the control time also had significant prognostic weights, whereas AST, ALT, and GGT had no apparent prognostic significance (Orrego *et al.*, 1983). Several markers of connective tissue metabolism and fibrogenesis, e.g., the aminoterminal propeptide of type III collagen and type IV collagen, and markers of basement membrane formation (laminin), also appear to have independent prognostic value (Niemelä *et al.*, 1990b). These markers will be discussed in detail in the following paragraphs.

Markers of fibrogenesis

It has been well established that not all alcohol abusers develop liver fibrosis even upon equal amounts of alcohol consumption. On the other hand, the appearance of early fibrosis in zone 3 hepatocytes may predict subsequent development for irreversible cirrhosis (Nakano *et al.*, 1982; Worner and Lieber, 1985). Therefore, it would be important to detect individuals at risk and to diagnose fibrogenesis in its early stages. It is also important to know whether fibrosis is affected by therapy without the need of biopsies.

Collagen in the liver mostly consists of type I and type III collagens although types IV, V and VI are also present (Rojkind *et al.*, 1979). In cirrhosis, all of these types are increased. Type III collagen is predominantly increased in early fibrosis, whereas type I collagen dominates at an advanced stage (Rojkind and Perez-Tamayo,

1983). Accumulation of basement membrane components, primarily type IV collagen and laminin, in the perisinusoidal space also takes place during fibrogenesis
disturbing liver function (capillarization of sinusoids).

Several methods are currently available to measure type I, III, IV and VI
collagen metabolism (Table 17.4) (Niemelä, 1996). The mechanisms by which the
alterations in serum collagen markers reflect actual collagen metabolism have,
however, remained a subject of debate. The concentrations of collagen-derived
peptides in serum apparently derive from a complex interaction of collagen biosynthesis, degradation, or both. Collagen production in alcoholic livers is active
since hepatic stellate cells (Ito cells), which are the primary source of the extracellular matrix, are readily stimulated by ethanol-induced oxidative stress and lipid
peroxidation (Friedman, 1990; Bedossa et al., 1994; Pares et al., 1994). The rate of
collagen degradation regulates the amount of collagen deposition in tissues and
thereby, may also influence the concentrations of the collagen-derived peptides
in circulation (Maruyama et al., 1982; Woessner, 1991; Lieber, 1994). Decreased
activities of collagen degrading enzymes have been reported in advanced cirrhosis, whereas in early fibrosis, collagenase activities may be stimulated (Maruyama
et al., 1982). In keeping with the above views, the levels of the tissue inhibitor of
metalloproteinase seem to correlate with the development of fibrosis (Lieber, 1994).

Table 17.4 Laboratory methods for quantifying connective tissue metabolism

Marker	Assay	Method	Clinical significance
Collagen-derived fragments			
Type I	C-Propeptide (PICP)	RIA	Marker of collagen type I metabolism. Bone and liver diseases.
	N-Propeptide (PINP)	RIA	Marker of collagen type I metabolism. Bone and liver diseases.
	C-Telopeptide (ICTP)	RIA	Marker of collagen type I degradation. Bone and liver diseases.
Type III	N-Propeptide (PIIINP) and its fragments	RIA	Marker of collagen type III metabolism. Assessment of fibrogenesis and disease prognosis.
Type IV	7-S Domain	RIA	Assessment of type IV collagen (basement membrane) metabolism.
	NCI Domain	RIA	
Type VI		RIA	Assessment of type VI collagen metabolism.
Other connective tissue components			
Laminin		RIA, TRFIA	Marker of basement membrane metabolism.
Hyaluronic acid		RIA, Radiometric assay	Marker of connective tissue metabolism.
Tissue inhibitor of metalloproteinase (TIMP)		EIA	Differential diagnosis of alcoholics with fibrosis from those with steatosis.

The degradation rate of collagen in alcoholic livers may also be affected by qualitative changes in collagen crosslinking (Feinman *et al.*, 1979; Eyre, 1984).

When interpreting the concentrations of the connective tissue derived protein fragments in circulation, the clearance of these proteins should also be considered (Niemelä, 1996). Smedsrød and co-workers (1990) have shown that circulating C-terminal propeptide of type I procollagen is cleared via mannose receptors in liver endothelial cells. On the other hand, Melkko *et al.* (1994) have demonstrated that the N-terminal propeptides of type I and III procollagens go through a scavenger receptor, which is also used by other ligands, such as formaldehyde-treated albumin. Therefore, the increased propeptide concentrations in circulation may also reflect impaired endothelial cell function in severe liver disease.

Type I collagen markers

The methods which address the metabolism of type I collagen types are the assays for the carboxyterminal (PICP) and aminoterminal (PINP) propeptides and the crosslinked carboxyterminal telopeptide of type I collagen (ICTP) (Table 17.4). Normal values for the PICP antigen are different for males and females, 40–200 mg/L and 50–170 mg/L., respectively. Serum PICP measurements were primarily introduced for monitoring collagen metabolism in bone, since most type I collagen is present in bone, comprising 90% of its organic matrix. However, serum PICP also seems to be increased in ALD, although the changes are usually of rather small magnitude (Savolainen *et al.*, 1984; Niemelä *et al.*, 1992).

Serum PINP levels are elevated in patients with ALD (Niemelä, 1996; Schytte *et al.*, 1999; Melkko and Niemelä, unpublished data). PINP appears to be a more sensitive marker of type I collagen metabolism than PICP, since type I collagen is frequently deposited in the tissue as pC-collagen (collagen retaining its carboxyterminal end).

An assay for human ICTP is based on a cross-linked peptide purified from human bone (Risteli, 1993). This protein originates from mature type I collagen fibres and if it exists in serum, it should reflect collagen degradation. Theoretically, using combined measurements of the various fragments, it may be possible to reach conclusions on the balance between collagen degradation and synthesis at any given time point. However, no data is currently available to support this hypothesis. The assay for ICTP was also originally introduced for monitoring bone destruction. However, it appears that this protein also shows significant changes in liver diseases (Ricard-Blum *et al.*, 1996). Serum ICTP antigen is elevated in ALD and its concentration also relates to the clinical severity of the disease (Niemelä *et al.*, unpublished data).

Type III procollagen peptide (PIIINP)

To date, the most widely used serum marker for collagen turnover has been the aminoterminal propeptide of type III procollagen (PIIINP). A radioimmunoassay for this peptide is based on human PIIINP antigen (Niemelä *et al.*, 1985a; Niemelä *et al.*, 1985b; Risteli *et al.*, 1988). This antigen is immunologically heterogeneous consisting of different forms with different molecular sizes and affinities to anti-PIIINP antibodies (Niemelä *et al.*, 1982). The smallest molecular weight component (Col1) appears to represent the degradation products of PIIINP. This antigen can be measured either by purifying the Col1 protein for use as a standard antigen (Niemelä, 1985b) or by using monovalent antigen binding fragments (Fab) of the anti-PIIINP antibodies, which show a strong affinity for the Col1 peptide (Rohde *et al.*, 1983). Using the Fab assay, Sato *et al.* (1986) have been able to discriminate between simple fatty liver and early fibrosis in alcoholic patients suggesting the possibility of using such assays for screening of individuals who are at risk for developing cirrhosis.

PIIINP seems to be a useful marker of disease activity in a variety of fibrosing conditions. In ALD, PIIINP is elevated in patients with active hepatitis and cirrhosis (Niemelä *et al.*, 1983; Colombo *et al.*, 1985; Sotaniemi *et al.*, 1986; Surrenti *et al.*, 1987; Annoni *et al.*, 1989; Niemelä *et al.*, 1990b). It is elevated in ALD patients more frequently than the other collagen markers (Niemelä *et al.*, 1990b, 1992). The changes in serum concentrations of this marker may also serve as prognostic indicators (Niemelä *et al.*, 1990b; Blake and Orrego, 1991). Serum PIIINP strongly correlates with the clinical and histological severity of liver disease (Annoni *et al.*, 1989; Bell *et al.*, 1989; González-Reimers *et al.*, 1990; Niemelä *et al.*, 1990b). Interestingly, a weaker correlation between PIIINP and the severity of liver disease is observed when an assay variant devoid of specificity for the authentic PIIINP is used (Shahin *et al.*, 1992). Serum PIIINP concentration in ALD patients rapidly decreases if the patient remains abstinent, suggesting the importance of alcohol withdrawal for patients with ongoing fibrogenesis (Niemelä *et al.*, 1990b, 1992).

In other liver diseases, such as primary biliary cirrhosis, PIIINP values have also been found to correlate with the subsequent outcome of the disease (Babbs *et al.*, 1988; Niemelä *et al.*, 1988). In acute and chronic viral hepatitis, PIIINP also marks disease activity (Annoni *et al.*, 1986). Follow-up of PIIINP concentration may also be used for monitoring treatment after liver transplantation (Höckerstedt *et al.*, 1990), interferon (Teran *et al.*, 1994), or corticosteroid administration (McCullough *et al.*, 1987). Serum PIIINP is also elevated during the development of fibrosis in a variety of extrahepatic organs, most markedly in bone marrow fibrosis (Hasselbach *et al.*, 1990). In other conditions, such as lung fibrosis, serum PIIINP concentrations usually show only minimal changes. In addition, serum PIIINP is increased in various malignancies correlating with their clinical extent and behavior (Zhu *et al.*, 1994).

Type IV collagen markers

Type IV collagen is a component of basement membranes which has been suggested to undergo changes early during the pathogenesis of liver diseases. Assays for monitoring type IV collagen metabolism are available based on its 7-S and NC1 domains. The aminoterminal 7-S domain is elevated in alcoholic liver disease and correlates with its clinical severity (Niemelä *et al.*, 1985b, 1990b). Type IV collagen concentration in serum has also been observed to follow type IV collagen concentrations in the liver (Tsutsumi *et al.*, 1993).

A non-collagenous cross-linked region (NC1) from the carboxyterminal end of type IV collagen has also been detected from serum specimens (Brocks *et al.*, 1985; Schuppan, 1986). This marker may reflect the rates of type IV collagen degradation (Schuppan *et al.*, 1986).

Other markers of connective tissue metabolism

An assay has been developed for the measurement of type VI collagen concentrations in serum (Schuppan *et al.*, 1985). However, only few studies are available on its clinical usefulness in liver diseases (Shahin *et al.*, 1992).

The non-collagenous components of the extracellular matrix also undergo distinct qualitative and quantitative changes during progression of ALD. Increased serum laminin concentration is associated with hepatic fibrosis (Kropf *et al.*, 1988). Similarly to PIIINP and type IV collagen-related antigens, it also shows an association with hepatic inflammation and necrosis (Niemelä *et al.*, 1990b). Hyaluronan is one of the glycosaminoglycans, which can be detected radioimmunologically from serum specimens (Engström-Laurent *et al.*, 1985). Serum hyaluronate concentrations are increased in liver diseases, especially in ALD. Recent studies have suggested that the increase in serum hyaluronate in ALD may be associated with hepatic fibrosis and also with alcohol drinking (Tsutsumi *et al.*, 1997).

Alcoholic or non-alcoholic liver disease? Differential diagnosis

Viral liver disease

Serological tests are widely available to detect viral hepatitis (Rosman and Lieber, 1994). Measurements of viral proteins (antigens) or corresponding immunological responses (antibodies) towards the viral antigens during and after acute infection are used for the detection of hepatitis A, B, C, D (delta antigens), E, and G. For instance, serological diagnosis of hepatitis C can be achieved by an enzyme-linked immunoassay with antibodies to hepatitis C virus. Interestingly, there seems to be a significant association between viral hepatitis and ALD (Lieber, 2000). A large number of alcoholics are seropositive for hepatitis C. In viral hepatitis, ALT is characteristically as high or higher than AST (Table 17.1). Determinations of serum immunoglobulins may also be of value in the differential diagnosis. Increased serum IgA is typical of ALD (Johnson and Williams, 1986; van de Wiel *et al.*, 1987; Israel *et al.*, 1988; Brown and Kloppel, 1989; Kerr, 1990), whereas increased IgG levels are characteristic of viral hepatitis.

Hemochromatosis

Pathologic iron overload in the liver may be either hereditary or secondary (acquired) as a consequence of alcoholism, thalassemia, or repeated transfusion (Bacon, 2001). Secondary hemochromatosis should be distinguished from the primary form by the demonstration of a hereditary hemochromatosis-linked point mutation (Cys282Tyr) (Waheed *et al.*, 1997; George *et al.*, 1998; Bacon, 2001).

Discrimination between secondary hemochromatosis and ALD may, however, be difficult (Rosman and Lieber, 1994). The hepatic histopathologic findings in ALD may also include increased iron stores in hepatocytes and in reticuloendothelial cells, together with fibrosis. The absence of iron staining with Perl's Prussian blue stain usually excludes the diagnosis of hemochromatosis. The diagnosis of hemochromatosis may be achieved by documenting elevation of serum ferritin levels in conjunction with increased serum iron and per cent of transferrin saturation, together with decreased transferrin and total iron-binding capacity (Balisteri and Rej, 1994). Since the liver plays a major role in iron metabolism, including transferrin and ferritin synthesis, acute liver cell necrosis leads to increases in both serum iron and ferritin concentrations because the damaged hepatocytes cannot take up iron or retain ferritin. Interestingly, several studies have indicated that alcohol and iron together have a synergistic effect in producing liver pathology, probably due to excessive stimulation of lipid peroxidation (Bassett *et al.*, 1986; Irving *et al.*, 1988; Houglum *et al.*, 1990; Kukielka and Cederbaum, 1990; Tsukamoto *et al.*, 1995; Adams and Agnew, 1996; Parkkila *et al.*, 1996; Niemelä *et al.*, 1999).

Wilson's disease

Wilson's disease is an autosomal recessive disorder characterized by excessive copper deposition in tissues. Determination of serum ceruloplasmin, non-ceruloplasmin-bound (free) serum copper, and 24-h urinary copper excretion are useful laboratory tests (Rosman and Lieber, 1994). The best marker for screening is serum ceruloplasmin, since 96% of patients with Wilson's disease have levels <30 mg/dL. Total serum copper is high in early Wilson's disease and is present in serum unbound to ceruloplasmin. Urinary copper excretion exceeds 100 µg/d. Increased copper content of liver tissue is the most reliable diagnostic finding (Balisteri and Rej, 1994).

Non-alcoholic steatohepatitis

While ALD is currently the most common cause of steatohepatitis, increasing amount of evidence is available to indicate that non-alcoholic steatohepatitis (NASH) is another highly common form of chronic liver disease. To date, there are no specific serum markers to differentiate between alcoholic fatty liver and NASH. This condition may be suggested by histological features indistinguishable from those of ALD in patients who do not consume alcohol excessively. Such findings are common in obesity and in uncontrolled diabetes. The morphological features of NASH include steatosis with focal necroinflammatory change, often including polymorphonuclear as well as mononuclear leucocytes and pericellular fibrosis. The pathogenic mechanism of NASH may have several features, which are similar to those of alcoholic steatohepatitis, including cytochrome 2E1 induction (Weltman *et al.*, 1998; Niemelä *et al.*, 2000). Interestingly, patients with NASH and mild iron overload often present with the hemochromatosis-related Cys282Tyr mutation (George *et al.*, 1998; Bonkovsky *et al.*, 1999).

Drug-induced liver disease

Several drugs or their metabolites, for example acetaminophen and isoniazid, are able to generate a dose-related hepatotoxic reaction. Such patients may suffer from protracted vomiting and nausea followed by an apparent recovery phase. Jaundice and hepatic tenderness are signs of the deterioration of liver function. Transaminase activities are markedly increased and prothrombin times are abnormal. The hepatotoxicity of acetaminophen, which like ethanol also uses microsomal cytochrome P-450 system for its metabolism, is known to be potentiated by alcohol consumption (Lieber, 1988a). Isoniazid, which is used in the treatment of tuberculosis, frequently produces transient aminotransferase elevations. This is typically 5–10 times normal and occurs within the first 2–3 months of therapy (Balisteri and Rej, 1994). Hepatotoxicity of glucocorticoids, methotrexate, valproic acid, tetracycline, salicylates, and nimesulide have also been documented.

Autoimmune hepatitis

Autoimmune hepatitis may be suspected in the presence of certain typical clinical features (female predominance, association with other autoimmune disorders), increased concentrations of serum globulins and the presence of portal inflammation on liver biopsy. Demonstration of antinuclear antibodies, liver-kidney-microsomal antibodies, or soluble liver antigen antibodies may be of additional diagnostic value (Rosman and Lieber, 1994).

Primary biliary cirrhosis

Primary biliary cirrhosis (PBC) can be recognized by characteristic clinical and histological features (progressive destruction of the intrahepatic bile ducts). The disease particularly affects middle aged women. The incidence in females is nine times higher than that in males. Serum anti-mitochondrial antibodies may be found in 90% of cases. There is usually a marked elevation in serum alkaline phosphatase concentrations, whereas transaminases are only modestly elevated and bilirubin elevations are variable. Antimitochondrial antibody (AMA) and antinuclear (ANA) and smooth muscle (SMA) autoantibodies may be found. Serum IgM levels are often high. A combination of a positive test for antimitochondrial antibody (AMA) in patients with elevated alkaline phosphatase, cholesterol, and high serum IgM strongly supports the diagnosis of PBC instead of extrahepatic obstruction (Balisteri and Rej, 1994).

α_1-antitrypsin deficiency

The laboratory diagnosis of liver disease as a result of α_1-antitrypsin deficiency may be based on the demonstration of low serum α_1-antitrypsin levels and the determination of the antitrypsin phenotype by isoelectric focusing or electrophoresis. However, liver histology is usually needed for confirmation (Rosman and Lieber, 1994).

ACKNOWLEDGEMENTS

The original studies in the author's laboratory were supported by the Finnish Foundation for Alcohol Studies. The expert assistance of Katja Viitala is gratefully acknowledged.

REFERENCES

Adams, P.C. and Agnew, S. (1996) Alcoholism in hereditary hemochromatosis revisited: Prevalence and clinical consequences among homozygous siblings. *Hepatology* **23**, 724–727.

Albano, E., Clot, P., Morimoto, M., Tomasi, A., Ingelman-Sundberg, M. and French, S.W. (1996) Role of cytochrome P4502E1-dependent formation of hydroxyethyl free radical in the development of liver damage in rats intragastrically fed with ethanol. *Hepatology* **23**, 155–163.

Allen, J.P., Fertig, J.B., Litten, R.Z., Sillanaukee, P. and Anton, R.F. (1997) Proposed recommendations for research on biochemical markers for problematic drinking. *Alcohol Clin Exp Res* **21**, 244–247.

Allen, J.P. and Litten, R.Z. (2001) The role of laboratory tests in alcoholism treatment. *J Subst Abuse Treat* **20**, 81–85.

Allen, J.P., Litten, R.Z., Anton, R.F. and Gross, G.M. (1994) Carbohydrate-deficient transferrin as a measure of immoderate drinking: Remaining issues. *Alcohol Clin Exp Res* **18**, 799–812.

Annoni, G., Caragnel, A., Colombo, M. and Hahn, E.G. (1986) Persistent elevation of the aminoterminal peptide of procollagen type III in serum of patients with acute viral hepatitis distinguishes chronic active hepatitis from resolving or chronic persistent hepatitis. *J Hepatol* **2**, 379–388.

Annoni, G., Colombo, M., Cantaluppi, M.C., Khlat, B., Lampertico, P. and Rojkind, M. (1989) Serum type III procollagen peptide and laminin (Lam-P1) detect alcoholic hepatitis in chronic alcohol abusers. *Hepatology* **9**, 693–697.

Anton, R. and Bean, P. (1994) Two methods for measuring carbohydrate-deficient transferrin in inpatient alcoholics and healthy controls compared. *Clin Chem* **40**, 364–368.

Anton, R.F. and Moak, D.H. (1994) Carbohydrate deficient transferrin and γ-glutamyltransferase as markers of heavy alcohol consumption: gender differences. *Alcohol Clin Exp Res* **18**, 747–754.

Babbs, C., Hunt, L.P., Haboubi, N.Y., Smith, A., Rowan, B.P. and Warnes, T.W. (1988) Type III procollagen peptide: a marker of disease activity and prognosis in primary biliary cirrhosis. *Lancet* **I**, 1021–1024.

Bacon, B.R. (2001) Hemochromatosis: diagnosis and management. *Gastroenterology* **120**, 718–725.

Balisteri, W.F. and Rej, R. (1994) Liver function. In *Tietz Textbook of Clinical Chemistry*, 2nd edn, edited by N.W. Tietz, pp. 1449–1512. Philadelphia: W.B. Saunders.

Bassett, M.L., Halliday, J.W. and Powell, L.W. (1986) Value of hepatic iron measurements in early hemochromatosis and determination of the critical iron level associated with fibrosis. *Hepatology* **6**, 24–29.

Bean, P. and Peter, J. (1994) Allelic D variants of transferrin in evaluation of alcohol abuse: differential diagnosis by isoelectric focusing-immunoblotting-laser densitometry. *Clin Chem* **40**.

Bean, P. and Peter, J.B. (1993) A new approach to quantitate carbohydrate-deficient transferrin isoforms in alcohol abusers: partial iron saturation in isoelectric focusing/immunoblotting and laser densitometry. *Alcohol Clin Exp Res* **17**, 1163–1170.

Bean, P., Liegmann, K., Løvli, T., Westby, C. and Sundrehagen, E. (1997) Semiautomated procedures for evaluation of carbohydrate-deficient transferrin in the diagnosis of alcohol abuse. *Clin Chem* **43**, 983–989.

Bedossa, P., Houglum, K., Trautwein, C., Holstege, A. and Chojkier, M. (1994) Stimulation of collagen alpha-1(I) gene expression is associated with lipid peroxidation in hepatocellular injury: a link to tissue fibrosis? *Hepatology* **19**, 1262–1271.

Behrens, U.J., Hoerner, M., Lasker, J.M. and Lieber, C.S. (1988b) Formation of acetaldehyde adducts with ethanol-inducible P450IIE1 *in vivo. Biochem Biophys Res Commun* **154**, 584–590.

Behrens, U.J., Worner, T.M., Braly, L.F., Schaffner, F. and Lieber, C.S. (1988a) Carbohydrate-deficient transferrin, a marker for chronic alcohol consumption in different ethnic populations. *Alcohol Clin Exp Res* **12**, 427–432.

Bell, H., Raknerud, N., Orjaseter, H. and Haug, E. (1989) Serum procollagen III peptide in alcoholic and other chronic liver diseases. *Scand J Gastroenterol* **24**, 1217–1222.

Bell, H., Tallaksen, C., Sjåheim, T., Weberg, R., Raknerud, N., Ørjaseter, H., Try, K. and Haug, E. (1993) Serum carbohydrate-deficient transferrin as a marker of alcohol consumption in patients with chronic liver diseases. *Alcohol Clin Exp Res* **17**, 246–252.

Bell, H., Tallaksen, C.C.M., Haug, E. and Try, K. (1994) A comparison between two commercial methods for determining carbohydrate deficient transferrin (CDT). *Scand J Clin Lab Invest* **54**, 453–457.

Blake, J. and Orrego, H. (1991) Monitoring treatment of alcoholic liver disease: evaluation of various severity indices. *Clin Chem* **37**, 5–13.

Bonford, A.B. and Munro, H.N. (1985) Transferrin and its receptors: their roles in cell function. *Hepatology* **5**, 870–875.

Bonkovsky, H.L. (1992) Detection of alcoholism and problem drinking. *Liver update, American Liver Foundation* **5**, 1–2.

Bonkovsky, H.L., Jawaid, Q., Tortorelli, K., LeClair, P., Cobb, J., Lambrecht, R.W. and Banner, B.F. (1999) Non-alcoholic steatohepatitis and iron: increased prevalence of mutations of the HFE gene in non-alcoholic steatohepatitis. *J Hepatol* **31**, 421–429.

Braun, K.P., Cody, R.B., Jones, D.R. and Peterson, C.M. (1995) A structural assignment for a stable acetaldehyde-lysine adduct. *J Biol Chem* **270**, 11263–11266.

Braun, K.P., Pavlovich, J.G., Jones, D.R. and Peterson, C.M. (1997) Stable acetaldehyde adducts: structural characterization of acetaldehyde adducts of human hemoglobin N-terminal beta-globin chain peptides. *Alcohol Clin Exp Res* **21**, 40–43.

Brocks, D., Neubauer, H. and Strecker, H. (1985) Type IV collagen antigens in serum of diabetic rats: a marker for basement membrane collagen biosynthesis. *Diabetologia* **28**, 928–932.

Brown, W.R. and Kloppel, T.M. (1989) The liver and IgA: immunological, cell biological and clinical implications. *Hepatology* **9**, 763–784.

Cederbaum, A.I. (1989) Role of lipid peroxidation and stress in alcohol toxicity. *Free Rad Biol Med* **7**, 537–539.

Chedid, A., Mendenhall, C.L., Garside, P., French, S.W., Chen, T., Rabin, L. and the VA Cooperative Group (1991) Prognostic factors in alcoholic liver disease. *Am J Gastroenterology* **82**, 210–216.

Chen, H.M., Scott, B.K., Braun, K.P. and Peterson, C.M. (1995) Validated fluorimetric HPLC analysis of acetaldehyde in hemoglobin fractions separated by cation exchange chromatography: three new peaks associated with acetaldehyde. *Alcohol Clin Exp Res* **19**, 939–944.

Clot, P., Albano, E., Eliasson, E., Tabone, M., Aricò, S., Israel, Y., Moncada, C. and Ingelman-Sundberg, M. (1996) Cytochrome P4502E1 hydroxyethyl radical adducts as the major antigen in autoantibody formation among alcoholics. *Gastroenterology* **111**, 206–216.

Clot, P., Bellomo, G., Tabone, M., Aricò, S. and Albano, E. (1995) Detection of antibodies against proteins modified by hydroxyethyl free radicals in patients with alcoholic cirrhosis. *Gastroenterology* **108**, 201–207.

Colombo, M., Annoni, G., Donato, M.I., Conte, D., Martines, D., Zaramella, M.G., Bianchi, P.A., Piperno, A. and Tiribelli, C. (1985) Serum type III procollagen peptide in alcoholic liver disease and idiopathic hemochromatosis: its relationship to hepatic fibrosis, activity of the disease and iron overload. *Hepatology* **5**, 475–479.

Crabb, D.W. (1990) Biological markers for increased risk of alcoholism and for quantitation of alcohol consumption. *J Clin Invest* **85**, 311–315.

de Jong, G., van Dijk, J.P. and van Eijk, H.G. (1990) The biology of transferrin. *Clin Chim Acta* **190**, 1–46.

Diehl, A.M. (1989) Alcoholic liver disease. *Med Clin North Am* **73**, 815–830.

Donohue, T.M., Tuma, D.J. and Sorrell, M.F. (1983) Acetaldehyde adducts with proteins: Binding of [^{14}C] acetaldehyde to serum albumin. *Arch Biochem Biophys* **220**, 239–246.

Engström-Laurent, A., Laurent, U.B.G., Lilja, K. and Laurent, T.C. (1985) Concentration of sodium hyaluronate in serum. *Scand J Clin Lab Invest* **45**, 497–504.

Eriksson, C.J.P. (1983) Human blood acetaldehyde concentration during ethanol oxidation (update 1982). *Pharmacol Biochem Behav* **18** (suppl), 141–150.

Eriksson, C.J.P. and Fukunaga, T. (1993) Human blood acetaldehyde (update 1992). *Alcohol Alcoholism* **2** (suppl), 9–25.

Esterbauer, H., Schaur, R.J. and Zolner, H. (1991) Chemistry and biochemistry of 4-hydroxy-nonenal, malonaldehyde, and related aldehydes. *Free Rad Biol Med* **11**, 81–128.

Eyre, D.R. (1984) Crosslinking in collagen and elastin. *Ann Rev Biochem* **53**, 717–748.

Feinman, L., Fecher, R., Lue, S.-L. and Lieber, C.S. (1979) Aldehyde content of collagen from alcoholic cirrhotic and noncirrhotic human livers. *Exp Mol Pathol* **30**, 271–278.

Fletcher, L.M., Kwoh-Gain, I., Powell, E.E., Powell, L.W. and Halliday, J.W. (1991) Markers of chronic alcohol ingestion in patients with nonalcoholic steatohepatitis: An aid to diagnosis. *Hepatology* **13**, 455–459.

Fowles, L.F., Beck, E., Worrall, S., Shanley, B.C. and de Jersey, J. (1996) The formation and stability of imidazolidinone adducts from acetaldehyde and model peptides: a kinetic study with implications for protein modification in alcohol abuse. *Biochem Pharmacol* **51**, 1259–1267.

French, S.W. (1989) Biochemical basis for alcohol-induced liver injury. *Clin Biochem* **22**, 41–49.

French, S.W., Wong, K., Jui, L., Albano, E., Hagbjörk, A.-L. and Ingelman-Sundberg, M. (1993) Effect of ethanol on cytochrome P450 (CYP2E1), lipid peroxidation and serum protein adduct formation in relation to liver pathology. *Exp Mol Pathol* **58**, 61–75.

Friedman, S.L. (1990) Acetaldehyde and alcoholic fibrogenesis: fuel to the fire, but not the spark. *Hepatology* **12**, 609–612.

Gaines, K., Salhany, J., Tuma, D. and Sorrell, M. (1977) Reactions of acetaldehyde with human erythrocyte membrane proteins. *Febs Lett* **75**, 115–119.

George, D.K., Goldwurm, S., MacDonald, G.A., Cowley, L.L., Walker, N.I., Ward, P.J., Jazwinska, E.C. and Powell, L.W. (1998) Increased hepatic iron concentrations in non-alcoholic steatohepatitis is associated with increased fibrosis. *Gastroenterology* **114**, 311–318.

Ghosh, P., Okoh, G., Liu, D.H. and Lakshman, M.R. (1993) Effects of chronic ethanol on enzymes regulating sialylation and desialylation of transferrin in rats. *Alcohol Clin Exp Res* **17**, 576–579.

Gonzalez-Reimers, E., Brajin-Rodríquez, M.M., Rodríguez-Moreno, F., Santolaria-Fernandez, F., Batista-Lopez, N., Alvarez-Arguelles, H., Milena, A., Rodríguez-Hernandez, A. (1990) Clinical and prognostic value of serum procollagen levels in chronic alcoholic liver disease. *Drug Alcohol Depend* **25**, 91–95.

Gross, M.D., Gapstur, S.M., Belcher, J.D., Scarlan, G. and Potter, J.D. (1992) The identification and partial characterization of acetaldehyde adducts of hemoglobin occurring *in vivo*: a possible marker of alcohol consumption. *Alcohol Clin Exp Res* **16**, 1093–1097.

Grønbæk, M., Henriksen, J.H. and Becker, U. (1995) Carbohydrate-deficient transferrin – A valid marker of alcoholism in population studies? Results from the Copenhagen City heart study. *Alcohol Clin Exp Res* **19**, 457–461.

Haberland, M.E., Fong, D. and Cheng, L. (1988) Malondialdehyde-altered protein occurs in atheroma of Watanabe heritable hyperlipidemic rabbits. *Science* **241**, 215–218.

Halsted, C.H., Villanueva, J., Chandler, C.J., Ruebner, B., Munn, R.J., Parkkila, S. and Niemelä, O. (1993) Centrilobular distribution of acetaldehyde and collagen in the ethanol-fed micropig. *Hepatology* **18**, 954–960.

Hasselbach, H., Junker, P., Horslev-Petersen, K., Lisse, I. and Bentsen, K.D. (1990) Procollagen type III aminoterminal peptide in serum in idiopatic myelofibrosis and allied conditions: relation to disease activity and effect of chemotherapy. *Am J Hematol* **33**, 18–26.

Heggli, D.-E., Aurebekk, A., Granum, B., Westby, C., Løvli, T. and Sundrehagen, E. (1996) Should tri-sialo-transferrins be included when calculating carbohydrate-deficient transferrin for diagnosing elevated alcohol intake? *Alcohol* **31**, 381–384.

Helander, A. (1999) Absolute or relative measurement of carbohydrate-deficient transferrin in serum? Experiences with three immunological assays. *Clin Chem* **45**, 131–135.

Helander, A., Tabakoff, B. and the WHO/ISBRA study centers (1997) Biochemical markers of alcohol use and abuse: Experiences from the pilot study of the WHO/ISBRA collaborative project on state and trait markers of alcohol. *Alcohol and Alcoholism* **32**, 133–144.

Hoerner, M., Behrens, U.J., Worner, T.M., Blacksberg, I., Braley, R., Schaffner, F. and Lieber, C.S. (1988) The role of alcoholism and liver disease in the appearance of serum antibodies against acetaldehyde adducts. *Hepatology* **8**, 569–574.

Holstege, A., Bedossa, P., Poynard, T., Kollinger, M., Chaput, J.C., Houglum, K. and Chojkier, M. (1994) Acetaldehyde-modified epitopes in liver biopsy specimens of alcoholic and non-alcoholic patients: localization and association with progression of liver fibrosis. *Hepatology* **19**, 367–374.

Houglum, K. (1996) Alcohol and iron: A radical combination. *Hepatology* **23**, 1700–1703.

Houglum, K., Filip, M., Witztum, J.L. and Chojkier, M. (1990) Malondialdehyde and 4-hydroxynonenal protein adducts in plasma and liver of rats with iron overload. *J Clin Invest* **86**, 1991–1998.

Hui-Min, C., Scott, B.K., Braun, K.P. and Peterson, C.M. (1995) Validated fluorimetric HPLC analysis of acetaldehyde in hemoglobin fractions separated by cation exchange chromatography: Three new peaks associated with acetaldehyde. *Alcohol Clin Exp Res* **19**, 939–944.

Hurme, L., Seppä, K., Rajaniemi, H. and Sillanaukee, P. (1998) Chromatographically identified alcohol-induced hemoglobin adducts as markers of alcohol abuse among women. *Eur J Clin Invest* **28**, 87–94.

Höckerstedt, K., Risteli, L., Salmela, K. and Risteli, J. (1990) Serum type III procollagen as a marker in liver transplantation. *Transplant Proc* **22**, 1574–1575.

Iimuro, Y., Frankenberg, M.V., Arteel, G.E., Bradford, B.U., Wall, C.A. and Thurman, R.G. (1997) Female rats exhibit greater susceptibility to early alcohol-induced liver injury than males. *Am J Physiol* **35**, G1186–G1194.

Irving, M.G., Halliday, J.W. and Powell, L.W. (1988) Association between alcoholism and increased hepatic iron stores. *Alcohol Clin Exp Res* **12**, 7–13.

Israel, Y., Hurwitz, E., Niemelä, O. and Arnon, R. (1986) Monoclonal and polyclonal antibodies against acetaldehyde-containing epitopes in acetaldehyde-protein adducts. *Proc Natl Acad Sci USA* **83**, 7923–7927.

Israel, Y., Macdonald, A., Niemelä, O., Zamel, D., Shami, E., Zywulko, M., Klajner, F. and Borgono, C. (1992) Hypersensitivity to acetaldehyde-protein adducts. *Mol Pharmacol* **42**, 711–717.

Israel, Y., Orrego, H. and Niemelä, O. (1988) Immune responses to alcohol metabolites: Pathogenic and diagnostic implications. *Semin Liver Dis* **8**, 81–90.

Izumi, N., Sakai, Y., Koyama, W. and Hasumura, Y. (1989) Clinical significance of serum antibodies against alcohol-altered hepatocyte membrane in alcoholic liver disease. *Alcohol Clin Exp Res* **13**, 762–765.

Jennett, R.B., Sorrell, M.F., Saffari-Fard, A., Ockner, J.L. and Tuma, D.J. (1989) Preferential covalent binding of acetaldehyde to the α-chain of purified rat liver tubulin. *Hepatology* **9**, 57–62.

Jeppsson, J.-O., Kristensson, H. and Fimiani, C. (1993) Carbohydrate-deficient transferrin quantified by HPLC to determine heavy consumption of alcohol. *Clin Chem* **39**, 2115–2120.

Johnson, R.D. and Williams, R. (1986) Immune responses in alcoholic liver disease. *Alcohol Clin Exp Res* **10**, 471–485.

Jukkola, A. and Niemelä, O. (1989) Covalent binding of acetaldehyde to type III collagen. *Biochem Biophys Res Commun* **159**, 163–169.

Kapur, A., Wild, G., Milford-Ward, A. and Triger, D.R. (1989) Carbohydrate deficient transferrin: A marker for alcohol abuse. *BMJ* **299**, 427–431.

Kerr, M.A. (1990) The structure and function of human IgA. *Biochem J* **271**, 285–296.

Klassen, L.W., Tuma, D.J., Sorrell, M.F., McDonald, T.L., DeVasure, J.M. and Thiele, G.M. (1994) Detection of reduced acetaldehyde protein adducts using a unique monoclonal antibody. *Alcohol Clin Exp Res* **18**, 164–171.

Koskinas, J., Kenna, J.G., Bird, G.L., Alexander, G.J.M. and Williams, R. (1992) Immunoglobulin A antibody to a 200-kilodalton cytosolic acetaldehyde adduct in alcoholic hepatitis. *Gastroenterology* **103**, 1860–1867.

Kropf, J., Gressner, A.M. and Negwer, A. (1988) Efficacy of serum laminin measurement for diagnosis of fibrotic liver disease. *Clin Chem* **34**, 2026–2030.

Kukielka, E. and Cederbaum, A.I. (1990) NADPH- and NADH-dependent oxygen radical generation by rat liver nuclei in the presence of redox cycling agents and iron. *Arch Biochem Biophys* **283**, 326–333.

Kwoh-Gain, I., Fletcher, M., Price, J., Powell, L.W. and Halliday, J.W. (1990) Desialylated transferrin and mitochondrial aspartate aminotransferase compared as laboratory markers of excessive alcohol consumption. *Clin Chem* **36**, 841–845.

Larsen, M.L., Horder, M. and Morgensen, E.F. (1990) Effect of long-term monitoring of glycosylated hemoglobin levels in insulin-dependent diabetes mellitus. *N Engl J Med* **323**, 1021–1025.

Lieber, C.S. (1988a) Biochemical and molecular basis of alcohol-induced injury to liver and other tissues. *N Engl J Med* **319**, 1639–1650.

Lieber, C.S. (1988b) Metabolic effects of acetaldehyde. *Biochem Soc Trans* **16**, 241–247.

Lieber, C.S. (1994) Alcohol and the liver: 1994 update. *Gastroenterology* **106**, 1085–1105.

Lieber, C.S. (1995) Medical disorders of alcoholism. *N Engl J Med* **333**, 1058–1065.

Lieber, C.S. (2000) Alcoholic liver disease: new insights in pathogenesis lead to new treatments. *J Hepatol* **32**, 113–128.

Lin, R.C., Fillenwarth, M.J. and Du, X. (1998) Cytotoxic effect of 7-alpha-hydroxy-4-cholesten-3-one on hepG2 cells: Hypothetical role of acetaldehyde-modified delta[4]-3-ketosteroid-5-beta reductase (the 37 kD-liver-protein) in the pathogenesis of alcoholic liver injury in the rat. *Hepatology* **27**, 100–107.

Lin, R., Lumeng, L., Shahidi, S., Kelly, T. and Pound, D.C. (1990) Protein-acetaldehyde adducts in serum of alcoholic patients. *Alcohol Clin Exp Res* **14**, 438–443.

Lin, R.C., Dai, J., Lumeng, L. and Zhang, M.Y. (1995b) Serum low density lipoprotein of alcoholic patients is chemically modified *in vivo* and induces apolipoprotein E synthesis by macrophages. *J Clin Invest* **95**, 1979–1986.

Lin, R.C., Shahidi, S., Kelly, T.J., Lumeng, C. and Lumeng, L. (1993) Measurement of hemoglobin-acetaldehyde adduct in alcoholic patients. *Alcohol Clin Exp Res* **17**, 669–674.

Lin, R.C., Shahidi, S. and Lumeng, L. (1993) Production of antibodies that recognize the heterogeneity of immunoreactive sites in human hemoglobin chemically modified by acetaldehyde. *Alcohol Clin Exp Res* **17**, 882–886.

Lin, R.C., Sidner, R.A., Fillenwarth, M.J. and Lumeng, L. (1992) Localization of protein-acetaldehyde adducts on cell surface of hepatocytes by flow cytometry. *Alcohol Clin Exp Res* **16**, 1125–1129.

Lin, R.C., Smith, J.B., Radtke, D.B. and Lumeng, L. (1995a) Structural analysis of peptide acetaldehyde adducts by mass spectrometry and production of antibodies directed against non-reduced protein-acetaldehyde adducts. *Alcohol Clin Exp Res* **19**, 314–319.

Lindenbaum, J. (1977) Metabolic effects of alcohol on the blood and bone marrow. In *Metabolic Aspects of Alcoholism*, edited by C.S. Lieber, pp. 215–247. Baltimore: University Park Press.

Lindenbaum, J. (1987) Hematologic complications of alcohol abuse. *Semin Liver Dis* **7**, 169–181.

Löf, K., Lindros, K., Seppä, K., Fukunaga, T., Badger, T., Ronis, M. and Sillanaukee, P. (1996) The effect of ethanol or hepatotoxin exposure on rat transferrin desialylation. *Alcohol Alcohol* **31**, 445–451.

Löf, K., Seppä, K., Itälä, L., Koivula, T., Turpeinen, U. and Sillanaukee, P. (1994) Carbohydrate-deficient transferrin as an alcohol marker among female heavy drinkers: a population based study. *Alcohol Clin Exp Res* **18**, 889–894.

MacKenzie, D., Langa, A. and Brown, T.M. (1996) Identifying hazardous or harmful alcohol use in medical admissions: a comparison of AUDIT, CAGE and brief MAST. *Alcohol Alcohol* **6**, 591–599.

Marshall, J.B., Burnett, D.A., Zetterman, R.K. and Sorrell, M.F. (1983) Clinical and biochemical course of alcoholic liver disease following sudden discontinuation of alcoholic consumption. *Alcohol Clin Exp Res* **7**, 312–315.

Maruyama, K., Feinman, L., Fainsilber, Z., Nakano, M., Okazaki, I. and Lieber, C.S. (1982) Mammalian collagenase increases in early alcoholic liver disease and decreases with cirrhosis. *Life Sci* **30**, 1379–1384.

Mauch, T.J., Donohue, T.M., Zetterman, R.K., Sorrell, M.F. and Tuma, D.J. (1986) Covalent binding of acetaldehyde selectively inhibits the catalytic activity of lysine dependent enzymes. *Hepatology* **6**, 263–269.

McCullough, A.J., Stassen, W.N., Weisner, R.H. and Czaja, A.J. (1987) Serum type III procollagen peptide concentrations in severe chronic active hepatitis: relationship to cirrhosis and disease activity. *Hepatology* **15**, 49–54.

Melkko, J., Hellevik, T., Risteli, L., Risteli, J. and Smedsrød, B. (1994) Clearance of circulating NH_2-terminal propeptides of type I and type III procollagens is a physiological function of the scavenger receptor in liver endothelial cells. *J Exp Med* **179**, 405–412.

Melkko, J., Parkkila, S., Sorvajärvi, K., Smedsrød, B. and Niemelä, O. (1996) Aldehyde-protein adducts *in vivo*. *Alcohol Clin Exp Res* **20**, 136A.

Miller, J.A., Tuma, D.J., Miller, C.C., Klassen, L.W. and Thiele, G.M. (1996) The effects of chronic ethanol consumption on the degradation of malondialdehyde-acetaldehyde (MAA) modified albumin by liver endothelial cells. *Alcohol Clin Exp Res* **20**, 124A.

Moncada, C., Torres, V., Varghese, G., Albano, E. and Israel, Y. (1994) Ethanol-derived immunoreactive species formed by free radical mechanisms. *Mol Pharmacol* **46**, 786–791.

Morgan, M.Y., Camil, M.E., Luck, W., Sherlock, S. and Hoffbrand, A.V. (1981) Macrocytosis in alcohol-related liver disease: its value for screening. *Clin Lab Haematol* **3**, 35–44.

Moussavian, S.N., Becker, R.C., Piepmayer, J.L., Mezey, E. and Bozian, R.C. (1985) Serum gamma-glutamyl transpeptidase and chronic alcoholism. Influence of alcohol ingestion and liver disease. *Dig Dis Sci* **30**, 211–214.

Nakano, M., Worner, T.M. and Lieber, C.S. (1982) Perivenular fibrosis in alcoholic liver injury: ultrastructure and histologic progression. *Gastroenterology* **83**, 777–785.

Nalpas, B., Vassault, A., Charpin, S., Lacour, B. and Berthelot, P. (1986) Serum mitochondrial aspartate aminotransferase as a marker of chronic alcoholism: Diagnostic value and interpretation in a liver unit. *Hepatology* **6**, 608–614.

Niemelä, O. (1985b) Radioimmunoassays for type III procollagen aminoterminal peptides in humans. *Clin Chem* **31**, 1301–1304.

Niemelä, O. (1996) Collagen breakdown products as markers of fibrosis and cirrhosis. In *The Biology of Alcohol Problems*, edited by J.B. Saunders and J.B. Whitfield, pp. 345–352. Wheaton Exeter: Pergamon Press.

Niemelä, O. (1999) Acetaldehyde-protein adducts in the liver as a result of ethanol-induced oxidative stress. *Front Biosci* **4**, D506–D513.

Niemelä, O., Blake, J. and Orrego, H. (1992) Serum type I procollagen peptide and severity of alcoholic liver disease. *Alcohol Clin Exp Res* **16**, 1064–1067.

Niemelä, O., Halmesmäki, E. and Ylikorkala, O. (1991) Hemoglobin-acetaldehyde adducts are elevated in women with alcohol-damaged fetuses. *Alcohol Clin Exp Res* **15**, 1007–1010.

Niemelä, O. and Israel, Y. (1992) Hemoglobin-acetaldehyde adducts in human alcohol abusers. *Lab Invest* **67**, 246–252.

Niemelä, O., Israel, Y., Mizoi, Y., Fukunaga, T. and Eriksson, C.J.P. (1990a) Hemoglobin-acetaldehyde adducts in human volunteers following acute ethanol ingestion. *Alcohol Clin Exp Res* **14**, 838–841.

Niemelä, O., Juvonen, T. and Parkkila, S. (1991) Immunohistochemical demonstration of acetaldehyde-modified epitopes in human liver after alcohol consumption. *J Clin Invest* **87**, 1367–1374.

Niemelä, O., Klajner, F., Orrego, H., Vidins, E., Blendis, L. and Israel, Y. (1987) Antibodies against acetaldehyde-modified protein epitopes in human alcoholics. *Hepatology* **7**, 1210–1214.

Niemelä, O., Parkkila, S., Britton, R.S., Brunt, E., Janney, C. and Bacon, B. (1999) Hepatic lipid peroxidation in hereditary hemochromatosis and alcoholic liver injury. *J Clin Lab Med* **133**, 451–460.

Niemelä, O., Parkkila, S., Juvonen, R.O., Gelboin, H.V. and Pasanen, M. (2000) Cytochromes P450, 2A6, 2E1 and 3A and production of protein-aldehyde adducts in the liver of patients with alcoholic and non-alcoholic liver diseases. *J Hepatol* **33**, 893–901.

Niemelä, O., Parkkila, S., Ylä-Herttuala, S., Halsted, C., Witztum, J.L., Lanca, A. and Israel, Y. (1994) Covalent protein adducts in the liver as a result of ethanol metabolism and lipid peroxidation. *Lab Invest* **70**, 537–546.

Niemelä, O., Parkkila, S., Ylä-Herttuala, S., Villanueva, J., Ruebner, B. and Halsted, C.H. (1995b) Sequential acetaldehyde production, lipid peroxidation and fibrogenesis in a micropig model of alcoholic liver disease. *Hepatology* **22**, 1208–1214.

Niemelä, O., Risteli, J., Blake, J., Risteli, L., Compton, K.V. and Orrego, H. (1990b) Markers of fibrogenesis and basement membrane formation in alcoholic liver disease: relation to severity, presence of hepatitis and alcohol intake. *Gastroenterology* **98**, 1612–1619.

Niemelä, O., Risteli, L., Parkkinen, J. and Risteli, J. (1985a) Purification and characterization of the N-terminal propeptide of human type III procollagen. *Biochem J* **232**, 145–150.

Niemelä, O., Risteli, L., Sotaniemi, E.A. and Risteli, J. (1982) Heterogeneity of the antigens related to the aminoterminal propeptide of type III procollagen. *Clin Chim Acta* **124**, 39–44.

Niemelä, O., Risteli, L., Sotaniemi, E.A. and Risteli, J. (1983) Aminoterminal propeptide of type III procollagen in serum in alcoholic liver disease. *Gastroenterology* **85**, 254–259.

Niemelä, O., Risteli, L., Sotaniemi, E.A. and Risteli, J. (1985b) Type IV collagen and laminin-related antigens in human serum in alcoholic liver disease. *Eur J Clin Invest* **15**, 132–137.

Niemelä, O., Risteli, L., Sotaniemi, E.A., Stenbäck, F. and Risteli, J. (1988) Serum basement membrane and type III procollagen related antigens in primary biliary cirrhosis. *J Hepatol* **6**, 307–314.

Niemelä, O., Sorvajärvi, K., Blake, J.E. and Israel, Y. (1995a) Carbohydrate-deficient trans-ferrin as a marker of alcohol abuse: relationship to alcohol consumption, severity of liver disease and fibrogenesis. *Alcohol Clin Exp Res* **19**, 1203–1208.

Nordmann, R., Ribière, C. and Rouach, H. (1992) Implication of free radical mechanisms in ethanol induced cellular injury. *Free Rad Biol Med* **12**, 219–240.

Nuutinen, H., Lindros, K.O. and Salaspuro, M. (1983) Determinants of blood acetaldehyde level during ethanol oxidation in chronic alcoholics. *Alcohol Clin Exp Res* **7**, 163–168.

Nyström, M., Peräsalo, J. and Salaspuro, M. (1992) Carbohydrate deficient transferrin (CDT) in serum as a possible indicator of heavy drinking in young university students. *Alcohol Clin Exp Res* **16**, 93–97.

Orrego, H., Blake, J.E., Blendis, L.M. and Medline, A. (1987) Prognosis of alcoholic cirrhosis in the presence and absence of alcoholic hepatitis. *Gastroenterology* **92**, 208–214.

Orrego, H., Israel, Y., Blake, J.E. and Medline, A. (1983) Assessment of prognostic factors in alcoholic liver disease: toward a global quantitative expression of severity. *Hepatology* **3**, 896–905.

Palinski, W., Rosenfeld, M.E., Ylä-Herttuala, S., Gartner, G.C., Socher, S.S., Butler, S., Parthasarathy, S., Carew, T.E. and Steinberg, J.L. (1989) Low density lipoprotein under-goes oxidative modification *in vivo*. *Proc Natl Acad Sci USA* **86**, 1372–1376.

Palinski, W., Ylä-Herttuala, S., Rosenfeld, M.E., Butler, S.W., Socher, S.A., Parthasarathy, S., Curtiss, L.K. and Witztum, J.L. (1990) Antisera and monoclonal antibodies specific for epitopes generated during oxidative modification of low density lipoprotein. *Arteriosclerosis* **10**, 325–335.

Paradis, V., Kollinger, M., Fabre, M., Holstege, A., Poynard, T. and Bedossa, P. (1997). *In situ* detection of lipid peroxidation by-products in chronic liver diseases. *Hepatology* **26**, 135–142.

Pares, A., Potter, J.J., Rennie, L. and Mezey, E. (1994) Acetaldehyde activates the promoter of the mouse α2(I) collagen gene. *Hepatology* **19**, 498–503.

Parkkila, S., Niemelä, O., Britton, R.S., Brown, K.E., Ylä-Herttuala, S., O'Neill, R. and Bacon, B.R. (1996) Vitamin E decreases hepatic levels of aldehyde-derived peroxidation products in rats with iron overload. *Am J Physiol* **270**, G376–G384.

Peterson, C.M. and Polizzi, C.M. (1987) Improved method for acetaldehyde in plasma and hemoglobin-associated acetaldehyde: Results in teetotalers and alcoholics reporting for treatment. *Alcohol* **4**, 477–480.

Peterson, C.M. and Scott, B.K. (1989) Studies of whole blood associated acetaldehyde as a marker of alcohol intake in mice. *Alcohol Clin Exp Res* **13**, 845–847.

Poikolainen, K. (1985) Underestimation of recalled alcohol intake in relation to actual consumption. *Br J Addict* **80**, 215–216.

Potter, B.J., Chapman, R.W.G., Nunes, R.M., Sorrentino, D. and Sherlock, S. (1985) Trans-ferrin metabolism in alcoholic liver disease. *Hepatology* **5**, 714–721.

Pullarkat, R.K. and Raguthu, S. (1985) Elevated urinary dolichol levels in chronic alcoholics. *Alcohol Clin Exp Res* **9**, 28–30.

Ricard-Blum, S., Bresson-Hadni, S., Guerret, S., Grenard, P., Volle, P.J., Risteli, L., Grimaud, J.A. and Vuitton, D.A. (1996) Mechanism of collagen network stabilization in human irreversible granulomatous liver fibrosis. *Gastroenterology* **111**, 172–182.

Risteli, J., Elomaa, I., Niemi, S., Novamo, A. and Risteli, L. (1993) Radioimmunoassay for the pyridinoline cross-linked carboxy-terminal telopeptide of type I collagen: a new serum marker of bone collagen degradation. *Clin Chem* **39**, 635–640.

Risteli, J., Niemi, S., Trivedi, P., Mäentausta, O., Mowat, A.P. and Risteli, L. (1988) Rapid equilibrium radioimmunoassay for the amino-terminal propeptide of human type III procollagen. *Clin Chem* **34**, 715–718.

Risteli, L. (1993) *Assay of collagen metabolism*. Helsinki: Orion Diagnostica.

Rohde, H., Langer, I., Krieg, T. and Timpl, R. (1983) Serum and urine analysis of the aminoterminal procollagen peptide type III by radioimmunoassay with antibody Fab fragment. *Collagen Rel Res* **3**, 371–379.

Roine, R.P., Turpeinen, U., Ylikahri, R. and Salaspuro, M. (1987) Urinary dolichol – a new marker of alcoholism. *Alcohol Clin Exp Res* **11**, 525–527.

Rojkind, M., Giambrone, M.-A. and Biempica, L. (1979) Collagen types in normal and cirrhotic liver. *Gastroenterology* **76**, 710–719.

Rojkind, M. and Perez-Tamayo, R. (1983) Liver fibrosis. *Int Rev Conn Tissue Res* **10**, 333–393.

Rolla, R., Vay, D., Mottaran, E., Parodi, M., Traverso, N., Arico, S., Sartori, M., Bellomo, G., Klassen, L.W., Thiele, G.M., Tuma, D.J. and Albano, E. (2000) Detection of circulating antibodies against malondialdehyde-acetaldehyde adducts in patients with alcohol-induced liver disease. *Hepatology* **31**, 878–884.

Rosman, A.S. and Lieber, C. (1994) Diagnostic utility of laboratory tests in alcoholic liver disease. *Clin Chem* **40**, 1641–1651.

Rosman, A.S. and Lieber, C.S. (1992) On overview of current and emerging markers of alcoholism. In *Measuring Alcohol Consumption*, edited by R. Litten and J. Allen, pp. 99–134. Totowa, New Jersey: Humana Press.

Rubin, E. and Farber, J.L. (1994) The liver and biliary system. In *Pathology*, 2nd edn, edited by E. Rubin and J.L. Farber, pp. 705–784. Philadelphia: J.B. Lippincott Company.

Salaspuro, M. (1986) Conventional and coming laboratory markers of alcoholism and heavy drinking. *Alcohol Clin Exp Res* **10** (suppl) 5S–12S.

Salaspuro, M. (1989) Characteristics of laboratory markers in alcohol-related organ damage. *Scand J Gastroenterol* **24**, 769–780.

San George, R.C. and Hoberman, H.D. (1986) Reaction of acetaldehyde with hemoglobin. *J Biol Chem* **261**, 6811–6821.

Sato, S., Nouchi, T., Worner, T.M. and Lieber, C.S. (1986) Liver fibrosis in alcoholics. Detection by Fab radioimmunoassay of serum procollagen III peptides. *JAMA* **256**, 1471–1473.

Savolainen E.R., Goldberg, B., Leo, M.A., Velez, M. and Lieber, C.S. (1984) Diagnostic value of serum procollagen peptide measurements in alcoholic liver disease. *Alcohol Clin Exp Res* **8**, 384–389.

Savolainen, M.J., Baraona, E. and Lieber, C.S. (1987) Acetaldehyde binding increases the catabolism of rat serum low-density lipoprotein. *Life Sci* **40**, 841–846.

Scheig, R. (1991) That demon rum. *Am J Gastroenterol* **86**, 150–152.

Schenker, S. (1997) Medical consequences of alcohol abuse: is gender a factor? *Alcohol Clin Exp Res* **21**, 179–181.

Schuppan, D., Besser, M., Schwarting, R. and Hahn, E.G. (1986) Radioimmunoassay for the carboxy-terminal cross-linking domain of type IV (basement membrane) procollagen in body fluids: characterization and application to collagen type IV metabolism in fibrotic liver disease. *J Clin Invest* **78**, 241–248.

Schuppan, D., Rühlman, T. and Hahn, E.G. (1985) Radioimmunoassay for human type VI collagen and its application to tissue and body fluids. *Anal Biochem* **148**, 238–247.

Schytte, S., Hansen, M., Moller, S., Junker, P., Henriksen, J.H., Hillingso, J. and Teisner, B. (1999) Hepatic and renal extraction of circulating type I procollagen aminopropeptide in patients with normal liver function and in patients with alcoholic cirrhosis. *Scand J Lab Invest* **59**, 627–633.

Seppä, K., Laippala, P. and Saarni, M. (1991) Macrocytosis as a consequence of alcohol abuse among patients in general practice. *Alcohol Clin Exp Res* **15**, 871–876.

Seppä, K., Sillanaukee, P. and Koivula, T. (1990) The efficiency of a questionnaire in detecting heavy drinkers. *Br J Addict* **85**, 1639–1645.

Shahin, M., Schuppan, D., Waldherr, R., Risteli, J., Risteli, L., Savolainen, E.R. Oesterling, C., Abdel Rahman, H.M., el Sahly, A.M., Abdel Razek, S.M. and Seitz, H.K. (1992) Serum procollagen peptides and collagen type VI for the assessment of activity and degree of hepatic fibrosis in schistosomiasis and alcoholic liver disease. *Hepatology* **15**, 637–644.

Sillanaukee, P. (1996) Laboratory markers of alcohol abuse. *Alcohol and Alcoholism* **6**, 613–616.

Sillanaukee, P., Löf, K., Härlin, A., Mårtensson, O., Brandt, K. and Seppä, K. (1994) Comparison of different methods for detecting carbohydrate-deficient transferrin. *Alcohol Clin Exp Res* **18**, 1150–1155.

Sillanaukee, P., Massot, N., Jousilahti, P., Vartiainen, E., Sundvall, J., Olsson, U., Poikolainen, K., Ponnio, M., Allen, J.P. and Alho, H. (2000) Dose response of laboratory markers to alcohol consumption in a general population. *Am J Epidemiol* **152**, 747–751.

Sillanaukee, P., Seppä, K., Koivula, T., Israel, Y. and Niemelä, O. (1992) Acetaldehyde-modified hemoglobin as a marker of alcohol consumption: Comparison of two new methods. *J Lab Clin Med* **120**, 42–47.

Sillanaukee, P., Seppä, K., Löf, K. and Koivula, T. (1993) CDT by anion-exchange chromatography followed by RIA as a marker of heavy drinking among men. *Alcohol Clin Exp Res* **17**, 230–233.

Sillanaukee, P., Strid, N., Allen, J.P. and Litten, R.Z. (2001) Possible reasons why heavy drinking increases carbohydrate-deficient transferrin. *Alcohol Clin Exp Res* **25**, 34–40.

Skinner, H.A., Holt, S., Sheu, W.J. and Israel, Y. (1986) Clinical versus laboratory detection of alcohol abuse: the alcohol index. *Br Med J* **292**, 1703–1708.

Smedsrød, B., Melkko, J., Risteli, L. and Risteli, J. (1990) Circulating C-terminal propeptide of type I procollagen is cleared mainly via the mannose receptor in liver endothelial cells. *Biochem J* **271**, 345–350.

Smith, S.L., Jennett, R.B., Sorrell, M.F. and Tuma, D.J. (1989) Acetaldehyde substoichiometrically inhibits bovine neurotubulin polymerization. *J Clin Invest* **84**, 337–341.

Sorrell, M. and Tuma, D.J. (1985) Hypothesis: Alcoholic liver injury and the covalent binding of acetaldehyde. *Alcohol Clin Exp Res* **9**, 306–309.

Sorrell, M.F. and Tuma, D.J. (1987) The functional implications of acetaldehyde binding to cell constituents. *Ann NY Acad Sci* **492**, 50–62.

Sorvajärvi, K., Blake, J.E., Israel, Y. and Niemelä, O. (1996) Sensitivity and specificity of carbohydrate-deficient transferrin as a marker of alcohol abuse are significantly influenced by alterations in serum transferrin: Comparison of two methods. *Alcohol Clin Exp Res* **20**, 449–454.

Sotaniemi, E.A., Niemelä, O., Risteli, L., Stenbäck, F., Pelkonen, R.O., Lahtela, J.T. and Risteli, J. (1986) Fibrotic process and drug metabolism in alcoholic liver disease. *Clin Pharmacol Ther* **40**, 46–55.

Stadtman, E.R. (1992) Protein oxidation and aging. *Science* **257**, 1220–1224.

Steinberg, D., Parthasarathy, S., Carew, T.F., Khoo, J.C. and Witztum, J.L. (1989) Beyond cholesterol. Modifications of low-density lipoprotein that increase its atherogenicity. *N Engl J Med* **320**, 915 924.

Steinbrecher, U.P., Fisher, M., Witztum, J.L. and Curtiss, L.K. (1984) Immunogenicity of homologous low density lipoprotein after methylation, ethylation, acetylation, or carbamylation: generation of antibodies specific for the derivatized lysine. *J Lipid Res* **25**, 1109–1116.

Stevens, V.J., Fantl, W.J., Newman, C.B., Sims, R.V., Cerami, A. and Peterson, C.M. (1981) Acetaldehyde adducts with hemoglobin. *J Clin Invest* **67**, 361–369.

Stibler, H. (1991) Carbohydrate-deficient transferrin in serum: a new marker of potentially harmful alcohol consumption reviewed. *Clin Chem* **37**, 2029–2037.

Stibler, H. and Borg, S. (1986) Carbohydrate composition of serum transferrin in alcoholic patients. *Alcohol Clin Exp Res* **10**, 61–64.

Stibler, H. and Borg, S. (1991) Glycoprotein glycosyltransferase activities in serum in alcohol-abusing patients and healthy controls. *Scand J Clin Lab Invest* **51**, 43–51.

Stibler, H., Borg, S. and Joustra, M. (1986) Micro anion exchange chromatography of carbohydrate-deficient transferrin in serum as a marker of high alcohol consumption. *Alcohol Clin Exp Res* **10**, 535–544.

Stibler, H. and Kjellin, K.G. (1976) Isoelectric focusing and electrophoresis of the CSF proteins in tremor of different origins. *J Neurol Sci* **30**, 269–285.

Storey, E.L., Anderson, G.J., Mack, U., Powell, L.W.P. and Halliday, J.W. (1987) Desialy-lated transferrin as a serological marker of chronic excessive alcohol ingestion. *Lancet* **i**, 1292–1294.

Stowell, L.I., Fawcett, J.P., Brooke, M., Robinson, G.M. and Stanton, W.R. (1997) Comparison of two commercial test kits for quantification of serum carbohydrate-deficient transferrin. *Alcohol Alcohol* **32**, 507–516.

Surrenti, C., Casini, A., Milani, S., Ambu, S., Ceccatelli, P. and D'Agata, A. (1987) Is determination of serum N-terminal procollagen type III peptide (sPIIINP) a marker of hepatic fibrosis? *Dig Dis Sci* **32**, 705–709.

Teran, J.C., Mullen, K.D., Hoofnagle, J.H. and McCullough, A.J. (1994) Decrease in serum levels of markers of hepatic connective tissue turnover during and after treatment of chronic hepatitis B with interferon-α. *Hepatology* **19**, 849–856.

Thiele, G.M., Miller, J.A., Klassen, L.W. and Tuma, D.J. (1996) Long-term ethanol administration alters the degradation of acetaldehyde adducts by liver endothelial cells. *Hepatology* **24**, 643–648.

Trudell, J.R., Ardies, C.M. and Anderson, W.R. (1990) Crossreactivity of antibodies raised against acetaldehyde adducts of protein with acetaldehyde adducts of phosphatidyl-ethanolamine: possible role in alcoholic cirrhosis. *Mol Pharmacol* **38**, 587–593.

Trudell, J.R., Ardies, C.M., Green, C.E. and Allen, K. (1991) Binding of anti-acetaldehyde IgG antibodies to hepatocytes with an acetaldehyde-phosphatidylethanolamine adduct on their surface. *Alcohol Clin Exp Res* **15**, 295–299.

Tsukamoto, H., Horne, W., Kamimura, S., Niemelä, O., Parkkila, S., Ylä-Herttuala, S. and Brittenham, G.M. (1995) Experimental liver disease induced by alcohol and iron. *J Clin Invest* **96**, 620–630.

Tsutsumi, M., Urashima, S., Matzuela, Y., Takase, S. and Takada, A. (1993) Changes in type IV collagen content in livers of patients with alcoholic liver disease. *Hepatology* **17**, 820–827.

Tsutsumi, M., Urashima, S., Takase, S., Ueshima, Y., Tsuchishima, M., Shimanaka, K. and Kawahara, H. (1997) Characteristics of serum hyaluronate concentrations in patients with alcoholic liver disease. *Alcohol Clin Exp Res* **21**, 1716–1721.

Tsutsumi, M., Wang, J.-S. and Takada, A. (1994) Microheterogeneity of serum glycoproteins in alcoholics: Is desialo-transferrin the marker of chronic alcohol drinking or alcohol liver injury? *Alcohol Clin Exp Res* **18**, 392–397.

Tuma, D.J. and Klassen, L.W. (1992) Immune responses to acetaldehyde-protein adducts: role in alcoholic liver disease. *Gastroenterology* **103**, 1969–1973.

Tuma, D.J., Newman, M.R., Donohue, T.M. and Sorrell, M.F. (1987) Covalent binding of acetaldehyde to proteins: participation of lysine residues. *Alcohol Clin Exp Res* **11**, 579–584.

Tuma, D.J. and Sorrell, M.F. (1995) The role of acetaldehyde adducts in liver injury. In *Alcoholic Liver Disease: Pathology and Pathogenesis*, 2nd edn, edited by P. Hall, pp. 89–99. London: Edward Arnold.

Tuma, D.J., Thiele, G.M., Xu, D., Klassen, L.W. and Sorrell, M.F. (1996) Acetaldehyde and malondialdehyde react together to generate distinct protein adducts in the liver during long-term ethanol administration. *Hepatology* **23**, 872–880.

van de Wiel, A., Schuurman, H.J. and Kater, L. (1987) Alcoholic liver disease: an IgA associated disorder. *Scand J Gastroenterol* **22**, 1025–1030.

van Eijk, H.G., van Noort, W.L., de Jong, G. and Koster, J.F. (1987) Human serum sialo transferrin in diseases. *Clin Chim Acta* **165**, 141–145.

Viitala, K., Israel, Y., Blake, J.E. and Niemelä, O. (1997) Serum IgA, IgG, and IgM antibodies directed against acetaldehyde-modified epitopes: Relationship to liver disease severity and alcohol consumption. *Hepatology* **25**, 1418–1424.

Viitala, K., Lähdesmäki, K. and Niemelä, O. (1998) Comparison of the Axis %CDT TIA and the CDTect method as laboratory tests of alcohol abuse. *Clin Chem* **44**, 1209–1215.

Viitala, K., Makkonen, K., Israel, Y., Lehtimäki, T., Jaakkola, O., Koivula, T., Blake, J.E. and Niemelä, O. (2000) Autoimmune responses against oxidant stress and acetaldehyde-derived epitopes in human alcohol consumers. *Alcohol Clin Exp Res* **24**, 1103–1109.

Watson, R.R., Mohs, M.E., Eskelson, C., Sampliner, R.E. and Hartmann, B. (1986) Identification of alcohol abuse and alcoholism with biological parameters. *Alcohol Clin Exp Res* **10**, 364–385.

Waheed, A., Parkkila, S., Zhou, X.Y., Tomatsu, S., Tsuchihashi, Z., Feder, J.N., Schatzman, R.C., Britton, R.S., Bacon, B.R. and Sly, W.S. (1997) Hereditary hemochromatosis: effects of C282Y and H63D mutations on association with beta2-microglobulin, intracellular processing, and cell surface expression of the HFE protein in COS-7 cells. *Proc Natl Acad Sci USA* **94**, 12384–12389.

Wehr, H., Rodo, M., Lieber, C.S. and Baraona, E. (1993) Acetaldehyde adducts and autoantibodies against VLDL and LDL in alcoholics. *J Lipid Res* **34**, 1237–1244.

Weltman, M.D., Farrell, G.C., Hall, P., Ingelman-Sundberg, M. and Liddle, C. (1998) Hepatic cytochrome P450 2E1 is increased in patients with non-alcoholic steatohepatitis. *Hepatology* **27**, 128–133.

Wickramasinghe, S.N., Gardner, B. and Barden, G. (1986) Cytotoxic protein molecules generated as a consequence of ethanol metabolism *in vitro* and *in vivo*. *Lancet* **ii**, 823–826.

Woessner, J.F. (1991) Matrix metalloproteinases and their inhibitors in connective tissue remodelling. *FASEB J* **5**, 2145–2154.

Worner, T.M. and Lieber, C.S. (1985) Perivenular fibrosis as precursor lesion of cirrhosis. *JAMA* **254**, 627–630.

Worrall, S., de Jersey, J., Shanley, B.C. and Wilce, P.A. (1991) Antibodies against acetaldehyde-modified epitopes: an elevated IgA response in alcoholics. *Eur J Clin Invest* **21**, 90–95.

Worrall, S., de Jersey, J., Shanley, B.C. and Wilce, P.A. (1994) Antiacetaldehyde-adduct antibodies generated by ethanol-fed rats react with reduced and unreduced acetaldehyde-modified proteins. *Alcohol Alcohol* **29**, 43–50.

Xin, Y., Lasker, J.M. and Lieber, C.S. (1995) Serum carbohydrate-deficient transferrin: mechanism of increase after chronic alcohol intake. *Hepatology* **22**, 1462–1468.

Xin, Y., Lasker, J.M., Rosman, A.S. and Lieber, C.S. (1991) Isoelectric focusing/Western blotting: A novel and practical method for quantitation of carbohydrate-deficient transferrin in alcoholics. *Alcohol Clin Exp Res* **15**, 814–821.

Xu, D., Thiele, G.M., Beckenhauer, J.L., Klassen, L.W., Sorrell, M.F. and Tuma, D.J. (1998) Detection of circulating antibodies to malondialdehyde-acetaldehyde adducts in ethanol-fed rats. *Gastroenterology* **115**, 686–692.

Yamauchi, M., Hirakawa, J., Maezawa, Y., Nishikawa, F., Mizuhara, Y., Ohata, M., Nakajima, H. and Toda, G. (1994) Serum level of carbohydrate-deficient transferrin as a marker of alcoholic liver disease. *Alcohol Alcohol* **1B** (Suppl), 3–8.

Yokoyama, H., Ishii, H., Nagata, S., Moriya, S., Ito, T., Kato, S. and Tsuchiya, M. (1993) Heterogeneity of hepatic acetaldehyde adducts in guinea-pigs after chronic ethanol administration: an immunohistochemical analysis with monoclonal and polyclonal antibodies against acetaldehyde-modified protein epitopes. *Alcohol Alcohol* **1A** (Suppl), 91–97.

Yokoyama, H., Ishii, H., Nagata, S., Kato, S., Kamegaya, K. and Tsuchiya, M. (1993) Experimental hepatitis induced by ethanol after immunization with acetaldehyde adducts. *Hepatology* **17**, 14–19.

Yokoyama, H., Nagata, S., Moriya, S., Kato, S., Ito, K., Kamegaya, K. and Ishii, H. (1995b) Hepatic fibrosis produced in guinea pigs by chronic ethanol administration and immunization with acetaldehyde adducts. *Hepatology* **21**, 1438–1442.

Zhu, G.G., Puistola, U., Risteli, J., Risteli, L. and Kauppila, A. (1994) Type I and type III procollagen metabolism and CA 125 in epithelial ovarian cancer. *Int J Oncol* **4**, 669–674.

Zhu, X., Fillenwarth, M.J., Crabb, D., Lumeng, L. and Lin, R.C. (1996) Identification of the 37 kD rat liver protein that forms an acetaldehyde adduct *in vivo* as delta 4-3-ketosteroid 5-beta-reductase. *Hepatology* **23**, 115–122.

Part V

Extrahepatic effects

Chapter 18

Extrahepatic effects of alcohol: an overview

Helen L. Reeves and Christopher P. Day

Acute and chronic alcohol abuse is associated with a wide range of effects outside the liver which contribute significantly to its enormous impact on mortality and morbidity. In the UK alone, alcohol has been estimated to cause 40,000 deaths and half a million admissions to medical wards per year. The effect on mortality is principally due to an increase in cardiovascular and cerebrovascular deaths despite the now established protective effect of moderate alcohol consumption on mortality from ischemic heart disease. Alcohol-related mortality is also attributable to its association with a number of cancers, principally those of the oropharynx, esophagus, larynx and breast, and to an increase in suicide and traumatic deaths.

The morbidity associated with alcohol abuse affects virtually every system in the body. The most important effects from a clinical point of view relate to diseases of the gastrointestinal, circulatory and nervous systems. In the gastrointestinal tract the effects range from increased intestinal transit time and gastritis, leading to classical early morning nausea and diarrhea, through to significant malabsorption and chronic pancreatitis. In the cardiovascular system, alcohol is associated with hypertension, cardiomyopathy, arrhythmias and sudden cardiac death. Reports of an increased risk of cerebrovascular accidents are probably explained by the association between alcohol and other known risk factors. Alcohol is associated with other neurological diseases including those of the brain and the peripheral and autonomic nervous systems. Many of these diseases are due to the associated nutritional effects of alcohol abuse rather than to alcohol *per se*. Alcohol also has prominent effects on the blood, bones and endocrine system and maternal consumption during pregnancy can severely damage the fetus.

KEYWORDS: alcohol (ethyl) malabsorption, pancreas, hypertension, stroke, arrhythmias

INTRODUCTION

Alcohol abuse and dependence are major public health problems throughout the Western World. Alcohol related illness has a significant impact on morbidity and mortality. In the UK alone it has been estimated to cause 40,000 excess deaths per year and accounts for between a fifth to a third of medical admissions to hospital – around half a million admissions per year (Lloyd *et al.*, 1986). The range of health problems associated with excess alcohol consumption is enormous, with virtually every system in the body affected. This chapter will give an overview of the effects of alcohol on some of these systems, focusing specifically on those systems not covered elsewhere in this book.

GASTROINTESTINAL EFFECTS

The effects of alcohol on the liver have been discussed extensively in previous chapters. Alcohol can also affect most other parts of the gastrointestinal system and these effects are summarized in Figure 18.1.

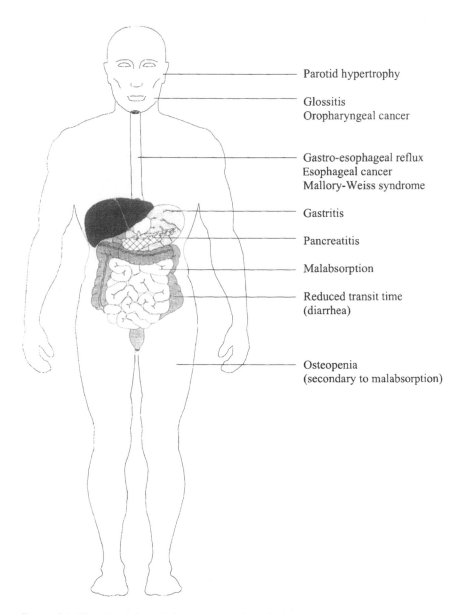

Figure 18.1 The effect of alcohol on the gastrointestinal system.

Salivary glands and oropharynx

Parotid enlargement is commonly observed in heavy drinkers with and without chronic liver disease (Bode, 1980). The precise mechanism is unclear, although a histological study of the major salivary glands at necropsy demonstrated an increase in adipose tissue at the expense of acinar tissue in patients with alcoholic cirrhosis compared to controls (Scott *et al.*, 1988). This may contribute to the reduction in both basal and stimulated parotid gland salivary flow reported in these patients (Dutta *et al.*, 1989). Whether reduced secretion and altered gland structure in patients with alcoholic cirrhosis is primarily associated with liver disease, or the effects of prolonged alcohol consumption *per se* is not entirely clear, however, reports of *increased* resting salivary flow in alcoholics without liver disease would suggest that the development of liver disease is the primary factor leading to reduced secretion.

The prevalence of glossitis and stomatitis is higher in alcoholics than controls (Larato, 1972), presumably reflecting their poor nutritional status which includes deficiencies in B vitamins and iron. Diseases of the oropharynx associated with alcohol abuse include a highly significant increase in the incidence of oropharyngeal tumors. Tobacco and alcohol are the principal etiological factors associated with the development of head and neck malignancies and appear to act in synergy. One recent study reported a history of alcohol and tobacco use in more than 75% of patients with tumors of the oropharynx (Erisen *et al.*, 1996). A history of alcoholism or alcohol-related disease is also associated with a worse prognosis in patients with head and neck malignancy.

Esophagus

Chronic alcohol ingestion can result in both gastro-esophageal reflux and peptic esophagitis. These effects are thought to be the result of esophageal motor dysfunction and enhanced mucosal penetration by cytotoxic agents in the presence of alcohol. The Mallory-Weiss syndrome (esophageal mucosal tears occurring during vomiting or retching) is also seen more frequently in alcoholics. Esophageal cancer is the sixth commonest cancer in the world, and smoking and alcohol have been identified as the major risk factors for the development of this neoplasm in industrialized countries. Alcohol associated nutritional deficiencies and the enhanced bioactivation of dietary mycotoxins and nitrosamines and tobacco related carcinogens may be the important factors (Launoy *et al.*, 1997).

Stomach

Acute alcohol consumption can cause an erosive hemorrhagic form of gastritis, with loss of surface epithelial cells and neutrophil infiltration, whereas chronic ethanol consumption is more likely to result in a superficial or atrophic type of gastritis. Whether alcohol abuse *per se* can result in classical chronic gastritis with a mononuclear cell infiltrate and glandular atrophy is unclear. However, it undoubtedly leads to delayed gastric emptying, altered acid secretion and diminished mucosal and submucosal integrity, all of which may play a role in the development of "alcoholic" gastritis (Korsten and Lieber, 1992). Recent studies have highlighted the importance of *Helicobacter pylori* infection in the gastrointestinal tract. A role for alcohol intake in the pathogenesis of *H. pylori* associated gastritis is suggested by a recent study demonstrating the presence of significant cytosolic alcohol dehydrogenase activity within *H. pylori* (Roine *et al.*, 1995). These authors have hypothesized that the generation of the toxic metabolite acetaldehyde during ethanol consumption plays a role in mucosal injury. However this hypothesis is not supported by a study showing that chronic active antral gastritis is not more severe in *H. pylori* infected alcoholics compared to similarly infected controls (Hauge *et al.*, 1994).

Small intestine

Alcohol is considered one of the main causes of malnutrition in Western Societies. It can be severe and is associated with neurological problems, skin abnormalities and glossitis, and may also contribute to increased susceptibility to infection and malignancy (Lieber, 1991). Malnutrition in an alcoholic can be both primary, due to inadequate nutrient intake, or secondary, due to malabsorption or maldigestion resulting from gastrointestinal complications. Pancreatic and hepatic dysfunction play a role, but the most important cause of malabsorption is probably altered small bowel function. Several factors contribute to alcohol-related intestinal dysfunction, including the effects of alcohol on gut motility, cellular structure and function and blood flow. Significant increases in motility in most regions of the bowel have been reported, the most obvious clinical manifestation of which is reduced transit time and diarrhea (Keshavarzian *et al.*, 1986). Cellular changes observed in the jejuno-ileal epithelium of alcoholics include abnormal mitochondria, dilated endoplasmic reticulum, altered membrane fluidity and focal cytoplasmic degradation (Rubin *et al.*, 1972). These changes are manifest macroscopically by a decrease in villous height (Hermos *et al.*, 1972), biochemically by a decrease in the activity of mucosal disaccharidases (Perlow *et al.*, 1977) and functionally by an increase is permeability to water and solutes (Robinson *et al.*, 1981). Intraluminal ethanol also causes regional changes in blood flow within the jejunal mucosa (Buell and Beck, 1983). Together, these various effects of alcohol intake impair the absorption of a variety of nutrients and minerals including glucose, amino acids, trace elements and vitamins such as thiamine, B_{12}, B_6 and folic acid. Thus, intestinal malabsorption can lead to overall weight loss and multiple deficiencies of micronutrients. The role of oxidative stress in the pathogenesis of many alcohol-related diseases implies that the most important micronutrient deficiencies are probably those of the antioxidant vitamins and trace elements such as zinc, manganese and selenium (Seal *et al.*, 1998).

Colon

The effects of alcohol on gut motility are also observed in the colon, with alcohol increasing propulsive activity and contributing to alcohol-induced diarrhea. This effect can be observed following alcohol withdrawal when colorectal transit time increases significantly from approximately 25 to 33 h (Bouchoucha *et al.*, 1991). Whether, as is the case for the oropharynx and esophagus, alcohol consumption is an important etiological factor in large bowel malignancy remains controversial. There are reports of an increased incidence of colorectal adenomatous polyps and tumors in heavy drinkers (Potter and McMicheal, 1986; Cope *et al.*, 1991), but this has not been confirmed in recent large epidemiological studies (Thomas, 1995; Longnecker *et al.*, 1996).

Pancreas

There is an established association between excessive alcohol intake and both acute and chronic pancreatitis. Indeed, the impact of pancreatic disease on health care is second only to liver disease in countries with a high prevalence of alcoholism. The precise mechanisms of alcohol-related pancreatic damage are unclear, certainly alcohol *per se* is not directly toxic (Wilson and Pirola, 1997). As in alcohol-induced liver disease one of the most important pathogenic mechanisms leading to alcoholic pancreatitis is oxidative stress (Braganza, 1996). This results from a combination of free radical generation during ethanol metabolism by pancreatic ethanol-inducible cytochrome P450 CYP2E1 (Norton *et al.*, 1998) and the concomitant depletion of antioxidant defences observed in heavy drinkers (Tanner *et al.*, 1986). Oxidative injury leads to a block in exocytosis, leading to the shunting of secretions into the interstitium. These diverted secretions contain potent chemoattractants derived from the oxidation of proteins and lipids including malondialdehyde and 4-hydroxynonenal (Curzio *et al.*, 1985). The resulting inflammatory response leads initially to acute pancreatitis and, if the insult (excess alcohol intake) persists, eventually to chronic pancreatitis as the acini de-differentiate into tubular structures, losing their secretory capacity and fibrosis commences. The fibrosis is particularly prominent in areas of fat necrosis (Kloppel and Maillet, 1991), presumably reflecting the direct fibrogenic effect of lipid peroxidation products. More recent studies have implicated a role for fatty acid ethyl esters, arising from the non-oxidative metabolism of ethanol, in the pathogenesis of acute alcohol-related pancreatitis (Werner *et al.*, 1997).

Typically, the first attack of pancreatitis occurs after 10 to 15 years of heavy drinking and is most often seen in middle aged men. If alcohol abuse continues the majority of patients will suffer from recurrent attacks of pain occurring at intervals of weeks or months. Eventually, with progressive loss of acinar tissue, patients develop clinical features of chronic pancreatitis. These include diabetes mellitus, reflecting impaired endocrine function, and malabsorption associated with steatorrhea due to impaired exocrine function. It remains controversial whether or not alcohol abuse is a risk factor for pancreatic cancer independent of its association with chronic pancreatitis – an established pre-malignant condition. Some studies have reported a positive association (Harnack *et al.*, 1997), while others have not (Tavani *et al.*, 1997). Whatever its role in the etiology of the disease, however, it is clear that heavy drinkers with pancreatic cancer have a worse prognosis than those who are abstinent or light drinkers (Yu *et al.*, 1997).

THE CARDIOVASCULAR SYSTEM

Acute and chronic alcohol ingestion lead to a variety of effects on the heart and vascular system. Importantly these may be beneficial as well as deleterious. There now seems little doubt that moderate alcohol intake is associated with a decreased risk of ischemic heart disease while excessive alcohol intake can lead to hypertension, disordered cardiac rhythm including sudden cardiac death, cardiomyopathy and cerebrovascular accidents ("strokes") (Figure 18.2). This dual effect of alcohol on the cardiovascular system is largely responsible for the well-known U- or J-shaped curve describing the relationship between alcohol intake and total as well as cardiovascular related mortality (Marmot and Brunner, 1991). This shows that

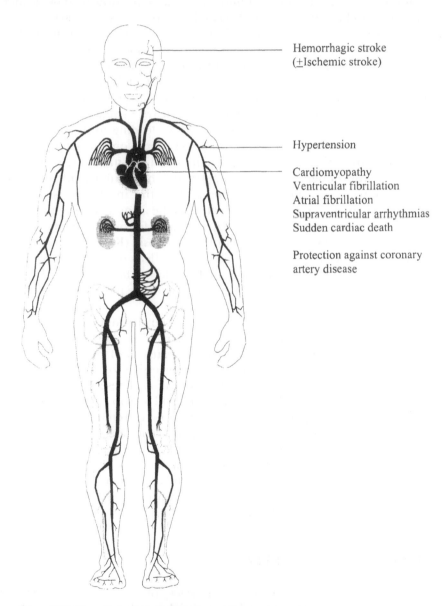

Figure 18.2 The effect of alcohol on the cardiovascular system.

mortality amongst light (1–9 drinks per week) and moderate (10–34 drinks per week) drinkers is lower than in abstainers and heavy drinkers. The left hand part of the curve is due to an inverse relationship between death from coronary artery disease and alcohol intake, while the right hand portion is attributable to a greater risk of non-ischemic cardiovascular and non-cardiovascular deaths (accidents, suicide, cancer, liver disease) in heavy drinkers. Importantly, contrary to popular belief, almost 50% of the excess deaths occurring in heavy drinkers are attributable to circulatory diseases rather than to liver disease (Ashley and Rankin, 1980).

Hypertension

A number of epidemiological studies, controlling the variables such as diet and smoking, have clearly established an association between chronic alcohol consumption and elevated blood pressure (MacMahon, 1987). It has been estimated that 30% of all cases of hypertension may be attributable to alcohol with females apparently less susceptible (Klatsky et al., 1986). The threshold for alcohol-associated hypertension appears to be around three standard drinks per day, with some studies showing a dose-response relationship with higher levels of intake (Paulin et al., 1985). Findings from short-term studies have suggested that cessation of alcohol consumption in hypertensive patients results in a decrease in blood pressure (Klatsky et al., 1986). Whether alcohol-induced hypertension remains reversible in the long term is unknown. The mechanisms underlying the association between alcohol and hypertension are unclear, but suggestions have included activation of the sympathetic nervous system during withdrawal, a direct effect on the central nervous system and abnormal glucocorticoid metabolism (Kaplan, 1995).

Coronary artery disease

As discussed, in recent years a number of epidemiological studies have demonstrated a negative correlation between moderate consumption of alcohol and fatal coronary artery disease (Rimm et al., 1991). Case control studies have also shown a lower incidence of myocardial infarction in moderate drinkers compared to abstainers (Lazarus et al., 1991). In these studies "moderate" drinking was no more than two drinks per day in men and one drink per day in women. Supportive evidence for a protective effect of alcohol on ischemic heart disease is provided by its biological plausibility (Friedman and Klatsky, 1993). Moderate alcohol consumption increases the plasma levels of the protective high-density lipoprotein cholesterol by as much as 33% (Gaziano et al., 1993). The mechanism is likely to be a result of altered hepatic synthesis and secretion of lipoproteins. Alcohol intake is also associated with impaired platelet aggregation (Haut and Cowan, 1974; Rubin, 1989) and lower levels of fibrinogen, thereby reducing the risk of thrombo-occlusive events.

Cerebrovascular disease

All types of strokes have been associated with alcohol consumption. This is perhaps not surprising in view of the association between alcohol and most of the established stroke risk factors, including hypertension, cardiomyopathy, arrhythmias, diabetes and cigarette smoking (Taylor, 1982). In view of its negative association with coronary heart disease, it might be expected that moderate consumption would be associated with a reduced risk of ischemic strokes. The consumption of one drink per day has been associated with a reduced risk of ischemic stroke in one study (Stampfer *et al.*, 1988) but this has not been confirmed in other similar studies (Donahue *et al.*, 1986) with some reporting a positive association between heavy alcohol intake and cerebral infarction in young men following alcohol "binges" (Lee, 1979; Wilkins and Kendall, 1985). This may be attributed either to dehydration or to the occurrence of alcohol-related supraventricular arrhythmias with resulting embolic events. The expected positive association with hemorrhagic strokes has been reported (Donahue *et al.*, 1986) but it remains unclear whether this association is independent of alcohol's effect on other risk factors, particularly hypertension.

Cardiomyopathy

Cardiomyopathy, due to a direct effect of alcohol rather than to associated thiamine deficiency or to toxins present in beverages, has been recognized since the early 1960s (Regan, 1984). Post-mortem and endomyocardial biopsy studies performed in chronic alcoholics both with and without cardiac symptoms have shown dilation of the atria and ventricles, increased myocardial mass, interstitial fibrosis and small vessel coronary artery disease (Schenk and Cohen, 1970). The putative mechanisms of alcohol-related myocardial toxicity will be discussed elsewhere in this book. Subclinical alcoholic cardiomyopathy, characterized by left ventricular hypertrophy and mild systolic and diastolic dysfunction appears to be relatively common in heavy drinkers. However clinical presentation is relatively uncommon and appears to require at least 10–20 years of excessive intake. The onset is usually insidious with non-specific fatigue and chest pain associated with palpitations, most commonly due to atrial fibrillation. As the disease progresses features of biventricular failure develop. With continued drinking, death from cardiac failure or arrhythmias usually occurs within 4 years of presentation although in the early stages of disease dramatic recovery can occur with abstention (Jacob *et al.*, 1991).

Arrhythmias and sudden cardiac death

Heavy drinking increases the risk of cardiac arrhythmias whether or not heart disease is present. This evidence has come from clinical observations, retrospective case-control studies, controlled studies of consecutive admissions for supraventricular tachyarrhythmias and prospective epidemiological studies (Koskinen and Kupari, 1992). The association is best established for atrial fibrillation, although in one study individuals drinking more than six drinks per day had a higher risk of all supraventricular tachyarrhythmias than those drinking less than one drink per day when matched for age, sex and smoking (Cohen *et al.*, 1988). The tendency of these arrhythmias to present following weekend or holiday "binges" has led to the term "holiday heart syndrome" (Ettinger *et al.*, 1978). Alcohol has also been shown to promote the onset of ventricular tachyarrhythmias (Greenspon and Schaal, 1983) and this presumably explains the increased incidence of sudden cardiac death observed in heavy when compared to occasional or light drinkers (Wannamethee and Shaper, 1992).

The mechanism of alcohol-related arrhythmogenesis is almost certainly multi-factorial. Factors that may play a role include subclinical cardiomyopathy producing conduction delays, potassium and magnesium depletion, the hyperadrenergic state accompanying alcohol withdrawal, autonomic neuropathy and a direct effect of ethanol on cardiac conduction (Greenspon and Schaal, 1983). The mechanism of ventricular tachyarrhythmias is most likely early after-depolarizations provoked by catecholamine release and potassium depletion during withdrawal in the presence of a prolonged action potential due to the autonomic neuropathy. In support, patients with a prolonged action potential, manifest on the surface electrocardio-gram as QT interval prolongation, have been shown to be at risk of sudden cardiac death (Day et al., 1993).

EFFECTS ON THE NERVOUS SYTEM

Acute and chronic alcohol intake is associated with a wide range of effects on the nervous system (Figures 18.3 and 18.4). Alcohol intoxication, which in its mild to moderate form is very common, can lead to blackouts and even coma. The with-drawal syndrome of tremulousness, hallucinations, seizures and delerium tremens is also frequently seen. Alcohol and its metabolite acetaldehyde are almost cer-tainly directly neurotoxic, but associated nutritional deficiencies undoubtedly con-tribute to the pathogenesis of some, if not all, alcohol-related neurological diseases (Butterworth, 1995). Alcoholic myopathy and the specific cerebral consequences of alcoholic liver disease are discussed elsewhere in this book.

The Wernicke-Korsakoff syndrome

The Wernicke-Korsakoff syndrome is a nutritional disorder caused by thiamine deficiency predominantly observed in alcoholics. Wernicke's encephalopathy represents its acute phase, while Korsakoff's psychosis represents the chronic continuation of the disease. The major pathologic changes of this syndrome are predominantly in the paraventricular parts of the thalamus and hypothalamus, the mammillary bodies, the periaqueductal grey matter, and the floor of the fourth ventricle. An abrupt onset and the triad of oculomotor disturbances, cerebellar ataxia and mental confusion characterize classical Wernicke's encephalopathy. The most common ocular abnormality is nystagmus (vertical or horizontal), but bilateral sixth nerve palsy, palsies of conjugate gaze and complete opthalmoplegia are also seen. Ptosis and pupillary abnormalities may also occur. Mental inatten-tion is characterized by disorientation, inattention and unresponsiveness which progresses to coma if untreated. Treatment is with parenteral thiamine, but it can be aggravated by giving intravenous dextrose before thiamine supplementation is administered. Patients either recover within 48–72 h or progress to Korsakoff's psychosis. Korsakoff's psychosis is characterized by various degrees of both

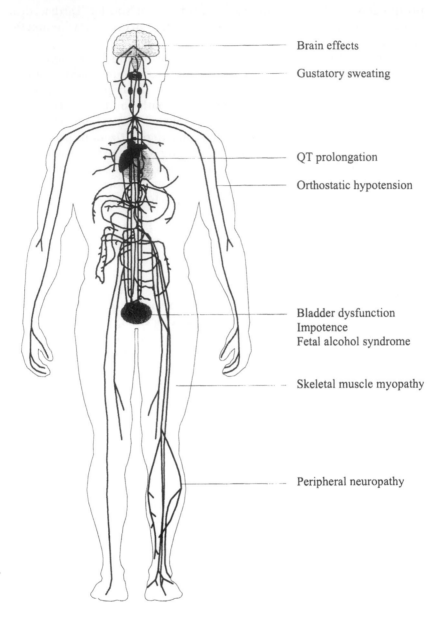

Figure 18.3 The effect of alcohol on the nervous system.

retrograde and anterograde amnesia, with relative preservation of other intellectual functions. The Korsakoff state is potentially reversible by early intervention with thiamine and prompt treatment of Wernicke's encephalopathy. Unfortunately recovery is incomplete in more than 50% of cases and individuals may be left with devastating chronic memory deficits (reviewed in Victor *et al.*, 1989).

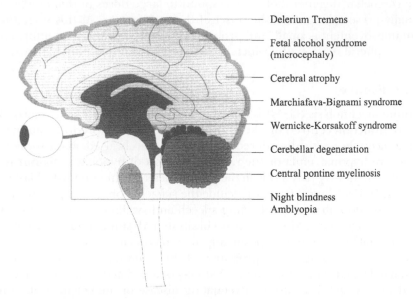

Delerium Tremens

Fetal alcohol syndrome
(microcephaly)

Cerebral atrophy

Marchiafava-Bignami syndrome

Wernicke-Korsakoff syndrome

Cerebellar degeneration

Central pontine myelinosis

Night blindness
Amblyopia

Figure 18.4 The effect of alcohol on the brain.

Alcoholic dementia

Recent studies indicate that a high level of alcohol consumption may be a contributing factor in 21–24% of cases of dementia (Smith and Atkinson, 1995). Computed tomography (CT) studies have shown a substantially higher incidence of cerebral cortical atrophy in alcoholics and brain weights in chronic alcoholics at autopsy are less than half that of age matched controls. However, no correlation has been demonstrated between either the CT or histological changes and the neuropsychological impairment frequently seen in chronic alcoholics. For example, ventricular and sulcal enlargements are often seen on CT in alcoholics with no clinical evidence of cerebral dysfunction. Furthermore, there is little firm evidence of any histological abnormality in the brains of alcoholics other than that related to the complications of alcoholism such as Wernicke's encephalopathy, post-traumatic changes and chronic hepatocerebral degeneration. Thus, cerebral atrophy is common in alcoholics and dementia may occur as a result of the direct toxic effect of ethanol on the brain. There is, however, no defined clinico-pathological entity which constitutes "alcoholic dementia" and the mental disturbances are more likely to be related to other established complications of alcohol abuse (Will, 1989).

Cerebellar disease

Alcoholic cerebellar degeneration is characterized clinically by an ataxic gait (Charness, 1993). Pathologically there is degeneration of the cerebellar cortex, predominantly of the vermis and anterior lobes. In most cases the syndrome evolves over a period of several weeks or months, after which it remains unchanged for years. Acute cerebellar degeneration may respond to large doses of thiamine, but patients usually present long after the onset of their symptoms. At this stage the likelihood of improvement is small, and probably occurs as a result of an improvement in the peripheral neuropathy which is present in around half the patients.

Brain stem disease

Central pontine myelinolysis (CPM) is a rare demyelinating disease characterized by neuronal dysfunction centred on the pons. It is encountered predominantly in malnourished alcoholics with disordered electrolytes. Cerebral edema associated with either severe hyponatremia or the rapid correction of hyponatremia during electrolyte replacement may play a role in the pathogenesis (Kleinschmidt-DeMasters and Norenberg, 1981). Clinical features include the subacute onset of a progressive quadriparesis, pseudobulbar palsy affecting speech and swallowing, and paralysis of horizontal eye movements. More extensive brain stem dysfunction may result in pupillary abnormalities, decerebrate posturing, altered conscious level and respiratory paralysis. Not surprisingly, the prognosis of this condition is poor with the diagnosis often only made at post-mortem. CPM may be associated with Marchiafava-Bignani syndrome, which is a rare demyelinating disease of the corpus callosum also occurring predominantly in alcoholics (Koeppen and Barron, 1978).

Neuropathies

Peripheral neuropathy is another common nutritional complication in alcoholics. The precise mechanism is unclear but histology reveals a non-inflammatory degeneration of myelin sheaths and axon cylinders, which is more intense in distal segments (D'Amour and Butterworth, 1994). In advanced cases, degeneration may also be observed in the anterior and posterior roots of the spinal cord. Patients with electrophysiological evidence of peripheral neuropathy can be asymptomatic, or, more typically, present with pain, parasthesia and weakness, initially affecting the lower limbs. With continued drinking the symptoms progress relentlessly, so that in advanced cases significant distal motor deficits with atrophy may be seen. Treatment consists of abstinence and nutritional supplementation, particularly with B vitamins. Recovery is slow and may be incomplete.

An association between alcoholism and autonomic neuropathy was first reported by Duncan and colleagues (1980). The subsequent observation that it was more common in alcoholics with liver disease than those without suggested that the liver disease rather than alcohol *per se* might be the primary cause (Barter and Tanner, 1987). This hypothesis was supported by a report that the incidence of autonomic neuropathy was similar (45%) in patients with alcohol and non alcohol-related liver disease (Thuluvath and Triger, 1989). More recently, evidence for a reversible metabolic effect of liver disease on autonomic function has been provided by a study demonstrating an improvement in autonomic function 3 months after successful liver transplantation (Mohamed *et al.*, 1996). Importantly, autonomic neuropathy is associated with an adverse prognosis in patients with liver disease, attributed either to an impaired response to stresses such as sepsis or bleeding (Fleckenstein *et al.*, 1996) or to the associated QT interval prolongation and subsequent risk of ventricular arrhythmias (Day *et al.*, 1993). As many as 50% of patients with liver disease experience typical symptoms of autonomic neuropathy, including postural dizziness, abnormal sweating and impotence (Thuluvath and Triger, 1989).

THE FETAL ALCOHOL SYNDROME

Fetal alcohol syndrome (FAS) is the leading cause of mental retardation in the USA, affecting around 4,000 infants annually, with an additional 7,000 children suffering from various alcohol related effects not amounting to the full syndrome. A similar *per capita* frequency is likely to occur in other industrialized countries, but little data is available on the magnitude of this problem in the developing or third world (Shibley and Pennington, 1997). FAS is caused by excessive alcohol consumption during pregnancy which results in a variety of abnormalities in the fetus thought to be due to a direct effect of alcohol and its metabolite acetaldehyde, rather than to associated nutritional deficiencies or other drugs (Fisher and Karl, 1988). The severity of the syndrome depends on both the timing and severity of maternal alcohol consumption during gestation. The diagnostic criteria include features of growth retardation and developmental delay, central nervous involvement and characteristic facial dysmorphology in the presence of a maternal alcohol consumption of more than two drinks per day. The central nervous system involvement typically presents as behavioral dysfunction and mental retardation. The characteristic facial features include short palpebral fissures, an elongated mid-face, an indistinct philtrum, a thin vermilion, and a foreshortened maxilla. The tragedy of this irreversible syndrome is that it is completely preventable. Complete abstention prior to conception or at least as early as possible in the prenatal period should be strongly advised (Bratton, 1995).

ALCOHOL AND CANCER

Results from several large epidemiological studies have firmly established that alcohol is associated with a higher cancer incidence and mortality (Longnecker and Enger, 1996). Alcohol consumption is most strongly associated with cancers of the esophagus, oropharynx and larynx, with the increased risk particularly prominent in smokers (Stinson and DeBakey, 1992). More recently the controversy over the association between alcohol and breast cancer has been resolved by a meta-analysis of six prospective cohort studies (Smith-Warner *et al.*, 1998). This has clearly demonstrated that for intakes less than 60 g per day, breast cancer risk increases linearly with intake. A daily intake of 30–60 g was associated with a relative risk of 1.41 (1.18–1.69) when compared to non-drinkers and this risk was independent of other known risk factors. The association between colorectal cancer and alcohol remains controversial and has been discussed previously. The associations between alcohol and liver and pancreatic cancers are almost certainly indirect, due to alcohol causing cirrhosis and chronic pancreatitis respectively.

CAUSE

EFFECT

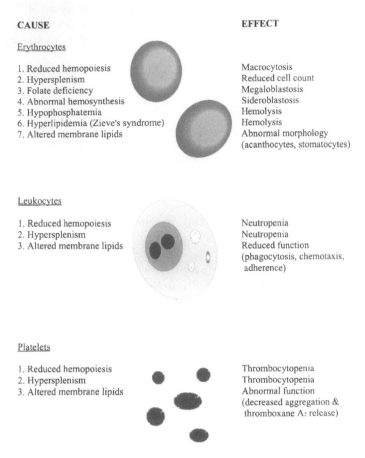

Erythrocytes

1. Reduced hemopoiesis
2. Hypersplenism
3. Folate deficiency
4. Abnormal hemosynthesis
5. Hypophosphatemia
6. Hyperlipidemia (Zieve's syndrome)
7. Altered membrane lipids

Macrocytosis
Reduced cell count
Megaloblastosis
Sideroblastosis
Hemolysis
Hemolysis
Abnormal morphology
 (acanthocytes, stomatocytes)

Leukocytes

1. Reduced hemopoiesis
2. Hypersplenism
3. Altered membrane lipids

Neutropenia
Neutropenia
Reduced function
 (phagocytosis, chemotaxis,
  adherence)

Platelets

1. Reduced hemopoiesis
2. Hypersplenism
3. Altered membrane lipids

Thrombocytopenia
Thrombocytopenia
Abnormal function
 (decreased aggregation &
  thromboxane A$_2$ release)

Figure 18.5 The effect of alcohol on the blood.

The mechanisms underlying alcohol-related cancers are unclear but several factors have been suggested to play a role. Alcohol may be important in the initiation of cancer, either by increasing the expression of certain oncogenes (Kharbanda *et al.*, 1993), or by impairing the cell's ability to repair DNA thereby increasing the likelihood that oncogenic mutations will occur (Espina *et al.*, 1988). Alcohol may act as a co-carcinogen by enhancing the effect of direct carcinogens such as those found in tobacco and the diet. This effect of alcohol is at least in part via induction of the cytochrome P450 family of enzymes that are found in the liver, lung and intestine and are capable of metabolizing various tobacco and dietary constituents into cancer promoting free radicals (Eskelson *et al.*, 1993). Since reduced levels of iron, zinc and vitamins A, B and E have been experimentally associated with some cancers, the nutritional deficiencies associated with chronic alcohol intake may also play a role in alcohol-related cancers possibly by increasing the magnitude of free radical related oxidative stress (Garro and Lieber, 1990). Finally, alcoholism is associated with immunosuppresion which makes chronic alcoholics more susceptible to infection and theoretically to cancer (Roselle, 1992).

OTHER SYSTEMS

Other prominent extra-hepatic manifestations of alcohol include osteopenia (reviewed in Sampson, 1997), hyperuricemia and gout, and hematological effects. The hematological effects of alcohol abuse have been the subject of two extensive reviews (Larkin and Watson-Williams, 1984; Lindenbaum, 1987) and are depicted schematically in Figure 18.5.

REFERENCES

Ashley, M.J. and Rankin, J.G. (1980) Hazardous alcohol consumption and diseases of the circulatory system. *Journal of Studies on Alcohol* **41**, 1040–1070.

Barter, F. and Tanner, A.R. (1987) Autonomic neuropathy in an alcoholic population. *Postgraduate Medical Journal* **63**, 1033–1036.

Bode, J.C. (1980) Alcohol and the gastrointestinal tract. *Ergebnisse der Inneren Medizin und Kinderheilkunde* **45**, 1–75.

Bouchoucha, M., Nalpas, B., Berger, M., Cugnenc, P.H. and Barbier, J.P. (1991) Recovery from disturbed colonic transit time after alcohol withdrawal. *Diseases of the Colon & Rectum* **34**, 111–114.

Braganza, J.M. (1996) The pathogenesis of chronic pancreatitis. *Quarterly Journal of Medicine* **89**, 243–250.

Bratton, R.L. (1995) Fetal alcohol syndrome. How you can help prevent it? *Postgraduate Medicine* **98**, 197–200.

Buell, M.G. and Beck, I.T. (1983) Effect of ethanol on jejunal regional blood flow in the rabbit. *Gastroenterology* **84**, 81–89.

Butterworth, R.F. (1995) Pathophysiology of alcoholic brain damage: synergistic effects of ethanol, thiamine deficiency and alcoholic liver disease. *Metabolic Brain Disease* **10**, 1–8.

Charness, M.E. (1993) Brain lesions in alcoholics. *Alcoholism Clinical and Experimental Research* **17**, 2–11.

Cohen, E.J., Klatsky, A.L. and Armstrong, M.A. (1988) Alcohol use and supraventricular arrhythmia. *American Journal of Cardiology* **62**, 971–973.

Cope, G.F., Wyatt, J.I., Pinder, I.F., Lee, P.N., Heatley, R.V. and Kelleher, J. (1991) Alcohol consumption in patients with colorectal adenomatous polyps. *Gut* **32**, 70–72.

Curzio, M., Esterbauer, H. and Dianzani, M.U. (1985) Chemotactic activity of hydroxy-alkenals on rat neutrophils. *International Journal of Tissue Reactions* **7**, 137–142.

D'Amour, M.L. and Butterworth, R. (1994) Pathogenesis of alcoholic peripheral neuropathy: direct effect of ethanol or nutritional deficit? *Metabolic Brain Disease* **9**, 133–142.

Day, C.P., James, O.F.W., Butler, T.J. and Campbell, R.W.F. (1993) QT prolongation and sudden cardiac death in patients with alcoholic liver disease. *Lancet* **341**, 1423–1428.

Donahue, R.P., Abbott, R.D., Reed D.M. and Yano K. (1986) Alcohol and hemorrhagic stroke. The Honolulu heart programme. *Journal of the American Medical Association* **255**, 2311–2314.

Duncan, G., Johnson, R.H., Lambie, D.G. and Whiteside, E.A. (1980) Evidence of vagal neuropathy in chronic alcoholics. *Lancet* **2**, 1053–1057.

Dutta, S.K., Dukehart, M., Narang, A. and Latham, P.S. (1989) Functional and structural changes in parotid glands of alcoholic cirrhotic patients. *Gastroenterology* **96**, 510–518.

Erisen, L., Basut, O., Tezel, I., Onart, S., Arat, M., Hizalan, I. and Coskun, H. (1996) Regional epidemiological features of lip, oral cavity, and oropharyngeal cancer. *Journal of Environmental Pathology, Toxicology & Oncology* **15**, 225–229.

Eskelson, C.D., Odeeye, O.E., Watson, R.R., Earnest, D.L. and Mufti, S.I. (1993) Modulation of cancer growth by vitamin E and alcohol. *Alcohol & Alcoholism* **28**, 117–125.

Espina, N., Lima, V., Lieber, C.S. and Garro, A.J. (1988) *In vitro* and *in vivo* inhibitory effect of ethanol and acetaldehyde on O_6-methylguanine transferase. *Carcinogenesis* **9**, 761–766.

Ettinger, P.O., Wu, C.F., De La Cruz Jr., C., Weisse, A.B., Ahmed, S.S. and Regan, T.J. (1978) Arrhythmias and the "Holiday Heart": alcohol-associated cardiac rhythm disorders. *American Heart Journal* **95**, 555–562.

Fisher, S.E. and Karl, P.I. (1988) Maternal ethanol use and selective fetal malnutrition. *Recent Developments in Alcoholism* **6**, 277–289.

Fleckenstein, J.F., Frank, S.M. and Thuluvath, P.J. (1996) Presence of autonomic neuropathy is a poor prognostic indicator in patients with advanced liver disease. *Hepatology* **23**, 471–475.

Friedman, G.D. and Klatsky, A.L. (1993) Is alcohol good for your health? *New England Journal of Medicine* **329**, 1882–1883.

Garro, A.J. and Lieber, C.S. (1990) Alcohol and cancer. *Annual Reviews in Pharmacology and Toxicology* **30**, 219–249.

Gaziano, J.M., Buring, J.E., Breslow, J.L., Goldhaber, S.Z., Rosner, B., VanDenburgh, M., Willett, W. and Hennekens, C.H. (1993) Moderate alcohol intake, increased levels of high-density lipoprotein and its subfractions, and decreased risk of myocardial infarction. *New England Journal of Medicine* **329**, 1829–1834.

Greenspon, A.J. and Schaal, S.F. (1983) The "holiday heart": electrophysiologic studies of alcohol effects in alcoholics. *Annals of Internal Medicine* **98**, 135–139.

Harnack, L.J., Anderson, K.E., Zheng, W., Folsom, A.R., Sellers, T.A. and Kushi, L.H. (1997) Smoking, alcohol, coffee, and tea intake and incidence of cancer of the exocrine pancreas: the Iowa Women's Health Study. *Cancer Epidemiology, Biomarkers & Prevention* **6**, 1081–1086.

Hauge, T., Persson, J. and Kjerstadius, T. (1994) Helicobacter pylori, active chronic antral gastritis, and gastrointestinal symptoms in alcoholics. *Alcoholism, Clinical & Experimental Research* **18**, 886–888.

Haut, M.J. and Cowan, D.H. (1974) The effect of ethanol on hemostatic properties of human blood platelets. *American Journal of Medicine* **56**, 22–33.

Hermos, J.A., Adams, W.H., Liu, Y.K., Sullivan, L.W. and Trier, J.S. (1972) Mucosa of the small intestine in folate-deficient alcoholics. *Annals of Internal Medicine* **76**, 957–965.

Jacob, A.J., McLaren, K.M. and Boon, N.A. (1991) Effects of abstinence on alcoholic heart muscle disease. *American Journal of Cardiology* **68**, 805–807.

Kaplan, N.M. (1995) Alcohol and hypertension. *Lancet* **345**, 1588–1589.

Keshavarzian, A., Iber, F.L., Dangleis, M.D. and Cornish, R. (1986) Intestinal-transit and lactose intolerance in chronic alcoholics. *American Journal of Clinical Nutrition* **44**, 70–76.

Kharbanda, S., Nakamura, T. and Kufe, D. (1993) Induction of the c-jun proto-oncogene by a protein kinase C dependent mechanism during exposure of human epidermal keratinocytes to ethanol. *Biochemical Pharmacology* **45**, 675–681.

Klatsky, A.L., Friedman, G.D. and Armstrong, M.A. (1986) The relationships between alcoholic beverage use and other traits to blood pressure: a new Kaiser Permanente study. *Circulation* **73**, 628–636.

Kleinschmidt-DeMasters, B.K. and Norenberg, M.D. (1981) Rapid correction of hyponatremia causes demyelination: relation to central pontine myelinolysis. *Science* **211**, 1068–1070.

Kloppell, G. and Maillet, B. (1991) Chronic pancreatitis: evolution of the disease. *Hepato-gastroenterology* **38**, 408–412.

Koeppen, A.H. and Barron, K.D. (1978) Marchiafava-Bignami disease. *Neurology* **28**, 290–294.

Korsten, M.A. and Lieber, C.S. (1992) The gastrointestinal effects of alcohol. In *Medical diagnosis and treatment of alcoholism*, edited by J.H. Mendelson and N.K. Mello, pp. 289–339. New York: McGraw-Hill, Inc.

Koskinen, P. and Kupari, M. (1992) Alcohol and cardiac arrhythmias. *British Medical Journal* **304**, 1394–1395.

Larato, D.C. (1972) Oral tissue changes in the chronic alcoholic. *Journal of Periodontology* **43**, 772–773.

Larkin, E.C. and Watson-Williams, E.J. (1984) Alcohol and the blood. *Medical Clinics of North America* **68**, 105–120.

Launoy, G., Milan, C.H., Faivre, J., Pienkowski, P., Milan, C.I. and Gignoux, M. (1997) Alcohol, tobacco and oesophageal cancer: effects of the duration of consumption, mean intake and current and former consumption. *British Journal of Cancer* **75**, 1389–1396.

Lazarus, N.B., Kaplan, G.A., Cohen, R.D. and Leu, D.J. (1991) Change in alcohol consumption and risk of death from all causes and from ischaemic heart disease. *British Medical Journal* **303**, 553–556.

Lee, K. (1979) Alcoholism and cerebrovascular thrombosis in the young. *Acta Neurologica Scandanavia* **59**, 270–274.

Lieber, C.S. (1991) Alcohol, liver, and nutrition. *Journal of the American College of Nutrition* **10**, 602–632.

Lindenbaum, J. (1987) Haematologic complications of alcohol abuse. *Seminars in Liver Disease* **7**, 169–181.

Lloyd, G., Chick, J., Crombie, E. and Anderson, S. (1986) Problem drinkers in medical wards: consumption patterns and disabilities in newly identified male cases. *British Journal of Addiction* **81**, 789–795.

Longnecker, M.P. and Enger, S.M. (1996) Epidemiologic data on alcoholic beverage consumption and risk of cancer. *Clinica Chimica Acta* **246**, 121–141.

Longnecker, M.P., Chen, M.J., Probst-Hensch, N.M., Harper, J.M., Lee, E.R., Frankl, H.D. and Haile, R.W. (1996) Alcohol and smoking in relation to the prevalence of adenomatous colorectal polyps detected at sigmoidoscopy. *Epidemiology* **7**, 275–280.

MacMahon, S. (1987) Alcohol consumption and hypertension. *Hypertension* **9**, 111–121.

Marmot, M. and Brunner, E. (1991) Alcohol and cardiovascular disease: the status of the U-shaped curve. *British Medical Journal* **303**, 565–568.

Mohamed, R., Forsey, P.R., Davies, M.K. and Neuberger, J.M. (1996) Effect of liver transplantation on QT interval prolongation and autonomic dysfunction in end-stage liver disease. *Hepatology* **23**, 1128–1134.

Norton, I.D., Apte, M.V., Haber, P.S., McCaughan, G.W., Pirola, R.C. and Wilson, J.S. (1998) Cytochrome P4502E1 is present in rat pancreas and is induced by chronic ethanol administration. *Gut* **42**, 426–430.

Paulin, J.M., Simpson, F.O. and Waal-Manning, H.J. (1985) Alcohol consumption and blood pressure in a New Zealand community study. *New Zealand Medical Journal* **98**, 425–428.

Perlow, W., Baraona, E. and Lieber, C.S. (1977) Symptomatic intestinal disaccharidase deficiency in alcoholics. *Gastroenterology* **72**, 680–684.

Potter, J.D. and McMicheal, A.J. (1986) Diet and cancer of the colon and rectum: a case control study. *Journal of the National Cancer Institute* **76**, 557–569.

Regan, T.J. (1984) Alcoholic cardiomyopathy. *Progress in Cardiovascular Diseases* **28**, 141–152.

Rimm, E.B., Giovannucci, E.L., Willett, W.C., Colditz, G.A., Ascherio, A., Rosner, B. and Stampfer, M.J. (1991) Prospective study of coronary disease in men. *Lancet* **338**, 464–468.

Robinson, G.M., Orrego, H., Israel, Y., Devenyi, P. and Kapur, B.M. (1981) Low-molecular-weight polyethylene glycol as a probe of gastrointestinal permeability after alcohol ingestion. *Digestive Diseases & Sciences* **26**, 971–977.

Roine, R.P., Salmela, K.S. and Salaspuro, M. (1995) Alcohol metabolism in Helicobacter pylori-infected stomach. *Annals of Medicine* **27**, 583–588.

Roselle, G. (1992) Alcohol and the immune system. *Alcohol Health & Research World* **16**, 16–22.

Rubin, E. (1989) Ethanol interferes with collagen-induced platelet activation by inhibition of arachidonic acid mobilization. *Archives of Biochemistry and Biophysics* **270**, 99–103.

Rubin, E., Rybak, B.J., Lindenbaum, J., Gerson, C.D., Walker, G. and Lieber, C.S. (1972) Ultrastructural changes in the small intestine induced by ethanol. *Gastroenterology* **63**, 801–814.

Sampson, H.W. (1997) Alcohol, osteoporosis, and bone regulating hormones. *Alcoholism, Clinical & Experimental Research* **21**, 400–403.

Schenk, E.A. and Cohen, J. (1970) The heart in chronic alcoholism. *Pathologica et Microbiologica* **35**, 96–104.

Scott, J., Burns, J. and Flower, E.A. (1988) Histological analysis of parotid and submandibular glands in chronic alcohol abuse: a necropsy study. *Journal of Clinical Pathology* **41**, 837–840.

Seal, C.J., Ford, C.L. and Day, C.P. (1998) Alcoholism: effects on nutritional status. In *Encyclopedia of Human Nutrition*, edited by N. Fallon, in press. London: Academic Press Ltd.

Shibley Jr., I.A. and Pennington, S.N. (1997) Metabolic and mitotic changes associated with the fetal alcohol syndrome. *Alcohol & Alcoholism* **32**, 423–434.

Smith, D.M. and Atkinson, R.M. (1995) Alcoholism and dementia. *International Journal of the Addictions* **30**, 1843–1869.

Smith-Warner, S.A., Spiegelman, D., Yaun, S.-S., van den Brandt, P.P., Folsom, A.R., Goldbohm, R.A., Graham, S., Howe, G.R., Marshall, J.R., Miller, B., Potter, J.D., Speizer, F.E., Willett, W.C., Wolk, A. and Hunter, D.J. (1998) Alcohol and breast cancer in women: a pooled analysis of cohort studies. *Journal of the American Medical Association* **279**, 535–540.

Stampfer, M.J., Colditz, G.A., Willett, W.C., Speizer, F.E. and Hennekens, C.H. (1988) A prospective study of moderate alcohol consumption and the risk of coronary disease and stroke in women. *New England Journal of Medicine* **319**, 267–273.

Stinson, F.S. and De Bakey, S.F. (1992) Alcohol-related mortality in the United States, 1979–1988. *British Journal of Addiction* **87**, 777–783.

Tanner, A.R., Bantock, I., Hinks, L., Lloyd, B., Turner, N.R. and Wright, R. (1986) Depressed selenium and vitamin E levels in an alcoholic population. Possible relationship to hepatic injury through increased lipid peroxidation. *Digestive Diseases and Sciences* **31**, 1307–1312.

Tavani, A., Pregnolato, A., Negri, E. and La Vecchia, C. (1997) Alcohol consumption and risk of pancreatic cancer. *Nutrition & Cancer* **27**, 157–161.

Taylor, J.R. (1982) Alcohol and strokes [letter]. *New England Journal of Medicine* **306**, 1111.

Thomas, D.B. (1995) Alcohol as a cause of cancer. *Environmental Health Perspectives* **103**, 153–160.

Thuluvath, P.J. and Triger, D.R. (1989) Autonomic neuropathy and chronic liver disease. *Quarterly Journal of Medicine* **72**, 737–747.

Wannamethee, G. and Shaper, A.G. (1992) Alcohol and sudden cardiac death. *British Heart Journal* **68**, 443–448.

Werner, J., Laposta, M., Fernandez-Del Castillo, C., Saghir, M., Iozzo, R.V., Lewandrowski, K.B. and Warshaw, A.L. (1997) Pancreatic injury in rats induced by fatty acid ethyl ester, a nonoxidative metabolite of alcohol. *Gastroenterology* **113**, 286–294.

Wilkins, M.R. and Kendall, M.J. (1995) Stroke affecting young men after alcoholic binges. *British Medical Journal* **291**, 1342.

Will, R.G. (1989) Alcohol and cerebral function. *Proceedings of the Royal College of Physicians of Edinburgh* **19**, 270–272.

Wilson, J.S. and Pirola, R.C. (1997) The drinker's pancreas: molecular mechanisms emerge. *Gastroenterology* **113**, 355–358.

Victor, M., Adams, R.D. and Collins, G.H. (1989) *The Wernicke-Korsakoff Syndrome: A clinical and pathological study of 245 patients, 82 with postmortem examinations*, 2nd edn, Philadelphia: Davis.

Yu, G.P., Ostroff, J.S., Zhang, Z.F., Tang, J. and Schantz, S.P. (1997) Smoking history and cancer patient survival: a hospital cancer registry study. *Cancer Detection & Prevention* **21**, 497–509.

Chapter 19

Endocrine system

Christian Gluud

The effects of acute and chronic alcohol exposure on the major endocrine systems of human adults are complex. Acute exposure affects the hypothalamic-pituitary axis resulting in, for example, decreased vasopressin and thyroid stimulating hormone secretion. The effects of chronic alcohol consumption seem to depend on the amounts of alcohol consumed. Moderate alcohol consumption may have beneficial effects, such as reducing the risk of type II diabetes mellitus and increasing estrogen levels in pre- and post-menopausal women, which could be associated with a lower risk of diseases such as cardiovascular disease and osteoporosis. However, chronic alcohol abuse profoundly and negatively affects: glucose metabolism (hypo- and hyperglycemia); decrease in vasopressin producing neurons; hypothalamic-pituitary-thyroidal axis (blunted thyroid stimulating hormone response, changes in thyroid hormone concentration, and decreased thyroid volume); hypothalamic-pituitary adrenal axis (blunted adrenocorticotropic hormone responses, increased cortisol production, and pseudo-Cushing's syndrome); and hypothalamic-pituitary-gonadal axis of men and women (sex hormone changes, feminization of men, and sexual dysfunction). Further, alcohol abuse changes the metabolism of endocrine organs through alcohol effects on binding proteins (e.g., raised thyroxine-binding globulin and sex hormone-binding globulin) and alcohol-induced organ damage (β-cell destruction in chronic pancreatitis and metabolic consequences of alcoholic liver disease). The remedy for these changes is significant reduction of alcohol consumption.

KEYWORDS: alcohol, diabetes mellitus, vasopressin, hypothalamic-pituitary-thyroidal axis, hypothalamic-pituitary-adrenal axis, hypothalamic-pituitary-gonadal axis

INTRODUCTION

Alcohol may profoundly affect all endocrine systems of the human body. The pathogenic mechanisms are complex and are still incompletely understood. The complexity arises from the following facts. First, alcohol has direct effects on the neuro-endocrine systems, i.e., the hypothalamic-pituitary axis, and the peripheral endocrine organs. Second, alcohol – because of the multiple metabolic effects – attacks the endocrine system through exertion of its effects on other organs, especially the liver. Third, the effects of alcohol on the endocrine systems may be highly influenced by the drinking pattern and quantity of alcohol and type of alcoholic beverage consumed. Fourth, personal (genetic?) susceptibility as well as external co-factors (e.g., smoking) and deficiencies (e.g., trace elements) may be involved in the endocrine defects. Fifth, a number of clinical studies trying to elucidate the way alcohol influences the endocrine systems have been flawed by small patient samples and inappropriate study designs. Sixth, a number of studies performed in animals are difficult to interpret due to interspecies difference, and to apply the results to humans may be misleading.

Despite the difficulties, a number of studies have increased our understanding of how acute and chronic exposure to alcohol may influence the endocrine systems of man. This chapter will focus on some of the major impacts, alcohol has on the important endocrine systems of adult humans, highlighting the clinical endocrine syndromes connected – directly or indirectly – with alcohol consumption and alcohol abuse.

ALCOHOL AND GLUCOSE METABOLISM AND DIABETES MELLITUS

Studies have shown that moderate alcohol consumption may exert a beneficial influence on the risk of developing type II diabetes mellitus. However, alcohol abuse affects glucose and insulin metabolism in a number of ways and should be considered a risk factor for diabetes mellitus. Alcohol consumption is among the risk factors for impaired glucose tolerance in humans (Selby *et al.*, 1987; Umeki *et al.*, 1989) and the control of diabetes is complicated by concurrent alcohol consumption.

Hypoglycemia

Ethanol is a common cause of hypoglycemia (Binder and Bendtson, 1992). The consumption of moderate amounts of ethanol may lead to hypoglycemia in healthy persons and type I diabetics (Kerr *et al.*, 1990; Lange *et al.*, 1991), the hypoglycemia being caused by reduced hepatic glucogenesis (Yki-Järvinen and Nikkilä, 1985). The reduced hepatic glucogenesis is a consequence of the metabolism of ethanol in the liver, increasing the ratio of NADH/NAD+. The raised NADH/NAD+ prevents gluconeogenesis from substrates such as amino acids, glycerophosphate and pyruvate. The risk of hypoglycemia increases when hepatic glycogen stores become depleted, e.g., during fasting and malnutrition.

In type II diabetics such a hypoglycemic effect of moderate doses of alcohol is rarely seen, but moderate doses of alcohol cause increased insulin resistance when ethanol is taken with a small carbohydrate load (Christiansen *et al.*, 1993). In the absence of such a carbohydrate load, type II diabetics show neither hypoglycemia nor increased insulin resistance following moderate amounts of ethanol (Christiansen *et al.*, 1996). The reason for the reduced risk of hypoglycemia in type II diabetics is probably the combination of larger hepatic glycogen stores, impaired insulin sensitivity (and hence a reduced ability to dispose of glycogen), and a higher rate of glycogenolysis (Christiansen *et al.*, 1996).

Larger amounts of alcohol, together with long stand fasting, may cause severe hypoglycemia in all patient groups. Therefore, intoxicated patients should have their serum glucose concentration checked and have glucose administered (after thiamine) in order to prevent central nervous system damage.

Type I diabetes mellitus

Type I diabetes mellitus is an organ-specific autoimmune disease in which the insulin-secreting β-cells are destroyed. Environmental agents (viruses, diet) as well as genetic factors (linked to the major histocompatibility complex (MHC)) appear to be involved in the etiology. It is, therefore, of interest that ethanol influences the expression of class I and class II MHC products of human fetal islet-like cell clusters (Ruhland *et al.*, 1991). On the other hand, there seems to be a paucity of data linking alcohol problems with the development of type I diabetes.

Once type I diabetes has developed and insulin treatment has been instituted, the combination of alcohol abuse and insulin cause the risk of hypoglycemia. Further, both alcohol consumption and hypoglycemia affect cognitive function negatively. Among type I diabetics and healthy controls, Kerr *et al.* (1990) observed less awareness of hypoglycemia after moderate alcohol drinking despite exaggerated physiologic changes (slowing of reaction time and increasing sweating) during hypoglycemia.

Moss *et al.* (1992), in a case-control study, observed a decreased risk of proliferative diabetic retinopathy among patients with higher alcohol consumption compared to those with lower alcohol consumption. In spite of these findings, it is generally assumed that diabetic control is significantly reduced by high alcohol consumption, due to the high caloric value of ethanol, the poorer diet control among patients with a high consumption of alcohol, and decreased rigor with metabolic control.

Type-II diabetes mellitus

Type II diabetes is characterized by impairment of insulin secretion as well as insulin resistance. Prospective epidemiological studies have shown that moderate alcohol consumption is associated with a decreased risk of developing type II diabetes mellitus in both women (Stampfer *et al.*, 1988) and men (Rimm *et al.*, 1995). After adjustment for body mass index, family history of diabetes, total caloric intake, and age, the relative risk of diabetes in female alcohol consumers of 5–15 g per day was 0.8 (95% confidence interval 0.6–1.2). In females who drank >15 g per day, the relative risk was 0.6 (95% confidence interval 0.3–0.9) compared to women with less alcohol consumption (Stampfer *et al.*, 1988). In men, almost similar observations have been made (Rimm *et al.*, 1995).

However, relatively few people with alcohol abuse were included in these studies and other studies have suggested that the risk of type II diabetes is increased in heavy drinkers (Holbrook *et al.*, 1990; Rimm *et al.*, 1995).

Alcohol may increase the risk of hypoglycemia in type II diabetes patients treated with sulfonylurea hypoglycemic agents.

Among patients with type II diabetes, chronic alcohol intake is known to be associated with higher fasting and postprandial glucose concentrations and higher hemoglobin A1c values when compared to non-alcohol consuming patients with type II diabetes (Ben *et al.*, 1991). Accordingly, alcohol abuse should be suspected in diabetics showing poor metabolic control.

Diabetes mellitus in alcoholic pancreatitis

The most direct mechanism by which alcohol can cause diabetes is through pancreatic destruction. Most cases of acute alcoholic pancreatitis seem to be associated with development of chronic alcoholic pancreatitis (Skinazi *et al.*, 1995).

Among patients with chronic alcoholic pancreatitis, about half have raised fasting glucose concentration and about three quarters have abnormal oral glucose tolerance tests (Nealon *et al.*, 1988). Unlike patients with type II diabetes, patients with chronic alcoholic pancreatitis do not have raised insulin release after an oral glucose tolerance test (Nealon *et al.*, 1988), and the impaired insulin secretion is due to a loss of β-cell mass in the pancreas. Furthermore, such patients often demonstrate insulin resistance (Cavallini *et al.*, 1993).

Diabetes mellitus in alcoholic cirrhosis

Insulin is subjected to a high first-pass metabolism in the normal liver, with about 50% being extracted (Nygren *et al.*, 1985). With decreasing liver function and increasing intrahepatic and extrahepatic portal-systemic shunting of cirrhosis, the fractional hepatic extraction of insulin is significantly decreased to about 13% (Nygren *et al.*, 1985).

Accordingly, cirrhotic patients have about six times higher peripheral fasting insulin concentrations than normal controls (Kruszynska *et al.*, 1995). This hyperinsulinemia is found irrespective of the development of diabetes (Kruszynska *et al.*, 1995). Despite the hyperinsulinemia, the blood glucose concentration is generally higher than normal after glucose loading, implying decreased insulin sensitivity in alcoholic cirrhosis (Iversen *et al.*, 1983). Moreover, alcoholic cirrhotics display changes in the maximal insulin secretory capacity rather than altered β-cell sensitivity to glucose (Kruszynska *et al.*, 1998). Compared to normal controls, non-diabetic alcoholic cirrhotics have significantly increased maximal insulin secretion (measured by the *C*-peptide response to arginine), whereas diabetic alcoholic cirrhotics demonstrate impaired maximal insulin secretion (Kruszynska *et al.*, 1998).

In conclusion, glucose intolerance in alcoholic cirrhosis results from insulin resistance and impaired insulin secretion. However, overt diabetes is relatively rare in alcoholic cirrhosis, found in about 10% of these patients.

Prognostic impact of diabetes mellitus in alcoholics

The interaction between alcohol abuse and diabetes has not been extensively studied. In Japanese alcoholics, however, Yokoyama *et al.* (1994) demonstrated an estimated odds ratio for death of 3.27 in alcoholic cirrhotics, of 3.70 in diabetic and cirrhotic alcoholics, and of 4.38 in diabetic alcoholics (without cirrhosis) compared to alcoholics without alcohol abuse after discharge. The 4.4-year survival rate among non-abstinent alcoholics without diabetes and cirrhosis was 73% compared to 26% in non-abstinent alcoholics with diabetes ($p < 0.0005$) and 35% in non-abstinent alcoholics with cirrhosis ($p < 0.0001$). Among those who died, 56% of the alcoholic diabetics died unexpectedly, whereas 71% of alcoholic cirrhotics died from liver failure during hospitalization. These figures highlight the danger of concurrent alcohol problems and diabetes and suggest that diabetic alcoholics should be intensively offered treatment for their diseases.

ALCOHOL-INDUCED "DIABETES INSIPIDUS"

The ethanol-induced acute diuresis involves suppressed production of vasopressin (Eisenhofer and Johnson, 1982; Ishizawa *et al.*, 1990; Gulya *et al.*, 1991; Gianoulakis *et al.*, 1997) in spite of the concurrent dehydration and plasma hyperosmolality. Further, a sharp increase in atrial natriuretic peptide production is observed (Colantonio *et al.*, 1991; Gianoulakis *et al.*, 1997). As a consequence, the "hangover dehydration" occurs.

In chronic alcoholic men, Harding *et al.* (1996) has observed a significant decrease in the number of vasopressin-immunoreactive neurones in the magno-cellular hypothalamic nuclei of the brain at consumption levels greater than 100 g of ethanol per day. The neurone loss also seemed to relate to the length of alcohol history, as neurone loss also occurred in the paraventricular nucleus in patients with long histories of alcohol consumption. These findings – confirming previous studies in animals – underscore the dramatic influence alcohol may have on fluid balance regulation.

HYPOTHALAMIC-PITUITARY-THYROID AXIS

The hypothalamic-pituitary-thyroid axis is influenced by alcohol consumption, alcohol abuse, and alcohol withdrawal in a number of ways. This influence encompasses direct effects of alcohol on the neuro-endocrine axis as well as changes in the concentration of thyroid hormone binding proteins and indirect changes in the metabolism of thyroid hormones secondary to liver damage. However, the impression is that alcoholics seem to stay euthyroid, irrespective of most of the abnormal hormonal findings. Therefore, therapeutic actions directed towards the abnormal findings are seldom warranted.

Acute effects of alcohol on the hypothalamic-pituitary-thyroid axis

Thyroid stimulating hormone (TSH) exhibits, like other pituitary hormones, diurnal rhythms in adult humans. The plasma concentration of TSH is elevated during the night and the mean TSH pulse amplitude at night is increased by 80% to 90% (Samuels *et al.*, 1990). The rhythmic pattern of TSH release depends on endogenous oscillations in the brain of various neurotransmitters and thyroid releasing hormone (TRH) as well as on environmental cues.

During daytime, alcohol does not seem to influence TSH concentrations in plasma or the TSH response to TRH (Leppäluoto *et al.*, 1975; Ylikahri *et al.*, 1978). Moreover, moderate doses of alcohol (0.8 g ethanol/kg body weight), ingested late in the evening, produced no effects on plasma TSH levels during the following night (Linnoila *et al.*, 1980).

However, Ekman *et al.* (1996) have demonstrated that alcohol ingested by healthy subjects (0.5 or 1.0 g/kg of body weight) between 19:00–19:45 hour produced a significant suppression of nocturnal TSH rise. According to the area under the curve analyses, the suppression in the nocturnal TSH was 32% in the 0.5 g ethanol/kg group and 45% in the 1.0 g ethanol/kg group, compared to subjects receiving no alcohol. The decreased TSH secretion is apparently due to an effect of alcohol on central mechanisms, as plasma concentrations of thyroxine (T4), free T4, triiodothyronine (T3) and free T3 did not exhibit significant changes before inhibition of TSH. Alcohol, however, was without significant effect on the plasma TSH response to TRH (Garbutt *et al.*, 1991a; Ekman *et al.*, 1996).

The interaction between alcohol and the central hypothalamic-pituitary axis may not only influence metabolism, but may also have interesting consequences for some of the cerebral-effects of ethanol. TRH has been reported to antagonize the hypnotic, hypothermic, and motor-impairing properties of alcohol in animals (Nemeroff *et al.*, 1984). In normal humans, TRH (500 μg given intravenously) failed to counteract most of the ethanol-induced effects on subjective measures, memory, time estimation and disinhibition, with the exception of free recall (Garbutt *et al.*, 1991a). However, Knutsen *et al.* (1989) pre-treated normal human subjects with TRH tablets (20 mg ingested five times) during the day before ethanol ingestion. Compared to similar testing after intake of placebo tablets, the TRH treated subjects displayed significantly reduced cerebral responses to alcohol, i.e., better performance for the counting test, finger–finger co-ordination test, and Romberg's test. It is tempting to speculate that alcohol may depress TRH in the human brain, but proof is lacking.

Effects of chronic alcohol abuse on the hypothalamic-pituitary-thyroid axis

Our knowledge about the activity of the hypothalamic-pituitary-thyroid axis during active drinking periods in chronic alcohol abusers is rudimentary. Heinz *et al.* (1996) measured TSH and thyroid hormone levels in 45 alcohol-dependent patients before detoxification. Compared to healthy controls, they observed decreased levels of T4 and thyroxine-binding globulin (TBG), but no differences were seen in T3, reverse T3 and TSH levels.

During withdrawal from alcohol, 39% of the patients with acute withdrawal symptoms demonstrated a blunted TSH response to TRH compared to 17% of alcoholic patients after 5–8 weeks of abstinence (Pienaar *et al.*, 1995). Further, the severity of withdrawal symptoms correlated with the T4 levels after 8 days of alcohol abstinence (Heinz *et al.*, 1996). Other investigators (Garbutt *et al.*, 1991b; Ekman *et al.*, 1996) have observed reduced basal TSH concentrations as well as reduced TSH response to TRH stimulation in male alcoholics being abstinent for a minimum of 28 days.

Kaptein (1997) investigated the effects of recent alcohol withdrawal on T4, T3 and reverse T3 metabolism by comparing patients with recent ethanol abstinence to normal controls. He observed an increased T4 fractional transfer rate from serum to rapidly equilibrating tissues (122%), an increased T4 binding to rapidly (195%) and slowly (190%) equilibrating tissues, and reduced serum total reverse T3 levels (69%) and reverse T3 degradation rates (61%). However, T3 kinetics were not significantly altered.

Heinz *et al.* (1996) observed slight elevation of the free T4 and free T3 levels in alcoholics abstinent for one week compared to healthy controls. During longer abstinence, the TBG and T3 levels increased and became higher in six months abstinent alcoholics than in healthy controls.

However, among alcoholics having been abstinent for more than one to two years, the TRH-TSH response appeared normal (Marchesi *et al.*, 1992; Piennaar *et al.*, 1995). Further, the TRH concentrations of cerebrospinal fluid did not differ significantly between alcoholics and normal controls (Roy *et al.*, 1990) and abstinent male alcoholics showed the same degree of T3-suppression of the TSH response to TRH as normal controls (Garbutt *et al.*, 1992).

In conclusion, chronic alcohol abuse and withdrawal from alcohol are accompanied by a number of changes in the regulation of the hypothalamic-pituitary-thyroid axis as well as changes in the metabolism of thyroid hormones. It appears that alcoholics without major organ damage may show alleviation of some, if not all, of the metabolic changes after prolonged abstention from alcohol.

The hypothalamic-pituitary-thyroid axis in alcoholic liver disease

The hormonal findings pertaining to the hypothalamic-pituitary-thyroid axis in alcoholic liver disease (ALD) demonstrate highly complex patterns, probably reflecting the effects of alcohol, abstinence, and the degree of liver dysfunction. Patients with ALD of sufficient severity to influence the hypothalamic-pituitary-thyroid axis, often display changes of this axis seen also in other forms of severe liver disease. The most frequent observations encompass normal to increased T4, normal free T4, normal to decreased T3, reduced free T3 levels, decreased or increased reverse T3, and increased TSH levels (Noth and Walter 1984; Hegedus 1984; Becker *et al.*, 1988; Burra *et al.*,, 1992; Vagenakis 1998). The increased T4 levels are mainly due to an elevation of serum TBG levels. It has been proposed that the inflammatory processes in the liver may increase TBG synthesis (Yamanaka *et al.*, 1980). Further, patients with alcoholic liver cirrhosis have significantly decreased thyroid volume, measured ultrasonically (11 ml (range 6–16 ml) versus 20 ml (range 10–31 ml) in healthy controls) (Hegedus, 1984). However, this low volume of the thyroid gland may be due to a toxic effect of alcohol as it is also seen in alcoholics without liver cirrhosis but it is not found in patients with non-alcoholic liver cirrhosis (Hegedus *et al.*, 1988).

In spite of the fact, that most studies find elevated TBG concentrations in patients with alcoholic cirrhosis, such patients may have normal T4 concentrations. The concentrations of T4 and T3 seem to correlate with the degree of liver dysfunction, i.e., the greater the liver dysfunction, the lower concentrations of these hormones (Burra *et al.*, 1992; Rumilly *et al.*, 1983; Grun and Kaffarnik, 1985; Becker *et al.*, 1988).

HYPOTHALAMIC-PITUITARY-ADRENAL AXIS

Acute effects of alcohol on the hypothalamic-pituitary-adrenal axis

Alcohol (0.8 g/kg body weight) taken at bedtime – even each night for nine days – does not seem to influence plasma cortisol concentrations during night-time in healthy men (Prinz et al., 1980). Further, no evidence for changes of plasma cortisol circadian rhythm and adrenocorticotropic hormone (ACTH) plasma concentrations have been reported after both oral and intravenous alcohol administration during the morning and afternoon hours (Davis and Jeffcoate, 1983; Waltman et al., 1993). Similar observations have been achieved in non-alcoholic volunteers without gastrointestinal complaints following 1.1 ml of 95% ethanol/kg body weight. In addition, these volunteers did not show significant changes in plasma concentrations of corticotropin-releasing hormone (CRH) and ACTH (Inder et al., 1995). In volunteers exposed to the same amount of ethanol, but experiencing significant gastrointestinal adverse effects (nausea and vomiting), plasma concentrations of both ACTH and cortisol rose significantly, but no significant changes were observed in CRH concentrations (Inder et al., 1995).

Effects of chronic alcohol abuse on the hypothalamic-pituitary-adrenal axis

Berman et al. (1990) studied non-depressed, actively drinking male alcoholics and normal controls. They observed an insignificant trend towards increased cortisol levels in the alcoholic group, but the 24 hours urinary free cortisol levels were 2-fold higher in actively drinking alcoholics than in controls (Wand and Dobs, 1991). In spite of a marked deficiency of 11-β-hydroxysteroid dehydrogenase activity (converting active cortisol to cortisone) in patients with chronic ALD, a normal counterregulatory down-regulation of cortisol production was not exhibited (Stewart et al., 1993). Following insulin-induced hypoglycemia, the alcoholic group displayed a significantly blunted plasma ACTH stress response (Berman et al., 1990). Further, actively drinking alcoholics demonstrate a significantly blunted ACTH response to the CRH stimulation test (Wand and Dobs, 1991). These studies suggest that actively drinking alcoholics have increased basal cortisol production as well as an ethanol-induced hypothalamic-pituitary-adrenal axis injury, resulting in an inappropriately reduced response to non-ethanol-induced stress.

During withdrawal from ethanol, 17–25% of alcoholics show non-suppression of cortisol in a dexamethasone suppression test (Muller et al., 1989; Costa et al., 1996) and plasma cortisol concentrations are almost twice as high during acute alcohol withdrawal as following recovery (Adinoff et al., 1991). Further, the duration of the cortisol diurnal cycle on the first day of withdrawal seems to be negatively correlated with the severity of withdrawal symptoms (Adinoff et al., 1991) and patients with moderate and severe withdrawal symptoms demonstrate elevated cortisol levels throughout the day (Risher-Flowers et al., 1988). Following CRH-stimulation and insulin-induced hypoglycemia, ACTH and cortisol responses were markedly reduced (Costa *et al.*, 1996). The blunted ACTH response does not appear to be the result of increased endogenous CRH activity, but rather appears to be secondary to an intrinsic defect in the CRH responsiveness of the pituitary corticotrope (Loosen *et al.*, 1993).

Alcohol induced pseudo-Cushing's syndrome

Patients with alcohol problems often display one or more of the symptoms of moon face, truncal obesity, impaired glucose tolerance, hypertension, hypogonadism, muscle weakness, etc. – all symptoms commonly found in high frequencies in patients with Cushing's syndrome (von Werder and Müller, 1998). It is possible that some of these symptoms may be at least partly linked to the increased cortisol production found in connection with repeated withdrawal symptoms and during chronic alcohol exposure (Heaney *et al.*, 1997), although some studies have not found a relationship (Duane and Peters, 1987).

Occasionally, alcoholic patients may develop the full blown clinical picture of Cushing's syndrome with several of these symptoms present in the same patient together with elevated basal cortisol concentrations, increased cortisol production rate, and increased urinary free cortisol excretion. These patients exhibit insufficient suppression of plasma cortisol with dexamethasone. After abstinence from alcohol, the clinical and laboratory abnormalities will tend to normalize within 1 to 2 months (von Werder and Müller, 1998; Proto *et al.*, 1985). This alcohol induced pseudo-Cushing's syndrome is, however, rare among alcoholics (Kirkman and Nelson, 1988) and an alcohol etiology of Cushing's syndrome is only found in about 5% of patients with Cushing's syndrome (Caduff *et al.*, 1991).

HYPOTHALAMIC-PITUITARY-GONADAL AXIS IN MEN

Acute effects of alcohol on the hypothalamic-pituitary-gonadal axis

Under experimental conditions in normal men, alcohol ingestion or infusion either decreases plasma testosterone concentrations (about 15–30% after 0.4–1.5 g ethanol/kg body weight) (Bertello *et al.*, 1983; Ellingboe, 1987; Välimäki *et al.*, 1990; Heikkonen *et al.*, 1996) or produces no substantial changes (Andersson *et al.*, 1986; Gluud, 1988; Ida *et al.*, 1992; Eriksson *et al.*, 1994). In studies showing a testosterone lowering effect of acute alcohol administration, plasma testosterone concentrations normalize within 24 hours. The decreased testosterone concentrations have been found in the absence of changes in pulsatility of luteinizing hormone (LH) or changes in the concentration of sex-hormone-binding-globulin (SHBG) (Ellingboe, 1987; Välimäki *et al.*, 1990; Ida *et al.*, 1992; Heikkonen *et al.*, 1996). This suggests a direct effect of alcohol on the testes (i.e., the Leydig cells) (Van Thiel and Gavaler, 1990) and/or increased degradation of testosterone together with an inappropriate pituitary response. Studies suggest that the type of alcohol consumed (beer or wine) and duration of drinking (fast or slow) may be related to the hormonal effects (Couwenbergs, 1988).

When normal men were given a pharmacological dose of gonadotropin releasing hormone, the LH or follicle stimulating hormone (FSH) responses were not changed by the ingestion of alcohol (0.7 g/kg body weight). However, the testosterone concentrations increased significantly compared to the same dose of gonadotropin releasing hormone without alcohol (Phipps *et al.*, 1987). In chronic alcoholics, unlimited alcohol consumption during one week led to a 19–27% decrease in testosterone levels (Persky *et al.*, 1977).

Even after low doses of alcohol (0.3 g/kg body weight) – in the absence of any effect of alcohol on unconjugated fractions of testosterone, androstenedione, estradiol, and estrone – a significant increase in the ratio of plasma estradiol/estrone monosulphates (and glucoronides) was observed during ethanol metabolism (Andersson *et al.*, 1986). In view of the effects of alcohol on the NADH/NAD+ ratio in the liver and the presence of a NAD-dependent 17-β-hydroxysteroid oxidoreductase, the results indicate that the two steroid sulphate redox couples are equilibrated with a common pool of NADH/NAD+. Further, the change from estrone to estradiol may have feminizing effects in tissues with sulphatase activity (Andersson *et al.*, 1986) despite the lack of effect of acute alcohol on plasma concentrations of unconjugated estradiol and estrone (Välimäki *et al.*, 1984a).

Effects of chronic alcohol use and abuse on the hypothalamic-pituitary-gonadal axis

Epidemiological assessments of the relationship between alcohol consumption in normal men and plasma testosterone concentrations have revealed contradictory results. A negative correlation between alcohol consumption and free testosterone in Japanese men (Shono *et al.*, 1996), no association in African-American, Caucasian and Asian men (Kato *et al.*, 1992; Gluud, 1988; Wu *et al.*, 1995) and a positive correlation in college students (La Grange *et al.*, 1995) have been observed. The observed correlations have generally been weak.

Serum testosterone concentrations do not differ significantly from normal controls in patients with chronic alcohol problems but without significant liver damage, during active drinking or after abstinence (Lindholm *et al.*, 1978a; Gluud, 1988; Markianos *et al.*, 1987; Martínez-Riera *et al.*, 1995; Iturriaga *et al.*, 1995). However, such patients had significantly increased SHBG levels compared to normal controls (Gluud, 1988; Martínez-Riera *et al.*, 1995; Iturriaga *et al.*, 1995), implying that these patients have significantly decreased free testosterone levels. In spite of this, the LH concentration is not significantly increased (Martínez-Riera *et al.*, 1995; Iturriaga *et al.*, 1995). This could be due both to a direct depressing effect of alcohol on the hypothalamic-pituitary region or secondary to the raised estradiol concentrations observed in these patients (Martínez-Riera *et al.*, 1995).

During florid alcohol withdrawal syndrome, male patients demonstrate significantly decreased testosterone levels that increase towards normal during diazepam treatment (Castilla-García *et al.*, 1987). However, other studies have found mostly normal plasma testosterone concentrations during the withdrawal state (Välimäki *et al.*, 1984b; Gluud, 1988; Heinz *et al.*, 1995; Ruusa *et al.*, 1997).

In conclusion, patients with alcohol problems without significant liver disease demonstrate either reduced or normal plasma testosterone concentrations, normal or raised plasma estradiol concentrations, and normal or raised SHBG concentrations. The raised SHBG concentrations are probably due to the combined effects of raised circulating estrogen levels as well as increased hepatic estrogen receptor levels and decreased hepatic androgen receptor levels (Gluud, 1988). The increased SHBG levels lead to low free testosterone levels, which in conjunction with the raised estrogen levels, may explain some of the clinical findings of feminization and hypoandrogenism occasionally observed in men with alcohol problems without concomitant liver disease.

The hypothalamic-pituitary-gonadal axis in alcoholic liver disease

There are few studies examining the hypothalamic-pituitary-gonadal axis of patients with alcoholic fatty liver and alcoholic hepatitis without concomitant cirrhosis. Myking et al. (1987), studying 20 patients with alcoholic fatty liver, observed changes in accordance with findings in alcoholic cirrhotic men with well preserved liver function, i.e., normal plasma testosterone, raised SHBG, estrone and estradiol and low free testosterone concentrations.

In men with alcoholic cirrhosis, most studies find normal median plasma testosterone concentrations (Gluud et al., 1983, 1987; Gluud, 1988). However, both raised and depressed plasma testosterone concentrations are observed (Bannister et al., 1987; Gluud, 1988). In 216 men with alcoholic cirrhosis, plasma testosterone concentrations varied by a factor of 43.9 compared to a factor of 3.2 in normal men (Gluud et al., 1987). The background for this complex picture in cirrhotics is due both to the degree of liver dysfunction and the raised SHBG concentrations as well as other factors. The only significant background variables associated with the testosterone concentration were Child-Turcotte's group C, Child-Turcotte's group B, age, duration of hospitalization and SHBG concentration (Gluud et al., 1987). Accordingly, the more severe the liver dysfunction is, the lower are the plasma concentrations of testosterone (being supernormal in patients with well preserved liver function) and of non-protein bound testosterone and non-SHBG bound testosterone (being subnormal in patients with well preserved liver function) (Gluud, 1988).

Plasma concentrations of estrone and estradiol are significantly increased in patients with alcoholic cirrhosis (Gluud et al., 1983; Bannister et al., 1987; Martínez-Riera et al., 1995; Kaymakoglu et al., 1995), and estrone (Gluud et al., 1983) and estradiol (Kaymakoglu et al., 1995) may increase with decreasing liver function.

The basal concentrations of LH (and FSH) are significantly increased in alcoholic cirrhotic patients with well preserved liver function (Gluud et al., 1983; Martínez-Riera 1995). With decreasing liver function, however, and in spite of the decreasing testosterone concentrations, LH (and FSH) concentrations decrease, approaching the concentrations of normal controls. It is conceivable that the increased estrogen levels may depress a physiologic compensatory rise in LH (and FSH). In accordance with this view, dexamethasone suppression (leading to a significant fall in estrone and estradiol levels of alcoholic cirrhotic patients) was associated with a significant rise in LH concentrations, which increased with decreasing liver function (Gluud et al., 1983).

Attempts to relate levels of alcohol consumption to the hormonal levels found in alcoholic cirrhotics have not revealed significant associations (Gluud *et al.*, 1987). One study comparing matched alcoholic versus non-alcoholic cirrhotical patients demonstrates that the hormonal changes are more pronounced in the alcoholi parties group, suggesting that alcohol amplifies the hormonal changes caused by the liver dysfunction (Bannister *et al.*, 1987). Other studies, however, do not find significant differences between the different etiologic groups (Wang *et al.*, 1991; Guêchot *et al.*, 1994; Kaymakoglu *et al.*, 1995).

Following successful orthotopic liver transplantation for advanced ALD, plasma estrone, estradiol and SHBG decrease and LH, FSH, and testosterone increase towards normal levels (Van Thiel *et al.*, 1990; Guêchot *et al.*, 1994).

Clinical findings related to gonadal hormonal changes of alcoholic men

In accordance with the observed slight hormonal changes in alcoholics with well preserved liver function, such patients seldom present with signs of feminization and hypoandrogenization like gynecomastia and testicular atrophy.

With decreasing liver function in alcoholic cirrhotics, the prevalence of gynecomastia and testicular atrophy increase significantly (Gluud, 1988). In Child-Turcotte group C patients, about 50% have gynecomastia and about 75% have testicular atrophy (Gluud, 1988). During testosterone treatment of alcoholic cirrhotic men, which significantly increases the plasma testosterone/estradiol ratio (Gluud *et al.*, 1988a), the prevalence of gynecomastia decreases significantly (The Copenhagen Study Group for Liver Diseases, 1986). The high prevalence of testicular atrophy is in accordance with the significantly depressed spermatogenesis found in alcoholics with and without liver disease (Lindholm *et al.*, 1978a,b). Lindholm *et al.* (1978b) noticed that SHBG concentrations were significantly higher among patients with severely reduced spermatogenesis compared to patents with intact germinal epithelium, but were unable to find a relationship between clinical signs of hypogonadism and levels of sex hormones. The lack of an association between alterations in sperm quality from alcoholics on one hand and hormonal levels on the other has recently been re-examined by Villalta *et al.* (1997). Between 40% and 50% of alcoholics without liver disease displayed significantly reduced spermatozoa count, significant morphological spermatozoa abnormalities, or changed spermatozoa motility. In a multivariate analysis, the only independent factor that determined alterations in sperm quality was the total lifetime of ethanol intake. Considering the high prevalence of alcohol problems in Western societies, it is therefore surprising to find that an alcohol related etiology is found in less than 12% of infertile men (Martin-Du Pan *et al.*, 1997). One explanation could be that the abnormalities of spermatogenesis are reversible after alcohol abstinence (Brzek, 1987).

Men with alcoholic cirrhosis and chronic alcoholics without overt liver disease have an increased prevalence of sexual dysfunction, encompassing problems with reduced sexual desire, erectile dysfunction, and premature ejaculation (Jensen *et al.*, 1985; Fahrner, 1987). In one study comparing alcoholic cirrhotic men with sexual dysfunction to those without, serum testosterone concentrations did not differ significantly between the two groups (Jensen *et al.*, 1985). In a larger study, however, low plasma testosterone concentrations were significantly associated with sexual dysfunction (Gluud *et al.*, 1988b). When treating cirrhotic men (of whom 67% (95% confidence limits 61–74%) complained of sexual dysfunction) with testosterone in a randomized placebo-controlled trial, no significant effect of testosterone treatment could be found (Gluud *et al.*, 1988b). During follow-up the prevalence of complaints of sexual dysfunction decreased significantly in both testosterone and placebo treated patients, about half of the patients reporting improvement of libido, erectile function and ejaculatory function (Gluud *et al.*, 1988b). The potential reversibility of sexual dysfunction has also been observed in other studies. Abstinent alcoholics, without hepatic or gonadal failure, did not differ significantly from non-alcoholic volunteers regarding a number of variables of sexual function (Schiavi *et al.*, 1995).

HYPOTHALAMIC-PITUITARY-GONADAL AXIS IN WOMEN

Acute effects of alcohol on the hypothalamic-pituitary-gonadal axis

Some studies have been unable to detect any acute effects of alcohol on LH, FSH, testosterone, estrone and estradiol concentrations of normal premenstrual women (Gavaler, 1985; Becker *et al.*, 1988). However, exposing normal premenopausal women to alcohol (0.3–1.0 g/kg body weight) led to a significant increase in plasma testosterone concentrations during the menstrual cycle (Eriksson *et al.*, 1994) and plasma concentrations of estradiol may increase slightly (Välimäki *et al.*, 1983). The effect of alcohol on testosterone levels was even more marked in women using oral contraceptives (Eriksson *et al.*, 1994). Further, in both the follicular and the luteal phase, alcohol compared to placebo ingestion augments estradiol concentrations following LH releasing hormone administration (Mendelson *et al.*, 1989) and increases estradiol following human chorionic gonadotrophin administration (Teoh *et al.*, 1990).

In postmenopausal women, few studies have examined the effects of acute alcohol administration on sex hormone levels. However, Ginsburg and coworkers (Ginsburg *et al.*, 1995a,b, 1996) have found that alcohol ingestion increases estradiol concentrations in women using transdermal estradiol patches and may decrease estradiol clearance after removal of the patches. Further, postmenopausal women receiving oral estrogen replacement therapy got a 3-fold increase in plasma estradiol concentration following alcohol ingestion (0.7 g/kg body weight). The estradiol concentration achieved is substantially higher than that targeted with estrogen replacement therapy and potential health consequences ought to be explored (Ginsburg *et al.*, 1996).

Effects of chronic alcohol use and abuse on the hypothalamic-pituitary-gonadal axis

Contradictory results have been found relating alcohol consumption to the levels of sex hormones in premenopausal women. Some small epidemiological studies have found no significant associations (Cauley *et al.*, 1989; Dorgan *et al.*, 1994).

Other studies, comparing plasma concentrations of sex hormones of chronic alco-holic women without severe liver damage to those of healthy controls, have found 65% higher plasma testosterone concentrations, but no significant changes in estrone, estradiol, LH, and FSH concentrations (Välimäki *et al.*, 1995). However, in a randomized crossover study evaluating sex hormones in three menstrual cycles during alcohol consumption of 30 g/day per participant versus no alcohol for the other three cycles, it was demonstrated that the cycles with alcohol consumption were associated with significantly higher (15–27%) estrone and estradiol levels (Reichman *et al.*, 1993). These findings have been supported by recent observations (Muti *et al.*, 1998). Contrary to what has been observed in men, alcohol-misusing women have significantly decreased SHBG concentrations and hence significantly increased free testosterone levels (Petterson *et al.*, 1990).

Also in postmenopausal women contradictory observations on alcohol and sex hormones have been made (Gavaler, 1988; Becker, 1993). In an international study, Gavaler *et al.* (1991) demonstrated a significant correlation between weekly alcohol consumption and serum estradiol concentrations in 244 postmenopausal women. Later studies of the same cohort, employing stepwise multiple linear regres-sion analyses, demonstrated positive associations between alcohol intake and plasma concentrations of testosterone, LH and FSH (Gavaler, 1993). However, other studies have been unable to confirm a relationship between alcohol consumption and plasma concentrations of estrogens, testosterone, and gonadotropins in non-alcoholic post-menopausal women (London *et al.*, 1991; Newcomb *et al.*, 1995) as well as alcoholic women (Becker *et al.*, 1991a).

Apart from the potential consequences induced by alcohol, other constituents of alcoholic beverages may affect hormonal levels. In accordance, Van Thiel *et al.* (1991) have demonstrated that de-ethanolized bourbon produces hormonal changes in a postmenopausal woman consistent with the presence of a biologically active estrogenic substance (phytoestrogen) in the bourbon extract.

The hypothalamic-pituitary-gonadal axis in alcoholic liver disease

Few studies have examined sex hormone metabolism in premenopausal women with ALD (Becker and Gluud, 1991; Gavaler and Van Thiel, 1992). Carlström *et al.* (1986) examined a mixture of pre- and postmenopausal women and reported normal testosterone levels in ALD patients.

In postmenopausal women with alcoholic cirrhosis, studies have observed nor-mal testosterone, LH, and FSH concentrations (Becker *et al.*, 1991a), while estrone and estradiol as well as SHBG concentrations generally are raised significantly compared to normal controls (Becker *et al.*, 1991a; Gavaler *et al.*, 1993a). Other studies have, however, shown decreased LH and FSH concentrations (Gavaler *et al.*, 1993a; Bell *et al.*, 1995). Similar to the findings in males, testosterone, LH, and FSH concentrations decrease in postmenopausal women with alcoholic cirrhosis with increasing Child's score (Gavaler and Van Thiel, 1992), which may explain the discrepant findings.

In deciding the relative impact of alcohol and alcoholic cirrhosis on the effects on sex hormone concentrations, it is noteworthy that women with non-alcoholic cirrhosis, e.g., primary biliary cirrhosis, demonstrate similar hormonal changes as found in alcoholic cirrhotics (Becker *et al.*, 1991b; Becker, 1993).

Clinical findings related to gonadal hormonal changes of alcoholic women

Moderate alcohol consumption is associated with higher estradiol levels in premenopausal women as well as a delayed menopausal development (Torgerson *et al.*, 1997). However, a higher frequency of menstrual disturbances (70% versus 55%) and uterine currettages (38% versus 16%) is observed in chronic alcoholic women compared to normal controls, and menopausal age is significantly decreased in alcohol abusers and alcoholic cirrhotics (Becker *et al.*, 1989, 1991a; Becker, 1993).

Heavy alcohol consumption is associated with sexual dysfunction (Beckman and Ackerman, 1995), but abstinence in alcoholic premenopausal women is associated with an apparently quick recovery of sexual function (Gavaler *et al.*, 1993b). Alcoholic postmenopausal women, being abstinent for more than a year, report greater sexual satisfaction than alcoholics abstinent for a shorter period of time (Gavaler *et al.*, 1994).

The hormonal changes observed in female alcohol consumers, female alcoholics as well as women with ALD may have consequences (positive and negative) for the development of diseases in women such as cardiovascular disease, osteoporosis, and breast cancer (Grodstein *et al.*, 1997; Kimble, 1997; Thomas *et al.*, 1997).

Based on the present evidence, alcohol abusing women may be treated with contraceptive pills and postmenopausal hormonal substitution. However, the possibility of adverse events cannot be excluded.

REFERENCES

Adinoff, B., Risher-Flowers, D., De Jong, J., Ravitz, B., Bone, G.H., Nutt, D.J., Roehrich, L., Martin, P.R. and Linnoila, M. (1991) Disturbances of the hypothalamic-pituitary-adrenal axis functioning during ethanol withdrawal in six men. *American Journal of Psychiatry* **148**, 1023–1025.

Andersson, S.H., Cronholm, T. and Sjövall, J. (1986) Effects of ethanol on the levels of unconjugated and conjugated androgens and estrogens in plasma of men. *Journal of Steroid Biochemistry* **24**, 1193–1198.

Bannister, P., Oakes, J., Sheridan, P. and Losowsky, M.S. (1987) Sex hormone changes in chronic liver disease: a matched study of alcoholic versus non-alcoholic liver disease. *Quarterly Journal of Medicine, New Series* **63**, 305–313.

Becker, U., Gluud, C. and Bennett, P. (1988a) Thyroid hormones and thyroxine-binding globulin in relation to liver function and serum testosterone in men with alcoholic cirrhosis. *Acta Medica Scandinavica* **224**, 367–373.

Becker, U., Gluud, C., Bennett, P., Micic, S., Svenstrup, B., Winkler, K., Christensen, N.J. and Hardt, F. (1988b) Effect of alcohol and glucose infusion on pituitary-gonadal hormones in normal females. *Drug and Alcohol Dependence* **22**, 141–149.

Becker, U., Tønnesen, H., Kaas-Claesson, N. and Gluud, C. (1989) Menstrual disturbances and fertility in chronic alcoholic women. *Drug and Alcohol Dependence* **24**, 75–82.

Becker, U., Gluud, C., Farholt, S., Bennett, P., Micic, S., Svenstrup, B. and Hardt, F. (1991a) Menopausal age and sex hormones in postmenopausal women with alcoholic and non-alcoholic liver disease. *Journal of Hepatology* **13**, 25–32.

Becker, U., Almdal, T., Christensen, E., Gluud, C., Farholt, S., Bennett, P., Svenstrup, B. and Hardt, F. (1991b) Sex hormones in postmenopausal women with primary biliary cirrhosis. *Hepatology* **13**, 865–869.

Becker, U. and Gluud, C. (1991) Sex, sex hormones and chronic liver diseases. *Digestive Diseases* **9**, 9–16.

Becker, U. (1993) The influence of ethanol and liver disease on sex hormones and hepatic oestrogen receptors in women. ScD Thesis. *Danish Medical Bulletin* **40**, 447–459.

Beckman, L.J. and Ackerman, K.T. (1995) Women, alcohol, and sexuality. *Recent Developments in Alcoholism* **12**, 267–285.

Bell, H., Raknerud, N., Falch, J.A. and Haug, E. (1995) Inappropriately low levels of gonadotrophins in amenorrhoeic women with alcoholic and non-alcoholic cirrhosis. *European Journal of Endocrinology* **132**, 444–449.

Ben, G., Gnudi, L., Maran, A., Gigante, A., Duner, E., Iori, E., Tiengo, A. and Avogaro, A. (1991) Effects of chronic alcohol intake on carbohydrate and lipid metabolism in subjects with type II (non-insulin-dependent) diabetes. *American Journal of Medicine* **90**, 70–76.

Berman, J.D., Cook, D.M., Buchman, M. and Keith, L.D. (1990) Diminished adrenocorticotropin response to insulin-induced hypoglycemia in nondepressed, actively drinking male alcoholics. *Journal of Clinical Endocrinology and Metabolism* **71**, 712–717.

Bertello, P., Gurioli, L., Faggiuolo, R., Veglio, F., Tamagnone, C. and Angeli, A. (1983) Effect of ethanol infusion on the pituitary-testicular responsiveness to gonadotropin releasing hormone and thyrotropin releasing hormone in normal males and in chronic alcoholics presenting with hypogonadism. *Journal of Endocrinological Investigation* **6**, 413–420.

Binder, C. and Bendtson, I. (1992) Hypoglycaemia. *Baillièr's Clinical Endocrinology and Metabolism* **6**, 23–39.

Brzek, A. (1987) Alcohol and male fertility (preliminary report). *Andrologia* **19**, 32–36.

Burra, P., Franklyn, J.A., Ramsden, D.B., Elias, E. and Sheppard, M.C. (1992) Severity of alcoholic liver disease and markers of thyroid and steroid status. *Postgraduate Medical Journal* **68**, 804–810.

Caduff, F., Staub, J.J., Nordmann, A., Radu, E.W. and Landolt, H. (1991) The diagnosis of Cushing's syndrome. Results of diagnostic assessment of 20 patients with Cushing's syndrome of variable etiology (1979–1989). *Schweizerische Medizinische Wochenschrift* **121**, 10–20.

Carlström, K., Eriksson, S. and Rannevik, G. (1986) Sex steroids and steroid binding proteins in female alcoholic liver disease. *Acta Endocrinologica* **111**, 75–79.

Castilla-Garcia, A., Santolaria-Fernandez, F.J., Gonzalez-Reimers, C.E., Batista-Lopez, N., Gonzalez-Garcia, C., Jorge-Hernandez, J.A. and Hernandez-Nieto, L. (1987) Alcohol-induced hypogonadism: reversal after ethanol withdrawal. *Drug and Alcohol Dependence* **20**, 255–260.

Cauley, J.A., Gutai, J.P., Kuller, L.H., LeDonne, D. and Powell, J.G. (1989) The epidemiology of serum sex hormones in postmenopausal women. *American Journal of Epidemiology* **129**, 1120–1131.

Cavallini, G., Vaona, B., Bovo, P., Cigolini, M., Rigo, L., Rossi, F., Tasani, E., Brunori, M.P., Di Francesco, V. and Frulloni, L. (1993) Diabetes in chronic alcoholic pancreatitis. Rose of residual beta cell function and insulin resistance. *Digestive Diseases and Sciences* **38**, 497–501.

Christiansen, C., Thomsen, C., Rasmussen, O., Glerup, H., Berthelsen, J., Hansen, C., Ørskov, H. and Hermansen, K. (1993) Acute effects of graded alcohol intake on glucose, insulin and free fatty acid levels in non-insulin-dependent diabetic subjects. *European Journal of Clinical Nutrition* **47**, 648–652.

Christiansen, C., Thomsen, C., Rasmussen, O., Hansen, C. and Hermansen, K. (1996) The acute impact of ethanol on glucose, insulin, triacylglycerol, and free fatty acid responses and insulin sensitivity in type 2 diabetes. *British Journal of Nutrition* **76**, 669–675.

Colantonio, D., Casale, R., Desiati, P., De Michele, G., Mammarella, M. and Pasqualetti, P. (1991) A possible role of atrial natriuretic peptide in ethanol-induced acute diuresis. *Life Sciences* **48**, 635–642.

Costa, A., Bono, G., Martignoni, E., Merlo, P., Sances, G. and Nappi, G. (1996) An assessment of hypothalamic-pituitary-adrenal axis functioning in non-depressed, early abstinent alcoholics. *Psychoneuroendocrinology* **21**, 263–275.

Couwenbergs, C.J. (1988) Acute effects of drinking beer or wine on the steroid hormones of healthy men. *Journal of Steroid Biochemistry* **31**, 467–473.

Davis, J.R. and Jeffcoate, W.J. (1983) Lack of effect of ethanol on plasma cortisol in man. *Clinical Endocrinology* **19**, 461–466.

Dorgan, J.F., Reichman, M.E., Judd, J.T., Brown, C., Longcope, C., Schatzkin, A., Campbell, W.S., Franz, C., Kahle, L. and Taylor, P.R. (1994) The relation of reported alcohol ingestion to plasma levels of estrogens and androgens in premenopausal women (Maryland, United States). *Cancer Causes and Control* **5**, 53–60.

Duane, P. and Peters, T.J. (1987) Glucocorticosteroid status in chronic alcoholics with and without skeletal muscle myopathy. *Clinical Science* **73**, 601–603.

Eisenhofer, G. and Johnson, R.H. (1982) Effect of ethanol ingestion on plasma vasopressin and water balance in humans. *American Journal of Physiology* **242**, R522–R527.

Ekman, A.-C., Vakkuri, O., Ekman, M., Leppäluoto, J., Ruokonen, A. and Knip, M. (1996) Ethanol decreases nocturnal plasma levels of thyrotropin and growth hormone but not those of thyroid hormones or prolactin in man. *Journal of Clinical Endocrinology and Metabolism* **81**, 2627–2632.

Ellingboe, J. (1987) Acute effects of ethanol on sex hormones in non-alcoholic men and women. *Alcohol and Alcoholism* **1** (Suppl), 109–116.

Eriksson, C.J., Fukunaga, T. and Lindman, R. (1994) Sex hormone response to alcohol. *Nature* **369**, 711.

Fahrner, E.M. (1987) Sexual dysfunction in male alcohol addicts: prevalence and treatment. *Archives of Sexual Behavior* **16**, 247–257.

Garbutt, J.C., Hicks, R.E., Clayton, C.J., Andrews, R.T. and Mason, G.A. (1991a) Behavioural and endocrine interactions between thyrotropin-releasing hormone and ethanol in normal subjects. *Alcoholism, Clinical and Experimental Research* **15**, 1045–1049.

Garbutt, J.C., Mayo, Jr. J.P., Gillette, G.M., Little, K.Y., Hicks, R.E., Mason, R.E. and Prange, Jr., A.J. (1991b) Dose-response studies with thyrotropin-releasing hormone (TRH) in abstinent male alcoholics: evidence for selective thyrotroph dysfunction? *Journal of Studies on Alcohol* **52**, 275–280.

Garbutt, J.C., McDavid, J., Mason, G.A., Quade, D. and Loosen, P.T. (1992) Evidence for normal feedback inhibition of triiodothyronine on the thyrotropin (TSH) response to thyrotropin-releasing hormone (TRH) in abstinent male alcoholics. *Alcoholism, Clinical and Experimental Research* **16**, 881–883.

Gavaler, J.S. (1985) Effects of alcohol on endocrine function in postmenopausal women: a review. *Journal of Studies on Alcohol* **46**, 495–516.

Gavaler, J.S. (1988) Effects of moderate consumption of alcoholic beverages on endocrine function in postmenopausal women. Bases for hypotheses. *Recent Developments in Alcoholism* **6**, 229–251.

Gavaler, J.S., Love, K., Van Thiel, D., Farholt, S., Gluud, C., Monteiro, E., Galvao-Teles, A., Ortega, T.C. and Cuervas-Mons, V. (1991) An international study of the relationship between alcohol consumption and postmenopausal estradiol levels. *Alcohol and Alcoholism* **1** (Suppl), 327–330.

Gavaler, J.S. and Van Thiel, D.H. (1992) Hormonal status of postmenopausal women with alcohol-induced cirrhosis: further findings and a review of the literature. *Hepatology* **16**, 312–319.

Gavaler, J.S. (1993) Alcohol and nutrition in postmenopausal women. *Journal of the American College and Nutrition* **12**, 349–356.

Gavaler, J.S., Deal, S.R., Van Thiel, D.H., Arria, A. and Allan, M.J. (1993a) Alcohol and estrogen levels in postmenopausal women: the spectrum of effect. *Alcoholism, Clinical and Experimental Research* **17**, 786–790.

Gavaler, J.S., Rizzo, A., Rossaro, L., Van Thiel, D.H., Brezza, E. and Deal, S.R. (1993b) Sexuality of alcoholic women with menstrual cycle function: effects of duration of alcohol abstinence. *Alcoholism, Clinical and Experimental Research* **17**, 778–781.

Gavaler, J.S., Rizzo, A., Rossaro, L., Van Thiel, D.H., Brezza, E. and Deal, S.R. (1994) Sexuality of alcoholic postmenopausal women: effects of duration of alcohol abstinence. *Alcoholism, Clinical and Experimental Research* **18**, 269–271.

Gianoulakis, C., Guillaume, P., Thavundayil, J. and Gutkowska, J. (1997) Increased plasma atrial natriuretic peptide after ingestion of low doses of ethanol in humans. *Alcoholism, Clinical and Experimental Research* **21**, 162–170.

Ginsburg, E.S., Walsh, B.W., Gao, X., Gleason, R.E., Feltmate, C. and Barbieri, R.L. (1995a) The effect of acute ethanol ingestion on estrogen levels in postmenopausal women using transdermal estradiol. *Journal of the Society for Gynecologic Investigation* **2**, 26–29.

Ginsburg, E.S., Walsh, B.W., Shea, B.F., Gao, X., Gleason, R.E. and Barbieri, R.L. (1995b) The effects of ethanol on the clearance of estradiol in postmenopausal women. *Fertility and Sterility* **63**, 1227–1230.

Ginsburg, E.S., Mello, N.K., Mendelson, J.H., Barbieri, R.L., Teoh, S.K., Rothman, M., Gao, X. and Sholar, J.W. (1996) Effects of alcohol ingestion on estrogens in postmenopausal women. *JAMA* **276**, 1747–1751.

Gluud, C., Bahnsen, M., Bennett, P., Brodthagen, U.A., Dietrichson, O., Johnsen, S.G., Nielsen, J., Micic, S., Svendsen, L.B. and Svenstrup, B. (1983) Hypothalamic-pituitary-gonadal function in relation to liver function in men with alcoholic cirrhosis. *Scandinavian Journal of Gastroenterology* **18**, 939–944.

Gluud, C. and The Copenhagen Study Group for Liver Diseases (1987) Serum testosterone concentrations in men with alcoholic cirrhosis: background for variation. *Metabolism* **36**, 373–378.

Gluud, C. (1988) Testosterone and alcoholic cirrhosis. Epidemiologic, pathophysiologic and therapeutic studies in men. ScD Thesis. *Danish Medical Bulletin* **35**, 564–575.

Gluud, C., Bennett, P., Svenstrup, B., Micic, S. and The Copenhagen Study Group for Liver Diseases. (1988a) Effect of oral testosterone treatment on serum concentrations of sex steroids gonadotrophins and prolactin in alcoholic cirrhotic men. *Alimentary Pharmacology and Therapeutics* **2**, 119–128.

Gluud, C., Wantzin, P., Eriksen, J. and The Copenhagen Study Group for Liver Diseases (1988b) No effect of oral testosterone treatment on sexual dysfunction in alcoholic cirrhotic men. *Gastroenterology* **95**, 1582–1587.

Grodstein, F., Stampfer, M.J., Colditz, G.A., Willett, W.C., Manson, J.E., Joffe, M., Rosner, B., Fuchs, C., Hankinson, S.E., Hunter, D.J., Hennekens, C.H. and Speizer, F.E. (1997) Postmenopausal hormone therapy and mortality. *New England Journal of Medicine* **336**, 1769–1775.

Grun, R. and Kaffarnik, H. (1985) Thyroid hormones in women with liver cirrhosis. *Klinische Wochenschrift* **63**, 752–761.

Guêchot, J., Chazouillerés, O., Loria, A., Hannoun, L., Balladur, P., Parc, R., Giboudeau, J. and Poupon, R. (1994) Effect of liver transplantation on sex-hormone disorders in male patients with alcohol-induced or post-viral hepatitis advanced liver disease. *Journal of Hepatology* **20**, 426–430.

Gulya, K., Dave, J.R. and Hoffman, P.L. (1991) Chronic ethanol ingestion decreases vasopressin mRNA in hypothalamic and extrahypothalamic nuclei of mouse brain. *Brain Research* **557**, 129–135.

Harding, A.J., Halliday, G. M., Ng, J.L., Harper, C.G. and Kril, J.J. (1996) Loss of vasopressin-immunoreactive neurons in alcoholics is dose-related and time-dependent. *Neuroscience* **72**, 699–708.

Heaney, A.P., Harper, R., Ennis, C., Rooney, D.P., Sheridan, B., Atkinson, A.B. and Bell, P.M. (1997) Insulin action and hepatic glucose cycling in Cushing's syndrome. *Clinical Endocrinology* **46**, 735–743.

Hegedus, L. (1984) Decreased thyroid gland volume in alcoholic cirrhosis of the liver. *Journal of Clinical Endocrinology and Metabolism* **58**, 930–933.

Hegedus, L., Rasmussen, N., Ravn, V.,Kastrup, J., Krogsgaard, K. and Aldershvile, J. (1988) Independent effects of liver disease and chronic alcoholism on thyroid function and size: the possibility of a toxic effect of alcohol on the thyroid gland. *Metabolism* **37**, 229–233.

Heikkonen, E., Ylikahri, R., Roine, R., Välimäki, M., Härkönen, M. and Salaspuro, M. (1996) The combined effect of alcohol and physical exercise on serum testosterone, luteinizing hormone, and cortisol in males. *Alcoholism, Clinical and Experimental Research* **20**, 711–716.

Heinz, A., Rommelspacher, H., Gräf, K.J., Kürten, I., Otto, M. and Baumgartner, A. (1995) Hypothalamic-pituitary-gonadal axis, prolactin, and cortisol in alcoholics during withdrawal and after three weeks of abstinence: comparison with healthy control subjects. *Psychiatry Research* **56**, 81–95.

Heinz, A., Bauer, M., Kuhn, S., Kruger, F., Graf, K.J., Rommelspacher, H. and Schmidt, L.G. (1996) Long-term observation of the hypothalamic-pituitary-thyroid (HPT) axis in alcohol-dependent patients. *Acta Psychiatrica Scandinavica* **93**, 470–476.

Holbrook, T.L., Barret-Connor, E. and Wingard, D.L. (1990) A prospective population-based study of alcohol use and non-insulin-dependent diabetes mellitus. *American Journal of Epidemiology* **132**, 902–909.

Ida, Y., Tsujimaru, S., Nakamaura, K., Shirao, I., Mukasa, H., Egami, H. and Nakazawa, Y. (1992) Effects of acute and repeated alcohol ingestion on hypothalamic-pituitary-gonadal and hypothalamic-pituitary-adrenal functioning in normal males. *Drug and Alcohol Dependence* **31**, 57–64.

Inder, W.J., Joyce, P.R., Wells, J.E., Evans, M.J., Ellis, M.J., Mattioli, L. and Donald, R.A. (1995) The acute effects of oral ethanol on the hypothalamic-pituitary-adrenal axis in normal human subjects. *Clinical Endocrinology* **42**, 65–71.

Ishizawa, H., Dave, J.R., Liu, L.I., Tabakoff, B. and Hoffman, P.L. (1990) Hypothalamic vasopressin mRNA levels in mice are decreased after chronic ethanol ingestion. *European Journal of Pharmacology* **189**, 119–127.

Iturriaga, H., Valladares, L., Hirsch, S., Devoto, E., P'erez, C., Bunout, D., Lioi, X. and Petermann, M. (1995) Effects of abstinence on sex hormone profile in alcoholic patients without liver failure. *Journal of endocrinological investigation* **18**, 638–644.

Iversen, J., Vilstrup, H. and Tygstrup, N. (1983) Insulin sensitivity in alcoholic cirrhosis. *Scandinavian Journal of Clinical Laboratory Investigation* **43**, 565–573.

Jensen, S.B., Gluud, C. and The Copenhagen Study Group for Liver Diseases (1985) Sexual dysfunction in men with alcoholic liver cirrhosis. A comparative study. *Liver* **5**, 94–100.

Kaptein, E.M. (1997) Hormone-specific alterations of T4, T3, and reverse T3 metabolism with recent ethanol abstinence in humans. *American Journal of Physiology* **272**, E191–E200.

Kato, I., Nomura, A., Stemmermann, G.N. and Chyou, P.H. (1992) Determinants of sex hormone levels in men as useful indices in hormone-related disorders. *Journal of Clinical Epidemiology* **45**, 1417–1421.

Kaymakoglu, S., Okten, A., Cakaloglu, Y., Boztas, G., Besisik, F., Tascioglu, C. and Yalcin, S. (1995) Hypogonadism is not related to the etiology of liver cirrhosis. *Journal of Gastroenterology* **30**, 745–750.

Kerr, D., Macdonald, I.A., Heller, S.R. and Tattersall, R.B. (1990) Alcohol causes hypoglycaemic unawareness in healthy volunteers and patients with Type 1 (insulin- dependent) diabetes. *Diabetologia* **33**, 216–221.

Kimble, R.B. (1997) Alcohol, cytokines, and estrogen in the control of bone remodeling. *Alcoholism, Clinical and Experimental Research* **21**, 385–391.

Kirkman, S. and Nelson, D.H. (1988) Alcohol-induced pseudo-Cushing's disease: a study of prevalence with review of the literature. *Metabolism* **37**, 390–394.

Knutsen, H., Dolva, L.Ø., Skrede, S., Bjørklund, R. and Mørland, J. (1989) Thyrothopin-releasing hormone antagonism of ethanol inebriation. *Alcoholism, Clinical and Experimental Research* **13**, 365–370.

Kruszynska, Y.T., Harry, D.S., Mohamed-Ali, V., Home, P.D., Yudkin, J.S. and McIntyre, N. (1995) The contribution of proinsulin and *des*-31,32 proinsulin to the hyperinsulinemia of diabetic and nondiabetic cirrhotic patients. *Metabolism* **44**, 254–260.

Kruszynska, Y.T., Goulas, S., Wollen, N. and McIntyre, N. (1998) Insulin secretory capacity and the regulation of glucagon secretion in diabetic and non-diabetic alcoholic cirrhotic patients. *Journal of Hepatology* **28**, 280–291.

La Grange, L., Jones, T.D., Erb, L. and Reyes, E. (1995) Alcohol consumption: biochemical and personality correlates in a college student population. *Addictive Behaviors* **20**, 93–103.

Lange, J., Arends, J. and Willms, B. (1991) Alcohol-induced hypoglycemia in type I diabetic patients. *Medizinische Klinik* **86**, 551–554.

Leppäluoto, J., Rapeli, M., Varis, R. and Ranta, T. (1975) Secretion of anterior pituitary hormones in man: effects of ethyl alcohol. *Acta Physiologica Scandinavia* **95**, 400–406.

Lindholm, J., Fabricius-Bjerre, N., Bahnsen, M., Boiesen, P., Bangstrup, L., Pedersen, M.L. and Hagen, C. (1978a) Pituitary-testicular function in patients with chronic alcoholism. *European Journal of Clinical Investigation* **8**, 269–272.

Lindholm, J., Fabricius-Bjerre, N., Bahnsen, M., Boiesen, P., Hagen, C. and Christensen, T. (1978b) Sex steroids and sex-hormone binding globulin in males with chronic alcoholism. *European Journal of Clinical Investigation* **8**, 273–276.

Linnoila, M., Prinz, P.N., Wonsowics, C.J. and Leppäluoto, J. (1980) Effects of moderate doses of ethanol and phenobarbital on pituitary and thyroid hormones and testosterone. *British Journal of Addiction* **75**, 207–212.

London, S., Willett, W., Longcope, C. and McKinlay, S. (1991) Alcohol and other dietary factors in relation to serum hormone concentrations in women at climacteric. *American Journal of Clinical Nutrition* **53**, 166–171.

Loosen, P.T., Chambliss, B., Ekhator, N., Burns, D., Geracioti, T.D. and Orth, D.N. (1993) Thyroid and adrenal dysfunction in abstinent alcoholic men: locus of disturbance. *Neuropsychopharmacology* **9**, 255–266.

Marchesi, C., De Riso, C., Campanini, G., Maggini, C., Piazza, P., Grassi, M., Chiodera, P. and Coiro, V. (1992) TRH test in alcoholics: relationship of the endocrine results with neuroradiological and neuropsychological findings. *Alcohol and Alcoholism* **27**, 531–537.

Markianos, M., Moussas, G. and Lykouras, L.L. (1987) Normal testosterone plasma levels in non-abstinent alcoholics. *Drug and Alcohol Dependence* **20**, 81–85.

Martin-Du Pan, R.C., Bischof, P., Campana, A. and Morabia, A. (1997) Relationship between etiological factors and total motile sperm count in 350 infertile patients. *Archives of Andrology* **39**, 197–210.

Martinez-Riera, A., Santolaria-Fernandez, F., Gonzalez Reimers, E., Milena, A., Gomez-Sirvent, J.L., Rodriguez-Moreno, F., Gonzalez-Martin, I. and Rodriguez-Rodriguez, E. (1995) Alcoholic hypogonadism: hormonal response to clomiphene. *Alcohol* **12**, 581–587.

Mendelson, J.H., Lukas, S.E., Mello, N.K., Amass, L., Ellingboe, J. and Skupny, A. (1988) Acute alcohol effects on plasma estradiol levels in women. *Psychopharmacology (Berl)* **94**, 464–467.

Mendelson, J.H., Mello, N.K., Teoh, S.K. and Ellingboe, J. (1989) Alcohol effects on luteinizing hormone releasing hormone-stimulated anterior pituitary and gonadal hormones in women. *The Journal of Pharmacology and Experimental Therapeutics* **250**, 902–909.

Moss, S.E., Klein, R. and Klein, B.E. (1992) Alcohol consumption and the prevalence of diabetic retinopathy. *Ophthalmology* **99**, 926–932.

Muller, N., Hoehe, M., Klein, H.E., Nieberle, G., Kapfhammer, H.P., May, F., Muller, O.A. and Fichter, M. (1989) Endocrinological studies in alcoholics during withdrawal and after abstinence. *Psychoneuroendocrinology* **14**, 113–123.

Muti, P., Trevisan, M., Micheli, A., Krogh, V., Bolelli, G., Sciajno, R., Schunemann, H.J. and Berrino, F. (1998) Alcohol consumption and total estradiol in premenopausal women. *Cancer Epidemiology, Biomarkers and Prevention* **7**, 189–193.

Myking, O., Aakvaag, A. and Digranes, O. (1987) Androgen-oestrogen imbalance in men with chronic alcoholism and fatty liver. *Alcohol and Alcoholism* **22**, 7–15.

Nealon, W.H., Townsend, C.M. and Thompson, J.C. (1988) The time course of beta cell dysfunction in chronic ethanol-induced pancreatitis: A prospective analysis. *Surgery* **104**, 1074–1079.

Nemeroff, C.B., Kalivas, P.W., Golden, R.N. and Prange, A.J. Jr. (1984) Behavioral effects of hypothalamic hypophysiotropic hormones, neurotensin, substance P and other neuropeptides. *Pharmacology and Therapeutics* **24**, 1–56.

Newcomb, P.A., Klein, R., Klein, B.E., Haffner, S., Mares-Perlman, J., Cruickshanks, K.J. and Marcus, P.M. (1995) Association of dietary and life-style factors with sex hormones in postmenopausal women. *Epidemiology* **6**, 318–321.

Noth, R.H. and Walter, R.M. (1984) The effects of alcohol on the endocrine system. *Medical Clinics of North America* **68**, 133–146.

Nygren, A., Adner, N., Sundblad, L. and Wiechel, K.L. (1985) Insulin uptake by the human alcoholic liver. *Metabolism* **34**, 48–52.

Persky, H., O'Brien, C.P., Fine, E., Howard, W.J., Khan, M.A. and Beck, R.W. (1977) The effect of alcohol and smoking on testosterone function and aggression in chronic alcoholics. *American Journal of Psychiatry* **134**, 621–625.

Pettersson, P., Ellsinger, B.M., Sjöberg, C. and Björntorp, P. (1990) Fat distribution and steroid hormones in women with alcohol abuse. *Journal of Internal Medicine* **228**, 311–316.

Phipps, W.R., Lukas, S.E., Mendelson, J.H., Ellingboe, J., Palmieri, S.L. and Schiff, I. (1987) Acute ethanol administration enhances plasma testosterone levels following gonadotropin stimulation in men. *Psychoneuroendocrinology* **12**, 459–465.

Pienaar, W.-P., Roberts, M.C., Emsley, R.A., Aalbers, C. and Taljaard, F.J. (1995) The thyrotropin releasing hormone stimulation test in alcoholism. *Alcohol and Alcoholism* **30**, 661–667.

Prinz, P.N., Roehrs, T.A., Vitaliane, P.P., Linnoila, M. and Weitzman, E.D. (1980) Effect of alcohol on sleep and night time plasma growth hormone and cortisol concentrations. *Journal of Clinical Endocrinology and Metabolism* **51**, 759–764.

Proto, G., Barberi, M. and Bertolissi, F. (1985) Pseudo-Cushing's syndrome: an example of alcohol-induced central disorder in corticotropin-releasing factor-ACTH release? *Drug and Alcohol Dependence* **16**, 111–115.

Reichman, M.E., Judd, J.T., Longcope, C., Schatzkin, A., Clevidence, B.A., Nair, P.P., Campbell, W.S. and Taylor, P.R. (1993) Effects of alcohol consumption on plasma and urinary hormone concentrations in premenopausal women. *Journal of the National Cancer Institute* **85**, 722–727.

Rimm, E.B., Chan, J., Stampfer, M.J., Colditz, G.A. and Willett, W.C. (1995) Prospective study of cigarette smoking, alcohol use, and the risk of diabetes in men. *British Medical Journal* **310**, 555–559.

Risher-Flowers, D., Adinoff, B., Ravitz, B., Bone, G.H., Martin, P.R., Nutt, D. and Linnoila, M. (1988) Circadian rhythms of cortisol during alcohol withdrawal. *Advances in Alcohol and Substance Abuse* **7**, 37–41.

Roy, A., Bissette, G., Nemeroff, C.B., DeJong, J., Ravitz, B., Adinoff, B. and Linnoila, M. (1990) Cerebrospinal fluid thyrotropin-releasing hormone concentrations in alcoholics and normal controls. *Biological Psychiatry* **28**, 767–772.

Ruhland, B., Walker, L., Wollitzer, A.O. and Peterson, C.M. (1991) Ethanol influences class I and class II MHC antigen expression on human foetal islet-like cell clusters. *Alcoholism, Clinical and Experimental Research* **15**, 745–747.

Rumilly, F., Bigard, M.A., Dupuis, D. and Gaucher, P. (1983) Thyroid hormones in alcoholic cirrhosis before and after alcohol withdrawal. *Semaine des Hopitaux* **59**, 390–396.

Ruusa, J., Bergman, B. and Sundell, M.L. (1997) Sex hormones during alcohol withdrawal: a longitudinal study of 29 male alcoholics during detoxification. *Alcohol and Alcoholism* **32**, 591–597.

Samuels, M.H., Veldhuis, J.D., Henry, P. and Ridgway, E.C. (1990) Pathophysiology of pulsatile and copulsatile release of thyroid-stimulating hormone, luteinizing hormone, follicle stimulationg hormone, and α-subunit. *Journal of Clinical Endocrinology and Metabolism* **71**, 425–432.

Schiavi, R.C., Stimmel, B.B., Mandeli, J. and White, D. (1995) Chronic alcoholism and male sexual function. *American Journal of Psychiatry* **152**, 1045–1051.

Selby, J.V., Newman, B., King, M.C. and Friedman, G.D. (1987) Environmental and behavioural determinants of fasting plasma glucose in women. *American Journal of Epidemiology* **125**, 979–988.

Shono, N., Kumagai, S., Higaki, Y., Nishizumi, M. and Sasaki, H. (1996) The relationships of testosterone, estradiol, dehydroepiandrosterone-sulfate and sex hormone-binding globulin to lipid and glucose metabolism in healthy men. *Journal of Atherosclerosis and Thrombosis* **3**, 45–51.

Skinazi, F., Levy, P. and Bernades, P. (1995) Does acute alcoholic pancreatitis always reveal chronic pancreatitis? *Gastroenterologie Clinique et Biologique* **19**, 266–269.

Stampfer, M.J., Colditz, G.A., Willett, W.C., Manson, J.E., Arky, R.A., Hennnekens, C.H. and Speizer, F.E. (1988) A prospective study of moderate alcohol drinking and risk of diabetes in women. *American Journal of Epidemiology* **128**, 549–558.

Stewart, P.M., Burra, P., Shackleton, C.H., Sheppard, M.C. and Elias, E. (1993) 11-β-Hydroxysteroid dehydrogenase deficiency and glucocorticoid status in patients with alcoholic and non-alcoholic chronic liver disease. *Journal of Clinical Endocrinology and Metabolism* **76**, 748–751.

Teoh, S.K., Mendelson, J.H., Mello, N.K., Skupny, A. and Ellingboe, J. (1990) Alcohol effects on hCG-stimulated gonadal hormones in women. *The Journal of Pharmacology and Experimental Therapeutics* **254**, 407–411.

The Copenhagen Study Group for Liver Diseases (1986) Testosterone treatment of men with alcoholic cirrhosis: a double-blind study. *Hepatology* **6**, 807–813.

Thomas, H.V., Reeves, G.K. and Key, T.J. (1997) Endogenous estrogen and postmenopausal breast cancer: a quantitative review. *Cancer Causes and Control* **8**, 922–928.

Torgerson, D.J., Thomas, R.E., Campbell, M.K. and Reid, D.M. (1997) Alcohol consumption and age of maternal menopause are associated with menopause onset. *Maturitas* **26**, 21–25.

Umeki, S., Hisamoto, N. and Hara, Y. (1989) Study on background factors associated with impaired glucose tolerance and/or diabetes mellitus. *Acta Endocrinologica* **120**, 729–734.

Vagenakis, A.G. (1998) Alterations of thyroid function in non-thyroideal illness: the 'euthyroid sick' syndrome. In *Clinical Endocrinology*, edited by A. Grossman, pp. 383–391. Oxford: Blackwell Science.

Van Thiel, D.H. and Gavaler, J.S. (1990) Endocrine consequences of alcohol abuse. *Alcohol and Alcoholism* **25**, 341–344.

Van Thiel, D.H., Kumar, S., Gavaler, J.S. and Tarter, R.E. (1990) Effect of liver transplantation on the hypothalamic-pituitary-gonadal axis of chronic alcoholic men with advanced liver disease. *Alcoholism, Clinical and Experimental Research* **14**, 478–481.

Van Thiel, D.H., Galvao-Teles, A., Monteiro, E., Rosenblum, E. and Gavaler, J.S. (1991) The phytoestrogens present in de-ethanolized bourbon are biologically active: a preliminary study in a postmenopausal woman. *Alcoholism, Clinical and Experimental Research* **15**, 822–823.

Villalta, J., Ballesca, J.L., Nicolas, J.M., Martinez de Osaba, M.J., Antunez, E. and Pimentel, C. (1997) Testicular function in asymptomatic chronic alcoholics: relation to ethanol intake. *Alcoholism, Clinical and Experimental Research* **21**, 128–133.

von Werder, K. and Müller, O.A. (1998) Cushing's syndrome. In *Clinical Endocrinology*, edited by A. Grossman, pp. 415–431. Oxford: Blackwell Science.

Välimäki, M., Härkönen, M. and Ylikahri, R. (1983) Acute effects of alcohol on female sex hormones. *Alcoholism, Clinical and Experimental Research* **7**, 289–293.

Välimäki, M.J., Härkönen, M., Eriksson, C.J. and Ylikahri, R.H. (1984a) Sex hormones and adrenocortical steroids in men acutely intoxicated with ethanol. *Alcohol* **1**, 89–93.

Välimäki, M., Pelkonen, R., Härkönen, M. and Ylikahri, R. (1984b) Hormonal changes in noncirrhotic male alcoholics during ethanol withdrawal. *Alcohol and Alcoholism* **19**, 235–242.

Välimäki, M., Tuominen, J.A., Huhtaniemi, I. and Ylikahri, R. (1990) The pulsatile secretion of gonadotropins and growth hormone, and the biological activity of luteinizing hormone in men acutely intoxicated with ethanol. *Alcoholism, Clinical and Experimental Research* **14**, 928–931.

Välimäki, M.J., Laitinen, K., Tiitinen, A., Steman, U.H. and Ylostalo, P. (1995) Gonadal function and morphology in non-cirrhotic female alcoholics: a controlled study with hormone measurements and ultrasonography. *Acta Obstetricia et Gynecologica Scandinavica* **74**, 462–466.

Waltman, C., Blevins, L.S. Jr., Boyd, G. and Wand, G.S. (1993) The effects of mild ethanol intoxication on the hypothalamic-pituitary-adrenal axis in nonalcoholic men. *Journal of Clinical Endocrinology and Metabolism* **77**, 518–522.

Wand, G.S. and Dobs, A.S. (1991) Alterations in the hypothalamic-pituitary-adrenal axis in actively drinking alcoholics. *Journal of Clinical Endocrinology and Metabolism* **72**, 1290–1295.

Wang, Y.J., Wu J.C., Lee, S.D., Tsai, Y.T. and Lo, K.J. (1991) Gonadal dysfunction and changes in sex hormones in postnecrotic cirrhotic men: a matched study with alcoholic cirrhotic men. *Hepatogastroenterology* **38**, 531–534.

Wu, A.H., Whittemore, A.S., Kolonel, L.N., John, E.M., Gallagher, R.P., West, D.W., Hankin, J., Teh, C.Z., Dreon, D.M. and Paffenbarger, R.S. Jr. (1995) Serum androgens and sex hormone-binding globulins in relation to lifestyle factors in older African-American, white, and Asian men in the United States and Canada. *Cancer Epidemiology, Biomarkers and Prevention* **4**, 735–741.

Yamanaka, T., Ido, K., Kimura, K. and Saito, T. (1980) Serum levels of thyroid hormone in liver disease. *Clinica Chimica Acta* **101**, 45–55.

Yki-Järvinen, H. and Nikkilä, E.A. (1985) Ethanol decreases glucose utilisation in healthy man. *Journal of Clinical Endocrinology and Metabolism* **61**, 941–945.

Ylikahri, R.H., Huttunen, M.O., Härkönen, M., Leino T., Helenius, T., Liewendahl, K. and Karonen, S.L. (1978) Acute effects of alcohol on anterior pituitary secretion of the tropic hormones. *Journal of Clinical Endocrinology and Metabolism* **46**, 715–720.

Yokoyama, A., Matsushita, S., Ishii, H., Takagi, T., Maruyama, K. and Tsuchiya, M. (1994) The impact of diabetes mellitus on the prognosis of alcoholics. *Alcohol and Alcoholism* **29**, 181–186.

Chapter 20

Cardiomyopathy and skeletal muscle myopathy

Alvaro Urbano-Márquez, Joaquim Fernández-Solà and Ramon Estruch

Alcohol consumption may induce skeletal and cardiac myopathies, well defined entities related to a direct effect of ethanol on striated muscle. The development of these diseases is clearly not related to nutritional factors or ionic and vitamin deficiencies, although the coexistence of these factors may increase the degree of muscle damage. The physiopathological mechanisms of these diseases are probably related to ethanol-induced changes in membrane permeability, channels, pumps and ionic (Ca^{2+}) transients. Protein synthesis may also be acutely disturbed, contributing to this damage. The role of genetic factors and apoptosis is currently under discussion. Multiorgan involvement is frequent in alcoholism and dilated cardiomyopathy is more frequently seen in patients with skeletal myopathy and and in those with cirrhosis. Thus, it is important to rule out the presence of alcoholic myopathy or cardiomyopathy in patients with other ethanol-related diseases. Women seem to be more sensitive to the toxic effects of ethanol on cardiac and skeletal muscle than men. Most patients with alcoholic myopathy or cardiomyopathy improve with abstinence, although the improvement is often partial. On the other hand, those patients who maintain ethanol intake present progressive functional and structural impairment of the previous muscle damage. In alcoholic skeletal myopathy, mortality is exceptional and only related to fatal cases of myoglobinuric-induced acute renal failure. In alcoholic cardiomyopathy, mortality is due to progression of left ventricular failure or arrhythmias and is related to the persistence of high ethanol intake or baseline end-stage disease.

KEYWORDS: alcohol, heart, skeletal muscle, alcoholic cardiomyopathy, alcoholic myopathy, ethanol

INTRODUCTION

Alcohol misuse may be deleterious for cardiac and skeletal striated muscle, inducing acute or chronic damage and leading to the development of the alcoholic cardiomyopathy and skeletal myopathy (Urbano-Márquez *et al.*, 1989; Preedy *et al.*, 1994a; Fernández-Solà *et al.*, 1996, 1997a). Since striated skeletal and cardiac muscle have close structural, functional and molecular similarities and the noxious effect of alcohol on these organs is very similar, cardiomyopathy and skeletal myopathy may develop simultaneously and synchronically in the same patient (Urbano-Márquez *et al.*, 1989; Fernández-Solà *et al.*, 1994).

Although the potential toxic effect of ethanol on cardiac muscle has been considered for millennia, modern descriptions of alcoholic cardiomyopathy date from the nineteenth century when the first cases of this disease were described and the first pathological data was reported in the heart of beer drinkers. Scientific recognition of alcoholic skeletal myopathy was first achieved in 1882, when Jackson observed the decrease of muscle strength in alcoholics with recovery after abstention. However, specific descriptions of alcoholic myopathy are still more recent. A series of Scandinavian authors, Hed (1955), Fahlgren (1957) and Ekbom (1964), reported the acute and chronic development of muscle damage due to the deleterious effects of alcohol. After these clinical descriptions, some researchers attributed the cause of alcoholic striated muscle damage to other factors such as malnutrition, vitamin deficiencies and/or alcohol-induced peripheral neuropathy. In several clinical and pathological series from the 1950s/60s, the specific characteristics of these entities were stated and the differentiation of alcoholic myopathy from alcoholic peripheral neuropathy, malnutrition or vitamin deficiencies, specially Beri-beri disease, was established.

Recently, the distinction of acute from chronic effects and the understanding of some pathogenic molecular and genetic mechanisms of alcohol-mediated muscle damage has allowed improvement in the scientific knowledge of these diseases. At present, alcoholic cardiomyopathy and skeletal myopathy are clearly defined and are well recognized clinical and histological entities, which usually develop in longstanding chronic alcoholics in a dose-dependent manner, regardless of causes other than alcohol consumption itself (Urbano-Márquez *et al.*, 1989; Regan, 1990; Rubin and Urbano-Márquez, 1994).

The relative high prevalence of these diseases among alcoholic misusers, the functional impairment produced by the reduction of muscle and cardiac strength and the increased mortality of chronic alcoholics due to alcoholic cardiomyopathy has made these diseases of ever greater interest.

PHYSIOPATHOLOGY

The physiopathological aspects of skeletal and cardiac alcohol-related damage are quite similar. Thus, we will discuss the two together. Complete knowledge of the specific mechanisms leading alcohol to produce striate muscle damage remains unknown and many questions still need to be answered (Fernández-Solà *et al.*, 1996; Preedy *et al.*, 1994). Ethanol is a lipophilic substance with a rapid diffusion through biological membranes and, consequently, may act at different cellular targets (membranes, mitochondria, structural and contractile proteins), modifying these different molecular mechanisms (channels, pumps, cell energy and genetic control of the cell) (Lieber, 1988). In addition, these effects may be produced in synchrony, being difficult to differentiate one from the another (Thomas *et al.*, 1994). On the other hand, it is still unknown whether the chronic effect is just a sum of repeated acute effects or whether it develops in a different manner, with different pathogenic mechanisms and cell targets than the acute effect (Fernández-Solà *et al.*, 1997).

The usefulness of animal models to solve these problems is very limited (Thomas *et al.*, 1994). There are reproducible acute *in vivo* and *in vitro* models of alcoholic cardiac and skeletal myopathy. However, the chronic effects of ethanol on cardiac and striated muscle are limited by the difficulties in maintaining the animals or the cells for a long enough period of ethanol intake, as it occurs in humans. Since these diseases need a minimum of 10 years to develop in the human being, it is quite difficult to assert whether 6 months of ethanol intake is enough time to perform similar changes in the animal model. In our opinion, acute animal models may be plausible, but chronic models do not reproduce the low output form of congestive cardiomyopathy seen in alcoholic patients.

Nutritional factors

After the clinical recognition of alcoholic skeletal and cardiac myopathies, some authors have suggested that malnutrition may lead to the development of striated muscle damage in alcoholics (Sherlock, 1984). Later, the confusion of Western Beri-beri with alcoholic cardiomyopathy also led some authors to suggest that vitamin B_1 deficiency was the cause of alcoholic cardiomyopathy. Finally, the co-existence of some ionic deficiencies (K^+, Ca^{2+}, Mg^{2+}, P^{5+}), which are common in alcoholics, with skeletal or cardiac damage, led to the supposition that alcohol-mediated striated muscle damage was induced by ionic deficiencies. However, at present this idea has been completely excluded, since several clinical controlled series have demonstrated the development of both alcoholic skeletal and cardiac myopathy regardless of nutritional, vitamin or ionic deficiencies (Urbano-Márquez et al., 1989; Moushmoush et al., 1991; Estruch et al., 1993).

Recently, a dose-related effect of ethanol on the production of skeletal or cardiac damage has been described, the lifetime dose of ethanol being the main etiologic factor (Urbano-Márquez et al., 1989, 1995). Therefore, at present, it has been well established that ethanol exerts a direct deleterious effect on cardiac and skeletal striated muscle, leading to alcohol myopathy in alcohol misusers.

Free radicals and acetaldehyde

It has been postulated that acetaldehyde plays a role in the pathogenesis of alcohol-induced muscle damage (Haller and Knochel, 1984). In fact, in experimental models, acetaldehyde may increase the negative effect that ethanol exerts in inhibiting muscle protein synthesis. However, acetaldehyde is not synthesized in the striated muscle, since there is no local activity of alcohol-dehydrogenase in the myocardium and skeletal striated muscle. In addition, the amount of acetaldehyde which reaches the muscle through the plasma is not great enough to cause pathological changes in the muscle (Thomas et al., 1994). Thus, acetaldehyde does not seem to be as important in the muscle as it is in the liver.

The production of free-radicals and lipid peroxidation products has also been suggested to intervene in the pathogenesis of alcohol-induced muscle damage (Ward and Peters, 1992). They may cause peroxidation of membrane phospholipids, alteration of myosin heavy-chain and excitation-contraction uncoupling. However, the relationship between oxidative injury and alcohol-induced muscle damage is not well established and may be a consequence, rather than a cause, of this disease.

Finally, acetaldehyde-protein adducts may lead to immunologically mediated organ damage, by inducing antibody formation, enzyme inactivation and DNA disruption. However, this mechanism has not been demonstrated to be deleterious in striated muscle.

Direct toxic effect of ethanol

In previous studies involving well-nourished chronic alcoholic patients of both sexes, we have found a highly significant correlation between left ventricular dysfunction parameters (ejection fraction, left ventricular mass) and parameters of alcohol consumption, especially the total lifetime dose of ethanol (Urbano-Márquez *et al.*, 1989, 1995). We observed a negative correlation between the left ventricular ejection fraction and the total lifetime dose of ethanol both in chronic alcoholic women and men (Figure 20.1) and a positive correlation of this parameter with the left ventricular mass. Similarly, in the skeletal striated muscle, we found a negative correlation between muscle strength and total lifetime dose of ethanol (Urbano-Márquez *et al.*, 1989) (Figure 20.2). This dose-related response between ethanol consumption and the induction of cardiac and skeletal muscle damage suggest a direct toxic effect of ethanol on the striated muscle. Thus, ethanol itself could be the main pathogenic factor of these diseases. The next question is how does ethanol specifically cause striated muscle damage?

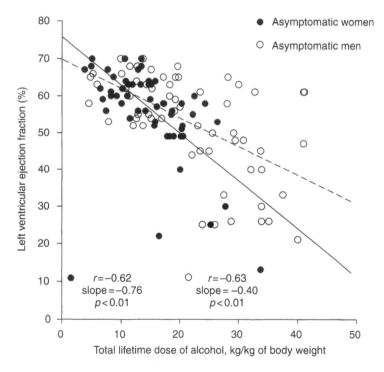

Figure 20.1 Inverse correlation between the total lifetime consumption of alcohol and left ventricular ejection fraction in 50 asymptomatic alcoholic women (solid line) and 100 asymptomatic alcoholic men (dashed line). The slope of this regression was significantly steeper in asymptomatic women than in asymptomatic men. (Reproduced with permission from JAMA, Urbano-Márquez *et al.*, 1995)

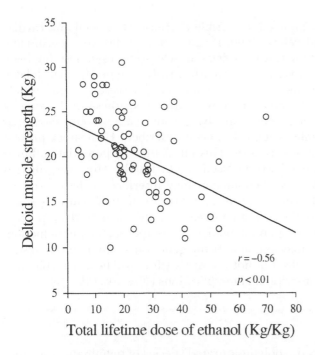

Figure 20.2 Inverse relationship between deltoid muscle strength measured by myometry and the total lifetime dose of ethanol consumed in a series of 68 chronic alcoholic men.

With respect to the molecular and genetic basis of ethanol-induced muscle damage, different hypotheses have emerged. Some are plausible and are based on the correlations observed between muscle disturbances and functional impairment, especially in regard to the main function of the striated muscle, which is contraction.

Metabolic and energetic disturbances

In preliminary studies, mitochondrial damage was suggested as the main cause of alcohol-induced muscle damage. However, we have found normal mitochondrial function in striated skeletal muscle in alcoholics with or without myopathy, thereby discounting this hypothesis (Cardellach *et al.*, 1992). Ethanol may induce an increase of the muscular anaerobic glycolytic metabolism by decreasing the activity of pyruvate kinase and altering the glycogen content of the muscle. However, there is no evidence of any functional disturbance related to this metabolic phenomenon. Ethanol may also disturb the function of some hormones, specially testosterone, the growth hormone and somatomedins. Although these hormonal disturbances may indirectly modify muscle protein synthesis and trophism, there is no evidence of their direct pathogenic effect. Little or no effect in cardiac nucleotide status has been observed in acute or chronic alcohol exposure (Piano and Schwertz, 1997).

Protein synthesis

Acute ethanol exposure may induce a reversible decrease of skeletal and cardiac protein synthesis (Preedy and Peters, 1990; Preedy *et al.*, 1994a). In experimental studies, a 15–30% decrease in the rate of skeletal muscle protein synthesis has been described after acute exposure to ethanol, primarily involving type II_B fibers (Slavin *et al.*, 1983). Specific muscle ribonuclease activities are increased in chronically ethanol fed rats, contributing to the alterations in protein synthesis. A decrease of 10% of 400 identifiable cardiac proteins, involving contractile proteins (actin), as well as fibrillary non-contractile proteins has been described. Heat-shock protein synthesis increases with ethanol exposure. This effect may be potentiated, but is absolutely independent of acetaldehyde (Preedy *et al.*, 1994b). However, there is no direct demonstration that this phenomenon may interfere in the contractile function. In chronic ethanol exposure, this alteration in protein synthesis is not maintained. In this situation there is an increase in the myofibrillary protein synthesis rate, probably indicating an adaptative or compensatory phenomenon. Chronic ethanol consumption may also modify the gene transcription mechanisms. In this situation, total mRNA falls, but not the mRNA for specific contractile proteins, implicating a role of transcriptional modifications (Preedy *et al.*, 1994c).

Transduction mechanisms

Acute ethanol exposure alters the polyunsaturated species of membrane phospholipids (phosphatidilinositol), perturbs its arrangement and has a fluidizing effect (Hoek and Rubin, 1990). This effect interferes with membrane channels and pumps as well as with transduction signals. Acute ethanol exposure produces a clear depression of muscle and cardiac contractile function of myocytes. This effect does not seem to be related to alterations in the myocardial phosphoinositide signaling system (Piano and Scwertz, 1997). Presently, the most relevant mechanisms to explain this phenomenon are related to the changes that ethanol induces in membrane permeability, channels and ionic fluxes. The basis of this phenomenon is related to both Ca^{2+} dependent and Ca^{2+} independent mechanisms (Thomas *et al.*, 1994). In animal and human experimental studies, ethanol induces a decrease in the activity of the voltage-sensitive Ca^{2+} and Na^+ sarcolemmal channels and decreases the sarcolemmal ATP Na^+/K^+ pump and the sarcoplasmic Ca^{2+} pump, leading to a decrease in cytosolic and sarcoplasmic Ca^{2+} content. It also decreases calcium transients in a dose-dependent manner through the sarcolemma both in skeletal and cardiac myocytes (Cofan *et al.*, 1995). Moreover, this decrease of the electrically-induced Ca^{2+} transients in cardiac myocytes parallels a decrease of myocyte contraction, which is dose-dependent and reversible when ethanol is removed from the media. Protein kinase C, a key intermediary in the control of Ca^{2+} transients, may also be directly modified by ethanol exposure. Therefore, ethanol exposure results in a loss of cell-Ca^{2+} storage, a decrease of Ca^{2+} after depolarization and a final reduction of myofibrillar contractility. We consider that this is presently the clearest demonstration of a cause-effect phenomenon in the decrease of muscle contractility induced by ethanol. Furthermore, ethanol reduces the efficacy of this Ca^{2+} signal by a direct interference of actin-myosin coupling mediated by

Ca^{2+}-independent mechanisms, probably by interfering with the calcium coupling to troponin. In the chronic model of ethanol exposure, intracytosolic resting Ca^{2+} normalizes, probably because of an adaptive phenomenon. In this situation, an increase in the density of sarcolemmal Ca^{2+} dihydropiridine-binding receptors and the Na^+/K^+ pump have been described, a up-regulation phenomenon that may justify the tolerance effect of chronic ethanol exposure on biological membranes (Guppy *et al.*, 1994). Ethanol also acutely inhibits the binding of actin to myosin, probably by interfering with the binding of calcium to troponin.

Other mechanisms

Since myocyte death is the final event of alcoholic skeletal and cardiac myopathy, the histological basis of this disease is a non-phagocytic, noninflammatory necrosis and given that ethanol has been demonstrated to produce apoptosis in other cells (lymphocytes), it is possible to assume that apoptosis may be a pathogenic mechanism in alcohol-induced striated muscle damage. The role of apoptosis in alcohol-induced muscle damage has not yet been demonstrated and some controversial evidence has been reported. In an experimental study of acute alcoholic myopathy in rats, no evidence of apoptosis was detected (Paice *et al.*, 1997). However, in end-stage heart failure not related to alcohol, apoptosis has been observed in most of the myocytes.

Ethanol may directly activate intermediate early-genes (*c-myc*, *fos*, *jun*) which regulate transcription and may subsequently induce changes in cell growth and differentiation. These changes may explain the alteration in protein synthesis induced by ethanol and may also lead to the indirect promotion of apoptosis.

Finally, a genetic susceptibilty to ethanol-induced heart and skeletal muscle damage may be taken into account. In fact, although there is a dose-related effect between ethanol consumption and muscle damage, some alcoholics with a high lifetime dose of ethanol, similar to that of the alcoholics with cardiomyopathy or skeletal myopathy, do not show muscle damage. This suggests that, apart from alcohol itself, other factors may be implicated in this individual susceptibility. Some evidence supports this assertion. In a previous study (Urbano-Márquez *et al.*, 1995), we observed that the decline of the left ventricular ejection fraction and that of deltoid muscle strength observed in alcoholic women were significantly steeper than those observed in men (see Figure 20.1). In another study comparing women and men with alcoholic cardiomyopathy (Fernández-Solà *et al.*, 1997c), we observed that women develop left ventricular failure as frequently as men, but after consumption of a significantly lower total lifetime dose of ethanol than men. These studies suggest that women are more sensitive to the toxic effects of ethanol, both in skeletal and cardiac muscle, than men.

ALCOHOLIC CARDIOMYOPATHY

Ethanol consumption may induce acute and chronic effects on the myocardium (Fernández-Solà *et al.*, 1996), which may produce a decrease in cardiac contractility and/or a variety of supraventricular and ventricular arrhythmias.

Acute cardiomyopathy

Acute binge ethanol consumption produces a direct negative inotropic effect, which is dose-dependent and reversible within hours (Thomas *et al.*, 1994). Acute ethanol decreases the rate and peak of systolic pressure and volume, and increases the end-diastolic pressure of the left ventricle, resulting in a decrease in cardiac output. This acute negative effect on cardiac contractility may be masked by an indirect positive chronotropic effect, related to the release of catecholamines and other neurohormones. The most important consequences of this acute effect have been described in patients with previous cardiac disease, where an acute alcohol binge may produce a rapid development of heart failure. Patients without under-lying cardiac disease may be more resistant to the acute depression of cardiac contractility induced by ethanol.

A large variety of arrhythmias may be produced by acute ethanol binge con-sumption, the most frequent being atrial fibrillation or flutter, paroxysmal atrial tachycardia and ventricular premature depolarizations (Ettinger *et al.*, 1978). Although acute arrhythmias related to ethanol intake have been described both in alcoholic and non-alcoholic patients, they are more frequent and dangerous in alcoholics with underlying cardiac disease (Greenberg *et al.*, 1982). The coexistence of electrolyte (Potasium, Phosphate, Magnesium) depletion or the development of ethanol abstinence, with catecholamine release, may increase the possibility of ethanol-induced arrhythmias.

Chronic cardiomyopathy

Chronic alcoholics with dilated cardiomyopathy may remain asymptomatic (sub-clinical cardiomyopathy) or exhibit signs and symptoms of heart failure (clinical cardiomyopathy). Subclinical left ventricular (LV) hypertrophy and dysfunction are frequent findings in chronic alcoholics (Kupari *et al.*, 1990; Bertolet *et al.*, 1991; Estruch, 1995). Both systolic and diastolic LV function may be affected by ethanol. An inverse relationship has been described between LV function parameters and alcohol even in the range of moderate consumption (Kupari *et al.*, 1993). In a pre-vious study (Urbano-Márquez *et al.*, 1989), we observed that the prevalence of alcoholic cardiomyopathy in well-nourished asymptomatic alcoholic men entering an outpatient treatment program for alcohol detoxification was 13%.

Most patients with high ethanol intake may remain asymptomatic for a long period of time. However, most patients with subclinical cardiomyopathy who main-tain a high ethanol intake finally develop dyspnea on exertion, orthopnea and paroxysmal nocturnal dyspnea, leading to a situation of congestive cardiomyopathy, similar to what happens in other causes of low-output dilated cardiomyopathy. Peripheral edema or anasarca as signs of right ventricular failure develop later in the course of disease. In some cases, atypical chest pain may appear. The incidence of atrial or ventricular arrhythmias with high risk of sudden death is also more fre-quent in these patients with alcoholic cardiomyopathy, specially if ethanol intake persists.

There are no specific laboratory, functional or pathologic findings of alcoholic cardiomyopathy, with all being similar to those obtained in idiopathic dilated cardiomyopathy (Fernández-Solà *et al.*, 1996). In laboratory blood analysis, a moderate rise in serum muscular enzymes (creatine kinase, aldolase) and proteins (myoglobin) may be detected in over one third of the patients, probably related to a coexistance of alcoholic skeletal myopathy. Moderate hypoxemia may be found as a manifestation of LV failure. Some of these patients may disclose increased plasma transaminases (sGOT and sGPT) and a decreased prothrombin activity as a reflection of liver cirrhosis or chronic liver failure, a finding frequent in alcoholics with cardiomyopathy. Global cardiac or LV enlargement and signs of pulmonary hypertension are frequent findings on chest X-ray. Electrocardiography is usually abnormal, the most relevant abnormalities being signs of left ventricular hypertrophy, conduction or repolarization defects and atrial or ventricular arrhythmias.

The diagnosis of alcoholic cardiomyopathy should be based on the epidemiological data (long history of high ethanol intake) and the results of echocardiography and radionuclide scanning. In echocardiography, a progressive enlargement of the LV diameters and a decrease in the shortening and ejection fractions are usually found. In radionuclide scanning, the LV ejection fraction is usually lower than 50%, in some cases being much lower than 15%. Since a high percentage of alcoholics smoke and exhibit risk factors for ischemic cardiopathy such as arterial hypertension and hypercholesterolemia, coronary cardiomyopathy must be ruled out in all alcoholics with dilated cardiomyopathy. Although there is no specific marker for the diagnosis of preclinical damage of the myocardium in chronic alcoholics, decrease of LV ejection fraction and impaired early filling of the LV have been suggested as early signs of systolic and diastolic LV dysfunction, respectively. Interestingly, a close correlation beteween ejection fraction and ethanol consumption (total lifetime dose of ethanol) has been observed in chronic alcoholics. Patients who have drunk more show a lower LV ejection fraction than alcoholics who have drunk less. Usually patients with alcoholic cardiomyopathy have drunk more than 20 Kg of ethanol/Kg of body weight.

Alcohol-related diseases affect both male and female chronic alcoholics, but the latter have been reported to be more sensitive to some of these effects than the former. In fact, women had the same prevalence of cardiomyopathy than men, despite women requiring a lower total lifetime dose of ethanol to develop the disease (Fernández-Solà *et al.*, 1997c). This susceptibility is confirmed by the steeper dose-response curve with respect to the ejection fraction of the women compared to men (Urbano-Márquez *et al.*, 1995) (see Figure 20.1).

Histological data of the myocardium of alcoholic cardiomyopathy may be found in autopsies or ventricular biopsies (Teragaki *et al.*, 1993). Patients with alcoholic cardiomyopathy show heart enlargement, weighing from 400 to 900 g, and a global enlargement of the heart chambers. The endocardium is usually thick, with frequent scars in the ventricles. The main histological findings are myocyte hypertrophy, myocytolysis and interstitial fibrosis (Figure 20.3). All these findings are more prominent in alcoholics with more advanced heart dysfunction. Nuclear and cellular hypertrophy of some myocytes and a variability in the size of the nuclear and myocytes are frequent and may be a compensatory phenomenon of myocyte death. Myocytolysis is a frequent finding manifested as a dissolution of myofibers and cell vacuolization. Interstitial or subendocardial fibrosis are frequent findings specially in advanced stages. The volume fraction of myocytes, an histomorphometric

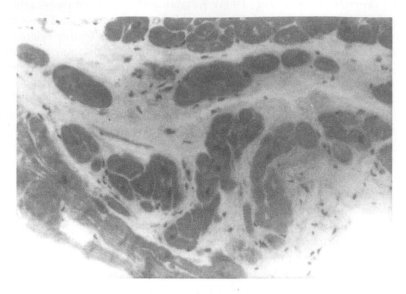

Figure 20.3 Endomyocardial biopsy of the left ventricle of an alcoholic patient with dilated cardiomyopathy. Myocytolysis, myocyte and nuclei hypertrophy and interstitial fibrosis are present. (Toluidine blue stain × 600)

parameter related to the degree of myocytolysis, has been described to be in inverse correlation with the total lifetime dose of ethanol consumed by the patient. A direct correlation has been described between LV dysfunction parameters and myocardial myocytolysis and myocyte hypertrophy in alcoholics with cardiomyopathy (Fernández-Solà *et al.*, 1994). No data of myocarditis have been observed in the histological studies of patients with alcoholic cardiomyopathy, although it is not possible to rule out previous viral infections of the myocardium.

As occurs in most toxic diseases, the cardiac damage induced by ethanol is reversible with alcohol abstinence. In most of the cases, this reversibility may be rapid, within a few months (Estruch *et al.*, 1989). In other patients, this may not be complete with persistence of residual functional and structural damage. In patients with end-stage skeletal or cardiac muscle damage, the reversal is not possible despite complete abstinence. The coexistence of muscle or cardiac diseases other than alcohol, may delay functional and structural recovery. The possibility of improvement despite maintaining low ethanol intake is currently under discussion.

Although no study has analyzed the natural history of alcoholic cardiomyopathy, its prognosis is clearly related to the persistence and degree of ethanol intake. The persistence of high-dose ethanol intake is usually related with a progressive left-ventricular functional impairment and a higher mortality (approximately 10 percent/ year) because of progression of heart failure or sudden death due to arrhythmias. Complete abstinence is followed by functional improvement in most cases, with the exception of patients with basal LV ejection fraction lower than 15%. In a prospective study of 54 patients with alcoholic cardiomyopathy, 7 out of 12 patients with persistent high ethanol intake died due to cardiac disease, compared to 5 out of 22 with alcohol intake lower than 80 grams and none of the 20 abstinent patients died. The main factors for mortality in alcoholic cardiomyopathy were the persistence of ethanol intake and the degree of left-ventricle enlargement at the time of diagnosis (Fernández-Solà *et al.*, 1997b).

The therapeutic approach to alcoholic cardiomyopathy does not differ from that of other causes of dilated cardiomyopathy, with rest and salt restriction being indicated during acute episodes of heart failure. Diuretics and angiotensin-converting enzyme inhibitors are the first-choice pharmacological treatment. Digoxin is only necessary if atrial fibrillation coexists. Because of the frequent coexistence of cirrhosis, the administration of anticoagulation therapy should be evaluated in each case. Heart transplantation should be considered in patients with end-stage cardiac disease, without other coexisting systemic diseases and with a long period of alcohol abstinence.

Sudden death

Alcohol misusers appear to have an increased risk of sudden death. Epidemiologic studies have observed an increased incidence of sudden, unexpected death in chronic alcoholics (Klatsky *et al.*, 1979; Estruch, 1995). In a Russian study (Vikhert *et al.*, 1986), alcoholic cardiomyopathy was found in 127 out of 752 cases of sudden cardiac death, predominantly in men under age 50 (73%). Another study (Randall, 1980) reported the occurrence of sudden death in individuals in their third to fifth decade of life whose only remarkable finding at autopsy was the presence of hepatic fatty metamorphosis. The sudden occurrence of death without pathologic explanation suggests an arrhythmic event. Cardiac arrthythmias have been related to alcohol abuse. This association has been popularized under the term of "holiday heart" (Ettinger *et al.*, 1978). This disease may be manifested as episodes of ventricular and atrial arrthymias, being more frequent in patients with preclinical or clinical cardiomyopathy. However, some cases of sudden death exhibited a relatively low blood ethanol concentration, less than 50 mg/dL. Therefore, these cases may be related to causes other than ethanol itself such as an increased left ventricular mass commonly found in alcoholics, an intense sympathoadrenal response to alcohol withdrawal or an electrolyte imbalance, such as hypokalemia or hypomagnesemia. Finally, alcohol abuse may also contribute to the occurrence of sudden death in individuals with coronary heart disease. In a multivariate analysis of variables associated with sudden death in coronary disease, heavy alcohol consumption emerged as an independent predictor of such events (Fraser and Upsell, 1981).

ALCOHOLIC SKELETAL MUSCLE MYOPATHY

Alcoholic skeletal myopathy is an evolving toxic myopathy which involves the proximal muscles of both girdles, producing weakness, myalgia and muscle atrophy (Urbano-Márquez *et al.*, 1989; Sacanella *et al.*, 1995; Preedy and Peters, 1990). Although there is no specific marker for this disease, diagnosis may be obtained from evidence of a toxic myopathy syndrome, with histological data of myocytolysis and fiber atrophy, in the absence of causes of skeletal myopathy other than alcohol. In alcohol-induced skeletal muscle damage, two different clinical pictures may be differentiated: acute and chronic alcoholic myopathies. Acute alcoholic myopathy is usually seen after binges of ethanol. In chronic myopathy, consumption of high doses of alcohol during a long period of time is required.

Acute skeletal myopathy

This is a syndrome of acute toxic myocytolysis which develops sporadically in binge drinking alcoholics, although it is more frequent in patients with persistent chronic alcohol intake (Biscaldi *et al.*, 1994). Its incidence has been estimated as 0.5 to 2% among alcohol misusers. In fact, alcoholism is one of the most prominent causes of acute rhabdomyolysis in Western countries. Proximal muscle pain (myalgia) of abrupt onset and local muscle swelling are the main clinical features. Weakness may develop progressively, predominantly involving the proximal zone of the legs and functional impairment going up stairs. The patient may notice a transitory darkness of the urine as a reflection of myoglobinuria. The symptoms usually resolve within a few days with ethanol abstinence, but may recur after acute ethanol reingestion. Acute renal failure is a potential serious complication induced by tubular necrosis due to massive myoglobinuria (Fernández-Reyes *et al.*, 1995).

High peak of blood creatine kinase is a frequent feature, returning to normal values in three to five days on discontinuation of alcohol intake. Other muscle enzymes, such as aldolase and lactate dehydrogenase, or proteins such as myoglobin may also increase. The coexistence of hypopotassemia or hypomagnesemia, alcohol abstinence syndrome and/or convulsions may increase acute alcohol induced-muscle damage. Electrophysiological studies reveal a proximal myopathic pattern in 10 to 50% of the cases, but during the first days of evolution, this study may be normal. The most relevant histological feature is the presence of myocytolysis. The histological picture is similar to that of acute toxic rhabdomyolysis and, thus, is non-specific (Fernández-Solà *et al.*, 1996). Myocytolysis may involve from 10 to 50% of the muscle fibers and resolves completely after abstinence within a few days. Occasional descriptions of cases of severe acute necrotizing myopathy with widespread muscle involvement have been reported.

Acute alcoholic skeletal myopathy resolves spontaneously within a few days with alcohol abstinence and resting in most cases. Mortality is exceptional in this disease and the only fatal cases have been described in cases of rhabdomyolysis and myoglubinuric-induced acute renal failure.

Chronic skeletal myopathy

This entity may develop progressively in high-dose chronic alcoholics, who report proximal muscle weakness, atrophy and slight myalgia (Preedy *et al.*, 1994a; Sacanella *et al.*, 1995). It is usually found in middle aged people, with a similar incidence in women and men, with equal involvement of the upper and lower limbs. Since there are many subclinical cases, its incidence depends on the parameter used for achieving diagnosis. Among chronic alcoholics, one third report muscle weakness or myalgia. A significant decrease in muscle strength is evident by myometry in 42% of these patients, and histological changes are present in half of the cases on light microscopy, although most of them have ultrastructural muscle changes (Urbano-Márquez *et al.*, 1989). In the chronic form of alcoholic myopathy, the histological findings are not specific, with the most prominent being fiber atrophy and myocytolysis. Myocytolysis is still the most prominent feature, sometimes preceded by intracellular edema and hypercontracted fibers. In advanced cases, myofilament dissolution is very apparent, involving 1 to 30% of the myocytes, with or without phagocytoses. Fiber atrophy is present in 30–50% of the cases and specially involves type II_b fibers (Slavin *et al.*, 1983; Fernández-Solà *et al.*, 1995). Other findings are moth-eaten fibers, subsarcolemmal deposition, internal nuclei, type I fiber predominance, interstitial fibrosis and presence of fat in endomysia in a proportion of 5 to 20% of the cases, respectively.

The diagnosis of chronic alcoholic myopathy should be based on the histological findings of skeletal muscle biopsy. However, since there is a highly significant correlation between low muscle strength and histological findings of alcoholic myopathy, this diagnosis may be made in all alcoholics who show a significant muscle weakness (usually deltoid muscle strength lower than 20 Kg measured by myometry) (Urbano-Márquez *et al.*, 1989).

The evolution of chronic alcoholic myopathy was analyzed in a 5-year follow-up study (Urbano-Márquez *et al.*, 1993). Most of the cases resolved with abstinence over a period of 2–12 months, although some patients did not achieve normalization of their previous muscle strength. On the other hand, 83% of actively drinking alcoholics presented a decrease in muscle strength and those who persisted in ethanol intake may develop progression in the severity of the histological muscle damage.

RELATION OF ALCOHOLIC MYOPATHY TO CARDIOMYOPATHY

Based on the evidence that skeletal and cardiac alcohol-induced striated muscle damage are dose-dependent and on the histological and molecular similarities of both tissues, there is reason to consider that a correlation may exist between both diseases.

In a previous study of 24 alcoholic patients with dilated cardiomyopathy, 20 (83%) presented histological findings of skeletal myopathy compared with only 1 out of 24 (4%) alcoholic patients with normal cardiac function (Fernández-Solà *et al.*, 1994). In the patients with alcoholic cardiomyopathy, the relation with skeletal myopathy was shown at a clinical level, with a relationship observed between the NYHA functional class and the presence of muscle weakness. This relationship was also evident at a functional level. In this respect, the patients with more advanced skeletal damage presented significantly greater left-ventricular dysfunction. Finally, we also found a correlation between these two diseases at an histological level, since patients with more advanced signs of skeletal myopathy also presented greater cardiac histological damage (myocytolysis, interstitial fibrosis and myocyte atrophy). Since skeletal muscle weakness may serve as a surrogate for myocardial damage, screening of alcoholic patients by evaluation of muscle strength has been proposed to detect those with high risk of developing cardiomyopathy.

RELATION TO OTHER ETHANOL-RELATED DISORDERS

Since the systemic toxic effects of ethanol on different organs seem to be dose-dependent, it is rational to expect the presence of other organ damage such as liver disease in patients with ethanol-induced striated muscle damage. Although a previous anecdotal perception of an inverse relationship between cirrhosis and cardiomyopathy in chronic alcoholism have been suggested (Leftowitch and Fenoglio, 1983), in a prospective study including alcoholics with cardiomyopathy, alcoholics without cardiomyopathy, actively drinking alcoholics with cirrhosis, abstaining alcoholics with cirrhosis and nonalcoholics with cirrhosis of other etiologies, a positive association was observed between cardiomyopathy and liver disease (Estruch *et al.*, 1995). Thus, alcoholics admitted solely for cardiomyopathy have a higher prevalence of cirrhosis than unselected alcoholics without heart disease. Cardiac studies of patients with nonalcoholic cirrhosis were normal. Finally, the prevalence of cardiomyopathy among actively drinking alcoholics with cirrhosis was higher than that of abstaining alcoholics with cirrhosis (Figure 20.4).

Thus, all these alcohol dose-related diseases seem to be associated and an increase in their incidence may be expected in patients with specific alcohol-induced organ

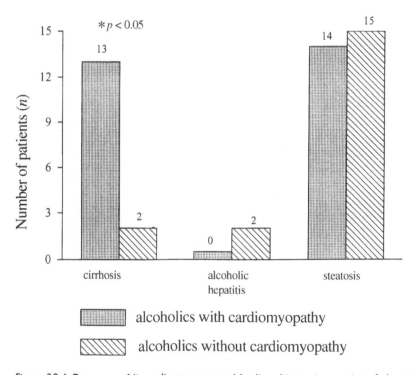

Figure 20.4 Presence of liver disease assessed by liver biopsy in a series of chronic alcoholics with and without alcoholic cardiomyopathy. Patients with cardiomyopathy presented a higher incidence of liver cirrhosis than alcoholic patients without cardiomyopathy.

damage. Therefore, screening for the presence of the full-spectrum of diseases should be carried out in this high-risk group of patients with chronic high ethanol intake.

CONCLUSIONS

At present, acute and chronic alcoholic skeletal and cardiac myopathies are well characterized clinical and histological entities, which seem to be dose-dependent. Although some cases remain asymptomatic, others progress to the development of muscle weakness and atrophy (skeletal myopathy) and exertional dyspnea and congestive heart failure (cardiomyopathy). Since the prevalence of alcoholic myopathy is high (one third to half of chronic alcoholic patients), whereas the prevalence of alcoholic cardiomyopathy is lower (13%), early diagnosis is always important, particularly in patients with accumulated high-doses of alcohol or with other alcoholic systemic diseases such as cirrhosis. Early detection is essential to avoid disease progression and mortality related to alcoholic cardiomyopathy. Both diseases are partially reversible with abstinence. Present pathogenic theories are based on the direct effect of ethanol on membrane fluidity and the interference which ionic Na^+ and Ca^{2+} channels and transients produce together with a disruption of protein synthesis and myocyte contraction mechanisms. Personal or gender susceptibility may also play a role in the development of these diseases. Women seem to be more sensitive to toxic alcohol effects on striated muscle. Future trends in alcohol-induced muscle damage are directed at improving the knowledge of molecular and genetic mechanisms of the disease.

REFERENCES

Bertolet, B.D., Freund, G., Martin, C.A., Perchalski, D.L., Williams, C.M. and Pepine, C.J. (1991) Unrecognized left ventricular dysfunction in apparently health alcohol abuse population. *Drug Alcohol Depend* **28**, 113–119.

Biscaldi, G., Guarnone, F., Fonte, R., Finozzi, E., Grossi, R. and Taglione, L. (1994) Miopatia alcolica acuta. *Recent Progress in Medicina* **85**, 537–539.

Cardellach, F., Galofré, J., Grau, J.M., Casademont, J., Hoeck, J.B., Rubin, E. and Urbano-Márquez, A. (1992) Oxidative metabolism in skeletal muscle mitochondria from patients with chronic alcoholism is normal. *Ann Neurol* **31**, 515–518.

Cofán, M., Fernández-Solà, J., Nicolás, J.M., Poch, E. and Urbano-Márquez, A. (1995) Ethanol decreases basal cytosolic-free calcium concentration in cultured skeletal muscle cells. *Alcohol & Alcoholism* **30**, 617–621.

Ekbon, K., Hed, R., Kistein, L. and Astron, K. (1964) Muscular affections in chronic alcoholism. *Arch Neurol* **10**, 449–458.

Estruch, R., Fernández-Solà, J., Grau, J.M., Mont, L. and Urbano-Márquez, A. (1989) Reversibilidad precoz mediante abstinencia de las manifestaciones clínicas en la miocardiopatía alcohólica. *Med Clin (Bar)* **92**, 69–71.

Estruch, R., Nicolás, J.M., Villegas, E., Junqué, A. and Urbano-Márquez, A. (1993) Relationship between ethanol-related diseases and nutritional status in chronic alcoholic men. *Alcohol & Alcoholism* **28**, 543–550.

Estruch, R. (1995) Efectos cardiovasculares del alcohol. *Med Clin (Bar)* **105**, 628–631.

Estruch, R., Fernández-Solà, J., Sacanella, E., Paré, J.C., Rubin, E. and Urbano-Márquez, A. (1995) Relationship between cardiomyopathy and liver disease in chronic alcoholism. *Hepatology* **22**, 532–538.

Ettinger, P.O., Wu, C.F., De la Cruz Jr., C., Weisse, A.B., Ahmed, S.S. and Regan, T.J. (1978) Arrhytmias and the "holiday heart": alcohol-associated cardiac Ruth disorders. *Am Heart J* **95**, 555–562.

Fahlgren, H., Hed, R. and Lundmank, K. (1957) Myonecrosis and myoglobinuria in alcohol and barbiturate intoxication. *Acta Med Scand* **158**, 405–412.

Fernández-Reyes, J.L., Navarro-Herrera, J., Bianchi, J.L., Gálvez, E. and Salguero, E. (1995) Miopatía guda etílica rabdomiolítica asociada a hepatitis alcohólica aguda. *Ann Med Interna (Spain)* **12**, 136–142.

Fernández-Solà, J., Estruch, R., Grau, J.M., Paré, J.C., Urbano-Márquez, A. and Rubin, E. (1994) The relation of alcoholic myopathy to cardiomyopathy. *Ann Intern Med* **120**, 529–536.

Fernández-Solà, J., Sacanella, E., Estruch, R., Nicolás, J.M., Grau, J.M. and Urbano-Márquez, A. (1995) Significance of type II fiber atrophy in chronic alcoholic myopathy. *J Neurol Sci* **130**, 69–76.

Fernández-Solà, J., Grau, J.M. and Urbano-Márquez, A. (1996) Alcoholic Myopathies. *Curr Opin Neurol* **9**, 400–405.

Fernández-Solà, J., Estruch, R. and Urbano-Márquez, A. (1997a) Alcohol and heart muscle disease. *Addiction Biology* **2**, 9–17.

Fernández-Solà, J., Estruch, R., Nicolás, J. and Urbano-Márquez, A. (1997b) Molecular and genetic basis of ethanol-related cardiac damage. *Alcohol Clin Exp Res* **32**, 3 (abst).

Fernández-Solà, J., Estruch, R., Nicolás, J.M., Paré, J.C., Sacanella, E., Antúnez, E. and Urbano-Márquez, A. (1997c) Comparison of alcoholic cardiomyopathy in women versus men. *Am J Cardiol* **80**, 481–485.

Fraser, G.E. and Upsell, M. (1981) Alcohol and other discriminants between cases of sudden death and myocardial infarction. *Am J Epidemiol* **114**, 462–476.

Greenberg, B.H., Schutz, R., Grunkemeier, G.L. and Griswold, H. (1982) Acute effects of alcohol in patients with congestive heart failure. *Ann Intern Med* **31**, 515–518.

Guppy, L.J. and Littleton, J.M. (1994) Binding characteristics of the calcium channel antagonist (3H)-nitrendipine in tissues from ethanol-dependent rats. *Alcohol & Alcoholism* **29**, 283–293.

Haller, R.G. and Knochel, J.P. (1984) Skeletal muscle disease in alcoholism. *Med Clin N Am* **68**, 91–103.

Hed, R., Larsson, H., Wahlgren, F. and Owell, J. (1955) Acute myoglobinuria: report of a case with fatal outcome. *Acta Med Scand* **152**, 459–463.

Hoek, J.B. and Rubin, E. (1990) Alcohol and membrane associated signal transduction. *Alcohol & Alcoholism* **25**, 143–156.

Jackson, O. (1882) On peculiar disease resulting from the use of ardent spirits. *N Engl J Med Surg* **21**, 351–353.

Klatsky, A.L., Friedman, G.D. and Siegelaub, A.B. (1979) Alcohol use, myocardial infarction, sudden cardiac death and hypertension. *Alcohol Clin Exp Res* **3**, 33–39.

Kupari, M., Koskinen, P., Suokas, A. and Ventila, M. (1990) Left ventricular filling impairment in asymptomatic chronic alcoholics. *Am J Cardiol* **66**, 473–477.

Kupari, M. and Koskinen, P. (1993) Relation of left ventricular function to habitual alcohol consumption. *Am J Cardiol* **72**, 1418–1424.

Leftowitch, J.H. and Fenoglio, J.J. (1983) Liver disease in alcoholic cardiomyopathy. Evidence against cirrhosis. *Hum Pathol* **14**, 457–463.

Lieber, C.S. (1988) Biochemical and molecular basis of ethanol-induced injury to the liver and other tissues. *N Engl J Med* **219**, 1639–1650.

Moushmoush, B. and Abi-Manour, P. (1991) Alcohol and the heart: the long-term effects of alcohol on cardiovascular system. *Arch Intern Med* **151**, 36–42.

Paice, A.G., Hirako, M., Peters, T.J. and Preedy, V.R. (1997) Alcohol's deleterious effect on skeletal muscle is not mediated by apoptosis. *Alcohol Clin Exp Res* **32**, 403 (abst).

Piano, M. and Schwertz, D.W. (1997) Effect of chronic ethanol exposure on myocardial phosphoinositide turnover. *Alcohol Clin Exp Res* **21**, 721–727.

Preedy, V.R. and Peters, T.J. (1990) Alcohol and skeletal muscle disease. *Alcohol & Alcoholism* **25**, 177–187.

Preedy, V.R., Salisbury, J.R. and Peters, T.J (1994a) Alcoholic muscle disease: features and mechanisms. *J Pathol* **173**, 309–315.

Preedy, V.R., Siddiq, T. and Richardson, P.J. (1994b) The deleterious effects of alcohol on the heart: involvement of protein turnover. *Alcohol & Alcoholism* **29**, 141–147.

Preedy, V.R., Peters, T.J., Patel, V.D. and Meill, J.P. (1994c) Chronic alcoholic myopathy: transcriptional and translational alterations. *FASEB J* **8**, 1146–1151.

Randall, B. (1980) Sudden death and hepatic fatty metamorphosis. *JAMA* **243**, 1723–1725.

Regan, T.J. (1990) Alcohol and the cardiovascular system. *JAMA* **264**, 337–381.

Rubin, E. and Urbano-Márquez, A. (1994) Alcoholic cardiomyopathy. *Alcohol Clin Exper Res* **18**, 111–114.

Sacanella, E., Fernández-Solà, J., Cofan, M., Nicolás, J.M., Estruch, R., Antúnez, E. and Urbano-Márquez, A. (1995) Chronic alcoholic myopathy: diagnostic clues and relationship with other ethanol-related diseases. *Quarterly Journal of Medicine* **88**, 811–817.

Sherlock, S. (1984) Nutrition and the alcoholic. *Lancet* **1**, 436–438.

Slavin, G., Martin, F., Ward, P., Levi, J. and Peters, T.J. (1983) Chronic alcohol excess associated with selective but reversible injury to type 2B fibres. *J Clin Pathol* **36**, 772–777.

Teragaki, M., Takeuchi, K. and Takeda, T. (1993) Clinical and histological features of alcohol drinkers with congestive heart failure. *Am Heart J* **125**, 808–817.

Thomas, A., Rozanski, D.J., Renard, D.C. and Rubin, E. (1994) Effects of ethanol on contractile function of the heart: A review. *Alcohol Clin Exp Res* **18**, 121–131.

Urbano-Márquez, A., Estruch, R., Navarro-López, F., Grau, J.M., Mont, L. and Rubin, E. (1989) The effects of alcoholism on skeletal and cardiac muscle. *N Engl J Med* **320**, 409–411.

Urbano-Márquez, A., Estruch, R., Sacanella, E., Fernández-Solà, J., Nicolás, J.M. and Antúnez, E. (1993) Partial reversibility of alcoholic myopathy with ethanol abstinence: a five-year follow-up study. *Alcohol & Alcoholism* **28**, 251 (abst).

Urbano-Márquez, A., Estruch, R., Fernández-Solà, J., Nicolás, J.M., Paré, J.C. and Rubin, E. (1995) The greater risk of alcoholic cardiomyopathy and myopathy in women compared with men. *JAMA* **274**, 149–154.

Vikhert, A.M., Tsiplenkova, V.G. and Cherpachenko, N.M. (1986) Alcoholic cardiomyopathy and sudden cardiac death. *J Am Coll Cardiol* **8**, 3A–11A.

Ward, R.J. and Peters, T.J. (1992) The antioxidant status of patients with either alcohol-induced liver damage or myopathy. *Alcohol & Alcoholism* **27**, 359–365.

Chapter 21

Cerebral consequences of alcoholic liver disease

Roger F. Butterworth

Alcoholic Liver Disease (ALD) and its consequences play an important role in the pathogenesis of cerebral dysfunction in chronic alcoholism. There is convincing evidence that Portal-Systemic Encephalopathy (PSE), the predominant neuropsychiatric abnormality resulting from ALD, is caused by the accumulation of neurotoxins such as ammonia and manganese in brain. Both toxins are normally eliminated almost exclusively by the liver. Ammonia exerts its deleterious effects on cerebral function by an array of direct and indirect mechanisms including effects of the ammonium ion (NH_4^+) on inhibitory and excitatory neurotransmission as well as effects on cerebral energy metabolism. Existing treatment of PSE relies on ammonia-lowering strategies including reduction of dietary protein and the use of lactulose, neomycin and, and more recently, L-ornithine-aspartate. Proton Magnetic Resonance Spectroscopy reveals increased brain concentrations of the ammonia detoxification product glutamine in patients with PSE. Magnetic Resonance Imaging, on the other hand, shows bilateral signal hyperintensity in globus pallidus in a large majority of patients with ALD. Neurochemical and neuropathological examination of pallidal tissue from these patients reveals several-fold increases of manganese and the appearance of Alzheimer-type II astrocytes, the cardinal neuropathological feature of PSE. Neurochemical studies of postmortem brain tissue from patients with ALD who died in hepatic coma demonstrate modifications of glutamate and serotonin synthesis and metabolism as well as increased expression of "peripheral-type" benzodiazepine receptors (PTBRs). Studies in experimental animal models of PSE reveal alterations in expression of PTBRs and of neuronal nitric oxide synthase. Further elucidation of these neurotransmitter changes could provide potential targets for pharmacological manipulation and thus afford new approaches to the prevention and treatment of PSE in patients with ALD.

KEYWORDS: alcoholic liver disease, cerebral consequences, hepatic encephalopathy, portal-systemic encephalopathy, ammonia, manganese, neutrotransmitters

INTRODUCTION

There is a growing body of evidence to suggest that alcoholic liver disease (ALD) and its consequences, play an important role in the pathogenesis of cerebral dysfunction commonly encountered in chronic alcoholics. Evidence may be summarized as follows:

1   Non-invasive imaging techniques demonstrate that the presence of cirrhosis in chronic alcoholics is associated with increased brain atrophy. For example,

in one Computed Tomographic (CT) study of brain changes as a function of liver status (determined by liver biopsy) in 41 chronic alcoholics, greater topographical brain changes were associated with greater severity of liver disease (Acker *et al.*, 1982);

2   Greater EEG slowing is observed in alcoholics with cirrhosis compared to alcoholics without cirrhosis (Kardel and Stigsby, 1975);

3   Measures of hepatic function correlate significantly with neuropsychologic test scores in alcoholics with biopsy-proven cirrhosis (Tarter *et al.*, 1993).

The cerebral consequences of ALD have generally been underestimated. As reported by Tarter and colleagues (1985), "where there is a conjoint alcoholism disorder and liver pathology, the effects of the latter have not been recognized generally or incorporated into overall rehabilitation planning. Indeed, the possibility remains that the cirrhosis, being a permanent disorder, perpetuates and possibly magnifies the encephalopathy due to alcohol abuse over time. This may be true even if drinking has been discontinued, particularly if the liver disease is advanced."

The most common form of cerebral disorder in ALD is Portal-Systemic Encephalopathy (PSE) which results from shunting of portal blood into the systemic circulation. Shunting may be spontaneous (resulting from portal-systemic collaterals) or from shunt procedures. One such procedure, the Transjugular Intrahepatic Portosystemic Stent Shunt (TIPS) is a non-surgical technique used for the prevention of rebleeding of variceal hemorrhages as well as for the treatment of intractible ascites in cirrhotic patients with portal hypertension. Although effective in the lowering of portal pressure in these patients, the TIPS procedure has been found to result in new PSE episodes or worsening of existing PSE in up to 44% of cases (Pomier Layrargues, 1996).

Prior to the development of overt PSE, cirrhotic patients manifest a high incidence of so-called "subclinical PSE". In one study, groups of patients with ALD or non-alcoholic liver disease were studied using an extensive battery of tests used in part to assess the patients' fitness to drive an automobile. One hundred per cent of alcoholic cirrhotics were found to be unfit to drive (Schomerus *et al.*, 1981). In another study, 22 patients with ALD and 20 non-alcoholics matched for Pugh score were compared to 42 control subjects matched for age and educational background and subjected to a battery of psychometric tests. Seventy six per cent of patients with ALD failed at least one test and the degree of neuropsychological impairment was comparable in alcoholic and non-alcoholic cirrhotics (Table 21.1) (Pomier Layrargues *et al.*, 1991). These findings again suggest that liver disease and its sequelae may play an important role in the cognitive disturbances in chronic alcoholism.

Clinical and diagnostic aspects

The clinical features of PSE include a spectrum of neuropsychiatric symptoms ranging from personality changes and altered sleep patterns through shortened attention span, temporal and spatial disorientation and finally stupor and coma (Butterworth, 1995a). Neuromuscular signs are frequently evident and include asterixis ("flapping tremor"), gait ataxia and Parkinsonian symptoms, particularly rigidity.

Table 21.1 Results of neuropsychological tests in control subjects and cirrhotic patients

Test	Controls (n = 42)	Cirrhotics Alcoholic (n = 22)	Cirrhotics nonalcoholic (n = 20)	Cirrhotics Total (n = 42)
Delayed recall (number of words)	2.7 ± 0.5	2.2 ± 0.9*	2.3 ± 0.9*	2.2 ± 0.9*
Serial threes (s)	57 ± 28	81 ± 45*	78 ± 39*	79 ± 42*
Arithmetic (number of errors)	0.6 ± 0.9	2.5 ± 1.9*	2.2 ± 1.9*	2.3 ± 1.9*
Months backward (s)	14 ± 6	33 ± 34*	28 ± 30	31 ± 32*
Digit span forward (number)	6.5 ± 1.2	5.7 ± 1.1*	5.9 ± 1.2*	5.8 ± 1.1*
Digit span backward (number)	4.7 ± 0.9	3.9 ± 1*	4.2 ± 1.4*	4.1 ± 1.2*
Alphabet (s)	9.4 ± 4.2	17 ± 13*	17 ± 11*	17 ± 12*
Digit symbol (number)	39.6 ± 11.4	25.7 ± 6.3*	27.7 ± 10.2*	26.7 ± 9.2*
Reitan trail making tests				
Part A (s)	38.9 ± 13.5	61.6 ± 24.3*	59.7 ± 22.1*	60.7 ± 23.0*
Part B (s)	83.9 ± 31.8	140.1 ± 50.1*	153.5 ± 50.2*	146.5 ± 50.0*
Clock drawing (normal/abnormal)	40/2	17/5	16/4	33/9

* Significantly different from control group (p < 0.01); no significant difference was found between alcoholic and nonalcoholic cirrhotic patients.

As with other severe metabolic encephalopathies, electroencephalographic (EEG) changes encountered in PSE consist initially of a bilaterally synchronous decrease in wave frequency and an increase in wave amplitude associated with the disappearance of normal alpha rhythm. Triphasic waves are characteristic paroxysmal waves in the EEG trace which frequently appear at severe stages of PSE. Although not adequate for a definitive diagnosis of PSE, EEG assessment may be useful for monitoring the evolution of PSE in a given patient.

Diagnosis of PSE in alcoholic patients can be difficult. No single clinical or laboratory measure has been found to be useful in the establishment of a specific diagnosis (Tarter *et al.*, 1993). Misdiagnosis most often occurs in the early stages of hepatic failure where symptoms common to a number of psychiatric disorders including euphoria, depression, inappropriate affect and sleep disorders may occur. The following characteristics have been proposed to be helpful in the diagnosis of PSE (from Tarter *et al.*, 1993):

1   History of hepatic disease;
2   EEG slowing particularly in association with triphasic wave pattern;
3   Neuropsychological impairment revealed by tests measuring visuospatial, perceptual-motor and fine motor control;
4   Asterixis;
5   Fetor hepaticus;
6   Hyperventilation;
7   Elevated fasting serum ammonia level;
8   Reduced consciousness or awareness.

It should be noted that the above signs and symptoms are not specific to PSE and that they may fluctuate and manifest to a greater or lesser degree depending upon fluctuations in medical status, diet and recent drinking history (Tarter *et al.*, 1993).

NEUROPATHOLOGY

Histopathologic studies of brain sections from patients with ALD who died in hepatic coma reveal astrocytic changes known as Alzheimer type II astrocytosis in which astrocytes take on a characteristic swollen appearance with a large pale nucleus, prominent nucleolus and margination of the chromatin pattern (Figure 21.1).

In addition to these characteristic morphologic changes, Alzheimer type II astrocytes appear to lose their immunoreactivity for glial fibrillary acidic protein (GFAP) (Sobel *et al.*, 1981). GFAP is the major protein of intermediate filaments in differentiated astrocytes (Eng, 1985) and antisera to GFAP are routinely used for identification of astrocytes in tissue sections. Astrocytes from cerebral cortex, basal ganglia and diencephalic structures from patients with PSE manifest reduced GFAP-immunostaining (Sobel *et al.*, 1981). On the other hand, the Bergmann glia,

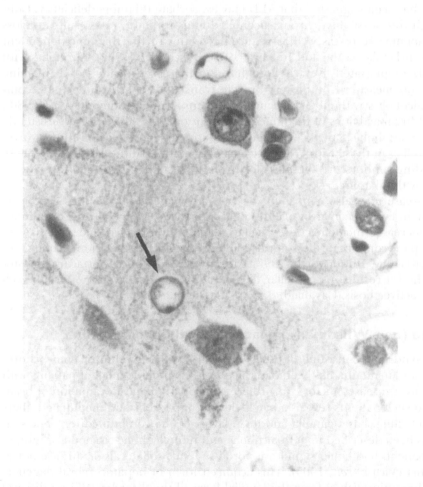

Figure 21.1 Alzheimer type II astrocytosis in basal ganglia of a 39 year-old patient with ALD who died in hepatic coma. Note enlarged pale astrocyte nucleus (arrow) with prominent nucleolus and margination of the chromatin pattern.

a specialized group of cerebellar astrocytes, do not show alterations of GFAP (Kril *et al.*, 1997). Changes in the expression of other astrocytic proteins have also been described in human PSE. Such changes include loss of activities of glutamine synthetase (Lavoie *et al.*, 1987b), increased activities of monoamine oxidase (MAO-B) (Raghavendra Rao *et al.*, 1993) and increased densities of "peripheral-type" (mitochondrial) benzodiazepine receptors (Lavoie *et al.*, 1990).

Relationship of ALD to alcoholic brain damage

Neuropathologic studies reveal that the incidence of Wernicke-type lesions and of cerebellar degeneration is increased two-fold in alcoholic patients with liver disease (Kril and Butterworth, 1997). Wernicke encephalopathy is caused by thiamine deficiency and in the case of alcoholics, this results from the effects of poor nutrition and diminished gastrointestinal absorption of thiamine. (Butterworth, 1995b). It has been suggested that ALD may exacerbate thiamine deficiency. Consistent with this possibility, chronic alcohol administration to rats results in a loss of liver thiamine stores as well as reduced activities of the thiamine-dependent enzyme transketolase (Abe and Itokawa, 1977; Bitsch *et al.*, 1982). Alcoholics with severely decompensated liver cirrhosis have an increased incidence of thiamine deficiency (as measured by the erythrocyte transketolase activation assay) compared to alcoholics without significant hepatic impairment (Somogyi *et al.*, 1980). Decreased brain activities of thiamine-dependent enzymes have been consistently described in alcoholic patients who died in hepatic coma (Lavoie and Butterworth, 1995) as well as in those with Wernicke encephalopathy (Butterworth *et al.*, 1993). These findings underscore the need for prompt, sustained treatment of patients with ALD with thiamine.

Liver disease may also contribute to the pathogenesis of alcoholic cerebellar degeneration. Evidence in favor of a role of liver disease *per se* is provided by findings of a 50% increased incidence of cerebellar degeneration in cirrhotic patients who died in hepatic coma regardless of the etiology (alcoholic versus non-alcoholic) of cirrhosis (Kril and Butterworth, 1997). Moreover, end-to-side portacaval anastomosis in the rat results in cerebellar degeneration characterized by Purkinje cell loss and reactive gliosis (Cavanagh *et al.*, 1972; Diemer *et al.*, 1977).

Acquired (non-Wilsonian) hepatocerebral degeneration

A clinical syndrome consisting of dysarthria, gait ataxia, intention tremor, choreoathetosis and dementia has been described in a small percentage of patients with end-stage liver disease (Victor *et al.*, 1965). Neuropathological evaluation of brain tissue from such patients reveals a patchy loss of nerve cells and medullated fibers in the cerebellum, basal ganglia and deep layers of the cerebral cortex. The syndrome has been described in both alcoholic and non-alcoholic cirrhotics where, in all cases, patients had either significant portal-systemic collaterals or surgical portacaval shunts (Victor *et al.*, 1965). This acquired form of hepatocerebral degeneration can be distinguished from the familial form of the disorder (Wilson disease) by the findings of normal serum and urinary copper, normal ceruloplasmin levels and the absence of Kayser-Fleischer rings.

Neurological sequelae of liver transplantation in patients with ALD

Neurological sequelae including encephalopathy, seizures, gait ataxia, memory impairment, central pontine myelinolysis and acquired (non-Wilsonian) hepato-cerebral degeneration have been described in alcoholic and non-alcoholic patients with advanced liver disease following liver transplantation (Arria *et al.*, 1991; Hockerstedt *et al.*, 1992; Menegaux *et al.*, 1994; Soffer *et al.*, 1995). Such complications have been generally attributed to irreversible brain damage which developed either during or after the transplant procedure caused by portal vein thrombosis, immunosuppressant neurotoxicity or electrolyte imbalances. On the other hand, these "sequelae" may result, in some cases, from alcohol-related neuropathology present prior to liver transplant surgery (Kril and Butterworth, 1997).

PATHOPHYSIOLOGY OF PORTAL-SYSTEMIC ENCEPHALOPATHY IN ALD

Despite several decades of intensive investigations, the precise pathophysiologic mechanisms responsible for PSE are incompletely understood. Theories involving the action of neurotoxic substances such as ammonia and manganese (substances which are normally removed by the liver) as well as impaired cerebral energy metabolism and neurotransmitter-related cerebral dysfunction have all been advanced. The recent advent of noninvasive techniques has provided novel additional approaches to the study of cerebral blood flow and metabolism in cirrhotic patients and the results of such studies have provided important new clues of possible pathophysiological importance in PSE (Lockwood *et al.*, 1997).

Clues from non-invasive techniques

In Positron Emission Tomography (PET) studies using $[^{18}F]$-2-fluoro-2-deoxyglucose for assessment of regional cerebral glucose metabolic rate ($CMR_{glucose}$) and $[^{15}O]H_2O$ as tracer for the study of cerebral blood flow (CBF), Lockwood *et al.* (1991a) demonstrated a redistribution of flow and metabolism from cerebral cortical regions to subcortical grey matter and cerebellar structures in cirrhotic patients with decompensated liver failure and mild PSE. A similar redistribution of CBF was reported by O'Carroll *et al.* (1991) using Single Photon Emission Tomography and in this latter study, a significant correlation was observed between the CBF changes and the degree of cognitive impairment in these patients. Lockwood *et al.* (1991a) proposed that the alterations of CBF and $CMR_{glucose}$ observed in PSE patients were the consequences of ammonia neurotoxicity. One process whereby ammonia could alter CBF is via nitric oxide-related mechanisms. Recent studies have demonstrated that portacaval anastomosis in the rat results in increased activities of nitric oxide synthase (NOS) (Raghavendra Rao *et al.*, 1995), an effect which appears to result from an ammonia-induced increase in uptake of *L*-arginine, the obligate precursor for NOS (Raghavendra Rao *et al.*, 1997a) as well as from increased NOS gene expression (Raghavendra Rao *et al.*, 1997b).

In a subsequent PET study using $[^{13}N]NH_3$ in 5 cirrhotic patients, Lockwood *et al.* (1991b) demonstrated a significant increase in the cerebral metabolic rate for ammonia (CMRA), i.e., the rate at which ammonia is taken up and metabolized by brain. Furthermore, this increased rate of ammonia uptake and metabolism by brain was found to be accompanied by increases in the permeability-surface area product (PS), a measure of blood-brain barrier permeability to ammonia, in these patients (Figure 21.2).

It was suggested that the apparent ease with which ammonia is transported into brain in chronic liver failure could explain both the hypersensitivity of cirrhotic patients to ammoniagenic conditions (such as protein loading or gastrointestinal hemorrhage) as well as the sometimes imperfect correlations observed between blood ammonia concentrations and neuropsychiatric status in these patients (Lockwood *et al.*, 1991b).

Further clues to pathophysiologic mechanisms in PSE have been provided by Magnetic Resonance Spectroscopy (MRS). ^{1}H-MRS studies in cirrhotic patients reveal a characteristic pattern of changes consisting of reduced choline and myo-inositol signals and a concomitant increase in intensity of signals assigned to the amino acids glutamate plus glutamine (Taylor-Robinson *et al.*, 1994, 1996). A significant advance in ^{1}H-MRS technology resulted in resolution of the glutamate/glutamine resonance and permitted the direct measurement of brain glutamine in cirrhotic patients (Laubenberger *et al.*, 1997). Typical patterns of the ^{1}H-MR spectra from a normal healthy volunteer compared to a cirrhotic patient with no

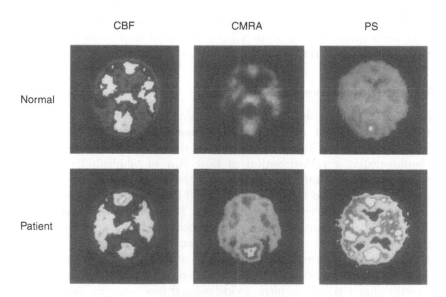

Figure 21.2 Typical PET images from a normal subject and a cirrhotic patient with mild PSE showing increased cerebral metabolic rate for ammonia (CMRA) and increased permeability-surface area product (PS). Mean values for groups of $n = 5$ controls and patients were: CMRA, controls: 0.35 ± 0.5 µmole/100 g/min; PSE patients: 0.91 ± 0.36 µmole/100 g/min $p < 0.01$; PS, controls: 0.13 ± 0.03 ml/g/min; PSE patients: 0.22 ± 0.07 ml/g/min $p < 0.05$ (From Lockwood *et al.*, 1991, with permission).

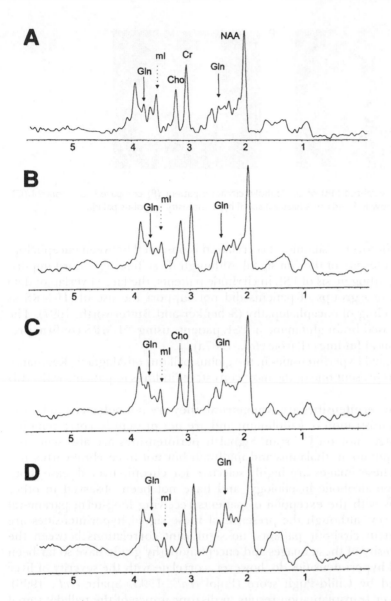

Figure 21.3 ¹H-MR spectra of gray matter structure from A: healthy control, B: asymptomatic cirrhotic patient, C: cirrhotic patient with subclinical hepatic encephalopathy, D: cirrhotic patient with overt encephalopathy. Note the progressive increase in the glutamine (Gln) resonance at 2.50 ppm with increasing severity of encephalopathy (From Laubenberger et al., 1997, with permission).

neuropsychiatric impairment, a patient with subclinical hepatic encephalopathy and a patient with overt hepatic encephalopathy are shown in Figure 21.3.

Increased intensity of the glutamine (Gln) resonance at 2.50 ppm is observed together with concomitant decreases in the myoinositol resonance at 3.60 ppm

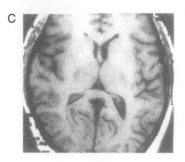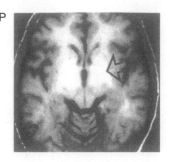

Figure 21.4 T₁ weighted MRI of an alcoholic cirrhotic patient (P) compared to a control (C). Arrow in P indicates bilateral signal hyperintensity in globus pallidus.

(Figure 21.3). Moreover, a significant correlation is observed between encephalopathy grade and intensity of the Gln signal. Although these findings afford important clues to the pathogenesis of PSE in cirrhotic patients, the large overlap of data between the various groups of patients did not support the use of ^{1}H-MRS as a tool for the grading of encephalopathy (Schenker and Butterworth, 1997). The findings of increased brain glutamine in PSE patients using ^{1}H-MRS confirm previous neurochemical findings (Lavoie *et al.*, 1987a).

T_1-weighted signal hyperintensities in the globus pallidus on Magnetic Resonance Imaging (MRI) represent one of the most consistent findings in patients with ALD (Figure 21.4).

The pallidal hyperintensities are symmetrical, they are not enhanced following intravenous administration of gadolinium and are not present in corresponding T_2-weighted images nor on CT scan. Signal hyperintensities are also seen to a lesser extent in putamen, thalamus and midbrain but not in cerebral cortex nor hippocampus. These images are highly selective for chronic liver disease (both alcoholic and non-alcoholic in etiology) and have not been observed in other clinical situations with the exception of patients receiving long-term parenteral nutrition. However, although the presence of these signal hyperintensities are highly consistent in cirrhotic patients, no significant correlations between the presence or intensity of these images and encephalopathy grade have so far been observed. Signal hyperintensities do, however, correlate with the severity of liver disease estimated by Child-Pugh score (Pujol *et al.*, 1993; Spahr *et al.*, 1996). Furthermore, liver transplantation results in disappearance of the pallidal signal hyperintensities (Pujol *et al.*, 1993), again suggesting that liver dysfunction is the primary cause.

ACCUMULATION OF NEUROTOXINS IN BRAIN IN ALD

Chronic liver disease and portal-systemic shunting result in increased blood concentrations of substances which are potentially neurotoxic. Such substances include ammonia and manganese.

Ammonia

Blood (particularly arterial) ammonia concentrations are frequently increased in alcoholic patients with PSE (see, for example, Lockwood *et al.*, 1991b). Studies in animal models of chronic liver failure reveal that brain ammonia concentrations at coma stages of encephalopathy are in the millimolar range (Butterworth, 1991). PET studies in humans with ALD and mild encephalopathy reveal increased ammonia uptake and metabolism by brain (see Figure 21.2) accompanied by alterations of regional cerebral glucose metabolism (Lockwood *et al.*, 1991a,b) where it was suggested that the altered cerebral glucose metabolism was the consequence of a toxic effect of ammonia. Ammonia may exert a deleterious effect on cerebral metabolism and function by a variety of mechanisms, both direct and indirect. Concentrations of ammonia in the 0.5 to 5 mM range directly impair postsynaptic inhibition in several brain preparations and *in vivo*; an action which results in part from a blocking action of NH_4^+ on chloride extrusion from the postsynaptic neuron (Raabe, 1989). Millimolar concentrations of ammonia also inhibit excitatory neurotransmission. In one series of experiments, synaptic transmission from Schaffer collaterals to CA1 neurons in the hippocampus was found to be depressed by 1 mM NH_4^+ (Szerb and Butterworth, 1992).

If present in sufficiently high concentrations, ammonia may ultimately result in impaired cerebral energy metabolism. Addition of ammonia in concentrations of 0.1 to 5 mM to brain preparations results in inhibition of α-ketoglutarate dehydrogenase, (Lai and Cooper, 1986) a rate-limiting tricarboxylic acid cycle enzyme. The IC_{50} for enzyme inhibition is 2 mM, well within the concentration range observed in brain in experimental PSE (Butterworth, 1991). Consistent with decreased tricarboxylic acid cycle flux, lactate concentrations are increased in brain and CSF in both human and experimental PSE (Yao *et al.*, 1987; Therrien and Butterworth 1991).

However, although glucose oxidation appears to be reduced in brain in chronic liver disease, attempts to identify an early deficit in high energy phosphates have so far yielded negative results. Studies in patients with mild PSE using ^{31}P-MRS did not show significant alterations of high energy phosphates (Taylor-Robinson *et al.*, 1994). Administration of ammonium salts to portacaval-shunted rats results in coma and in decreased brain ATP content (Hindfelt *et al.*, 1977). However, the cerebral energy deficit is only apparent after a prolonged period of coma suggesting that it is a late (preterminal) event in PSE.

Manganese

The hepatobiliary system is the major system involved in the removal of manganese. Serum manganese concentrations are increased in post-hepatitic cirrhosis and significant correlations have been observed between serum manganese concentrations and liver enzyme activities in cirrhotic patients (Versiek *et al.*, 1974; Spahr *et al.*, 1996). Serum manganese concentrations are increased in cirrhotic patients who manifest MR signal hyperintensities in globus pallidus (see Figure 21.4). Furthermore, similar pallidal MR signal hyperintensities were reported in a patient with Alagille Syndrome, an autosomal dominant disorder characterized by cholestasis, intrahepatic bile duct paucity, end-stage liver disease and increased blood manganese (Devenyi *et al.*, 1994). Similar MR signal hyperintensities have been reported in patients during total parenteral nutrition where manganese was again proposed as the causative factor (Mirowitz *et al.*, 1991). Direct measurement in pallidal samples obtained at autopsy from cirrhotic patients who died in hepatic coma reveal several-fold increases of manganese concentrations (Pomier Layrargues *et al.*, 1995a; Butterworth *et al.*, 1995); concentrations of other divalent metal ions were increased two-fold (in the case of copper) or within normal limits (in the case of zinc) (Pomier Layrargues *et al.*, 1995b). Furthermore, repeated administration of manganese to non-human primates results in T_1-weighted MR signal hyperintensity in globus pallidus similar to that observed in cirrhotic patients (Newland *et al.*, 1989) and results in Alzheimer type II astrocytosis (Pentschew *et al.*, 1963), the characteristic neuropathologic finding in PSE. Taken together, these findings strongly suggest that manganese deposition in brain is the cause of the MR signal hyperintensities and may also contribute to the neuropathologic characteristics of PSE in human ALD.

NEUROTRANSMITTER CHANGES IN BRAIN IN ALD

In common with other metabolic and degenerative disorders of the central nervous system, PSE is characterized by alterations of several neurotransmitter systems in brain. Some of these neurotransmitter changes result from a toxic effect of ammonia or manganese while others have no apparent link to either of these neurotoxins. Studies in autopsied brain tissue from patients with ALD who died in hepatic coma together with studies using material from appropriate animal models of PSE reveal alterations in expression of gene coding for key proteins involved in neurotransmitter regulation (Butterworth, 1998). Significant alterations of glutamatergic, serotoninergic and opioid neurotransmitter systems have been described in PSE (Butterworth, 1996).

It is of particular interest that these same neurotransmitter systems have consistently been implicated in the mediation of the toxic effects of chronic ethanol *per se* (in the absence of significant liver impairment) on CNS function (Shanley and Wilce, 1993). It is not surprising, therefore, that the typical alcoholic patient with end-stage liver disease may manifest a complex pattern of neuropsychiatric abnormalities. Some of these, no doubt, result from the deleterious effects of chronic ethanol consumption (and associated nutritional factors such as thiamine deficiency), while others result from the effects of liver failure.

Glutamate

In 1990, Schmidt and co-workers reported a dose-dependent inhibition of uptake of D-aspartate (a non-metabolizable analog transported by the *L*-glutamate transport system) into rat hippocampal slices exposed to blood extracts from patients with PSE. Furthermore, the relative potency of inhibition of *D*-aspartate uptake was significantly correlated with ammonia concentrations of the blood extracts from these patients. Other studies demonstrated increased glutamate concentrations in the extracellular fluid of brain in rats following end-to-side portacaval anastomosis (Moroni *et al.*, 1983; Butterworth *et al.*, 1991) a finding which again suggested a deficit of glutamate uptake in PSE. Alterations of glutamate receptors have been reported in experimental animal models of PSE. In dogs with PSE resulting from congenital portosystemic shunts, increased cerebrospinal fluid glutamate concentrations (Butterworth *et al.*, 1997) and a significant loss of glutamate receptor densities (Maddison *et al.*, 1991) were reported. Portacaval-shunted rats manifest a selective loss of *N*-methyl-*D*-aspartate (NMDA) receptors in brain (Peterson *et al.*, 1990).

Serotonin

Many of the neuropsychiatric symptoms in early PSE such as personality changes, altered affect and sleep disorders are signs which have classically been attributed to changes in serotonin (5HT)-mediated neurotransmission. The degree of reduction of CBF in alcoholic cirrhotic patients with subclinical PSE is negatively correlated with plasma concentrations of free tryptophan (Rodriguez *et al.*, 1987), the amino acid precursor of 5HT. Cerebrospinal fluid concentrations of *L*-tryptophan are increased in alcoholic patients in hepatic coma (Young *et al.*, 1995) and increased concentrations of 5-hydroxyindoleacetic acid (5HIAA), the final metabolite of 5HT, are increased in the brains of alcoholic patients who died in hepatic coma (Bergeron *et al.*, 1989). These latter changes were accompanied by increased activities ((Raghavendra Rao *et al.*, 1993) and gene expression (Mousseau *et al.*, 1997)) of the 5HT-metabolizing enzyme MAO_A (Raghavendra Rao *et al.*, 1993) and increased binding sites for the postsynaptic $5HT_2$ binding site ligand ^{3}H-ketanserin (Raghavendra Rao and Butterworth, 1994). Taken together, these findings suggest that ALD results in alterations of 5HT receptor-mediated neurotransmission.

The opioid system

Patients with ALD are hypersensitive to morphine (Laidlaw *et al.*, 1961) and portacaval anastomosis in the rat results in increased pain sensitivity (Salomon *et al.*, 1976), a phenomenon in which the endogenous opioid system is implicated. Brain extracts from portacaval-shunted rats contain a modified distribution of the endogenous opioid peptide β-endorphin (Panerai *et al.*, 1982). β-endorphin is synthesized mainly in neurons of the arcuate nucleus of the hypothalamus with projections to nuclei involved in pain modulation, memory function as well as in the mediation of the positive-reinforcing effects of alcohol (Routtenberg, 1976). Portacaval-shunted rats drink significantly more alcohol in a free-choice drinking paradigm (Figure 21.5), a behavior which starts within 1 week of portacaval anastomosis surgery (De Waele *et al.*, 1996, 1997).

Autoradiographic studies of brain sections from shunted animals revealed region-selective alterations of μ and δ opioid receptors (De Waele *et al.*, 1996). Furthermore, the increased alcohol preference ratio resulting from portacaval shunting was found to be significantly attenuated by administration of the opioid antagonist naloxone (De Waele *et al.*, 1997). It was proposed that the increased

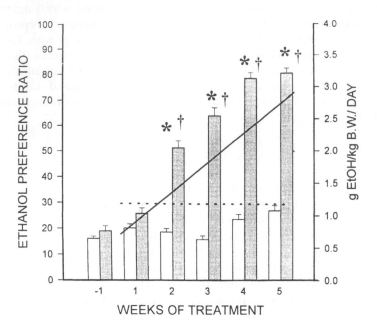

Figure 21.5 Portacaval anastomosis (PCA) results in increased alcohol consumption in rats in a free choice paradigm. Data indicate the ethanol preference ratio (5% ethanol solution versus water) at various times prior to and following PCA surgery (filled bars) or sham operation (open bars). Solid and broken lines indicate the slope of the changes. Significant difference between PCA and sham-operated values indicated by * $p < 0.01$. Significant differences from pre-surgery values indicated by † $p < 0.01$ by analysis of variance (from De Waele *et al.*, 1997, with permission).

alcohol preference following portacaval shunting was the consequence of modifications of the endogenous opioid system. Extrapolation of these findings to humans would suggest that the development of significant ALD could lead to increased alcohol consumption via a mechanism involving the endogenous opioid system.

The "peripheral-type" benzodiazepine receptor

The "peripheral-type" benzodiazepine receptor (PTBR) in brain is a hetero-oligomeric complex located predominantly on the outer mitochondrial membrane of astrocytes. The PTBR is not allosterically coupled to GABA receptors nor to chloride channels. Densities of binding sites for the PTBR ligand ^{3}H-PK11195 are significantly increased in autopsied brain tissue from patients with ALD who died in hepatic coma (Lavoie *et al.*, 1990). Increased ^{3}H-PK11195 binding sites have also been reported in the brains of rats following portacaval anastomosis where both increased binding densities (Raghavendra Rao *et al.*, 1994) and increased PTBR gene expression (Desjardins *et al.*, 1997) have been described.

There is evidence to suggest that both ammonia and manganese may be the causative factors in the increased PTBR expression in brain in PSE. Chronic hyperammonemia resulting from an inherited defect of the urea cycle enzyme ornithine transcarbamylase results in increased PTBR sites in brain (Raghavendra Rao *et al.*, 1993) and exposure of primary astrocytes to pathophysiologic concentrations of ammonia (Itzhak and Norenberg, 1994) or manganese (Hazell *et al.*, 1997) likewise result in increased densities of PTBR sites.

Although the precise role of increased PTBRs in the pathogenesis of PSE remains unclear, one possibility may involve the production of neurosteroids (Figure 21.6). Diazepam Binding Inhibitor (DBI) is an endogenous neuropeptide which is elevated in concentration in the CSF of patients with severe ALD and a positive correlation has been described between CSF DBI levels and severity of encephalopathy in these patients (Rothstein *et al.*, 1989). DBI acts on the PTBR to stimulate cholesterol transport and hence facilitates the synthesis of neurosteroids, some of which are potent GABA receptor agonists (Puia *et al.*, 1989). DBI is stored in selective populations of astrocytes in the central nervous system where it is colocalized with PTBR and, as both DBI concentrations as well as PTBR sites are increased in human ALD, it is likely that neurosteroids are produced in brain in ALD which may act as endogenous modulators of GABAergic neurotransmission. In this way, PTBR activation by ammonia or manganese could contribute to the pathogenesis of PSE in patients with ALD.

DBI expression in brain is also increased during alcohol withdrawal and it has been suggested that this may relate to the withdrawal signs as well as to the abstinence syndrome characterized by anxiety and insomnia (Katsura *et al.*, 1995).

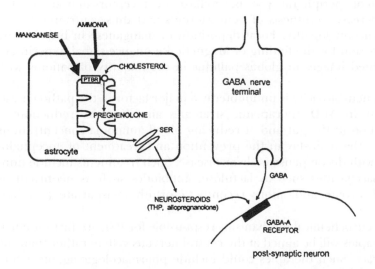

Figure 21.6 Schematic representation of the action of ammonia or manganese on the mitochondrial "peripheral-type" benzodiazepine receptor (PTBR) to stimulate cholesterol uptake and hence the synthesis of neurosteroids, some of which are potent positive allosteric modulators of the GABA$_A$ receptor in brain.

Nitric oxide

Portacaval anastomosis in the rat results in increased neuronal nitric oxide synthase (nNOS) gene expression (Raghavendra Rao *et al.*, 1997a). Increased nNOS nRNA was accompanied by increased nNOS protein (Raghavendra Rao *et al.*, 1997b) and increased NOS catalytic activities (Raghavendra Rao *et al.*, 1995). The cause of increased NOS activities in brain in chronic liver failure is unknown but evidence suggests that ammonia may be implicated. Exposure of synaptosomal preparations to ammonia results in increased high affinity uptake of *L*-arginine, the obligate precursor for NOS (Raghavendra Rao *et al.*, 1997b). Alterations of NOS activity could be responsible for the redistribution of cerebral blood flow in ALD (Lockwood *et al.*, 1991a).

SUMMARY AND THERAPEUTIC IMPLICATIONS

In summary, there is a growing body of evidence that liver disease *per se* contributes to the cognitive dysfunction in chronic alcoholism. Severe ALD and its associated portal-systemic shunting results in the accumulation of toxic subtances such as manganese and ammonia in brain. Recent studies using non-invasive techniques reveal significant redistribution of cerebral blood flow and metabolism in patients with ALD together with evidence of increased permeability of the blood-brain barrier to ammonia in these patients. Studies in autopsied brain tissue from patients with ALD provide evidence for alterations of both excitatory and inhibitory neurotransmitter systems, particularly the glutamate, serotonin and opioid systems. Activation of "peripheral-type" benzodiazepine receptors in brain in ALD could result in increased synthesis of neurosteroids and thus contribute to the pathogenesis of encephalopathy. Focal deposition of manganese in brain is the most likely explanation for the finding of Magnetic Resonance signal hyperintensities on T_1-weighted images in globus pallidus in the majority of patients with severe ALD.

Since ammonia neurotoxicity is undoubtedly a major factor in the pathogenesis of encephalopathy in ALD, therapeutic strategies aimed at the reduction of ammonia production in the gut and at reducing blood ammonia concentrations remain, therefore, the mainstay in the prevention and treatment of encephalopathy in patients with decompensated liver disease. Such treatments include non-metabolizable disaccharides such as lactulose, antibiotics such as neomycin as well as sodium benzoate and, more recently, *L*-ornithine-aspartate (Kircheis *et al.*, 1997).

As the precise neurochemical mechanisms responsible for PSE are further elucidated, future therapies will be aimed at the central nervous system rather than the gastrointestinal tract. Such therapies could include pharmacologic agents acting on monoaminergic and amino acid neurotransmitter systems. Additional studies are therefore required to more precisely define these neurotransmitter systems and to develop appropriate pharmacologic agents. Chelation therapy to remove manganese has also been suggested.

ACKNOWLEDGMENTS

Studies from the author's research unit were funded by grants from CIHR and the Canadian Liver Foundation. The author is grateful to Dominique D. Roy for her help with the preparation of the manuscript.

REFERENCES

Abe, T. and Itokawa, Y. (1977) Effect of ethanol administration on thiamine metabolism and transketolase activity in rats. *Int J Vit Nutr Res* **47**, 307–314.

Acker, W., Aps, E.J., Majumdar, S.K., Shaw, G.K. and Thomson, A.D. (1982) The relationship between brain and liver damage in chronic alcoholic patients. *J Neurol Neurosurg Psychiat* **45**, 984–987.

Arria, A.M., Tarter, R.E., Starzl, T.W. and Van Thiel, D.H. (1991) Improvement in cognitive functioning of alcoholics following orthotopic liver transplantation. *Alcoholism Clin Exp Res* **15**, 956–962.

Bergeron, M., Reader, T.A., Pomier Layrargues, G. and Butterworth, R.F. (1989) Monoamines and metabolites in autopsied brain tissue from cirrhotic patients with hepatic encephalopathy. *Neurochem Res* **14**, 853–859.

Bitsch, R., Hansen, J. and Hotzel, D. (1982) Thiamin metabolism in the rat during long-term alcohol administration. *Int J Vit Nutr Res* **52**, 125–132.

Butterworth, R.F., Le, O., Lavoie, J. and Szerb, J.C. (1991) Effect of portacaval anastomosis on electrically-stimulated release of glutamate from rat hippocampal slices. *J Neurochem* **56**, 1481–1484.

Butterworth, R.F. (1992) Pathogenesis and treatment of portal-systemic encephalopathy: an update. *Digest Dis Sci* **37**, 321–327.

Butterworth, R.F., Kril, J.J. and Harper, C.G. (1993) Thiamine-dependent enzyme changes in the brains of alcoholics: relationship to the Wernicke-Korsakoff Syndrome. *Alcohol Clin Exp Res* **17**, 1084–1088.

Butterworth, R.F. (1995a) Hepatic Encephalopathy. *The Neurologist* **1**, 95–104.

Butterworth, R.F. (1995b) Pathophysiology of alcoholic brain damage: synergistic effects of ethanol, thiamine deficiency and alcoholic liver disease. *Metab Brain Dis* **10**, 1–9.

Butterworth, R.F., Spahr, L., Fontaine, S. and Pomier Layrargues, G. (1995) Manganese toxicity, dopaminergic dysfunction and hepatic encephalopathy. *Metab Brain Dis* **4**, 259–267.

Butterworth, R.F. (1996) The neurobiology of hepatic encephalopathy. *Semin Liver Dis* **16**, 235–244.

Butterworth, J., Gregory, C.R. and Aronson, L.R. (1997) Selective alterations of cerebrospinal fluid amino acids in dogs with congenital portosystemic shunts. *Metab Brain Dis* **12**, 299–306.

Butterworth, R.F. (1998) Alterations of neurotransmitter-related gene expression in human and experimental portal-systemic encephalopathy. *Metab Brain Dis* **13**, 339–347.

Cavanagh, J.B., Lewis, P.D., Blakemore, W.F. and Kyu, M. (1972) Changes in the cerebellar cortex in rats after portocaval anastomosis. *J Neurol Sci* **15**, 13–26.

Desjardins, P., Bandeira, P., Raghavendra Rao, V.L., Ledoux, S. and Butterworth, R.F. (1997) Increased expression of the peripheral-type benzodiazepine receptor-isoquinoline carboxamide binding protein in mRNA brain following portacaval anastomosis. *Brain Res* **758**, 255–258.

Devenyi, A.G., Barron, T.F. and Mamourian, A.C. (1994) Dystonia, hyperintense basal ganglia, and high whole blood manganese levels in Alagille's syndrome. *Gastroenterology* **106**, 1068–1071.

De Waele, J.P., Audet, R.M., Leong, D.K. and Butterworth, R.F. (1996) Portacaval anastomosis induces region-selective alterations of the endogenous opioid system in the rat brain. *Hepatology* **24**, 895–901.

De Waele, J.P., Audet, R.M., Rose, C. and Butterworth, R.F. (1997) The portacaval-shunted rat: a new model for the study of the mechanisms controlling voluntary ethanol consumption and ethanol dependence. *Alcoholism Clin & Exp Res* **21**, 305–310.

Diemer, N.H., Klee, J., Schroder, H. and Klinken, L. (1977) Glial and nerve cell changes in rats with porto-caval anastomosis. *Acta Neuropath (Berl.)* **39**, 59–68.

Eng, L.F. (1985) Glial fibrillary acidic protein (GFAP): the major protein of glial intermediate filaments in differentiated astrocytes. *J Neuroimmunol* **8**, 203–214.

Hazell, A.S., Desjardins, P. and Butterworth, R.F. (1999) Chronic exposure of primary astrocyte cultures to manganese results in increased binding sites for "peripheral-type" benzodiazepine receptor ligands ^{3}H-PK 11195. *Neurosci Lett* **271**, 5–8.

Hindfelt, B., Plum, F. and Duffy, T.E. (1977) Effects of acute ammonia intoxication on cerebral metabolism in rats with portacaval shunts. *J Clin Invest* **59**, 386–396.

Hockerstedt, K., Kajaste, S., Muuronen, A., Raininko, R., Seppalainen, A.-M. and Hillbom, M. (1992) Encephalopathy and neuropathy in end-stage liver disease before and after liver transplantation. *J Hepatol* **16**, 31–37.

Itzhak, Y. and Norenberg, M.D. (1994) Ammonia-induced upregulation of peripheral-type benzodiazepine receptors in cultured astrocytes labeled with ^{3}H-PK11195. *Neurosci Lett* **177**, 35–38.

Kardel, T. and Stigsby, B. (1975) Period-amplitude analysis of the electroencephalogram correlated with liver function in patients with cirrhosis of the liver. *Electroenceph Clin Neurophysiol* **38**, 605–609.

Kircheis, G., Nilius, R., Held, C., Berndt, H., Buchner, M., Görtelmeyer, R., Hendricks, R., Kruger, B., Kuklinski, B., Meister, H., Otto, H.-J., Rink, C., Rosch, W. and Stauch, S. (1997) Therapeutic efficacy of *L*-ornithine-*L*-aspartate infusions in patients with cirrhosis and hepatic encephalopathy: results of a placebo-controlled, double-blind. *Hepatology* **25**, 1351–1360.

Katsura, M., Ohkuma, S., Tsujimura, A. and Kuriyama, K. (1995) Increase of diazepam binding inhibitor mRNA levels in the brains of chronically ethanol-treated and -withdrawn mice. *J Pharmacol Exp Therap* **273**, 1529–1533.

Kril, J.J. and Butterworth, R.F. (1997) Diencephalic and cerebellar pathology in alcoholic and nonalcoholic patients with end-stage liver disease. *Hepatology* **26**, 837–841.

Kril, J.J., Flowers, D. and Butterworth, R.F. (1997) Distinctive pattern of Bergmann glial pathology in human hepatic encephalopathy. *Mol Chem Neuropathol* **31**, 279–287.

Lai, J.C.K. and Cooper, A.J.L. (1986) Brain α-ketoglutarate dehydrogenase: kinetic properties, regional distribution and effects of inhibitors. *J Neurochem* **47**, 1376–1386.

Laidlaw, R., Read, A.E. and Sherlock, S. (1961) Morphine tolerance in hepatic cirrhosis. *Gastroenterology* **40**, 389–396.

Lavoie, J., Giguère, J.F., Pomier Layrargues, G. and Butterworth, R.F. (1987a) Amino acid changes in autopsied brain tissue from cirrhotic patients with hepatic encephalopathy. *J Neurochem* **49**, 692–697.

Lavoie, J., Giguère, J.F., Pomier Layrargues, G. and Butterworth, R.F. (1987b) Activities of neuronal and astrocytic marker enzymes in autopsied brain tissue from patients with hepatic encephalopathy. *Metab Brain Dis* **2**, 283–290.

Lavoie, J., Pomier Layrargues, G. and Butterworth, R.F. (1990) Increased densities of peripheral-type benzodiazepine receptors in brain autopsy samples from cirrhotic patients with hepatic encephalopathy. *Hepatology* **11**, 874–878.

Lavoie, J. and Butterworth, R.F. (1995) Reduced activities of thiamine-dependent enzymes in brains of alcoholics in the absence of Wernicke's Encephalopathy. *Alcohol Clin & Exp Res* **19**, 1073–1077.

Laubenberger, J., Haussinger, D., Boyer, S., Guffer, H., Henning, J. and Lange, M. (1997) Proton magnetic resonance spectroscopy of brain in symptomatic and asymptomatic patients with liver cirrhosis. *Gastroenterology* **112**, 1610–1616.

Lockwood, A.H., Yap, E.W.H., Rhoades, H.M. and Wong, W. (1991a) Altered cerebral blood flow and glucose metabolism in patients with liver disease and minimal encephalopathy. *J Cerebral Blood Flow Metab* **11**, 331–336.

Lockwood, A.H., Yap, E.W.H. and Wong, W.-H. (1991b) Cerebral ammonia metabolism in patients with severe liver disease and minimal hepatic encephalopathy. *J Cerebral Blood Flow Metab* **11**, 337–341.

Lockwood, A., Weissenborn, K. and Butterworth, R.F. (1997) An image of the brain in patients with liver disease. *Current Opinion in Neurology* **10**, 525–533.

Maddison, J.E., Watson, W.E.J., Dodd, P.R. and Johnston, G.A.R. (1991) Alterations in cortical ^{3}H-kainate and α-^{3}H-amino-3-hydroxy -5-methyl-4-isoxazolepropionic acid binding in a spontaneous canine model of chronic hepatic encephalopathy. *J Neurochem* **56**, 1881–1888.

Menegaux, F., Keeffe, E.B., Andrews, B.T., Egawa, H., Monge, H., Concepcion, W. So, S.K. *et al.* (1994) Neurological complications of liver transplantation in adult versus pediatric patients. *Transplantation* **58**, 447–450.

Mirowitz, S.A., Westrich, J.J. and Hirsch, J.D. (1991) Hyperintense basal ganglia on T_1-weighted MR images in patients receiving parenteral nutrition. *Radiology* **181**, 177–120.

Moroni, F., Lombardi, G., Moneti, G. and Cortesini, C. (1983) The release and neosynthesis of glutamic acid are increased in experimental models of hepatic encephalopathy. *J Neurochem* **40**, 850–854.

Mousseau, D.D., Baker, G.B. and Butterworth, R.F. (1997) Increased density of catalytic sites and expression of brain monoamine oxidase A in humans with hepatic encephalopathy. *J Neurochem* **68**, 1200–1208.

Newland, M.C., Ceckler, T.L., Kordower, J.H. and Weiss, B. (1989) Visualizing manganese in the primate basal ganglial with magnetic resonance imaging. *Exp Neurol* **106**, 251–258.

O'Carroll, R.E., Hayes, P.C., Ebmeier, K.P., Dougall, N., Murray, C., Best, J.J.K., Bouchier, I.A.D. and Goodwin, G.W. (1991) Regional cerebral blood flow and cognitive function in patients with chronic liver disease. *Lancet* **337**, 1250–1253.

Panerai, A.E., Salerno, F., Baldissera, F., Martini, A., DiGiulio, A.M. and Mantegazza, P. (1982) Brain β-endorphin concentrations in experimental chronic liver disease. *Brain Res* **247**, 188–190.

Pentschew, A., Ebner, F. and Kovatch, R. (1963) Experimental manganese encephalopathy in monkeys: a preliminary report. *J Neuropathol Exp Neurol* **22**, 488–499.

Peterson, C., Giguère, J.F., Cotman, C.W. and Butterworth, R.F. (1990) Selective loss of *N*-methyl-*D*-aspartate-sensitive *L*-^{3}H-glutamate binding sites in rat brain following portacaval anastomosis. *J Neurochem* **55**, 386–390.

Pomier Layrargues, G., Huu Nguyen, N., Faucher, C., Giguère, J.F. and Butterworth, R.F. (1991) Subclinical hepatic encephalopathy in cirrhotic patients: prevalence and relationship to liver function. *Can J Gastroenterol* **5**, 121–125.

Pomier Layrargues, G., Spahr, L. and Butterworth, R.F. (1995a) Increased manganese concentrations in pallidum of cirrhotic patients: cause of magnetic resonance hyperintensity? *Lancet* **345**, 735.

Pomier Layrargues, G., Shapcott, D., Spahr, L. and Butterworth, R.F. (1995b) Accumulation of manganese and copper in pallidum of cirrhotic patients: Role in the pathogenesis of the hepatic encephalopathy? *Metab Brain Dis* **4**, 351–354.

Pomier Layrargues, G. (1996) TIPS and hepatic encephalopathy. In *Semin Liver Dis*, edited by M.A. Rothschild, P.D. Berk, A.T. Blei and R.F. Butterworth. New York: Thieme Medical Publishers, Inc.

Pujol, A., Pujol, J., Graus, F., Rimola, A., Peri, J., Mercader, J.M., Garcia-Pagan, J.C., Bosch, J. Rodés, J. and Tolosa, E. (1993) Hyperintense globus pallidus on T_1-weighted MRI in cirrhotic patients is associated with severity of liver failure. *Neurology* **43**, 65–69.

Puia, G., Santi, M.R., Vicini, S., Pritchett, D.B., Seeburg, P.H. and Costa, E. (1989) Differences in the negative allosteric modulation of GABA receptors elicited by 4'-chlorodiazepam and by a β-carboline-3-carboxylate ester: a study with natural and reconstituted receptors. *Proc Nat Acad Sci USA* **86**, 7275–7279.

Raabe, W.A. (1989) Neurophysiology of ammonia intoxication. In *Hepatic Encephalopathy: Pathophysiology and Treatment*, edited by R.F. Butterworth and G. Pomier Layrargues, pp. 49–77. Clifton, NJ: Humana Press.

Raghavendra Rao, V.L., Giguère, J.F., Pomier Layrargues, G. and Butterworth, R.F. (1993) Increased activities of MAO_A and MAO_B in autopsied brain tissue from cirrhotic patients with hepatic encephalopathy. *Brain Res* **621**, 349–352.

Raghavendra Rao, V.L., Audet, R., Therrien, G. and Butterworth, R.F. (1994) Tissue specific alterations of binding sites for the peripheral-type benzodiazepine receptor ligand ^{3}H-PK11195 in rats following portacaval anastomosis. *Digest Dis Sci* **39**, 1055–1063.

Raghavendra Rao, V.L. and Butterworth, R.F. (1994) Alterations of [^{3}H]8-OH-DPAT and [^{3}H]-ketanserin binding sites in autopsied brain tissue from cirrhotic patients with hepatic encephalopathy. *Neurosci Lett* **182**, 69–72.

Raghavendra Rao, V.L., Audet, R.M. and Butterworth, R.F. (1995) Selective alterations of extracellular brain amino acids in relation to function in experimental portal-systemic encephalopathy: results of an *in vivo* microdialysis study. *J Neurochem* **65**, 1221–1228.

Raghavendra Rao, V.L., Audet, R.M. and Butterworth, R.F. (1997a) Increased neuronal nitric oxide synthase expression in brain following portacaval anastomosis. *Brain Res* **765**, 169–172.

Raghavendra Rao, V.L., Audet, R.M. and Butterworth, R.F. (1997b) Portacaval shunting and hyperammonemia stimulate the uptake of L-^{3}H-arginine but not of L-^{3}H-nitroarginine into rat brain synaptosomes. *J Neurochem* **68**, 337–343.

Raghavendra Rao, V.L. and Butterworth, R.F. (1998) Neuronal nitric oxide synthase and hepatic encephalopathy. *Metab Brain Dis* **12**, 175–189.

Rodriguez, G., Testa, R., Celle, G. *et al.* (1987) Reduction of cerebral blood flow in subclinical hepatic encephalopathy and its correlation with plasma-free tryptophan. *J Cereb Blood Flow Metab* **7**, 768–772.

Rothstein, J.D., McKhann, G., Guarneri, P., Barbaccia, M.L., Guidotti, A. and Costa, E. (1989) Hepatic encephalopathy and cerebrospinal fluid content of diazepam binding inhibitor (DBI). *Ann Neurol* **26**, 57–62.

Routtenberg, A. (1976) Self-stimulation pathways: orgins and terminations – a three stage technique. In *Brain-Stimulation Reward*, edited by A. Wauquier and B.J. Rolls, pp. 31–39. Amsterdam: Elsevier.

Salomon, F., Beaubernard, C., Thangapregassam, M.J., Grange, D. and Bismuth, H. (1976) Encéphalopathie hépatique expérimentale. II – Étude de la réaction à la douleur chez le rat avec anastomose porto-cave. *Biol Gastroenterol* **9**, 105–108.

Schenker, S. and Butterworth, R.F. (1997) Proton magnetic resonance spectroscopy in the diagnosis and pathogenesis of hepatic encephalopathy of cirrhosis, are we there yet? *Gastroenterology* **112**, 2758–2761.

Schomerus, H., Hamster, W., Blunck, H. *et al.* (1981) Latent portasystemic encephalopathy. I. Nature of cerebral function defects and their effect on fitness to drive. *Dig Dis Sci* **26**, 622–630.

Shanley, B.C. and Wilce, P.A. (1993) Receptor changes associated with ethanol-induced brain damage. In *Alcohol-Induced Brain Damage*, edited by W.A. Hunt and S.J. Nixon, NIAAA Research Monograph **22**, 299–324.

Sobel, R.A., DeArmond, S.J., Forno, L.S. and Eng, L.F. (1981) Glial fibrillary acidic protein in hepatic encephalopathy. An immunohistochemical study. *J Neuropathol Exp Neurol* **40**, 625–632.

Soffer, D., Sherman, Y., Tur-Kaspa, R. and Eid, A. (1995) Acquired hepatocerebral degeneration in a liver transplant recipient. *Acta Neuropathol* **90**, 107–111.

Somogyi, J.C., Kopp, P.M., Filippini, L. and Monnat, A. (1980) Transketolase-TPP-effect in chronic alcoholics with various degrees of liver cirrhosis. *J Nutr Sci Vitaminol* **26**, 221–229.

Spahr, L., Butterworth, R.F., Fontaine, S., Bui, L., Therrien, G., Milette, P.C., Lebrun, L.H., Zayed, J., Leblanc, A. and Pomier Layrargues, G. (1996) Increased blood manganese in cirrhotic patients: relationship to pallidal magnetic resonance signal hyperintensity and neurological symptoms. *Hepatology* **24**, 1116–1120.

Szerb, J.C. and Butterworth, R.F. (1992) Effect of ammonium ions on synaptic transmission in the mammalian central nervous system. *Progress in Neurobiology* **39**, 135–153.

Tarter, R.E., Hegedus, A.M., van Thiel, D.H. and Schade, R.R. (1985) Portal-systemic encephalopathy: neuropsychiatric manifestations. *Int J Psychiatr In Med* **15**, 1985–1986.

Tarter, R.E., Arria, A. and Van Thiel, D.H. (1993) Liver-brain interactions in alcoholism. In *Mechanisms and Therapeutic Strategies*, NIAAA Monograph **21**, 415–429.

Taylor-Robinson, S.D., Sargentoni, J., Mallalieu, R.J., Bell, J.D., Bryant, D.J., Coutts, G.A. and Morgan, M.Y. (1994) Cerebral phosphorus[31] magnetic resonance spectroscopy in patients with chronic hepatic encephalopathy. *Hepatology* **20**, 1173–1178.

Taylor-Robinson, S.D., Sargentoni, J., Oatridge, A., Bryant, D.J., Hajnal, J.V., Marcus, C.D., Seery, J.P., Hodgson, H.J.F. and deSouza, N.M. (1996) MR Imaging and spectroscopy of the basal ganglia in chronic liver disease: correlation of T_1-weighted contrast measurements with abnormalities in proton and phosphorus-[31] MR spectra. *Metab Brain Dis* **11**, 249–268.

Therrien, G. and Butterworth, R.F. (1991) Cerebrospinal fluid amino acids in relation to neurological status in experimental portal-systemic encephalopathy. *Metab Brain Dis* **6**, 65–74.

Versieck, J., Barbier, F., Speecke, A. and Hoste, J. (1974) Manganese, copper and zinc concentrations in serum and packed blood cells during acute hepatitis, chronic hepatitis and posthepatic cirrhosis. *Clin Chem* **20**, 1141–1145.

Victor, M., Adams, R.D. and Cole, M. (1965) The Acquired (non-Wilsonian) type of chronic hepatocerebral degeneration. *In Medicine* **44**, 345–396.

Yao, H., Sadoshima, S., Fujii, K., Kusada, K., Ishitsuka, T., Tamaki, K. and Fujishima, M. (1987) Cerebrospinal fluid lactate in patients with hepatic encephalopathy. *Eur Neurol* **27**, 182–187.

Young, S.N., Lal, S., Feldmuller, F., Aranoff, A. and Martin, J.B. (1975) Relationships between tryptophan in serum and CSF and 5-hydroxyindoleacetic acid in CSF of man: effects of cirrhosis of the liver and probenecid administration. *J Neurol Neurosurg Psychiat* **38**, 322–330.

Part VI

Management

Chapter 22

General management of alcoholic liver disease

Martin Phillips and John O'Grady

Alcoholic liver disease is increasing in incidence in hospital and general practice. The management strategies for ascites, varices and variceal hemorrhage have all undergone important changes in recent years. We discuss the current use of therapeutic paracentesis, variceal banding ligation and transjugular intrahepatic porto-systemic shunting. Nutritional support is recommended early for many hospitalized patients with alcoholic liver disease. In particular, it is now recognized that protein restriction is not necessary in the vast majority of patients with encephalopathy. Many patients also have coexisting other end organ damage. We briefly discuss cardiac and pancreatic disease due to alcohol excess. These factors are important in the patient who is being considered for orthotopic liver transplantation. Critically ill patients with alcoholic liver disease are perceived to fare poorly in the intensive care unit. We review the data on this and share some of our own observations. Finally, we have some suggestions concerning the challenge of general medical and nursing care of patients with alcoholic liver disease. It should be stressed that the fundamental aspect of the management of alcoholic liver disease remains abstinence from alcohol.

KEYWORDS: alcoholic liver disease, portal hypertension, hepatic encephalopathy, nutrition, intensive care, general medical care

INTRODUCTION

The complications of alcohol excess and alcoholism are common underlying causes of referral to a wide variety of medical services. It has been estimated that in the United States approximately 40% of medical and surgical admissions to hospital have alcohol problems accounting for more than 15% of healthcare costs, and that there are 100,000 deaths annually directly related to alcohol abuse (Lieber, 1995). Alcoholic cirrhosis accounts for approximately 11,500 of these deaths (McCullough and O'Connor, 1998). In England and Wales, an estimated 33,000 premature deaths occur related to alcohol consumption annually. In 1994, there were approximately 1,300 deaths from alcoholic liver disease in patients under the age of 65 (Davies *et al.*, 1992). In the UK, it was recently reported that 1.3% of general practice consultations and 12.5% of emergency department attendances had a recognized alcohol problem, and 25% of intensive care unit admissions were alcohol-related (Pirmohamed and Gilmore, 2000). The estimated economic cost to the UK is approximately £10 billion per year. Some of these admissions are the result of acute "binge" drinking episodes. Others represent those with chronic alcoholism of which many will display features of problem drinking behavior or alcohol dependency. Clinically significant alcoholic liver disease (ALD) will only develop in a minority of chronic alcoholics.

Epidemiological studies consistently show that the prevalence of ALD is related to the availability and affordability of alcohol (Lelbach, 1976; Corrao *et al.*, 1997). Almost every chronic heavy alcohol user will develop alcoholic fatty liver but this is a relatively benign condition. Only 10–35% will ever experience a recognized episode of acute alcoholic hepatitis and only 8–20% will go on to develop cirrhosis (Lelbach, 1976). The vast majority of patients presenting with these more serious forms of ALD have had several previous attendances to general practitioners or hospital with alcohol-related problems. In many of these cases the role of alcohol was not recognized by the attending physician. Patients with ALD are often difficult to manage and demand extensive practitioner time and health service resources.

DIAGNOSIS OF ALD

The diagnosis of ALD is often not straightforward. Many patients are less than forthcoming with regard to their level of alcohol consumption. Medical practitioners in general are poor at eliciting and recording an accurate alcohol history (Kitchens, 1994). In addition it is increasingly clear that there is great inter-individual variation in the amount of alcohol consumption required to place a patient at risk of ALD. This probably occurs due to genetic predisposition to ALD although this hypothesis has not yet been proven. There is also a tendency to make a presumed diagnosis of ALD in a patient with significant alcohol consumption that often transpires to be incorrect on subsequent investigation.

From epidemiological studies it has been estimated that alcohol consumption of 80 g/day for 10–12 years is necessary for cirrhosis to develop in men, but the threshold is only 60 g/day in women (Lelbach, 1976). The average "cirrhotogenic" dose has been calculated to be 180 g ethanol/day consumed regularly over 25 years. One standard unit contains approximately 10 g of alcohol. The diagnosis can only be made in the absence of other causes of chronic liver disease. This usually entails clinical examination, blood tests and abdominal ultrasound as screening tests. Classical clinical features include parotid enlargement, pseudo-Cushingoid appearance, hypertension, gout, Dupuytren's contractures, prominent spider nevi, gynecomastia, testicular atrophy and proximal myopathy. Characteristic laboratory features of ALD include elevated gamma-glutamyltransferase, macrocytosis, plasma aspartate transaminase greater than alanine transaminase (ratio 2:1), hypertriglyceridemia, hyperuricemia, elevated immunoglobulin A levels and fatty hepatomegaly on ultrasound. Usually the transaminases are relatively low and even in a severe alcoholic hepatitis rarely rise to more than 400 IU/l.

Ultimately the diagnosis of ALD can only be confirmed on liver biopsy. Many patients who are assumed to have ALD will turn out to have cofactors for liver disease, the most common examples being viral hepatitis (hepatitis B or C), auto-immune hepatitis, homozygous or heterozygous state for hereditary hemochromatosis, and alpha 1-antitrypsin deficiency. Often these diagnoses are missed in the absence of liver histology. In addition there is notoriously poor correlation between clinical features, biochemical results and liver histology. For example, relatively asymptomatic patients may be found to have histologically advanced cirrhosis or severe alcoholic hepatitis. Clearly liver biopsy is not always necessary, particularly in end-stage chronic liver disease (CLD) associated with coagulopathy, thrombocytopenia or ascites when the risks of the procedure may outweigh the potential benefits. Clinically decompensated disease carries a poor prognosis irrespective of the histological features, but particularly in the context of severe alcoholic hepatitis liver biopsy may be desirable in order to confirm the diagnosis prior to the commencement of corticosteroid therapy which may have potentially serious complications. Many would argue that where the clinical diagnosis is secure liver biopsy is not mandatory (McCullough and O'Connor, 1998). However, when there is any doubt about the diagnosis, or in early presentations of ALD, histology is recommended to confirm the diagnosis, accurately stage the disease and to be able to give a prognosis (McCullough and O'Connor, 1998).

Once a diagnosis has been made abstinence from alcohol must be strongly advised. Despite modern advances in the medical management of CLD, abstinence remains the key to the management of ALD. The reason for this is clear from the natural history of cirrhosis. In a six year follow up study of 1,155 patients presenting with cirrhosis (33% due to ALD), continued alcohol abuse was identified as an independent predictor of death in those patients presenting with decompensated CLD (D'Amico et al., 1986).

MANAGEMENT OF PORTAL HYPERTENSION

The management of portal hypertension complicating ALD is similar to that for other causes of CLD with one exception: portal hypertension improves significantly with abstinence from alcohol. The mechanisms behind this phenomenon remain to be fully elucidated. Clinically portal hypertension is complicated by the development of ascites and variceal hemorrhage.

Pathogenesis of portal hypertension

The mechanisms involved in the formation of ascites in CLD are complex and there are 3 hypotheses to explain the phenomenon. The traditional "underfilling hypothesis" suggests that mechanical obstruction to blood flow through the fibrotic liver results in increased portal pressure leading to increased formation of lymph. Ascites develops when the rate of production of lymph exceeds the rate of removal (Witte et al., 1980).

Increased plasma volume was demonstrated in cirrhosis with retention of sodium predating the development of ascites (Lieberman and Reynolds, 1967), leading to the "overflow theory" of ascites formation (Lieberman et al., 1970). According to this hypothesis, the initiating event in patients with portal hypertension is renal sodium and water retention triggered by a hepatorenal reflex. This leads to an expanded circulating blood volume, compensatory decreased peripheral vascular resistance and increased pressure in the splanchnic circulation with overflow formation of ascites.

These theories could not explain the frequent finding of arterial hypotension despite high cardiac index, increased blood volume and activation of many vasoconstrictor systems. The "peripheral arterial vasodilation hypothesis" was subsequently proposed to address the deficiencies in the previously described theories (Schrier *et al.*, 1988). In this theory, the initial event is splanchnic arteriolar vasodilation secondary to portal hypertension. This leads to pooling of blood in the splanchnic vascular bed with a consequent reduction of the central arterial blood volume (Henriksen *et al.*, 1989). As a result there is activation of baroceptors and stimulation of the sympathetic nervous system, renin-angiotensin-aldosterone system and release of antidiuretic hormone (ADH), all of which contributes to renal sodium retention (Arroyo and Gines, 1992; Henriksen *et al.*, 1992). This model explains how there can be underfilling of the central arterial blood volume but increased total blood volume as there is pooling of blood in the splanchnic circulation. This may also lead to elevated hydrostatic pressure in the splanchnic circulation and explain in part the development of ascites.

In recent years, much has been learnt about the mechanisms involved in the formation of ascites. Sodium retention and free water retention are thought to be particularly important. One of the earliest changes is a reduction in the ability of the renal tubules to excrete sodium (Bernardi *et al.*, 1993). The renin-angiotensin-aldosterone system is implicated as plasma aldosterone levels are increased in cirrhosis with ascites and inversely correlated with renal sodium excretion. The aim of treatment of cirrhotic patients with ascites is to achieve a natriuresis which is best achieved with the aldosterone antagonist spironolactone (Perez-Ayuso *et al.*, 1983). The sympathetic nervous system is also important as there is a high plasma concentration of norepinephrine in patients with ascites but this is not seen in cirrhotic patients without ascites (Henriksen and Ring-Larsen, 1994). Deficiency of atrial natriuretic peptides is not implicated as plasma levels are elevated in cirrhotic patients with ascites (Wong and Blendis, 1994).

At a later stage cirrhotic patients with ascites develop impaired ability to excrete free water eventually resulting in dilutional hyponatremia. Increased plasma levels of ADH are frequently observed and correlate with the reduction in free water excretion (Bichet *et al.*, 1982). ADH levels are elevated due to increased hypothalamic secretion of ADH that is released even in the presence of hyponatraemia and low plasma osmolality which would normally inhibit ADH. Fluid restriction is appropriate in these circumstances.

Management of ascites

The accumulation of ascites is often the first clinical sign of decompensated alcoholic cirrhosis. It is also a common feature of acute alcoholic hepatitis of moderate or severe degree. The therapeutic approach to the management of ascites is a logical stepwise one which follows the physiological changes seen in portal hypertension. In the early stages, abstinence from alcohol may be enough to control accumulation of ascites. Simple bedrest is also associated with improvement in ascites as a result of postural changes in portal pressure. However this is not a practical long-term solution. Restriction of sodium intake is the single most important intervention in the management of ascites. Sodium restriction to less than 40 mmol/day is desirable but usually not achievable as these diets become unpalatable such that compliance is poor. In practice a diet containing less than 80 mmol/day of sodium is usually sufficient to control ascites and likely to be better tolerated. Although, conventionally, fluids are restricted to 1–1.5 liters/day in the treatment of ascites, this is only necessary when there is dilutional hyponatremia (serum sodium less than 130 mmol/l). In such cases water restriction of 800 ml/day may be required in resistant cases (serum sodium less than 125 mmol/l).

Diuretics are used when simple measures are not satisfactory in order to achieve a natriuresis. The diuretics most commonly used are spironolactone and frusemide. These drugs should not be used in the presence of hyponatremia (serum sodium less than 130 mmol/l). Treatment is often begun with spironolactone monotherapy at a low dose of 50 mg daily but can be increased if necessary up to 400 mg daily. Higher doses of spironolactone are usually combined with the loop diuretic frusemide. This is also usually started at low dose and titrated to achieve desired weight loss up to a maximum of 160 mg daily. In patients with peripheral edema fluid can be mobilized rapidly. Patients without peripheral edema are more prone to diuretic-induced electrolyte disturbance and renal impairment. Weight loss of 0.5 kg/day should be the target in these patients.

An alternative approach is the use of therapeutic paracentesis. Therapeutic paracentesis with appropriate monitoring and intravascular repletion has been shown to be quick, well tolerated, associated with less complications and cost effective when compared to diuretic therapy (Quintero et al., 1985; Salerno et al., 1987). Patients can undergo daycase therapeutic paracentesis leading to reduced healthcare costs. Diuretics should be commenced post-paracentesis to prevent reaccumulation of ascites.

Hemodynamic complications can occur post-paracentesis and may in some cases precipitate the hepatorenal syndrome. However these complications are unusual in Childs-Pugh Grade A or B patients and can usually be prevented by the use of intravenous volume replacement immediately after paracentesis. The choice of replacement remains controversial. Traditionally, human albumin solution has been used (Gines et al., 1988). Optimal colloid replacement appears to be 8 g albumin/liter ascites removed. The use of other less expensive plasma expanders such as polygelin and dextran-70 has also been advocated, but these are reported to be less effective in the prevention of post-paracentesis circulatory dysfunction than albumin (Gines et al., 1996). Transjugular intrahepatic portosystemic shunt (TIPS) is a relatively new addition to the armamentarium for the treatment of ascites. TIPS is usually performed by interventional radiologists and in experienced hands the complication rate is acceptable. In a study of 50 patients treated with TIPS more than 75% had resolution or substantial improvement in ascites after 3 months and there was an associated reduction in serum creatinine (Ochs et al., 1995). There were no cases of cardiac failure after TIPS possibly because all patients underwent large volume paracentesis prior to TIPS. Patients under 60 years of age and with less advanced liver disease had better survival rates. Natriuresis is often delayed by several weeks after TIPS such that resolution of ascites may be delayed. In a randomized trial comparing TIPS with large volume paracentesis in 25 patients with refractory ascites, the ascites was easier to control in the TIPS group (Lebrec et al., 1996). However, in the patients with Child-Pugh Grade C disease ascites control was not improved and mortality was higher in the TIPS group. TIPS was only beneficial in Child-Pugh Grade B patients but without improvement in survival. By contrast, a recently reported larger randomized trial of 60 patients with refractory or recurrent ascites comparing of TIPS versus large-volume paracentesis revealed no difference in overall survival without liver transplantation or in frequency of hepatic encephalopathy (Rossle *et al.*, 2000). In this study almost 80% had ALD but had better baseline liver function and renal function than in previous studies.

Although TIPS has been effective in the control of ascites and variceal hemorrhage in ALD, there are potential problems with its use in these patients. As experience with TIPS is accumulating it is becoming clear that patients who have received TIPS need frequent follow up to detect the common problem of shunt stenosis and occlusion. Follow up of 100 cirrhotic patients after TIPS showed that within 6 months stent occlusion had occurred in 5 patients, stent retraction in 2 patients and stent stenosis in 51 patients resulting in recurrent portal hypertension (Sanyal *et al.*, 1997a). In a prospective study of 122 patients undergoing TIPS for variceal hemorrhage 77% of patients required balloon angioplasty or restenting within the first year (Casado *et al.*, 1998). This is time consuming and costly. There is also a high rate of encephalopathy post-TIPS. Data from the same study showed that 31% had developed hepatic encephalopathy within the first year. In 15–30% chronic encephalopathy results. Many centers only consider elective TIPS for ascites as a bridge to transplantation, i.e., as a temporary measure in suitable candidates for orthotopic liver transplantation who are likely to be transplanted within the next 6 months (Kamath and McKusick, 1994).

Spontaneous bacterial peritonitis (SBP) is a serious complication of end-stage ALD. It is defined as positive ascitic fluid culture, ascitic fluid neutrophil count greater than 250 cells/ml (or total white cell count greater than 500 cells/ml) and no other obvious intra-abdominal source of sepsis. In clinical practice positive culture of ascitic fluid occurs in 40% of clinical SBP cases when standard culture is performed of ascitic fluid in a sterile container, but is considerably improved when ascites is inoculated directly into blood culture bottles at the bedside. Therefore, in the appropriate clinical context, an ascitic neutrophil count greater than 250 cells/ml is highly suggestive of the diagnosis of SBP and is enough to commence antibiotic treatment before ascitic culture results are available. Mortality following an episode of SBP is approximately 40% usually as a result of hepatorenal failure or variceal hemorrhage (Follo *et al.*, 1994). The 1-year mortality after an episode of SBP is reported to be as high as 75%. Recently published data suggests that patients with SBP treated with intravenous albumin and antibiotics survive longer than those treated with antibiotics alone (Sort *et al.*, 1999). The median survival period following the first episode of SBP has been extended from 6 to 18 months.

SBP is often asymptomatic without systemic leucocytosis, fever, or abdominal pain. Any patient with ALD who presents with ascites for the first time, or at any time when they are unwell or have decompensated should undergo diagnostic ascitic tap to exclude SBP.

Hydrothorax is another complication of ascites and usually accumulates in the right pleural cavity through a diaphragmatic defect. Often symptoms are respiratory and the ascites is not troublesome. Management should be optimization of ascites treatment and symptomatic drainage of hydrothorax as required. In recurrent and resistant cases TIPS placement has been successfully deployed (Shiffman et al., 1995).

Finally, it should be appreciated that the development of ascites, SBP and recurrent hydrothorax are all indicators of deteriorating liver function and poor prognosis. Patients with cirrhosis who develop ascites have a mortality of 50% at 2 years. This is an ideal time to establish whether the patient is a candidate for liver transplantation.

Orthotopic liver transplantation is an established and well-tolerated therapy in end-stage ALD. Diuretic resistant ascites is frequently the major indication for transplantation. Results for patients transplanted for ALD are comparable to those for other etiologies of CLD (Everson et al., 1997). However, there is a long-term risk of relapse to alcohol.

Management of varices

Patients with cirrhosis develop esophageal varices at the rate of approximately 8% per year (Christensen et al., 1981). Mortality from an acute variceal hemorrhage is 30–50%, most deaths resulting from early rebleeding in the first 7–10 days after the initial bleed (D'Amico et al., 1995). The development of varices and variceal hemorrhage is associated with the severity of liver dysfunction and ongoing alcohol abuse. Increasing portal pressure causes increasing size of varices which is accompanied by thinning of the variceal wall and increasing variceal wall tension. Variceal rupture occurs when the intravariceal pressure can no longer be neutralized by the variceal wall tension. A recent hypothesis, as yet unproven, is that a common precipitant of acute elevations in portal pressure resulting in variceal hemorrhage is sepsis, particularly SBP (Goulis et al., 1999). Non-steroidal anti-inflammatory drugs are also a recognized precipitant of variceal bleeding.

The clinical management of varices in the ALD patient is similar to that in other causes of cirrhosis. Once again abstinence from alcohol is vitally important and can result in significant reduction in portal pressure over a period of weeks without any other intervention. In fact abstinence from alcohol with improvement in liver function may be accompanied by the disappearance of varices in ALD (Vorobioff et al., 1996).

The management of varices has undergone significant changes in recent years. This is a result of improved understanding of the pathophysiology of varices and better methods of monitoring portal pressure. Portal hypertension in patients with CLD is caused by increased portal blood flow and increased intrahepatic resistance. Both of these phenomena are amenable to therapeutic manipulation.

Increased portal blood flow occurs as a result of peripheral and splanchnic arteriolar dilatation which is the underlying cause of the hyperdynamic state of cirrhosis (Vorobioff et al., 1983). The portal system adapts to increased flow by the formation of portosystemic collaterals and varices. Intrahepatic resistance is partly due to the underlying parenchymal liver disease with fibrosis and partly to increased vascular tone. Recent work has revealed some of the functions of the hepatic stellate cell. It has myofibroblastic properties and is involved in the laying down of collagen during fibrosis, but when activated can also transform into a contractile cell which may be important in the dynamic regulation of intrahepatic resistance and portal blood flow. Active alcohol consumption is known to activate hepatic stellate cells and may explain the increased portal pressure in such individuals as well as the decrease in portal pressure observed with abstinence from alcohol.

The characteristic histological lesions of ALD also contribute to increased intrahepatic resistance and portal hypertension. Sinusoidal resistance is increased by hepatocyte ballooning, perisinusoidal fibrosis, sinusoidal capillarization and collagen deposition in the space of Disse, all early events in the pathogenesis of ALD which may result in portal hypertension in the pre-cirrhotic stage (Schaffner and Popper, 1963; Reynolds *et al.*, 1969). Hepatic vein fibrosis may add a post-hepatic element. Later when cirrhosis is established, regenerating nodules and intrahepatic venous thrombosis increase vascular resistance further.

Portal pressure can now be measured indirectly using hepatic vein wedge pressure measurements. This invasive procedure involves the radiological passage of a balloon into the hepatic vein and measurement of the free and wedged hepatic vein pressures, the latter being an approximation for the pre-hepatic sinusoidal pressure. The difference gives a hepatic venous pressure gradient (HVPG) or portal pressure gradient (equivalent to the pressure gradient between portal pressure and inferior vena cava pressure). It is now clear that varices only form when the HVPG is greater than 10 mmHg (Viallet *et al.*, 1975; Lebrec *et al.*, 1980). However not all patients with HVPG > 10 mmHg have varices (Garcia-Tsao *et al.*, 1985). Increases in HVPG are associated with increasing size of varices endoscopically. Varices enlarge in 10–20% of patients during the first 2 years after detection (Cales, 1990). There is now good evidence that variceal bleeding does not occur when the HVPG falls to below 12 mmHg (Viallet *et al.*, 1975; Garcia-Tsao *et al.*, 1985; Groszmann *et al.*, 1990).

There are several aspects of the management of varices that need to be addressed (Figure 22.1). Firstly, there is the issue of primary prophylaxis against variceal hemorrhage, i.e., the prevention of first bleed after initial detection of varices. This is important as the mortality rate with the first variceal hemorrhage is as high as 30–50% (D'Amico and Luca, 1997). In addition, the management of actively bleeding varices, the prevention of rebleeding, the management of rebleeding and secondary prevention of variceal hemorrhage are important. In survivors of the first bleed there is still a 60% rebleed rate and 30% mortality at one year (D'Amico *et al.*, 1995).

Primary prophylaxis

Initial clinical assessment of patients with ALD and clinical or histological evidence of cirrhosis should include gastroscopy to screen for varices. Patients who are found to have significant varices and have no previous history of variceal hemorrhage should commence primary prophylaxis therapy. The risk of first variceal hemorrhage increases with the severity of liver disease (Child-Pugh grade), size of varices and the presence of endoscopic stigmata of cherry red spots and red weals (NIEC, 1988; Kleber *et al.*, 1991). Patients with Child-Pugh grade A cirrhosis and small esophageal varices without stigmata are at low risk of variceal hemorrhage. In clinical

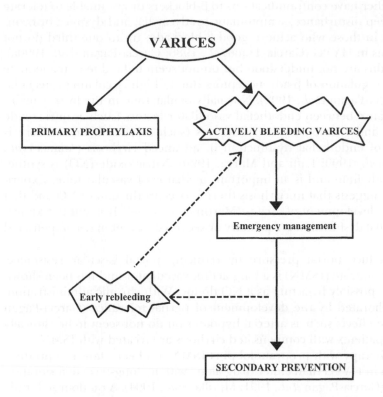

Figure 22.1 Management of varices.

practice the platelet count is a reasonable surrogate marker for the presence of varices, in that low platelet counts are associated with more severe portal hypertension and larger varices. The most common cause of thrombocytopenia in actively drinking alcoholics is direct alcohol-induced bone marrow toxicity. Patients with suspected ALD and cirrhosis with persistently low platelet counts despite abstinence from alcohol should be offered gastroscopy to screen for varices.

There is now good evidence that the primary prophylaxis of choice is a non-selective β-blocker. Most published data used propranolol but nadolol is an acceptable alternative. Propranolol must be administered 12 hourly but nadolol has the advantage of once daily dosing. Meta-analysis of 9 controlled trials including almost 1,000 patients showed significant reduction of bleeding episodes with β-blocker therapy and a trend towards reduction in mortality (D'Amico *et al.*, 1995). The protective effects seem to be lost when treatment is stopped suggesting that treatment should be lifelong (Grace *et al.*, 1990).

Non-selective β-blockers work in two ways: β1-receptor blockade results in negative inotropic effect with reduced cardiac output, whereas β2-receptor blockade causes splanchnic vasoconstriction. Both these actions result in reduced portal blood flow and lowering of portal pressure (Bosch *et al.*, 1984; Mastai *et al.*, 1987).

Propranolol therapy is usually introduced at low dose (e.g., 20 mg bd) and increased to a target of 80 mg bd or a 25% reduction in baseline heart rate. Unfortunately many patients either have contraindications to β-blockers or are unable to tolerate them (fatigue, sleep disturbance, symptomatic bradycardia, and dyspnea or bronchospasm). Even in those who achieve good β-blockade, up to one third do not achieve reductions in HVPG (Garcia-Tsao *et al.*, 1986; Garcia-Pagan *et al.*, 1990a). The reasons for this are not understood but do not seem to be due to inadequate dosing, or down-regulation of β-adrenoceptors due to high circulating catecholamine levels (Garcia-Pagan *et al.*, 1992). Normal vascular tone in the liver is maintained by the balance between endothelial vasodilator factors (such as nitric oxide or prostacyclins) and vasoconstrictor substances (such as endothelins). There is recent evidence of endothelial dysfunction in advanced cirrhosis (Adams *et al.*, 1994; Albornoz *et al.*, 1999; Laffi and Marra, 1999). Nitric oxide (NO) is synthesized in the endothelium and is an important mediator of vascular tone. Experimental evidence suggests that in cirrhosis there is overproduction of NO and that this precedes the development of ascites (Martin *et al.*, 1998). It is still not known whether endothelial dysfunction is a primary or secondary event in decompensated cirrhosis.

Vasodilators reduce portal pressure by reducing portal vascular resistance. Isosorbide-5-mononitrate (ISMN) is a long-acting vasodilator and has been shown to reduce HVPG, possibly by acting as a NO donor. With chronic administration, the effect is ameliorated by the development of partial tolerance (Garcia-Pagan *et al.*, 1990b). Side effects such as arterial hypotension do not seem to be clinically significant when patients with compensated cirrhosis are treated with ISMN.

Combination therapy with propranolol plus ISMN has been shown to produce greater reduction in HVPG than either drug alone with no long-term deterioration in renal function (Garcia-Pagan *et al.*, 1991; Morillas *et al.*, 1994). A randomized study comparing nadolol plus ISMN against nadolol alone reported that combination therapy was more effective in preventing first bleed (Merkel *et al.*, 1996). One study directly compared ISMN with propranolol and found no difference in efficacy as primary prophylaxis (Angelico *et al.*, 1993). Although this study was underpowered, it does suggest that in patients unable to tolerate β-blockers, ISMN is an alternative as monotherapy.

An alternative strategy is prophylactic endoscopic therapy for large esophageal varices. This was recently addressed by a trial of primary endoscopic banding ligation versus propranolol as primary prevention of variceal hemorrhage in 89 patients with large esophageal varices at endoscopy (Sarin *et al.*, 1999). At 18 months follow up bleeding rate in the propranolol group was 43% compared to 15% in the banding ligation group. This reported significant benefit from banding ligation has been criticized because of the extremely high rate of bleeding in the propranolol group.

In summary, all patients with clinically significant ALD should be offered gastroscopy to screen for varices. If present all except those of lowest risk should be considered for primary prophylactic therapy to prevent first variceal hemorrhage. Many clinicians use propranolol alone but the most efficacious therapy is propranolol plus ISMN. Ideally therapy should be guided by HVPG measurements. Endoscopic therapy as primary prophylaxis is not currently advocated except perhaps for those patients with contraindications to or intolerance of pharmacological prophylaxis.

Active variceal hemorrhage

The management of acute variceal hemorrhage comprises several often-complementary modalities. These can be broadly divided into pharmacotherapeutic interventions, endoscopic procedures and balloon tamponade. The initial management plan is often determined by the local availability of these modalities.

Once a diagnosis of probable variceal hemorrhage has been made, urgent resuscitation (with blood, fresh frozen plasma, colloid and crystalloid as required) guided by central venous pressure monitoring is indicated. Early therapeutic endoscopy remains the treatment of choice. However, there is usually some delay before emergency endoscopy can be organized, in some cases as long as 12–24 hours. Pharmacotherapy can be useful in these situations and can be started early in the emergency department and does not require personnel experienced in variceal hemorrhage.

Variceal sclerotherapy is an established endoscopic therapy. Meta-analysis of trials comparing sclerotherapy with pharmacotherapy, balloon tamponade or combination therapy included 2,338 patients and reported improved control of bleeding and short-term mortality with sclerotherapy (De Franchis, 1994). Endoscopic banding ligation of varices is a more recently introduced technique which appears to have several advantages over variceal sclerotherapy. In a study of 71 acute esophageal variceal bleeds where 37 patients were randomized to banding ligation and 34 to sclerotherapy, banding ligation was found to be associated with lower rebleeding and 1 month mortality rates (19% versus 35%) (Lo et al., 1997). Control of oozing varices was similar but for the spurting esophageal varix banding ligation was superior. Meta-analysis of randomized controlled trials including 547 patients showed reduced mortality rates and rebleeding rates with banding ligation compared to sclerotherapy (Laine and Cook, 1995). There is also evidence that banding ligation results in fewer long-term complications of endoscopic eradication of varices (such as esophageal stricture formation) and that variceal eradication can be achieved in fewer endoscopic sessions than with sclerotherapy (Laine and Cook, 1995; Lo et al., 1997; Tait et al., 1999). However, the technique of banding ligation requires specialized advanced endoscopic expertise, skills that need updating regularly. Therefore, it may be better for endoscopists inexperienced in banding ligation to continue to use sclerotherapy in the emergency situation. Both techniques are equally effective in controlling the initial hemorrhage (Tait et al., 1999). In cases where control of hemorrhage cannot be achieved with these methods, balloon tamponade can be a life-saving temporizing procedure prior to definitive therapy. An alternative approach to the treatment of active variceal hemorrhage is the use of vasoactive drug therapy. Pharmacologically active agents useful in variceal hemorrhage are shown in Table 22.1.

Table 22.1 Pharmacotherapy in acute variceal hemorrhage

vasopressin (+ nitroglycerin)
somatostatin
octreotide
terlipressin

Vasopressin is a natural hormone that acts on specific receptors and causes vasoconstriction in many vascular beds including the splanchnic circulation. The efficacy of vasopressin is questionable (Patch and Burroughs, 1995) and there are serious side effects (abdominal colic, angina, cerebrovascular ischemia). These effects can be ameliorated with co-administration of nitroglycerin. Four clinical trials with a total of 131 patients have compared vasopressin versus placebo (Merigan et al., 1962; Conn et al., 1975; Mallory et al., 1980; Fogel et al., 1982). Meta-analysis showed significant improvement in control of bleeding but no effect on mortality. However, vasopressin is no longer widely used chiefly because of the development of alternative drugs with better side effect profiles.

Somatostatin, a natural 14 amino acid peptide, decreases splanchnic blood flow with few side effects (Tyden et al., 1979). Unfortunately studies of portal pressure effects have been variable (Bosch et al., 1981; Kleber et al., 1988). Similarly, the three randomized placebo-controlled trials using somatostatin in acute variceal hemorrhage, with a total of 308 patients, have given conflicting results. The single trial reporting improved control of bleeding used somatostatin at a dose of 250 μg/hour for 5 days (Burroughs et al., 1990). Neither this trial nor a later meta-analysis of these trials showed a survival advantage with the use of somatostatin. The favorable side effect profile and probable efficacy make somatostatin an attractive therapy, although it is currently rarely used.

Octreotide is a synthetic 8 amino acid analog of somatostatin with similar biological activity and longer half-life. Some studies show reduced portal pressures with octreotide but others show no difference. Clinical trials of somatostatin or octreotide in acute variceal hemorrhage have shown conflicting results, probably as a result of differences in patient selection, methodology and end-point definitions (Valenzuela et al., 1989; Burroughs et al., 1990). Overall, it is likely that octreotide is useful for control of acute variceal hemorrhage but that there is no proven survival advantage over placebo. Direct comparison of octreotide with sclerotherapy in acute variceal hemorrhage showed no differences in control of bleeding but a non-significant trend towards increased mortality with octroetide (Jenkins et al., 1997). Studies using octreotide in addition to sclerotherapy or banding ligation suggest that this approach is better than endoscopic therapy alone (Besson et al., 1995; Sung et al., 1995).

Terlipressin (or triglycyl-lysine vasopressin) is a synthetic analog of vasopressin with longer half-life than vasopressin. Terlipressin is slowly cleaved into vasopressin *in vivo* but has fewer side effects even when compared to vasopressin plus nitroglycerin (D'Amico et al., 1994). However, there is still a risk of cardiac arrhythmia and ischemia with terlipressin. It is also the only one of these agents which has been shown to reduce mortality in acute variceal hemorrhage (Walker et al., 1986; Soderlund et al., 1990). However, there have been criticisms of these studies and further trials are awaited to confirm these findings.

Balloon tamponade remains a useful technique in situations where other treatments are not available or have failed, or when bleeding is catastrophic. There are however numerous potentially serious complications of balloon tamponade. These include aspiration pneumonia, esophageal mucosal injury and esophageal rupture. Most complications can be avoided with good technique and deflation of the balloon within 24 hours. Inflation of the esophageal balloon found with some devices is rarely indicated. There have been several studies which have compared balloon tamponade to drug therapy in acute variceal hemorrhage. Unfortunately these studies use differing end-points and are difficult to interpret. None have demonstrated significant differences between these modalities in terms of control of bleeding or mortality (D'Amico *et al.*, 1995). However, in view of the complication rate of balloon tamponade it is not recommended as first line therapy and should be reserved for life threatening situations or for safe transfer of patients to specialist units.

Gastric variceal hemorrhage

The management of gastric varices deserves special mention, as there are some important differences from that of esophageal varices. The prevalence of gastric varices in patients with portal hypertension is reported to be approximately 20% (Sarin *et al.*, 1992). Gastric varices which are in continuity with esophageal varices may be treated in a similar fashion as esophageal varices. Isolated gastric varices appear to bleed less frequently than esophageal varices, but when they do rupture bleeding is more difficult to control and mortality rates are higher (Sarin *et al.*, 1992; Kim *et al.*, 1997). Isolated gastric varices do not respond well to endoscopic techniques, which are successful for esophageal varices. Small studies report better results with injection of tissue adhesives (e.g., histoacryl) and bovine thrombin. In general isolated gastric varices are technically difficult to treat endoscopically especially in the context of acute variceal hemorrhage. Pharmacotherapy should be instituted early in these situations and facilities for TIPS or surgical shunts should be considered earlier than is usually practised for esophageal hemorrhage, probably by the time of the first rebleed.

Variceal rebleeding

Those who survive the initial variceal bleed have a 70% risk of a rebleed in the first year if left untreated. Much of the mortality associated with acute variceal hemorrhage is related to early rebleeding within the first 5 days after the initial bleed. There is some evidence that continuation of vasoactive drug therapy over this time period reduces early rebleeding from varices (Burroughs *et al.*, 1990). However, this is not currently standard practice.

Clinical practice for the management of rebleeding varies with local preference and availability of expertise. The most common policy is to treat the first rebleed in a similar manner to the initial bleed. However, further bleeding episodes are increasingly being treated with emergency TIPS. In some centers surgical shunt placement is an alternative. In approximately 10% of patients with acute variceal hemorrhage the bleeding cannot be controlled despite 2 endoscopic treatments within the first 24 hours (Burroughs *et al.*, 1989). Emergency TIPS can control bleeding in the majority of these patients more effectively than endoscopic therapy (Papatheodoridis *et al.*, 1999). TIPS is equally as effective for gastric fundal variceal bleeding as it is for esophageal variceal bleeding (Chau *et al.*, 1998). However, survival rates are not improved by TIPS placement. Patients requiring emergency TIPS are often critically ill with severe coagulopathy, poor liver function, and/or sepsis prior to TIPS. In such patients TIPS can precipitate or worsen encephalopathy, result in deterioration in liver function, and induce cardiac failure and multiple organ failure. Until more data become available the place of TIPS will remain as a rescue therapy when endoscopy and pharmacotherapy have failed to control bleeding.

Secondary prevention of variceal hemorrhage

In ALD the most important factor in the secondary prevention of variceal hemorrhage is abstinence from alcohol. This alone will lead to substantial fall in portal pressure and often to the eradication of varices. Eradication of esophageal varices is usually achieved by regular follow-up sclerotherapy or band ligation. Band ligation is proven to be superior to sclerotherapy in this regard (Laine and Cook, 1995). Band ligation requires fewer session of endoscopy to achieve eradication and there are fewer serious complications such as esophageal stricture (Laine and Cook, 1995; Tait et al., 1999). Endoscopic sessions are usually performed at 1–3 weekly intervals until eradication is achieved. This interval allows banding-induced ulceration to heal prior to further treatment. After this the patient should remain under 6 monthly endoscopic surveillance as varices may recur, in which event a further programme of variceal eradication will be required.

TIPS has been evaluated in secondary prevention and found to be more effective than sclerotherapy at preventing variceal hemorrhage but at an increased risk of encephalopathy (Cabrera et al., 1996). Again, there was no difference in survival. However, Sanyal et al. (1997b) randomized 80 patients with recent variceal hemorrhage to TIPS or sclerotherapy and found no significant difference in rebleeding rate over a mean follow up of 3 years. In addition, there was more encephalopathy and reduced survival in the TIPS group. Comparison of TIPS with endoscopic therapy (sclerotherapy and/or banding) plus propranolol in 126 patients showed significantly less rebleeding in the TIPS group but at a cost of double the incidence of hepatic encephalopathy at 1 year (Rossle et al., 1997). Again, there was no difference in survival. A study comparing TIPS with small diameter surgical portocaval shunts reported less rebleeding and improved survival in the surgical group (Rosemurgy et al., 1996). Recent meta-analysis of 11 randomized clinical trials involving 811 patients comparing TIPS to endoscopic therapy for secondary prevention of variceal hemorrhage showed that although recurrent variceal hemorrhage was reduced in the TIPS group, there was a much higher incidence of encephalopathy post-TIPS and no difference in mortality (Papatheodoridis et al., 1999). Currently available data do not advocate TIPS in the secondary prevention of variceal hemorrhage.

There is strong evidence that non-selective β-blockers (propranolol or nadolol) are effective in the secondary prevention of variceal hemorrhage. Very few patients enrolled into such trials were Child-Pugh grade C, so the effectiveness of β-blockers in this setting is uncertain. Meta-analysis of 11 randomized controlled trials revealed a 32% reduction in the risk of rebleeding (Bernard et al., 1997a). However, the effect of these drugs on mortality is less clear. D'Amico et al. (1995) found no statistical improvement in survival with β-blockers in their meta-analysis, but Bernard et al. (1997a) reported a significant result in favor of β-blockers. Several trials have compared propranolol with sclerotherapy for secondary prevention of variceal hemorrhage. Meta-analysis of 9 of these trials showed that sclerotherapy was more effective in preventing rebleeding but at a cost of higher incidence of adverse effects (Bernard *et al.*, 1997b). There was no difference in survival. These results recommend propranolol as first choice therapy for secondary prophylaxis of variceal hemorrhage. In view of the high early rebleeding risk, β-blocker therapy should probably be instituted once a period of stability has been observed within the first few days. In patients unable to tolerate β-blockers, ISMN may be a reasonable alternative, although there is no good data to support this. Ideally the doses of these drugs should be titrated to clinical effectiveness as monitored by formal portal pressure studies in order to keep HVWP < 12 mmHg.

MANAGEMENT OF ENCEPHALOPATHY

Hepatic encephalopathy is a neuropsychiatric condition that is common in patients with advanced ALD. The cause of this condition remains unknown. One hypothesis suggests that ammonia accumulates as a result of liver failure with disruption of the urea cycle, crosses the blood brain barrier and is the cause of the syndrome of hepatic encephalopathy. However, ammonia levels do not correlate well with the clinical severity of encephalopathy. Other theories implicate as yet unidentified endogenous gut-derived nitrogenous toxins, alterations in central neurotransmitter systems (e.g., endogenous benzodiazepine receptor ligands), manganese toxicity or zinc deficiency.

The patient with hepatic encephalopathy may present with an acute episode associated with a precipitating factor (Table 22.2). The most common precipitants are infections including SBP, gastrointestinal hemorrhage, constipation, electrolyte disturbance, dehydration, and overuse of sedative drugs (especially benzodiazepines) and narcotics, e.g., codeine. Overaggressive therapy for ascites can often precipitate encephalopathy by means of fluid restriction, diuretics and excessive paracentesis. In addition the utilization of surgical shunts or TIPS is frequently accompanied by the development or worsening of encephalopathy and is the most significant complication of these procedures. Hepatic encephalopathy can also

Table 22.2 Hepatic encephalopathy – common precipitating factors in ALD

Factor	Common causes
infection	SBP
gastrointestinal hemorrhage	peptic ulcer, varices
constipation	fluid restriction
hypokalaemia	diuretics, renal tubular leak
uraemia	diuretics, NSAIDs, hepatorenal syndrome post-paracentesis
dehydration	diuretics, fluid restriction, post-paracentesis
drugs	benzodiazepines, other CNS depressants e.g., in alcohol withdrawal programmes, general anesthetics
post-TIPS	
hepatocellular carcinoma	

herald the emergence of hepatocellular carcinoma. Alternatively, hepatic encephalopathy may be present as a subclinical state. This usually occurs in the context of early CLD and requires the use of formal psychometric testing to confirm. However, the number connection time test is still a useful and easy to use bedside assessment for such cases.

Less commonly encephalopathy may develop spontaneously without an obvious precipitant. This is presumed to be due to the development of porto-systemic shunts. These patients often go on to suffer debilitating chronic encephalopathy despite relatively well preserved liver function in many cases.

Hepatic encephalopathy can usually be controlled simply by removal or treatment of the precipitating factor. The disaccharide lactulose is also a simple and effective therapy. Although the effectiveness of lactulose has never been the subject of a randomized controlled trial, it is considered the "gold standard" therapy for hepatic encephalopathy (Ferenci et al., 1996). It is not digested in the small bowel but is metabolised by colonic bacterial flora with the formation of organic acids and a lowering of colonic pH which inhibits the growth of ammonia producing bacteria. There is also a laxative effect which helps to increase nitrogen excretion. The dose is titrated aiming for 2–3 soft stools per day. Usual doses required are 45–90 g daily.

In resistant cases antibiotic therapy can be considered. Neomycin is relatively non-absorbable and is usually given in doses of 2–8 g daily in 4 divided doses. 70–80% of patients improve on neomycin. It has been shown to be as effective as lactulose (Conn et al., 1977). However, a small proportion of neomycin is absorbed and is potentially nephrotoxic and ototoxic. It should not be given for more than one month.

The benzodiazepine antagonist flumazenil has been used in the treatment of hepatic encephalopathy. The studies done so far have been difficult to compare because of methodological differences. Similarly the results have been conflicting and are difficult to interpret. It would appear that some patients benefit from flumazenil therapy but this is transient with encephalopathy returning or worsening soon after discontinuation of therapy. Currently, flumazenil is only of use in the differentiation of hepatic encephalopathy from benzodiazepine-induced coma.

Protein restriction has traditionally been used in the treatment of hepatic encephalopathy. However, this is not necessary except in the most severe cases of chronic spontaneous encephalopathy. Therefore, once the patient is able to recommence feeding the dietary protein content should be gradually increased as tolerated. Indeed most ALD patients are malnourished and should have nutritional supplementation including at least 1 g/kg body weight of protein daily.

Zinc deficiency is common in alcoholics and is associated with neurological complications. However, in only one of three randomized controlled trials of zinc supplementation was there an improvement in subclinical hepatic encephalopathy. Recently there has been much interest in the use of new non-invasive functional brain imaging techniques (e.g., magnetic resonance imaging and spectroscopy, single photon and positron emission tomography) in hepatic encephalopathy. T1-weighted magnetic resonance images show hyperintensity in the globus pallidus in hepatic encephalopathy (Morgan, 1996). This is thought to be due to deposition of manganese in the basal ganglia. Further research continues to elucidate the significance of these findings.

In clinical practice, the most difficult aspect of management of this condition is making a correct diagnosis. In the recently drinking alcoholic with suspected CLD, the usual diagnostic problem is differentiation from the alcohol withdrawal syndrome. Disoriented patients with alcohol still on the breath are not likely to be withdrawing. However, in other patients this differentiation can be extremely difficult. Patients suffering withdrawal symptoms have been drinking heavily up to 6–72 hours before presentation. There is usually prominent fine tremor, tachycardia, fever and sweating. Encephalopathic patients characteristically have the slower and coarser flapping tremor of asterixis, but may also have tachycardia and fever particularly if the episode has been precipitated by infection. In unclear cases treatment should be started for the most likely clinical diagnosis but frequent clinical review is recommended.

NUTRITION

Malnutrition is present in the vast majority of patients with ALD, and is reported at 100% in patients presenting with alcoholic hepatitis (Mendenhall *et al.*, 1995). There are two common presentations of malnutrition in ALD: those which appear marasmic with reduction in body fat and protein; and those with protein-calorie malnutrition with reasonable fat stores but decreased skeletal muscle mass and peripheral edema and/or ascites. Chronic alcohol abuse results in malnutrition in several ways. Many alcoholics do not eat regular meals because of their drinking behavior and anorexia induced by alcoholism. Alcohol can also cause malabsorption and can impair the metabolism of many ingested nutrients. There is evidence of steatorrhea in up to 50% of cirrhotic patients with ALD due to subclinical pancreatic insufficiency and reduced bile secretion (Roggin *et al.*, 1972).

Traditional nutritional assessment techniques are often difficult in patients with ALD as body water distribution in the form of ascites and peripheral edema makes dry weight calculations difficult. Simple measurements such as anthropometric studies (e.g., triceps skinfold thickness) and tissue function tests (e.g., hand grip strength) are reasonable for everyday clinical use. However, simple subjective "end of the bed" assessment by an experienced physician has been found to be a reliable indicator of nutritional status. Patients with ALD have reductions in both fat and muscle mass (Italian Multicentre Co-operative Project on Nutrition in Liver Cirrhosis, 1994).

Resting energy expenditure has consistently been found to be increased by up to 60% in patients with alcoholic hepatitis or end-stage ALD (John *et al.*, 1989; Schneeweiss *et al.*, 1990). Studies on protein metabolism in compensated cirrhotics demonstrate increased protein synthesis to compensate for increased protein breakdown but with overall negative nitrogen balance (Swart *et al.*, 1988). In addition, malnourished ALD patients often show signs of hypermetabolism with insulin resistance, reduced ability to store glycogen, increased skeletal muscle breakdown for gluconeogenesis and greater reliance on fatty acids in the fasting state. Patients with cirrhosis appear to tolerate prolonged periods of fasting poorly. After an overnight fast cirrhotic patients utilize fat much earlier than normal subjects (McCullough and Tavill, 1991). It has also been shown that frequent meals, in particular an evening snack, improve nitrogen balance in cirrhotic patients (Swart *et al.*, 1989).

Nutritional status is correlated with survival in hospitalized patients with a variety of medical conditions (Naber *et al.*, 1997), including patients with cirrhosis and ALD patients with moderate to severe alcoholic hepatitis (Mendenhall *et al.*, 1995). However, severity of liver disease also correlates well with the degree of malnutrition in cirrhotic patients, so that nutritional status is not an independent predictor of mortality in cirrhosis. However, nutritional status may be a good pre-operative predictor of outcome after liver transplantation. In a study of 150 transplant patients for various etiologies of chronic liver disease nutritional parameters were found to be better predictors of post-operative survival than standard markers of liver function such as the Child-Pugh score (Selberg *et al.*, 1997).

Enteral nutritional support in ALD

Clinical studies on the use of nutritional therapy in ALD suffer from a number of methodological and design faults resulting in inconclusive data. Many studies are in small numbers of patients of varying severity and etiology of liver disease, poorly controlled, and with very short follow-up periods. It is now recognized that in cirrhotics 1–1.5 g/kg body weight/day protein is required to achieve neutral nitrogen balance but that this increases significantly in those with severe disease such as severe alcoholic hepatitis. Several studies of oral dietary protein and calorie supplementation show improved nutritional status in stable ALD cirrhotics but had varying effects on liver function. In patients hospitalized for severe alcoholic hepatitis oral supplements are unlikely to be of benefit as these patients are anorectic with severe negative nitrogen balance. Such patients often require more aggressive nutritional support. This was borne out by a study of nutritional support in 64 patients with severe alcoholic hepatitis: the mortality rate was 3.3% for those who achieved positive nitrogen balance compared to 57.9% for those who did not (Calvey *et al.*, 1985).

Total enteral nutrition can be administered via a nasogastric tube. This is generally well tolerated except in some patients with hepatic encephalopathy. In a study of 35 patients with alcoholic cirrhosis, a subgroup tolerated 3 weeks tube feeding with enteral nutrition supplemented by branched-chain amino acids (BCAA) and resulted in improved Child-Pugh scores and improved survival with 12% hospital mortality compared to 47% mortality in a matched control group consuming only half the calories and protein by mouth (Cabre *et al.*, 1990). Meta-analysis of 835 patients, mostly with severe ALD, showed that enteral feeding was well tolerated, does not worsen encephalopathy, is of most benefit to those with moderate to severe protein-calorie malnutrition and often improves liver function (Nompleggi and Bonkovsky, 1994). Formulas enriched in BCAA were not found to be beneficial.

Parenteral nutritional support in ALD

Parenteral nutrition has been used in many small studies of hospitalized ALD patients. Most of these studies were performed on patients with alcoholic hepatitis using treatment periods of one month. This is a very short time in which to expect to see major improvement in nutritional status. Nonetheless there have been reports of improvements in liver histology (Diehl *et al.*, 1985) and nitrogen balance (Bonkovsky *et al.*, 1991). Analysis of all of these studies including 239 patients concluded that treatment with parenteral nutrition in ALD patients improves nitrogen balance, liver function tests and short-term survival (Nompleggi and Bonkovsky, 1994). Long-term survival remains uncertain. Despite these findings there are practical concerns about the use of parenteral nutrition in severely ill ALD patients. The major concern is the risk of infection associated with long-term central intravenous cannulae.

Antioxidant therapy in ALD

There are well documented micronutrient deficiencies in chronic alcoholics including folate, thiamine, pyridoxine, zinc, selenium and vitamins A, C and E. Many of the clinical findings in chronic alcoholics are caused by these deficiencies, e.g., anemia (folate, pyridoxine), Wernicke-Korsakoff syndrome (thiamine) (Butterworth *et al.*, 1993), poor cell-mediated immunity and hypogonadism (zinc) (McClain *et al.*, 1979). Selenium is a precursor of glutathione peroxidase, one of the most important intracellular antioxidants. Vitamin E is the most important natural antioxidant in cellular membranes and is recycled by vitamin C. Deficiencies of these nutrients in chronic alcoholics is thought to be a significant factor in the development of oxidant stress and hepatic injury leading to the development of ALD.

Recently preliminary results of newer nutritional therapies have been reported. Fifty six patients with alcoholic hepatitis and advanced cirrhosis were treated with antioxidants (600 mg vitamin E, 200 mg selenium, and 12 mg zinc) or placebo. In this trial there was a significant improvement in bilirubin, markers of oxidative damage (serum malondialdehyde) and mortality (6.5% versus 40%) in the antioxidant treated group (Wenzel *et al.*, 1993). Silymarin has antioxidant properties by acting as a free radical scavenger and iron chelator. Clinical studies in ALD have shown conflicting results but a large study is due to be completed and reported later this year. S-adenosylmethionine (SAM) is essential in the synthesis of methionine and glutathione. Administration of SAM has been shown to reduce the depletion of glutathione seen in a variety of animal models of liver diseases including alcohol-induced hepatotoxicity. Treatment of 123 patients with alcoholic cirrhosis in a placebo-controlled trial of SAM for 2 years showed no significant difference in mortality in the group as a whole, but a significant survival advantage in patients with Child-Pugh Grade A and B treated with SAM (Mato *et al.*, 1999). Confirmatory studies are awaited. Lack of SAM also results in reductions in membrane phospholipids particularly in mitochondrial membranes. Supplementation of phosphatidylcholine in the baboon model of ALD prevents alcohol-induced fibrosis and cirrhosis (Lieber *et al.*, 1994). Clinical studies are nearing completion. Other antioxidant trials are currently under way, including one in severe alcoholic hepatitis from our own unit, the final results of which should be available in the near future.

ALCOHOLIC PANCREATITIS

Alcohol remains the most important cause of acute and chronic pancreatitis. Chronic pancreatitis usually presents in the 4th decade of life, the vast majority of patients are male, and the mean alcohol consumption of such patients is approximately 150 g daily for 10–15 years (Ammann *et al.*, 1996). As with ALD, pancreatitis only occurs in a minority of alcoholics but the incidence increases in proportion to the level of alcohol consumption. Chronic pancreatitis appears to be less common in patients with ALD (1%) than in alcoholics without liver disease (5%) (Dreiling and Koller, 1985). These epidemiological data suggest that there is both an environmental element (alcohol consumption) and an inherited genetic susceptibility to the disease (which is distinct from that for ALD).

The "necrosis-fibrosis" hypothesis is currently favored to explain the pathogenesis of this condition. This suggests that repeated attacks of acute pancreatitis occur which are initially reversible but later develop into a chronic irreversible state (Ammann and Muellhaupt, 1994). Attacks may be precipitated by plugs of protein and calcium carbonate which then obstruct the ducts. Oxidative stress has been implicated in the pathogenesis of pancreatitis (Tsai *et al.*, 1998). Recently described pancreatic stellate cells may be activated by oxidative stress and promote pancreatic fibrogenesis in a mechanism similar to that thought to occur in ALD. Duodenal juice from patients with acute and chronic pancreatitis has increased levels of lipid peroxidation products (Guyan *et al.*, 1990). Antioxidant therapy is reported to be of therapeutic benefit for chronic pancreatitis in uncontrolled trials (Whitely *et al.*, 1993). In addition, other possible mechanisms implicated in the pathogenesis of pancreatitis include biliary-pancreatic reflux due to spasm of the sphincter of Oddi and the direct toxic effects of metabolites of alcohol such as acetaldehyde.

Autopsy data from 1022 patients who died from ALD showed significantly more evidence of pancreatitis compared to a control group of 352 patients who died from cardiac or pulmonary disease (Renner *et al.*, 1984). Similarly, undiagnosed pancreatic insufficiency due to subclinical chronic pancreatitis is a relatively common finding in patients with end-stage ALD being evaluated for liver transplantation. This complicates surgery significantly in view of the associated malnutrition, glucose intolerance and increased technical difficulty.

CARDIAC DISEASE IN ALD

Acute alcohol intoxication may cause alterations in cardiac contractility and rhythm disturbances. In high concentration alcohol exerts a direct negative inotropic effect but this is often masked by an increased release of catecholamines (Fernandez-Sola *et al.*, 1997). This effect of acute alcohol ingestion may only be clinically significant in patients with established heart disease in whom it may induce acute cardiac failure. Rhythm disturbances are common in acute alcohol ingestion and are multifactorial. Electrolyte disturbances, in particular hypokalemia and hypomagnesemia which are common in heavy drinkers, may predispose to arrhythmia. A variety of arrhythmias are reported including atrial and ventricular extrasystoles, atrial fibrillation, atrial flutter, junctional tachycardia and ventricular tachycardia (Greenspon and Schaal, 1983). This led to the term "holiday heart syndrome" which was later discovered to be due to subclinical alcoholic cardiomyopathy (Greenspon and Schaal, 1983). Arrhythmia is also commonly seen in severe alcohol withdrawal reactions with delirium tremens where electrolyte depletion is combined with high endogenous catecholamine release.

Patients with ALD frequently have coexisting significant heart disease as a result of alcoholic cardiomyopathy or coronary artery disease. In chronic heavy alcohol drinkers the presentation of alcoholic cardiomyopathy is similar to that of idiopathic cardiomyopathy and is the most common cause of acquired dilated cardiomyopathy in the developed world, accounting for 21–36% of cases (Urbano-Marquez et al., 1989). There is a strong correlation between total lifetime alcohol consumption and the development of alcoholic cardiomyopathy. In men who drank the equivalent of 60 g of alcohol per day (or 6 units) for 20 years, 36% had reduced left ventricular function (Urbano-Marquez et al., 1989). Women seem to be more susceptible to alcoholic cardiomyopathy, raising the possibility that hormonal or genetic factors may be important in the pathogenesis of the condition. Arrhythmias are common in patients with alcoholic cardiomyopathy who continue to drink. This may explain the high incidence of sudden death in this population (Klatsky et al., 1979).

In the context of a compatible alcohol history, the diagnosis is made by the presence of left ventricular enlargement on echocardiography, left ventricular ejection fraction < 50% on radionucleotide imaging, and the exclusion of other causes of dilated cardiomyopathy (coronary artery disease, valvular or hypertensive heart disease). In addition there is diastolic dysfunction with impaired left ventricular relaxation. Symptoms are generally attributable to left ventricular failure, peripheral edema due to right ventricular failure being uncommon.

The early recognition of alcoholic cardiomyopathy is crucial, as the condition is reversible with abstinence from alcohol if intervention occurs prior to the development of severe heart failure. Follow up of 57 patients with alcoholic cardiomyopathy for a mean of 40.5 months indicated that those who improved clinically were much more likely to have been abstinent (73%) compared to those who remained unchanged (25%) or deteriorated (13%) (Demakis et al., 1974). A later study in asymptomatic patients with alcoholic cirrhosis showed that 50% of the cohort who were actively drinking had evidence of the disease compared with only 6% of patients abstinent for > 2 years (Estruch et al., 1989). The maintenance of abstinence remains the most beneficial therapy for this condition.

Pharmacological treatment is similar to other causes of cardiomyopathy with diuretics, angiotensin-converting enzyme inhibitors and digoxin in those with atrial fibrillation. There is less enthusiasm for anticoagulation therapy particularly when there is coexisting liver disease with portal hypertension and varices, coagulopathy and platelet dysfunction.

In many cases cardiac disease is asymptomatic and may only come to light during the evaluation of such patients for liver transplantation. Coronary artery disease is reported to occur less often in moderate or heavy alcohol consumers than in abstainers. However it is a relatively common finding in patients being considered for liver transplantation for ALD, usually because of coexisting diabetes mellitus and cigarette smoking. It is generally agreed that coronary artery disease should be treated first as liver transplantation places a major stress on the myocardium. Percutaneous balloon angioplasty is the treatment of choice as bypass surgery may be poorly tolerated and lead to severe hepatic decompensation. Recent data shows overall 50% mortality and 81% morbidity in 32 patients with coronary artery disease undergoing liver transplantation (Plotkin et al., 1996). Preliminary data suggests a poor outcome for those patients with significant coronary artery disease whether it is treated prior to liver transplantation or not (Keefe, 1997).

ALD IN THE INTENSIVE CARE UNIT

Patients with ALD have reduced physiological reserves and may fall seriously ill either due to decompensation of CLD or to other common illnesses such as sepsis. Active alcohol consumption and cirrhosis both compromise immune function. There is some evidence that although cirrhosis is associated with portal hypertension and splenomegaly, splenic function is suboptimal. This could leave cirrhotic patients susceptible to infections with encapsulated organisms, especially pneumococcus. In a case-control study of hospitalized patients with community acquired pneumonia, alcohol ingestion of greater than 80 g/day was found to be an independent risk factor indicating severity of disease as judged by need for admission to the intensive care unit (ICU) (Ruiz et al., 1999). The most frequent pathogen was *Streptococcus Pneumoniae*. In a prospective study of 170 hospitalized patients with cirrhosis the most common types of infection were SBP (31%), urinary tract infections (25%) and pneumonia (21%) (Caly and Strauss, 1993). In this and similar studies, risk of infection appears to be related to the severity of liver disease (Child-Pugh grade) and to the presence of gastrointestinal bleeding rather than etiology of cirrhosis (Caly and Strauss, 1993; Deschenes and Villeneuve, 1999). However, in other studies hospitalized patients with alcoholic cirrhosis have been reported to have higher bacterial infection rates than patients with other causes of CLD (Rosa et al., 2000). These factors contribute to the high mortality amongst ALD patients who become critically ill.

Traditionally there has been reluctance on the part of ICU physicians to admit patients with ALD. This is based on the reported poor outcome of patients with CLD in the ICU. In a study of 216 consecutive ICU admissions, 26 (12%) were found to abuse alcohol. These patients had higher mortality of 50% compared to 26% for non-alcohol abusers (Jensen et al., 1988). In another small study, 12 patients with cirrhosis and septic shock had 100% mortality as compared to 23 patients in septic shock but without cirrhosis who had 43% mortality (Moreau et al., 1992). Out of 100 cirrhotic patients needing mechanical ventilation in a single ICU the overall mortality rate was 89% and 100% in those with septic shock or end-stage CLD (Goldfarb et al., 1983). A retrospective analysis of 100 patients with CLD in a single medical ICU showed overall mortality of 64%, but this rose to 91% in those requiring mechanical ventilation, 89% for those in Child-Pugh class C, and 93% for those with renal failure (creatinine > 1.3 mg/dl). Child-Pugh class C patients with renal failure receiving mechanical ventilation had a mortality rate of 98% (Shellman *et al.*, 1988). A retrospective analysis of 198 patients with cirrhosis admitted to a single medical ICU demonstrated that the Acute Physiology and Chronic Health Evaluation (APACHE) III scoring system was the most reliable predictor of outcome at admission and after 48 hours as it includes physiological parameters (Zauner *et al.*, 1996). In the APACHE III database of 17,440 ICU admissions, 537 patients were known to have cirrhosis. Of these 117 were ventilated on the first day of ICU admission which from previous studies placed them at high risk of death. Analysis of these patients showed that APACHE III accurately stratified these patients into high, medium and low risk groups for hospital mortality (Zimmerman *et al.*, 1996). These authors further suggest that serial daily APACHE III data may be of additional benefit for clinicians to assess the effectiveness of ICU treatment. In a study from Pittsburgh 54 ICU admissions in 40 patients with cirrhosis were analyzed (Singh *et al.*, 1998). Overall ICU mortality was 43%. The best independent predictors of mortality were pulmonary infiltrates on chest radiography and renal dysfunction (serum creatinine > 1.5 mg/dl). In this study mortality in patients with cirrhosis due to ALD was significantly lower than that in cirrhosis of other etiologies.

Recent data from our own institution confirmed several findings of earlier studies. This is a tertiary referral unit which results in a degree of selection of better candidates. We retrospectively analyzed 173 admissions for patients with CLD (excluding elective liver transplants) to our specialist liver ICU over a 2 year period (Phillips *et al.*, 1999). Seventy per cent of these admissions were for patients with ALD. ICU and hospital outcome was poor (49% and 62% mortality respectively). None of these patients were transplanted from the ICU or within the same hospital admission. We found that patients with ALD did not have any worse outcome compared to other etiologies of CLD. All but 1 of 46 patients (98%) treated with mechanical ventilation, inotropes and renal replacement therapy died in the ICU. Similarly two organ support was associated with very poor outcome (21% ICU survival). However, mechanical ventilation alone, particularly in the context of variceal hemorrhage was associated with a good outcome.

Current evidence indicates that patients with end-stage CLD with severe decompensation, septic shock, or renal failure have high mortality when admitted to ICU. In many such cases ICU admission may be considered a poor use of resources. On the other hand those needing ICU therapy for single organ support or for variceal hemorrhage seem to have an acceptable outcome. In addition, patients with ALD fare no worse than those with other causes of CLD. These factors should be considered carefully when deciding on whether to admit critically ill patients with ALD to the ICU.

GENERAL MEDICAL WARD CARE

Patients with ALD often represent a challenge to medical and nursing staff. Many patients come from difficult social circumstances. There are frequently serious psychological and personality problems. It is important to treat patients with ALD in a non-judgmental manner, and to gain trust in order to treat effectively what is a complex and challenging disease. In addition, many patients admitted with ALD are seriously ill with multiple medical, surgical and psychiatric problems. These need to be assessed promptly and treated with meticulous care by appropriate healthcare professionals.

As discussed earlier, specific attention should concentrate on the nutritional deficiencies of patients with ALD, particularly those still drinking. Early parenteral therapy with thiamine and multivitamins should be considered on admission of all ALD patients, as well as parenteral vitamin K for those with coagulopathy. Many patients are also folate deficient and this can be given orally. Drug prescriptions should avoid preparations tolerated poorly in ALD. In particular non-steroidal anti-inflammatory drugs should be avoided if at all possible in view of hepatic and renal toxicity. Sedative drugs may precipitate encephalopathy in advanced ALD and need to be kept to the lowest possible doses or avoided. Difficulty arises in patients being treated for alcohol withdrawal with significant ALD. These patients should not be treated prophylactically unless there is previous history of severe withdrawal reactions or previous withdrawal seizures. In the latter, prophylactic carbamazepine should be considered.

SUMMARY

Alcohol excess is widespread within our society, a common underlying factor in a wide variety of medical consultations, and frequently unrecognized by medical practitioners. If the consequences of alcohol abuse are to be avoided the problem must be identified early and treatment plans instituted. Sadly all too often these programs are unsuccessful and patients present with serious end organ damage. In order to diagnose ALD other causes of CLD must be excluded. Liver biopsy is important in ALD to confirm the diagnosis, stage of the disease, and to determine prognosis. Liver biopsy should be deferred in end-stage disease where there are contraindications and the risk outweighs potential benefit.

In the patient with ALD presenting with ascites SBP should be excluded. Diuretics and paracentesis are useful therapies. Once varices appear primary prophylaxis against variceal hemorrhage with propranolol should be considered. Variceal hemorrhage is best managed with a combination of endoscopic therapy and pharmacotherapy. TIPS or open shunt surgery are currently best reserved as a rescue therapies.

Management of the ALD patient requires attention to detail and meticulous medical and nursing care. Nutrition should be supplemented early, drug prescribing needs particularly careful attention and the optimal management of coexisting medical problems such as alcoholic cardiomyopathy and chronic pancreatitis must not be neglected. ALD patients with end-stage disease who deteriorate and become critically ill often have a poor outcome. However selected patients may do well with intensive therapy and should be referred to ICU physicians. Lastly, survival rates after liver transplantation are as good for ALD patients as other etiologies of CLD. Current evidence suggests that many patients with ALD who would be good surgical candidates are not offered to liver transplant centers (Davies *et al.*, 1992). Referral for assessment should be considered for all ALD patients developing signs of decompensated cirrhosis.

REFERENCES

Adams, D.H., Burra, P., Hubscher, S.G., Elias, E. and Newman, W. (1994) Endothelial activation and circulating vascular adhesion molecules in alcoholic liver disease. *Hepatology* **19**, 588–594.

Albornoz, L., Alvarez, D., Otaso, J.C., Gadano, A., Salviu, J., Gerona, S., Sorroche, P., Villamil, A. and Mastai, R. (1999) Von Willebrand factor could be an index of endothelial dysfunction in patients with cirrhosis: relationship to degree of liver failure and nitric oxide levels. *Journal of Hepatology* **30**, 451–455.

Ammann, R.W. and Muellhaupt, B. (1994) Progression of alcoholic acute to chronic pancreatitis. *Gut* **35**, 552–556.

Ammann, R.W., Heitz, P.U. and Kloppel, G. (1996) Course of alcoholic chronic pancreatitis: a prospective clinicomorphological long-tern study. *Gastroenterology* **111**, 224–231.

Angelico, M., Carli, L., Piat, C., Gentile, S., Rinaldi, V., Bologna, E. and Capocaccia, L. (1993) Isosorbide-5-mononitrate versus propranolol in the prevention of first bleed in cirrhosis. *Gastroenterology* **104**, 1460–1465.

Arroyo, V. and Gines, P. (1992) Arteriolar vasodilation and the pathogenesis of the hyperdynamic circulation and renal sodium and water retention in cirhosis. *Gastroenterology* **102**, 1077–1079.

Bernard, B., Lebrec, D., Mathurin, P., Opolon, P. and Poynard, T. (1997a) Beta-adrenergic antagonists in the prevention of gastrointestinal rebleeding in patients with cirrhosis: a meta-analysis. *Hepatology* **25**, 63–70.

Bernard, B., Lebrec, D., Mathurin, P., Opolon, P. and Poynard, T. (1997b) Propranolol and sclerotherapy in the prevention of gastrointestinal rebleeding in patients with cirrhosis: a meta-analysis. *Journal of Hepatology* **26**, 312–324.

Bernardi, M., Di Marco, C., Trevisani, F., Fornale, L., Andreone, P., Cursaro, C., Baraldini, M., Ligabue, A., Tame, M.R. and Gasbarrini, G. (1993) Renal sodium retention during upright posture in preascitic cirrhosis. *Gastroenterology* **105**, 188–193.

Besson, I., Ingrand, P., Person, B., Boutroux, D., Heresbach, D., Bernard, P., Hochain, P., Larricq, J., Gourlaouen, A., Ribard, D., Kara, N.M., Legoux, J.L., Pillegand, B., Becker, M.C., Di Constanzo, J., Metreau, J.M., Silvain, C. and Beauchant, M. (1995) Sclerotherapy with or without octreotide for acute variceal bleeding. *New England Journal of Medicine* **333**, 555–560.

Bichet, D.G., Szatalowicz, V., Chaimovitz, C. and Schrier, R.W. (1982) Role of vasopressin in abnormal water excretion in cirrhotic patients. *Annals of Internal Medicine* **96**, 413–417.

Bonkovsky, H.L., Singh, R.H., Jafri, I.H., Fiellin, D.A., Smith, G.S., Simon, D., Cotsonis, G.A. and Slaker, D.P. (1991) A randomized, controlled trial of treatment of alcoholic hepatitis with parenteral nutrition and oxandrolone. II. Short-term effects on nitrogen metabolism, metabolic balance, and nutrition. *American Journal of Gastroenterology* **86**, 1209–1218.

Bosch, J., Kravetz, D. and Rodes, J. (1981) Effects of somatostatin on hepatic and systemic hemodynamics in patients with cirrhosis of the liver: comparison with vasopressin. *Gastroenterology* **80**, 518–525.

Bosch, J., Mastai, R., Kravetz, D., Bruix, J., Gaya, J., Rigau, J. and Rodes, J. (1984) Effects of propranolol on azygous blood flow and hepatic and systemic hemodynamics in cirrhosis. *Hepatology* **4**, 1200–1205.

Burroughs, A.K., Hamilton, G., Phillips, A., Mezzanotte, G., McIntyre, N. and Hobbs, K.E. (1989) A comparison of sclerotherapy with staple transection of the esophagus for the emergency control of bleeding from esophageal varices. *New England Journal of Medicine* **321**, 857–862.

Burroughs, A.K., McCormick, P.A., Hughes, M.D., Sprengers, D., D'Heygere, F. and McIntyre, N. (1990) Randomized, double blind, placebo controlled trial of somatostatin for variceal bleeding: emergency control and prevention of early variceal rebleeding. *Gastroenterology* **99**, 1388–1395.

Butterworth, R.F., Kril, J.J. and Harper, C.G. (1993) Thiamine-dependent enzyme changes in the brains of alcoholics: relationship to the Wenicke-Korsakoff syndrome. *Alcoholism, Clinical and Experimental Research* **17**, 1084–1088.

Cabre, E., Gonzalez-Huix, F., Abad-Lacruz, A., Esteve, M., Acero, D., Fernandez-Banares, F., Xiol, X. and Gassull, M.A. (1990) Effect of total enteral nutrition on the short-term outcome of severely malnourished cirrhotics. A randomized controlled trial. *Gastroenterology* **98**, 715–720.

Cabrera, J., Maynar, M., Granados, R., Gorriz, E., Reyes, R., Pulido-Duque, J.M., Rodriguez SanRoman, J.L., Guerra, C. and Kravetz, D. (1996) Transjugular intrahepatic portosystemic shunt versus sclerotherapy in the elective treatment of variceal hemorrhage. *Gastroenterology* **110**, 832–839.

Cales, P. (1990) Incidence of large oesophageal varices in patients with cirrhosis: application to prophylaxis of first bleeding. *Gut* **31**, 1298–1302.

Calvey, H., Davis, M. and Williams, R. (1985) Controlled trial of nutritional supplmentation, with and without branched chain amino acid enrichment, in treatment of acute alcoholic hepatitis. *Journal of Hepatology* **1**, 141–151.

Caly, W.R. and Strauss, E. (1993) A prospecive study of bacterial infections in patients with cirrhosis. *Journal of Hepatology* **18**, 353–358.

Casado, M., Bosch, J., Garcia-Pagan, J.C., Bru, C., Banares, R., Bandi, J.C., Escorsell, A., Rodriguez-Laiz, J.M., Gilabert, R., Feu, F., Schorlemer, C., Echenagustia, A. and Rodes, J. (1998) Clinical events after transjugular intrahepatic portosystemic shunt: correlation with hemodynamic findings. *Gastroenterology* **114**, 1296–1303.

Chau, T.N., Patch, D., Chan, Y.W., Nagral, A., Dick, R. and Burroughs, A.K. (1998) "Salvage" transjugular intrahepatic portosystemic shunts: gastric fundal compared with esophageal variceal bleeding. *Gastroenterology* **114**, 981–987.

Christensen, E., Fauerholdt, L., Schlichting, P., Juhl, E., Poulsen, H. and Tygstrup, N. (1981) Aspects of natural history of gastrointestinal bleeding in cirrhosis and the effect of prednisolone. *Gastroenterology* **81**, 944–952.

Conn, H.O., Ramsby, G.R., Storer, E.H., Mutchnick, M.G., Joshi, P.H., Phillips, M.M., Cohen, G.A., Fields, G.N. and Petroski, D. (1975) Intra arterial vasopressin in the treatment of upper gastrointestinal haemorrhage: a prospective, controlled clinical trial. *Gastroenterology* **68**, 211–221.

Conn, H.O., Leevy, C.M., Vlahcevic, Z.R., Rodgers, J.B., Maddrey, W.C., Seeff, L. and Levy, L.L. (1977) Comparison of lactulose and neomycin in the treatment of chronic portal-systemic encephalopathy. *Gastroenterology* **72**, 573–583.

Corrao, G., Ferrari, P., Zambon, A. and Torchio, P. (1997) Are the recent trends in liver cirrhosis mortality affected by the changes in alcohol consumption? Analysis of latency period in European countries. *Journal of Studies on Alcohol* **58**, 486–494.

D'Amico, G., Morabito, A., Pagliaro, L., Marubini, E., and the Liver Study Group of "V. Cervello" Hospital (1986) Survival and prognostic indicators in compensated and decompensated cirrhosis. *Digestive Diseases and Sciences* **31**, 468–475.

D'Amico, G., Traina, M., Vizzini, G., Tine, F., Politi, F., Montalbano, L., Luca, A., Pasta, L., Pagliaro, L. and Morabito, A. (1994) Terlipressin or vasopressin plus transdermal nitroglycerin in a treatment strategy for digestive bleeding in cirrhosis. A randomized clinical trial. *Journal of Hepatology* **20**, 206–212.

D'Amico, G., Pagliaro, L. and Bosch, J. (1995) The treatment of portal hypertension: a meta analytical review. *Hepatology* **22**, 332–354.

D'Amico, G. and Luca, A. (1997) Natural history: clinical-haemodynamic correlations: prediction of the risk of bleeding. *Baillieres Clinical Gastroenterology* **11**, 243–256.

Davies, M.H., Langman, M.J., Elias, E. and Neuberger, J.M. (1992) Liver disease in a district hospital remote from a transplant centre: a study of admissions and deaths. *Gut* **33**, 1397–1399.

De Franchis, R. (1994) Treatment of bleeding oesophageal varices: a meta-analysis. *Scandinavian Journal of Gastroenterology* **207** (suppl.), 29–33.

Demakis, J.G., Proskey, A., Rahimtoola, S.H., Jamil, M., Sutton, G.C., Rosen, K.M., Gunnar, R.M. and Tobin, J.R. (1974) The natural course of alcoholic cardiomyopathy. *Annals of Internal Medicine* **80**, 293–297.

Deschenes, M. and Villeneuve, J.P. (1999) Risk factors for the development of bacterial infections in hospitalized patients with cirrhosis. *American Journal of Gastroenterology* **94**, 2193–2197.

Diehl, A.M., Boitnott, J.K., Herlong, H.F., Potter, J.J., Van Duyn, M.A., Chandler, E. and Mezey, E. (1985) Effect of parenteral amino acid supplementation in alcoholic hepatitis. *Hepatology* **5**, 57–63.

Dreiling, D.A. and Koller, M. (1985) The natural history of alcoholic pancreatitis: Update 1985. *Mount Sinai Journal of Medicine* **52**, 340–342.

Estruch, R., Fernandez-Sola, J., Sacanella, E., Pare, C., Rubin, E. and Urbano-Marquez, A. (1989) Relationship between cardiomyopathy and liver disease in chronic alcoholism. *Hepatology* **22**, 532–538.

Everson, G., Bharadhwaj, G., House, R., Talamantes, M., Bilir, B., Shrestha, R., Kam, I., Wachs, M., Karrer, F., Fey, B., Ray, C., Steinberg, T., Morgan, C. and Beresford, T.P. (1997) Long-term follow-up of patients with alcoholic liver disease who underwent hepatic transplantation. *Liver Transplantation and Surgery* **3**, 263–274.

Ferenci, P., Herneth, A. and Steindl, P. (1996) Newer approaches to therapy of hepatic encephalopathy. *Seminars in Liver Disease* **16**, 329–338.

Fernandez-Sola, J., Estruch, R. and Urbano-Marquez, A. (1997) Alcohol and heart muscle disease. *Addiction Biology* **2**, 1–9.

Fogel, M.R., Knauer, C.M. and Andress, L.L. (1982) Continuous intravenous vasopressin in active upper gastrointestinal bleeding: a placebo controlled trial. *Annals of Internal Medicine* **96**, 565–569.

Follo, A.,Llovet, J.M., Navasa, M., Planas, R., Forns, X., Francitorra, A., Rimola, A., Gassull, M.A., Arroyo, V. and Rodes, J. (1994) Renal impairment after spontaneous bacterial peritonitis in cirrhosis: incidence, clinical course, predictive factors and prognosis. *Hepatology* **20**, 1495–1501.

Garcia-Pagan, J.C., Navasa, M., Bosch, J., Bru, C., Pizcueta, P. and Rodes, J. (1990a) Enhancement of portal pressure reduction by the association of isosorbide-5-mononitrate to propranolol administration in patients with cirrhosis. *Hepatology* **11**, 230–238.

Garcia-Pagan, J.C., Feu, F., Navasa, M., Bru, C., Ruiz del Arbol, L., Bosch, J. and Rodes, J. (1990b) Long-term hemodynamic effects of isosorbide-5-mononitrate in patients with cirrhosis and portal hypertension. *Journal of Hepatology* **11**, 189–195.

Garcia-Pagan, J.C., Feu, F., Bosch, J. and Rodes, J. (1991) Propranolol compared with propranolol plus isosorbide-5-mononitrate for portal hypertension in cirrhosis. A randomized controlled study. *Annals of Internal Medicine* **114**, 869–873

Garcia-Pagan, J.C., Navasa, M., Rivera, F., Bosch, J. and Rodes, J. (1992) Lymphocyte b-2-adrenoceptors and plasma catecholamines in patients with cirrhosis. Relationship with the hemodynamic response to propranolol. *Gastroenterology* **102**, 2015–2023.

Garcia-Tsao, G., Groszmann, R.J., Fisher, R.L., Conn, H.O., Atterbury, C.E. and Glickman, M. (1985) Portal pressure, presence of gasrtoesophageal varices and variceal bleeding. *Hepatology* **5**, 419–424.

Garcia-Tsao, G., Grace, N.D., Groszmann, R.J., Conn, H.O., Bermann, M.M., Patrick, M.J., Morse, S.S. and Alberts, J.L. (1986) Short term effects of propranolol on portal venous pressure. *Hepatology* **6**, 101–106.

Gines, P., Tito, L., Arroyo, V., Planas, R., Panes, J., Viver, J., Torres, M., Humbert, P., Rimola, A., Llach, J. *et al.* (1988) Randomized comparative study of therapeutic paracentesis with and without intravenous albumin in cirrhosis. *Gastroenterology* **94**, 1493–1502.

Gines, A., Fernandez-Esparrach, G., Monescillo, A., Vila, C., Domenech, E., Abecasis, R., Angeli, P., Ruiz-Del-Arbol, L., Planas, R., Sola, R., Gines, P., Terg, R., Inglada, L., Vaque, P., Salerno, F., Vargas, V., Clemente, G., Quer, J.C., Jiminez, W., Arroyo, V. and Rodes, J. (1996) Randomized trial comparing albumin, dextran-70, and polygelin in cirrhotic patients with ascites treated by paracentesis. *Gastroenterology* **111**, 1002–1010.

Goldfarb, G., Nouel, O., Poynard, T. and Rueff, B. (1983) Efficiency of respiratory assistance in cirrhotic patients with liver failure. *Intensive Care Medicine* **9**, 271–273.

Goulis, J., Patch, D. and Burroughs, A.K. (1999) Bacterial infection in the pathogenesis of variceal bleeding. *Lancet* **353**, 139–142.

Grace, N.D., Conn, H.O., Groszmann, R.J., Richardson, C.R., Matloff, D.S., Garcia-Tsao, G., Wright, S.C., Drewniak, S.J., Bosch, J., Rodes, J. and Fisher, R.L. (1990) Propranolol for prevention of first esophageal variceal hemorrhage: A lifetime commitment? *Hepatology* **12**, 407.

Greenspon, A.J. and Schaal, S.F. (1983) The "holiday heart": electrophysiologic studies of alcohol effects in alcoholics. *Annals of Internal Medicine* **98**, 135–139.

Groszmann, R.J., Bosch, J., Grace, N.D., Conn, H.O., Garcia-Tsao, G., Navasa, M., Alberts, J., Rodes, J., Fischer, R., Bermann, M. *et al.* (1990) Hemodynamic events in a prospective randomized trial of propranolol versus placebo in the prevention of a first variceal hemorrhage. *Gastroenterology* **99**, 1401–1407.

Guyan, P.M., Uden, S. and Braganza, J.M. (1990) Heightened free radical activity in pancreatitis. *Free Radical Biology and Medicine* **8**, 347–354.

Henriksen, J.H., Bendtsen, F., Sorensen, T.I, Stadeager, C. and Ring-Larsen, H. (1989) Reduced central blood volume in cirrhosis. *Gastroenterology* **97**, 1506–1513.

Henriksen, J.H., Bendtsen, F., Gerbes, A.L., Christensen, N.J., Ring-Larsen, H. and Sorensen, T.I. (1992) Estimated central blood volume in cirrhosis: relationship to sympathetic nervous activity, β-adrenergic blockade and atrial natriuretic factor. *Hepatology* **5**, 1163–1170.

Henriksen, J.H. and Ring-Larsen, H. (1994) Hepatorenal disorders: role of the sympathetic nervous system. *Seminars in Liver Disease* **14**, 35–43.

Italian Multicentre Cooperative Project on Nutrition in Liver Cirrhosis (1994) Nutritional status in cirrhosis. *Journal of Hepatology* **21**, 317–325.

Jenkins, S.A., Shields, R., Davies, M., Elias, E., Turnbull, A.J., Bassendine, M.F., James, O.F., Iredale, J.P., Vyas, S.K., Arthur, M.J., Kingsnorth, A.N. and Sutton, R. (1997) A multicentre randomised trial comparing octreotide and injection sclerotherapy in the management and outcome of acute variceal haemorrhage. *Gut* **41**, 526–533.

Jensen, N.H., Dragsted, L., Christensen, J.K., Jorgensen, J.C. and Qvist, J. (1988) Severity of illness and outcome of treatment in alcoholic patients in the intensive care unit. *Intensive Care Medicine* **15**, 19–22.

John, W.J., Phillips, R., Ott, L., Adams, L.J. and McClain, C.J. (1989) Resting energy expenditure in patients with alcoholic hepatitis. *Journal of Parenteral and Enteral Nutrition* **13**, 124–127.

Kamath, P.S. and McKusick, M.A. (1994) Transjugular intrahepatic portosystemic shunts: a note of caution. *Gastroenterology* **106**, 1384–1387.

Keefe, E.B. (1997) Comorbidities of alcoholic liver disease that affect outcome of orthotopic liver transplantation. *Liver Transplantation and Surgery* **3**, 251–257.

Kitchens, J. (1994) Does this patient have an alcohol problem? *Journal of the American Medical Association* **272**, 1782–1787.

Kim, T., Shijo, H., Kokawa, H., Tokumitsu, H., Kubara, K., Ota, K., Akiyoshi, N., Iida, T., Yokoyama, M. and Okumura, M. (1997) Risk factors for hemorrhage from gastric fundal varices. *Hepatology* **25**, 307–312.

Klatskin, G. (1961) Alcohol and its relation to liver damage. *Gastroenterology* **41**, 443–451.

Klatsky, A.L., Friedman, G.D. and Siegelaub, A.B. (1979) Alcohol use, myocardial infarction, sudden cardiac death and hypertension. *Alcoholism, Clinical and Experimental Research* **3**, 33–39.

Kleber, G., Sauerbruch, T., Fischer, G. and Paumgartner, G. (1988) Somatostatin does not reduce oesophageal variceal pressure in liver cirrhosis. *Gut* **29**, 153–156.

Kleber, G., Sauerbruch, T., Ansari, H. and Paumgartner, G. (1991) Prediction of variceal hemorrhage in cirrhosis: a prospective follow-up study. *Gastroenterology* **100**, 1332–1337.

Laffi, G. and Marra, F. (1999) Complications of cirrhosis: is endothelium guilty? *Journal of Hepatology* **30**, 532–535.

Laine, L. and Cook, D. (1995) Endoscopic ligation compared with sclerotherapy for treatment of esophageal variceal bleeding. A meta-analysis. *Annals of Internal Medicine* **123**, 280–287.

Lebrec, D., De Fleury, P., Rueff, B., Nahum, H. and Benhamou, J.P. (1980) Portal hypertension, size of esophageal varices, and risk of gastrointestinal bleeding in alcoholic cirrhosis. *Gastroenterology* **79**, 1139–1144.

Lebrec, D., Giuily, N., Hadengue, A., Vilgrain, V., Moreau, R., Poynard, T., Gadano, A., Lassen, C., Benhamou, J.P. and Erlinger, S. (1996) Transjugular intrahepatic portosystemic shunts: comparison with paracentesis in patients with cirrhosis and refractory ascites: a randomized trial. *Journal of Hepatology* **25**, 135–144.

Lelbach, W.K. (1976) Epidemiology of alcoholic liver disease. In *Progress in Liver Disease*, Vol. 5, edited by H. Popper and F. Schaffner, pp. 494–515. New York: Grune and Stratton.

Lieber, C.S., Robins, S.J., Li, J., DeCarli, L.M., Mak, K.M., Fasulo, J.M. and Leo, M.A. (1994) Phospatidylcholine protects against fibrosis and cirrhosis in the baboon. *Gastroenterology* **106**, 152–159.

Lieber, C.S. (1995) Medical disorders of alcoholism. *New England Journal of Medicine* **333**, 1058–1065.

Lieberman, F.L. and Reynolds, T.B. (1967) Plasma volume in cirrhosis of the liver: its relation to portal hypertension, ascites, and renal failure. *Journal of Clinical Investigation* **46**, 1297–1308.

Lieberman, F.L., Denison, E.K. and Reynolds, T.B. (1970) The relationship of plasma volume, portal hypertension, ascites and renal sodium retention in cirrhosis. The "overflow" theory of ascites formation. *Annals of the New York Academy of Sciences* **170**, 202–212.

Lo, G.H., Lai, K.H., Cheng, J.S., Lin, C.K., Huang, J.S., Hsu, P.I. and Chiang, H.T. (1997) Emergency banding ligation versus sclerotherapy for the control of active bleeding from esophageal varices. *Hepatology* **25**, 1101–1104.

Mallory, A., Schaefer, J.E. and Cohen, J.R. (1980) Selective intra arterial vasopressin infusion for upper gastrointestinal haemorrhage. A controlled trial. *Archives of Surgery* **115**, 30–32.

Martin, P.Y., Gines, P. and Schrier, R.W. (1998) Nitric oxide as a mediator of hemodynamic abnormalities and sodium and water retension in cirrhosis. *New England Journal of Medicine* **339**, 533–541.

Mastai, R., Bosch, J., Navasa, M., Kravetz, D., Bruix, J., Viola, C. and Rodes, J. (1987) Effects of alpha-adrenergic stimulation and beta-adrenergic blockade on azygous blood flow and splanchnic hemodynamics in patients with cirrhosis. *Journal of Hepatology* **4**, 71–79.

Mato, J.M., Camara, J., Fernandez de Paz, J., Caballeria, L., Coll, S., Caballero, A. *et al.* (1999) S-Adenosylmethionine in alcoholic liver cirrhosis: a randomized, placebo-controlled, double-blind, multicentre clinical trial. *Journal of Hepatology* **30**, 1081–1089.

McClain, C.J., Van Thiel, D.H., Parker, S., Badzin, L.K. and Gilbert, H. (1979) Alterations in zinc, vitamin A, and retinol-binding protein in chronic alcoholics: a possible mechanism for night blindness and hypogonadism. *Alcoholism, Clinical and Experimental Research* **3**, 135–141.

McCullough, A.J. and O'Connor, J.F. (1998) Alcoholic liver disease: proposed recommendations for the American College of Gastroenterology. *American Journal of Gastroenterology* **93**, 2022–2036.

McCullough, A.J. and Tavill, A.S. (1991) Disordered protein and energy metabolism in liver disease. *Seminars in Liver Disease* **11**, 265–277.

Mendenhall, C., Roselle, G.A., Gartside, P. and Moritz, T. (1995) Relationship of protein calorie malnutrition to alcoholic liver disease: a reexamination of data from two Veterans Administration Cooperative Studies. *Alcoholism, Clinical and Experimental Research* **19**, 635–641.

Merigan Jr., T.C., Poltkin, J.R. and Davidson, C.S. (1962) Effect of intravenously administered posterior pituitary extract on haemorrhage from bleeding oesophageal varices. *New England Journal of Medicine* **266**, 134–135.

Merkel, C., Marin, R., Enzo, E., Donada, C., Cavallarin, G., Torboli, P., Amodio, P., Sebastianelli, G., Sacerdoti, D., Felder, M., Mazzaro, C., Beltrame, P. and Gatta, A. (1996) Randomized trial of nadolol alone or with isosorbide mononitrate for primary prophylaxis of variceal bleeding in cirrhosis. *Lancet* **348**, 1677–1681.

Moreau, R., Hadengue, A., Soupison, T., Kirstetter, P., Mamzer, M.F., Vanjak, D., Vanquelin, P., Assous, M. and Sicot, C. (1992) Septic shock in patients with cirrhosis: hemodynamic and metabolic characteristics and intensive care unit outcome. *Critical Care Medicine* **20**, 746–750.

Morgan, M.Y. (1996) Noninvasive neuroinvestigation in liver disease. *Seminars in Liver Disease* **16**, 293–314.

Morillas, R.M., Planas, R., Cabre, E., Galan, A., Quer, J.C., Feu, F., Garcia-Pagan, J.C., Bosch, J. and Gassull, M.A. (1994) Propranolol plus isosorbide-5-mononitrate for portal hypertension in cirrhosis: long-term hemodynamic and renal effects. *Hepatology* **20**, 1502–1508.

Naber, T.H., Schermer, T., de Bree, A., Nusteling, K., Eggink, L., Kruimel, J.W., Bakkeren, J., van Heereveld, H. and Katan, M.B. (1997) Prevalence of malnutrition in nonsurgical hospitalized patients and its association with disease complications. *American Journal of Clinical Nutrition* **66**, 1232–1239.

NIEC (North Italian Endoscopic Club for the Study and Treatment of Esophageal Varices) (1988) Prediction of the first variceal hemorrhage in patients with cirrhosis of the liver and esophageal varices. *New England Journal of Medicine* **319**, 989–989.

Nompleggi, D.J. and Bonkovsky, H.L. (1994) Nutritional supplementation in chronic liver disease: an analytical review. *Hepatology* **19**, 518–533.

Ochs, A., Rossle, M., Haag, K., Hauenstein, K.H., Deibert, P., Siegerstetter, V., Huonker, M., Langer, M. and Blum, H.E. (1995) The transjugular intrahepatic portosystemic stent-shunt procedure for refractory ascites. *New England Journal of Medicine* **332**, 1192–1197.

Papatheodoridis, G.V., Goulis, J., Leandro, G., Patch, D. and Burroughs, A.K. (1999) Transjugular intrahepatic portosystemic shunt compared with endoscopic treatment for prevention of variceal rebleeding: A meta-analysis. *Hepatology* **30**, 612–622.

Patch, D. and Burroughs, A.K. (1995) Pharmacological treatment of portal hypertension. *Progress in Liver Diseases* **13**, 269–292.

Perez-Ayuso, R.M., Arroyo, V., Planas, R., Gaya, J., Bory, F., Rimola, A., Rivera, F. and Rodes, J. (1983) Randomized comparative study of efficacy of furosemide versus spironolactone in nonazotemic cirrhosis with ascites. Relationship between the diuretic response and the activity of the renin-aldosterone system. *Gastroenterology* **84**, 961–968.

Phillips, M.G., Bernal, W. and Wendon, J.A. (1999) Determinants of survival of patients with chronic liver disease in the intensive therapy unit. *Hepatology* **30**, 420A.

Pirmohamed, M. and Gilmore, I.T. (2000) Alcohol abuse and the burden on the NHS – time for action. *Journal of the Royal College of Physicians of London* **34**, 161–162.

Plotkin, J.S., Scott, V.L., Pinna, A., Dobsch, B.P., De Wolf, A.M. and Kang, Y. (1996) Morbidity and mortality in patients with coronary artery disease undergoing liver transplantation. *Liver Transplantation and Surgery* **2**, 436–430.

Quintero, E., Gines, P., Arroyo, V., Rimola, A., Bory, F., Planas, R., Viver, J. and Rodes, J. (1985) Paracentesis versus diuretics in the treatment of cirrhotics with tense ascites. *Lancet* **1**, 611–612.

Renner, I.G., Savage, W.T., Stace, N.H., Pantoja, J.L., Schultheis, W.M. and Peters, R.L. (1984) Pancreatitis associated with alcoholic liver disease. A review of 1022 autopsy cases. *Digestive Diseases and Sciences* **29**, 593–599.

Reynolds, T.B., Hidmura, R., Michel, H. and Peters, R. (1969) Portal hypertension without cirrhosis in alcoholic liver disease. *Annals of Internal Medicine* **70**, 497–506.

Roggin, G.M., Iber, F.L. and Linscheer, W.G. (1972) Intraluminal fat digestion in the chronic alcoholic. *Gut* **13**, 107–111.

Rosa, H., Siverio, A.O., Perini, R.F. and Arrunda, C.B. (2000) Bacterial infection in cirrhotic patients and its relationship with alcohol. *American Journal of Gastroenterology* **95**, 1290–1293.

Rosemurgy, A.S., Goode, S.E., Zweibel, B.R., Black, T.J. and Brady, P.G. (1996) A prospective trial of transjugular intrahepatic portosystemic stent shunts versus small diameter prosthetic H-graft portocaval shunts in the treatment of bleeding varices. *Annals of Surgery* **224**, 378–384.

Rossle, M., Deibert, P., Haag, K., Ochs, A., Olschewski, M., Siegerstetter, V., Hauenstein, K.H., Geiger, R., Stiepak, C., Keller, W. and Blum, H.E. (1997) Randomised trial of transjugular-intrahepatic-portosystemic shunt versus endoscopy plus propranolol for prevention of variceal rebleeding. *Lancet* **349**, 1043–1049.

Rossle, M., Ochs, A., Gulberg, V., Siegerstetter, V., Holl, J., Deibert, P., Olschewski, M., Reiser, M. and Gerbes, A.L. (2000) A comparison of paracentesis and transjugular intrahepatic portosystemic shunting in patients with ascites. *New England Journal of Medicine* **342**, 1701–1707.

Ruiz, M., Ewig, S., Torres, A., Arancibia, F., Marco, F., Mensa, J., Sanchez, M. and Martinez, J.A. (1999) Severe community-acquired pneumonia. Risk factors and follow-up epidemiology. *American Journal of Respiratory and Critical Care Medicine* **160**, 923–929.

Salerno, F., Badalamenti, S., Incerti, P., Tempini, S., Restelli, B., Bruno, G. and Roffi, L. (1987) Repeated paracentesis and iv albumin infusion to treat "tense" ascites in cirrhotic patients: A safe alternative therapy. *Journal of Hepatology* **5**, 102–108.

Sanyal, A.J., Freedman, A.M., Luketic, V.A., Purdam, P.P., Shiffman, M.L., DeMeo, J., Cole, P.E. and Tisnado, J. (1997a) The natural history of portal hypertension after transjugular intrahepatic portosystemic shunts. *Gastroenterology* **112**, 889–898.

Sanyal, A.J., Freedman, A.M., Luketic, V.A., Purdam, P.P., Shiffman, M.L., Cole, P.E., Tisnado, J. and Simmons, S. (1997b) Transjugular intrahepatic portosystemic shunts compared with endoscopic sclerotherapy for the prevention of recurrent variceal hemorrhage. A randomized, controlled trial. *Annals of Internal Medicine* **126**, 849–857.

Sarin, S.K., Lahoti, D., Saxena, S.P., Murthy, N.S. and Makwana, U.K. (1992) Prevalence, classification and natural history of gastric varices: a long-term follow-up study in 568 portal hypertension patients. *Hepatology* **16**, 1343–1349.

Sarin, S.K., Lamba, G.S., Kumar, M., Misra, A. and Murthy, N.S. (1999) Comparison of endoscopic ligation and propranolol for the primary prevention of variceal bleeding. *New England Journal of Medicine* **340**, 988–993.

Schaffner, F. and Popper, H. (1963) Capillarization of the hepatic sinusoids in man. *Gastroenterology* **44**, 239–251.

Schneeweiss, B., Graninger, W., Ferenci, P., Eichinger, S., Grimm, G., Schneider, B., Laggner, A.N., Lenz, K. and Kleinberger, G. (1990) Energy metabolism in patients with acute and chronic liver disease. *Hepatology* **11**, 387–393.

Schrier, R.W., Arroyo, V., Bernardi, M., Epstein, M., Henriksen, J.H. and Rodes, J. (1988) Peripheral arteriolar vasodilation hypothesis: a proposal for the initiation of renal sodium and water retention in cirrhosis. *Hepatology* **8**, 1151–1157.

Selberg, O., Bottcher, J., Tusch, G., Pichlmayr, R., Henkel, E. and Muller, M.J. (1997) Identification of high and low-risk patients before liver transplantation: a prospective cohort study of nutritional and metabolic parameters in 150 patients. *Hepatology* **25**, 652–657.

Shellman, R.G., Fulkerson, W.J., DeLong, E. and Piantadosi, C.A. (1988) Prognosis of patients with cirrhosis and chronic liver disease admitted to the medical intensive care unit. *Critical Care Medicine* **16**, 671–678.

Shiffman, M.L., Jeffers, L., Hoofnagle, J.H. and Tralka, T.S. (1995) The role of transjugular intrahepatic portosystemic shunt for the treatment of portal hypertension and its complications: A conference sponsored by the National Digestive Diseases Advisory Board. *Hepatology* **22**, 1591–1597.

Singh, N., Gayowski, T., Wagener, M.M. and Marino, I.R. (1998) Outcome of patients with cirrhosis requiring intensive care unit support: Prospective assessment of predictors of mortality. *Journal of Gastroenterology* **33**, 73–79.

Soderlund, C., Magnusson, I., Torngren, S. and Lundell, L. (1990) Terlipressin (triglycyl-lysine vasopressin) controls acute bleeding oesophageal varices. A double blind, randomized, placebo-controlled trial. *Scandinavian Journal of Gastroenterology* **25**, 622–630.

Sort, P., Navasa, M., Arroyo, V., Aldeguer, X., Planas, R., Ruiz-del-Arbol, L., Castells, L., Vargas, V., Soriano, G., Guevara, M., Gines, P. and Rodes, J. (1999) Effect of intravenous albumin on renal impairment and mortality in patients with cirrhosis and spontaneous bacterial peritonitis. *New England Journal of Medicine* **341**, 403–409.

Sung, J.J., Chung, S.C., Yung, M.Y., Lai, C.W., Lau, J.Y., Lee, Y.T., Leung, V.K., Li, M.K. and Li, A.K. (1995) Prospective randomized study of effect of octreotide on rebleeding from oesophageal varices after endoscopic ligation. *Lancet* **346**, 1666–1669.

Swart, G.R., van der Berg, J.W., Wattimena, J.L., Rietveld, T., van Vuure, J.K. and Frenkel, M. (1988) Elevated protein requirements in cirrhosis of the liver investigated by whole body protein turnover studies. *Clinical Science* **75**, 101–107.

Swart, G.R., Zillikens, M.C., van Vurre, J.K. and van den Berg, J.W. (1989) Effect of late evening meal on nitrogen balance in patients with cirrhosis of the liver. *British Medicial Journal* **299**, 1202–1203.

Tait, I.S., Krige, J.E. and Terblanche, J. (1999) Endoscopic band ligation of oesophageal varices. *British Journal of Surgery* **86**, 437–446.

Tsai, K., Wang, S.S., Chen, T.S., Kong, C.W., Chang, F.Y., Lee, S.D. and Lu, F.J. (1998) Oxidative stress: an important phenomenon with pathogenetic significance in the progression of acute pancreatitis. *Gut* **42**, 850–855.

Tyden, G., Samnegaard, H., Thulin, L., Muhrbeck, O. and Efendic, S. (1979) Circulatory effects of somatostatin in anaesthetized man. *Acta Chirugica Scandinavica* **145**, 443–446.

Urbano-Marquez, A., Estruch, R., Navarro-Lopez, F., Grau, J.M., Mont, L. and Rubin, E. (1989) The effects of alcoholism on skeletal and cardiac muscle. *New England Journal of Medicine* **320**, 409–415.

Valenzuela, J.E., Schubert, T., Fogel, M.R., Strong, R.M., Levine, J., Mills, P.R., Fabry, T.L., Taylor, L.W., Conn, H.O. and Posillico, J.T. (1989) Amulticenter, randomized, double-blind trial of somatostatin in the management of acute haemorrhage from oesophageal varices. *Hepatology* **10**, 958–961.

Viallet, A., Marleau, D., Huet, M., Martin, F., Farley, A., Villeneuve, J.P. and Lavoie, P. (1975) Hemodynamic evaluation of patients with intrahepatic portal hypertension: relationship between bleeding varices and the portohepatic gradient. *Gastroenterology* **69**, 1297–1300.

Vorobioff, J., Bredfeldt, J.E. and Groszmann, R.J. (1983) Hyperdynamic splanchnic circulation in portal hypertensive rat model: a primary factor for maintenance of chronic portal hypertension. *American Journal of Physiology* **244**, G52-G57.

Vorobioff, J., Groszmann, R.J., Picabea, E., Gamen, M., Villavicencio, R., Bordato, J., Morel, I., Audano, M., Tanno, H., Lerner, E. and Passamonti, M. (1996) Prognostic value of hepatic venous pressure gradient measurements in alcoholic cirrhosis: a 10-year prospective study. *Gastroenterology* **111**, 701–709.

Walker, S., Stiehl, A., Raedseh, R. and Kommerell, B. (1986) Terlipressin in bleeding oesophageal varices: a placebo controlled double blind study. *Hepatology* **6**, 112–115.

Wenzel, G., Kuklinski, B., Ruhlmann, C. and Ehrhardt, D. (1993) Alcohol toxic hepatitis – a free radical associated disease. Decreased mortality by adjuvant antioxidant therapy. *Zeitschrift fur die Gesamte Innere Medizin und ihre Grenzgebiete* **48**, 490–496.

Whitely, G.S.W., Kienle, A.P.B., McCloy, R.F. and Braganza, J.M. (1993) Long-term pain relief without surgery in chronic pancreatitis: value of antioxidant therapy. *Gastroenterology* **A343**.

Witte, C.L., Witte, M.H. and Dumont, A.E. (1980) Lymph imbalance in the genesis and perpetuation of the ascites syndrome in hepatic cirrhosis. *Gastroenterology* **78**, 1059–1069.

Wong, F. and Blendis, L. (1994) Pathophysiology of sodium retention and ascites formation in cirrhosis: role of atrial natriuretic factor. *Seminars in Liver Disease* **14**, 59–70.

Zauner, C.A., Apsner, R.C., Kranz, A., Kramer, L., Madl, C., Schneider, B., Schneeweiss, B., Ratheiser, K., Stockenhuber, F. and Lenz, K. (1996) Outcome prediction for patients with cirrhosis of the liver in a medical ICU: a comparison of the APACHE scores and liver-specific scoring systems. *Intensive Care Medicine* **22**, 559–563.

Zimmerman, J.E., Wagner, D.P., Seneff, M.G., Becker, R.B., Sun, X. and Knaus, W.A. (1996) Intensive care unit admissions with cirrhosis: risk-stratifying patient groups and predicting individual survival. *Hepatology* **23**, 1393–1401.

Chapter 23

The role of the psychiatrist in the treatment of alcoholic liver disease

José Martínez-Raga and E. Jane Marshall

It is estimated that between 15–30% of male and 8–15% female medical admissions to general hospitals have significant alcohol problems. Successful management of patients with alcoholic liver disease (ALD) is complex, involving multiple specific treatments within a multidisciplinary team setting. Psychiatric management is often an important and crucial element. The role of the psychiatrist is not limited to managing intoxication and withdrawal states. It also involves monitoring the patient's mental state, developing and facilitating adherence to a treatment plan, preventing relapse, providing education about alcohol use disorders and diagnosing and treating associated psychiatric disorders. Finally, psychiatrists are also specifically trained in the clinical use of psychopharmacological agents. In this chapter, we shall review the role of the psychiatrist in the management of patients with alcohol-induced liver disease. This will include an overview of psychiatric problems associated with ALD and a discussion of the role of psychiatrists in managing such problems in the general hospital and in outpatient settings. The assessment of alcohol use disorder in individuals with liver disease will be reviewed, with a discussion of appropriate psychopharmacological and psychological interventions.

KEYWORDS: alcohol use disorders – hazardous/harmful use, alcohol dependence, abstinence, psychopathology, drinking history, screening instruments, "stages of change" model, brief interventions, motivational enhancement therapy, cognitive behavioral therapy, relapse prevention, psychopharmacological interventions, alcohol withdrawal syndrome, anti-craving agents, comorbid affective disorders/anxiety/sleep disorders, comorbid psychotic disorders, comorbid substance use disorders, liver transplantation

PSYCHIATRIC ASPECTS OF ALCOHOLIC LIVER DISEASE

The psychiatrist in alcoholic liver disease

Psychiatrists care for patients with alcohol use disorders in a variety of clinical settings, frequently working in collaboration with members of other professional disciplines. The role of the psychiatrist will vary according to the specific clinical situation and the physical and mental state of the individual patient. Psychiatric care should be tailored to meet the needs of each patient. Its frequency, intensity and focus is likely to vary over time (American Psychiatric Association, 1995). The contribution of psychiatry to the management of patients with ALD includes assessment and clinical diagnosis of the alcohol use disorder, the mental state and the presence of any concurrent mental illness. Much of this work falls to the consultation-liaison psychiatrist attached to the general hospital. General psychiatrists may have a role in areas where liaison psychiatry services are poorly developed. Specialist Liver Units should, ideally, have access to and close links with a Specialist Addiction Service. Addiction psychiatrists can facilitate harm reduction and relapse prevention techniques. They also have a role in policy development, education, training and research.

The treatment of patients with alcohol-induced liver injury is best provided within a multidisciplinary team approach. Management must be directed at achieving complete abstinence from alcohol, as well at treating the hepatic impairment. Most mild cases of alcoholic hepatitis improve with abstinence and even those with moderately advanced cirrhosis can have a remarkable improvement of quality of life and increased survival rates with complete abstinence (Harris and Brunt, 1995). Complete abstinence from alcohol doubles the five year survival rate for patients with compensated alcohol-induced liver cirrhosis (Saunders *et al.*, 1981). Unfortunately, at least 25% of patients with ALD will continue to drink irrespective of therapy (Sherlock, 1995).

Psychiatrists, however, cannot see and treat everyone with ALD. Physicians and nurses who deal with such patients in their day-to-day work should be able to distinguish between hazardous/harmful drinking and alcohol dependence. It is not enough merely to tell these patients to stop drinking. This just gives health-care professionals the excuse to do nothing. Individuals drinking in a hazardous or harmful way should be offered a "brief intervention" and their alcohol consumption monitored at out-patient follow-up. Many liver units are supraregional, and can only offer infrequent follow-up. Good communication with the primary healthcare team is critical in this situation. Here the role of the psychiatrist is as educator and motivator. Psychiatrists should support the implementation of standardized screening instruments for alcohol consumption in the general hospital and devise guidelines for brief interventions. Nurses in particular have a significant role to play in such interventions.

Referral to psychiatrists should be reserved for patients who are alcohol dependent, have other psychiatric, social or physical problems, and who are unable to maintain abstinence. It could be argued that women with ALD should always be referred for psychiatric assessment, because they are more likely than men to have a comorbid psychiatric problem.

Alcohol use disorder and alcoholic liver disease

Individuals with ALD are a heterogeneous population. Not only do they differ in the degree and severity of the liver injury as outlined in previous chapters, but the severity of their drinking problem also varies markedly. Alcohol consumption is determined by a complex interaction of a variety of factors: genetic, economic, dietary, social and cultural. Individuals vary enormously in the amounts they consume and there is no clear boundary between "normal" and "heavy" drinkers. The interaction between genetic vulnerability and environmental factors determines whether a person goes on to develop a drinking problem or not. The risk of developing a drinking problem rises with the amount of alcohol consumed. Men drinking 3–4 units and women drinking 2–3 units per day are unlikely to damage their health. However, men drinking above 50 units and women drinking above 35 units per week are drinking in a "harmful" way and are likely to be experiencing problems as a result. Harmful drinkers may come to a point where they can no longer control their drinking as they once did. These individuals drink in order to maintain a constant blood alcohol level and usually show evidence of the other key elements of the alcohol dependence syndrome. Table 23.1 shows the diagnostic criteria for alcohol dependence according to the two main psychiatric classification systems, the Diagnostic and Statistical Manual (DSM-IV) of the American Psychiatric Association (1994) and the International Classification of Disorders (ICD-10) of the World Health Organisation (1992). These classifications also include an alcohol abuse (DSM-IV) or harmful alcohol use (ICD-10), which is defined primarily on the basis of adverse consequences that result from alcohol use (Table 23.2).

Table 23.1 ICD-10 and DSM-IV diagnostic criteria for alcohol dependence

ICD-10 Symptoms[§]	DSM-IV Symptoms[§]
Tolerance: need for increased doses of alcohol to achieve effects originally produced by lower doses, or markedly reduced effect with continued use of the same amount	
Withdrawal, as evidenced by the characteristic withdrawal syndrome, or alcohol use is taken to relieve or avoid withdrawal symptoms	
	Alcohol is taken in larger amounts or over a longer period of time than was intended
	Persistent desire or repeated unsuccessful efforts to cut down or control alcohol use
A strong desire or compulsion to use	
Difficulties in controlling alcohol-using behavior in terms of its onset, termination or levels of use	
	A great deal of time is spent in activities necessary to obtain or use alcohol, or recover from its effects
Progressive (important) neglect of alternative pleasures interests or activities in favour of drinking	
Persistence with alcohol despite clear evidence of overtly harmful consequences (social, physical or psychological)	

[§] A diagnosis of dependence should only be made if three or more items have been experienced or exhibited at some time during the previous 12-month period.

Table 23.2 ICD-10 and DSM-IV diagnostic criteria for harmful alcohol use and alcohol abuse

ICD-10 criteria – harmful alcohol use
Clear evidence that alcohol use was responsible for causing actual psychological or physical harm

DSM-IV criteria – alcohol abuse
A maladaptive pattern of alcohol use indicated by at least one of the following:
1 recurrent alcohol use resulting in inability to fulfil major role obligations at work, school, or home
2 recurrent alcohol-related legal or interpersonal problems
3 important social, occupational or recreational activities given up or reduced because of drinking
4 recurrent alcohol use in situations in which it is physically hazardous

Neither the abuse/harmful use category, nor the diagnosis of alcohol dependence can be viewed as all or nothing phenomena, but rather should be viewed as existing along a continuum of severity. Similarly, not all alcohol dependent patients develop hepatic impairment; some individuals appear to be more susceptible. It is estimated that between 8 and 30% of chronic drinkers will develop alcoholic cirrhosis typically after a 10–20 year history of daily excessive alcohol intake (Sherman and Williams, 1994). Conversely, about 33% of heavy drinkers have no hepatic consequences. It has been suggested that genetic factors contribute to an increased risk of liver damage (Lumeng and Crabb, 1994). Environmental factors such as hepatitis B and C also may contribute to the development of ALD and continuing heavy alcohol consumption may worsen hepatic injury associated with viral hepatitis (Sherlock, 1995). In addition, women are more susceptible than men to alcoholic hepatic damage (Mello *et al.*, 1992).

Psychopathology in patients with alcoholic liver disease

An important aspect of patients with ALD is the well recognized association of alcohol use disorder with several forms of psychopathology. Patients with alcohol abuse or dependence have higher rates of comorbid psychiatric disorders than the general population, especially affective disorders, anxiety disorders, antisocial personality disorders, post-traumatic stress disorder and other substance use disorders (Regier *et al.*, 1990; Marshall and Alam, 1997). Patients with alcohol-induced liver injury have been shown to have a higher prevalence of psychiatric disorders, especially mood and anxiety disorders, than patients with other forms of chronic liver disease of comparable severity (Ewusi-Mensah *et al.*, 1984). Many patients with ALD continue to drink after discharge from hospital (Saunders *et al.*, 1981) and underlying psychiatric illness may contribute to this. The presence of a comorbid psychiatric disorder is associated with poor drinking outcomes (Rounsaville *et al.*, 1987) and the more severe the psychiatric disorder, the less favorable the outcome (McLellan *et al.*, 1983). Patients with alcohol use disorder should therefore be screened for psychiatric disorders and have access to appropriate treatment. Psychiatric assessment and intervention have the potential to improve overall treatment outcome and, more specifically, abstinence rates.

CLINICAL RECOGNITION AND ASSESSMENT

Taking a history

It is well documented that hospital doctors do not routinely screen for alcohol problems (Canning *et al.*, 1999), often citing their excessive workload as the reason. About a third of physicians neglect to take a history of alcohol use from their patients (Sherlock, 1995). Specialist workers identify more cases (Tolley and Rowland, 1991) and nurses have been shown to be more cost-effective than doctors at screening admissions for problem drinkers. Patients may feel that they can speak more openly to a nurse than to a doctor and nurses may have more time to do this work. The public health case for employing alcohol liaison nurses in the general hospital is therefore very strong.

It is important to remember that patients with ALD often feel ashamed about their drinking problem and may initially deny any excessive alcohol use. They may find it difficult to discuss their drinking openly, are likely to evade alcohol-related questions and can even become hostile. This difficulty will only be overcome if the therapist (nurse, physician, psychiatrist) can convey an empathic and non-judgemental attitude. Rather than confronting the patient with questions on quantity consumed and frequency of consumption and risking a defensive reply, it is generally more useful to open with non-specific questions, such as what they perceive as the main problem. It can be helpful to set the scene with a casual introductory remark, such as, "I always ask everyone about drinking." This implies that it is a routine question in this area and the patient is not left feeling that he/she is a single case.

As well as a drinking history, the assessment should include information on the patient's personal, marital, social, psychiatric and medical background, with emphasis on elucidating those features that are likely to be of particular relevance to the understanding of the drinking problems. The assessment should also include information on the patient's family background, with details on the family attitudes to alcohol and the family history of alcoholism and other psychiatric illness. Finally, a detailed drinking history is essential in order to understand the patient's alcohol in longitudinal perspective (Edwards *et al.*, 1997). For such purposes it may be relevant to explore the evolution of drinking and current drinking patterns, the evolution of alcohol-related problems and an outline of a typical recent heavy drinking day.

Screening instruments and questionnaires

Routine alcohol use screening questionnaires are of enormous potential value in the general hospital setting. Several instruments have been developed for the detection of heavy drinking or alcohol-related problems. These can be made more acceptable if they are included as part of a health and lifestyle assessment focusing on smoking, diet, exercise and stress (Graham, 1991). The 4-item CAGE questionnaire (Ewing, 1984), the 24-item Michigan Alcoholism Screening Test (MAST) (Selzer *et al.*, 1971) and its shorter version, the 13-item Short MAST (sMAST) (Selzer *et al.*, 1975), are all helpful in identifying individuals with severe and obvious alcohol problems.

The more recently developed 10-item Alcohol Use Disorders Identification Test (AUDIT), detects both "at risk" (hazardous) drinking and dependence (Table 23.3) (Saunders *et al.*, 1993; Bohn *et al.*, 1995). The AUDIT has been shown to be a good predictor of both alcohol-related social and medical problems (Conigrave *et al.*, 1995b). The AUDIT can be self-administered or administered by non-clinical staff. Each item is scored on a scale of 0–4 giving a possible maximum score of 40. Different cut-off points can be used, but a score of 8 or more appears to produce the highest sensitivity (Conigrave *et al.*, 1995a; MacKenzie *et al.*, 1996). The AUDIT appears to be a good adjunct to obtaining additional information from other sources, the records or a full clinical assessment. A shortened version of the AUDIT, using 5 items (1;2;4;5;10) has now been validated for screening purposes (Piccinelli *et al.*, 1997). A score of 5 or more on these items detects "at risk" drinking.

Table 23.3 The AUDIT questionnaire

1 How often do you have a drink containing alcohol?
( ) Never   ( ) Less than monthly   ( ) Monthly   ( ) Two to three   ( ) Four or more
                                                          times a week   times a week

2 How many drinks containing alcohol do you have on a typical day when you are drinking?
( ) 1 or 2   ( ) 3 or 4   ( ) 5 or 6   ( ) 7 to 9   ( ) 10 or more

3 How often do you have six or more drinks on one occasion?
( ) Never   ( ) Less than monthly   ( ) Monthly   ( ) Two to three   ( ) Four or more
                                                          times a week   times a week

4 How often during the last year have you found that you were not able to stop drinking once
   you had started?
( ) Never   ( ) Less than monthly   ( ) Monthly   ( ) Two to three   ( ) Four or more
                                                          times a week   times a week

5 How often during the last year have you failed to do what was normally expected from you
   because of drinking?
( ) Never   ( ) Less than monthly   ( ) Monthly   ( ) Two to three   ( ) Four or more
                                                          times a week   times a week

6 How often during the last year have you needed a first drink in the morning to get yourself
   going after a heavy drinking session?
( ) Never   ( ) Less than monthly   ( ) Monthly   ( ) Two to three   ( ) Four or more
                                                          times a week   times a week

7 How often during the last year have you had a feeling of guilt or remorse after drinking?
( ) Never   ( ) Less than monthly   ( ) Monthly   ( ) Two to three   ( ) Four or more
                                                          times a week   times a week

8 How often during the last year have you been unable to remember what happened the night
   before because you had been drinking?
( ) Never   ( ) Less than monthly   ( ) Monthly   ( ) Two to three   ( ) Four or more
                                                          times a week   times a week

9 Have you or someone else been injured as a result of your drinking?
( ) No   ( ) Yes, but not in the last year   ( ) Yes, during the last year

10 Has a relative or friend, or a doctor or other health worker been concerned about your
    drinking or suggested you cut down?
( ) No   ( ) Yes, but not in the last year   ( ) Yes, during the last year

In addition to screening questionnaires, a number of standardized instruments have been developed which can be employed to assess the severity of alcohol dependence, or alcohol-related problems. The Severity of Alcohol Dependence Questionnaire or SADQ (Stockwell *et al.*, 1979) has been widely used both for clinical and research purposes to rate the patient's degree of alcohol dependence. On the SADQ's 60-point scale, scores of around 20–30 suggest that the patient is entering a range of severe dependence. The Alcohol Problems Questionnaire or APQ (Drummond, 1989) is another self-report instrument, which can be valuable for measuring intensity of alcohol-related problems.

TREATMENT/MANAGEMENT

The treatment goal for individuals with ALD is complete abstinence from alcohol. In order to achieve and maintain abstinence, psychological support, help to initiate motivation, ongoing support and monitoring, often combined with pharmacotherapies, are required. The recent diagnosis of ALD or exacerbation of known ALD can be used to engage patients in treatment and to motivate them to consider abstinence. Heavy drinkers are not only concerned about their own health. Often a relative or friend may have died from alcoholic cirrhosis. However, interventions are only likely to produce movement when used alongside the real possibilities for change within the individual, the family and the social setting (Edwards *et al.*, 1997). In addition, the patient with ALD has to be presented with the unambiguous message that dealing with the drinking problem is an absolute priority. In this context, it might be useful to assess the patient's motivation to stop drinking. This can be carried out within Prochaska and DiClemente's transtheoretical model of change, often associated with motivational counseling (Prochaska and DiClemente, 1992).

Prochaska and DiClemente's "stages of change" model, which acknowledges the pivotal role of the individual in the process of behavioral change, describes five discrete stages of change: *precontemplation, contemplation, determination, action* and *maintenance*. Under this model, motivation is operationalized by assessing the stage at which the patient finds himself/herself. In the *precontemplation* stage individuals are not currently considering a change in their drinking habits. Individuals in the *contemplation* stage recognize that they have a problem and begin to consider the implications for change, but remain ambivalent to change. In the *determination* stage individuals are intending to take action and may already have tried to reduce their alcohol consumption. They move to the *action* stage when they make a decision and commitment to change. In the *maintenance* stage individuals seek to maintain the changes in order to prevent relapse. The model is best viewed a spiral, as individuals usually relapse and re-enter the cycle, often moving through the stages several times before achieving long-term maintenance (Prochaska and DiClemente, 1992). This model helps healthcare professionals to meet drinkers "where they are" and to choose the appropriate treatment strategies. Thus, patients in the precontemplation stage who deny that they have a problem will not respond to interventions designed to produce behavior change. Non-confrontational motivational techniques would be best used here. The model is possibly best viewed as a model of ideal change that may be helpful in the design of interventions (Sutton, 1996).

Psychological interventions

A number of psychological interventions have been shown to be effective in the treatment of drinking problems. Five broad approaches, summarized in Table 23.4 will be discussed.

Brief interventions

Brief interventions are simple, easily administered treatments that have been shown to yield significant reductions in alcohol use and related drinking problems

Table 23.4 Psychological interventions for drinking problems

- Brief interventions
- Motivational enhancement therapy
- Cognitive-behavioral therapy
- Relapse prevention
- Individual and group psychotherapies

in a variety of settings, including primary care, accident and emergency departments and medical wards (Dunn and Ries, 1997; Wilk *et al.*, 1997). The aim is to raise awareness of problems and promote behavioral change. Brief interventions are particularly useful for individuals with problem or hazardous drinking rather than alcohol dependence. They consist of an assessment of alcohol intake and related problems, clarification of triggers for drinking, feedback, advice about sensible drinking and negotiation of realistic aims. Evidence suggests that brief interventions following opportunistic screening in primary care and in the general hospital are effective in reducing alcohol intake particularly in men (Wallace *et al.*, 1988). They may also have a similar impact to more intensive, longer term programs and can increase the effectiveness of subsequent treatment (Bien *et al.*, 1993; WHO Brief Intervention Study Group, 1996; Wilk *et al.*, 1997). They focus on raising problem awareness and advising change and have the advantage that they can be implemented by non-specialists.

Brief interventions incorporate six common elements that have been summarized by the acronym FRAMES: Feedback, Responsibility, Advice, Menu, Empathy and Self-efficacy (Miller and Sanchez, 1994) (Table 23.5). Although brief interventions are typically used and have been reported to be more successful in less severely affected individuals who have not received previous treatment for an alcohol use disorder, a recent meta-analysis of randomized controlled trials of brief interventions found that heavy alcohol drinkers in outpatient settings who

Table 23.5 The FRAMES elements of brief interventions

F	**FEEDBACK** to patient about personal risk or impairment, which may produce a strong motivational impact through the inherent feedback involved.
R	Emphasis on personal **RESPONSIBILITY** for change. Brief interventions commonly advise patients that their drinking is their own responsibility and choice. Perceived personal control has been recognized as an element of motivation for behavior change and maintenance (Miller, 1985).
A	**ADVICE** to change. Explicit verbal or written advice to reduce or stop drinking.
M	**MENU** of alternative options for change. Brief interventions tend to advise either a general goal or a range of options. Apparently, this increases the likelihood that the patient will find a strategy acceptable to his or her own situation.
E	**EMPATHIC** interviewing. A warm, reflective, empathic and understanding counseling style has been described as most effective.
S	Enhancement of patients **SELF-EFFICACY**. Rather than emphasising helplessness or powerlessness, brief interventions encourage the patient's self-efficacy for change. The patient must believe that he or she can change.

received a brief intervention were twice as likely to moderate their drinking 6 to 12 months after an intervention when compared with heavy drinkers who received no intervention (Wilk *et al.*, 1997). A general medical setting such as a liver unit can provide the right environment for initiating brief interventions. Hospitalized general medical patients with alcohol-related physical damage may be particularly receptive to counseling. They might come to see a link between their alcohol abuse and their health problems after brief, opportunistic interventions (Dyehouse and Sommers, 1998). The role of the psychiatrist here should be to train Liver Unit staff to implement these interventions on a routine basis.

Motivational enhancement therapy (MET)

Since its original description as a therapeutic technique for use with problem drinkers (Miller, 1985), MET has emerged as a practical and acceptable treatment approach in a wide range of disorders, including alcohol and drug problems and eating disorders (Miller and Rollnick, 1991). The concept of MET emerged from the clinical experience of dealing with ambivalence and motivation for change in individuals with alcohol and other problems. MET is a useful counseling approach for individuals who are reluctant to change and ambivalent about changing. The therapist does not assume an authoritarian role within the sessions but seeks to create a positive atmosphere conducive to change. The overall goal is to increase the intrinsic motivation of the client. It is helpful to view MET in the context of the stages of change model, as it is a very useful treatment tool to deal with precontemplation.

In MET the therapist uses empathic warmth and reflective listening to establish a therapeutic relationship with the patient, by using open-ended questions, reflective listening, affirmation and listening. Overtly confrontational tactics and arguments are deliberately avoided. The therapist does not oppose resistance but tries to use it to good advantage. Self-motivational statements are elicited from patients in order to help them develop a perceived discrepancy or dissonance between their behavior and their stated goals. MET develops and amplifies this discrepancy, ultimately allowing the patient to present the reasons for change without feeling coerced. Another key element in motivation for change is self-efficacy. MET can be applied within specialist liver units by appropriately trained staff.

Cognitive-behavioral therapy (CBT)

Evidence suggests that CBT consistently leads to reduced drinking (Holder *et al.*, 1991). CBT is a short-term, comparatively brief approach well suited to the resource capabilities of most clinical programs. It has been extensively evaluated in rigorous clinical trials and has solid empirical support as treatment for depression and anxiety disorders, as well as in the treatment of alcohol misuse and other addictive behaviors. CBT is a flexible, structured, individualized approach that can be adapted to a wide range of patients as well as a variety of settings (inpatient, outpatient) and formats (group, individual), focused on the immediate problems faced by alcohol abusers who are struggling to control their drinking (Carroll, 1996).

CBT is compatible with a range of other treatments the patient may receive, such as pharmacotherapy. Cognitive-behavioral therapies refer to a broad spectrum of approaches, which include social skills training and assertiveness training, training of problem-solving skills, relaxation techniques, anger management, cognitive restructuring, behavioral self-control, cue-exposure therapy and relapse prevention therapy (American Psychiatric Association, 1995; Botvin *et al.*, 1990; Marlatt and Gordon, 1985). Overall, cognitive behavioral therapies focus on altering the cognitive processes that lead to maladaptive behaviors in alcohol abusers, intervening in the behavioral chain of events that lead to alcohol use, helping patients deal successfully with craving, and promoting and reinforcing the development of social skills and behaviors compatible with remaining abstinent. Cognitive behavioral strategies are based on the assumption that problem drinking is substantially a learned behavior and the treatment involves replacing the maladaptive pattern of drinking behavior with more appropriate drinking or like in the case of patients of ALD, complete abstinence.

Relapse prevention

The term relapse prevention refers to a wide range of techniques, many or all of which are based on cognitive or behavioral strategies. This approach has its origin in a theoretical model of relapse proposed by Marlatt and Gordon (1985). Within this perspective, relapse is not viewed as a catastrophe, but as an event that takes place through a series of cognitive, behavioral and affective processes. Relapse prevention is a self-management approach based on social-learning theory, which considers drinking behavior to be substantially a learned behavior, designed to teach individuals who are trying to change their behavior how to anticipate and cope with the problem of relapse. One of the main objectives of the program is preventing a lapse from becoming a relapse. Relapse is viewed as an untoward event, which is to be avoided by careful forward planning and by the design of an individual relapse prevention program. Patients are active in identifying high-risk situations that are associated with a potential for relapse. Patients are taught more effective coping mechanisms, including cognitive strategies and personally planned alternative activities. Strategies will thus involve both learning how to avoid unnecessary risks and how to deal positively and confidently with inevitable risks and consequently increase the patient's sense of self-efficacy. Relapse prevention procedures can be applied either in the form of a specific maintenance strategy to prevent relapse or as a more general programme of lifestyle change. The aim is for the patient to improve/change his lifestyle by identifying sources of stress, to identify and change unhealthy habit patterns, to discover and take up positive activities, to learn more effective time management and to arrive at a moderate or balanced lifestyle (Carroll, 1996).

Psychopharmacological interventions

Because of the multifaceted nature of alcohol problems, it is not surprising that drugs from a number of different pharmacological classes have been used to treat abuse and dependence syndromes. The pharmacological treatments can be classified according to the following major categories (Liskow and Goodwin, 1987; Litten and Allen, 1991):

a   Medications used to treat the alcohol withdrawal syndrome;
b   Agents that block the desire and compulsion to drink, the preoccupation with acquiring alcohol, the desire to use or continue to use alcohol and to deter alcohol consumption. This category includes anticraving medications and alcohol sensitizing or aversive agents;
c   Agents to treat comorbid psychiatric disorders;
d   Medications to treat concurrent substance use disorders.

In liver disease, psychotropic drugs need to be used with caution. The severity and degree of liver impairment will determine the use of these agents. This relates specifically to those drugs metabolized by the liver as is the case for most psychopharmacological agents. In severe liver disease, sedative drugs may adversely affect cerebral function and may precipitate or mask hepatic encephalopathy. In addition, even in moderate liver disease renal function may be affected. Consequently, lower doses of renally cleared drugs may therefore be required.

Treatment of alcohol withdrawal symptoms

Only patients who are dependent on alcohol develop withdrawal symptoms. In this case medically assisted withdrawal represents the first therapeutic intervention. Patients with alcohol withdrawal must be detoxified in a setting that provides for frequent clinical assessment. Outpatient settings can accommodate these requirements and may be appropriate for individuals considered to be at low risk of a complicated withdrawal. However, patients with a past history of severe withdrawal symptoms, such as seizures or delirium tremens, as well as patients with medical and psychiatric disorders may need to be hospitalized for medically assisted detoxification. Specifically, in alcohol dependent patients with severe medical complications, such as liver damage, an intense and closely supervized inpatient medically assisted alcohol withdrawal may be associated with more favorable mortality outcomes (Bunn *et al.*, 1994). In patients with ALD it can be carried out within the setting of a Liver Unit or a Specialist Addiction Unit.

The withdrawal syndrome

The alcohol withdrawal syndrome results from abrupt cessation of drinking in alcohol dependent patients. Symptoms of alcohol withdrawal typically begin within 4–12 hours after cessation or reduction of alcohol use, peak in intensity during the second day of abstinence and generally resolve within 4–5 days. The severity of this syndrome differs greatly. The patient may initially experience a variety of milder withdrawal symptoms, such as anxiety, mild gastrointestinal symptoms (e.g., nausea and vomiting), tremulousness, sweating, irritability, tachycardia, systolic hypertension and insomnia. More severe symptoms include generalized seizures (usually grand mal), which may appear singly or as a series, usually within 24–48 hours after the last drink (Edwards *et al.*, 1997). Delirium tremens, the most serious form of the alcohol withdrawal syndrome, is characterized by a state of profound confusion, delusions, vivid hallucinations, tremor and agitation, with a pronounced loss of insight, sleeplessness, as well as signs of increased autonomic nervous system activity (hyperthermia, tachycardia and profuse sweating). Several neurotransmitter and receptor systems have been implicated in the development of alcohol withdrawal symptoms, including noradrenergic hyperactivity, gamma-aminobutyric acid (GABA)-benzodiazepine receptor alteration, hyperactivation of the hypothalamic-pituitary-adrenal axis and changes in the N-methyl-D-aspartate (NMDA) receptors (Adinoff et al., 1988; Litten and Allen, 1991).

Although the severity of withdrawal symptoms is generally proportional to the duration of the preceding levels of alcohol consumption, other factors are involved, such as prior experience of withdrawal symptoms. A concurrent medical illness may accelerate the withdrawal, or increase its severity. In addition, liver disease can also affect the duration and severity of the withdrawal symptoms. Individuals with liver damage may experience a prolonged withdrawal syndrome and often experience cognitive problems such as increased drowsiness or lethargy, memory impairment or temporo-spatial disorientation during the course of alcohol withdrawal.

Pharmacotherapy of the alcohol withdrawal syndrome

A wide variety of pharmacological agents, such as benzodiazepines, beta-adrenergic blockers, alpha-2 adrenergic agonists, dopamine receptor blockers such as haloperidol, phenytoin, calcium channel blockers and carbamazepine (Malcolm et al., 1989; Leslie et al., 1990; Williams and McBride, 1998; Garbutt et al., 1999) have been used during the last three decades to treat the alcohol withdrawal syndrome.

BENZODIAZEPINES

Benzodiazepines are the drugs most widely used to suppress alcohol withdrawal symptoms. They appear effective in preventing and treating withdrawal seizures and delirium tremens (Nutt et al., 1989). There is no empirical evidence to suggest that any one benzodiazepine is significantly superior to another, but most of clinical studies comparing benzodiazepines to placebo and other drugs in alcohol withdrawal have used diazepam and chlordiazepoxide. These long-acting benzodiazepines are the established treatments in Europe and in the USA (Williams and McBride, 1998). As both drugs are metabolized by the liver, their use is problematic in patients suffering from severe liver impairment, since side effects of benzodiazepines, such as memory impairment, drowsiness, lethargy or ataxia are more likely to occur. Reduced clearance in patients with ALD means that the active metabolites, desmethylchlordiazepoxide and demoxepam can be prolonged for up to 346 hours and 150 hours respectively (Barton et al., 1989). Metabolites may be detectable in urines of patients with hepatic encephalopathy two months after stopping treatment (Meier et al., 1991). Benzodiazepines that are not significantly oxidized by the liver are indicated in liver disease. These include lorazepam, temazepam and particularly oxazepam, all of which have shorter half-lives (Sellers et al., 1979; Peppers, 1996). It is, however, important to note that that lorazepam and temazepam have greater abuse potential than chlordiazepoxide or oxazepam (Griffiths and Wolf, 1990).

CHLORMETHIAZOLE

Chlormethiazole, a sedative-hypnotic with anticonvulsant activity, has enjoyed widespread use in Europe as an alcohol withdrawal agent, but has never been licensed for use in the USA. Its major disadvantage is its potential interaction with alcohol, causing respiratory depression and arrest (McInnes, 1987). Higher plasma concentrations of chlormethiazole (up to ten-fold) occur in severe liver disease as a result of increased bioavailability and reduced clearance occurs in severe liver disease. Chlormethiazole-induced sedation can mask the onset of liver coma or even precipitate hepatic encephalopathy or coma in patients with liver disease (Pentikainen *et al.*, 1980). It is therefore not recommended in patients with liver impairment.

ANTICONVULSANTS

Carbamazepine, an anticonvulsant with mood-stabilizing properties, has been shown to be effective in the treatment of severe alcohol withdrawal symptoms, including DT (Malcolm *et al.*, 1989). However, its use is not recommended when liver function tests are elevated and it must only be used with caution in hepatic disease. Jaundice, hepatitis and liver function disorders have been reported after carbamazepine use (Sillanpaa, 1981). In addition, although rare, serious hepato-toxicity from carbamazepine has been recognized (Forbes *et al.*, 1992).

TIAPRIDE

Tiapride is a selective dopamine D_2-receptor blocker, with anxiolytic properties, that is used in some countries to facilitate management of alcohol withdrawal (Ramos Castellanos *et al.*, 1982). However, like other dopaminergic blockers, tiapride is metabolized in the liver and should be used with caution in patients with liver damage. It is not recommended in cases of severe liver impairment.

Anticraving and alcohol sensitising agents

Anticraving agents

NALTREXONE

The opiate receptor antagonist naltrexone hydrochloride has been shown to be an effective pharmacological adjunct to psychosocial intervention in preventing relapse for alcohol-dependent subjects following detoxification, by reducing alcohol craving and the number of days in which any alcohol was consumed (O'Malley *et al.*, 1992; Volpicelli *et al.*, 1992). Due to its high hepatic extraction, questions have been raised regarding its hepatotoxic potential. Consequently, naltrexone is best avoided in patients with severe ALD.

ACAMPROSATE

Acamprosate (or calcium acetylhomotaurinate) is a novel anti-craving agent derived from the amino acid taurine and structurally related to the neurotransmitters glutamate and gamma amino butyric acid (GABA) (Littleton, 1995). It has been hypothesized that acamprosate may act by mimicking the action or by modifying levels of taurine during withdrawal (Dahcour et al., 1994) when the experience of craving is severe, thus suppressing neuronal excitation in this period. Acamprosate has been reported to be an effective and well-tolerated pharmacological adjunct to psychosocial and behavioral treatment programs in the management of alcohol-dependent patients in several double-blind, placebo-controlled trials (Sass et al., 1996; Whitworth et al., 1996). This drug is contraindicated in severe hepatic failure (Childs-Pugh Classification C), but the pharmacokinetics are not altered by mild to moderate hepatic dysfunction (Delgrange et al., 1992). Indeed, although there is no systematic study of its use in less severe forms of liver disease, it appears that acamprosate can be safely used with appropriate supervision.

ALCOHOL SENSITISING AGENTS

Several drugs alter the breakdown of alcohol, thus resulting in an unpleasant or toxic reaction when alcohol is taken with them. Two such drugs, disulfiram and calcium carbimide, are currently used in the treatment of alcohol use disorders (Garbutt et al. 1999). Both, however, are known to induce hepatotoxicity (Peachey, 1981; Berlin, 1989) and their use is contraindicated in patients with moderate or severe ALD.

Treatment of individuals with alcoholic liver disease who have another psychiatric problem

Comorbid affective disorders

OVERVIEW

The relationship between depression and alcohol abuse and dependence is well documented (Regier et al., 1990), particularly the role of depression in relapse to drinking (Roy, 1996).

SELECTIVE SEROTONIN REUPTAKE INHIBITORS (SSRIs)

Some selective serotonin reuptake inhibitors (SSRIs), such as citalopram (Naranjo et al., 1995), fluvoxamine (Linnoila et al., 1987) and fluoxetine (Kranzler et al., 1995) appear to be effective in reducing alcohol related craving and improving abstinence rates. In addition, fluoxetine has been shown to be effective in reducing the depressive symptoms and alcohol consumption in alcohol dependent patients with comorbid depression (Cornelius et al., 1997).

Elimination of fluoxetine depends primarily on hepatic metabolism, with formation of a pharmacologically active demethylated product, norfluoxetine. In hepatic impairment, the manufacturers recommend alternate day dosing of fluoxetine. In one study, 14 cirrhotic patients with ALD were reported to have higher plasma levels of fluoxetine and norfluoxetine and longer half-lives. The dose should, therefore, be reduced by at least 50%, particularly if a low albumen is present (Schenker *et al.*, 1988). More recently, three cases of fluoxetine-induced hepatitis have been reported (Friedenberg and Rothstein, 1996). Sertraline is metabolized extensively by the liver and its elimination half-life is significantly prolonged in liver impairment (Demolis *et al.*, 1996); it is therefore contraindicated in liver disease. There is very little data available on citalopram, which is metabolized by the liver with three metabolites (Milne and Goa, 1991). Low doses are recommended in liver disease. Similarly, Dalhoff *et al.* (1991) reported higher plasma concentrations and reduced elimination of paroxetine in patients with cirrhosis, suggesting that in the latter the dose should be in the lower end of the therapeutic range. However, in a single dose study, pharmacokinetic data for paroxetine in patients with liver disease was similar to healthy volunteers and it has been suggested as the SSRI of first choice in ALD (Bazire, 1999).

TRICYCLIC ANTIDEPRESSANTS (TCAs)

TCAs have been widely prescribed for the treatment of patients with an alcohol use disorder. Sedative TCAs, such as amitriptyline, clomipramine and dothiepin are best avoided in liver disease, because decreased metabolism leads to increased sedation. In addition, increased blood concentration may also be caused by a reduced plasma protein binding if there is a decrease in albumen levels. Indeed, plasma levels of TCAs have been reported to double or triple in patients with cirrhosis (Hrdina *et al.*, 1985). Following case reports of hepatic toxicity with lofepramine, its use in liver disease is contraindicated (Kelly *et al.*, 1993). Overall, reduced doses of TCA in patients with hepatic impairment are generally recommended. Imipramine has been suggested as the recommended drug among the TCAs, starting at 10 mg tds for 2 weeks and then increased by 10 mg each week until a therapeutic effect is seen (Bazire, 1999).

NEWER ANTIDEPRESSANTS

Newer antidepressants, such as Nefazodone (serotonin reuptake inhibitor and serotonin blocker), Reboxetine (selective noradrenaline reuptake inhibitor), Venlafaxine (serotonin and noradrenaline reuptake inhibitor), Mirtazapine (noradrenergic and specific serotoninergic antidepressant), also should be used with caution in patients with ALD.

Nefazodone is metabolized in the liver to three active metabolites. Although the pharmacokinetics of nefazodone and its metabolites are not appreciably altered in patients with mild-to-moderate hepatic impairment, its plasma concentrations are significantly affected in severe hepatic impairment and in the elderly. Indeed, subjects with liver cirrhosis show approximately a 2-fold increase in levels of nefazodone and hydroxynefazodone compared with normal subjects after a single dose of nefazodone, the difference decreasing to approximately 25% at steady state (Barbhaiya *et al.*, 1995). Nefazodone should be used with caution in these groups and a lower daily dose of this antidepressant is recommended when treating patients with impairment of hepatic function (Ferry *et al.*, 1994). Similarly, the half-life and plasma levels of reboxetine appear to rise in severe hepatic insufficiency and dose reduction may be necessary, although mild to moderate liver insufficiency does not seem to have significant effects on its metabolism (Dostert *et al.*, 1997). Venlafaxine's clearance is reduced by about 35% in mild to moderate hepatic impairment and consequently doses need to be reduced by about 25–50% in such cases (Anonyme, 1993). It is not recommended in severe hepatic impairment. Transient asymptomatic raised liver function tests have been reported in a few patients in mirtazapine clinical trials; in addition, mirtazapine clearance is reduced in moderate to severe hepatic impairment and so care with higher doses is recommended (Montgomery, 1995). In all the newer antidepressants a dose reduction is generally necessary. Nefazodone, reboxetine, venlafaxine and venlafaxine are best avoided in severe liver disease.

MOOD STABILISERS

Mood stabilizing medications are effective in the treatment and prophylaxis of bipolar affective disorder. Although the general side effects must be considered, lithium does not pose any appreciable risk in liver disease and is therefore the mood stabilizer of choice in this group (Bazire, 1999). Lithium has also been postulated as an aid to reduce alcohol consumption, with rather disappointing results (Garbutt *et al.*, 1999). Other frequently used mood stabilizers, such as carbamazepine need also to be used with caution in hepatic impairment. Sodium valproate has been associated with liver toxicity, hence is contraindicated in severe liver disease and must be used with caution in mild to moderate impairment (Lammert and Matern, 1997).

Comorbid anxiety and sleep disorders

OVERVIEW

The relationship between alcohol use disorders and anxiety is complex. Feelings of nervousness and anxiety are to be expected during withdrawal and for several months thereafter. Since anxiety and sleep disturbances can persist for weeks or months following withdrawal, it is unclear where withdrawal ends and other causes of anxiety and disturbed sleep may begin. Clinical studies have estimated that about one-third of problem drinkers may experience anxiety symptoms in the context of alcohol withdrawal (Schuckit and Hesselbrock, 1994; Allan, 1995). In addition, rates of panic disorders, generalized anxiety disorders and social phobia have been described to be higher in alcohol abusers than in the general population (Schuckit and Hesselbrock, 1994). Prospective follow-up studies of individuals with alcohol dependence show that anxiety symptoms diminish in the early stages of abstinence and continue to improve with prolonged abstinence. It is also important to remember that some of the main clinical symptoms in patients with ALD are weakness, fatigue, lethargy, as well as somnolence and appearance of mild confusion in the more severe cases.

THE PHARMACOLOGICAL TREATMENT OF ANXIETY AND
SLEEP DISTURBANCES IN ALD

The use of benzodiazepines for the treatment of comorbid anxiety or panic disorder in alcohol-dependent patients is controversial. Considering the high abuse potential of these drugs, particularly so in patients with an alcohol use disorder, their use should be restricted to the period of immediate alcohol withdrawal. Their use in patients with ALD has already been discussed.

Buspirone, a partial serotonin 5-HT$_{1A}$-agonist, is a non-benzodiazepine anxiolytic with low abuse potential which has been shown to be helpful for patients with long-term generalized anxiety disorder. Buspirone plasma levels have been reported to be higher in patients with hepatic failure, with a good correlation between steady-state buspirone levels and serum albumin (Barbhaiya *et al.*, 1994). Caution is recommended in patients with a history of hepatic impairment and in severe hepatic disease.

Zolpidem is a non-benzodiazepine hypnotic with a rapid onset of action and a short (6–8 hours) duration. Reduced plasma protein binding of zolpidem in hepatic impairment has been reported (Pacifici *et al.*, 1988). Zolpidem is contraindicated in severe hepatic insufficiency and reduced doses are recommended in cirrhosis and other liver disease due to increases in half-life (up to 10 hours in cirrhosis) and peak plasma concentrations. Zopiclone is another non-benzodiazepine hypnotic which is widely used in the treatment of insomnia. In cirrhotic patients the response to zopiclone has been found to be delayed and exaggerated, in addition to a reduced elimination (Parker and Roberts, 1983). It should be therefore used with caution. Overall, anxiolytic and hypnotic medications are best avoided in patients with ALD.

Comorbid psychotic disorders

In patients with ALD, antipsychotic drugs should generally be restricted to the treatment of comorbid schizophrenic illness. However, alcoholic hallucinosis during or after prolonged alcohol use may also respond to antipsychotic medication. Sulpiride is often considered the neuroleptic of choice for patients with liver damage, because it is virtually unmetabolized with little or no biliary excretion and a transient rise in serum transaminase is the only reported effect on the liver (Harnryd *et al.*, 1984). Low dose haloperidol is also often recommended in liver disease, although it has been associated with acute and chronic cholestatic liver disease (Dincsoy *et al.*, 1982). Few problems have been reported with flupenthixol and zuclopenthixol and they remain therapeutic options. Phenothiazines, especially chlorpromazine, are best avoided because of their hepatotoxic properties (Dossing and Andreasen, 1982; Regal *et al.*, 1987). Of the newer atypical antipsychotic agents, risperidone and clozapine are contraindicated in severe hepatic disease. Transient, asymptomatic transaminase elevation has been noted in patients treated with olanzapine (Beasley *et al.*, 1997), therefore lower starting and maintenance doses of olanzapine may be required in patients with liver impairment.

Pharmacotherapies for comorbid substance use disorders

Individuals with ALD may have other substance use disorders. In addition, a significant of patients on methadone maintenance programmes develop an alcohol use disorder. Interactions of both a pharmacodynamic and also dispositional type may occur between alcohol and exogenous opioids, such as heroin or methadone (Kreek, 1984). Alcohol dependent patients who also abuse drugs intravenously have an increased risk of developing cirrhosis. However, while active viral hepatitis and chronic persistent hepatitis have been reported to be more prevalent in patients with exclusive intravenous drug abuse (HBV and HCV), cirrhosis is found most often in patients with a comorbid alcohol use disorder (Novick *et al.*, 1986).

It has been suggested that alcohol is a major factor in the development of irreversible liver disease in active heroin dependent patients and patients in methadone maintenance programs (Gelb *et al.*, 1977). However, while chronic liver disease is common in methadone-maintained patients, methadone maintenance treatment *per se* has not been associated with cirrhosis. Indeed, several reports have concluded that methadone-maintained patients who abuse alcohol and develop cirrhosis should remain on methadone and the usual methadone maintenance dose may be continued in patients with stable chronic liver disease (Novick *et al.*, 1985, 1986). Moreover, it is believed that continuation of methadone maintenance for heroin dependent patients is advisable during treatment for the alcohol problem (Bickel *et al.*, 1987).

LIVER TRANSPLANTATION

Liver transplantation is being increasingly used as a treatment for end stage alcohol-related cirrhosis and outcomes are as good as for other liver disease. Resource utilization appears to be equivalent to that for patients undergoing transplantation for non-alcohol-related cirrhosis (McCurry *et al.*, 1992). Psychiatric assessment of transplant patients has become an important element of the routine multidisciplinary screening process. In addition, the nature of the surgery and the need for intensive medical assessment and treatment are associated with significant neurological, emotional and psychiatric consequences (Devlin and O'Grady, 1999). Indeed, significant psychiatric problems, most commonly anxiety and depression, have been described in approximately a quarter of patients after liver transplantation (Surman, 1989; Collis *et al.*, 1995). Consequently, psychiatric intervention in the post-operative period is an essential part of the management of transplantation patients. Resumption of alcohol consumption after liver transplantation is of concern. Reported relapse rates vary from 14–80% (Douds and Neuberger, 1998), and drinking is usually reinstated at lower levels than previously. However, comparisons across studies are difficult because different instruments have been used and studies have not been prospective. An evidence-based approach calls for prospective studies with randomized treatment interventions (Howard *et al.*, 1994).

CONCLUSION

Abstinence from alcohol is the single most important component of treatment for ALD. In order to achieve and maintain abstinence, a combined effort of psychological and pharmacological strategies is often required. Successful management of patients with alcohol-induced liver injury is complex and is generally best provided in the context of a closely coordinated multidisciplinary treatment program. Psychiatric management is often an important and crucial component of such programs. The frequency, intensity and focus of psychiatric care must be tailored to meet each patient's needs and the type of management is likely to vary over time, depending on the patient's clinical condition. Psychiatric management includes assessment and treatment of the alcohol use disorder, managing intoxication and withdrawal states, diagnosis and treatment of associated psychiatric disorders, developing and facilitating adherence to a treatment plan, preventing relapse and providing education about alcohol use disorders, as well as psychiatric assessment and post-operative counseling of transplantation patients.

In patients with liver impairment all psychotropic drugs should be started at a low dose and dose adjustments should be made slowly. The total dose should generally be lower than that considered in normal circumstances.

REFERENCES

Adinoff, B., Bone, G.H.A. and Linnoila, M. (1988) Acute ethanol poisoning and the ethanol withdrawal syndrome. *Med Toxicol* **3**, 172–196.

Allan, C.A. (1995) Alcohol problems and anxiety disorders – a critical review. *Alcohol Alcohol* **30**, 145–151.

American Psychiatric Association (1994) *Diagnostic and Statistical Manual of Mental Disorders*, 4th edn. Washington: American Psychiatric Press.

American Psychiatric Association (1995) Practice guideline for the treatment of patients with substance use disorders: alcohol, cocaine, opioids. *Am J Psychiatry* **152** (Suppl), 1–59.

Anonyme (1993) Venlafaxine: a new dimension in antidepressant pharmacotherapy. *J Clin Psychiatry* **54**, 119–126.

Barbhaiya, R.H., Shukla, U.A., Pfeffer, M. *et al.* (1994) Disposition kinetics of buspirone in patients with renal or hepatic impairment after administration of single and multiple doses. *Eur J Clin Pharmacol* **46**, 41–47.

Barbhaiya, R.H., Shukla, U.A., Natarajan, C.S. *et al.* (1995) Single- and multiple-dose pharmacokinetics of nefazodone in patients with hepatic cirrhosis. *Clin Pharmacol Ther* **58**, 390–398.

Barton, K., Auld, P.W., Scott, M.G. and Nicholls, D.P. (1989) Chlordiazepoxide metabolite accumulation in liver disease. *Med Toxicol Adverse Drug Exp* **4**, 73–76.

Bazire, S. (1999) *Psychotropic drug directory 1999*. Dinton, UK: Quay Books.

Beasley Jr., C.M., Tollefson, G.D. and Tran, P.V. (1997) Safety of olanzapine. *J Clin Psychiatry* **58** (Suppl 10), 13–17.

Berg, B.J., Pettinati, H.M. and Volpicelli, J.R. (1996) A risk-benefit assessment of naltrexone in the treatment of alcohol dependence. *Drug Saf* **15**, 274–282.

Berlin, R.G. (1989) Disulfiram hepatotoxicity: a consideration of its mechanism and clinical spectrum. *Alcohol Alcohol* **24**, 241–246.

Bertolotti, M., Ferrari, A., Vitale, G. *et al.* (1997) Effect of liver cirrhosis on the systemic availability of naltrexone in humans. *J Hepatol* **27**, 505–511.

Bickel, W.K., Marion, I. and Lowinsin, J.H. (1987) The treatment of alcoholic methadone patients: a review. *J Subst Abuse Treat* **4**, 15–19.

Bien, T.H., Miller, W.R. and Tonigan, J.S. (1993) Brief interventions for alcohol problems: a review. *Addiction* **88**, 315–335.

Bohn, M.J., Babor, T.F. and Kranzler, H.R. (1995) The Alcohol Use Disorders Identification Test (AUDIT): validation of a screening instrument for use in medical settings. *J Stud Alcohol* **56**, 423–432.

Botvin, G.J., Baker, E., Filazzola, A.D. and Botvin, E.M. (1990) A cognitive-behavioral approach to substance abuse prevention: one-year follow-up. *Addict Behav* **15**, 47–63.

Bunn, J.Y., Booth, B.M., Cook, C.A.L. *et al.* (1994) The relationship between mortality and intensity of inpatient alcoholism treatment. *Am J Public Health* **84**, 211–214.

Canning, U.P., Kennell-Webb, S.A., Marshall, E.J. *et al.* (1999) Substance misuse in acute general medical admissions. *Q J Med* **92**, 319–326.

Carroll, K.M. (1996) Relapse prevention as a psychosocial treatment approach: a review of controlled clinical trials. *Exp Clin Psychopharmacol* **4**, 46–54.

Collis, I., Burroughs, A., Rolles, K. and Lloyd, G. (1995) Psychiatric and social outcome of liver transplantation. *Br J Psychiatry* **166**, 521–524.

Conigrave, K.M., Hall, W.D. and Saunders, J.B. (1995a) The AUDIT questionnaire: choosing a cut-off score. Alcohol Use Disorder Identification Test. *Addiction* **90**, 1349–1356.

Conigrave, K.M., Saunders, J.B. and Reznik, R.B. (1995b) Predictive capacity of the AUDIT questionnaire for alcohol-related harm. *Addiction* **90**, 1479–1485.

Cornelius, J.R., Salloum, I.M., Ehler, J.G. *et al.* (1997) Fluoxetine in depressed alcoholics. A double-blind, placebo-controlled trial. *Arch Gen Psychiatry* **54**, 700–705.

Dahcour, A., Queremont, E. and De Witte, P. (1994) Acute ethanol increases taurine, but neither GABA nor glutamate in the nucleus accumbens: a microdyalisis study in the male rat. *Pfluger's Arch Eur J Physiol* **427**, 3–4.

Dalhoff, K., Almdal, T.P., Bjerrum, K. *et al.* (1991) Pharmacokinetics of paroxetine in patients with cirrhosis. *Eur J Clin Pharmacol* **41**, 351–354.

Delgrange, T., Khater, J., Capron, D. *et al.* (1992) Effet de l'administration aigue d'acamprosate sur le risque d'encephalopathie et sur la pression arterielle chez les malades atteints de cirrhose alcoolique. *Gastroenterol Clin Biol* **16**, 687–691.

Demolis, J.L., Angebaud, P., Grange, J.D., *et al.* (1996) Influence of liver cirrhosis on sertraline pharmacokinetics. *Br J Clin Pharmacol* **42**, 394–397.

Devlin, J. and O'Grady. (1999) Indications for referral and assessment in adult liver transplantation: a clinical guideline. *Gut* **45** (Suppl VI), VI1–VI22.

Dincsoy, H.P. and Saelinger, D.A. (1982) Haloperidol-induced chronic cholestatic liver disease. *Gastroenterology* **83**, 694–700.

Dossing, M. and Andreasen, P.B. (1982) Drug-induced liver disease in Denmark. An analysis of 572 cases of hepatotoxicity reported to the Danish Board of Adverse Reactions to Drugs. *Scand J Gastroenterol* **17**, 205–211.

Dostert, P., Benedetti, M.S. and Poggesi, I. (1997) Review of the pharmacokinetics and metabolism of reboxetine, a selective noradrenaline reuptake inhibitor. *Eur Neuropsychopharmacol* **7** (Suppl 1), 23–35.

Douds, A. and Neuberger, J. (1998) Liver transplantation for alcoholic cirrhosis: current situation. *Hospital Medicine* **59**, 604–605.

Drummond, C.D. (1989) The relationship between alcohol dependence and alcohol-related problems in a clinical population. *Br J Addict* **85**, 357–366.

Dunn, C.W. and Ries, R. (1997) Linking substance abuse services with general medical care: integrated, brief interventions with hospitalized patients. *Am J Drug Alcohol Abuse* **23**, 1–13.

Dyehouse, J.M. and Sommers, M.S. (1998) Brief intervention after alcohol-related injuries. *Nurs Clin North Am* **33**, 93–104.

Edwards, G., Marshall, E.J. and Cook, C.C.H. (1997) *The treatment of drinking problems. A guide for the helping professionals*. Cambridge: Cambridge University Press.

Ewing, J.A. (1984) Detecting alcoholism: the CAGE questionnaire. *JAMA* **252**, 1905–1907.

Ewusi-Mensah, I., Saunders, J.B. and Williams, R. (1984) The clinical nature and detection of psychiatric disorders in patients with alcoholic liver disease. *Alcohol Alcohol* **19**, 297–302.

Ferry, N., Bernard, N., Cuisinaud, G. *et al*. (1994) Influence of hepatic impairment on the pharmacokinetics of nefazodone and two of its metabolites after single and multiple oral doses. *Fundam Clin Pharmacol* **8**, 463–473.

Forbes, G.M., Jeffrey, G.P., Shilkin, K.B. and Reed, W.D. (1992) Carbamazepine hepatotoxicity: another cause of the vanishing bile duct syndrome. *Gastroenterology* **102**, 1385–1388.

Friedenberg, F.K. and Rothstein, K.D. (1996) Hepatitis secondary to fluoxetine treatment. *Am J Psychiatry* **153**, 580.

Garbutt, J.C., West, S.I., Carey, T.S. *et al*. (1999) Pharmacological treatment of alcohol dependence: a review of the evidence. *JAMA* **281**, 1318–1325.

Gelb, A.M., Mildvan, D. and Stenger, R.J. (1977) The spectrum and causes of liver diseases in narcotic addicts. *Am J Gastroenterol* **67**, 314–318.

Graham, A.W. (1991) Screening for alcoholism by Life-style Risk Assessment in a community hospital. *Arch Int Med* **151**, 958–964.

Griffiths, R.R. and Wolf, B. (1990) Relative abuse liability of different benzodiazepines in drug abusers. *J Clin Psychopharmacol* **10**, 237–243.

Harnryd, C., Bjerkenstedt, L., Bjork, K. *et al*. (1984) Clinical evaluation of sulpiride in schizophrenic patients a double blind comparison with chlorpromazine. *Acta Psychiatr Scand* **311** (Suppl), 7–30.

Harris, D. and Brunt, P. (1995) Prognosis of alcoholic liver disease – 100 years on and the need for international standards and guidelines. *Alcohol Alcohol* **30**, 591–600.

Holder, H.D., Longabaugh, R., Miller, W.R. and Rubonis, A.V. (1991) The cost effectiveness of treatment for alcoholism: a first approximation. *J Stud Alcohol* **52**, 517–540.

Howard, L., Fahy, T., Wong, P., Sherman, D., Gane, E. and Williams, R. (1994) Psychiatric outcome in alcoholic liver transplant patients. *Quarterly Journal of Medicine* **87**, 731–736.

Hrdina, P.D., Lapierre, Y.D. and Koranyi, E.K. (1985) Altered amitriptyline kinetics in a depressed patient with porto-caval anastomosis. *Can J Psychiatry* **30**, 111–113.

Kelly, C., Roche, S., Naguib, M. *et al*. (1993) A prospective evaluation of the hepatotoxicity of lofepramine in the elderly. *Int Clin Psychopharmacol* **8**, 83–86.

Kranzler, H.R., Burleson, J.A., Korner, P. *et al*. (1995) Placebo-controlled trial of fluoxetine as an adjunct to relapse prevention in alcoholics. *Am J Psychiatry* **152**, 391–397.

Kreek, M.J. (1984) Opioid interactions with alcohol. *Adv Alcohol Subst Abuse* **3**, 35–46.

Lammert, F. and Matern, S. (1997) Hepatopathien durch Medikamente. *Schweiz Rundsch Med Prax* **86**, 1167–1171.

Linnoila, M., Eckardt, M., Duncan, M. *et al*. (1987) Interactions of serotonin with ethanol: clinical and animal studies. *Psychopharmacol Bull* **23**, 452–457.

Leslie, S.W., Brown, L.M., Dildy, J.E. and Sims, J.S. (1990) Ethanol and neuronal calcium channels. *Alcohol* **7**, 233–236.

Littleton, J. (1995) Acamprosate in alcohol dependence: how does it work? *Addiction* **90**, 1179–1188.

Litten, R.Z. and Allen, J.P. (1991) Pharmacotherapies for alcoholism: promising agents and clinical issues. *Alc Clin Exp Res* **15**, 620–633.

Liskow, B.I. and Goodwin, D.W. (1987) Pharmacological treatment of alcohol intoxication, withdrawal and dependence: a critical review. *J Stud Alcohol* **48**, 356–370.

Lumeng, L. and Crabb, D.W. (1994) Genetic aspects and risk factors in alcoholism and alcoholic liver disease. *Gastroenterology* **107**, 571–578.

MacKenzie, D.M., Langa, A. and Brown, T.M. (1996) Identifying hazardous or harmful alcohol use in medical admissions: a comparison of AUDIT, CAGE and brief MAST. *Alcohol Alcohol* **31**, 591–599.

Malcolm, R., Ballenger, J.C., Sturgis, E.T. and Anton, R. (1989) Double-blind controlled trial comparing carbamazepine to oxazepam treatment of alcohol withdrawal. *Am J Psychiatry* **146**, 617–621.

Marlatt, G. and Gordon, I. (1985) *Relapse Prevention*. New York: Guilford Press.

Marshall, E.J. and Alam, F. (1997) Psychiatric problems associated with alcohol misuse and dependence. *Br J Hosp Med* **58**, 44–46.

McCurry, K.R., Baliga, P., Merion, R.M. *et al.* (1992) Resource utilization and outcome of liver transplantation for alcoholic cirrhosis: a case-control study. *Arch Surg* **127**, 772–776.

McInnes, G.T. (1987) Chlormethiazole and alcohol: a lethal cocktail. *BMJ* **294**, 592.

McLellan, A.T., Luborsky, L., Woody, G.E. *et al.* (1983) Predicting response to alcohol and drug abuse treatments. Role of psychiatric severity. *Arch Gen Psychiatry* **40**, 620–625.

Meier, R., Gyr, K. and Scholer, A. (1991) Persisting benzodiazepine metabolites responsible for the reaction to the benzodiazepine antagonist flumazenil in patients with hepatic encephalopathy. *Gastroenterology* **101**, 274–275.

Mello, N.K., Mendelson, J.H. and Teoh, S.K. (1992) Alcohol and neuroendocrine function in women of reproductive age. In: *Medical diagnosis and treatment of alcoholism*, edited by J.H. Mendelson and N.K. Mello, pp. 575–621. New York: McGraw Hill.

Milne, R.J. and Goa, K.L. (1991) Citalopram. A review of its pharmacodynamic and pharmacokinetic properties, and therapeutic potential in depressive illness. *Drugs* **41**, 450–477.

Miller, W.R. (1985) Motivation for treatment: a review with special emphasis on alcoholism. *Psychol Bull* **98**, 84–107.

Miller, W.R. and Hester, R.K. (1986) Inpatient alcoholism treatment: who benefits? *Am Psychol* **41**, 794–805.

Miller, W.R. and Rollnick, S. (1991) *Motivational interviewing: Preparing people to change addictive behavior*. New York: Guilford Press.

Miller, W.R. and Sanchez, V.C. (1994) Motivating young adults for treatment and lifestyle change. In *Issues in alcohol use and misuse by young adults* edited by G. Howard, pp. 55–82. Notre Dame, IN: University of Notre Dame Press.

Montgomery, S.A. (1995) Safety of mirtazapine: a review. *Int Clin Psychopharmacol* **10** (Suppl 4), 37–45.

Naranjo, C.A., Bremner, K.E. and Lanctot, K.L. (1995) Effects of citalopram and a brief psycho-social intervention on alcohol intake, dependence and problems. *Addiction* **90**, 87–99.

Novick, D.M., Kreek, M.J., Arns, P.A. *et al.* (1985) Effect of severe alcoholic liver disease on the disposition of methadone in maintenance patients. *Alcohol Clin Exp Res* **9**, 349–354.

Novick, D.M., Stenger, R.J., Gelb, A.M. *et al.* (1986) Chronic liver disease in abusers of alcohol and parenteral drugs: a report of 204 consecutive biopsy-proven cases. *Alcohol Clin Exp Res* **10**, 500–505.

Nutt, D., Adinoff, B. and Linnoila, M. (1989) Benzodiazepines in the treatment of alcoholism. In *Recent developments in alcoholism: Treatment Research*, Vol 7, edited by M. Galanter, pp. 283–313. New York Plenum Press.

O'Malley, S.S., Jaffe, A.J., Chang, G. *et al.* (1992) Naltrexone and coping skills therapy for alcohol dependence. *Arch Gen Psychiatry* **49**, 881–887.

Pacifici, G.M., Viani, A., Rizzo, G. *et al.* (1988) Plasma protein binding of zolpidem in liver and renal insufficiency. *Int Clin Pharmacol Ther Toxicol* **26**, 439–443.

Parker, G. and Roberts, C.J. (1983) Plasma concentrations and central nervous system effects of the new hypnotic agent zopiclone in patients with chronic liver disease. *Br J Clin Pharmacol* **16**, 259–265.

Peachey, J.E., Brien, J.F., Roach, C.A. and Loomis, C.W. (1981) A comparative review of the pharmacological and toxicological properties of disulfiram and calcium carbimide. *J Clin Psychopharmacol* **1**, 21–26.

Peachey, J.E. and Sellers, E.M. (1981) The disulfiram and calcium carbimide acetaldehyde-mediated ethanol reactions. *Pharmacol Ther* **15**, 89–97.

Pentikainen, P.J., Neuvonen, P.J. and Jostell, K.G. (1980) Pharmacokinetics of chlormethiazole in healthy volunteers and patients with cirrhosis of the liver. *Eur J Clin Pharmacol* **17**, 275–284.

Peppers. (1996) Benzodiazepines in liver disease. *Pharmacotherapy* **16**, 49–58.

Prochaska, J.O., DiClemente, C.C. and Norcross, J.C. (1992) In search of how people change: applications to addictive behaviours. *Am Psychol* **7**, 1102–1114.

Ramos Castellanos, J.L., Lozano Suárez, M. and Hernández-García, P. (1982) Nuestra experiencia con tiapride en enfermos alcohólicos. *Actas Luso Esp Neurol Psiquiatr Cienc Afines* **10**, 235–256.

Regal, R.E., Billi, J.E. and Glazer, H.M. (1987) Phenothiazine-induced cholestatic jaundice. *Clin Pharm* **6**, 787–794.

Regier, D.A., Farmer, M.E., Rae, D.S. *et al.* (1990) Comorbidity of mental disorders with alcohol and other drug abuse. Results from the Epidemiologic Catchment Area (ECA) Study. *JAMA* **264**, 2511–2518.

Rounsaville, B.J., Dolinsky, Z.S., Babor, T.F. and Meyer, R.E. (1987) Psychopathology as a predictor of treatment outcome in alcoholics. *Arch Gen Psychiatry* **44**, 505–513.

Roy, A. (1996) Aetiology of secondary depression in male alcoholics. *Br J Psychiatry* **169**, 753–757.

Sass, H., Soyka, M., Mann, K. and Zieglgänsberger, W. (1996) Relapse prevention by acamprosate. Results from a placebo-controlled study on alcohol dependence. *Arch Gen Psychiatry* **53**, 673–680.

Saunders, J.B., Walters, J.R.F., Davies, P. and Paton, A. (1981) A 20-year prospective study of cirrhosis. *BMJ* **282**, 263–266.

Saunders, J.B., Asaland, O.G., Babor, T.F. *et al.* (1993) Development of the Alcohol Use Disorders Identification Test (AUDIT). WHO collaborative project on early detection of persons with harmful alcohol consumption – II. *Addiction* **88**, 791–804.

Selzer, M.L. (1971) The Michigan Alcoholism Screening Test: the search for a new diagnostic instrument. *Am J Psychiatry* **127**, 1653–1658.

Selzer, M.L., Vinokur, A. and Van Rooijen, L. (1975) A self-administered Short Michigan Alcoholism Screening Test (SMAST). *J Stud Alcohol* **36**, 117–126.

Schenker, S., Bergstrom, R.F., Wolen, R.L. and Lemberger, L. (1988) Fluoxetine disposition and elimination in cirrhosis. *Clin Pharmacol Ther* **44**, 353–359.

Schuckit, M.A. and Hesselbrock, V. (1994) Alcohol dependence and anxiety disorders. *Am J Psychiatry* **151**, 1723–1734.

Sellers, E.M., Greenblatt, D.J., Giles, H.G. *et al.* (1979) Chlordiazepoxide and oxazepam disposition in cirrhosis. *Clin Pharmacol Ther* **26**, 240–246.

Sherlock, S. (1995) Alcoholic Liver Disease. *Lancet* **345**, 227–229.

Sherman, D.I.N. and Williams, R. (1994) Liver damage: mechanisms and management. *Br Med Bull* **50**, 124–138.

Sillanpaa, M. (1981) Carbamazepine. Pharmacology and clinical uses. *Acta Neurol Scand* **88**(Suppl), 1–202.

Stockwell, T., Hodgson, R., Edwards, G., Taylor, C. and Rankin, H. (1979) The development of a questionnaire to measure severity of alcohol dependence. *Br J Addict* **74**, 79–87.

Surman, O.S. (1989) Psychiatric aspects of organ transplantation. *Am J Psychiatry* **146**, 972–982.

Sutton, S. (1997) Can "stages of change" provide guidance in the treatment of addictions? A critical examination of Prochaska and DiClemente's model. In *Psychotherapy, psychological treatments and the addictions*, edited by G. Edwards and C. Dare, pp.189–205. Cambridge: Cambridge University Press.

Tolley, K. and Rowland, N. (1991) Identification of alcohol-related problems in a general hospital: a cost-effectiveness evaluation. *Br J Addict* **86**, 429–438.

Volpicelli, J., Alterman, A., Hayashida, M. and O'Brien, C. (1992) Naltrexone in the treatment of alcohol dependence. *Arch Gen Psychiatry* **49**, 876–880.

Whitworth, A.B., Fischer, F., Lesch, O.M. *et al.* (1996) Comparison of acamprosate and placebo in long-term treatment of alcohol dependence. *Lancet* **347**, 1438–1442.

Wilk, A.I., Jensen, N.M. and Havighurst, T.C. (1997) Meta-analysis of randomized control trials addressing brief interventions in heavy alcohol drinkers. *J Gen Intern Med* **12**, 274–283.

Williams, D. and McBride, A.J. (1998) The drug treatment of alcohol withdrawal symptoms: A systematic review. *Alcohol Alcohol* **33**, 103–115.

World Health Organisation (1992) *The ICD-10 classification of mental and behavioural disorders: Clinical descriptions and diagnostic guidelines.* Geneva: World Health Organisation.

WHO Brief Intervention Study Group (1996) A cross-national trial of brief interventions with heavy drinkers. *Am J Public Health* **86**, 948–955.

Chapter 24

Pharmacological treatment for alcoholic hepatitis and cirrhosis: present practice and future strategies

Philippe Mathurin and Thierry Poynard

ABSTRACT

Controversies surrounding pharmacological treatments in patients with alcoholic hepatitis or alcoholic cirrhosis continue to persist. In the present chapter, we perform a critical review of pharmacological treatments which have been evaluated in randomized controlled trials. A meta-analysis was performed when a treatment modality was evaluated in 2 trials or more (published in article forms) using the same endpoint survival (short-term or long-term survival). The main limits of studies are the high dropout rate particularly in long-term therapy and the difficulties in evaluating abstinence of patients. Future studies will have to determine the effect of colchicine and propylthiouracil on long-term survival in patients with alcoholic cirrhosis. Preliminary and promising data concerning new drugs such as pentoxyfilline, S-adenosylmethionine and phosphatidylcholine have been published recently. Evaluation of pharmacological treatments which inhibit inflammatory cytokines will probably take place in the near future. This review observed that only corticosteroids improve short-term survival of patients suffering from severe alcoholic hepatitis. There was a significant short-term survival effect of corticosteroids, with a mean difference of 15% (CI: 6–24%, $p < 0.01$). Among all patients with encephalopathy, corticosteroids again had a significant short-term survival effect, with a mean difference of 27% (CI: 11–44%, $p < 0.0001$).

INTRODUCTION

Morphological changes in alcoholic patients are classified into fatty liver, fibrosis, alcoholic hepatitis and cirrhosis (see chapters 1, 2, 3). Among these lesions, alcoholic hepatitis and alcoholic cirrhosis are associated with an increase in mortality. It is well known that the pivotal treatment in alcoholic liver disease (ALD) is abstinence since abstinent patients have a longer survival than non-abstinent patients (Powell, 1968; Pande, 1978). However, to improve the survival of patients with ALD, pharmacological treatments for controlling alcohol-induced liver injury are required.

Several studies have led to major advances in the understanding of the mechanisms involved in alcoholic liver injury (see chapters 5, 6, 7, 8, 14, 15). Alcohol-induced cell injury develops as a consequence of several factors such as acetaldehyde production, free radicals generation, lipid peroxidation, glutathione depletion, pro-inflammatory cytokines, endotoxinemia, collagen production, immune disorders and malnutrition. Thus, the main objectives for therapies in ALD are reducing or reversing liver fibrosis, decreasing peroxidation products, improving immunological disorders, protecting hepatocytes from free radicals, reducing hypermetabolic state, increasing liver regeneration and correcting malnutrition. These rational bases have led the investigators to evaluate: (a) colchicine, which increases collagenase production, decreases collagen synthesis and prevents CCL4-induced liver cirrhosis in rats (Diegelmann, 1972; Ehrlich, 1974; Tanner, 1981); (b) propylthiouracil, as this drug depresses hypermetabolic state in ethanol treated animals (Israel, 1975); (c) silymarin, a drug which protects the liver from CCL4-induced injury (Cavallini, 1978; Leng-Preschlow, 1985); (d) d-Penicillamin, which alters collagen cross linkage (Nimmi, 1965); (e) free radical scavengers which reduce oxidative stress (Gajdos, 1972; Marshall, 1982; Tanner, 1986; Matsuda, 1988; Kawase, 1989); (f) nutritional supplementation, since many studies have shown a high incidence of malnutrition in patients with ALD (Mendenhall, 1986); (g) insulin and glucagon, which are believed to be hepatotrophic factors (Leffert, 1979); (h) anabolic steroids, which prevent liver injury associated with toxic chemicals and accelerate liver regeneration (Hirayama, 1970; Figueroa, 1973); (h) corticosteroids, which reduce inflammation in immune and non-immune disorders (Boumpas, 1993); (i) polyunsaturated phosphatidylcholine which protects from alcoholic liver fibrosis in the baboon model (Lieber, 1994) and (j) S-adenosyl-methionine, a precursor of glutathione (Cabrero, 1988; Duce, 1988).

Unfortunately, studies evaluating pharmacological treatments yield inconsistent results. No recommendation can be clearly proposed for patients suffering from ALD, since conflicting results have been published in several randomized trials (Maddrey, 1988; Mezey, 1993; Nompleggi, 1994).

Contradictory results may be attributed either to systematic bias, methodological deficiencies or insufficient sample size, resulting in a lack of power to detect clinically meaningful differences. Meta-analysis, a quantitative technique for therapeutic evaluation, may be used when controversy persists after several trials. It is particularly useful when several trials have insufficient statistical power, since the pooling of trials decreases random error (Sacks, 1987). In the present chapter, we performed a critical review of pharmacological treatments which have been evaluated in randomized controlled trials. For this purpose, we performed a meta-analytical review for a pharmacological treatment when this treatment was evaluated in 2 trials or more (published in article forms) using the same end-point survival (short-term or long-term survival). Treatment of ascites, gastrointestinal bleeding and hepatocellular carcinoma were not analyzed in the present chapter.

ANALYTICAL REVIEW OF MEDICAL TREATMENT IN ALCOHOLIC LIVER DISEASE

Literature research

Medline and manual searches were combined, since we had previously demonstrated that Medline search alone was not sensitive enough (Poynard, 1985). General reviews and references from published RCTs were also used (Gluud, 1984; Maddrey, 1986; Maddrey, 1988; Mezey, 1993; Nompleggi, 1994). For each meta-analysis, the following methods were used: (1) assessment of heterogeneity of results between control groups; (2) assessment of efficacy by Der Simonian and Laird method (Der Simonian, 1986).

Colchicine

Collagen synthesis in liver injury induced by CCL4, is inhibited by colchicine, an anti-inflammatory drug used for gout and Mediterranean fever. *In vitro*, colchicine increases collagenase production and inhibits collagen synthesis by preventing the assembly of tubulin subunits in microtubules (Diegelmann, 1972; Ehrlich, 1974).

Kershenobich *et al*. observed that long-term treatment with colchicine might be efficient. The results were presented successively in an interim analysis and in a final report (Kershenobich, 1979; Kershenobich, 1988). In the final report, 5 and 10 year survival were significantly higher in the colchicine group (75 and 56%, respectively) than in the placebo group (34 and 20%, $p < 0.001$). However, 20% of patients in this study were lost to follow up and the colchicine group had significantly better prognostic factors at the inclusion. The efficacy of colchicine was not confirmed by two later studies (Trinchet, 1989; Akriviadis, 1990). Nevertheless, comparison between these studies cannot be performed since: (a) Kershobich *et al*. assessed colchicine effect on long-term survival, whereas the other studies looked at short-term survival; and (b) evaluation was restricted to patients with cirrhosis in one study and to patients with alcoholic hepatitis in the other studies; (c) in Kershnobich's study, the mean duration of treatment (4.7 years) was longer than in Akriviadis' (1 month) and Trinchet's studies (6 months). Strong heterogeneity in disease severity may also explain the discrepancies. For example, mean serum bilirubin and prothrombin time were 30 µmol/l and 16 seconds in Kershnobich's study, whereas in Akriviadis' study, mean bilirubin and prothrombin time were 300 mmol/l and 20 seconds.

Among patients who underwent successive liver biopsies, the results concerning colchicine effect on liver fibrosis have been also controversial. In Kershnobich's study, histological analysis showed cirrhosis disappearance in the colchicine group. However, the disappearance of cirrhosis, usually an irreversible lesion, as observed in one study is a disquieting result (Kershenobich, 1988). In contrast, Trinchet *et al*. did not observe any effect of colchicine on fibrosis score (3 at the admission, 3.6 at 6 months). The discrepancies between the studies may be explained by the duration of treatment (4.7 years versus 6 months).

Therefore, based on these studies, we conclude that the data were insufficient to determine clearly colchicine effectiveness. In future randomized trials, evaluation of colchicine effect on short-term survival is not recommended. Additional randomized controlled trials are necessary for testing colchicine on long-term survival in patients with alcoholic cirrhosis. As non compliance with treatment in alcoholic patients is notorious, evaluation of colchicine on long-term survival will require randomized controlled trials with a sufficient number of patients.

Propylthiouracil

Hypoxic damage in ALD, particularly in the centrilobular region of the liver, is due at least in part to an hypermetabolic state (Israel, 1975). Treatment with propylthiouracil in a rat model for 3–10 days reduced the hypermetabolic state and diminished histological and biochemical abnormalities (Israel, 1975). For these reasons, the effectiveness of propylthiouracil was tested in alcoholic patients in 3 randomized controlled trials (Orrego, 1978; Halle, 1982; Orrego, 1987).

The effects of propylthiouracil were tested on biochemical and histological features in the first study, on short-term survival in the second and on long-term survival in the third. In their first study, Orrego *et al.* assessed the severity of liver disease with a scoring method (CCLI) combining abnormal clinical and laboratory findings (Orrego, 1978). For assessing the effects of treatment, a "normalization rate" was developed (difference between the highest and lowest CCLI scores divided by the number of days). The authors observed that the normalization rate was higher in the propylthiouracil-group than in the placebo-group. Sensitive analysis showed that this effect was significant only in patients with severe liver disease (CCLI $\geq$ 13). There was no significant difference for short-term survival between the propylthiouracil and placebo groups. Inefficiency of propylthiouracil on short term survival was confirmed by another group (Halle, 1982). Meta-analysis of the two randomized trials published as full papers were performed with the Der Simonian method. Assessment of survival between control groups did not show heterogeneity. There was no significant survival effect of propylthiouracil association on short-term survival, with a mean difference of 1% (CI: −7 to 9%). Thus, evaluation of propylthiouracil is not recommended in future studies evaluating short-term survival.

Orrego *et al.* analyzed the effect of propylthiouracil on long-term survival in alcoholic patients. This trial involved 310 alcoholic patients who received propylthiouracil ($n = 157$) or a placebo ($n = 153$) for 2 years. The placebo and propylthiouracil were mixed with riboflavin, a fluorescent compound that was used as a marker of compliance (Orrego, 1987). Urine samples were used for monitoring compliance and abstinence. Using this accurate method, the investigators observed that 70% of patients in both groups were compliant and abstinent. Two year-mortality rate was lower in the propylthiouracil-group than in the placebo group: 13% versus 26%, $p < 0.05$. Proportional-hazards stepwise regression showed that propylthiouracil treatment, prothrombin time, hemoglobin levels and mean daily urinary alcohol levels significantly affected mortality. Sensitivity analysis showed that (a) propylthiouracil did not protect patients with mean morning urinary alcohol concentrations >8 mM; and (b) a more striking effect of propylthiouracil was observed in the subgroup of patients with severe disease. However, the main difficulty with this study was the high dropout rate of patients (61%) during the follow-up period. Therefore evidence concerning the use of propylthiouracil remains unsettled. Future randomized trials should be recommended for testing the effect of propylthiouracil on long-term survival in alcoholic patients with cirrhosis.

D-Penicillamine

Only one randomized trial evaluated d-penicillamine in 40 patients with alcoholic liver disease. No survival difference was observed between the placebo and d-penicillamine groups (Resnick, 1974).

Silymarin

In animal models, Silymarin reduces liver injury induced with various hepato-toxins including phalloidin, α-amanitin, CCL4 and galactosamine (Leng-Preschlow, 1985; Morgan, 1985).

A randomized controlled trial was performed in 170 patients with cirrhosis (Ferenci, 1989). Cirrhosis was related to alcohol consumption in 42% of patients. Eighty seven patients received 140 mg of Silymarin 3 times daily and 83 patients a placebo. The mean duration of treatment was 41 months. Within the 2 year study period, survival rates were 67 and 77% ($p = 0.07$) in the placebo and Silymarin groups respectively. After 4 years, survival was 58 and 38% ($p = 0.04$) in the placebo and Silymarin groups respectively. No information was given concerning alcohol consumption in the 2 groups. Sensitivity analysis observed the survival benefit only in the subgroup of alcoholic cirrhosis. However, as the study was initially designed for 2 years, the number of patients at risk at 4 years was approximately 10 for each group. Thus, caution has to be taken when considering the results of 4 year survival. Another randomized double-blind trial was carried out in 116 patients with alcoholic hepatitis biopsy-proven (Trinchet, 1989). In this study, Silymarin effect during 3 months was tested on histologic scores of alcoholic hepatitis and fibrosis in patients who underwent successive liver biopsies. No significant differences were observed between the two groups. A recent study evaluated the survival effect of Silymarin in 200 patients with alcoholic cirrhosis (Pares, 1998). At 5 years, survival rate of control group ($75 \pm 6\%$) was similar to the survival of Silymarin group ($78 \pm 5\%$). Therefore, Silymarin seems to have no effect on long-term survival.

Vitamin E

Vitamin E, an important antioxidant, protects cells against lipid peroxidation injury. Hepatic vitamin E content was significantly lower in alcoholic rats than in control rats and hepatic lipid peroxidation was increased in a group receiving a low vitamin E diet (Kawase, 1989). Diminished hepatic vitamin E content was observed in patients with cirrhosis (Tanner, 1986). A randomized controlled trial was carried out in 67 alcoholic patients. Vitamin E did not influence survival or biochemical parameters (Pia de la Maza, 1995).

(+)-Cyanidanol-3

(+)-cyanidanol-3 reduces ATP levels, NADH/NAD ratio and membrane damage in the livers of rats with ALD (Gajdos, 1972). Cyanidanol-3 was tested in one randomized controlled trial (Colman, 1980). Forty patients were randomly allocated to receive (+)-cyanidanol-3 ($n = 20$) or placebo ($n = 20$) for 3 months. No appreciable effect of (+)-cyanidanol-3 was observed on biochemical or histological features. The investigators did not provide survival data. The future evaluation of (+)-cyanidanol-3 is not recommended.

Thioctic acid

Thioctic acid (α-lipoic acid) may reduce inflammation and oxidative stress. However, the mechanisms of its action remain unclear. A randomized controlled trial was carried out in 40 alcoholic patients with marked fibrosis (Marshall, 1982). Over a 6 month period, patients randomly received thioctic acid 300 mg/j ($n = 20$) or placebo ($n = 20$). At the end of the study, no significant differences were observed between the groups for biological features. Among the patients with successive liver biopsies, no significant improvement of liver injury was observed between thioctic acid-patients (70%) and placebo-patients (50%). Moreover, histological lesions diminished only in patients who abstained from alcohol consumption. Thus, future evaluation of thioctic acid is not recommended.

Malotilate

Malotilate (diisopropyl 1,3-dithiol-2-ylidenemalonate) reduces liver injury in animal models. In a multicenter study, 335 patients were randomized to receive 1500 mg Malotilate ($n = 171$) or placebo ($n = 164$). There were no significant differences in survival between the two groups (Multimer, 1988). The effect of malotilate was tested in a further randomized controlled trial of 407 alcoholic patients (140 received malotilate 1500 mg/day, 133 received 750 mg malotilate/day and 134 received placebo). Patients treated by malotilate 750 mg had a better survival rate than the other two groups. However, there was no significant long-term survival effect of malotilate using multivariate analysis (Keiding, 1994). Therefore, evaluation of malotilate is not recommended in future randomized controlled trials.

Nutritional supplementation

Severe protein malnutrition, a common feature in patients with advanced liver disease, not only inhibits liver regeneration and immune response but it also increases bacterial, viral and fungal infections. Moreover, protein malnutrition was correlated significantly with survival (Nompleggi, 1994). In a study of 352 patients with ALD, 31% had a mild protein-calorie malnutrition, 60% a moderate and 9% a severe (Mendenhall, 1986). At 1 year, survival in the groups with mild, moderate and severe protein-calorie malnutrition were significantly different: 86, 57 and 25% respectively ($p < 0.001$). Patients with improvement in their protein-malnutrition score over 30 days of hospitalization improved their survival.

For the reasons described above, randomized controlled trials were carried out to determine the effect of nutritional supplementation in patients with ALD. Eight randomized controlled trials evaluated nutritional supplementation in alcoholic patients (Nasrallah, 1980; Calvey, 1985; Dhiel, 1985; Naveau, 1986; Cabre, 1990; Bonkovski, 1991; Bonkovsky, 1991; Mezey, 1991; Kearns, 1992). Among these studies, only two studies observed a survival benefit due to nutritional supplementation (Nasrallah, 1980, Cabre, 1990). In the first randomized controlled trial, amino acid therapy was evaluated in 35 patients with alcoholic hepatitis (Nasrallah, 1980). All patients were offered a 3000 Kcal 100 g protein diet. The amino acid group received 70–85 g of amino acid intravenously. At the time of randomization, the two groups showed similar severity of liver disease. During the 28 day study period, 4 patients in the control group died but none in the amino acid group ($p < 0.02$). In the amino acid group, serum bilirubin decreased from 9.1 mg/dl at randomization to 2.9 mg/dl after therapy ($p < 0.01$) and albumin level increased from 28 g/l at randomization to 33 g/l after therapy ($p < 0.025$). In the other randomized controlled trial of 35 patients, survival rate was significantly higher in patients who received enteral-tube feeding than in control patients: 88% versus 53%, $p = 0.02$ (Cabre, 1990). No significant difference for short-term survival was observed in the other studies. In a randomized controlled trial of 15 patients with alcoholic hepatitis biopsy-proven, amino acid therapy was no more beneficial than control therapy for biological and clinical parameters (Dhiel, 1985). A randomized controlled trial of supplementary parenteral nutrition was carried out in 40 jaundiced alcoholic cirrhotic patients (Naveau, 1986). On day 28, serum bilirubin was lower in the supplementary parenteral nutrition group (2.5 versus 4.1 mg/dl, $p < 0.02$). No significant differences were observed for serum transferrin, serum prealbumin and retinol-binding protein concentrations. The investigators observed an increase of infections related to the central venous catheter. During the treatment period one patient died in each group. Similar results concerning survival data were observed in Calvey and Mezey's studies. No survival data were given in Bonkovsky's study. Meta-analysis of the 7 randomized trials published as full papers were performed with the Der Simonian method. Assessment of survival between control groups showed significant heterogeneity ($\chi^2 = 15.5$, $p = 0.02$). There was no significant survival effect of nutritional supplementation on short-term survival, with a mean difference of 6% (−4 to 15%). A recent randomized controlled trial compared the short- and long-term effects of total enteral tube feeding or steroids in patients with severe alcoholic hepatitis (Cabre, 2000). Interestingly, formula of the enteral diet was adapted after considering the data from animal models. It was a low-fat diet and medium-chain triglycerides and oleic acid accounted for most its lipid content. Indeed, deleterious effects of high-fat diet on alcoholic liver injury have been clearly established in experimental studies using animal models (Tsukamoto, 1985, 1986, 1996, 1998). Mortality occurred earlier in the enteral group: 7 days versus 23 days, $p = 0.025$. During follow-up after the treatment period, deaths were observed more frequently in the corticosteroids group (10/27) than in the enteral group (2/4, $p = 0.04$). Therefore the authors suggested that a possible synergistic effect of both treatments should be investigated (Cabre, 2000).

Therefore, we considered that even though there was no survival benefit associated with the nutritional supplementation, future evaluation of this treatment modality may be interesting. For this purpose, the investigators will have to focus on the study design. To identify a survival effect, only patients with malnutrition will have to be included and low-fat diet will have to be preferred to other formula in future trials. As recommended by the investigators of the last RCT, the synergistic effect of nutritional supplementation and corticosteroids will have to be tested (Cabre, 2000).

Insulin and glucagon association

In the animal model, the insulin-glucagon association has been shown to stimulate hepatic regeneration after partial hepatectomy (Leffert, 1979). In a mouse model of fulminant hepatitis, administration of insulin and glucagon reduced the mortality (Farivar, 1976). However, results in clinical situations concerning the insulin-glucagon association were disappointing.

Five randomized controlled trials (3 published in article form and 2 in abstract form) evaluated the insulin-glucagon association in patients with alcoholic hepatitis (Mirouze, 1981; Radvan, 1982; Feher, 1987; Bird, 1991; Trinchet, 1992). Feher *et al.* reported a significant reduction of mortality in the group treated by the insulin-glucagon association (15 versus 42%, $p < 0.02$). On the other hand, 4 studies did not show significant difference in short-term survival between the placebo and the insulin-glucagon groups. In Trinchet's trial, mortality rate was not significantly different in the placebo (14%) than in the insulin-glucagon groups (27%). In Bird's study, mortality rates of the placebo and insulin-glucagon groups were similar: 35 versus 33%. Meta-analysis of the 3 randomized trials published as full papers was performed with the Der Simonian method. Assessment of survival between control groups showed a trend toward heterogeneity ($\chi^2 = 7.1$, $p = 0.07$). There was no significant effect of insulin-glucagon association on short-term survival, with a mean difference of 5% (CI: −11 to 23%). Therefore, we considered that there was no survival benefit associated with the insulin-glucagon association and future evaluation of these drugs is not recommended.

Anabolic-androgenic steroids

The majority of men with alcoholic cirrhosis have low serum concentrations of non protein-bound testosterone. Anabolic steroids were tested in patients with alcoholic liver disease in the hope of reversing the patients' catabolic state and promoting hepatic regeneration (Gluud, 1984). The first studies evaluating anabolic steroids have methodological defects as follows (Wells, 1960; Islam, 1973; Puliyel, 1977): (a) most of the studies were not blind; (b) some patients were excluded after allocation; and (c) allocation was not always randomly performed. The last three randomized controlled trials were negative. A trial from Compenhagen evaluated 184 male patients (Gluud, 1986). There was no significant difference in long-term survival between the placebo and testosterone groups: 25 versus 18%. In a Veterans Administration study, oxandrolone had no effect on short-term or long-term survival (Mendenhall, 1984). In another study from the Veterans Administration, 136 male patients received placebo and 137 males oxandrolone (Mendenhall, 1993). On an intention-to-treat basis, no difference in mortality between the two groups was observed. The investigators performed a sensitivity analysis according to the nutrition status. In patients with moderate malnutrition, 6 month mortality in oxandrolone-group was significantly lower than in placebo-group: 9.4 versus 20.9%, $p = 0.001$. No significant effect of oxandrolone was observed in patients with severe malnutrition. However, these results are questionable as this analysis was performed retrospectively. Meta-analysis of the controlled trials published as full papers was performed with the Der Simonian method. Assessment of survival between control groups showed a significant heterogeneity ($\chi^2 = 9.99$, $p = 0.04$). There was no significant long-term survival effect of anabolic steroids, with a mean difference of 10% (−20 to 1%). We performed a sensitivity analysis after exclusion of the first two controlled trials and observed no significant effect of anabolic steroids on long-term survival, with a mean difference of −3% (−11 to 5%). Based on these results, anabolic steroids are not indicated in patients with ALD. Furthermore, development of hepatocellular carcinoma has been reported with the use of other anabolic-androgenic agents.

Corticosteroids

Alcoholic hepatitis is a necrotizing inflammatory lesion of alcoholic liver injury that, in its severe form, is associated with high mortality. Thirteen randomized control trials evaluated corticosteroids in patients with alcoholic hepatitis (Helman, 1971; Porter, 1971; Campra, 1973; Blitzer, 1977; Lesesne, 1978; Maddrey, 1978; Shumaker, 1978; Depew, 1980; Theodossi, 1982; Mendenhall, 1984; Bories, 1987; Carithers, 1989; Ramond, 1992). These trials yielded inconsistent results. Among them, only 4 trials showed a survival benefit in treated patients (Helman, 1971, Lesesne, 1978, Carithers, 1989, Ramond, 1992). These contradictory results may be attributed either to the wide variability of severity between the studies, the lack of histological analysis before enrollment of patients, the small sample size, or the presence of confounding factors at inclusion such as hepatorenal syndrome or gastrointestinal bleeding.

Some studies included only patients with severe alcoholic hepatitis whereas other studies did not take into account the severity of the illness. The wide variability in survival of patients enrolled in the RCTs was demonstrated by assessment of survival in untreated control arms (Figure 24.1). Moreover, no accurate criteria for assessing severity were available until Maddrey *et al.*, described a discriminant-function (Maddrey, 1978). This discriminant-function was as follows: 4.6 (prothrombin time − control time [in seconds]) + serum bilirubin (in micro moles per liter)/17. This function is now used for identifying a subgroup of patients with high risk of mortality. The last two randomized trials included only patients with either a discriminant-function ≥ 32 or spontaneous encephalopathy

Carithers, 1989	64%	
Ramond, 1992	55%	
Campra, 1973	64%	
Porter, 1971	22%	
Shumaker, 1978	54%	$p < 0.001$
Depew, 1980	46%	
Lesesne, 1978	0%	
Helman, 1971	65%	
Maddrey, 1986, 1988	81%	
Mendenhall, 1984	80%	
Bories, 1987	76%	
Blitzer, 1977	69%	

Figure 24.1 Survival of non-treated patients in the RCTs evaluating corticosteroids.

(Carithers, 1989; Ramond, 1992). In these trials, survival in corticosteroid groups was significantly higher than in placebo-groups: 94% versus 65% at 28 days in Carithers' study ($p = 0.006$) and 88% versus 45% at 66 days in Ramond's study ($p = 0.001$).

Diagnosis of alcoholic hepatitis depends on histological analysis as biological and clinical criteria classically used by the investigators were non specific. In alcoholic patients admitted with a presumed diagnosis of alcoholic hepatitis and a discriminant function above 32, we observed that only 70% of them suffered from an alcoholic hepatitis biopsy-proven (Mathurin, 1992). Among the 13 randomized control trials, only 3 used liver biopsy as an entry criteria (Helman, 1971; Bories, 1987; Ramond, 1992). Thus, inclusion of alcoholic patients without biopsy-proven alcoholic hepatitis, as observed in some previous randomized trials, may partially explain the contradictory results concerning corticosteroid efficacy.

Patients with gastrointestinal bleeding or hepatorenal syndrome may be less responsive to steroid treatment than patients without these complications. In these circumstances, the outcome of patients may be related to these cofactors rather than to alcoholic hepatitis itself (Imperiale, 1990). Based on this hypothesis, we performed a meta-analysis using the Der Simonian method (Mathurin, 1995). Among the randomized controlled trials which excluded patients with gastrointestinal bleeding, survival benefit in treated patients was significant (26%; CI:6–36%, $p < 0.01$); there was no survival benefit among the studies which did not exclude patients with gastrointestinal bleeding (1%).

Five meta-analyses observed a survival benefit in treated patients, especially in those with encephalopathy (Reynolds, 1989; Imperiale, 1990; Daures, 1991; Poynard, 1991; Mathurin, 1995). However, a recent meta-analysis, using weight logistic regression analysis concluded that corticosteroids are ineffective (Christensen, 1993; #7). The method used by the authors is questionable because the statistical weights attributed to negative trials had a wide influence in the results (Figure 24.2). Indeed, the statistical weight attributed to Mendenhall's study was 9.53 whereas the statistical weights attributed to Carithers' and Ramond's studies were 1.72 and 2.47 respectively.

Mendenhall, using a backward elimination logistic regression analysis on patients from his previous randomized controlled trial, recently observed that corticosteroids improve survival in the subgroup of patients with Maddrey's discriminant function higher than 35 (Mendenhall, 1995). Thus, as this RCT had the higher statistical weight and was considered as a negative trial in Cristensen's meta-analysis, the results of this meta-analysis are questionable. Recently, representatives of the American College of Gastroenterology published guidelines and recommended glucocorticosteroids for patients with severe AH as defined by the Maddrey (Imperiale, 1990; Mc Cullough, 1998). However, based on their negative meta-analysis, Christensen et al. criticized this recommendation and suggested that the proposed guidelines were not sufficiently evidence-based (Christensen, 1999). To end this controversy, the investigators of the last 3 randomized controlled trials (Mendenhall, Carithers, Ramond) combined their individual data. The authors restricted their analysis on patients with a disciminant function ≥ 32. Determination of discriminant function in each patient allow the authors to identify rigorously the patients in Mendenhall's study with severe alcoholic hepatitis. This study

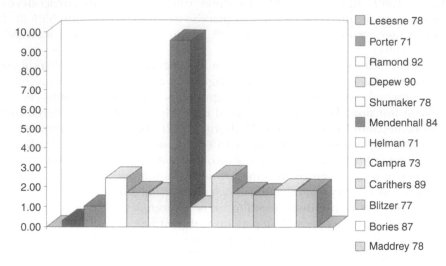

Figure 24.2 Statistical weights attributed to each RCTs in the study of Christensen *et al.*

clearly showed that corticosteroids improve short-term survival of patients with severe alcoholic hepatitis (Mathurin, 2001).

In the present chapter, a meta-analysis of the 13 randomized trials published as full papers was performed with the Der Simonian method. Assessment of survival between control groups showed significant heterogeneity ($\chi^2 = 34.6$, $p < 0.001$). There was a significant short-term survival effect of corticosteroids, with a mean

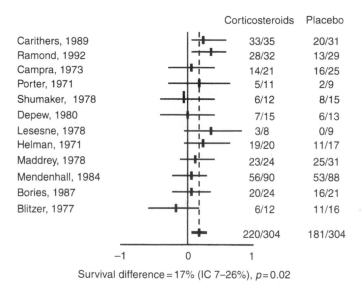

Figure 24.3 Meta-analysis of randomized controlled trials evaluating coricosteroids DerSimanian & Laird method.

difference of 15% (CI: 6–24%, $p < 0.01$) (Figure 24.3). Among all patients with encephalopathy, there was a significant short-term survival effect of corticosteroids, with a mean difference of 27% (CI:11–44%, $p < 0.0001$).

A study evaluated 122 alcoholic patients with severe biopsy-proven alcoholic hepatitis: 61 patients of the previous randomized controlled trial (32 prednisolone-randomized patients, 29 placebo-randomized patients), 61 prospectively treated with prednisolone until the end of this trial and 61 simulated-control patients using a previously validated prognostic model which enabled the prediction of the theoretical survival of each patient if he/she was not treated. This study observed that: (a) corticosteroids are associated with short-term survival benefit; (b) age, neutrophilia and polymorphonuclear infiltrate were useful prognostic factors for identifying a subgroup of patients who more strongly benefited from corticosteroid treatment; and (c) survival benefit due to corticosteroid treatment persisted for at least 1 year and disappeared at 2 years (Mathurin, 1996).

STUDIES ARE ASSOCIATED WITH METHODOLOGICAL DEFICIENCY

This analytic review observed that some randomized controlled trials evaluated the short-term effect of a drug whereas others evaluated the long-term effect. Thus, no comparisons between these studies can be done. For example, colchicine and propylthiouracil had no efficacy on short-term survival. On the other hand, their effects on long-term survival remain controversial. No data were available to contradict the long-term survival effects of these drugs which had been observed in two randomized controlled trials (Orrego, 1987; Kershenobich, 1988). Evaluation of these drugs in the same conditions as the 2 previous randomized trials may be an important step toward progress in the therapeutic field of ALD.

One of the main problems in the evaluation of pharmacological treatment in alcoholic patients is the high dropout rate, particularly in long-term therapy. For example, a randomized controlled trial of long-term treatment with propylthiouracil showed a 60% dropout (Orrego, 1987). Future trials evaluating long-term therapy need to take into account the high predicted dropout rate and would have to include a large number of patients.

Abstinence, a classic prognostic factor in alcoholic cirrhosis, is a confounding variable for studies, especially in long-term treatment. An imbalance in abstinence percentage may contribute, at least in part, to a negative or a positive result. No consensus was available for accurately assessing abstinence in alcoholic patients. However, a questionnaire on admitted daily alcohol consumption and mean daily urinary alcohol levels may be useful markers of abstinence. Future investigators will have to accurately determine the percentage of abstinence.

It is known that biological features are poorly correlated with histological outcome. It also has been demonstrated in some studies that histological analysis may be useful for identifying responder patients. Corticosteroids are efficient only in patients with severe alcoholic hepatitis whereas colchicine would be efficient only in patients without alcoholic hepatitis (Kershenobich, 1988; Akriviadis, 1990; Mathurin, 1996). Thus, lack of histological analysis probably explain, at least in part, the discrepancies between some studies. Therefore, study design evaluating pharmacological treatments in alcoholic patients will have to systematically include a liver biopsy as an inclusion criteria.

In patients with ALD, survival was clearly correlated with the severity of liver insufficiency. This analytical review observed an interaction between some treatments and the severity of the liver disease: corticosteroids are efficient only in a subgroup of patients with severe ALD whereas colchicine and propylthiouracil would be efficacious in patients with moderate liver disease. It appears that a precise definition of the subgroup according to the illness severity is essential for performing prognostic stratification. The use of prognostic functions such as Child-Pugh score, Beclere model and Maddrey discriminant function are recommended (Poynard, 1994). Using these functions, future trials can evaluate the drug in the same subgroup of patients. Thus, these future trials would be compared and pooled.

FUTURE STRATEGIES

Regulation of cytokines in alcoholic hepatitis

Frequent manifestations of alcoholic hepatitis are features of an acute phase response, immunological manifestations such as autoantibodies to liver-specific antigens, neoantigens, neutrophilia and neutrophil infiltration. Pro-inflammatory cytokines, such as interleukin-8 (IL-8), interleukin-6 (IL-6) and tumor necrosis alpha (TNFα), probably play a role in these manifestations (Olinger, 1993). Moreover, in animal models a convincing collection of data exists supporting a pivotal role of TNFα in alcohol-induced liver injury. Many studies observed that patients with alcoholic hepatitis had elevated serum TNFα, IL-1, IL-6 and IL-8 levels (Bird, 1990; Sheron, 1993). Serum levels of these three inflammatory cytokines are much higher in plasma of patients with alcoholic hepatitis than in alcoholic patients with inactive cirrhosis or without liver disease (Taïeb, 2000). Peripheral blood mononuclear cells isolated from patients with alcoholic cirrhosis disclosed higher IL-6, IL-8 and TNFα than peripheral blood mononuclear cells isolated from healthy controls (Taïeb, 2000). The prognostic values of IL-6, IL-8 and TNFα serum levels mainly have been evaluated. Serum levels of these cytokines were correlated with the severity of liver disease. It also appears that serum levels of these three cytokines were higher in deceased patients and univariate survival analysis suggested that serum IL-6, IL-8 and TNFα levels would be useful prognostic factors for predicting survival (for more details see chapter 8) (Bird, 1990; Felver, 1990). Based on these findings, pharmacological treatments which inhibit inflammatory cytokines would be efficient in patients with alcoholic hepatitis.

An imbalance of production of pro-inflammatory and anti-inflammatory cytokines has been demonstrated in patients with severe ALD. For example, a defective IL-10 release by human monocytes in alcoholic cirrhosis accounts for an increased production of TNFα by these cells upon LPS challenge (Le Moine, 1995). In an animal model, the hepatoprotective role of IL-10, an anti-inflammatory cytokine, was recently demonstrated (Louis, 1997). In Galactosamine/Lipopolysaccharide mouse liver injury, administration of recombinant IL-10 decreased TNFα and ALT levels. Conversely, anti-IL-10 increased TNFα and ALT concentrations. Therefore, a defective secretion of IL-10 may be involved in the pathogenesis of alcoholic hepatitis.

Progress in understanding the network of intercellular and intracellular signals among Kupffer cells, monocytes and neutrophils could provide new targets for therapeutic intervention. For example, administering TNFα receptors or antibodies anti-TNFα in animal models reduced the degree of liver injury and lowered mortality (Czaja, 1995; Limuro, 1997). In the future, soluble TNFα receptor and anti-TNFα antibodies should be evaluated in patients with alcoholic hepatitis.

Pentoxyfilline

Pentoxyfilline, an inhibitor of TNFα synthesis, was recently evaluated in a randomized controlled trial of patients with severe alcoholic hepatitis (discriminant function >32). One hundred and one patients were randomly allowed to receive pentoxyfilline ($n = 49$) or placebo ($n = 52$) (Akriviadis, 2000). Short-term mortality was significantly lower in the pentoxyfilline group than in the placebo group: 24.5% versus 46.1% ($p = 0.04$). There were no significant differences between the two groups during the study period for serum TNFα level. Hepatorenal syndrome was the cause of death in 6 pentoxyfille patients (50%) and in 22 placebo patients (92%, $p = 0.009$). In multivariate analysis, age, serum creatinine and pentoxyfilline treatment were the three variables independently associated with survival. There were no significant differences in serum TNFα during the study period between the pentoxyfilline and placebo groups. Some remarks can be made concerning this interesting trial: (a) the investigators compared pentoxyfilline to placebo instead of corticosteroids; (b) development of hepatorenal syndrome was quite higher than in other studies and no clear explanations were provided to this phenomenon; (c) approximately 20% of randomized patients had positive anti-HCV antibodies; and (d) during the study period, pentoxyfilline did not have any significant effect as compared to placebo on biological features of hepatic function (Akriviadis, 2000). In the future, evaluation of pentoxyfilline will require further studies evaluating this drug versus corticosteroids in patients with severe alcoholic hepatitis.

Phosphatidylcholine

It is known that membrane alteration induced by lipid peroxidation is one of the mechanisms involved in alcohol liver injury. Phosphatidylcholine may reduce membrane damage (Lieber, 1990). For these reasons, phosphatidylcholine effect was assessed by Lieber *et al.* in the baboon model (Lieber, 1994). Thirty-eight baboons were studied: 12 were fed a lecithin extract containing 55–60% phosphatidylcholine without alcohol, 12 were fed alcohol, 8 were fed alcohol and phosphatidylcholine, and 6 were fed phosphatidylcholine without alcohol. After 6 years, none of the alcohol-fed animals developed severe fibrosis or cirrhosis in the phosphatidylcholine supplemented group. On the other hand 80% of alcohol-fed baboons developed severe fibrosis or cirrhosis ($p < 0.001$). However, after a longer period of follow-up (8 years) the investigators observed the occurrence of severe fibrosis in the alcohol-fed baboons supplemented with phosphatidylcholine. As expected, transformation of Ito cells to transitional cells was significantly lower in the phosphatidylcholine group than in the alcohol group. In cultured lipocytes, phosphatidylcholine increases collagenase activity but has no effect on $\alpha 1$ procollagen mRNA (Li, 1992). The same group assessed the effectiveness of phosphatidylcholine on liver injury induced by CCL4 in rats (Ma, 1996). Phosphatidylcholine supplementation prevents lipid peroxidation, reduces the score of fibrosis and attenuates the hepatic collagen content. The authors also observed that phosphatidylcholine reduced established fibrosis when this treatment was given after 8 weeks of CCL4 injection. As phosphatidylcholine does not significantly modify $\alpha 1$ procollagen mRNA, an increase in collagenase activity may explain, at least in part, the phosphatidylcholine effect on liver fibrosis. Other mechanisms may be suggested. For example, phosphatidylcholine reduces *in vitro* the secretion of TNFα by rat Kupffer cells and suppresses the PDGF-mediated proliferation of stellate cells (Brady, 1997). Based on these promising results, the effectiveness of phosphatidylcholine is being evaluated in a multicenter randomized trial in humans (Veterans Administration Study 391).

S-adenosylmethionine

Glutathione is one of the most important scavenger of toxic free radicals. It has been shown that glutathione depletion, a common feature in patients with ALD, was involved in liver injury induced by alcohol (Speisky, 1985; Jewell, 1986). Although, glutathione depletion cannot by itself induce lipid peroxidation, it was demonstrated that it may increase the lipid peroxidation induced by ethanol (Shaw, 1981). S-adenosylmethionine plays a central role in the trans-sulfuration pathway. Through this route, S-adenosylmethionine acts as a precursor of glutathione. S-adenosylmethionine transferase, the main enzyme for S-adenosylmethionine synthesis, is reduced in human cirrhosis (Duce, 1988). In the baboon model, S-adenosylmethionine depletion can be partially corrected by the administration of S-adenosylmethionine, resulting in an attenuation of alcohol-induced liver injury (Lieber, 1990). However, in this model no regression or attenuation of liver fibrosis has been reported. Other mechanisms may be involved in the effects of S-adenosylmethionine. *In vitro*, S-adenosylmethionine decreases the amounts of TNFα protein and TNFα mRNA (Watson, 1997). *In vivo*, S-adenosylmethionine decreases serum TNFα in liver injury induced by LPS (Chawla, 1997).

In humans, oral S-adenosylmethionine therapy (1200 mg daily for 6 months) was evaluated in a placebo-controlled trial (Vendemiale, 1989). S-adenosylmethionine therapy significantly increases hepatic levels either in alcoholic and in non alcoholic patients with liver disease as compared with placebo control groups. A significant decrease of aspartate aminotransferase was observed in alcoholic patients treated with S-adenosylmethionine (from 32 IU/l to 21 IU/l, $p < 0.05$). However, the authors did not give information concerning the histological effects of S-adenosylmethionine. Another study showed that parenteral administration of S-adenosylmethionine increases glutathione content in erythrocytes (Loguercio *et al.*, 1994).

Recently, important results from a double randomized controlled trial were reported (Mato, 1999). Patients with alcoholic cirrhosis were randomly allocated for receiving 1200 mg S-adenosylmethionine daily ($n = 62$) or placebo ($n = 61$). There were no significant differences between the groups for sex ratio, age, bilirubin, albumin, aspartate aminotransferase, and prothrombin time. During the follow-up, approximately 50% of patients became abstinent and 5% dropout occurred. Overall survival in the adenosylmethionine group (90%) was significantly better than in the placebo group (73%, $p = 0.04$). However, using the log-rank test there was only a trend toward difference for cumulative survival at 2 years between the two groups ($p = 0.08$). Sensitivity analysis showed that adenosylmethionine effect on survival was observed only in the subgroup of patients with moderate liver disease (Child-Pugh A or B). These results, to our knowledge, are the first results suggesting a survival benefit due to S-adenosylmethionine in human subjects. In the future, further studies with a sufficient number of patients are recommended.

SUMMARY

In summary, only corticosteroids improve short-term survival in patients with severe alcoholic hepatitis (Maddrey discriminant function ≥ 32). Patients with gastrointestinal bleeding are less responsive to corticosteroids. Young patients with marked neutrophil infiltrate more strongly benefited from corticosteroid treatment. Colchicine and propylthiouracil may ameliorate long-term survival in patients with alcoholic cirrhosis. In the future, further studies evaluating the effects of these drugs are necessary. Preliminary and promising data concerning new drugs such as pentoxyfilline, S adenosylmethionine and phosphatidylcholine have been recently published. Randomized controlled trials for these drugs are ongoing.

REFERENCES

Akriviadis, E., Botla, R., Briggs, W., Han, S., Reynolds, T. and Shakil, O. (2000) Pentoxifylline improves short-term survival in severe acute alcoholic hepatitis: a double-blind, placebo-controlled trial. *Gastroenterology* **119**, 1637–1648.

Akriviadis, E.A., Steindel, H., Pinto, P.C., Fong, T.L., Kanel, G., Reynolds, T.B. and Gupta, S. (1990) Failure of colchicine to improve short-term survival in patients with alcoholic hepatitis. *Gastroenterology* **99**, 811–818.

Bird, G., Lau, J.Y.N., Koskinas, J., Wicks, C. and Williams, R. (1991) Insulin and glucagon infusion in acute alcoholic hepatits: a randomized controlled trial. *Hepatology* **14**, 1097–1101.

Bird, G.L.A., Sheron, N., Goka, A.K.J., Alexander, G.J. and Williams, R.S. (1990) Increased plasma tumor necrosis factor in severe alcoholic hepatitis. *Ann Intern Med* **112**, 917–920.

Blitzer, B.L., Mutchnick, M.G., Joshi, P.H., Phillips, M.M., Fessel, J.M. and Conn, H.O. (1977) Adrenocorticosteroid therapy in alcoholic hepatitis: A prospective, double-blind randomized study. *Am J Dig Dis* **22**, 477–484.

Bonkovski, H.L., Singh, R.H., Jafri, I.H., Fiellin, D.A., Smith, G.S., Simon, D., Citsonis, G.A. and Slaker, D.P. (1991) Randomized, controlled trial of treatment of alcoholic hepatitis with parenteral nutrition and oxandrolone. II. Short-term effects on nitrogen metabolism, metabolic balance, and nutrition. *Am J Gastroenterol* **86**, 1209–1218.

Bonkovsky, H.L., Fiellin, D.A., Smith, G.S., Slaker, D.P., Simon, D. and Galambos, J.T. (1991) A randomized, controlled trial of treatment of alcoholic hepatitis with parenteral nutrition and oxandrolone. Short-term effect on liver function. *Am J Gastroenterol* **86**, 1200–1208.

Bories, P., Guedj, J.Y., Mirouze, D., Yousfi, A. and Michel, H. (1987) Traitement de l'hépatite alcoolique aiguë par la prednisolone. *Presse Med* **16**, 769–772.

Boumpas, D.T. (1993) Glucocorticoid therapy for Immune-mediated Diseases: Basic and Clinical Correlates. *Ann Intern Med* **119**, 1198–1208.

Brady, L.M., Fimmel, C.J. and Fox, E.S. (1997) Phosphatidylcholine suppresses PDGF induced MAPK activation and proliferation in hepatic stellate cells (abstract). *Hepatology* **26**, 333A.

Cabre, E., Gonzalez-Huix, F., Abdad-Lacruz, A., Esteve, M., Acero, D., Fernades-Banares, Xiol, X. and Gassull, M.A. (1990) Effects of total enteral nutrition on the short-term outcome of severely malnourished cirrhotics: A randomized controlled trial. *Gastroenterology* **98**, 715–720.

Cabre, E., Rodriguez-Iglesias, P., Caballeria, J., Quer, J.C., Sanchez-Lombrana, J.L., Pares, A., Papo, M., Planas, R. and Gassul, M.A. (2000) Short- and long-term outcome of severe alcohol-induced hepatitis treated with steroids or enteral nutrition: a multicenter randomized trial. *Hepatology* **32**, 36–42.

Cabrero, C., Martin Duce, Q., Ortiz, P., Alemany, S. and Mato, J.M. (1988) Specific loss of the high-molecular-weight form of *S*-adenosyl-*L*-methionine synthetase in human liver cirrhosis. *Hepatology* **8**, 1530–1534.

Calvey, H., Davis, M. and Williams, R. (1985) Controlled trial of nutritional supplementation, with and without branched aminoacid enrichment, in treatment of acute alcoholic hepatitis. *J Hepatol* **1**, 141–151.

Campra, J.L., Hamlin, E.M., Kirshbaum, R.J., Olivier, M., Redeker, A.G. and Reynolds, T.B. (1973) Prednisone therapy of acute alcoholic hepatitis. *Ann Intern Med* **79**, 625–631.

Carithers Jr., R.L., Herlong, H.F., Diehl, A.M., Shaw, E.W., Combes, B., Fallon, H.J. and Maddrey, W.C. (1989) Methylprednisolone therapy in patients with severe alcoholic hepatitis: a randomized multicenter trial. *Ann Intern Med* **110**, 685–690.

Cavallini, L., Bindoli, A. and Silipirandi, N. (1978) Comparative evaluation of antiperoxidative action of silymarin and other flavonoids. *Pharmacol Res Commun* **10**, 133–136.

Chawla, R.K., Watson, W.H., Eastin, C.E., Lee, E.Y. and McClain, C.J. (1997) *S*-adenosylmethionine modulates serum TNF concentrations in lipopolysaccharide induced liver injury. *Hepatology* **26**, 227A.

Christensen, E. and Gluud, C. (1999) Glucocorticosteroids are not effective in alcoholic patients. *Am J Gastroenterol* **94**, 3065–3066.

Colman, J.C., Morgan, M.Y., Sheuer, P.J. and Sherlock, S. (1980) Treatment of alcohol-related liver disease with (+)-cyanidanol-3: a randomised double-blind trial. *Gut* **21**, 965–969.

Czaja, M.J., Xu, J. and Alt, E. (1995) Prevention of carbon tetrachloride-induced liver injury. *Gastroenterology* **108**, 1849–1854.

Daures, J.P., Peray, P., Bories, P., Blanc, P., Youfsi, A., Michel, H. and Gremy, F. (1991) Place de la corticothérapie dans le traitement des hépatites alcooliques aiguës. Résultats d'une méta-analyse. *Gastroenterol Clin Biol* **15**, 223–228.

Depew, W., Boyer, T., Omata, M., Redeker, A. and Reynolds, T. (1980) Double-Blind controlled trial of prednisolone therapy in patients with severe acute alcoholic hepatitis and spontaneous encephalopathy. **78**, 524–529.

Der Simonian, R. and Laird, N. (1986) Meta-analysis in clinical trials. *Control Clin Trials* **7**, 177–188.

Dhiel, A.M., Boinott, H., Herlong, H.F., Potter, J.J., Duyn, M.A., Chandmer, E. and Mezzey, E. (1985) Effect of parenteral amino acid supplementation in alcoholic hepatitis. *Hepatology* **5**, 57–63.

Diegelmann, R.F. and Peterkofsky, B. (1972) Inhibition of collagen secretion from bone and cultured fibroblasts by microtubular disruptive drugs. *Proc Natl Acad Sci USA* **69**, 892–896.

Duce, A.M., Ortiz, P., Cabrero, C. and Mato, M. (1988) S-adenosyl methionine synthetase and phospholipid methyltransferase are inhibited in human cirrhosis. *Hepatology* **8**, 65–68.

Ehrlich, H.P., Ross, R. and Bornstein, P. (1974) Effects of antimicrotubular agents on the secretion of collagen. A biological and morphological study. *J Cell Biol* **62**, 390–405.

Farivar, M., Wands, J.R., Isselbacher, K.J. and Bucher, N.L. (1976) Effect of insulin and glucagon on fulminant murine hepatitis. *N Engl J Med* **295**, 1517–1519.

Feher, J., Cornides, A., Romany, A., Karteszi, M., Szalay, L. and Gogl, Picazo, J. (1987) A prospective multicenter study of insulin and glucagon infusion therapy in acute alcoholic hepatits. *J Hepatol* **5**, 224–231.

Felver, M.E., Mezey, E., McGuire, M., Mitchell, M.C., Herlong, H.F., Veech, G.A. and Veech, R.L. (1990) Plasma tumor necrosis factor alpha predicts decreased long-term survival in severe alcoholic hepatitis. *Alcohol Clin Exp Res* **14**, 255–259.

Ferenci, P., Dragsics, B., Dittrich, H., Frank, H., Benda, L., Lochs, H., Meryn, S., Base, W. and Schneider, B. (1989) Randomized controlled trial of silymarin treatment in patients with cirrhosis of the liver. *J Hepatol* **9**, 105–113.

Figueroa, R.B. (1973) Mesterolone in steatosis and cirrhosis of the liver. *Br J Clin Pract* **20**, 282–290.

Gajdos, A., Gajdos-Török, M. and Horn, R. (1972) The effect of (+) catechin on the hepatic level of ATP and the lipid content of the liver during experimental cirrhosis. *Biochem Pharmacol* **21**, 594–600.

Gluud, C. (1984) Anabolic-androgenic steroid treatment of liver diseases. *Liver* **4**, 159–169.

Gluud, C. (1986) Copenhagen Study Group For Liver diseases. Testosterone treatment of men with alcoholic cirrhosis: A double-blind study. *Hepatology* **6**, 807–813.

Halle, P., Pare, P., Kaptein, K., Kanel, G., Redeker, A.G. and Reynolds, T.B. (1982) Double-blind controlled trial of propylthiouracyl in patients with severe acute alcoholic hepatitis. *Gastroenterology* **82**, 925–931.

Helman, R.A., Temko, M.H., Nye, S.W. and Fallon, H.J. (1971) Natural history and evaluation of prednisolone therapy. *Ann Intern Med* **74**, 311–321.

Hirayama, C., Kimura, N. and Massuya, T. (1970) Anabolic steroid effect of hepatic protein synthesis in patients with liver cirrhosis. *Digestion* **3**, 41–47.

Imperiale, T.F. and McCullough, A.J. (1990) Do corticosteroids reduce mortality from alcoholic hepatitis? *Ann Intern Med* **113**, 299–307.

Islam, N. and Islam, A. (1973) Testosterone propionate in cirrhosis of the liver. A controlled trial. *Br J Clin Pract* **27**, 125–128.

Israel, Y., Videla, L. and Bernstein, J. (1975) Experimental alcohol-induced hepatic necrosis: suppression by propylthiouracil. *Proc Nat Accad Sci USA* **72**, 1137–1141.

Israel, Y., Videla, L. and Bernstein, J. (1975) Liver hypermetabolic state after chronic ethanol consumption: hormonal interrelationships and pathogenic implications. *Fed Proc* **34**, 2052–2059.

Jewell, S.A., Di Monte, D., Gentile, A., Guglielmi, A., Altomare, E. and Albano, O. (1986) Decreased hepatic glutathione in chronic alcoholic patients. *J Hepatol* **3**, 1–6.

Kawase, T., Kato, S. and Lieber, C.S. (1989) Lipid peroxidation and antioxidant defense systems in rat liver after chronic ethanol feeding. *Hepatology* **10**, 815–821.

Kearns, P.J., Young, H., Garcia, G., Blaschke, T., O'Hanlon, G., Rinki, M. and Suher, K. (1992) Accelerated improvement of alcoholic liver disease with enteral nutrition. *Gastroenterology* **102**, 200–205.

Keiding, S., Badsberg, J.H., Becker, U., Bentsen, K.D., Bonnevie, O., Caballeria, J. *et al.* (1994) The prognosis of patients with alcoholic liver disease. An international randomized, placebo-controlled trial on the effect of malotilate on survival. *J Hepatol* **20**, 454–460.

Kershenobich, D., Uribe, M., Suarez, G.I., Mata, J.M., Perez-Tamayo, R. and Rojkind, M. (1979) Treatment of cirrhosis with colchicine. *Gastroenterology* **77**, 532–536.

Kershenobich, D., Vargas, F., Garcia-Tsao, G., Perez-Tamayo, R., Gent, M. and Rojkind, M. (1988) Colchicine in the treatment of cirrhosis of the liver. *N Engl J Med* **318**, 1709–1713.

Le Moine, O., Marchant, A., De Groote, D., Azar, C., Goldman, M. and Deviere, J. (1995) Role of defective monocyte interleukin-10 release in tumor necrosis factor-alpha over-production in alcoholic cirrhosis. *Hepatology* **22**, 1436–1439.

Leffert, H.L., Koch, K.S., Moran, T. and Rubalcava, B. (1979) Hormonal control of rat liver regeneration. *Gastroenterology* **76**, 1470–1482.

Leng-Preschlow (1985) Antagonization of CCL4 damage in isolated perfused rat liver by silibini. *J Hepatol* **1**, S81.

Lesesne, H.R., Bozymski, E.M. and Fallon, H.J. (1978) Treatment of alcoholic hepatitis with encephalopathy. Comparison of prednisolone with caloric supplements. *Gastroenterology* **74**, 169–173.

Li, J., Kim, C.I., Leo, M.A., Mak, K.M. and Lieber, C.S. (1992) Polyunsaturated lecithin prevents acetaldehyde-mediated hepatic collagen accumultion by stimulating collagenase activity in cultured lipocytes. *Hepatology* **15**, 373–381.

Lieber, C.S., Casini, A., Decarli, L.M., Kim, C.I., Lowe, N., Sasaki, R. and Leo, M.A. (1990) S-adenosylmethionine attenuates alcohol-induced liver injury in the baboon. *Hepatology* **11**, 165–172.

Lieber, C.S., DeCarli, L.M., Mak, K.M., Kim, C.I. and Leo, M.A. (1990) Attenuations of alcohol-induced hepatic fibrosis by polyunsaturated lecithin. *Hepatology* **12**, 1390–1398.

Lieber, C.S., Robins, S.J., Li, J., Decarli, L.M., Mak, K.M., Fasulo, J.M. and Leo, M.A. (1994) Phosphatidylcholine protects against fibrosis and cirrhosis in the baboon. *Gastroenterology* **106**, 152–159.

Limuro, Y., Gallucci, R.M., Luster, M.I., Khono, H. and Thurman, R.G. (1997) Antibodies to tumor necrosis factor alpha attenuate hepatic necrosis and inflammation due to chornic exposure to ethanol in rats. *Hepatology* **26**, 1530–1537.

Loguercio, C., Nardi, G., Argenzio, F., Aurilio, C., Petrone, E., Grella, A., Del Vecchio Blanco, C. and Coltorti, M. (1994) Effect of *S*-adenosyl-*L*-methionie administration on red blood cell cysteine and gluthatione levels in alcoholic patients with and without liver disease. *Alcohol & Alcoholism* **5**, 597–604.

Louis, H., Le Moine, O., Peny, M.O., Gulbis, B., Nisol, F., Goldman, M. and Devière, J. (1997) Hepatoprotective role of interleukin 10 in Galactosamine/Lipopolysaccharide mouse liver injury. *Gastroenterology* **112**, 935–942.

Ma, X., Zhao, J. and Lieber, C.S. (1996) Polyenylphosphatidylcholine attenuates non-alcoholic hepatic fibrosis and accelerates its regression. *J Hepatol* **24**, 604–613.

Maddrey, W.C. (1986) Is therapy with testosterone or anabolic-androgenic steroids useful in the treatment of alcoholic liver disease. *Hepatology* **6**, 1033–1035.

Maddrey, W.C. (1988) Alcoholic hepatitis: clinicopathologic features and therapy. *Semin Liv Dis* **8**, 91–102.

Maddrey, W.C., Boitnott, J.K., Bedine, M.S., Weber, F.L., Mezey, E. and White, R.I. (1978) Corticosteroid therapy of alcoholic hepatitis. *Gastroenterology* **75**, 193–199.

Marshall, A.W., Graul, R.S., Morgan, M.Y. and Sherlock, S. (1982) Treatment of alcohol-related liver disease with thioctic acid: a six month randomised double-blind trial. *Gut* **23**, 1088–1093.

Mathurin, P., Bernard, B., Quichon, J.P., Opolon, P. and Poynard, T. (1995) L'hémorragie digestive et l'insuffisance rénale: deux facteurs de confusion dans l'analyse de l'efficacité des corticoïdes dans l'hépatite alcoolique aiguë (abstract). *Gastroenterol Clin Biol* **19**, A162.

Mathurin, P., Duchatelle, V., Ramond, M.J., Degott, C., Bedossa, P., Erlinger, S., Benhamou, J.P., Chaput, J.C., Rueff, B. and Poynard, T. (1996) Survival and prognostic factors in patients with severe biopsy-proven alcoholic hepatitis treated by prednisolone: random-ized trial, new cohort, and simulation. *Gastroenterology* **110**, 1847–1853.

Mathurin, P., Mendenhall, C.L., Carithers Jr., R., Ramond, M.J., Maddrey, W.C., Garstide, P., Rueff, B., Naveau, S., Chaput, J.C. and Poynard, T. (2001) Severe alcoholic hepatitis (AH): individual data analysis of the last three randomized placebo controlled double blind trials. (submitted).

Mathurin, P., Poynard, T., Ramond, M.J., Degott, C., Bedossa, P. Cassard, T. *et al.* (1992) Intérêt de la biopsie hépatique pour la sélection des sujets suspects d'hépatite alcoolique aigue (abstract). *Gastroenterol Clin Biol* **16**, A231.

Mato, J.M., Camara, J., Fernandez de Paz, J., Caballiera, L., Coll, S., Caballero, A., Garcia-Buey, L., Beltran, J., Benita, V., Caballeria, J., Sola, R., Moreno-Otero, R., Barrao, F., Martin-Duce, A., Correa, J.A., Pares, A., Barrao, E., Garcia-Magaz, I., Puerta, J.L., Moreno, J., Boissard, G., Ortiz, P. and Rodes, J. (1999) S-adenosylmethionine in alcoholic liver cirrhosis: a randomized, placebo-controlled, double-blind, multicenter clinical trial. *J Hepatol* **30**, 1081–1089.

Matsuda, Y., Takada, A., Yasura, M. and Sato, H. (1988) Effects of malotilate on alcoholic liver injury in rats. *Alcohol Clin Exp Res* **12**, 665–670.

Mc Cullough, A.J. and O'Connor, J.F.B. (1998) Alcoholic liver disease: proposed recommendations for the american college of gastroenterology. *Am J Gastroenterol* **93**, 2022–2036.

Mendenhall, C., Roselle, G.A., Gartside, P. and Moritz, T. (1995) Relationship of protein calorie malnutrition to alcoholic liver disease: a reexamination of data from two veterans administration cooperative studies. *Alcohol Clin Exp Res* **19**, 635–641.

Mendenhall, C.L., Anderson, S., Garcia-Pont, P., Goldberg, S., Kiernan, T., Seef, L.B., Sorrell, M., Tamburro, C., Weesner, R., Zetterman, R., Chedid, A., Chen, T. and Rabin, L. (1984) Short-term and long-term survival in patients with alcoholic hepatitis treated with oxandrolone and prednisolone. *N Engl J Med* **311**, 1464–1470.

Mendenhall, C.L., Anderson, S., Weesner, R.E., Garcia-Pont, P., Goldberg, S., Kiernan, T., Seef, L.B., Sorell, M., Tamburro, C., Zetterman, R., Chedid, A., Chen, T. and Rabin, L. (1986) VA cooperative study in alcoholic hepatitis II: prognostic significance of protein-calorie malnutrition. *Am J Clin Nutr* **43**, 213–218.

Mendenhall, C.L., Moritz, T.E., Roselle, G.A., Morgan, T.R., Nemchausky, B.A., Tamburro, C.H., Schiff, E.R., McClain, C.J., Marsano, L.S., Allen, J.I., Samanta, A., Weesner, R.E., Henderson, W., Gartside, P., Chen, T.S., French, S.W. and Chedid, A. (1993) A study of oral nutritional support with oxandrolone in malnourished patients with alcoholic hepatitis: Results of a department of veterans affairs cooperative study. *Hepatology* **17**, 564–576.

Mezey, E. (1993) Treatment of alcoholic liver disease. *Semin Liver Dis* **13**, 210–216.

Mezey, E., Caballeria, J., Michell, M.C., Pares, A., Herlong, H.F. and Rodes, J. (1991) Effect of parenteral amino acid supplementation on short-term and long-term outcomes in severe alcoholic hepatitis: A randomized controlled trial. *Hepatology* **14**, 1090–1096.

Mirouze., Redeker, A.G., Reynolds, T.B. and Michel, H. (1981) Traitement de l'hépatite alcoolique aiguë grave par insulin et glucagon: étude contrôlée sur 26 malades (abstract). *Gastroenterol Clin Biol* **5**, 1187A–1188A.

Morgan, M.Y. (1985) Hepatoprotective agents in alcoholic liver disease. *Acta Med Scand* **703**, 225–233.

Multimer, D., Brunner, H., Berthelot, P., Portmann, B. and James, O. (1988) Malotilate in alcoholic hepatitis: lessons from 3 European controlled trials (abstract). *Hepatology* **8**, 1411.

Nasrallah, S.M. and Galambos, J.T. (1980) Aminoacid therapy of alcoholic hepatitis. *Lancet* **2**: 1276–1277.

Naveau, S., Pelletier, G., Poynard, T., Attali, P., Poitrine, A., Buffet, C., Etienne, J.P. and Chaput, J.C. (1986) A randomized clinical trial of supplementary parenteral nutrition in jaundiced alcoholic cirrhotic patients. *Hepatology* **6**, 270–274.

Nimmi, M.E. and Bavetta, L.A. (1965) Collagen deffect induced by penicillamine. *Science* **150**, 905–907.

Nompleggi, D. and Bonkovsky, H.L. (1994) Nutritional supplementation in chronic liver disease: An analytical review. *Hepatology* **19**, 518–533.

Olinger, W., Dinges, H.P., Zatloukal, K., Mair, S., Gollowitsch, F. and Denk, H. (1993) Immuno-histochemical detection of tumor necrosis factor-alpha, other cytokines and adhesion molecules in human livers with alcoholic hepatitis. *Virchows Archiv A Pathol Anat* **423**, 169–176.

Orrego, H., Blake, J.E., Blendis, L.M., Compton, K.V. and Israel, Y. (1987) Long-term treatment of alcoholic liver disease with propylthiouracil. *N Engl J Med* **317**, 1421–1427.

Orrego, H., Kalant, H., Israel, Y., Blake, J., Medline, A., Rankin, J.G., Armstrong, A. and Kapur, B. (1978) Effect of short-term therapy with propylthiouracil in patients with alcoholic liver disease. *Gastroenterogy* 105–115.

Pande, N., Resnick, R., Yee, W., Eckardt, V.F. and Shurberg, J.L. (1978) Cirrhotic portal hypertension: morbidity of continued alcoholism. *Gastroenterology* **74**, 64–69.

Pares, A., Planas, R., Torres, M., Caballeria, J., Viver, J.M., Acero, D., Panes, J., Rigau, J., Santos, J. and Rodes, J. (1998) Effects of silymarin in alcoholic patients with cirrhosis of the liver: results of a controlled, double-blind, randomized and multicenter trial. *J Hepatol* **28**, 615–621.

Pia de la Maza, M., Petermann, M., Bunout, D. and Hirsh, S. (1995) Effects of long-term vitamine E supplementation in alcoholic cirrhosis. *J Am Coll Nutr* **2**, 192–196.

Porter, H.P., Simon, F.R., Pope, C.E., Volwiler, W. and Fenster, F. (1971) Corticosteroid therapy in severe alcoholic hepatitis. *N Engl J Med* **284**, 1350–1355.

Powell Jr., W.J., and Klastin, G. (1968) Duration of survival in patients with Laennec's cirrhosis: influence of alcohol withdrawal, and possible effects of recent changes in general management of the disease. *Am J Med* **44**, 406–420.

Poynard, T., Barthelemy, P., Fratte, S., Boudjema, K., Doffoel, M., Vanlemmens, C. *et al.* (1994) Evaluation of liver transplantation in alcoholic cirrhosis by a case-control study and simulated controls. *Lancet* **344**, 502–507.

Poynard, T. and Conn, H.O. (1985) The retrieval of randomized clinical trials in liver disease from the medical literature. A comparison of medlars and manual methods. *Control Clin Trials* **6**, 271–279.

Poynard, T., Ramond, M.J., Rueff, B., Mathurin, P., Chaput, J.C. and Benhamou, J.P. (1991) Corticosteroids reduce mortality from alcoholic hepatitis in patients without encephalopathy. a meta-analysis of randomized control trials (abstract). *Hepatology* **14**, 234A.

Puliyel, M.M., Vyas, G.P. and Mehta, G.S. (1977) Testosterone in the management of cirrhosis of the liver. A controlled study. *Aust NZ J Med* **7**, 596–599.

Radvan, G., Kanel, G. and Redeker, A. (1982) Insulin and glucagon infusion in acute acoholic hepatitis (abstract). *Gastroenterology* **82**: 1154.

Ramond, M.J., Poynard, T., Rueff, B., Mathurin, P., Theodore, C., Chaput, J.C. and Benhamou, J.P. (1992) A randomized trial of prednisolone in patients with severe alcoholic hepatitis. *N Engl J Med* **326**, 507–512.

Resnick, R.H., Boinott, J., Iber, I.L., Makopour, H. and Cerda, J.J. (1974) Preliminary observations of d-penicillamine therapy in acute alcoholic liver disease. *Digestion* **11**, 257–365.

Reynolds, T.B., Benhamou, J.P., Blake, J., Naccarato, R. and Orrego, H. (1989) Treatment of alcoholic hepatitis. *Gastroenterology International* **2**, 208–216.

Sacks, H.S., Berrier, J., Reitman, D., Angoma-Berk, V.A. and Chalmers, T.C. (1987) Meta-analysis of randomized controlled trials. *N Engl J Med* **19**, 450–455.

Shaw, S.E., Jayatilleke, E., Ross, W.A., Gordon, E.R. and Lieber, C.S. (1981) Ethanol-induced lipid peroxidation: potentiation by long-term alcohol feeding and attenuation by methionine. *J Lab Clin Med* **98**, 417–424.

Sheron, N., Bird, G., Koskinas, J., Portmann, B., Ceska, M., Lindley, I. and Williams, R. (1993) Circulating and tissue levels of the neutrophil chemotaxin IL8 are elevated in severe acute alcoholic hepatitis, and tissue level correlate with neutrophil infiltration. *Hepatology* **18**, 41–46.

Shumaker, J.B., Resnick, R.H., Galambos, J.T., Makopour, H. and Iber, F.L. (1978) A controlled trial of 6-methylprednisolone in acute alcoholic hepatitis. *Am J Gastroenterol* **69**, 443–449.

Speisky, H., MacDonald, A., Giles, G., Orrego, H. and Israel, Y. (1985) Increased loss and decreased synthesis of hepatic glutathione after acute ethanol administration. *Biochem J* **225**, 565–572.

Taïeb, J., Mathurin, P., Elbim, C., Cluzel, P., Arce-Vicioso, M., Bernard, B., Opolon, P., Gougerot-Pocidalo, M.A., Poynard, T. and Chollet-Martin, S. (2000) Blood neutrophil functions and cytokine synthesis in severe alcoholic hepatitis. Effect of corticosteroids. *J Hepatol* **32**, 579–586.

Tanner, A.R., Bantcok, I., Hinks, L., Lloyd, B., Turner, N.R. and Wright, R. (1986) Depressed selenium and vitamine E levels in alcoholic population: possible relationship to hepatic injury through increased lipoperoxidation. *Dig Dis Sci* **31**, 1307–13112.

Tanner, M.S., Jackson, D. and Mowat, A.P. (1981) Hepatic collagen synthesis in a rat model of fibrosis and its modification by colchicine. *J Pathol* **135**, 179–187.

Theodossi, A., Eddleston, A.L.W.F. and Williams, R. (1982) Controlled trial of methyl-prednisolone therapy in severe acute alcoholic hepatitis. *Gut* **23**, 75–79.

Trinchet, J.C., Balkau, B., Poupon, R.E., Heintzmann, F., Callard, P., Gotheil, C., Grange, J.D. *et al.* (1992) Treatment of severe alcoholic hepatitis by infusion of insulin and glucagon: a multicenter sequential trial. *Hepatology* **15**, 76–81.

Trinchet, J.C., Beaugrand, M., Callard, P., Hartmann, D.J., Gotheil, C., Nusgens, B.V., Lapiere, C.M. and Ferrier, J.P. (1989) Treatment of alcoholic hepatitis with colchicine: results of a randomized double blind trial. *Gastroenterol Clin Biol* **13**, 551–555.

Trinchet, J.C., Coste, T., Levy, V.G., Vivet, F., Duchatelle, V., Legendre, C. *et al.* (1989) Traitement de l'hépatite alcoolique par la silymarine. Une étude comparative en double insu chez 116 malades. *Gastroenterol Clin Biol* **13**, 120–124.

Tsukamoto, H. (1998) Animal models of alcoholic liver injury. *Clinics in liver disease* **2**, 739–752.

Tsukamoto, H., Cheng, S. and Blanner, W.S. (1996) Effects of dietary polyunsaturated fat on ethanol-induced Ito cell activation. *Am J Physiol* **270**, G581–G586.

Tsukamoto, H., French, S.W., Benson, N., Delgado, G., Rao, G.A., Lzrkin, E.C. and Largman, C. (1985) Severe and progressive steatosis and focal necrosis in rat liver induced by continuous intragastric infusion of ethanol and low fat diet. *Hepatology* 5(224–232).

Tsukamoto, H., Towner, C., Ciofalo, L.M. and French, S.W. (1986) Ethanol induced liver fibrosis in rats fed high fat diet. *Hepatology* **6**, 814–822.

Vendemiale, G., Altomare, E., Trizio, T., Le Grazie, C., Di Padova, C., Salerno, M.T., Carrieri, V. and Albano, O. (1989) Effects of oral *S*-denosyl-*L*-methionine on hepatic glutathione in patients with liver disease. *Sand J Gastroenterol* **24**, 407–415.

Watson, W.H. and Chawla, R.K. (1997) *S*-adenosylmethionine modulates biosynthesis of tumor necrosis alpha in murine macrophages. *Hepatology* **26**, 227A.

Wells, R. (1960) Prednisolone and testosterone propionate in cirrhosis of the liver: a controlled trial. *Lancet* **2**, 1416–1419.

Chapter 25

Nutritional support in alcoholic liver disease: practical management and future strategies

Angela Madden

Many patients with alcoholic liver disease are malnourished and, as a consequence, have a higher morbidity and mortality than their better nourished counterparts. The prevalence of nutritional impairment increases with the severity of liver injury and therefore, a full nutritional assessment based on a combination of clinical, historical and anthropometric evaluation should be undertaken at an early stage. Subsequent nutritional management must then reflect the individual's nutrition status, the degree of alcohol-related liver damage and the presence of complications including ascites, encephalopathy and esophageal varices. The provision of an adequate nutrient intake must take into account altered requirements for energy, protein and some micronutrients and overcome the challenge of feeding patients who are frequently anorexic, nauseous and reluctant to eat. In such circumstances, the early instigation of enteral feeding with regular review is essential to arrest further nutritional deterioration with its attendant risks.

KEYWORDS: dietary modification, energy and nutrient requirements, liver diseases, nutritional assessment, nutritional support

INTRODUCTION

The nutritional management of patients with alcoholic liver disease (ALD) is not easy; assessing their nutritional status is difficult, evaluating nutritional requirements is complicated by the disease process itself and only limited work has been undertaken to determine the benefits of nutritional intervention. In view of these difficulties, it is reasonable to ask whether effort and resources should be directed towards this challenging area of hepatology which seems, at best, an inexact science and, at its worst, insuperable. The answer to this question must be undoubtedly "yes" and is supported by a growing body of evidence which shows a positive association between impaired nutritional status and adverse clinical outcome in patients with liver disease, including those with alcoholic disease (O'Keefe *et al.*, 1980; Mendenhall *et al.*, 1986; Abad *et al.*, 1987; Lautz *et al.*, 1992; Pikul *et al.*, 1994; Merli *et al.*, 1996). While a positive relationship has also been shown between nutritional status and the severity of liver disease (see below), it can be speculated that if feeding regimes are optimized and nutritional status improved, substantial benefits may ensue.

PREVALENCE OF NUTRITIONAL IMPAIRMENT

A substantial proportion of patients presenting with ALD have evidence of either obvious or subclinical nutritional impairment. The prevalence of malnutrition in chronic liver disease varies between 10 and 100% (McCullough and Tavill, 1991; Müller, 1995; Kalman and Saltzman, 1996) depending on the population investigated, the duration and extent of alcohol abuse, the severity of the liver injury and the methodology used to evaluate and define nutritional impairment (Patek *et al.*, 1948, 1975; Leevy *et al.*, 1965; Neville *et al.*, 1968; Morgan, 1981; Simko *et al.*, 1982; Bunout *et al.*, 1983; Mills *et al.*, 1983; Mendenhall *et al.*, 1984; Abad *et al.*, 1987; Lolli *et al.*, 1992; Wood *et al.*, 1992; Italian MCP, 1994; Nöel-Jorand and Bras, 1994; Thuluvath and Triger, 1994; Nielsen *et al.*, 1995; Caregaro *et al.*, 1996; Sarin *et al.*, 1997).

The patients investigated in these studies varied from indigent homeless people to those fully employed and living within a socialized family unit (Leevy *et al.*, 1965; Mendenhall *et al.*, 1984; Wood *et al.*, 1992) and with, consequently, diverse opportunities to consume an adequate nutrient intake. Although the adequacy of nutrient intake has been examined in a number of studies of patients with ALD, the results have usually been expressed in comparison with healthy volunteers and the prevalence of inadequate intake not reported (Morgan, 1981; Simko *et al.*, 1982; Mills *et al.*, 1983; Mendenhall *et al.*, 1984; Noël-Jorand and Bras, 1994; Thuluvath and Triger, 1994; Caregaro *et al.*, 1996; Sarin *et al.*, 1997). However, there is little doubt that some patients with ALD have a very poor nutrient intake.

The assessment techniques used to determine the prevalence of nutritional impairment, have included the evaluation of the status of individual vitamins (Leevy *et al.*, 1965; Wood *et al.*, 1992), patients' clinical condition (Patek *et al.*, 1948; Morgan, 1981; Italian MCP, 1994) and anthropometric measurements which have been compared with a variety of different reference values (Mills *et al.*, 1983; Lolli *et al.*, 1992; Wood *et al.*, 1992; Italian MCP, 1994; Thuluvath and Triger, 1994; Caregaro *et al.*, 1996). There is evidence of low body weight in up to 30% of patients (Table 25.1), although measurements may be confounded by the presence of fluid retention. Generally, the overall prevalence of muscle wasting, determined by depleted mid-arm muscle circumference, is greater than that of subcutaneous fat depletion (Tables 25.2 and 25.3). This differential is particularly noticeable in men, but less apparent in women (Italian MCP, 1994; Caregaro *et al.*, 1996).

While the role of malnutrition in the development and progression of ALD remains unclear (Mendenhall, 1992), there is considerable evidence from studies of patients with cirrhosis that the prevalence and severity of impaired nutritional status increase with the extent of the liver injury (Mendenhall *et al.*, 1984; Abad *et al.*, 1987; Italian MCP, 1994; Caregaro *et al.*, 1996) (Table 25.4).

The difficulties in defining the degree of nutritional depletion in patients with liver disease has been acknowledged (Porayko *et al.*, 1991) but it is clearly necessary for clinicians to be aware of potential nutritional problems in order that they may be identified and treated effectively.

Table 25.1 Body weight in patients with alcoholic liver disease

First author (year)	Population	Cirrhosis (%)	Fluid retention	Evidence of depletion	Prevalence of depletion (%)
Neville (1968)	34 alcoholics ± liver disease	9	minimal in 3%	"underweight"	9
Mills (1983)	32 alcoholic liver disease	38	NA	<80% reference[a]	3
Wood (1992)	39 alcoholics ± liver disease	41	NA	<90% reference[b]	22
Italian MCP (1994)	1402 chronic liver disease (38% alcoholic)	100	nil	<90% reference[c]	5
Thuluvath (1994)	132 chronic liver disease (39% alcoholic)	NA	minimal in 26%	<80% reference[d]	2
Caregaro (1996)	120 chronic liver disease (64% alcoholic)	100	65%	<90% reference[e]	30

NA, not available
[a] Jelliffe, 1966; [b] National Health & Medical Research Council, 1957; [c] FAO/WHO/UN, 1985; [d] Black, 1983; [e] Frisancho, 1981.

Table 25.2 Mid-arm muscle circumference in patients with alcoholic liver disease

First author (year)	Population	Cirrhosis (%)	Evidence of depletion	Prevalence of depletion (%)
Mills (1983)	32 alcoholic liver disease	38	<80% reference[a]	13
Lolli (1992)	200 chronic liver disease (39% alcoholic)	100	<5th percentile[b]	33
Wood (1992)	39 alcoholics ± liver disease	41	<90% reference[a]	22
Italian MCP (1994)	1402 chronic liver disease (38% alcoholic)	100	<5th percentile MAMA[b]	23
Thuluvath (1994)	132 chronic liver disease (39% alcoholic)	NA	<5th percentile[b]	32
Caregaro (1996)	120 chronic liver disease (64% alcoholic)	100	<5th percentile[b]	26

NA, not available; MAMA, mid-arm muscle area.
[a] Jellife, 1966; [b] Frisancho, 1984.

ASSESSMENT OF NUTRITIONAL STATUS

Although there is no consensus about the optimum methods of assessing nutritional status in patients with ALD (DiCecco *et al.*, 1989; Hasse *et al.*, 1993; Higashiguchi *et al.*, 1995), it is essential that some form of nutritional evaluation is undertaken before initiating nutritional support and at regular intervals to monitor the effects of dietary intervention and particularly to ensure that deficiencies do not arise as a result of inadequate or ill-conceived dietary advice. It is difficult to assess nutritional status in this patient population because liver disease *per se* may influence the validity and interpretation of standard tests (see below). However, a satisfactory and useful evaluation can be made by combining the results

Table 25.3 Triceps skinfold measurements in patients with alcoholic liver disease

First author (year)	Population	Cirrhosis (%)	Evidence of depletion	Prevalence of depletion (%)
Mills (1983)	32 alcoholic liver disease	38	<60% reference[a]	9
Lolli (1992)	200 chronic liver disease (39% alcoholic)	100	<5th percentile[b]	7
Wood (1992)	39 alcoholics ± liver disease	41	<90% reference[a]	55
Italian MCP (1994)	1402 chronic liver disease (38% alcoholic)	100	<5th percentile MAFA[b]	16
Thuluvath (1994)	132 chronic liver disease (39% alcoholic)	NA	<5th percentile[b]	12
Caregaro (1996)	120 chronic liver disease (64% alcoholic)	100	<5th percentile[b]	13

NA, not available; MAFA, mid-arm fat area.
[a] Jellife, 1966; [b] Frisancho, 1984.

from a clinical and diet history, a physical examination and anthropometric measurements. A global assessment scheme incorporating these variables has been externally validated in patients with chronic liver disease and shown to be reliable (Madden *et al.*, 1997) (Table 25.5).

Clinical observation

Clinical examination will indicate the presence of muscle wasting, loss of subcutaneous fat and the presence of ascites, edema and jaundice. A history of the presenting complaint will give an indication of the duration and severity of the patient's illness and should include details of any recent weight changes and whether these reflect fluctuations in fluid retention or lean tissue. Patients who report a gain in weight associated with an increase in abdominal girth and swollen lower limbs often recognize that they are also losing "flesh" even though they are becoming heavier.

Diet history

A diet history should be obtained by a registered dietitian although in some patients this may be unreliable; relatives may be able to provide some clarification (Watson *et al.*, 1984; Bingham 1987). Nevertheless, even a rough guide will facilitate the identification of nutrient deficiencies and serve as a useful guide for planning dietary advice. When evaluating the adequacy of intake it must be borne in mind that most patients with liver disease have increased nutritional requirements (see below).

Anthropometric measurements

Height and weight must be measured. In the presence of ascites and/or edema, an approximate "dry weight" may be estimated by deducting an estimated weight for fluid retention. This figure should be derived using published guidelines (Mendenhall, 1992), previously known accurate weight and clinical judgement

Table 25.4 Nutritional status and the severity of chronic alcoholic liver disease

First author (year)	Population n (% ALD)	Cirrhosis %	Categorization of severity of liver disease	Nutritional variable	Mean values or percentage prevalence, by severity of liver disease		
Mendenhall (1984)	361 (100)	59	mild, moderate and severe	Dry weight MAMC TSF	Mild: 67.7 kg Mild: 24.6 cm Mild: 8.9 mm	moderate: 63.3 kg moderate: 23.4 cm[+] moderate: 8.5 mm	severe: 61.1 kg[+] severe: 23.1 cm* severe: 7.5 mm*
Abad (1987)	125 (71)	100	Child's grade[a]	Adequate nutrition Moderate malnutrition Severe malnutrition	Child A: 22% Child A: 0% Child A: 0%	Child B: 66%** Child B: 27% Child B: 0%	Child C: 12% Child C: 73% Child C: 100%
Italian MCP (1994)	1402 (38)	100	Child's grade[a]	Adequate nutrition Moderate malnutrition Severe malnutrition	Child A: 81% Child A: 15% Child A: 4%	Child B: 61% Child B: 26% Child B: 13%	Child C: 42% Child C: 32% Child C: 26%
Caregaro (1996)	120 (64)	100	Child's grade[a]	MAMC <5th percentile[b] TSF <5th percentile[b]	Child A: 10% Child A: 1%	Child B: 22% Child B: 14%	Child C: 38%*** Child A: 19%

* $p < 0.05$ cf mild; ** $p < 0.05$ cf Child A; *** $p < 0.02$ cf Child A; [+] $p < 0.01$ cf mild.
ALD, alcoholic liver disease; MAMC, mid-arm muscle circumference; TSF, triceps skinfold thickness; [a] Child and Turcotte, 1964, [b] Frisancho, 1984.

Table 25.5 Key points for assessing global nutritional status in patients with chronic liver disease based on an externally validated and reliable scheme (Madden *et al.*, 1997)

Body mass index (derived from estimated dry weight) relative to 20 kg . m^{-2}
Mid-arm muscle circumference relative to the 5th percentile of gender- and age-matched reference values[a]
Recent nutrient intake relative to estimated requirements[b]
Other factors including recent change in body weight and the presence of symptoms likely to impair nutritional status (e.g., ascites, malabsorption)

[a] Bishop *et al.*, 1981; [b] Plauth *et al.*, 1997.

Table 25.6 Guidelines for estimating fluid weight in patients with ascites and peripheral edema (Mendenhall, 1992; Wicks and Madden, 1994)

	Ascites	*Edema*
Minimal	2.2 kg	1.0 kg
Moderate	6.0 kg	5.0 kg
Severe	14.0 kg	10.0 kg

(Wicks and Madden, 1994) (Table 25.6). An estimated dry weight, although of very limited accuracy in itself, will facilitate the calculation of an approximate body mass index value and provide some indication of current body stores. Mid-arm circumference and triceps skinfold thickness (TSF) should be measured by a trained observer using a standard technique (Durnin and Womersley, 1974) and mid-arm muscle circumference (MAMC) calculated:

$$MAMC = MAC - (TSF \times 3.142)$$

where all measurements are in centimetres. Values of TSF and MAMC are then compared with reference tables (Bishop *et al.*, 1981) and those below the 5th percentile of the appropriate age and gender indicate risk of nutritional depletion (Gray and Gray, 1979). Although peripheral edema may confound the measurement of skinfold thickness, this is rarely a problem in upper arm anthropometry which, in the practiced observer, provides one of the most useful and reliable measures of nutritional status in this patient population (Loguerico *et al.*, 1990; Lolli *et al.*, 1992; Naveau *et al.*, 1995). TSF and MAMC must be remeasured by the same observer at regular intervals to assess change.

Muscle function

Skeletal muscle function has been shown to be significantly and independently associated with nutritional status in patients with chronic liver disease (Lafleur *et al.*, 1996; Tarter *et al.*, 1997; Andersen *et al.*, 1998; Madden and Morgan, 1999a). Hand grip dynamometry can be undertaken quickly and easily in many patients although further studies are required to establish the value of such measurements in routine nutritional assessments. The confounding effects of disease severity and alcohol intake on muscle function also require clarification (Martin and Peters, 1985; Pacy *et al.*, 1991).

Biochemical variables

The transport proteins, including albumin, transferrin and retinol binding protein, which are frequently measured in nutritional assessment, are synthesized in the liver and are, therefore, invalid markers of nutritional status in patients with liver disease. Hepatorenal failure and a compromised urinary output may affect the validity of nitrogen balance while a low urinary creatinine excretion may reflect reduced hepatic degradation of its precursor, creatine, rather than loss of muscle. Laboratory evaluation of trace element and vitamin status is complex, not always available and difficult to interpret. Biochemical variables should not be used to assess nutritional status in patients with ALD.

Markers of immune function

The immune response is adversely affected by malnutrition and the evaluation of delayed cutaneous hypersensitivity has been used as an indicator of nutritional status (Meakins *et al.*, 1977). However, patients with chronic liver diseases have impaired reticuloendothelial and granulocyte function, reduced concentrations of complement and impaired cell-mediated immunity (Rimola, 1991) which are independent of their nutritional status. Thus evaluation of immune function should not be used to assess nutritional status in this patient population.

NUTRITIONAL SUPPORT IN DETOXIFICATION

Patients with ALD may initially present with symptoms of alcohol withdrawal. Appropriate nutritional evaluation and support at this early stage may help support recovery and reduce hypoglycemia and craving for alcohol (Pezzarosa *et al.*, 1986, 1999; Biery *et al.*, 1991). Micronutrient deficiency and an inadequate nitrogen intake may also be identified and appropriate treatment should be instigated. Some patients experience a rapid and striking increase in appetite within days of cessation of alcohol intake and are able to achieve an adequate nutrient intake without assistance. Oral intake may remain inadequate in others, particularly those with more severe problems and accompanying gastric or psychiatric symptoms, and thus additional oral supplements or enteral feeding are required.

NUTRITIONAL MANAGEMENT OF ALCOHOLIC STEATOHEPATITIS

Patients with the histological diagnosis of alcoholic steatohepatitis, even if asymptomatic, may benefit from a review of their nutritional status, particularly with regard to their current nutrient intake. Some individuals may be obese and, in alcoholics, obesity is associated with a greater independent risk of developing ALD possibly mediated by induction of the microsomal system or through increased levels of interleukin-1 (Iturriaga *et al.*, 1988; Bunout, 1999). It is of interest that obesity may also contribute to non-alcoholic steatohepatitis (James and Day, 1999). However, the nutritional management of obese patients with alcoholic steatosis must be nutrient-holistic and not focus on weight reduction alone. Abstinence from alcohol may result in a reduction in energy intake of up to 80% of values while drinking and thus replacing alcohol-derived calories with a well-balanced diet is a priority. Subsequent gradual weight loss of 1–3 kg per month should then be encouraged. Non-obese patients with steatohepatitis should be advised to eat a well-balanced but otherwise unrestricted diet.

NUTRITIONAL SUPPORT IN ACUTE ALCOHOLIC HEPATITIS

Most patients with mild to moderate alcoholic hepatitis improve following abstinence from alcohol and the instigation of an adequate nutrient intake (Morgan, 1996). However, those with severe disease may require more intensive nutritional support, the provision of which may be complicated by the gravity of their illness. The efficacy of nutritional support via the enteral route, either alone or in conjunction with steroid therapy, has been documented in a number of studies of patients with ALD (Galambos *et al.*, 1979; Mendenhall *et al.*, 1985, 1993; Soberon *et al.*, 1987; Cabre *et al.*, 1990; Kearns *et al.*, 1992; Hirsch *et al.*, 1993). In the few studies where no significant improvements in either nutritional status or clinical outcome were observed, no adverse effects of feeding were reported (Calvey *et al.*, 1985; Bunout *et al.*, 1989); in particular, nutritional supplements did not exacerbate encephalopathy, edema or fluid retention (Nompleggi and Bonkovsky, 1994). Parenteral nutrition support has also been evaluated in patients with alcoholic hepatitis but an analysis of seven studies by Nompleggi and Bonkovsky (1994) concluded that no favourable effects on either short- or long-term mortality were apparent.

Patients with alcoholic hepatitis should, therefore, undergo nutritional assessment and evaluation of their ability to achieve a spontaneously adequate intake. If this is deemed insufficient or in doubt, nasogastric feeding should be commenced as soon as possible. In the absence of clearly defined guidelines, it seems reasonable to base the minimum provision of energy and protein on values which have been well-tolerated in published studies, that is from 35 kcal and 1.2 g protein/kg body weight (Nompleggi and Bonkovsky, 1994). However, these values may be conservative, particularly in very malnourished individuals, and further studies are required to determine optimum feeding regimes. The practical issues of feeding acutely ill patients with alcoholic hepatitis must also be considered; actual nutrient intake rather than the prescribed quantity must be used to evaluate the patient's response to nutritional support.

NUTRITIONAL SUPPORT IN CIRRHOSIS

The nutritional management of patients with cirrhosis varies according to the functional severity of the liver injury. In asymptomatic patients with well-compensated disease, an unrestricted and well-balanced diet should be encouraged. Provided these individuals eat an adequate quantity (see below) of a variety of foods no other dietary modification is required. In particular, there is no therapeutic value in introducing dietary restrictions in an attempt to prevent the occurrence of the complications associated with cirrhosis, for example, fluid retention and encephalopathy. Indeed, in some instances, unnecessary restrictions may be of detriment to the individual by compromising their long-term nutritional status.

The nutritional priority for all patients with cirrhosis must be to achieve a nutrient intake which meets their requirements, which may be substantially increased. In patients with decompensated cirrhosis, who have specific symptoms, additional dietary manipulation may help to alleviate or control these problems. In all cases, a full nutritional assessment should be undertaken on presentation.

Dietary requirements

Energy

There is limited but increasing evidence to show that adults with liver disease have altered requirements of energy. Few studies have evaluated total energy expenditure in this patient population, but measurements of resting energy expenditure show a greater deviation from predicted values (Harris and Benedict, 1919; Schofield, 1985) than would be expected in a healthy population with more than 50% of patients outside the ±10% range (Müller et al., 1992; Madden and Morgan, 1999b). Although both hypo- and hypermetabolism exist in patients with chronic liver disease, increased resting energy expenditure has been more widely reported (Green et al., 1991; Campillo et al., 1992; Müller et al., 1999) and consequently, daily energy intakes of up to 40 kcal/kg body weight have been recommended (Plauth et al., 1997) (Table 25.7). However, these guidelines do not specify whether these weight-based requirements should be adjusted in the presence of fluid retention and/or emaciation. It is, therefore, suggested that in the

Table 25.7 Energy and protein intakes in chronic liver disease recommended by the ESPEN Consensus Group (Plauth et al., 1997)

Clinical condition	Non-protein energy (kcal/kg/day)	Protein (g/kg/day)
Compensated cirrhosis	25–35	1.0–1.2
Inadequate intake/malnutrition	35–40	1.5
Encephalopathy grade I–II	25–35	Transiently 0.5, then 1.0–1.5
Encephalopathy grade III–IV	25–35	0.5–1.2

presence of fluid retention, an estimated dry weight is used to calculate requirements, while in patients with severe weight loss, energy provision should be based on 45 kcal/kg of actual weight. Regular review of nutritional status will help facilitate the revision of intakes as necessary.

Protein

Increased protein requirements have been clearly demonstrated in adults with chronic liver disease and are substantially higher than in healthy individuals (Kondrup and Müller, 1997). The results from balance studies undertaken in patients with stable cirrhosis have shown a minimum daily requirement of 0.83 g protein/kg body weight suggesting that a safe intake of 1.2 g protein/kg body weight must be consumed to ensure that all patients achieve nitrogen balance (Swart et al., 1989a; Nielsen et al., 1993, 1995; Kondrup et al., 1997). The authors of these studies conclude that patients with cirrhosis have an increased requirement for protein rather than a decreased utilization. The European Society of Parenteral and Enteral Nutrition (ESPEN) Consensus Group have interpreted these results and published guidelines, with values extrapolated to include recommendations for patients with malnutrition (Plauth et al., 1997) (Table 25.7).

Micronutrients

All patients with ALD may be at risk from frank or subclinical deficiencies of vitamins, minerals and trace elements, irrespective of the severity of their condition. Deficiencies may arise secondary to a decreased intake, reduced intestinal absorption, impaired utilization and increased demands (Ryle and Thomson, 1984). However, limited work has been undertaken to elucidate the optimum requirements of all micronutrients in this patient population. While circulating concentrations of specific micronutrients can be measured, the results must be interpreted with caution as circulating levels may not reflect tissue stores, plasma binding may be abnormal and function may be impaired by the deficiency of co-factors. As a result, oral multivitamin therapy, which is cheap and harmless if recommended doses are not exceeded, is often instigated.

Patients misusing alcohol may present with a variety of psychiatric syndromes associated with deficiencies of the B vitamins including thiamine in Wernicke-Korsakoff syndrome and nicotinamide deficiency in alcoholic pellagra encephalopathy (Cook et al., 1998). Patients with such conditions require urgent parenteral supplementation with high-potency B-complex vitamins, as oral supplements may not be adequately absorbed. A prophylactic daily dose of one pair of ampoules of intramuscular or intravenous high-potency vitamins B and C is recommended for the first 3 to 5 days of inpatient alcohol detoxification (Cook et al., 1998).

Attention must also be given to the fat soluble vitamins, especially vitamin A, as a narrow therapeutic window exists between correcting depletion and avoiding an enhanced susceptibility to its toxic effects in alcoholic patients (Lieber, 1991) (Table 25.8). The administration of single agents should be avoided unless there is a good evidence of a specific need and then care should be taken to ensure that all other micronutrients are provided in adequate quantities.

Table 25.8 Supplementation of fat-soluble vitamins in adults with chronic liver disease and cholestasis (Morgan, 1999)

Vitamin	Route of administration	
	Oral	Intramuscular
A	25,000 IU daily	100,000 IU 3-monthly
D	400–4000 IU daily	100,000 IU monthly
E	α tocopherol acetate 50–200 IU/kg daily*	DL-α-tocopherol 1–2 IU/kg daily then at intervals
K	2.5–5.0 mg daily	10 mg monthly

* Paediatric dose

Ascites

Patients with ascites are often malnourished and, as a consequence of severe abdominal distension, frequently have an inadequate intake (Wicks *et al.*, 1995). There is limited evidence to show that ascites may also increase resting energy expenditure (Dolz *et al.*, 1991). The restriction of sodium intake, both dietary and pharmaceutical, may help alleviate symptoms.

Dietary sodium restriction

While sodium restriction alone may not be effective in treating ascites, it will enhance and hasten the effects of diuretics (Reynolds *et al.*, 1978; Gauthier *et al.*, 1986). Levels of restriction vary between a low sodium diet of 20 mmol Na^+/day and a No Added Salt regimen providing up to 100 mmol Na^+/day. The degree of sodium restriction advised should be based on the severity of the ascites, urinary sodium excretion and the practicality of providing a diet which is otherwise nutritionally adequate. Restrictions below 40 mmol Na^+/day are rarely required even in the presence of gross ascites and, because of the detrimental effects on nutrient intake (Soulsby *et al.*, 1997), should not be advocated for long-term use. If such diets are instigated, it should be for a limited period of time and managed under strict hospital supervision by a registered dietitian so that the adequacy of nutrient intake and its effect on nutritional status can be closely monitored. It is essential that both medical practitioners and dietitians advising dietary sodium restrictions understand exactly what they are asking their patients to undertake and appreciate the potential, nutritional and social consequences of what appears, at first, a straightforward and logical treatment.

Salt substitutes containing potassium compounds are available and, in small quantities, can be used to add flavor and improve palatability of a low sodium diet. However, careful monitoring of serum potassium concentration is required and the use of salt substitutes is contraindicated in patients with hyperkalemia and hepatorenal syndrome. All patients should be advised to avoid Lo Salt (Klinge, East Kilbride, UK) and other preparations which contain a substantial amount of sodium. Prescribed and "over the counter" medication, in particular antacids, effervescent tablets and some antibiotics, may also contribute a significant intake of sodium.

Nutritional support in sodium restriction

The sodium content of most standard, 1 kcal/ml sip feeds, with the exception of some savoury flavors, does not exceed 4 mmol/100 ml of supplement and, therefore, small volumes can be incorporated into a No Added Salt regime without exceeding the sodium restriction. However, severely ascitic patients with gross abdominal distension and a profoundly compromised food intake may require additional nutrient supplementation while restricted to a 40 mmol sodium diet. These patients require calorie-dense supplements providing at least 2 kcal/ml with minimal sodium. Nepro (Abbott Laboratories Ltd, Maidenhead, UK) and Nutrison Concentrated LE (Nutricia Clinical Care, Trowbridge, UK) fulfil these criteria and can be used both as an oral supplement or enteral feed. Alternatively, a standard feed supplemented with glucose polymers and/or a liquid fat source, or a homemade feed based on specific nutrient modules may be prepared for individual oral use. The adequacy of vitamin, mineral and trace element content must also be considered.

Paracentesis

The therapeutic benefits of large-volume paracentesis are immediate with improvements in appetite, mobility and sense of well-being (Ginés et al., 1987; Arroyo et al., 1999). However, the long-term nutritional consequences of repeated paracentesis have not been evaluated. It is probable that the protein content of the infused albumin does not adequately replace that lost in the drained ascitic fluid which exceeds 30 g/l in up to 30% of patients with uncomplicated ascites (Arroyo et al., 1999). Over several months, regular paracentesis may result in a significant accumulated loss of protein. It is, therefore, essential that the nutrient intake and protein stores of patients undergoing frequent large-volume paracentesis are reviewed regularly and that they are advised to increase their dietary protein intake accordingly.

Encephalopathy

The treatment of patients with ALD and encephalopathy consists of removing or treating the precipitating factors, bowel cleansing with enemata and medication with non-absorbable disaccharides such as lactulose. Dietary protein restriction, which was once considered a central pillar of treatment, is no longer considered optimum therapy and may in fact be detrimental to the patient's long-term well-being.

Low protein diets were first introduced in the 1950s in response to the implication of nitrogenous substances in the pathogenesis of encephalopathy (Sherlock et al., 1954). However, considerable variation was observed in the degree of tolerance of dietary protein and although only a small minority of patients were considered to be truly protein intolerant, dietary protein restriction became an accepted and widespread treatment. The subsequent development of non-absorbable antibiotics and disaccharides in the 1950s and 1960s provided effective alternative treatment for encephalopathy and yet low protein diets continued to be widely advocated and strictly implemented. A growing awareness of the high prevalence of malnutrition in patients with chronic liver disease (Mendenhall *et al.*, 1984; Lautz *et al.*, 1992; Italian MCP, 1994), the association between nutritional status and clinical outcome (Merli *et al.*, 1996) and the accumulating evidence of increased protein requirements (Kondrup and Müller, 1997) brought about a questioning of routine protein restriction (Soulsby and Morgan, 1999). There is an increasing evidence that patients with ALD and hepatic encephalopathy can tolerate intakes of up to 100 g protein/day without exacerbation of their symptoms and that supplemented patients receiving a higher protein intake actually show a significant improvement in their mental symptoms compared to unsupplemented patients (Kearns *et al.*, 1992; Morgan *et al.*, 1995).

This evidence is reflected in the ESPEN guidelines for recommended protein intakes (Plauth *et al.*, 1997) (see Table 25.7). The recommendation of 0.5 g protein/kg body weight should be undertaken for a very limited period and only until an acute episode of hepatic encephalopathy resolves. If the patient is acutely ill, for example after a variceal bleed, they may remain without nutritional support for 24 to 48 hours and thus effectively be protein restricted for this period. On commencement of nutritional support, it is therefore inappropriate to impose additional restrictions and protein intake should be increased steadily to a daily target of 1.2 g/kg body weight. Standard or high energy enteral feeds should be used if patients require nasogastric feeding.

Truly, protein intolerant patients are rarely encountered; although it is difficult to provide exact figures, it is likely that most specialist liver centers will treat only a handful or less per year. Dietary manipulation rather than restriction may reduce the need to impose strict low protein regimes. Dairy and vegetable derived protein may be tolerated better than meat protein (Fenton *et al.*, 1966; Greenburger, 1977; Bianchi *et al.*, 1993) and a high fiber diet will help to ensure that gastrointestinal transit time is reduced. Encouraging several smaller meals and a bedtime snack rather than a few larger meals may improve protein tolerance and optimize energy and nitrogen metabolism (Swart *et al.*, 1989b; Verboeket-van de Venne *et al.*, 1995; Chang *et al.*, 1997).

Branched chain amino acids

The use of branched chain amino acids (BCAA) in the treatment of encephalopathy remains controversial (Morgan, 1991). A large number of studies have been undertaken to investigate the effects of BCAA with varying results and a recent meta-analysis was unsuccessful because insufficient data was available (Fabbri *et al.*, 1996). Consequently, no recommendations can be made for the use of BCAA as treatment for encephalopathy in patients with ALD. If they are used, they should be reserved for malnourished patients with encephalopathy who are unable to tolerate an adequate protein intake using the dietary manipulations described above.

Malabsorption

Malabsorption occurs frequently in chronic alcohol abuse and may arise secondary to pancreatic insufficiency, abnormalities of biliary secretions, dietary protein and folate deficiency and the direct effects of alcohol on the gastrointestinal tract

(Green, 1983). However, although up to 50% of adults with chronic liver disease have increased fecal fat excretion, far fewer experience steatorrhoea and the majority of those who do are patients with biliary, rather than alcoholic liver disease (Romiti *et al.*, 1990). The need to restrict dietary fat intake is, therefore, limited to a small minority of alcoholic patients and may, if pancreatic in origin, be effectively treated with pancreatic enzyme supplements.

Non-pancreatic malabsorption of dietary fat, when it does occur, is idiosyncratic, highly individual and may have a significant impact on nutritional status, rapidly leading to severe malnutrition. Patients should be initially advised to reduce their fat intake to approximately 20 g per day for two weeks so that any potential benefit from the diet can be confirmed. If malabsorption improves, dietary fat should be slowly reintroduced with the patient keeping a food diary and recording their abdominal symptoms and bowel movements. A maintenance diet can then be developed by trial and error, supported by flexible advice. Restricting dietary fat may lead to an inadequate intake of energy and other nutrients and, therefore, additional advice and supplementation are required:

a   Total energy. Carbohydrate and protein intake should be increased and, if necessary, the calorie density of the diet augmented with additional sugar, glucose polymers or medium chain triglycerides (MCT). If enteral feeding is required, an MCT based feed should be used and feeding commenced slowly. Fruit juice-based oral supplements may provide a useful adjunct.
b   Fat soluble vitamins. Replacement vitamins A and D should be given orally or by intramuscular injection, depending on the degree of fat malabsorption (see Table 25.8). Prothrombin time should be monitored and, if prolonged, vitamin K is given.
c   Essential fatty acids. If total fat intake is limited, it must include a good source of essential fatty acids. Parenteral or topical administration has been advocated for the treatment of deficiency but there is little evidence to support this.

Gastrointestinal varices

Patients are kept "nil by mouth" while varices are actively bleeding and often until their clinical condition stabilizes. The presence of varices is no longer considered a contraindication to enteral feeding as fine-bore nasoenteric tubes are well tolerated (Nompleggi and Bonkovsky, 1994). Although a recent study failed to demonstrate the theoretical benefit of commencing nasogastric feeding on the first day after variceal bleeding, no significant differences in the incidence of re-bleeding, mortality or length of hospital stay were found between patients who were enterally fed and those permitted oral intake on the fourth day after bleeding (de Lédinghen *et al.*, 1997). Further studies are clearly needed.

After hematemesis, oral intake should be re-established as soon as possible. There is little objective evidence to show that eating rough foods, for example toast or biscuits, increases the incidence of bleeding in patients with esophageal or gastric varices. However, some patients may prefer to take a softer diet immediately after an episode of hematemesis or for short periods after endoscopic treatment and this is acceptable providing that their nutritional intake remains adequate. Some individuals may need help to overcome fears that swallowing food will provoke further hematemesis and require reassurance and encouragement to eat; regular monitoring of nutritional status is essential.

Transient, occasionally severe, encephalopathy may occur after variceal bleeding in some patients caused by the effects of large quantities of endogenous blood-derived protein in the gastrointestinal tract. Suppression of bleeding followed by enemata to remove residual blood are the principal treatments; protein restriction is not required.

NUTRITIONAL SUPPORT IN TRANSPLANTATION

Patients with ALD who are candidates for liver transplantation must undergo a detailed nutritional assessment as part of their pre-surgery work up. Such patients are frequently malnourished and, therefore, at greater perioperative risk (Pikul *et al.*, 1994; Selberg *et al.*, 1997). The identification of malnourished individuals should provide an opportunity to instigate active nutritional support if time before transplantation permits; malnutrition alone does not provide a reason for withholding surgery.

Many patients undergoing elective transplantation make a prompt recovery and are able to recommence oral intake by the third post-operative day and rapidly progress to a full diet. Nutritional support varies greatly between transplant centers (Weimann *et al.*, 1998) and there is little objective evidence on which to compare treatment. In some centers, early jejunal feeding is undertaken, either as routine practice or in selected patients, while others instigate parenteral support within the first two post-operative days and continue feeding until an adequate oral intake is achieved; in some cases, nutritional support is deferred until it is apparent that the reintroduction of oral nutrients will be delayed. Jejunal feeding within 24-hours of surgery, either via nasojejunal tube or jejunostomy, is practical and safe and may reduce the incidence of infection (Wicks *et al.*, 1994; Hasse *et al.*, 1995; Mehta *et al.*, 1995). Studies are required to support anecdotal evidence that early jejunal feeding is safe in patients who have undergone a Roux-en-Y anastomosis.

Patients who receive parenteral nutrition should be weaned to an enteral intake as soon as possible because of the additional risk of infection during immunosuppression. A high energy, high protein oral diet should be encouraged but if the appetite is slow to return and intake is inadequate, supplements and/or tube feeding are indicated. Patients should be allowed to consume an unrestricted diet and reassured that it is safe for them to do so; pre-transplant dietary restrictions are rarely required after surgery.

Hyperglycemia may occur during the first post-operative week and is controlled by insulin; dietary restrictions are not necessary. In some patients, steroid-induced diabetes may develop and additional dietary measures may then be needed. Increased appetite due to steroid therapy and the relaxation of dietary restrictions may result in excessive weight gain and appropriate advice should be given. Obesity and hyperlipidemia are common long-term problems which may require dietetic intervention (Munoz *et al.*, 1991; Palmer *et al.*, 1991). Unlike patients with non-alcoholic disease, those undergoing transplantation for ALD must be cautioned to remain abstinent and should receive appropriate alcohol counseling both before and after surgery (Tang *et al.*, 1998; Pageaux *et al.*, 1999; see Chapter 27).

ENTERAL NUTRITION

Patients with ALD who are unable to consume a nutritionally adequate oral intake should receive enteral supplementation via a nasogastric or nasojejunal tube. Prompt nutritional assessment and instigation of early enteral feeding is essential to arrest malnutrition and to initiate rehabilitation. The presence of esophageal varices is not a contraindication to enteral feeding providing fine-bore tubes are used (Nompleggi and Bonkovsky, 1994) (see above). A percutaneous endoscopic gastrostomy (PEG), which is regarded as the enteral feeding route of choice if nutritional support is required for more than 4 weeks (McAtear *et al.*, 1999), is considered contradicted in patients with poor clotting and ascites and thus unsuitable in many with ALD. However, satisfactory outcomes have been reported in a small number of patients with cirrhosis and portal hypertension who have been successfully fed via a PEG, suggesting that absolute contraindications for this procedure should be reviewed (Kynci *et al.*, 1995; Sawyerr *et al.*, 1995). The development of a device for securing nasogastric tubes out of sight when not in use by means of a Nasal Olive (Fresenius, Germany) offers a potential alternative for patients requiring long-term home enteral feeding.

Standard enteral feeding regimes may be adequate in some patients with ALD, although the need to restrict fluid and electrolytes may necessitate the use of formulae providing 2 kcal/ml (see above). Gastrointestinal tolerance is not improved by commencing enteral support with diluted feeds or reduced infusion rates and thus starter regimens, which limit the intake of feed in the first few days and prolong negative nitrogen balance, are not recommended (McAtear *et al.*, 1999). Some enterally-fed patients may develop diarrhea if also prescribed lactulose; a temporary reduction or cessation of the drug's administration may resolve the problem. Enteral nutrition should be continued until the patient is able to sustain an adequate oral intake, if necessary, including oral supplements.

PARENTERAL NUTRITION

Patients with ALD should receive total parenteral nutrition only if it is impossible to achieve an adequate nutrient intake via the gastrointestinal tract (McCullough and O'Connor, 1998). Parenteral nutrition is associated with many disadvantages which are not observed with enteral feeding, including the risks of catheter-related infection, thromboembolism, severe metabolic fluctuations and electrolyte disturbances (Weinsier *et al.*, 1982; Freund and Rimon, 1990). Hepatic complications with a high morbidity and mortality are also associated with long-term parenteral nutrition in approximately 15% of patients with no previous history of liver disease (Chan *et al.*, 1999). If parenteral nutrition is essential, and particularly if feeding is anticipated for less than 14 days, attempts should be made to provide sufficient nutrients via peripheral rather than central venous access (Payne-James and Khawaja, 1993). Intravenous feeding should be continued for the minimum period necessary.

Patients with ALD require a mixed energy source of carbohydrate and lipid and tolerate fat emulsions well (Forbes *et al.*, 1987; Druml *et al.*, 1995, 1998). Although both regular and branched-chain amino acid sources of nitrogen are well-tolerated in patients with chronic and acute liver disease, branched-chain solutions confer no additional benefit (Nompleggi and Bonkovsky, 1994). Conditionally indispensable amino acids, including choline, cystine, taurine and tyrosine may not be synthesized adequately in cirrhosis so care must be taken to ensure that these, as well as all other indispensable amino acids, are provided in parenteral formulae. Fluid and electrolyte requirements may differ in patients with ALD and must be individually assessed and regularly reviewed.

Unless contraindicated, parenterally fed patients should continue an oral or enteral intake to help to maintain the integrity of the gastrointestinal tract, minimize the risk of bacterial translocation, stimulate gall bladder contraction and, when clinically appropriate, assist weaning off intravenous nutrition (Korzenik and Fisher, 1995; Pennington *et al.*, 1996).

CONCLUSION AND FUTURE STRATEGIES

We enter the new millennium with clear evidence of the importance of nutrition in the management of patients with ALD. The prevalence of malnutrition increases with the severity of liver injury and is associated with increased morbidity and mortality. The first step in trying to prevent, arrest or reverse nutritional impairment must be to undertake a reliable assessment of nutritional status using a combination of clinical, historical and anthropometric evaluation. The instigation of nutritional support will then depend not only on the patient's nutritional status but also on the degree of liver damage and the presence of complications. Although energy and nutrient requirements are known to be altered in this patient population, with the exception of protein, little definitive data is available on what constitutes optimum nutritional support: we know these patients need feeding but not exactly what, how or when they should be fed.

Future research must, therefore, be directed in three key areas. Firstly, *what* to feed; more information is required about precise nutritional requirements and whether clinical outcome can be improved simply by meeting perceived needs quantitatively or whether more significant benefits can be achieved with specific agents or combinations of nutrients which support the metabolic disability observed in liver disease. Secondly, *how* to feed; the safety and efficacy of artificial feeding routes, including pre- and post-pyloric enteral tubes and PEGs, must be clearly delineated in this patient population, particularly in relation to varices and transplantation. Thirdly, *when* to feed; the benefits of manipulating the timing of nutrient delivery must be established so that optimum patterns of daily intake can be determined. Long-term and prophylactic nutritional support also require evaluation in both the acute and community setting and may be of particular interest to health economists.

Considerable effort, commitment and financial support is required to undertake such work and in order to command these, the science of nutrition must lose its undeserved "low tech" image and compete with other exciting innovations facing hepatologists from the fields of endoscopy, pharmacology and radiology. The nutritional management of patients with ALD may not be easy but may provide some of the most challenging work and potentially beneficial treatment of the future.

REFERENCES

Abad, A., Cabre, E., Gonzalez-Huix, F., Gine, J.J., Dolz, C., Xiol, X. and Gassull, M.A. (1987) Influence of the nutritional status in the prognosis and clinical outcome of hospitalized patients with liver cirrhosis. Preliminary report. *Journal of Clinical Nutrition and Gastroenterology* **2**, 63–68.

Andersen, H., Borre, M., Jakobsen, J., Andersen, P.H. and Vilstrup, H. (1998) Decreased muscle strength in patients with alcoholic liver cirrhosis in relation to nutrition status, alcohol abstinence, liver function, and neuropathy. *Hepatology* **27**, 1200–1206.

Arroyo, V., Ginés, P., Planas, R. and Rodés, J. (1999) Pathogenesis, diagnosis, and treatment of ascites in cirrhosis. In *Oxford Textbook of Clinical Hepatology*, edited by J. Bircher, J.P. Benhamou, N. McIntyre, M. Rizzetto and J. Rodés, pp. 697–731. Oxford: Oxford University Press.

Bianchi, G.P., Marchesini, G., Fabbri, A., Rondelli, A., Bugianesi, E., Zoli, M. and Pisi, E. (1993) Vegetable versus animal protein diet in cirrhotic patients with chronic encephalopathy: a randomized cross-over comparison. *Journal of International Medicine* **233**, 385–392.

Biery, J.R., Williford Jr., J.H. and McMullen, E.A. (1991) Alcohol craving in rehabilitation: assessment of nutrition therapy. *Journal of the American Dietetic Association* **91**, 463–466.

Bingham, S.A. (1987) The dietary assessment of individuals: Methods, accuracy, new techniques and recommendations. *Nutrition Abstracts and Reviews* **57**, 705–742.

Bishop, C.W., Bowen, P.E. and Ritchey, S.J. (1981) Norms for nutritional assessment of American adults by upper arm anthropometry. *American Journal of Clinical Nutrition* **34**, 2530–2539.

Black, D. (1983) Obesity. A report of the Royal College of Physicians. *Journal of the Royal College of Physicians of London* **17**, 5–65.

Bunout, D. (1999) Nutritional and metabolic effects of alcoholism: their relationship with alcoholic liver disease. *Nutrition* **15**, 583–589.

Bunout, D., Aicardi, V., Hirsch, S., Petermann, M., Kelly, M., Silva, G., Garay, P., Ugarte, G. and Iturriaga, H. (1989) Nutritional support in hospitalized patients with alcoholic liver disease. *European Journal of Clinical Nutrition* **43**, 615–621.

Bunout, D., Gattás, V., Iturriaga, H., Pérez, C., Pereda, T. and Ugarte, G. (1983) Nutritional status of alcoholic patients: its possible relationship to alcoholic liver damage. *American Journal of Clinical Nutrition* **38**, 469–473.

Cabre, E., Gonzalez-Huix, F., Abad-Lacruz, A., Esteve, M., Acero, D., Fernandez-Bañares, F., Xiol, X. and Gassull, M.A. (1990) Effect of total enteral nutrition on the short-term outcome of severely malnourished cirrhotics: a randomized controlled trial. *Gastroenterology* **98**, 715–720.

Calvey, H., Davis, M. and Williams, R. (1985) Controlled trial of nutritional supplementation, with and without branched chain amino acid enrichment, in treatment of acute alcoholic hepatitis. *Journal of Hepatology* **1**, 141–151.

Campillo, B., Bories, P.N., Devanlay, M., Sommer, F., Wirquin, E. and Fouet, P. (1992) The thermogenic and metabolic effects of food in liver cirrhosis: consequences on the storage of nutrients and the hormonal counterregulatory response. *Metabolism* **41**, 476–482.

Caregaro, L., Alberino, F., Amodio, P., Merkel, C., Bolognesi, M., Angeli, P. and Gatta, A. (1996) Malnutrition in alcoholic and virus-related cirrhosis. *American Journal of Clinical Nutrition* **63**, 602–609.

Chan, S., McCowen, K.C., Bistrian, B.R., Thibault, A., Keane-Ellison, M., Forse, R.A., Babineau, T. and Burke, P. (1999) Incidence, prognosis and etiology of end-stage liver disease in patients receiving home total parenteral nutrition. *Surgery* **126**, 28–34.

Chang, W.K., Chao, Y.C., Tang, H.S., Lang, H.F. and Hsu, C.T. (1997) Effects of extra-carbohydrate supplementation in the late evening on energy expenditure and substrate oxidation in patients with liver cirrhosis. *Journal of Parenteral and Enteral Nutrition* **21**, 96–99.

Child III, C.G. and Turcotte, J.G. (1964) Surgery and portal hypertension. In *The Liver and Portal Hypertension* edited by C.G. Child III, pp. 1–85. Philadelphia: WB Saunders & Company.

Cook, C.C., Hallwood, P.M. and Thomson, A.D. (1998) B vitamin deficiency and neuropsychiatric syndromes in alcohol misuse. *Alcohol and Alcoholism* **33**, 317–336.

de Lédinghen, V., Beau, P., Mannant, P.R., Borderie, C., Ripault, M.P., Silvain, C. and Beauchant, M. (1997) Early feeding or enteral nutrition in patients with cirrhosis after bleeding from esophageal varices? A randomized controlled study. *Digestive Diseases and Science* **42**, 536–541.

DiCecco, S.R., Wieners, E.J., Wiesner, R.H., Southorn, P.A., Plevak, D.J. and Krom, R.A.F. (1989) Assessment of nutritional status of patients with end-stage liver disease undergoing liver transplantation. *Mayo Clinic Proceedings* **64**, 95–102.

Dolz, C., Raurich, J.M., Ibáñez, J., Obrador, A., Marsé, P. and Gayá, J. (1991) Ascites increases the resting energy expenditure in liver cirrhosis. *Gastroenterology* **100**, 738–744.

Druml, W., Fischer, M., Pidlich, J. and Lenz, K. (1995) Fat elimination in chronic hepatic failure: Long-chain vs medium-chain triglycerides. *American Journal of Clinical Nutrition* **61**, 812–817.

Druml, W., Fischer, M. and Ratheiser, K. (1998) Use of intravenous lipids in critically ill patients with sepsis with and without hepatic failure. *Journal of Parenteral and Enteral Nutrition* **22**, 217–223.

Durnin, J.V.G.A. and Womersley, J. (1974) Body fat assessed from total body density and its estimation from skinfold thickness: Measurements on 481 men and women aged 16 to 72 years. *British Journal of Nutrition* **32**, 77–97.

Fabbri, A., Magrini, N., Bianchi, G., Zoli, M. and Marchesini, G. (1996) Overview of randomized clinical trials of oral branched-chain amino acid treatment in chronic hepatic encephalopathy. *Journal of Parenteral and Enteral Nutrition* **20**, 159–164.

FAO/WHO/UN Expert consultation (1985) *Energy and protein requirements*. Technical Report Series 724. Geneva: WHO.

Fenton, J.C.B., Knight, E.J. and Humpherson, P.L. (1966) Milk and cheese diet in portal-systemic encephalopathy. *Lancet* **i**, 164–165.

Forbes, A., Wicks, C., Marshall, W., Johnson, P., Forsey, P. and Williams, R. (1987) Nutritional support in fulminant hepatic failure: the safety of lipid solutions. *Gut* **28**, A1347–A1348.

Freund, H.R. and Rimon, B. (1990) Sepsis during total parenteral nutrition. *Journal of Parenteral and Enteral Nutrition* **14**, 39–41.

Frisancho, A.R. (1981) New norms of upper limb fat and muscle areas for assessment of nutritional status. *American Journal of Clinical Nutrition* **34**, 2540–2545.

Frisancho, A.R. (1984) New standards of weight and body composition by frame size and height for assessment of nutritional status of adults and the elderly. *American Journal of Clinical Nutrition* **40**, 808–819.

Galambos, J.T., Hersh, T., Fulenwider, J.T., Ansley, J.D. and Rudman, D. (1979) Hyperalimentation in alcoholic hepatitis. *American Journal of Gastroenterology* **72**, 535–541.

Gauthier, A., Levy, V.G., Quinton, A., Michel, H., Rueff, B., Descos, L., Durbec, J.P., Fermanian, J., Lancrenon, S. and the ENTAC group. (1986) Salt or no salt in the treatment of cirrhotic ascites: A randomised study. *Gut* **27**, 705–709.

Ginés, P., Arroyo, V., Quintero, E., Planas, R., Bory, F., Cabrera, J., Rimola, A., Viver, J., Camps, J., Jiménez, W., Mastai, R., Gaya, J. and Rodés, J. (1987) Comparison of paracentesis and diuretics in the treatment of cirrhosis with tense ascites. Results of a randomized study. *Gastroenterology* **93**, 234–241.

Gray, G.E. and Gray, L.K. (1979) Validity of anthropometric norms used in the assessment of hospitalized patients. *Journal of Parenteral and Enteral Nutrition* **3**, 366–368.

Green, J.H., Bramley, P.N. and Losowsky, M.S. (1991) Are patients with primary biliary cirrhosis hypermetabolic? A comparison between patients before and after liver transplantation and controls. *Hepatology* **14**, 464–472.

Green, P.H. (1983) Alcohol, nutrition and malabsorption. *Gut* **12**, 563–574.

Greenburger, N.J. (1977) Effect of vegetable and animal protein diets in chronic hepatic encephalopathy. *Digestive Diseases* **22**, 845–855.

Harris, J.A. and Benedict, T.G. (1919) *Biometric Studies of Basal Metabolism in Man.* Publication No 279. Washington, DC: Carnegie Institute of Washington.

Hasse, J., Strong, S., Gorman, M.A. and Liepa, G. (1993) Subjective global assessment: Alternative nutrition-assessment technique for liver transplant candidates. *Nutrition* **9**, 339–343.

Hasse, J.M., Blue, L.S., Liepa, G.U., Goldstein, R.M., Jennings, L.W., Mor, E., Husberg, B.S., Levy, M.F., Gonwa, T.A. and Klintmalm, G.B. (1995) Early enteral nutritional support in patients undergoing liver transplantation. *Journal of Parenteral and Enteral Nutrition* **19**, 437–443.

Higashiguchi, T., Yokoi, H., Noguchi, T., Kawarada, Y., Mizumoto, R. and Hasselgren, P.O. (1995) The preoperative nutritional assessment of surgical patients with hepatic dysfunction. *Japanese Journal of Surgery* **25**, 113–118.

Hirsch, S., Bunout, D., de la Maza, P., Iturriaga, H., Petermann, M., Icazar, G., Gattas, V. and Ugarte, G. (1993) Controlled trial on nutrition supplementation in outpatients with symptomatic alcoholic cirrhosis. *Journal of Parenteral and Enteral Nutrition* **17**, 119–124.

Italian Multicentre Cooperative Project on nutrition in liver cirrhosis (1994) Nutritional status in cirrhosis. *Journal of Hepatology* **21**, 317–325.

Iturriaga, H., Bunout, D., Hirsch, S. and Ugarte, G. (1988) Overweight as a risk factor or a predictive sign of histological liver damage in alcoholics. *American Journal of Clinical Nutrition* **47**, 235–238.

James, O. and Day, C. (1999) Non-alcoholic steatohepatitis: Another disease of affluence. *Lancet* **353**, 1634–1636.

Jelliffe, D.B. (1966) *The assessment of the nutritional status of the community (With special reference to field surveys in developing regions of the world).* WHO Monograph 53. Geneva: WHO.

Kalman, D.R. and Saltzman, J.R. (1996) Nutrition status predicts survival in cirrhosis. *Nutrition Reviews* **54**, 217–219.

Kearns, P.J., Young, H., Garcia, G., Blaschke, T., O'Hanlon, G., Rinki, M., Sucher, K. and Gregory, P. (1992) Accelerated improvement of alcoholic liver disease with enteral nutrition. *Gastroenterology* **102**, 200–205.

Kondrup, J., Nielsen, K. and Juul, A. (1997) Effect of long-term refeeding on protein metabolism in patients with cirrhosis of the liver. *British Journal of Nutrition* **77**, 197–212.

Kondrup, J. and Müller, M.J. (1997) Energy and protein requirements of patients with chronic liver disease. *Journal of Hepatology* **27**, 239–247.

Korzenik, J. and Fisher, R.L. (1995) Total parenteral nutrition and its possible complications in the gastrointestinal tract. *Current Opinion in Gastroenterology* **11**, 174–178.

Kynci, J.A., Chodash, H.B. and Tsang, T.K. (1995) PEG in a patient with ascites and varices. *Gastrointestinal Endoscopy* **42**, 100–101.

Lafleur, M., Labelle, F. and Lemoyne, M. (1996) Nutritional assessment in chronic liver disease patients: a comparison between skeletal muscle function and standard nutritional parameters. *Nutrition Research* **16**, 545–553.

Lautz, H.U., Selberg, O., Körber, J., Bürger, M. and Müller, M.J. (1992) Protein-calorie malnutrition in liver cirrhosis. *Clinical Investigator* **70**, 478–486.

Leevy, C.M., Baker, H., Ten Hove, W., Frank, O. and Cherrick, G.R. (1965) B-Complex vitamins in liver disease of the alcoholic. *American Journal of Clinical Nutrition* **16**, 339–346.

Lieber, C.S. (1991) Alcohol, liver and nutrition. *Journal of the American College of Nutrition* **10**, 602–632.

Loguerico, C., Sava, E., Marmo, R., Del Vecchio Blanco, C. and Coltorti, M. (1990) Malnutrition in cirrhotic patients: anthropometric measurements as a method of assessing nutritional status. *British Journal of Clinical Practice* **44**, 98–101.

Lolli, R., Marchesini, G., Bianchi, G., Fabbri, A., Bugianesi, E., Zoli, M. and Pisi, E. (1992) Anthropometric assessment of the nutritional status of patients with liver cirrhosis in an Italian population. *Italian Journal of Gastroenterology* **24**, 429–435.

Madden, A.M. and Morgan, M.Y. (1999a) Hand-grip strength in cirrhosis – its relationship to nutritional status and the degree of hepatic decompensation. *Clinical Nutrition* **18**, S1, 32 (Abstract).

Madden, A.M. and Morgan, M.Y. (1999b) Resting energy expenditure should be measured in patients with cirrhosis, not predicted. *Hepatology* **30**, 655–664.

Madden, A.M., Soulsby, C.T. and Morgan, M.Y. (1997) Assessment of nutrition in patients with cirrhosis. *Journal of Hepatology* **26**, 124 (Abstract P/C07/13).

Martin, F. and Peters, T.J. (1985) Alcoholic muscle disease. *Alcohol and Alcoholism* **20**, 125–136.

McAtear, C.A., Arrowsmith, H., McWhirter, J., Payne-James, J., Silk, D.B.A., Stanford, J. and Teahon, K. (1999) *Current Perspectives on Enteral Nutrition in Adults*. Maidenhead: British Association for Parenteral and Enteral Nutrition.

McCullough, A.J. and O'Connor, J.F. (1998) Alcoholic liver disease: Proposed recommendations for the American College of Gastroenterology. *American Journal of Gastroenterology* **93**, 2022–2036.

McCullough, A.J. and Tavill, A.S. (1991) Disordered energy and protein metabolism in liver disease. *Seminars in Liver Disease* **11**, 265–277.

Meakins, J.L., Pietsch, J.B., Bubenick, O., Kelly, R., Rode, H., Gordon, J. and MacLean, L.D. (1977) Delayed hypersensitivity: Indicator of acquired failure of host defences in sepsis and trauma. *Annals of Surgery* **186**, 241–249.

Mehta, P.L., Alaka, K.J., Filo, R.S., Leapman, S.B., Milgrom, M.L. and Pescovit, M.D. (1995) Nutritional support following liver transplantation: Comparison of jejunal versus parenteral routes. *Clinical Transplantation* **9**, 364–369.

Mendenhall, C.L. (1992) Protein-calorie malnutrition in alcoholic liver disease. In *Nutrition and Alcohol* edited by R.R. Watson and B. Watzl, pp. 363–384. Boca Raton: CRC Press.

Mendenhall, C.L., Anderson, S., Weesner, R.E., Goldberg, S.J. and Crolic, K.A. (1984) Protein-calorie malnutrition associated with alcoholic hepatitis. *American Journal of Medicine* **76**, 211–222.

Mendenhall, C.L., Bongiovanni, G., Goldberg, S., Miller, B., Moore, J., Rouster, S., Schneider, D., Tamburro, C., Tosch, T., Weesner, R., and the VA Cooperative Study Group on Alcoholic Hepatitis (1985) VA cooperative study on alcoholic hepatitis III. Changes in protein-calorie malnutrition associated with 30 days of hospitalization with and without enteral nutritional therapy. *Journal of Parenteral and Enteral Nutrition* **9**, 590–596.

Mendenhall, C., Moritz, T.E., Roselle, G.A., Morgan, T.R., Nemchausky, B.A., Tamburro, C.H., Schiff, E.R., McClain, C.J., Marsano, L.S., Allen, J.I., Samanta, A., Weesner, R.E.,

Henderson, W., Gartside, P., Chen, T.S., French, S.W., Chedid, A. and Veterans Affairs Cooperative Study Group 275 (1993) A study of oral nutritional support with oxandrolone in malnourished patients with alcoholic hepatitis: results of a Department of Veterans Affairs Cooperative Study. *Hepatology* **17**, 564–576.

Mendenhall, C.L., Tosch, T., Weesner, R.E., Garcia-Pont, P., Goldberg, S.J., Kiernan, T., Seeff, L.B., Sorrell, M., Tamburro, C., Zetterman, R., Chedid, A., Chen, T. and Rabin, L. (1986) VA cooperative study on alcoholic hepatitis II: Prognostic significance of protein-calorie malnutrition. *American Journal of Clinical Nutrition* **43**, 213–218.

Merli, M., Riggio, O., Dally, L. and PINC (Policentrica Italiana Nutrizione Cirrosi) (1996) Does malnutrition affect survival in cirrhosis? *Hepatology* **23**, 1041–1046.

Mills, P.R., Shenkin, A., Anthony, R.S., McLelland, A.S., Main, A.N.H., MacSween, R.N.M. and Russell, R.I. (1983) Assessment of nutritional status and *in vivo* immune responses in alcoholic liver disease. *American Journal of Clinical Nutrition* **38**, 849–859.

Morgan, M.Y. (1981) Enteral nutrition in chronic liver disease. *Acta Chirurgica Scandinavica Supplement* **507**, 81–90.

Morgan, M.Y. (1991) The treatment of chronic hepatic encephalopathy. *Hepato-Gastroenterology* **38**, 377–387.

Morgan, M.Y. (1996) The treatment of alcoholic hepatitis. *Alcohol and Alcoholism* **31**, 117–134.

Morgan, M.Y. (1999) Nutritional aspects of liver and biliary disease. In *Oxford Textbook of Clinical Hepatology*, edited by J. Bircher, J.P. Benhamou, N. McIntyre, M. Rizzetto and J. Rodés, pp. 1923–1981. Oxford: Oxford University Press.

Morgan, T.R., Moritz, T.E., Mendenhall, C.L., Haas, R. and VA Cooperative Study Group #275 (1995) Protein consumption and hepatic encephalopathy in alcoholic hepatitis. *Journal of the American College of Nutrition* **14**, 152–158.

Müller, M.J. (1995) Malnutrition in cirrhosis. *Journal of Hepatology* **23**, S1, 31–35.

Müller, M.J., Böttcher, J., Selberg, O., Weselmann, S., Böker, K.H.W., Schwarze, M., von zur Mühlen, A. and Manns, M.P. (1999) Hypermetabolism in clinically stable patients with liver cirrhosis. *American Journal of Clinical Nutrition* **69**, 1194–1201.

Müller, M.J., Lautz, H.U., Plogmann, B., Bürger, M., Körber, J. and Schmidt, F.W. (1992) Energy expenditure and substrate oxidation in patients with cirrhosis: The impact of cause, clinical staging and nutritional state. *Hepatology* **15**, 782–794.

Munoz, S.J., Deems, R.O., Moritz, M.J., Martin, P., Jarrell, P. and Maddrey, W.C. (1991) Hyperlipidaemia and obesity after orthotopic liver transplantation. *Transplant Proceedings* **23**, 1480–1483.

National Health and Medical Research Council (1957) *Standard Height-Weight Tables for Australians*. Canberra: Australian Institute of Anatomy.

Naveau, S., Belda, E., Borotto, E., Genuist, F. and Chaput, J.C. (1995) Comparison of clinical judgment and anthropometric parameters for evaluating nutritional status in patients with alcoholic liver disease. *Journal of Hepatology* **23**, 234–235.

Neville, J.N., Eagles, J.A., Samson, G. and Olson, R.E. (1968) Nutritional status of alcoholics. *American Journal of Clinical Nutrition* **21**, 1329–1340.

Nielsen, K., Kondrup, J., Martinsen, L., Dossing, H., Larsson, B., Stilling, B. and Jensen, M.G. (1995) Long-term oral refeeding of patients with cirrhosis of the liver. *British Journal of Nutrition* **74**, 557–567.

Nielsen, K., Kondrup, J., Martinsen, L., Stilling, B. and Wikman, B. (1993) Nutritional assessment and adequacy of dietary intake in hospitalized patients with alcoholic liver cirrhosis. *British Journal of Nutrition* **69**, 665–679.

Nöel-Jorand, M.C. and Bras, J. (1994) A comparison of nutritional profiles of patients with alcohol-related pancreatitis and cirrhosis. *Alcohol and Alcoholism* **29**, 65–74.

Nompleggi, D.J. and Bonkovsky, H.L. (1994) Nutritional supplementation in chronic liver disease: an analytical review. *Hepatology* **19**, 518–533.

O'Keefe, S.J.D., El-Zayadi, A.R., Carraher, T.E., Davis, M. and Williams, R. (1980) Malnutrition and immuno-incompetence in patients with liver disease. *Lancet* **2**, 615–617.

Pacy, P.J., Preedy, V.R., Peters, T.J., Read, M. and Halliday, D. (1991) The effect of chronic alcohol ingestion on whole body and muscle protein synthesis – A stable isotope study. *Alcohol and Alcoholism* **26**, 505–513.

Pageaux, G.P., Michel, J., Coste, V., Perney, P., Possoz, P., Perrigault, P.F., Navarro, F., Fabre, J.M., Domergue, J., Blanc, P. and Larrey, D. (1999) Alcoholic cirrhosis is a good indication for liver transplantation, even for cases of recidivism. *Gut* **45**, 421–426.

Palmer, M., Schaffner, F. and Thung, S.N. (1991) Excessive weight gain after liver transplantation. *Transplantation* **51**, 797–800.

Patek Jr., A.J., Post, J., Ratnoff, O.D., Mankin, H. and Hillman, R.W. (1948) Dietary treatment of cirrhosis of the liver. Results in one hundred and twenty-four patients observed during a ten year period. *Journal of the American Medical Association* **138**, 543–549.

Patek, A.J., Toth, I.G., Saunders, M.G., Castro, G.A.M. and Engel, J.J. (1975) Alcohol and dietary factors in cirrhosis. *Archives of Internal Medicine* **135**, 1053–1057.

Payne-James, J.J. and Khawaja, H.T. (1993) First choice for total parenteral nutrition: the peripheral route. *Journal of Parental and Enteral Nutrition* **17**, 468–478.

Pennington, C.R., Fawcett, H., Macfie, J, McWhirter, J., Sizer, T. and Whitney, S. (1996) *Current Perspectives on Parenteral Nutrition in Adults*. Maidenhead: British Association for Parenteral and Enteral Nutrition.

Pezzarossa, A., Cervigni, C., Ghinelli, F., Molina, E. and Gnudi, A. (1986) Glucose tolerance in chronic alcoholics after alcohol withdrawal: Effect of accompanying diet. *Metabolism* **35**, 984–988.

Pezzarosa, A., Dazzi, D., Negro, R., Cervigni, C. and Vescovi, P.P. (1999) Effects of alcohol consumption and accompanying diet on metabolic response to arginine in chronic alcoholics. *Journal of Studies on Alcohol* **60**, 581–585.

Pikul, J., Sharpe, M.D., Lowndes, R. and Ghent, C.N. (1994) Degree of preoperative malnutrition is predictive of postoperative morbidity and mortality in liver transplant recipients. *Transplantation* **57**, 469–472.

Plauth, M., Merli, M., Kondrup, J., Weimann, A., Ferenci, P. and Müller, M.J. (1997) ESPEN guidelines for nutrition in liver disease and transplantation. *Clinical Nutrition* **16**, 43–55.

Porayko, M.K., DiCecco, S. and O'Keefe, S.J.D. (1991) Impact of malnutrition and its therapy on liver transplantation. *Seminars in Liver Disease* **11**, 305–314.

Reynolds, T.B., Lieberman, F.L. and Goodman, A.R. (1978) Advantages of treatment of ascites without sodium restriction and without complete removal of excess fluid. *Gut* **19**, 549–553.

Rimola, A. (1991) Infections in liver disease. In *Oxford Textbook of Clinical Hepatology*, edited by N. McIntyre, J.P. Benhamou, J. Bircher, M. Rizzetto and J. Rodes, pp. 1272–1284. Oxford: Oxford University Press.

Romiti, A., Merli, M., Martorano, M., Parrilli, G., Martino, F., Riggio, O., Truscelli, A., Capocaccia, L. and Budillon, G. (1990) Malabsorption and nutritional abnormalities in patients with liver cirrhosis. *Italian Journal of Gastroenterology* **22**, 118–123.

Ryle, P.R. and Thomson, A.D. (1984) Nutrition and vitamins in alcoholism. *Contemporary Issues in Clinical Biochemistry* **1**, 188–224.

Sarin, S.K., Dhingra, N., Bansal, A., Malhotra, S. and Guptan, R.C. (1997) Dietary and nutritional abnormalities in alcoholic liver disease: a comparison with chronic alcoholics without liver disease. *American Journal of Gastroenterology* **92**, 777–783.

Sawyerr, A.M., Ghosh, S. and Eastwood, M.A. (1995) Satisfactory outcome of percutaneous endoscopic gastrostomy in two patients with cirrhosis and portal hypertension. *American Journal of Gastroenterology* **90**, 826–828.

Schofield, W.N. (1985) Predicting basal metabolic rate, new standards and review of previous work. *Human Nutrition: Clinical Nutrition* **39C**, S1, 5–41.

Selberg, O., Böttcher, J., Tusch, G., Pichlmayr, R., Henkel, E. and Müller, M.J. (1997) Identification of high- and low-risk patients before liver transplantation: A prospective cohort study of nutritional and metabolic parameters in 150 patients. *Hepatology* **25**, 652–657.

Sherlock, S., Summerskill, W.H.J., White, L.P. and Phear, E.A. (1954) Portal-systemic encephalopathy. Neurological complications of liver disease. *Lancet* **2**, 453–457.

Simko, V., Connell, A.M. and Banks, B. (1982) Nutritional status in alcoholics with and without liver disease. *American Journal of Clinical Nutrition* **35**, 197–203.

Soberon, S., Pauley M.P., Duplantier, R., Fan, A. and Halsted, C.H. (1987) Metabolic effects of enteral formula feeding in alcoholic hepatitis. *Hepatology* **7**, 1204–1209.

Soulsby, C.T., Madden, A.M. and Morgan, M.Y. (1997) The effect of dietary sodium restriction on energy and protein intake in patients with cirrhosis. *Hepatology* **26**, 382A (Abstract 1013).

Soulsby, C.T. and Morgan, M.Y. (1999) Dietary management of hepatic encephalopathy in cirrhotic patients: Survey of current practice in United Kingdom. *British Medical Journal* **318**, 1391.

Swart, G.R., van den Berg, J.W.O., van Vuure, J.K., Rietveld, T., Wattimena, D.L. and Frenkel, M. (1989a) Minimum protein requirements in liver cirrhosis determined by nitrogen balance measurements at three levels of protein intake. *Clinical Nutrition* **8**, 329–336.

Swart, G.R., Zillikens, M.C., van Vuure, J.K. and van den Berg, J.W.O. (1989b) Effect of a late evening meal on nitrogen balance in patients with cirrhosis of the liver. *British Medical Journal* **299**, 1202–1203.

Tang, H., Boulton, R., Gunson, B., Hubscher, S. and Neuberger J. (1998) Patterns of alcohol consumption after liver transplantation. *Gut* **43**, 140–145.

Tarter, R.E., Panzak, G., Switala, J., Lu, S., Simkevitz, H. and Van Thiel, D. (1997) Isokinetic muscle strength and its association with neuropsychological capacity in cirrhotic alcoholics. *Alcohol, Clinical and Experimental Research* **21**, 191–196.

Thuluvath, P.J. and Triger, D.R. (1994) Evaluation of nutritional status by using anthropometry in adults with alcoholic and nonalcoholic liver disease. *American Journal of Clinical Nutrition* **60**, 269–273.

Verboeket-van de Venne, W.P.H.G., Westerterp, K.R., van Hoek, B. and Swart, G.R. (1995) Energy expenditure and substrate metabolism in patients with cirrhosis of the liver: Effects of the pattern of food intake. *Gut* **36**, 110–116.

Watson, C.G., Tilleskjor, C., Hoodecheck-Schow, E.A., Pucel, J. and Jacobs, L. (1984) Do alcoholics give valid self-reports? *Journal of Studies on Alcohol* **45**, 344–348.

Weimann, A., Kuse, E.R., Bechstein, W.O., Neuberger, J.M., Plauth, M. and Pichlmayr, R. (1998) Perioperative and enteral nutrition for patients undergoing orthotopic liver transplantation. Results of a questionnaire from 16 European transplant units. *Transplant International* **11** (Suppl 1), S289–S291.

Weinsier, R.L., Bacon, J. and Butterworth, C.E. (1982) Central venous alimentation: A prospective study of the frequency of metabolic abnormalities among medical and surgical patients. *Journal of Parenteral and Enteral Nutrition* **6**, 421–425.

Wicks, C., Bray, G.P. and Williams, R. (1995) Nutritional assessment in primary biliary cirrhosis: The effect of disease severity. *Clinical Nutrition* **14**, 29–34.

Wicks, C. and Madden, A. (1994) *A Practical Guide to Nutrition in Liver Disease*, 2nd edn, p. 5. Birmingham: Liver Interest Group of the British Dietetic Association.

Wicks, C., Somasundaram, S., Bjarnason, I., Menzies, I.S., Routley, D., Potter, D., Tan, K.C. and Williams, R. (1994) Comparison of enteral feeding and total parenteral nutrition after liver transplantation. *Lancet* **344**, 837–840.

Wood, B., Nicholls, K.M. and Breen, K.J. (1992) Nutritional status in alcoholism. *Journal of Human Nutrition and Dietetics* **5**, 275–285.

Chapter 26

Alcohol and viral hepatitis: interactions and management

Albert Parés and Joan Caballería

Despite the close correlation between alcohol intake and liver disease, only a relatively low number of chronic alcoholics have severe liver damage, thus indicating that factors other than alcohol intake may contribute to the pathogenesis of liver disease in chronic alcoholics. Besides genetic, immunologic, nutritional and gender factors, environmental agents which are responsible for many chronic liver diseases, such as hepatitis B virus (HBV) and hepatitis C virus (HCV) could also have some influence in the development of liver damage in heavy drinkers. There is ample experience indicating that HBV as well as HCV are associated with liver disease in alcoholics, not only because of the frequent prevalence of serum markers of these viruses, but also because the presence of the virus is associated with more severe liver disease, particularly cirrhosis. HCV is also the factor responsible for most of the chronic hepatitis in alcoholics. Based on epidemiological, clinical and laboratory data both viruses are also important pathogenic cofactors for hepatocellular carcinoma in alcoholics.

KEYWORDS: alcoholic liver disease, liver cirrhosis, alcoholic hepatitis, hepatocellular carcinoma, chronic hepatitis, hepatitis A virus, hepatitis B virus, hepatitis C virus, hepatitis G virus

INTRODUCTION

Alcohol consumption misuse is wide spread throughout the world, and there is a close relationship between the amount and duration of alcohol intake and the prevalence of liver cirrhosis (Lelbach, 1985). Despite this correlation, only a relatively low number of chronic alcoholics develop severe liver damage, thereby indicating that factors other than alcohol intake may contribute to the development of liver disease (Patek *et al.*, 1975). Besides genetic, immunologic, nutritional and gender factors, environmental agents which are responsible for many chronic liver diseases, such as hepatitis B virus (HBV) and hepatitis C virus (HCV) may also have some influence in the liver damage of heavy drinkers. Thus, from the end of the 1970s until the middle of the 1980s, several studies focused on the association between a past or present HBV infection and liver disease in chronic alcoholic patients, as well as the potential contribution of this virus to the pathogenesis of hepatocellular carcinoma. The experience regarding the potential role of HCV in liver damage among alcoholics is more recent, because of the later discovery of the virus, and consequently, the lack of procedures for detecting antibodies against the virus and for assessing viral RNA in serum and liver samples. A large amount of information concerning the prevalence of past or current HCV infection in chronic alcoholics, as well as the implication of this virus in the pathogenesis of liver damage and hepatocellular carcinoma in these patients, has, however, emerged in the last decade. This chapter is focused on the interactions between alcohol and hepatitis viruses resulting in liver damage.

HEPATITIS B VIRUS MARKERS AND THE ROLE OF HBV IN THE DEVELOPMENT OF LIVER DISEASE IN ALCOHOLICS

The contribution of HBV to the pathogenesis of liver damage in chronic alcoholics was first suggested because approximately 10% of the patients diagnosed with alcoholic cirrhosis had HBV core antigen in the liver (Omata et al., 1978), a fact which presumes previous viral exposure. Later on, several studies from different parts of the world reported the high prevalence of HBV markers in alcoholics. Indeed, the prevalence of HBV markers is increased, not only in patients with alcoholic liver disease (ALD), but also in alcoholics without or with only minimal evidence of liver damage (Mills et al., 1979, 1981; Hislop et al., 1981; Orholm et al., 1981; Chalmers and Bullen, 1981; Gludd et al., 1982; Saunders et al., 1983; Chevillotte et al., 1983; Bassendine et al., 1983; Figus et al., 1984; Vetter et al., 1985; Brechot et al., 1987; Mendenhall et al., 1991; Renard et al., 1991) (Table 26.1). The prevalence of antibodies against different B virus particles (mainly HB surface and HB core antigens), ranges from 7 to 31% of the cases. In a sample of 110 alcoholics from Barcelona, the prevalence of at least one HBV marker in alcoholics was 35% (Parés and Caballería, 1996), a figure similar to that reported in other countries. The prevalence of the HBs antigen was similar in alcoholics and volunteer blood donors, while the prevalence of HBs and HBc antibodies was significantly higher in alcoholics than in controls (Figure 26.1), thus indicating previous exposure to

Table 26.1 Prevalence of hepatitis B virus markers in chronic alcoholics (results are expressed in %)

References	Normal	Fatty changes	Alcoholic liver disease	Cirrhosis	Overall alcoholics	Control
Orholm (1981)	nd	nd	nd	nd	31	nd
Mills (1981)	10	15	16	23	22	4
Chalmers (1981)	nd	nd	nd	15	nd	5
Hislop (1981)	nd	11	12	26	18	nd
Gluud (1982)	nd	27	nd	24	26	4
Saunders (1983)	nd	18	6	21	12	nd
Bassendine (1983)	nd	6.6	6	8	7	12
Vetter (1985)	nd	1.2	nd	10.5	nd	1
Parés (1996)	33	29	nd	49	34	21
Mendenhall (1991)	26	nd	29	nd	29	5
Renard (1991)	nd	nd	26.9	nd	nd	nd

nd, not done.

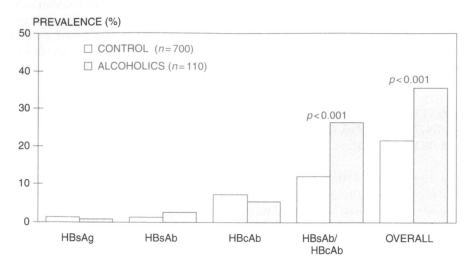

Figure 26.1 Prevalence of hepatitis B virus markers in chronic alcoholics and controls (Parés and Caballería, 1996).

HBV. Although no clear differences were found, the prevalence of HBV markers was much higher in alcoholics with liver cirrhosis (about 50%) than in those with alcoholic hepatitis and fibrosteatosis. The high prevalence observed in alcoholics without liver disease is probably an overestimation, since only 6 alcoholics with normal liver were included in this study. On the other hand, the HBc antigen was not found in any liver specimen by immunoperoxidase staining.

The reasons for the increased prevalence of HBV markers in alcoholics is unknown. It is perhaps related to the patients' lifestyles or their economic conditions. Thus, in a large study performed in patients from the Veterans Administration of the USA, the higher prevalence of HBV markers in alcoholics was associated with the low social and economic status of alcoholics, which may result in a higher chance of exposure to the virus (Mendenhall *et al.*, 1991). In other studies, the prevalence of previous hospitalizations and blood transfusions was higher in patients with HB virus markers than in those without (Parés and Caballería, 1996).

Besides markers of past HBV infection in alcoholics, the HBV-DNA in the blood, as an indicator of viral replication, has also been described in patients with ALD (Bréchot *et al.*, 1982; Nalpas *et al.*, 1985; Harrison *et al.*, 1986; Fong *et al.*, 1988). Nalpas *et al.* (1985) found HBV-DNA in the serum of 12% of the alcoholics with normal liver function, 10% of the alcoholics with non-cirrhotic and in 13% of the alcoholics with cirrhotic liver disease. In this series, the overall prevalence of HBV markers was similar in the three groups studied. They concluded that active HBV infection can exist in alcoholics in the absence of any usual marker, a fact which was attributed to impaired immune response and/or variation in the expression of the viral genes. By contrast, other attempts to demonstrate HBV-DNA in the liver of alcoholic subjects have yielded negative results (Fong *et al.*, 1988; Walter *et al.*, 1988; Horiike *et al.*, 1989). Despite these controversies, there is no doubt that alcoholics are at risk of acquiring HBV infection, although this infection only plays a role for developing liver damage in a small group of patients.

HEPATITIS C VIRUS INFECTION IN CHRONIC ALCOHOLICS: PREVALENCE AND RISK FACTORS

After the identification of HCV in 1989, several studies have evaluated the prevalence of past or present HCV-infection in chronic alcoholics. Although the first results (Parés et al., 1990) were questioned because the positivity of serum HCV-antibodies may be masked by the high immunoglobulin levels frequently found in patients with chronic liver diseases (MacFarlane et al., 1990), most reports from different parts of the world have confirmed the high prevalence of HCV-antibodies and also HCV-RNA in alcoholic patients, particularly in those with severe liver damage.

As summarized in Table 26.2 (Amitrano et al., 1990; Parés et al., 1990; Mendenhall et al., 1991; Nalpas et al., 1991; Bode et al., 1991; Halimi et al., 1991; Nishiguchi et al., 1991; Caldwell et al., 1991; Laskus et al., 1992; Deny et al., 1994; Bird et al., 1995; Coelho-Little et al., 1995; Sata et al., 1996), the prevalence of HCV antibodies ranges from 9% to 55% in the largest published series, and HCV antibodies are more prevalent in patients with, than in those without, cirrhosis. The studies showing the highest HCV antibody prevalences in non-cirrhotic alcoholics included many patients with histological features of chronic hepatitis, suggesting that, in most of these subjects, liver disease was secondary to viral infection but not due to alcohol abuse (Amitrano et al., 1990; Nishiguchi et al., 1991; Caldwell et al., 1991; Laskus et al., 1992; Deny et al., 1994; Bird et al., 1995; Sata et al., 1996). However, because there were high rates of false-positives using the first method for detecting

Table 26.2 Prevalence of hepatitis C virus markers in chronic alcoholic patients

	Total n	Total %	Cirrhosis %	Non cirrhosis %
Parés (1990)	144	24.3	42.6	13.0
Bode (1991)	73	26.0	35.5	8.8
Halimi (1991)	164	18.0	18	nd
Nalpas (1991)	174	25.8	35.9	17.7
Caldwell (1991)	37	29.7	nd	nd
Brillanti (1991)	41	37.0	36.6	69.0
Nichiguchi (1991)	80	46.2	64.5	34.6
Mendenhall (1991)	350	27.1	nd	nd
Amitrano (1990)	263	45.0	69	nd
Bird (1995)	60	0.0	nd	nd
Bode (1995)	130	9.2	11.3	6.8
Coelho-Little (1995)	100	23.0	nd	nd
Sata (1996)	252	55.5	nd	nd

nd: not done.

HCV antibodies, particularly in patients with hyperglobulinemia (MacFarlane *et al.*, 1990), these results were questioned if they were not confirmed by HCV-RNA detection. Actually, using the polymerase chain reaction procedure, HCV-RNA sequences have been detected in the sera of alcoholics (Nishiguchi *et al.*, 1991; Nalpas *et al.*, 1992; Caldwell *et al.*, 1993; Mendenhall *et al.*, 1993; Takase *et al.*, 1993; Zarski *et al.*, 1993). In this concern, most alcoholics with liver disease and anti-HCV also have HCV-RNA detectable in serum, therefore indicating that HCV replication is maintained in most alcoholics who score positive for anti-HCV antibodies in the RIBA2 tests, and that HCV viremia may be associated with histological features typical of ALD. The sensitivity and specificity of anti-HCV antibodies as an index of viral replication was demonstrated in another study, in which RNA amplification was only observed in patients who were anti-HCV positive in sera using second generation methods (Zarski *et al.*, 1993). The studies questioning the high prevalence of HCV infection in alcoholics were performed in restricted areas with a very low prevalence of HCV in the general population. Thus, in one study from Scotland, no patients with ALD were positive for HCV antibodies (Bird *et al.*, 1995), and in Germany no correlation was observed between the prevalence of anti-HCV antibodies and the severity of liver dysfunction (Bode *et al.*, 1995).

The epidemiology of HCV among alcoholic patients is not definitely characterized, since up to now a good explanation has not been reported for the disproportionately high prevalence of HCV-antibodies among alcoholic patients with liver disease without a history of intravenous drug abuse or other risk factors for HCV infection (Rosman *et al.*, 1996). In our series of patients from Spain, there was no relationship between the presence of HCV-antibodies and former drug abuse. However, previous blood transfusions or hospitalizations were more frequent in HCV-positive alcoholic patients. Thus, in alcoholic patients without liver disease or fibrosteatosis, two of the five (40%) anti-HCV positive, but only 3.3% of the anti-HCV negative patients had previously received transfusions. In the group of patients with alcoholic hepatitis and cirrhosis, the prevalence of previous blood transfusions was also higher in the HCV positive than in the HCV negative subjects. Moreover, the prevalence of previous hospitalizations was also higher in the HCV positive patients from both groups (Parés *et al.*, 1990). However, in larger series of patients having HCV chronic hepatitis, such a relationship is not as clear and in most cases no risk factors could be determined. Similar results have been reported in series from other geographical areas. One epidemiological study from Israel has not identified any risk factor for HCV infection in alcoholics, although a potential heterosexual transmission was suggested, as well as an impairment in the immune system by alcohol consumption which may predispose alcoholic patients to viral infection (Srugo *et al.*, 1998). Likewise, the prevalence of anti-HCV antibodies was similar in alcoholic patients with liver disease who had high risk factors compared with those without identifiable modes of parenteral transmission in a series from the USA (Rosman *et al.*, 1996). This, however, may depend on the demographic and social characteristics of the patients evaluated. In this respect, Fong *et al.* (1994) identified a parenteral risk factor for having concomitant hepatitis C infection in patients with ALD.

HEPATITIS C VIRUS AND THE SEVERITY OF
LIVER DISEASE IN CHRONIC ALCOHOLICS

Whether alcohol and HCV are synergistic in causing liver injury is a critical question. In this respect, most studies have demonstrated a higher prevalence of HCV antibodies or HCV-RNA in alcoholic patients with more advanced liver disease (Parés et al., 1990; Nalpas et al., 1991; Bode et al., 1991). In our series of 144 chronic alcoholics, the prevalence of HCV antibodies correlated with the severity of liver injury (2.2% of patients without liver disease, 20% of those with fibrosteatosis, 21.4% of those with alcoholic hepatitis and 42.6% of those with cirrhosis). Moreover, features of severe liver disease such as ascites, jaundice and liver enlargement were also higher in patients with, than in those without hepatitis C antibodies regardless of the severity of liver disease. Likewise, the presence of anti-HCV antibodies was associated with more impaired liver tests in patients with normal liver and fibrosteatosis, as well as in those with alcoholic hepatitis and cirrhosis. Accordingly, in both groups serum bilirubin and gamma-globulin were higher and albumin concentration and aminopyrine breath tests were lower in alcoholic patients who were HCV positive than in those without this antibody (Table 26.3). The histological features, evaluated in 76 of these patients, were similar in alcoholics with and without anti-HCV antibodies, except for the presence of cells within sinusoids, which was significantly more frequent in anti-HCV positive patients (30.4%) than in those who were anti-HCV negative (3.8%) (Figure 26.2).

HCV subtypes in chronic alcoholics have only been assessed in a few studies (Takada et al., 1992; Yokoama et al., 1995; Sherman et al., 1997). Data are scarce because of the limited number of patients included, although recent studies did not find any correlation between either the HCV subtypes and the severity of liver disease in chronic alcoholics, or any association with a particular genotype. Sherman et al. (1997) described similar genotype distributions in alcoholic and non-alcoholic patients, with the genotype 1 being present in 66% of non-alcoholic and in 74% of alcoholic patients. A subset analysis revealed, however, that samples identified as untypable were significantly more prevalent among the alcoholic patient cohort than among those not classified as alcohol abusers. Notwithstanding, the genotype depends

Table 26.3 Liver function tests in alcoholic patients according to the positivity of anti-HCV antibodies and the severity of liver disease

	Normal liver and/or fibrosteatosis		Alcoholic hepatitis & cirrhosis	
	HCV+ n = 5	HCV– n = 60	HCV+ n = 29	HCV– n = 46
Bilirubin (mg/dl)	2.8±4.0	0.8±0.1*	4.5±3.3	3.9±3.3
Albumin (g/l)	36.6±8.2	42.1±6.2*	29.9±6.9	32.3±6.2
γ-globulins (g/l)	13.4±3.3	10.1±2.9*	23.6±8.8	18.5±6.0*
Prothrombin (%)	89.4±16.9	96.6±7.5*	54.6±17.3	60.7±20.7
Aminopyrine (%2h)	3.3±2.0	6.0±2.0*	0.8±0.7	1.6±1.7*

* $p < 0.05$.

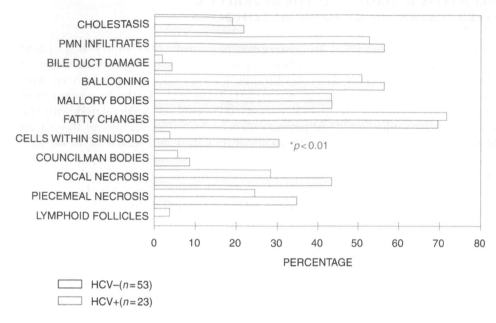

Figure 26.2 Histologic changes in patients with alcoholic liver disease according to the positivity of anti-HCV antibodies (Parés *et al.*, 1990).

on the geographical area of the patients, as well as the duration of the infection. Thus, it has been suggested that genotype 1b may not be a more aggressive viral strain, but it is associated with longer duration of the infection. Actually, the genotype 1b was the most prevalent in the 1960s, but in the last decade, the percentage of patients newly infected with genotype 1b has decreased, and genotypes 2 and 3 have now emerged as most prevalent genotypes in some geographical areas (Mita *et al.*, 1994; Yamada *et al.*, 1994).

INFLUENCE OF ALCOHOL INTAKE ON HCV-RNA LEVELS IN HEAVY DRINKERS

The amount of alcohol intake influences HCV-RNA levels. Thus, a highly significant correlation was found between the self-reported alcohol consumption and HCV viremia in patients with chronic hepatitis C, even in those cases with alcohol intake as low as 140 g per week. In a cross-sectional study, conducted in 233 chronic hepatitis C carriers, alcohol consumption correlated with serum HCV-RNA levels measured by a branched DNA technique (Pessione *et al.*, 1998). The results of this study suggest that in HCV carriers, alcohol consumption, even with low alcohol intake, increases hepatic fibrosis and viremia. This latter relation was also found in other studies in which the viremia was evaluated semi-quantitatively. Thus, habitual drinkers consuming more than 60 g/day of alcohol have been shown to have higher titers of HCV-RNA than non-habitual drinkers (Oshita *et al.*, 1994). The pathogenic mechanism of an alcohol-induced increase in serum HCV-RNA in patients with HCV infection is unclear. Increased release of HCV-RNA into the serum as a consequence of increased cell death or increased replication and delivery of virus from infected cells, as well as decreased clearance of viral RNA from serum as a consequence of alcohol-induced impaired macrophage function may play a role for such an effect. Thus, an interaction has been documented between alcohol consumption and virus infection for other viruses, such as the human immunodeficiency virus which highly replicates in patients with high alcohol intake (Bagasra *et al.*, 1993). Since alcohol intake results in increased viremia, chronic HCV carriers should be advised to abstain from consuming alcohol.

CHRONIC HEPATITIS IN ALCOHOLICS: ROLE OF HEPATOTROPIC VIRUSES

Previous observations have suggested that alcohol is responsible for certain morphologic pictures of chronic active hepatitis (Bruguera *et al.*, 1977; Goldberg *et al.*, 1977; Levin *et al.*, 1979; Nei *et al.*, 1983; Crapper *et al.*, 1983; Montull *et al.*, 1988). Indeed, we have observed that approximately 5% of chronic alcoholics have features of chronic hepatitis (Parés, 1995). In this concern, HCV antibodies and markers of hepatitis B were negative in three out of four patients with chronic hepatitis included in our series of 144 chronic alcoholics, in which anti-HCV antibodies were assessed (Parés *et al.*, 1990). We compared the clinical, biochemical and histologic features of 25 alcoholics showing changes in chronic hepatitis with a matched group of chronic hepatitis C. There were no clinical differences between the two groups, but serum alanine aminotransferase, total protein and albumin were lower in alcoholics, whereas γ-glutamyltransferase and mean erythrocyte volume were higher in alcoholics. The histological features were similar in both groups with respect to the severity of portal and periportal changes, lobular necrosis, cholestasis and bile duct dysplasia. However, portal fibrosis and fatty changes were more frequent in alcoholics than in non-alcoholics. Likewise, pericellular fibrosis was only observed in alcoholics and cells within the sinusoids and portal lymphoid follicles were more frequent in non-alcoholics (Montull *et al.*, 1988) (Figure 26.3). Furthermore, during two years of follow-up, the aminotransferase levels improved or normalized in 7 alcoholics who stopped drinking, while these levels did not change during follow-up in non-alcoholics. These results indicate that alcohol may induce a picture resembling chronic hepatitis. Additional information has been shown by a Japanese group (Takase *et al.*, 1991). This latter report confirmed the existence of a few alcoholic patients with chronic hepatitis who did not exhibit serum markers of HBV infection or antibodies to HCV or HCV-RNA detectable by PCR, thus indicating that in some patients alcohol may induce a picture resembling chronic active hepatitis. However, since the role of other still badly characterized hepatitis viruses cannot be excluded, further studies should be done in this respect.

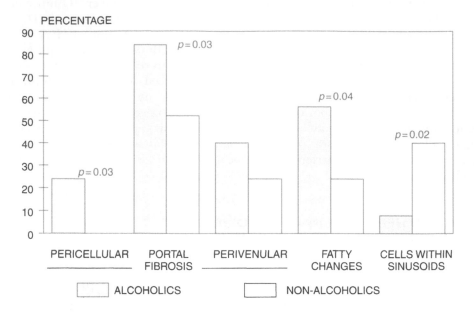

Figure 26.3 Prevalence of histologic abnormalities in alcoholic patients with chronic hepatitis and patients with confirmed viral chronic hepatitis C.

MANAGEMENT OF CHRONIC HEPATITIS C IN ALCOHOLIC PATIENTS: INFLUENCE OF HEAVY DRINKING ON THE EFFICACY OF INTERFERON

The rate of previous alcohol intake may have some influence in the treatment results as indicated in three studies addressed to evaluating the influence of alcohol intake on the efficacy of interferon therapy in patients with chronic hepatitis. In a series of 119 patients treated with interferon, the rate of HCV-RNA disappearance after a 6-month treatment period was of 27%, and the multivariate logistic analysis revealed that the rate of HCV-RNA negativity was affected by alcohol intake and the cumulative alcohol consumption, as well as the HCV-RNA levels (Mochida *et al.*, 1996). In another study, rates of sustained response to interferon were 53% among non-drinkers, 43% among drinkers of less than 70 g/day, and 0% among drinkers of more than 70 g/day. Importantly, abstinence for at least 3 years before the initiation of interferon therapy was associated with an improved therapeutic response to continued drinking up to the time of therapy (Okazaki *et al.*, 1994). The rate of responders after 6 months of interferon therapy is also affected by the amount of alcohol intake, as reported by Onhishi *et al.* (1996). Actually, alanine aminotransferase levels remained normal for 6 months after the end of the treatment in only 6% of the alcoholics consuming more than 70 g of ethanol daily. Since the amount of alcohol intake influences the rate of response to interferon in alcoholic patients with chronic hepatitis C, it is reasonable to offer treatment only to patients with a sustained period of alcohol restraint.

HEPATITIS B AND C VIRAL INFECTIONS AND THE DEVELOPMENT OF HEPATOCELLULAR CARCINOMA IN ALCOHOLICS

Hepatocellular carcinoma is a late event in most patients with chronic liver diseases, particularly in those with liver cirrhosis. In addition to the fact of having nodular regeneration, other factors such as alcohol intake, and especially the association of a viral etiology, play a relevant role in increasing the risk of having HCC, particularly in alcoholic patients. The contribution of HBV in the development of hepatocellular carcinoma in alcoholic patients is critical. Thus, in one study most alcoholic patients with cirrhosis and HCC had HBV markers and all cases had HBV-DNA integrated into the genome of the neoplastic liver cells (Brechot et al., 1982). These interesting results were not confirmed in other studies using similar techniques (Fong et al., 1988; Walter et al., 1988; Horiike et al., 1989). However, new evidence using polymerase chain reaction procedures have confirmed the initial results demonstrating the presence of integrated HBV-DNA in tumoral and non-tumoral cells (Partelini et al., 1990, 1993). From these results, it has been estimated that HBV may play a role in the pathogenesis of hepatocellular carcinoma in approximately 50% of the chronic alcoholics with liver cirrhosis.

The prevalence of HCV antibodies has also been found to be elevated in the sera of patients with HCC regardless of the etiology of liver cirrhosis (Bruix et al., 1989). Indeed, the prevalence of HCV antibodies was significantly higher in alcoholics with cirrhosis who had HCC than in those without, suggesting that the HCV could play an important role in the development of HCC as described for the HBV. To reinforce these findings another study described viral RNA in tumor and non-tumor cells and patients with liver cancer (Partelini et al., 1993). Likewise, HCC developed more frequently in HCV-marker positive alcoholic patients, than in those who were HCV negative. Thus, the cumulative rate for developing HCC in HCV positive alcoholics 6 years after diagnosis of liver disease, mainly cirrhosis, was 0.7, while the rate was only of about 0.3 in alcoholics without HCV markers. Moreover, the cumulative survival rates of cirrhotic patients were significantly lower in the HCV marker-positive patients than in those without HCV markers. From these results, it was concluded that HCV infection is a determining factor for the development of HCC and for the prognosis of cirrhosis in alcoholic patients who continue to drink (Takase et al., 1993).

Other studies have also demonstrated the close association between HCV and HCC in alcoholic patients. Thus, the probability of HCC in patients with alcoholic cirrhosis was significantly higher in anti-HCV positive versus negative patients. After 10 years of follow up, the cumulative occurrence rate was 81% in the HCV-infected patients as compared to 18.5% in the non-infected group. Furthermore, the converse is also true, since alcohol consumption in patients with HCV-related cirrhosis was an independent risk factor for development of HCC (Ikeda et al., 1993). Another epidemiological study from Italy also found a synergism between HCV infection and alcohol drinking in causing HCC (Donato et al., 1997). Heavy alcohol intake by itself was an independent risk factor for developing HCC, although HBV and HCV infection cooperate in more than additive effects of viral infections and alcohol drinking in increasing the risk for developing HCC.

HEPATITIS A AND ALCOHOLISM

Data concerning the prevalence of hepatitis A virus (HAV) in chronic alcoholic patients is scarce, probably because the HAV hepatitis does not cause chronic liver damage. However, as a consequence of the fecal-oral transmission route of the virus, which is related with poor hygiene and a low socio-economical status, it is reasonable to find high rates of past HAV infection in patients with chronic alcoholism, which in turn have low socio-economic and hygienic conditions. In this concern, there is a significantly higher prevalence of HAV antibodies in alcoholics than in controls suggesting that alcoholism may be a risk factor for HAV infection. Actually, in a French study performed in 258 heavy drinkers, the prevalence of serum HAV antibodies was 65% in alcoholics and 52% in controls (Aparicio et al., 1995). There were no clear associated-risk factors for such an increased rate of past HAV infection, since the positivity of HAV antibodies in alcoholics was not related to the severity of liver injury, amount of alcohol intake, sex and type of employment. HAV antibodies were not related to HBsAg positivity, the presence of any marker of prior HBV infection or to HCV antibodies in the same group of patients. The lack of association between the presence of HAV antibodies and the amount of alcohol intake suggests that the risk of contact with the HAV might be related to the fact of being alcoholic, but not to the severity of alcoholism.

The association of past HAV infection and alcoholism may depend on the geographical area and, moreover, the economic, social and hygienic conditions of the subjects. Thus, there is one report from Denmark performed in sera from 137 alcoholics (74 with cirrhosis and 63 with steatosis), showing that the prevalence of HAV antibodies was similar in alcoholic patients (46%) and controls (40%). The prevalence of HAV antibodies was not significantly increased in alcoholics with steatosis or cirrhosis compared with controls. (Gluud et al., 1982).

HEPATITIS G VIRUS AND LIVER DISEASE IN ALCOHOLIC PATIENTS

A new hepatitis virus, named virus G, was discovered in 1996. The virus is transmitted via the blood and it is probably involved in cases of acute and chronic hepatitis, similar to what has been reported for the HCV. This virus does not play a relevant role in causing chronic liver diseases at least in Western countries, and neither is it associated with chronic alcoholism. Thus, in a series of 104 alcoholic patients with a liver biopsy showing fatty liver (41%), fibrosis (13%), alcoholic hepatitis (22%), cirrhosis (20%) and chronic hepatitis (3%) HGV-RNA was only found in two cases (1.9%) (Guilera et al., 1998). All alcoholics were HBsAg and anti-HCV negative. One of the HGV-RNA positive patients was a 39-year-old woman without clinical evidence of liver disease and a slight aspartate aminotransferase increase, while liver biopsy showed mild fatty infiltration. The other was a 51-year-old man with cirrhosis on liver biopsy. Neither had a history of blood transfusion or intravenous drug misuse. One relevant fact is that HGV-RNA was not detected in the three patients with histological features of chronic hepatitis who were anti-HCV negative. In another series from Japan, the prevalence of HGV-RNA was found in

14% of patients with alcoholic liver disease, although most of the positive cases were also infected with the HCV (Sobue *et al.*, 1998). Therefore, HGV is not associated with the presence and severity of liver disease in alcoholic patients.

SUMMARY

Despite the close correlation between alcohol intake and liver disease, only a relatively low number of chronic alcoholics have severe liver damage, thus indicating that factors other than alcohol intake may contribute to the pathogenesis of liver disease in chronic alcoholics. Besides genetic, immunologic, nutritional and gender factors, environmental agents which are responsible for many chronic liver diseases, such as hepatitis B virus (HBV) and hepatitis C virus (HCV) could also have some influence in the development of liver damage in heavy drinkers. There is ample experience indicating that HBV as well as HCV are associated with liver disease in alcoholics, not only because of the frequent prevalence of serum markers of these viruses, but also because the presence of the virus is associated with more severe liver disease, particularly cirrhosis. HCV is also the factor responsible for most of the chronic hepatitis in alcoholics. Based on epidemiological, clinical and laboratory data, both viruses are also important pathogenic cofactors for hepatocellular carcinoma in alcoholics.

REFERENCES

Amitrano, L., Ascione, A., Canestrini, C., D'Agostino, S., Iaccarino, L., Vacca, C. and Gigliotti, T. (1990) Prevalence of antibody to hepatitis C virus (anti-HCV) in chronic liver diseases (CLD) in southern Italy. *Italian Journal of Gastroenterology* **22**, 16–18.

Aparicio, T., Driss, F., Thèpot, V., Hispard, E., Berthelot, P. and Nalpas, B. (1995) Séro-épidémiologie de l'hepatite A: les alcooliques son un groupe à risque. *Gastroenterologie Clinique et Biologique* **19**, 751–755.

Bagasra, O., Kajdacsy-Balla, A., Lischner, H.W. and Pomerantz, R.J. (1993) Alcohol intake increases human immunodeficiency virus type 1 replication in human peripheral blood mononuclear cells. *Journal of Infectious Diseases* **167**, 789–797.

Bassendine, M.F., Della Seta, L., Salmeron, J., Thomas, H.C. and Sherlock, S. (1983) Incidence of hepatitis B virus infection in alcoholic liver disease: HBsAg negative chronic active liver disease and primary liver cancer in Britain. *Liver* **3**, 65–70.

Bird, G.L., Tibbs, C.J., Orton, D., Hillan, K.J., MacSween, R.N., Williams, R. and Mills, P.R. (1995) Does hepatitis C contribute to liver injury in alcohol abusers in the west of Scotland? *European Journal of Gastroenterology and Hepatology* **7**, 161–163.

Bode, J.C., Biermann, J., Kohse, K.P., Walker, S. and Bode, C. (1991) High incidence of antibodies to hepatitis C virus in alcoholic cirrhosis: fact or fiction ? *Alcohol and Alcoholism* **26**, 111–114.

Bode, J.C., Alscher, D.M., Wisser, H. and Bode, C. (1995) Detection of hepatitis C virus antibodies and hepatitis C virus RNA in patients with alcoholic liver disease. *Alcohol and Alcoholism* **30**, 97–103.

Brechot, C., Nalpas, B., Courouce, A.M., Duhamel, G., Gallard, P., Carnot, F., Tiollais, P. and Berthelot, P. (1982) Evidence that hepatitis B virus has a role in liver-cell carcinoma in alcoholic liver disease. *New England Journal of Medicine* **306**, 1384–1387.

Brechot, C., Degos, F., Lugassy, C., Thiers, V., Zafrani, S., Franco, D. and Bismuth, H. (1987) Hepatitis B virus DNA in chronic liver disease. *New England Journal of Medicine* **317**, 116–117.

Brillanti, S., Masci, C., Siringo, S., DiFebo, G., Miglioli, M. and Barbara, L. (1991) Serological and histological aspects of hepatitic C virus infection in alcoholic patients. *Journal of Hepatology* **13**, 347–350.

Bruguera, M., Bordas, J.M. and Rodés, J. (1977) Asymptomatic liver disease in chronic alcoholics. *Archives of Pathology and Laboratory Medicine* **101**, 644–647.

Bruix, J., Barrera, J.M., Calvet, X., Costa, J., Sánchez-Tapias, J.M., Ventura, M., Vall, M., Bruguera, M., Bru, C., Castillo, R. and Rodés, J. (1989) Prevalence of antibodies to hepatitis C virus in Spanish patients with hepatocellular carcinoma and hepatic cirrhosis. *Lancet* **ii**, 1004–1006.

Caldwell, S.H., Jeffers, L.J., Ditomaso, A., Millar, A., Clark, R.M., Rabassa, A., Reddy, R., Medina, M. and Schiff, E.R. (1991) Antibody to hepatitis C is common among patients with alcoholic liver disease with or without risk factors. *American Journal of Gastroenterology* **86**, 1219–1223.

Caldwell, S.H., Li, X., Rourk, R.M., Millar, A., Sosnowski, K.M., Sue, M., Barritt, S., McCallum, R.W. and Schiff, E.R. (1993) Hepatitis C infection by polymerase chain reaction in alcoholics: false-positive ELISA results and the influence of infection on a clinical prognostic score. *American Journal of Gastroenterology* **88**, 1016–1021.

Chalmers, D.M. and Bullen, A.W. (1981) Evidence for previous B virus infection in alcoholic cirrhosis. *British Medical Journal* **282**, 819.

Chevillotte, G., Durbec, J.P., Gerolamio, A., Bethnezene, P., Bidart, J.M. and Camatte, R. (1983) Interaction between hepatitis B virus and alcohol consumption in liver cirrhosis: an epidemiological study. *Gastroenterology* **85**, 141–145.

Coelho-Little, M.E., Jeffers, L.J., Bernstein, D.E., Goodman, J.J., Reddy, K.R., de Medina, M., Li, X., Hill, M., La Rue, S. and Schiff, E.R. (1995) Hepatitis C virus in alcoholic patients with and without clinically apparent liver disease. *Alcoholism: Clinical and Experimental Research* **19**, 1173–1176.

Crapper, R.M., Bhathal, P.S. and Mackay, I.R. (1983) Chronic active hepatitis in alcoholic patients. *Liver* **3**, 327–337.

Deny, P., Halimi, C., Trinchet, J.C., Munoz, C., Bianchi, A., Mal, F. and Beaugrand, M. (1994) Role du virus de l'hepatite C dans la gènese des lesions hepatiques observees chez les malades alcooliques atteints de cirrhose. *Gastroenterologie Clinique et Biologique* **18**, 110–114.

Donato, F., Tagger, A., Chiesa, R., Ribero, M.L., Tomasoni, V., Fasola, M., Gelatti, U., Portera, G., Boffetta, P. and Nardi, G. (1997) Hepatitis B and C virus infection, alcohol drinking, and hepatocellular carcinoma: A case-control study in Italy. *Hepatology* **26**, 579–584.

Figus, A., Blum, H.E., Vyas, G.N., De Virgilis, S., Cao, A., Lippi, M. and Lai, E. (1984) Hepatitis B viral nucleotide sequences in non-A non-B or hepatitis B virus-related chronic liver disease. *Hepatology* **3**, 364–368.

Fong, T.L., Govindarajan, S., Valinluck, B. and Redeker, A.G. (1988) Status of hepatitis B virus DNA in alcoholic liver disease: a study of a large urban population in the United States. *Hepatology* **8**, 1602–1604.

Fong, T.L., Kanel, G.C., Conrad, A., Valinluck, B., Charboneau, F. and Adkins, R.H. (1994) Clinical significance of concomitant hepatitis C infection in patients with alcoholic liver disease. *Hepatology* **19**, 554–557.

Gluud, C., Aldershvile, J., Henriksen, J., Kryger, P. and Mathiesen, L. (1982) Hepatitis B and A virus antibodies in alcoholic cirrhosis and steatosis. *Journal of Clinical Pathology* **35**, 693–697.

Goldberg, S.J., Mendenhall, C.L., Connell, A.M. and Chedid, A. (1977) Nonalcoholic chronic hepatitis in the alcoholic. *Gastroenterology* **72**, 598–604.

Guilera, M., Sáiz, J.C., López-Labrador, F.X., Olmedo, E., Ampurdanés, S., Forns, S., Bruix, J., Parés, A., Sánchez-Tapias, J.M., Jiménez de Anta, M.T. and Rodés, J. (1998) Hepatitis G virus infection in chronic liver disease. *Gut* **42**, 107–111.

Halimi, C., Deby, P., Gotheil, C., Trinchet, J.C., Mal, F. and Scavrizzi, M. (1991) Pathogenesis of liver cirrhosis in alcoholic patients: Histologic evidence for hepatitis C responsibility. *Liver* **11**, 329–333.

Harrison, T.J., Anderson, M.G., Murray-Lyon, I.M. and Zuckerman, A.J. (1986) Hepatitis B virus DNA in the hepatocyte: A series of 160 biopsies. *Journal of Hepatology* **2**, 1–10.

Hislop, W.S., Follett, E.A.C., Bouchier, I.A.D. and MacSween, R.N.M. (1981) Serologic markers of hepatitis B in patients with alcoholic liver disease: a multicenter study. *Journal of Clinical Pathology* **34**, 1017–1019.

Horiike, N., Muchika, K., Onji, M., Murota, T. and Ohta, Y. (1989) HBV-DNA hybridization in hepatocellular carcinoma associated with alcohol in Japan. *Journal of Medical Virology* **28**, 189–192.

Ikeda, K., Saitoh, S., Koida, I., Arase, Y., Tsubota, A., Chayama, K., Kumada, H. and Kawanishi, M. (1993) A multivariate analysis of risk factors for hepatocellular carcinogenesis: a prospective observation of 795 patients with viral and alcoholic cirrhosis. *Hepatology* **18**, 47–53.

Laskus, T., Radkowski, M., Lupa, E., Horban, A., Cianciara, J. and Slusarczyk, J. (1992) Prevalence of markers of hepatitis viruses in out-patient alcoholics. *Journal of Hepatology* **15**, 174–178.

Lelbach, W.K. (1985) Epidemiology of alcoholic liver disease. Continental Europe. In *Alcoholic liver disease*, edited by P. Hall, pp. 130–166. London: Edward Arnold Pubs Ltd.

Levin, D.M., Baker, A.L., Riddell, R.H., Rochman, H. and Boyer, J.L. (1979) Nonalcoholic liver disease: overlooked causes of liver injury in patients with heavy alcohol consumption. *American Journal of Medicine* **66**, 429–434.

MacFarlane, I.M., Smith, H.M., Thomson, P.J. and Williams, R. (1990) Hepatitis C virus antibodies in chronic active hepatitis: pathogenetic factor or false-positive result. *Lancet* **i**, 754–757.

Mendenhall, C.L., Seeff, L., Diehl, A.M., Ghosn, S.J., French, S.W., Gartside, P.S. *et al.* (1991) Antibodies to hepatitis B virus and hepatitis C virus in alcoholic hepatitis and cirrhosis: their prevalence and clinical relevance. *Hepatology* **15**, 581–589.

Mendenhall, C.L., Moritz, T., Rouster, S.M., Roselle, G., Polito, A., Quan, S. and DiNelle, R.K. (1993) Epidemiology of hepatitis C among Veterans with alcoholic liver disease. *American Journal of Gastroenterology* **88**, 1022–1026.

Mills, P.R., Pennington, T.A., Kay, P., MacSween, R.N.M. and Watkinson, G. (1979) Hepatitis Bs antibody in alcoholic cirrhosis. *Journal of Clinical Pathology* **32**, 778–782.

Mills, P.R., Follett, E.A.C., Uruhart, G.R.D., Clements, G., Watkinson, G. and MacSween, R.N.M. (1981) Evidence for previous hepatitis B virus infection in alcoholic cirrhosis. *British Medical Journal* **282**, 730.438.

Mita, E., Hiyashi, N., Kanazawa, Y., Hagiwara, H., Ueda, K., Kasahara, A., Fusumato, H. and Kamada, T. (1994) Hepatitis C virus genotype and RNA titers in the progression of type C chronic liver disease. *Journal of Hepatology* **21**, 468–473.

Mochida, S., Ohnishi, K., Matsuo, S., Kakihara, K. and Fujiwara, K. (1996) Effect of alcohol intake on the efficacy of interferon therapy in patients with chronic hepatitis C as evaluated by multivariate logistic regression analysis. *Alcoholism: Clinical and Experimental Research* **20**, 371A–377A.

Montull, S., Parés, A., Bruguera, M., Caballería, L., Caballería, J. and Rodés, J. (1988) Chronic active hepatitis in alcoholics. A comparison study with non-A non-B chronic active hepatitis. *Journal of Hepatology* **7**, S153.

Nalpas, B., Berthelot, P., Thiers, V., Duhamel, G., Courouce, A.M., Tiollais, P. and Brechot, C. (1985) Hepatitis B Virus multiplication in the absence of usual serologic markers: a study of 146 chronic alcoholics. *Journal of Hepatology* **1**, 89–97.

Nalpas, B., Driss, F., Pol, S., Hamelin, B., Housset, C., Brechot, C. and Berthelot, P. (1991) Association between HCV and HBV infection in hepatocellular carcinoma and alcoholic liver disease. *Journal of Hepatology* **12**, 70–74.

Nalpas, B., Thiers, V., Pol, S., Driss, F., Thepot, V., Berthelot, P. and Brechot, C. (1992) Hepatitis C viremia and anti-HCV antibodies in alcoholics. *Journal of Hepatology* **14**, 381–384.

Nei, J., Matsuda, Y. and Takada, A. (1983) Chronic hepatitis induced by alcohol. *Digestive Diseases and Science*, **28**, 207–215.

Nishiguchi, S., Kuroki, T., Yabusako, T., Seki, S., Kobayashi, K., Monna, T., Otani, S., Sakurai, M., Shikata, T. and Yamamoto, S. (1991) Detection of hepatitis C virus antibodies and hepatitis C RNA in patients with alcoholic liver disease. *Hepatology* **14**, 985–989.

Ohnishi, K., Matsuo, S., Matsutani, K., Itahashi, M., Kakihara, K., Suzuki, K., Ito, S. *et al.* (1996) Interferon therapy for chronic hepatitis C in habitual drinkers: comparison with chronic hepatitis C in infrequent drinkers. *American Journal of Gastroenterology* **91**, 1374–1379.

Okazaki, T., Yoshihara, H., Suzuki, K., Yamada, Y., Tsujimura, T., Kawano, K., Yamada, Y. and Abe, H. (1994) Efficacy of interferon therapy in patients with chronic hepatitis C: Comparison between non-drinkers and drinkers. *Scandinavian Journal of Gastroenterology* **29**, 1039–1043.

Omata, M., Afroudakis, A., Liew, C.T., Asccavai, M. and Peters, R.L. (1978) Comparison of serum hepatitis B surface antigen and serum anticore with tissue HBsAg and hepatitis B core antigen (HBcAg). *Gastroenterology* **75**, 1003–1009.

Orholm, M., Aldershvile, J., Tage-Jensen, U., Schlichting, P., Nielse, J.O., Hardt, F. and Christoffersen, P. (1981) Prevalence of hepatitis B virus infection among alcoholic patients with liver disease. *Journal of Clinical Pathology* **34**, 1378–1380.

Oshita, M., Hayashi, N., Kashahara, A., Hagiwara, H., Mita, E., Naito, M.. Katayama, K., Fusamoto, H. and Kamada, T. (1994) Increased serum hepatitis C virus RNA levels among alcoholic patients with chronic hepatitis C. *Hepatology* **20**, 1115–1120.

Parés, A., Barrera, J.M., Caballería, J., Ercilla, G., Bruguera, M., Caballería, L., Castillo, R. and Rodés, J. (1990) Hepatitis C virus in chronic alcoholic patients: association with the severity of liver injury. *Hepatology* **12**, 1295–1299.

Parés, A. (1995) Epidemiología del consumo de alcohol y de la enfermedad hepática alcohólica. In *Actualidades en Gastroenterología y Hepatología*, edited by J. Rodés and R. Chantar, pp. 61–72. Barcelona: J.R. Prous Editores.

Parés, A. and Caballería, J. (1996) Virus de la hepatitis y enfermedad hepática alcohólica. *Gastroenterologia y Hepatologia* **19**, 383–389.

Partelini, P., Gerken, G., Nakajima, E., Terres, D., D'Errico, A. and Grignioni, W. (1990) Polymerase chain reaction for detection of hepatitis B virus DNA and RNA sequences in hepatitis B surface antigen negative patients with primary liver cancer: a study in high and low endemic areas. *New England Journal of Medicine* **323**, 80–85.

Parterlini, P., Driss, F., Nalpas, B., Pisi, E., Franco, O. and Bcrthclot, P. (1993) Persistence of hepatitis B and C viral genomes in primary liver cancers from HBsAg-negative patients: a study in low-endemic area. *Hepatology* **17**, 20–29.

Patek, A.J., Toth, I.G., Saunders, M.G., Castro, G.A.H. and Emgel, J.I. (1975) Alcohol and dietary factors in cirrhosis. An epidemiological study of 304 alcoholic patients. *Archives of Internal Medicine* **135**, 1053–1057.

Pessione, F., Degos, F., Marcellin, P., Duchatelle, V., Njapoum, C., Martinot-Peignoux, M., Degott, C., Valla, D., Erlinger, S. and Rueff, R. (1998) Effect of alcohol consumption on serum hepatitis C virus RNA and histological lesions in chronic hepatitis C. *Hepatology* **27**, 1717–1722.

Renard, P., Hillon, P., Bedenne, L., Fourot, M., Milan, C., Faivre, J. and Klepping, C. (1991) Markers of the hepatitis B virus and chronic alcoholism. Prevalence and risk factors. *Annals du Gastroenterologie et Hepatologie* (Paris) **27**, 7–12.

Rosman, A.S., Waraich, A., Galvin, K., Casiano, J., Paronetto, F. and Lieber, C.S. (1996) Alcoholism is associated with hepatitis C but not hepatitis B in an urban population. *American Journal of Gastroenterology* **91**, 498–505.

Sata, M., Fukuizumi, K., Uchimura, Y., Nakano, H., Ishii, K., Kumashiro, R., Mizokami, M., Lau, J.Y. and Tanikawa, K. (1996) Hepatitis C virus infection in patients with clinically diagnosed alcoholic liver diseases. *Journal of Viral Hepatology* **3**, 143–148.

Saunders, J.B., Wodak, A.D., Morgan-Capner, P., White, Y.S., Portmann, B., Davies, M. and Williams, R. (1983) Importance of markers of hepatitis B virus in alcoholic liver disease. *British Medical Journal* **11**, 1851–1854.

Sherman, K.E., Mendenhall, C., Thee, D.L., O'Brien, J. and Rouster, Ss.D. (1997) Hepatitis C serotypes in nonalcoholic and alcoholic patients. *Digestive Diseases and Science* **42**, 2285–2291.

Sobue, S., Higashi, K., Nakao, H., Takahashi, Y., Itoh, M. and Nakajima, K. (1998) Hepatitis G virus infection in patients with alcoholic liver disease. *Alcoholism: Clinical and Experimental Research* **22**, 156S–160S.

Srugo, I., Shinar, E., Bar-Shany, S. and Amos, L. (1998) Hepatitis B and C markers among alcoholics in Israel: High incidence of HCV infection. *European Journal of Epidemiology* **14**, 333–337.

Takada, N., Takase, S., Enomoto, N., Takada, A. and Date, T. (1992) Clinical backgrounds of the patients having different types of hepatitis C virus genomes. *Journal of Hepatology* **14**, 35–40.

Takase, S., Takada, N., Enomoto, N., Yasuhara, M. and Takada, A. (1991) Different types of chronic hepatitis in alcoholic patients. Does chronic hepatitis induced by alcohol exist? *Hepatology* **13**, 876–881.

Takase, S., Tsutsumi, M., Kawahara, H., Takada, N. and Takada, A. (1993) The alcohol-related membrane antibody and hepatitis C virus infection in the progression of alcoholic liver disease. *Hepatology* **17**, 9–13.

Vetter, D., Doffoel, M., Gut, J.P., Doffoel, S., North, M.L., Charrault, A., Ventre, G., Mayer, S. and Bockel, R. (1985) Hepatitis B virus, serological markers of viral infections and humoral immunity in alcoholic cirrhosis. *Gastroenterologie Clinique et Biologique* **9**, 389–395.

Walter, E., Blum, H.E., Meier, P., Huanker, M., Schmid, M. and Paier, K.P. (1988) Hepato-cellular carcinoma in alcoholic liver diseases: No evidence for a pathogenic role of hepatitis B virus infection. *Hepatology* **8**, 745–748.

Yamada, M., Kakumu, S., Yoshioka, K., Higashi, Y., Tanaka, K., Ishiwara, T. and Takayenegi, M. (1994) Hepatitis C virus genotypes are not responsible for development of serious liver disease. *Digestive Diseases and Science* **39**, 234–239.

Yokoama, H., Ishii, H., Moriya, S., Nagata, S., Watanabe, T., Kamegaya, K., Takahashi, H., Murayama, K., Haber, P. and Tsuchiya, M. (1995) Relationship between hepatitis C virus subtypes and clinical features of liver disease in alcoholics. *Journal of Hepatology* **22**, 130–134.

Zarski, J.P., Thelu, M.A., Moulin, C., Rachail, M. and Seigneurin, J.M. (1993) Interest of the detection of hepatitis C virus RNA in patients with alcoholic liver disease. Comparison with HBV status. *Journal of Hepatology* **7**, 10–14.

Chapter 27

Liver transplantation in alcoholic liver disease

Stephen P. Pereira and Roger Williams

The process by which patients with end-stage alcoholic liver disease (ALD) are selected for liver transplantation, in the presence of increasing donor shortages and rising transplantation requirements for most categories of liver disease, remains one of the most controversial areas in medicine today. Other questions such as the relationship between pre-transplant abstinence, alcohol relapse and quality of life after liver transplantation also remain unresolved. This chapter examines the indications and selection criteria for transplantation of patients with end-stage ALD, the issues of quality of life and recidivism post-transplant, and possible future directions for liver transplantation in ALD.

KEYWORDS: alcohol relapse, alcoholic liver disease, liver transplantation, quality of life

DEMAND FOR LIVER TRANSPLANTATION IN ALD

Alcoholic liver disease (ALD) is a major cause of cirrhosis and a leading cause of death due to end-stage liver disease. In the United States, where the age-standardized mortality rates from liver cirrhosis are approximately 12.5/100,000 men and 5.5/100,000 women respectively (La Vecchia *et al.*, 1994), liver disease accounts for about 26,000 deaths each year and ALD is thought to be the etiology in 40% to 50% of this total (Hoofnagle *et al.*, 1997); a consistent long-term trend relation between cirrhosis mortality and per capita consumption of distilled spirits has been reported recently (Roizen *et al.*, 1999). In the UK, which in 1985–1989 had lower (but rising) cirrhosis mortality rates of 6.3/100,000 men and 4.3/100,000 women (Corrao *et al.*, 1997), more than 4,000 people die due to end-stage chronic liver disease each year. Approximately two-thirds of these deaths are thought to be due to alcohol (Corrao *et al.*, 1997; Office for National Statistics, 1997), although there is considerable under-reporting (Davies *et al.*, 1992). In continental Europe, cirrhosis mortality figures vary widely, from 6–9/100,000 population per year in Norway, Sweden and the Netherlands to rates of 42–47/100,000 men and 13–16/100,000 women in Austria, Italy and Portugal (Corrao *et al.*, 1997).

Although ALD is now a major indication for liver transplantation in many countries, the number of potential transplant candidates with end-stage ALD far exceeds current liver transplant activity. In the USA, for example, the number of patients who were transplanted for ALD in 1995 represented less than 6% of the estimated 12,000 deaths from alcoholic cirrhosis (Hoofnagle *et al.*, 1997). In recent years, the proportion of transplants performed for ALD alone has fallen steadily, from 20% (508 of 2,568) of total adult transplant activity in 1992, to 16% (534 of 3,429) in 1995, and to 14% (549 of 4,043) in 1999 – although the percentage of patients transplanted for ALD with or without concomitant chronic viral hepatitis has remained steady at approximately 21%. In the USA, ALD is the next most common indication for liver transplantation in adults after chronic hepatitis C, which in 1999 made up over 27% of total adult transplant activity (Annual Report, 2000) (Figure 27.1a).

In the UK, the number of transplants performed for ALD has remained relatively small but is increasing, from 31 cases (6% of the total number of liver transplants) in 1992, to 71 (10%) in 1995, with a further rise to 80 (11%) in 1997 (Pereira and Williams, 1998). In 2000, 83 of the 709 liver transplants (12%) were for ALD. Of the 596 liver transplant recipients over 17 years of age in that year, 14% had a diagnosis of ALD while 15% ($n = 90$) had chronic hepatitis C cirrhosis (UK Transplant, 2001). Throughout Europe, there has been a similar rise in the number of patients undergoing liver transplantation for ALD. According to data from the European Liver Transplant Registry (1998), 385 (19%) of 2,063 adult patients were transplanted for ALD in Europe in 1992, rising to 589 (22%) of 2,710 transplants in 1995. In 1998, 631 (22%) of 2,824 adults' transplants were for ALD alone, while 577 patients (20%) were transplanted for chronic hepatitis C cirrhosis and a further 59 patients (2%) had dual diagnoses of ALD and chronic hepatitis C cirrhosis (Figure 27.1b).

Even if as few as 10% of patients with end-stage ALD were referred and fulfilled the criteria for transplantation, the demand would greatly exceed the number of available donors. According to one study of liver-related deaths in a district general hospital in England (Davies *et al.*, 1992), up to 250 alcoholic patients – more than double the current number transplanted – may be eligible for liver transplantation in the UK each year. In the USA, 3,644 of 8,383 listed patients (43%) underwent liver transplantation in 1994, but an estimated 6,000 other potentially eligible patients with end-stage chronic liver disease were never assessed (Evans, 1995). It is likely that this unrecognized need is particularly applicable to the subgroup of patients with end-stage ALD, and that only a small proportion of patients with alcoholic cirrhosis that might benefit from liver transplantation are currently being referred. There is also a growing disparity between the number of donated organs and the number of liver transplants that are performed each year. In the USA from 1988 to 1996, liver donor and transplant activity both increased by a factor of 2.4. Over the same period, the number of patients waiting for a liver transplant increased 12-fold and the number of deaths on the waiting list rose by a factor of five (Keeffe, 1998). In 2000, 4,934 patients underwent liver transplantation from an end-of-year waiting list of over 17,000 candidates, one-third of whom had been on the national liver transplant waiting list for more than two years (Annual Report, 2000) (Figure 27.2). In the UK, the waiting list for liver transplantation remains relatively short but increased by 30% over the two years to January 1998, with median times from listing to transplantation for chronic liver disease rising from 30 to 38 days over the same period (Pereira and Williams, 1998). These waiting times are still much lower than those of the USA and countries in continental Europe with a higher prevalence of liver disease than the UK. In the United States, the median waiting time for liver transplantation rose from 247 days in 1995 to

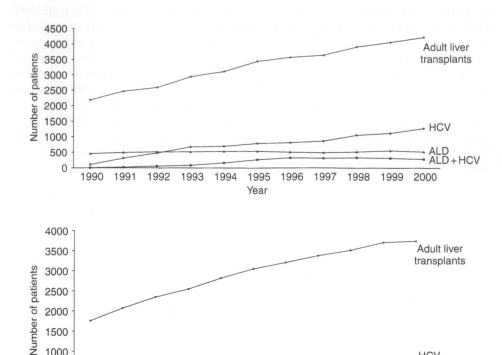

Figure 27.1 Liver transplantation among adult recipients in: (a) the United States, 1990 to 2000 and (b) Europe, 1990 to 2000, expressed as (♦) total number of adult transplants, (▲) alcoholic cirrhosis alone (ALD), (●) chronic hepatitis C cirrhosis (HCV), and (■) dual indications (ALD with HCV). Data from UNOS (*www.unos.org*) and ELTR (*www.eltr.org*).

477 days in 1997, and 7% of patients died while awaiting transplantation (Gilbert *et al.*, 1999). According to data from the Council of Europe (1996), 15–30% of patients listed for heart, lung or liver transplants in continental Europe will die while awaiting a donor organ.

There is some limited information about the reasons for referral or non-referral of patients with end-stage ALD who are potentially eligible for transplantation. The greatest selection biases probably occur at the time when the referring physician decides whether or not to send the patient to a transplant center (Lucey, 1997). However, the rising number of patients transplanted for ALD in many countries is also likely to be a reflection of improved physician awareness and referral patterns, rather than greater leniency by transplant programmes in listing patients with ALD; according to a survey of US transplant centers (Everhart and Beresford, 1997), 95% of programmes were at least as restrictive as they had been five years beforehand. In a prospective study of patients referred for liver transplantation in

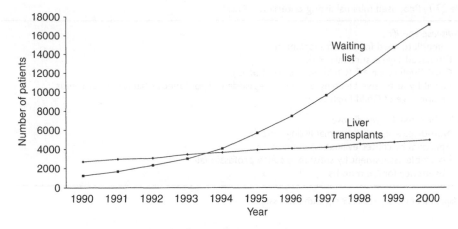

Figure 27.2 Total number of (■) registrations on the United States liver transplant waiting list, and (♦) liver transplants (all ages), at the year end 1990 to 2000. Data from UNOS.

1990–1993, analyzed as part of the NIDDK (National Institute of Diabetes and Digestive and Kidney Diseases) Liver Transplant Database, ALD represented 23% of 1,346 adult patients referred to three large transplant centers and 23% of the 805 who eventually underwent transplantation. After one year of follow-up, the rates of listing (overall 73%) and performance of liver transplantation (61%) were the same for patients with ALD as for those with other nonmalignant diagnoses (Wiesner *et al.*, 1997).

PRE-TRANSPLANT ASSESSMENT

Medical assessment

Eligibility for transplantation is usually based on the selection of abstinent patients with adequate social support who fulfill strict medical criteria. In most published series, patients are considered for transplantation, if there is a history of recurrent hospital admissions for the complications of advanced cirrhosis despite abstinence (corresponding to a Child-Pugh score of B or C), and/or small hepatocellular carcinomas are present. The most common symptoms are recurrent bleeding from esophageal or gastric varices, diuretic-resistant ascites with spontaneous bacterial peritonitis or requiring repeated paracentesis, and poor quality of life due to chronic encephalopathy or other features of end-stage liver disease. An American consensus conference held in 1996 set a general minimal listing criterion for a patient with chronic liver disease of any etiology at an estimated 90% or less chance of surviving one year (Lucey *et al.*, 1997a; Keeffe, 1998). Based on the results of large natural history studies of cirrhotic patients with estimated one- and five-year survival rates of 95% and 75%, respectively, for patients with Child-Pugh class B, and 85% and 50% for those with Child-Pugh class C cirrhosis (Propst *et al.*, 1995), this criterion would make all patients with Child's C or decompensated Child's B

Table 27.1 Proposed minimal listing criteria for ALD*

Non-disease-specific
- Immediate need for liver transplantation
- Estimated 1-year survival ≤ 90%
- Child-Pugh score ≥ 7 (Child-Pugh class B or C)
- Portal hypertensive bleeding or a single episode of spontaneous bacterial peritonitis, irrespective of Child-Pugh score

Specific for alcoholic liver disease
- Non-disease-specific minimal listing criteria
- Approval by center evaluation committee
- Favorable assessment by substance abuse professional
- Abstinence for ≥ 6 months

---

* Adapted from Lucey *et al.* (1997), with permission.

cirrhosis potentially eligible for transplant assessment. At the National Institutes of Health consensus conference, disease-specific minimal listing criteria for ALD also included favorable assessment by a substance abuse professional and abstinence from alcohol for at least 6 months (Keeffe, 1998).

Medical contraindications to transplantation include the presence of extra-hepatic disease such as cerebral dysfunction other than hepatic encephalopathy, alcoholic cardiomyopathy and/or ischemic heart disease, chronic pancreatitis, myopathy and severe undernutrition. The range of investigations performed during medical, surgical and anesthetic assessment to exclude these general medical contraindications varies between centers and depends to some extent on the clinical features of the individual patient. One retrospective analysis of additional tests performed specifically in patients with end-stage ALD undergoing transplant assessment at a single center in the UK concluded that, in the absence of clinical signs and symptoms, routine cardiac echocardiography or computerized tomography of the head did not significantly affect the selection process (Anand *et al.*, 1997). A recent American review of comorbid medical conditions in alcoholic patients undergoing transplant assessment made broadly similar conclusions (Keeffe, 1997).

There are limited data regarding the prevalence of alcohol-induced extrahepatic disease in patients with end-stage ALD. Both alcoholic cardiomyopathy and myopathy are related to the total lifetime amount of alcohol ingested (Urbano-Marquez *et al.*, 1989), but generally improve when alcohol is discontinued. Overall, these conditions seem to be uncommon in abstinent alcoholics referred for transplantation (Keeffe, 1997). Coronary artery disease is found more often in patients with end-stage chronic liver disease than in the general population, but whether patients with alcoholic cirrhosis are at particular risk of peroperative ischemic complications remains unclear. Clinically unsuspected moderate or severe coronary artery disease has been reported in 2% to 13% of patients being assessed for transplantation, depending on whether non-invasive testing (dobutamine stress echocardiography or multiple equilibrium-gated radionuclide echocardiography) or coronary arteriography were performed (Keeffe, 1997). A retrospective study from the University of Pittsburgh reported an overall mortality rate of 50% in 32 patients with known coronary artery disease who underwent liver transplantation for end-stage chronic

Table 27.2 Comorbid conditions associated with ALD

Alcoholic cardiomyopathy
Ischemic heart disease
Myopathy
Neurological dysfunction
    Korsakoff's psychosis
    Chronic cerebral dysfunction
    Alcoholic cerebellar degeneration
    Peripheral sensorimotor neuropathy
Chronic pancreatitis
Malnutrition
Hypothalamic-pituitary-gonadal dysfunction
Osteoporosis
Other liver diseases
    Chronic hepatitis C
    Hepatocellular carcinoma

liver disease, 20 of whom had undergone coronary artery bypass grafting 6 months to 12 years beforehand (Plotkin *et al.*, 1996). Referral bias probably excludes most patients with these or other conditions such as severe chronic pancreatitis from consideration for transplantation. Osteoporosis has been reported in 10% to 48% of patients with alcoholic cirrhosis, with a prevalence rate of spinal and peripheral fractures approximately twice that of controls (Diamond *et al.*, 1989; Bonkovsky *et al.*, 1990). Although there are few comparable post-transplant data in ALD, studies in patients with cholestatic liver disease suggest that bone strength worsens in the initial 3 to 6 months after transplantation but improves to baseline by 1 year (Hay, 1993; Lowowsky and Hussaini, 1996). Irreversible organic brain disease may be difficult to distinguish from reversible hepatic encephalopathy, and imaging studies of the brain and possibly psychometric testing are warranted in patients with atypical hepatic encephalopathy or findings suggestive of organic brain dysfunction.

Predicting post-transplant abstinence

In most transplant centers in Europe and the USA, patients are generally not considered for transplantation unless they have been abstinent from alcohol for an arbitrary period before listing. Although some studies have suggested that lack of abstinence for a defined period is predictive of alcohol relapse (Kumar *et al.*, 1990; Osorio *et al.*, 1994; Gerhardt *et al.*, 1996), other authors have concluded that there is little evidence to support the 6-month rule alone in selecting ALD patients for liver transplantation (Howard *et al.*, 1994b; Beresford, 1997; Foster *et al.*, 1997; DiMartini *et al.*, 1998; Yates *et al.*, 1998b; Pereira *et al.*, 2000). An analysis of four studies involving 167 ALD patients estimated that the predictive value of a pre-transplant abstinence period of less than 6 months in identifying post-transplant relapse was only 41% (Foster *et al.*, 1997). Other potential predictors of a return to alcohol abuse, such as severity of alcohol dependence, levels of social support and psychiatric morbidity, have been less well-studied. Nevertheless, in a questionnaire survey of US transplant programs published in 1997, there was general agreement among centers concerning: (i) a defined period of abstinence (85% of centers required 6 months), in addition to (ii) stable social support for the patient, and (iii) the absence of other substance abuse or psychiatric disability (Everhart and Beresford, 1997). Virtually all centers required a formal psychosocial assessment during the pre-transplant workup to try to establish the likelihood of long-term abstinence, and all centers monitored patients for evidence of alcohol use and removed patients from the list if they were found to be drinking. Although there have been no prospective studies of the value of signed contracts in establishing long-term abstinence, more than a third of centers utilized a signed contract committing the patient to compliance prior to acceptance into the transplant program (Gish *et al.*, 1993; Everhart and Beresford, 1997).

Similar selection criteria were reported in a questionnaire survey of 20 European transplant centers (Neuberger and Tang, 1997), accounting for over a third of transplant activity in Europe at the time – 16 centers (80%) required patients to be abstinent before transplantation and 15 of these used the 6-month rule. Post-transplant, all but one center advised continued abstinence and about half routinely screened for alcohol relapse, ranging from simply asking the patient if they were drinking again to regular estimations of blood or urinary alcohol.

Although there is uncertainty concerning the 6-month rule as a predictor of future abstinence, a defined period of abstinence does allow time for the patient's clinical condition to stabilize or improve following the withdrawal of alcohol and sometimes avoids the need for transplantation. Conversely, others have argued that the imposition of an arbitrary period of abstinence prior to transplantation is potentially punitive to a deteriorating candidate with a limited life expectancy (Lucey *et al.*, 1992; DiMartini *et al.*, 1998; Weinrieb *et al.*, 2000) and there have been recent calls for definitive studies to test this practice (Beresford and Everson, 2000). Other controversial issues are how to define and monitor pre-transplant abstinence and whether a return to drinking after transplantation necessarily has a poor outlook. The experience of most centers is that only a few per cent of patients return to heavy drinking after transplantation, but those that do so may progress to early cirrhosis and graft failure very rapidly. Of 60 patients transplanted for ALD at King's College Hospital between 1990–1995, 2 patients – both of whom claimed to have been abstinent for 6 months pre-transplant – died from recurrent alcoholic hepatitis and liver failure at 10 and 24 months, respectively (Pereira and Williams, 1997). In two other studies comprising a total of 223 patients transplanted for ALD, alcohol was considered to be a major contributing factor to death in 6 patients (3%) within 5 years post-transplant (Foster *et al.*, 1997; Wiesner *et al.*, 1997). Currently, most programs place some emphasis on the severity of prior alcohol dependence, the acceptance of the alcohol problem by the patient and his or her family, the presence of substitute activities, the absence of concomitant psychiatric disease, and a stable work and family environment (Beresford, 1997). There is some evidence that patients with alcohol-related liver disease are less severely dependent on alcohol, and more likely to remain abstinent, than those attending alcohol clinics alone, which generally report relapse rates at one year after completion of treatment of 30% to 60% (Wodak *et al.*, 1983; Beresford *et al.*, 1990; O'Brien and McLellan, 1996).

Psychiatric assessment

There are relatively few data on the prevalence of psychiatric disorder in ALD transplant candidates and its influence on alcohol relapse and quality of life post-transplant. In an early series, Beresford *et al.* (1990) reported that only one of 34 liver transplant candidates with a history of alcohol dependence syndrome or drug dependence had a non-substance related psychiatric diagnosis. Osorio *et al.* (1994) found that 6 of 37 patients transplanted for ALD had a pre-transplant history of psychiatric symptoms, although this was not predictive of a return to drinking. In contrast, Gish *et al.* (1993), in reviewing the outcome of 47 patients evaluated for liver transplantation, regarded a previous psychiatric diagnosis as a risk factor for post-transplant relapse. In another study of 73 subjects with alcohol-related liver disease (Yates *et al.*, 1998a), the subgroup with severe personality disorder had higher rates of divorce and comorbid drug abuse or dependence, but personality disorder was not associated with an increased risk of alcohol relapse over a 6-month period. Three of the patients with personality disorder underwent liver transplantation without subsequent behavioral or substance abuse complications (Yates *et al.*, 1998a). A history of other drug use, in addition to alcohol, has been regarded as predictive of alcohol relapse and substance abuse post-transplant. However, this supposition was not substantiated in an American study of 91 successfully transplanted alcoholic patients, 33 of whom also had a pre-transplant history of substance abuse (Coffman *et al.*, 1997). In this study, psychiatric comorbidity, particularly a history of antisocial behavior or eating disorder, did correlate with a return to drinking. These results may reflect referral bias of a particularly psychologically robust group, and there is a need for further research to determine the prevalence and nature of psychiatric morbidity in alcoholic transplant candidates and how such disorders influence outcome. Although social stability is a potent factor in predicting treatment compliance among non-transplanted alcoholics (Beresford, 1997), the relevance of social support to drinking outcome post-transplant has also not been established; putative predictive factors such as marital status, education and employment do not correlate well with abstinance after transplantation (Osorio *et al.*, 1994; Berlakovich *et al.*, 1994; Gerhardt *et al.*, 1996).

Liver transplantation for acute alcoholic hepatitis

The question of transplantation for severe acute alcoholic hepatitis remains controversial, and it is currently regarded as a contraindication to liver transplantation in most centers. Patients with this condition are usually actively drinking just before or at the time of presentation, and even if such patients were listed and survived the waiting period prior to transplantation, they are also at an increased operative risk due to the severity of their liver disease and associated multiorgan failure. Although patients with mild or moderate alcoholic hepatitis will usually recover with medical management, mortality rates in those with severe acute alcoholic hepatitis complicated by acute renal failure and hepatic encephalopathy may be as high as 80% or more despite intensive care support (Theodossi *et al.*, 1982; Mutimer *et al.*, 1993). Liver transplantation would be expected to improve on these figures, but there are relatively few data on the long-term outcome of such

Table 27.3 UNOS liver status for patients ≥ 18 years of age according to disease severity*

Status 1	Fulminant liver failure with life expectancy < 7 days
	• Fulminant hepatic failure as traditionally defined
	• Primary graft dysfunction < 7 days of transplantation
	• Hepatic artery thrombosis < 7 days of transplantation
	• Acute decompensated Wilson's disease
Status 2A	Hospitalised in ICU for chronic liver failure with life expectancy < 7 days, with a Child-Pugh score of ≥ 7 and one of the following:
	• Unresponsive active variceal haemorrhage
	• Hepatorenal syndrome
	• Refractory ascites/hepatic hydrothorax
	• Stage 3 or 4 hepatic encephalopathy
Status 2B	Requiring continuous medical care, with a Child-Pugh score of ≥ 10, or a Child-Pugh score of ≥ 10 and one of the following:
	• Unresponsive active variceal haemorrhage
	• Hepatorenal syndrome
	• Refractory ascites/hepatic hydrothorax
	• Spontaneous bacterial peritonitis
Status 3	Requiring continuous medical care, with a Child-Pugh score of ≥ 7 but not meeting criteria for status 2B
Status 7	Temporarily inactive

* From (Keeffe, 1998), with permission.
  Data from UNOS; initially implemented – July 1997, modified – January 1998.

patients after transplantation, particularly with respect to alcohol relapse. In an early series from King's College Hospital (Bird *et al.*, 1990), three non-abstinent patients with alcoholic hepatitis plus cirrhosis were transplanted on the basis of their young age and the rapid progression of liver disease. However, within a year post-transplant, all three had evidence of a return to harmful drinking (as suggested by laboratory indices and liver histology), although they denied a return to alcohol and also gave negative responses to a screening questionnaire for alcohol misuse (Mayfield *et al.*, 1974).

More recent studies have confirmed that liver transplantation improves the expected survival of selected patients with acute alcoholic hepatitis, with reported alcohol relapse rates ranging from less than 10% to more than 50%. Of 41 patients with ALD transplanted at the University of Wisconsin (Knechtle *et al.*, 1992), one-third had presented with life-threatening decompensated liver disease and underwent transplantation without meeting the 6-month abstinence requirement. One- and five-year patient survival rates in the ALD group were 83% and 71%, respectively, compared with 83% and 65% in 93 non-alcoholic patients. Four of the patients returned to some alcohol post-transplant, but none claimed to drink more than three units (30 g) daily. Of 221 ALD patients transplanted at the University of Pittsburgh Medical Centre over a 6 year period (Van Thiel *et al.*, 1995), the survival of the 64 patients transplanted for alcoholic hepatitis plus cirrhosis (80%) was similar to that of those transplanted for cirrhosis alone (84%), at a mean follow-up of 4.4 years. Recurrent alcohol use was detected in 52% of patients transplanted for alcoholic hepatitis plus cirrhosis, compared with 15% of those transplanted for endstage alcoholic cirrhosis alone. Of the 9 patients with severe acute alcoholic hepatitis, as defined by a discriminant function of Maddrey *et al.* (1978) of greater than 32, 8 survived for more than 6 months, and follow-up regarding alcohol consumption was available in 6; 3 remained abstinent for at least 7 years but 3 relapsed within 1 year, one of whom died due to graft failure 8 months after receiving the transplant (Shakil *et al.*, 1997). In another report from the same center (DiMartini *et al.*, 1998), of 78 patients with alcohol-related liver disease who were United Network for Organ Sharing status IIA (critically ill) at the point of transplantation, there was a trend towards poorer survival in patients with the shortest length of sobriety (less than 1 month), but these patients were also most likely to be on dialysis, on vasopressor support and severely encephalopathic. Pre-transplant dialysis requirement was the only variable that predicted poorer survival.

Survival of patients not accepted for transplantation

As discussed above, most centers use the Child-Pugh score as a guide to liver disease severity in selecting ALD patients for transplantation, together with some form of individual assessment. This selection process would seem to be fairly accurate, as indicated by post-transplant survival and quality of life indicators, but there is less information about the outcome of those who are not accepted for transplantation. In an early series from the USA, (Lucey *et al.*, 1992), 99 patients were subjected to both medical and psychiatric assessment, the latter consisting of a scoring system based on: (a) acceptance of their drinking problem; (b) the presence of favorable prognostic indices for future abstinence; and (c) social stability and family support. Of the 19 patients (18 of whom were Child's grade C) considered to be unsuitable for transplantation because of sepsis, malignancy, cardiac or renal failure, only a third survived to 3 months and none was alive at 12 months. In contrast, 16 of 17 patients (12 Child's B or C) who were "too well" for a transplant were still alive at 18 months, although survival had fallen to 59% at 2 years. One-third of those excluded on psychiatric grounds were alive at 1 year – in this group many deaths were not liver-related. Overall, approximately 50% of the alcoholics referred for assessment were considered suitable for transplantation. In a more recent prospective study of 342 ALD patients evaluated for liver transplantation at three American centers (Wiesner *et al.*, 1997), 139 (41%) were eventually transplanted, while 56 patients (16%) were thought to be too well and 118 (35%) were considered to have a medical, financial or psychological contraindication to liver transplantation. Survival data in the non-transplanted patients were not given. Of 104 alcoholic liver transplant candidates evaluated at another American center (Coffman *et al.*, 1997), 38 were initially rejected, generally because they continued to drink or did not cooperate with the medical work-up; one-third were dead within two months of evaluation and 50% were dead within 13 months. Those who survived remained abstinent, and nine of these patients eventually received liver transplants.

Somewhat lower acceptance rates were reported in a study of ALD patients referred to a single UK transplant center between 1987 and 1994 (Anand *et al.*, 1997). Of 180 patients referred for transplantation, 39 (22%) were transplanted,

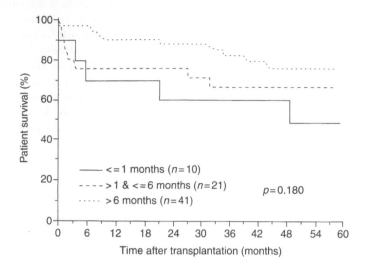

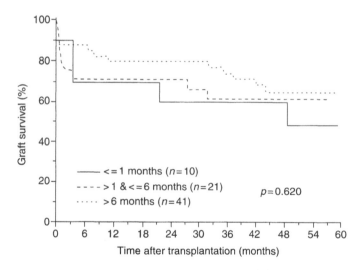

Figure 27.3 (a) Kaplan-Meier patient and (b) graft survival after liver transplantation of 72 critically ill (UNOS Status IIA) patients with ALD, according to length of pre-transplant
sobriety. From DiMartini *et al.* (1998), with permission.

with a 1-year actuarial survival of 79%. Of the 137 in whom case records were sufficiently complete for analysis, a further 4 patients were still on the waiting list
and 7 others refused transplantation, giving an overall acceptance rate of 30%. Of
the 29 patients who were medically unsuitable for transplantation, the 1-year
survival was 44%, compared with 65% in the 16 thought to be psychologically
unsuitable and 94% in 19 considered too well for transplantation.

A large case-control study using combined results from 12 French transplant
centers (Poynard *et al.*, 1994) has provided further data on which patients benefit

most from transplantation. The outcome after transplantation of 169 patients with alcoholic cirrhosis was compared to that of 169 matched controls who were of similar age and liver disease severity to the transplant cohort but who were treated conservatively. A simulated control group – derived by statistical modeling of a database of 797 patients with alcoholic cirrhosis – was also used to derive a proportional hazards prognostic model (the Beclere model), incorporating age and three of the five variables of the Child-Pugh classification (serum bilirubin and albumin levels, and the presence or absence of encephalopathy). The results of a 2-year follow-up showed that transplantation conferred a significant survival advantage only in the 40 "high-risk" patients with severe liver disease. The 2-year survival of transplanted patients was 64%, compared with 41% in matched controls and 23% in the simulated control group. In contrast, there was little difference in outcome in 59 "medium-risk" and 70 "low-risk" patients. Subsequent data from this study indicate that the 5-year survival of patients transplanted for severe ALD (comparable to Child-Pugh grade C) is improved to approximately double that of non-transplanted disease controls, but that Child's A or B cirrhotics fare just as well with conservative management (Poynard et al., 1996). However, these data may not be universally applicable to liver units in other countries. In a retrospective analysis of 137 patients referred to a single transplant center in the UK, the Beclere model overestimated the expected risk of early death in those who were not transplanted (Anand et al., 1997). It should also be noted that consideration of survival of cirrhotic patients with medical treatment alone takes no account of the improved quality of life afforded by a liver transplant (Pereira et al., 2000).

Table 27.4 Prognostic models for patients with ALD

Child-Pugh Score	I Point	2 Points	3 Points
Bilirubin (μmol/L)	<34	34–51	>51
Albumin (g/L)	>35	28–35	<28
INR	<1.3	1.3–1.5	>1.5
Ascites	None	Mild	Moderate
Encephalopathy	None	I/II	III/IV

Child-Pugh class: A, 5–6 points; B, 7–9 points; C, 10–15 points

Beclere risk score (Poynard et al., 1994)
= 0.537 $\log_e$ (serum bilirubin μmol/L)
−0.052 (albumin g/L)
+0.048 (age in year)
+0.469 (if encephalopathy)

Survival function S (2 years) = $0.643^{R-3.058}$

Birmingham relative risk (Anand et al., 1997)
= 2.07 $\log_e$ (serum bilirubin μmol/L)
+2.33 $\log_e$ (blood urea mmol/L)
−0.07 (serum albumin g/L)
−2.49 (if ascites present)
+4.31 (if bacterial peritonitis)
−9.61

OUTCOME AFTER LIVER TRANSPLANTATION FOR ALD

Published graft and patient survival figures

Patient survival rates after liver transplantation for ALD compare favorably with those for other chronic liver diseases, being somewhat lower than those for patients with chronic cholestatic liver disease but higher than the rates for patients with chronic viral hepatitis (Starzl et al., 1988; Kumar et al., 1990; Knechtle et al., 1992; Lucey et al., 1992; Berlakovich et al., 1994). Recent data from the UNOS (United Network for Organ Sharing) Registry gave a 7-year survival after liver transplantation of approximately 76% for patients with primary biliary cirrhosis, 60% for those with ALD, and 57% and 49% for those with chronic hepatitis C and B, respectively (Belle et al., 1997). These trends are also evident in 1997 data from the European Liver Transplant Registry, which reported a one-year patient survival rate for primary biliary cirrhosis of 81%, compared with 80% for ALD and 78% for viral-related cirrhosis. At 5 years, the patient survival rate was 75% for primary biliary cirrhosis, 69% for ALD and 67% for viral-related cirrhosis (Douds and Neuberger, 1998).

As in non-ALD recipients, infection and graft failure are the two most common causes of death in the early post-transplant period. Compared with patients transplanted for other conditions, an increased incidence of bacterial and fungal infections has been reported in some studies of patients transplanted for ALD (Farges et al., 1996; Wiesner et al., 1997). The reasons for this are unclear, but may be due in part to alcoholic patients being transplanted at a more advanced stage of liver disease than are non-alcoholic patients, and to a nonspecific inhibitory effect of previous heavy alcohol intake on the immune response (Farges et al., 1996; Wiesner et al., 1997). Alcohol-induced immunosuppression is also one explanation why patients with ALD may suffer fewer episodes of acute (but not chronic) rejection than those transplanted for other chronic liver diseases (Van Thiel et al., 1995; Farges et al., 1996; Wiesner et al., 1997; Neuberger, 1998). A study of 209 alcoholic patients transplanted for ALD reported that the rate of acute cellular rejection was three times as great in those who remained alcohol-abstinent than in those who admitted to continued alcohol use after transplantation (Van Thiel et al., 1995), although these data have not been confirmed by other studies (Lucey et al., 1997b). In contrast, the risks of de novo skin, oropharyngeal and pulmonary malignancies appear to be higher in patients transplanted for ALD than in those transplanted for nonalcoholic cirrhosis, and these conditions represent an important cause of death beyond 2 years (Wiesner et al., 1997; Duvoux et al., 1999; Jain et al., 2000). Nevertheless, long-term survival after liver transplantation for ALD is similar to that for non-alcoholic cirrhosis, despite a possible reluctance to retransplant patients with ALD as the primary diagnosis (Belle et al., 1997; Wiesner et al., 1997).

Quality of life and return to work

Survival is the major outcome variable for assessing the success of liver transplantation, but also important is whether the quality of life attained after liver transplantation is equivalent among patients with ALD compared with those with other causes of liver disease. In general, patients with chronic liver disease show an improvement after transplantation in mood state, cognitive functioning and quality of life indicators, with no such improvements in waiting list controls (Lowe *et al.*, 1990; Moore *et al.*, 1992; Price *et al.*, 1995). Although there have been relatively few studies using standardized quality of life markers in patients transplanted for ALD, early reports suggested that 75% or more of alcoholic patients were able to return to normal occupational and social functioning after transplantation, which compared well with patients transplanted for other liver diseases (Starzl *et al.*, 1988; Kumar *et al.*, 1990). Similar results were obtained in an early series of 24 patients (21 men and 3 women) transplanted for ALD in the combined King's/ Cambridge programme from 1980 to 1989 (Bird *et al.*, 1990). At the time of transplantation, 21 of the patients had been abstinent from alcohol for a median of two years. Three-quarters of the patients had Child's C cirrhosis, and 6 had superimposed hepatocellular carcinoma as the indication for transplantation. Of the 18 patients who survived for at least 3 months, 17 (94%) were able to return to full activity at home and/or at work.

Other more recent studies have not reported such favorable outcomes in terms of return to work, with only 13% of alcoholics returning to full-time employment in one study, compared with 27% of those transplanted for other indications (Knechtle *et al.*, 1992). In two other series, employment rates ranged from 25% (Beresford *et al.*, 1992) to 59% (Osorio *et al.*, 1994) within 3 years post-transplant – comparable figures to those in the non-alcoholic transplant controls. However, few of these series gave details of objective measures of social and occupational functioning and most had relatively short follow-up periods. In a study from King's College Hospital (Howard *et al.*, 1994a), scores in the Medical Outcomes Survey (a 20-item questionnaire to assess physical functioning, role and social functioning, mental health, health perceptions and pain (Stewart *et al.*, 1988)) were comparable between those transplanted for ALD and other indications – similar findings to those of other recent studies (Coffman *et al.*, 1997; Gledhill *et al.*, 1999). However, the patients transplanted for ALD had slightly poorer perceptions of their health, possibly due to guilt about their drinking or to their relatively low levels of occupational functioning. Post-transplant, only 6 of the 20 alcoholic patients studied returned to full-time employment (Howard *et al.*, 1994a). It has been argued that employment status may not be an accurate indicator of quality of life, since patients who have been unable to work due to their previous chronic ill health may have difficulty in being accepted back into the workforce after transplantation (Knechtle *et al.*, 1992; Adams *et al.*, 1995). In one study of transplanted patients who were asked to classify themselves as able or unable to work, 89% felt able to work but only a minority were in the active workforce (Berlakovich *et al.*, 1994). In a recent prospective study from three American transplant centers (Wiesner *et al.*, 1997), 80% of 66 ALD patients were unable to work before transplantation, compared with 63% of 257 non-ALD cirrhotics ($p = 0.07$). However, at 1 year post-transplant, the percentages of patients who were not able to work (42% vs. 38%) and those with improved ability to work (51% vs. 50%), were similar in the alcoholic and nonalcoholic groups – similar findings to a recent American study with 2- and 5-years follow-up (Cowling *et al.*, 2000). In contrast, a recent

French study (Pageaux *et al.*, 1999) reported that only 30% of long-term surviving ALD transplant patients regained employment, compared with 60% of non-alcoholic patients. In a recent systematic review of alcohol use or employment in transplant recipients, Bravata *et al.* (2001) analyzed the combined data from 68 available studies, comprising a total of 1,992 ALD and 3,028 non-ALD patients. The overall results of the analysis suggested that non-ALD recipients worked in significantly greater proportions than ALD recipients before transplantation (29% vs. 59%) and at most time points thereafter, but the (arguably stronger) data from the eight comparative studies showed no difference in the rates of employment post-transplantation. Pretransplantation employment was not a significant predictor of post-transplantation employment among either ALD or non-ALD recipients, and there was no association between post-transplant alcohol use and employment in either group. The implications of these findings were discussed in an accompanying editorial (Pereira and Williams, 2001).

Few studies have compared the post-transplant psychological outcome of alcoholic patients with nonalcoholic transplant recipients. House *et al.* (1983) reported that all 20 of the liver transplant patients that they studied had some form of psychological distress after transplantation (depression was diagnosed in 17), but no standardized instruments were used. In another early report, 24% of liver transplant patients were referred post-operatively for treatment of depressive disorder, usually associated with medical deterioration or cancer recurrence (Surman *et al.*, 1987). Such studies will obviously miss non-referred cases so that it is difficult to draw conclusions on the incidence of psychiatric illness post-transplant. One center that did screen all liver transplant patients post-operatively, using standardized measures including the General Health Questionnaire, found a prevalence of psychiatric disorder comparable to general population surveys (Commander *et al.*, 1992).

In a 7-year prospective study of patients undergoing liver transplantation at three American centers (Wiesner *et al.*, 1997), quality of life indices among 82 patients transplanted for ALD and 340 non-ALD transplant patients had improved equally after 1 year. However, by the third year post-transplant, patients with ALD had somewhat diminished quality of life scores compared with non-alcoholic patients, as measured by the following parameters: (i) general health perception; (ii) well-being; (iii) affect score; and (iv) degree of distress due to psychological symptoms. Whether or not this fall in quality of life indices was attributable to the 16% alcohol relapse rate, or to other factors such as progression of extra-hepatic disease, may become more apparent with further follow-up. Although some studies have suggested that a return to drinking correlates highly with low quality of life scores (Coffman *et al.*, 1997), a recent study from King's College Hospital reported that the subgroup of patients who had returned to potentially harmful drinking (more than 3 units daily) had similar Nottingham Health Profile and Short Form-36 Health Survey scores to those with continued abstinence or mild relapse, at a median of 2.5 years post-transplant (Pereira *et al.*, 2000).

Improvement in cognitive ability may in itself improve the prognosis for psychosocial adjustment. Preoperative hepatic encephalopathy usually reverses after transplantation for liver disease of any etiology (Tarter *et al.*, 1984). In patients with alcoholic cirrhosis, cognitive function improves substantially after liver transplantation, although memory disturbance shows less improvement (Arria *et al.*, 1991). However, there have been no controlled studies comparing cognitive improvement in alcoholic and nonalcoholic liver transplant recipients and few studies have investigated the effects of subsequent drinking on any improvement that may occur. Overall, alcoholic cirrhosis does not seem to be associated with greater cognitive impairment than that found in patients with nonalcoholic cirrhosis (Tarter *et al.*, 1988). Patients with ALD have more gross pathology on magnetic resonance imaging than nonalcoholic patients (Barthauer *et al.*, 1992) – possibly because their liver disease is more advanced at the time of transplantation – but it is not known whether this means they are at an increased risk of irreversible cognitive deficits.

Alcohol relapse post-transplant

A return to alcohol consumption after liver transplantation is a highly emotive issue and is often perceived as a treatment failure, even though the intake may be low and graft function normal. A large number of studies have monitored the rate of alcohol relapse after liver transplantation, but the definitions have varied considerably and methods to monitor patients have ranged from telephone surveys to the use of structured interviews. Other common methodological problems have included reliance to a greater or lesser extent on patients' accounts of their alcohol intake (Orrego *et al.*, 1979), the use of investigators who are not independent of the transplant team, the cross-sectional design of studies preventing an accurate prospective analysis of drinking behavior, and the lack of standardized validated instruments of psychosocial outcome and alcohol consumption. The numerous confounding factors influencing alcohol abuse (for example, social problems and medical complications) have sometimes not been considered, and there are few comparative data on alcohol intake in patients transplanted for other indications – despite the finding from one center that 46% of nonalcoholic patients occasionally consumed alcohol although they had been advised not to do so by the transplant team (Beresford *et al.*, 1992). Addiction specialists have also made the point that the 30% to 60% success rates reported for the treatment of alcoholism and other addictive disorders such as nicotine and opiate dependence are at least as good as drug compliance rates in patients with common medical conditions such as insulin-dependent diabetes, hypertension or asthma (O'Brien and McLellan, 1996).

Reported rates of alcohol relapse vary considerably between centers, partly as a consequence of differing selection criteria and the ways of looking for recidivism. Several early single-center studies from the USA and Europe reported 10% to 15% relapse rates in the first year, with up to 30% returning to some alcohol use 2 to 3 years after transplantation (Starzl *et al.*, 1988; Kumar *et al.*, 1990; Knechtle *et al.*, 1992; Lucey *et al.*, 1992; Gish *et al.*, 1993; Osorio *et al.*, 1994; Berlakovich *et al.*, 1994). In a questionnaire survey of US transplant centers, the overall relapse rate at 2 years was 14% (Hoofnagle *et al.*, 1997), while in a comparable survey of 20 European transplant centers, the median relapse rate in patients receiving transplants for ALD was 28% (range, 5% to 60%), with 17% of the relapsers drinking more than 20 units per week (Neuberger and Tang, 1997). In the systematic review of alcohol use or employment in transplant recipients by Bravata *et al.* (2001) discussed earlier, only 8 of the 37 studies with alcohol use data included both ALD and non-ALD patients, with a similar proportion in each group reporting any alcohol use at 1 year post-transplantation (17% vs. 16%). Inclusion of the 29 other studies without comparative data suggested that non-ALD recipients were more likely to drink regularly (4 to 7 drinks/week) and ALD recipients to drink either occasionally or excessively, but only 19 of the 37 studies actually reported how alcohol use was determined and the non-ALD data were derived from three small studies comprising a total of 35 patients. Data on graft dysfunction or compliance with clinical protocols and immunosuppressive drug regimens were not included in the analysis, although there is little evidence that alcohol relapse leads to non-compliance in liver transplant recipients (Everson *et al.*, 1997; Berlakovich *et al.*, 2000).

Although there are relatively few long-term data in alcoholic transplant recipients, the risk of alcohol relapse appears to decrease if abstinence is maintained for more than 3 to 5 years post-transplant (Gerhardt *et al.*, 1996; Campbell *et al.*, 1998) – similar findings to those in non-transplanted alcoholics, in whom alcohol relapse is rare after more than five years of continued abstinence (Vaillant, 1996). Nevertheless, there is still a potential for long-term transplant survivors to return to problem drinking after as long as 4 to 5 years post-transplant (Pereira *et al.*, 2000). Recent studies using objective markers of alcohol relapse, such as urinary alcohol levels (Fabrega *et al.*, 1998), serum carbohydrate-deficient transferrin concentrations (Heinemann *et al.*, 1998; Berlakovich *et al.*, 1999), or the degree of fat in liver biopsy specimens (Wiesner *et al.*, 1997), suggest that there may also be considerable under-reporting.

It should be noted that admitted relapse rates of less than 30% at two to three years are low compared with rates after conventional alcohol rehabilitation programs (Yates *et al.*, 1993; Project MATCH Research Group, 1997). Possible reasons for this are the strong selection factors involved during transplant evaluation, as well as the "sobering effect" of the liver transplant itself (Vaillant, 1997). Furthermore, most studies suggest that only a few per cent of patients will return to heavy or uncontrolled drinking. The results of a single-center study from the UK (Howard *et al.*, 1994a), where the drinking behavior and psychiatric outcome of patients transplanted for ALD were assessed exhaustively by a psychiatrist independent of the transplant team, are of some interest. At least 1 year after transplantation, 20 English-speaking patients transplanted for ALD underwent semi-structured interviews and standardized questionnaires to assess physical and psychiatric morbidity, depression and neurosis, social functioning and alcohol dependence. Corroborative information was obtained from their partners, close relatives and friends, and general practitioners, and the results were compared with a control group of 54 patients who received transplants during the same period for non-alcoholic cirrhosis. At the time of pre-transplant assessment, all but 2 patients had been abstinent for an average of 26 months. However, at a mean of 2 years after transplantation, only one patient remained totally abstinent. Sixteen consumed alcohol regularly, with a mean consumption of 3.5 units daily. Forty per cent of the group were drinking above the recommended safe levels for the general population, while a further 50% were "binge"-drinking and three were drinking heavily (over 20 units daily). Nevertheless, the patients remained compliant with their immunosuppressants and outpatient visits, and the majority did not have higher levels of physical or psychiatric morbidity than the controls.

During a median 7-year follow-up of 13 of these patients (Pereira et al., 2000), seven still indulged in potentially harmful drinking (more than 3 units daily), of whom two had developed alcoholic cirrhosis and one had abnormal liver function tests. Five of the other six patients had occasionally ingested small amounts of alcohol when first interviewed and continued to do so during long-term follow-up. One patient who had been drinking heavily with features of alcohol dependence at the time of the initial study had reduced his alcohol intake to less than one unit weekly at the time of the second follow-up. Despite the high frequency of continued harmful drinking in over half of the patients, health dimension scores remained high and were comparable to those of UK community controls.

In a recent questionnaire study from the same center (Pereira et al., 2000), 27% of 56 patients transplanted for ALD were found to have had an episode of harmful drinking during a median follow-up of 2.5 years (range, 0.5 to 10 years) post-transplant, and a further 23% admitted to drinking a smaller amount of alcohol at least once. The patients with harmful drinking had begun regular or heavy drinking at a younger age, had shorter pre-transplant abstinence periods and were transplanted longer ago than those with no or mild alcohol relapse. Over half of the harmful drinkers also admitted to regular benzodiazepine use, compared with less than 10% of those with no or mild alcohol relapse, suggesting that patients who report difficulty in sleeping post-transplant may be at particular risk of a return to harmful drinking. Given that postal questionnaires are insensitive tools to detect very low levels of alcohol exposure (Howard et al., 1994b), compared with a multidisciplinary approach to the detection of alcohol relapse (Howard et al., 1994a; Burra et al., 2000; DiMartini et al., 2001), it is likely that even this 50% relapse rate is still an underestimate of the true frequency of recidivism in these patients.

A similar 48% relapse rate was reported in 59 patients transplanted for ALD at Queen Elizabeth Hospital, Birmingham. At a median of 16 months post-transplant (range, 3–49 months), 28 patients said they had drunk some alcohol after the transplant: nine were classified as heavy drinkers (over 20 units/week) and 19 were moderate drinkers (less than 20 units/week). The median time to alcohol relapse was less than 8 months; all of the moderate or heavy relapsers had claimed abstinence for at least five months before transplantation. Alcohol consumption was also assessed in 39 age- and sex-matched non-ALD transplant recipients: 23 (59%) consumed alcohol in moderation after their transplant, but none were heavy drinkers (Tang et al., 1998).

In some patients with continued problematic drinking, severe recurrent alcoholic hepatitis and progression to cirrhosis has been reported within 2 to 5 years post-transplant (Coffman et al., 1997; Pereira and Williams, 1997). The mechanisms underlying this rapid development of cirrhosis with graft failure are unknown, but are intriguing in view of the long latency for cirrhosis in the native liver. As discussed earlier, the risks of acute or chronic rejection in patients transplanted for ALD are lower than or similar to those transplanted for other conditions, and there is little evidence that alcohol relapse leads to non-compliance in liver transplant

Table 27.5 Published rates of survival and alcohol relapse in liver transplantation for ALD

Author	Center	No. of ALD transplants	Child's C cirrhosis (%)	Pre-transplant abstinence >6 months (%)	One-year survival (%)	Returned to full activity (%)	Any alcohol relapse (%)				Death attributable to alcohol (%)
							1 year	2 years	3 years	5 years	
Starzl et al. (1988)	Pittsburgh	41	–	–	73	90	3	3	–	–	3
Kumar et al. (1990)	Pittsburgh	73	64	85	74	79	–	12	–	–	2
Bird et al. (1990)	London	24	75	88 (>3 months)	66	94	–	23	–	–	0
Knechtle et al. (1992)	Madison, Wis.	41	95	66 (>3 months)	83	57	–	13	–	–	0
Lucey et al. (1992)	Ann Arbor, Mich.	45	73	–	78	–	–	15	–	–	0
Gish et al. (1993)	San Francisco	29	–	93	93	80	–	21	–	–	0
Goldstein et al. (1993)	Dallas	41	–	–	86	–	–	14	–	–	0
Howard et al. (1994)	London	20	70	90	79	30	–	95	–	–	0
Poynard et al. (1994)	France multicentre	169	40 "high-risk"	99	76	–	–	12	–	–	1
Osorio et al. (1994)	San Francisco	43	–	93	100	59	8	19	–	–	0
Berlakovich et al. (1994)	Vienna	58	77	–	71	89	15	27	31	–	5

Study	Location									
Raakow et al. (1995)	Berlin	78	–	96	98	–	22	–	–	3
Gerhardt et al. (1996)	Dallas	67	–	90	67	12	22	40	–	0
Foster et al. (1997)	Chicago	84	–	79	–	10	22	–	–	5
Pereira et al. (1997)	London	111	58	79	68	–	–	40	–	2
Wiesner et al. (1997)	USA multicenter	139	44	84	58	–	–	16	–	2
Lucey et al. (1997)	Ann Arbor, Mich.	59	67	80	–	–	–	–	34	3
Everson et al. (1997)	Colorado	68	–	91	33	8	17	20	30	6
Tang et al. (1998)	Birmingham, UK	70	70	83	52	–	48	–	–	1
Pageaux et al. (1999)	Montpellier	53	81	75	75	–	–	–	32	2

(–, data not given)

recipients. In a study by Beresford *et al.* (1992), 5 of 22 patients transplanted for ALD reported missing doses of cyclosporin compared with 13 of 39 nonalcoholic patients – similar findings to a more recent study from the same group (Everson *et al.*, 1997). It is conceivable that alcoholic patients may be less likely to report noncompliance, although studies monitoring tacrolimus or cyclosporin A levels have generally reported good drug compliance in patients with recurrent alcohol use post-transplant (Berlakovich *et al.*, 1994; Van Thiel *et al.*, 1995; Fabrega *et al.*, 1998; Tang *et al.*, 1998).

ETHICAL CONSIDERATIONS

Given the current interest in priority setting and the fact that society inevitably regards alcoholics as bearing some moral responsibility for their condition (Neuberger *et al.*, 1998), it is important that medical and psychiatric selection criteria be further refined so that those who are most likely to benefit receive liver transplants. Although there are few data to support a predetermined period of abstinence as an accurate predictor of future sobriety, most centers continue to use the 6-month rule as a prerequisite for selection for transplantation in ALD, and remove patients from the transplant waiting list after a single relapse for further alcoholism treatment and re-evaluation at a later date. However, others have argued that a single relapse does not necessarily predict continuing relapses in the future and that alcoholism, viewed as a chronic, relapsing disorder, means that the most reasonable expectation should be a significant decrease in alcohol use and long periods of abstinence, with only occasional relapses. Lucey's group (Weinrieb *et al.*, 2000) have argued that it is unethical to force ALD patients who have resumed alcohol use while waiting for transplantation to choose between hiding their drinking to remain suitable candidates for transplantation or risk death by asking for treatment of alcoholism. This approach makes a reasonable standard for treatment success – as is the case for other chronic illnesses – the management of the illness rather than anticipation of a cure (Beresford, 1997; Leshner, 1997; Weinrieb and O'Brien, 1997; O'Connor and Schottenfeld, 1998).

On the basis of medical utility and given the difficulty in predicting post-transplant relapse, it can be argued that liver transplantation may also be indicated in some non-abstinent patients with life-threatening decompensated alcoholic cirrhosis or severe acute alcoholic hepatitis, in whom there may be insufficient time to assess a commitment to future abstinence. Transplanting such patients results in outcomes only marginally inferior to those in more elective cases, with 50% or more of patients remaining abstinent from alcohol post-transplant. Wider acceptance by transplant centers of these less rigid selection criteria would stimulate further debate about the ethics of using a scarce resource in patients with ALD. In a community-wide study of the need for liver transplantation in Israel (Modan *et al.*, 1995), the addition of patients with non-reformed alcoholism and end-stage liver disease, originally set as an exclusion criterion, would have added 20% to the annual estimate of 10–15.5 transplants per million population.

The ethical issues raised by providing or withholding liver transplants to alcoholic patients have been reviewed recently by a number of authors (Benjamin,

1997; Ubel, 1997; Weinrieb *et al.*, 2000). Whether an ALD patient's not having sought prior treatment for alcoholism should place him or her at a comparative disadvantage in competing for an allograft with nonalcoholic patients, whose liver failure is more obviously beyond their control, remains controversial. Clearly, not all patients with a diagnosis of alcohol dependence will have been explicitly fore-warned about the possibility of end-stage liver disease and advised to abstain from alcohol or seek counseling. As noted in previous chapters, there are major genetic, psychosocial, and environmental factors which determine the response of the indi-vidual to ingested alcohol so that there is no one-to-one correlation between alco-holism and ALD. Only 10–30% of chronic alcohol abusers will progress to cirrhosis, and women develop cirrhosis at lower levels of intake than men (Grant *et al.*, 1988). Furthermore, individuals may have ALD diagnosed without having met standard diagnostic criteria for alcoholism. In one study of 267 patients with apparent ALD, 74% were determined to be alcohol-dependent, 13% qualified for the lesser diagnosis of alcohol abuse, and 13% failed to meet any psychiatric diagnosis for alcoholism (Beresford, 1994).

Given the increasing discrepancy between the availability of suitable donor organs and eligible patients listed for transplantation, donor livers will of neces-sity continue to be rationed to a decreasing percentage of potential candidates. The rapidity with which better therapeutic agents are introduced that can defer or delay the need for liver transplantation – for example, continued refinements in the development of bioartificial livers and the use of new or combination antiviral therapies – will be other factors affecting the demand for liver grafting in coming years. Parallel efforts to increase the availability of transplants, for example, increased use of split livers, adult-to-adult living-related liver trans-plantation and xenotransplantation will also play a role. In response to the widening gap between supply and demand, a variety of methods have been pro-posed and instituted for increasing public awareness, liberalizing donor criteria, educating health professionals in organ donation and improving request and consent practices for donor organs (Council of Europe, 1996; Briggs *et al.*, 1997; Pereira and Williams, 1998; Gralnek *et al.*, 1999). The medium-term comparative outcome data in ALD and non-ALD transplant recipients, including the low reported incidence of graft dysfunction due to severe alcohol use in either group (Bravata *et al.*, 2001) are reassuring. However, there is ongoing concern that alcoholic patients who have drinking "slips" are still removed from waiting lists based on the arbitrary 6-month rule, without proper evidence that they would have had a poor outcome if allowed transplantation (Weinrieb *et al.*, 2000; Pereira and Williams, 2001). Properly designed, multicenter studies of alcohol use and functional outcome in such patients, using a more flexible, multidisciplinary approach to clinical decision making, together with better interventional studies of the treatment of alcohol relapse before and after trans-plantation, are needed. These initiatives, together with the establishment of uni-form minimal listing criteria for liver transplantation in ALD, improvements in the recognition and early referral of potentially eligible patients with end-stage ALD to liver centers, and continuous monitoring of the quality of liver trans-plant programs, may all contribute to improvement in outcome of patients with end-stage ALD.

REFERENCES

Adams, P.C., Ghent, C.N., Grant, D.R. and Wall, W.J. (1995) Employment after liver transplantation. *Hepatology* **21**, 140–145.

Anand, A.C., Ferraz-Neto, B.H., Nightingale, P., Mirza, D.F., White, A.C., McMaster, P. and Neuberger, J.M. (1997) Liver transplantation for alcoholic liver disease: evaluation of a selection protocol. *Hepatology* **25**, 1478–1484.

Annual Report of the U.S. Scientific Registry for Transplant Recipients and the Organ Procurement and Transplantation Network: Transplant Data: 1990–1999 (2000) U.S. Department of Health and Human Services, Health Resources and Services Administration, Office of Special Programs, Division of Transplantation, Rockville, MD; UNOS, Richmond, VA (*www.unos.org*).

Arria, A.M., Tarter, R.E., Starzl, T.E. and Van Thiel, D.H. (1991) Improvement in cognitive functioning of alcoholics following orthotopic liver transplantation. *Alcohol Clin Exp Res* **15**, 956–962.

Barthauer, L., Tarter, R., Hirsch, W. and Van Thiel, D. (1992) Brain morphologic characteristics of cirrhotic alcoholics and cirrhotic nonalcoholics: an MRI study. *Alcohol Clin Exp Res* **16**, 982–985.

Belle, S.H., Beringer, K.C. and Detre, K.M. (1997) Liver transplantation for alcoholic liver disease in the United States: 1988 to 1995. *Liver Transpl Surg* **3**, 212–219.

Benjamin, M. (1997) Transplantation for alcoholic liver disease: the ethical issues. *Liver Transpl Surg* **3**, 337–342.

Beresford, T.P. (1994) Overt and covert alcoholism. In *Liver Transplantation and the Alcoholic Patient*, edited by M.R. Lucey, R.M. Merion and T.P. Beresford, pp. 6–28. Cambridge: Cambridge University Press.

Beresford, T.P. (1997) Predictive factors for alcoholic relapse in the selection of alcohol-dependent persons for hepatic transplant. *Liver Transpl Surg* **3**, 280–291.

Beresford, T.P. and Everson, G.T. (2000) Liver transplantation for alcoholic liver disease: bias, beliefs, 6-month rule, and relapse – But where are the data? *Liver Transpl* **6**, 777–778.

Beresford, T.P., Schwartz, J., Wilson, D., Merion, R. and Lucey, M.R. (1992) The short-term psychological health of alcoholic and non-alcoholic liver transplant recipients. *Alcohol Clin Exp Res* **16**, 996–1000.

Beresford, T.P., Turcotte, J.G., Merion, R., Burtch, G., Blow, F.C., Campbell, D., Brower, K.J., Coffman, K. and Lucey, M.R. (1990) A rational approach to liver transplantation for the alcoholic. *Psychosomatics* **31**, 241–254.

Berlakovich, G.A., Langer, F., Freundorfer, E., Windhager, T., Rockenschaub, S., Sporn, E., Soliman, T., Pokorny, H., Steininger, R. and Muhlbacher, F. (2000) General compliance after liver transplantation for alcoholic cirrhosis. *Transpl Int* **13**, 129–135.

Berlakovich, G.A., Steininger, R., Herbst, F., Barlan, M., Mittlbock, M. and Muhlbacher, F. (1994) Efficacy of liver transplantation for alcoholic cirrhosis with respect to recidivism and compliance. *Transplantation* **58**, 560–565.

Berlakovich, G.A., Windhager, T., Freundorfer, E., Lesch, O.M., Steininger, R. and Muhlbacher, F. (1999) Carbohydrate deficient transferrin for detection of alcohol relapse after orthotopic liver transplantation for alcoholic cirrhosis. *Transplantation* **67**, 1231–1235.

Bird, G.L., O'Grady, J.G., Harvey, F.A., Calne, R.Y. and Williams, R. (1990) Liver transplantation in patients with alcoholic cirrhosis: selection criteria and rates of survival and relapse. *Br Med J* **301**, 15–17.

Bonkovsky, H.L., Hawkins, M., Steinberg, K., Hersh, T., Galambos, J.T., Henderson, J.M., Millikan, W.J. and Galloway, J.R. (1990) Prevalence and prediction of osteopenia in chronic liver disease. *Hepatology* **12**, 273–280.

Bravata, D.M., Olkin, I., Barnato, A.E., Keeffe, E.B. and Owens, D.K. (2001) Employment and alcohol use after liver transplantation for alcoholic and nonalcoholic liver disease: a systematic review. *Liver Transplantation* **7**, 191–203.

Briggs, J.D., Crombie, A., Fabre, J., Major, E., Thorogood, J. and Veitch, P.S. (1997) Organ donation in the UK: a survey by a British Transplantation Society working party. *Nephrol Dial Transplant* **12**, 2251–2257.

Burra, P., Mioni, D., Cillo, U., Fagiuoli, S., Senzolo, M., Naccarato, R. and Martines, D. (2000) Long-term medical and psycho-social evaluation of patients undergoing orthotopic liver transplantation for alcoholic liver disease. *Transpl Int* **13**, S174–S178.

Campbell Jr., D.A., Magee, J.C., Punch, J.D., Merion, R.M., Turcotte, J.G. and Bromberg, J.S. (1998) One center's experience with liver transplantation: alcohol use relapse over the long-term. *Liver Transpl Surg* **4**, S58–S64.

Coffman, K.L., Hoffman, A., Sher, L., Rojter, S., Vierling, J. and Makowka, L. (1997) Treatment of the post-operative alcoholic liver transplant recipient with other addictions. *Liver Transpl Surg* **3**, 322–327.

Commander, M., Neuberger, J. and Dean, C. (1992) Psychiatric and social consequences of liver transplantation. *Transplantation* **53**, 1038–1040.

Corrao, G., Ferrari, P., Zambon, A., Torchio, P., Aricò, S. and Decarli, A. (1997) Trends of liver cirrhosis mortality in Europe, 1970–1989: age-period-cohort analysis and changing alcohol consumption. *Internat J Epidemiol* **26**, 100–109.

Council of Europe (1996) Select Committee of Experts on the Organisational Aspects of Cooperation in Organ Transplantation. Meeting the organ shortage: current status and strategies for improvement of cadaveric organ donation. ONT, Madrid, 1996.

Cowling, T., Jennings, L.W., Jung, G.S., Goldstein, R.M., Molmenti, E., Gonwa, T.A., Klintmalm, G.B. and Levy, M.F. (2000) Comparing quality of life following liver transplantation for Laennec's versus non-Laennec's patients. *Clin Transplant* **14**, 115–120.

Davies, M.H., Langman, M.J., Elias, E. and Neuberger, J.M. (1992) Liver disease in a district hospital remote from a transplant centre: a study of admissions and deaths. *Gut* **33**, 1397–1399.

Diamond, T., Stiel, D., Lunzer, M., Wilkinson, M. and Posen, S. (1989) Ethanol reduces bone formation and may cause osteoporosis. *Am J Med* **86**, 282–288.

DiMartini, A., Day, N., Dew, M., Lane, T., Fitzgerald, M., Magill, J. and Jain, A. (2001) Alcohol use following liver transplantation: a comparison of follow-up methods. *Psychosomatics* **42**, 55–62.

DiMartini, A., Jain, A., Irish, W., Fitzgerald, M.G. and Fung, J. (1998) Outcome of liver transplantation in critically ill patients with alcoholic cirrhosis: survival according to medical variables and sobriety. *Transplantation* **66**, 298–302.

Douds, A. and Neuberger, J. (1998) Liver transplantation for alcoholic cirrhosis: current situation. *Hosp Med* **59**, 604–605.

Duvoux, C., Delacroix, I., Richardet, J.P., Roudot-Thoraval, F., Metreau, J.M., Fagniez, P.L., Dhumeaux, D. and Cherqui, D. (1999) Increased incidence of oropharyngeal squamous cell carcinomas after liver transplantation for alcoholic cirrhosis. *Transplantation* **67**, 418–421.

European Liver Transplant Registry (1998) Data analysis 05/1968–12/1998, ELTR, Villejuif (*www.eltr.org*).

Evans, R.W. (1995) Need for liver transplantation. *Lancet* **346**, 1169.

Everhart, J.E. and Beresford, T.P. (1997) Liver transplantation for alcoholic liver disease: a survey of transplantation programs in the United States. *Liver Transpl Surg* **3**, 220–226.

Everson, G., Bharadhwaj, G., House, R., Talamantes, M., Bilir, B., Shrestha, R., Kam, I., Wachs, M., Karrer, F., Fey, B., Ray, C., Steinberg, T., Morgan, C. and Beresford, T.P. (1997) Long-term follow-up of patients with alcoholic liver disease who underwent hepatic transplantation. *Liver Transpl Surg* **3**, 263–274.

Fabrega, E., Crespo, J., Casafont, F., De las Heras, G., de la Pena, J. and Pons-Romero, F. (1998) Alcoholic recidivism after liver transplantation for alcoholic cirrhosis. *J Clin Gastroenterol* **26**, 204–206.

Farges, O., Saliba, F., Farhamant, H., Samuel, D., Bismuth, A., Reynes, M. and Bismuth, H. (1996) Incidence of rejection and infection after liver transplantation as a function of the primary disease: possible influence of alcohol and polyclonal immunoglobulins. *Hepatology* **23**, 240–248.

Foster, P.F., Fabrega, F., Karademir, S., Sankary, H.N., Mital, D. and Williams, J.W. (1997) Prediction of abstinence from ethanol in alcoholic recipients following liver transplantation. *Hepatology* **25**, 1469–1477.

Gerhardt, T.C., Goldstein, R.M., Urschel, H.C., Tripp, L.E., Levy, M.F., Husberg, B.S., Jennings, L.W., Gonwa, T.A. and Klintmalm, G.B. (1996) Alcohol use following liver transplantation for alcoholic cirrhosis. *Transplantation* **62**, 1060–1063.

Gilbert, J.R., Pascual, M., Schoenfeld, D.A., Rubin, R.H., DelMonico, F.L. and Cosimi, A.B. (1999) Evolving trends in liver transplantation. *Transplantation* **67**, 246–253.

Gish, R.G., Lee, A.H., Keeffe, E.B., Rome, H., Concepcion, W. and Esquivel, C.O. (1993) Liver transplantation for patients with alcoholism and end-stage liver disease. *Am J Gastroenterol* **88**, 1337–1342.

Gledhill, J., Burroughs, A., Rolles, K., Davidson, B., Blizard, B. and Lloyd, G. (1999) Psychiatric and social outcome following liver transplantation for alcoholic liver disease: a controlled study. *J Psychosom Res* **46**, 359–368.

Gralnek, I.M., Liu, H., Shapiro, M.F. and Martin, P. (1999) The United States liver donor population in the 1990s. *Transplantation* **67**, 1019–1023.

Grant, B.F., Dufour, M.C. and Harford, T.C. (1988) Epidemiology of alcoholic liver disease. *Semin Liver Dis* **8**, 12–25.

Hay, J.E. (1993) Bone disease in liver transplant recipients. *Gastroenterol Clin North Am* **22**, 337–349.

Heinemann, A., Sterneck, M., Kuhlencordt, R., Rogiers, X., Schulz, K.H., Queen, B., Wischhusen, F. and Puschel, K. (1998) Carbohydrate-deficient transferrin: diagnostic efficiency among patients with end-stage liver disease before and after liver transplantation. *Alcohol Clin Exp Res* **22**, 1806–1812.

Hoofnagle, J.H., Kresina, T., Fuller, R.K., Lake, J.R., Lucey, M.R., Sorrell, M.F. and Beresford, T.P. (1997) Liver transplantation for alcoholic liver disease: executive statement and recommendations. Summary of a National Institutes Health Workshop held December 6–7, 1996, Bethesda, Maryland. *Liver Transpl Surg* **3**, 347–350.

House, R., Dubovsky, S.L. and Penn, I. (1983) Psychiatric aspects of hepatic transplantation. *Transplantation* **36**, 146–150.

Howard, L., Fahy, T., Wong, P., Sherman, D., Gane, E. and Williams, R. (1994a) Psychiatric outcome in alcoholic liver transplant patients. *Quart J Med* **87**, 731–736.

Howard, L.M., Williams, R. and Fahy, T.A. (1994b) The psychiatric assessment of liver transplant patients with alcoholic liver disease: a review. *J Psychosom Res* **38**, 643–653.

Jain, A., DiMartini, A., Kashyap, R., Youk, A., Rohal, S. and Fung, J. (2000) Long-term follow-up after liver transplantation for alcoholic liver disease under tacrolimus. *Transplantation* **70**, 1335–1342.

Keeffe, E.B. (1997) Comorbidities of alcoholic liver disease that affect outcome of orthotopic liver transplantation. *Liver Transpl Surg* **3**, 251–257.

Keeffe, E.B. (1998) Summary of guidelines on organ allocation and patient listing for liver transplantation. *Liver Transpl Surg* **4**, S108–S114.

Knechtle, S.J., Fleming, M.F., Barry, K.L., Steen, D., Pirsch, J.D., Hafez, G.R., Am, D.A., Reed, A., Sollinger, H.W., Kalayoglu, M. and Belzer, F.O. (1992) Liver transplantation for alcoholic liver disease. *Surgery* **112**, 694–701.

Kumar, S., Stauber, R.E., Gavaler, J.S., Basista, M.H., Dindzans, V.J., Schade, R.R., Rabinovitz, M., Tarter, R.E., Gordon, R., Starzl, T.E. and Van Thiel, D.H. (1990) Orthotopic liver transplantation for alcoholic liver disease. *Hepatology* **11**, 159–164.

La Vecchia, C., Levi, F., Lucchini, F., Franceschi, S. and Negri, E. (1994) Worldwide patterns and trends in mortality from liver cirrhosis, 1955 to 1990. *Ann Epidemiol* **4**, 480–486.

Leshner, A.I. (1997) Addiction is a brain disease, and it matters. *Science* **278**, 45–47.

Lowe, D., O'Grady, J.G., McEwen, J. and Williams, R. (1990) Quality of life following liver transplantation: a preliminary report. *J R Coll Physicians Lond* **24**, 43–46.

Lowowsky, M.S. and Hussaini, S.H. (1996) Bone disease after liver transplantation. *Gut* **39**, 505–507.

Lucey, M.R. (1997) Issues in selection for and outcome of liver transplantation in patients with alcoholic liver disease. *Liver Transpl Surg* **3**, 227–230.

Lucey, M.R., Brown, K.A., Everson, G.T., Fung, J.J., Gish, R., Keeffe, E.B., Kneteman, N.M., Lake, J.R., Martin, P., McDiarmid, S.V., Rakela, J., Shiffman, M.L., So, S.K. and Wiesner, R.H. (1997a) Minimal criteria for placement of adults on the liver transplant waiting list: a report of a national conference organized by the American Society of Transplant Physicians and the American Association for the Study of Liver Diseases. *Liver Transpl Surg* **3**, 628–637.

Lucey, M.R., Carr, K., Beresford, T.P., Fisher, L.R., Shieck, V., Brown, K.A., Campbell, D.A. and Appelman, H.D. (1997b) Alcohol use after liver transplantation in alcoholics: a clinical cohort follow-up study. *Hepatology* **25**, 1223–1227.

Lucey, M.R., Merion, R.M., Henley, K.S., Campbell, D.A. Jr., Turcotte, J.G., Nostrant, T.T., Blow, F.C. and Beresford, T.P. (1992) Selection for and outcome of liver transplantation in alcoholic liver disease. *Gastroenterology* **102**, 1736–1741.

Maddrey, W.C., Boitnott, J.K., Bedine, M.S., Weber Jr., F.L., Mezey, E. and White Jr., R.I. (1978) Corticosteroid therapy of alcoholic hepatitis. *Gastroenterology* **75**, 193–199.

Mayfield, D., MacLeod, G. and Hall, P. (1974) The CAGE questionnaire: validation of a new alcoholism screening instrument. *Am J Psych* **131**, 1121–1123.

Modan, B., Shpilberg, O., Baruch, Y., Sikuler, E., Anis, E., Ashur, Y., Chetrit, A., Luxenburg, O., Rosenberg, E., Rosenthol, N., Sadetzki, S., Benaim, H., Eckstein, H. and Shouval, D. (1995) The need for liver transplantation: a nationwide estimate based on consensus review. *Lancet* **346**, 660–662.

Moore, K.A., Burrows, G., Jones, R.M. and Hardy, K. (1992) Control evaluation of cognitive functioning, mood state, and quality of life post-liver transplant. *Transplant Proc* **24**, 202.

Mutimer, D., Burra, P., Neuberger, J.M., Hubscher, S., Buckels, J.A., Mayer, A.D., McMaster, P. and Elias, E. (1993) Managing severe alcoholic hepatitis complicated by renal failure. *Quart J Med* **86**, 649–656.

Neuberger, J. (1998) Transplantation for alcoholic liver disease: a perspective from Europe. *Liver Transpl Surg* **4**, S51–S57.

Neuberger, J., Adams, D., MacMaster, P., Maidment, A. and Speed, M. (1998) Assessing priorities for allocation of donor liver grafts: survey of public and opinions. *Br Med J* **317**, 172–175.

Neuberger, J. and Tang, H. (1997) Relapse after transplantation: European studies. *Liver Transpl Surg* **3**, 275–279.

O'Brien, C.P. and McLellan, A.T. (1996) Myths about the treatment of addiction. *Lancet* **347**, 237–240.

O'Connor, P.G. and Schottenfeld, R.S. (1998) Patients with alcohol problems. *N Engl J Med* **338**, 592–602.

Office for National Statistics (1997) Series DH2 no. 22. Mortality statistics: review of the Registrar General on deaths, by cause, sex and age, in England and Wales, 1995. *The Stationary Office*, London.

Orrego, H., Blake, J.E., Blendis, L.M., Kapur, B.M. and Israel, Y. (1979) Reliability of assessment of alcohol intake based on personal interviews in a liver clinic. *Lancet* **2**, 1354–1356.

Osorio, R.W., Ascher, N.L., Avery, M., Bacchetti, P., Roberts, J.P. and Lake, J.R. (1994) Predicting recidivism after orthotopic liver transplantation for alcoholic liver disease. *Hepatology* **20**, 105–110.

Pageaux, G.-P., Michel, J., Coste, V., Perney, P., Possoz, P., Perrigault, P.-F., Navarro, F., Fabre, J.-M., Domergue, J., Blanc, P. and Larrey, D. (1999) Alcoholic cirrhosis is a good indication for liver transplantation, even for cases of recidivism. *Gut* **45**, 421–426.

Pereira, S.P., Howard, L.M., Muiesan, P., Rela, M., Heaton, N. and Williams, R. (2000) Quality of life after liver transplantation for alcoholic liver disease. *Liver Transpl* **6**, 762–768.

Pereira, S.P. and Williams, R. (1997) Liver transplantation for alcoholic liver disease at King's College Hospital: survival and quality of life. *Liver Transpl Surg* **3**, 245–250.

Pereira, S.P. and Williams, R. (1998) Limits to liver transplantation in the UK. *Gut* **42**, 883–885.

Pereira, S.P. and Williams, R. (2001) Alcohol relapse and functional outcome after liver transplantation for alcoholic liver disease. *Liver Transpl* **7**, 204–205.

Plotkin, J.S., Scott, V.L., Pinna, A., Dobsch, B.P., De Wolf, A.M. and Kang, Y. (1996) Morbidity and mortality in patients with coronary artery disease undergoing orthotopic liver transplantation. *Liver Transpl Surg* **2**, 426–430.

Poynard, T., Barthelemy, P., Fratte, S., Boudjema, K., Doffoel, M., Vanlemmens, C., Miguet, J.P., Mantion, G., Messner, M., Launois, B., Naveau, S. and Chaput, J.C. (1994) Evaluation of efficacy of liver transplantation in alcoholic cirrhosis by a case-control study and simulated controls. *Lancet* **344**, 502–507.

Poynard, T., Naveau, S., Doffoel, M., Boudjema, K., Vanlemmens, C., Mantion, G., Messner, M., Launois, B., Samuel, S., Cherqui, D., Pageaux, G.P., Bernard, P.H., Calmus, Y., Zarski, J.P., Miguet, J.P., Balian, A. and Chaput, J.C. (1996) Evaluation of liver transplantation in alcoholic cirrhosis by comparison with matched and simulated controls' 5-year survival. *Hepatology* **24**, 184A.

Price, C.E., Lowe, D., Cohen, A.T., Reid, F.D., Forbes, G.M., McEwen, J. and Williams, R. (1995) Prospective study of the quality of life in patients assessed for liver transplantation: outcome in transplanted and not transplanted groups. *J R Soc Med* **88**, 130–135.

Project MATCH Research Group (1997) Matching alcoholism treatments to client heterogeneity: Project MATCH post-treatment drinking outcomes. *J Stud Alcohol* **58**, 7–29.

Propst, A., Propst, T., Zangeri, G., Ofner, D., Judmaier, G. and Vogel, W. (1995) Prognosis and life expectancy in chronic liver disease. *Dig Dis Sci* **40**, 1805–1815.

Roizen, R., Kerr, W.C. and Fillmore, K.M. (1999) Cirrhosis mortality and per capita consumption of distilled spirits, United States, 1949–1994: trend analysis. *BMJ* **319**, 666–670.

Shakil, A.O., Pinna, A., Demetris, J., Lee, R.G., Fung, J.J. and Rakela, J. (1997) Survival and quality of life after liver transplantation for acute alcoholic hepatitis. *Liver Transpl Surg* **3**, 240–244.

Starzl, T.E., Van Thiel, D., Tzakis, A.G., Iwatsuki, S., Todo, S., Marsh, J.W., Koneru, B., Staschak, S., Stieber, A. and Gordon, R.D. (1988) Orthotopic liver transplantation for alcoholic cirrhosis. *JAMA* **260**, 2542–2544.

Stewart, A.L., Hays, R.D. and Ware, J.E. (1988) The MOS short-form general health survey. *Medical Care* **26**, 465–486.

Surman, O.S., Dienstag, J.L., Cosimi, A.B., Chauncey, S. and Russell, P.S. (1987) Psychosomatic aspects of liver transplantation. *Psychother Psychosom* **48**, 26–31.

Tang, H., Boulton, R., Gunson, B., Hubscher, S. and Neuberger, J. (1998) Patterns of alcohol consumption after liver transplantation. *Gut* **43**, 140–145.

Tarter, R.E., Van Thiel, D., Arria, A.M., Carra, J. and Moss, H. (1988) Impact of cirrhosis on the neuropsychological test performance of alcoholics. *Alcohol Clin Exp Res* **12**, 619–621.

Tarter, R.E., Van Thiel, D.H., Hegedus, A.M., Schade, R.R., Gavaler, J.S. and Starzl, T.S. (1984) Neuropsychiatric status after liver transplantation. *J Lab Clin Med* **103**, 776–782.

Theodossi, A., Eddleston, A.W. and Williams, R. (1982) Controlled trial of methylprednisolone therapy in severe acute alcoholic hepatitis. *Gut* **23**, 75–79.

Ubel, P.A. (1997) Transplantation in alcoholics: separating prognosis and responsibility from social biases. *Liver Transpl Surg* **3**, 343–346.

UK Transplant (2001) Statistics prepared by UK Transplant from the National Transplant Database maintained on behalf of transplant services in the UK and Republic of Ireland (*www.uktransplant.org.uk*).

Urbano-Marquez, A., Estruch, R., Navarro-Lopez, F., Grau, J.M., Mont, L. and Rubin, E. (1989) The effect of alcoholism on skeletal and cardiac muscle. *N Engl J Med* **320**, 409–415.

Vaillant, G.E. (1996) A long-term follow-up of male alcohol abuse. *Arch Gen Psychiatr* **53**, 243–249.

Vaillant, G.E. (1997) The natural history of alcoholism and its relationship to liver transplantation. *Liver Transpl Surg* **3**, 304–310.

Van Thiel, D.H., Bonet, H., Gavaler, J. and Wright, H.I. (1995) Effect of alcohol use on allograft rejection rates after liver transplantation for alcoholic liver disease. *Alcohol Clin Exp Res* **19**, 1151–1155.

Weinrieb, R.M. and O'Brien, C.P. (1997) Current research in the treatment of alcoholism in liver transplant recipients. *Liver Transpl Surg* **3**, 328–336.

Weinrieb, R.M., Van Horn, D.H., McLellan, A.T. and Lucey, M.R. (2000) Interpreting the significance of drinking by alcohol-dependent liver transplant patients: fostering candor is the key to recovery. *Liver Transpl* **6**, 769–776.

Wiesner, R.H., Lombardero, M., Lake, J.R., Everhart, J. and Detre, K.M. (1997) Liver transplantation for end-stage alcoholic liver disease: an assessment of outcomes. *Liver Transpl Surg* **3**, 231–239.

Wodak, A.D., Saunders, J.B., Ewusi-Mensah, I., Davis, M. and Williams, R. (1983) Severity of alcohol dependence in patients with alcoholic liver disease. *BMJ Clin Res Ed* **287**, 1420–1422.

Yates, W.R., Booth, B.M., Reed, D.A., Brown, K. and Masterson, B.J. (1993) Descriptive and predictive validity of a high-risk alcoholism relapse model. *J Stud Alcohol* **54**, 645–651.

Yates, W.R., LaBrecque, D.R. and Pfab, D. (1998a) Personality disorder as a contraindication for liver transplantation in alcoholic cirrhosis. *Psychosomatics* **39**, 501–511.

Yates, W.R., Martin, M., LaBrecque, D., Hillebrand, D., Voigt, M. and Pfab, D. (1998b) A model to examine the validity of the 6-month abstinence criterion for liver transplantation. *Alcohol Clin Exp Res* **22**, 513–517.

Index

Page numbers in **bold** refer to illustrations and tables